Atlas of Practical Genitourinary Pathology

Notice

Atlas of Practical Genitourinary Pathology

Ximing J. Yang, MD, PhD

Marie A. Fleming Research Professor of Pathology
Chief, Urological Pathology
Medical Director, Immunohistochemistry Laboratory
Northwestern Memorial Hospital
Northwestern University
Feinberg School of Medicine
Chicago, Illinois

Mc Graw Hill Education | Medical

New York Chicago San Francisco Athens London Madrid Mexico City
Milan New Delhi Singapore Sydney Toronto

Atlas of Practical Genitourinary Pathology

1 2 3 4 5 6 7 8 9 0 CTP/CTP 18 17 16 15 14

ISBN 978-0-07-179882-2
MHID 0-07-179882-X

This book was set in Adobe Jenson by MPS Limited.
The editors were Alyssa K. Fried and Cindy Yoo.
The production supervisor was Catherine Saggese.
Project management was provided by Asheesh Ratra of MPS Limited.
The designer was Diana Andrews; the cover designer was Thomas De Pierro.
China Translation & Printing Services, Ltd. was printer and binder.

This book is printed on acid-free paper.

Library of Congress Cataloging-in-Publication Data
Yang, Ximing J., author.
Atlas of practical genitourinary pathology / Ximing Yang.
p. ; cm.
ISBN 978-0-07-179882-2 (hardcover : alk. paper)—ISBN 0-07-179882-X (hardcover : alk. paper)
I. Title.
[DNLM: 1. Urologic Diseases—pathology. 2. Genital Diseases, Male—pathology. WJ 140]
RC871
616.6—dc23

2014022182

This book is dedicated to my loving wife Jan,
and my two wonderful children, Julie and Jason.
I am profoundly grateful for their understanding
and support for the countless hours I spent on this book.

Contents

Contributors

Pauline M. Chou, MD
Director, Anatomic Pathology
Lurie Children Hospital
Professor of Pathology
Northwestern University
Feinberg School of Medicine
Chicago, Illinois
Chapters 34 [*Autosomal Recessive Polycystic Kidney Disease*] ***and 37***

Laurie Eisengart, MD
Attending Pathologist
Arlington Heights Pathologists
Chicago, Illinois
Chapter 40 [*Tubulocystic carcinoma*]

Rajen Goyal, MD
Genitourinary Pathology Fellow
Northwestern University
Feinberg School of Medicine
Chicago, Illinois
Chapter 60

Huiying He, MD
Associate Professor of Pathology
Peking University Health Center
Beijing, China
Chapters 35 and 39

Ondrej Hes, MD, PhD
Professor of Pathology
Charles University
Pilzen, Czech Republic
Chapters 35, 37 [*Wilms Tumor*]***, 38 and 40***

Liwei Jia, MD
Resident Pathologist
Case Western Reserve University Hospital
Cleveland, Ohio
Chapters 36 and 40 [*Renal Medullary Carcinoma, and Renal Cell Carcinoma, Unclassified*]

Yashpal Kanwar, MD, PhD
Professor of Pathology
Northwestern University
Feinberg School of Medicine
Chicago, Illinois
Chapter 32

William Laskin, MD
Associate Professor of Pathology
Northwestern University
Feinberg School of Medicine
Chicago, Illinois
Chapter 40

Fan Lin, MD, PhD
Director of Anatomic Pathology and Attending Pathologist
Geisinger Health System
Danville, Pennsylvania
Chapters 36 and 39

Ning Lu, MD
Chair and Professor of Pathology
Cancer Institute & Hospital
Chinese Academy of Medical Sciences
Beijing, China
Chapter 23

Sanjiv V. Prabhu, MD
Genitourinary Pathology Fellow
Northwestern University
Feinberg School of Medicine
Chicago, Illinois
Chapters 41 and 55

Kirtee Raparia, MD
Assistant Professor of Pathology
Northwestern University
Feinberg School of Medicine
Chicago, Illinois
Chapter 32

Nedjema Sustento-Reodica, MD
Assistant Professor of Pathology
Northwestern University
Feinberg School of Medicine
Chicago, Illinois
Chapter 32

Bin Tean Teh, MD
Senior Principal Investigator
Cancer Science Institute of Singapore
Professor, Duke-NUS Graduate Medical School
Singapore
Chapter 40 [*Hybrid Oncocytic Tumor In Birt-Hogg-Dube Patients*]

Celina Villa, MD
Resident Pathologist
Northwestern University
Feinberg School of Medicine
Chicago, Illinois
Chapters 56, 57, 58, and 59

Sean K. Wang, BS
Stanford University
Palo Alto, California
Chapters 14 and 20

Anjana Yeldandi, MD
Associate Professor of Pathology
Northwestern University
Feinberg School of Medicine
Chicago, Illinois
Chapters 56, 57, 58, and 59

Shan Zheng, MD
Assistant Professor of Pathology
Cancer Institute & Hospital
Chinese Academy of Medical Sciences
Beijing, China
Chapter 23

Minghao Zhong, MD, PhD
Assistant Professor of Pathology
Westchester Medical Center
Valhalla, New York
Chapter 40 [*Renal Cell Carcinoma Associated With XP11.2 Translocation and TFE3-Gene Fusion*]

Bing Zhu, MD, PhD
Pathology Fellow
University of Illinois
Chicago, Illinois
Chapters 34 [*Autosomal Recessive Polycystic Kidney Disease, Mixed Epithelial and Stromal Tumor*], ***37 and 40*** [*Clear Cell Papillary Renal Cell Carcinoma*]

Preface

The genitourinary (GU) system is one of most complicated systems in the body, composed of multiple organs with different structures and functions. In this system, a wide range of diseases from common benign conditions and malignant neoplasms such as prostate cancer to rare diseases may develop. A surgical pathologist has to be familiar with these pathologic conditions in order to make the correct diagnosis and provide useful guidance for clinical management.

Looking back on my past 20 years of experience in practicing pathology, I am very fortunate to have had the opportunity to receive training and to work at some of the most prestigious medical institutions in the world—including the University of California, University of Chicago, Johns Hopkins University, and Weill Cornell Medical College. Most recently, I have had the pleasure of spending the last 10 years as a faculty member and attending physician at Northwestern University Feinberg School of Medicine and Northwestern Memorial Hospital. By working with some of the finest urological surgeons and medical oncologists in the country, I have learned a great deal about how much a pathology diagnosis can impact the clinical management of patients with genitourinary diseases. I have had not only the chance to see the full spectrum of common and rare pathological conditions in the GU system, but also the capacity to study many of these GU diseases by morphological characterization as well as by immunohistochemical and molecular analyses in a great academic environment. The 1,400 color images in this book are just a small subset of a large digital photo library containing more than 20,000 images that I have collected from GU cases encountered over the years.

This book is almost exclusively based on our firsthand experience of more than 20 years. It is intended to provide a reference to common and rare GU conditions for practicing pathologists. It can also be used as a teaching guide for pathology and urology residents, as well as medical students.

Ximing J. Yang
Chicago
2014

Acknowledgments

I would like to take this opportunity to thank my teachers and colleagues in the Departments of Pathology, Urology, and Medicine, who contributed to my knowledge of genitourinary diseases and completion of this book. I also want to thank my current and former residents and fellows who studied these diseases with me and worked on these illustrated cases. The vast majority of outstanding gross photos were taken by our residents at Northwestern. Finally, I am grateful to my fellow Dr. Sanjiv Prabhu who helped me immensely with editing the text.

PART I
Male Reproductive Surgical Pathology

INTRODUCTION

Male reproductive organs include several functional units which are the following:

Testes

- A pair of male gonads
- Function: production of male gametes, spermatozoa (sperm), and secretion of male hormones, mostly testosterone
- Scrotum: the sacs for protection of the testes

Ducts

- Function: storage and transportation of sperm
- Ductuli efferentes
- Epididymis (pair: epididymides)
- Vas (ductus) deferens (pair: vasa deferentia, ductus deferentes)
- Ejaculatory duct (pair)
- Urethra

Exocrine glands

- Function: secretion combined as seminal fluid
- Seminal vesicle (pair)
- Prostate

Penis

- Function: organ of copulation and passage for sperm and urine through penile urethra
- Cowper gland (pair) secretes lubricant to the urethra during ejaculation

SECTION 1
The Prostate

CHAPTER 1 Normal Histology of the Prostate and Related Structures

PROSTATE

Location

- The prostate is located within the pelvis, underneath the bladder, and anterior to the rectum
- The urethra (prostatic urethra) courses through the center of the prostate
- Right and left seminal vesicles enter the posterior superior prostate as two ejaculatory ducts opening to the prostatic urethra

Adjacent organs

- Bladder (superior aspect)
- Prostatic urethra with urothelium lining (middle portion of the prostate)
- Seminal vesicles (posterior lateral aspect of the prostate)

Anatomy

- Shape: inverted chestnut
- Size: of a walnut
- Weight: normally 30 to 40 g
- There are two lobes, right and left, but without a clear boundary
- Anatomic divisions of the prostate
  - Base (top portion)
  - Mid (middle portion)
  - Apex (bottom portion) merging with pelvic floor muscle, not defined capsule
- Zoning
  - Peripheral zone (70%), where most prostatic adenocarcinoma develops
  - Central zone (25%), base of the prostate next to ejaculatory ducts
  - Transition zone (5%), anterior to the prostatic urethra where most cases of benign prostatic hyperplasia (BPH) develop
  - Anterior fibromuscular zone, composed of smooth and skeletal muscle

Histology

- Capsule: there is no true capsule for the prostate, rather a dense fibromuscular tissue that separates the prostatic parenchyma from the loose extraprostatic fibroadipose tissue
- The epithelial components of the prostate are large convoluted glands (Figs. 1-1 to 1-5) including ducts and acini; normally they cannot be distinguished
- The prostatic glands in the central zone are large and more complex (Fig. 1-5)
- There are at least three populations of prostatic epithelial cells
- Secretory cells (luminal cells)
  - The most dominant population lining the glandular lumen (Fig. 1-2)
  - Corpus amylacea present in the lumen (Fig. 1-3)
  - Some fixatives may particularly enhance the nuclear details. In this situation, the diagnosis of high-grade prostatic neoplasia and adenocarcinoma should be made with caution because of the frequent presence of prominent nucleoli (Fig. 1-4)

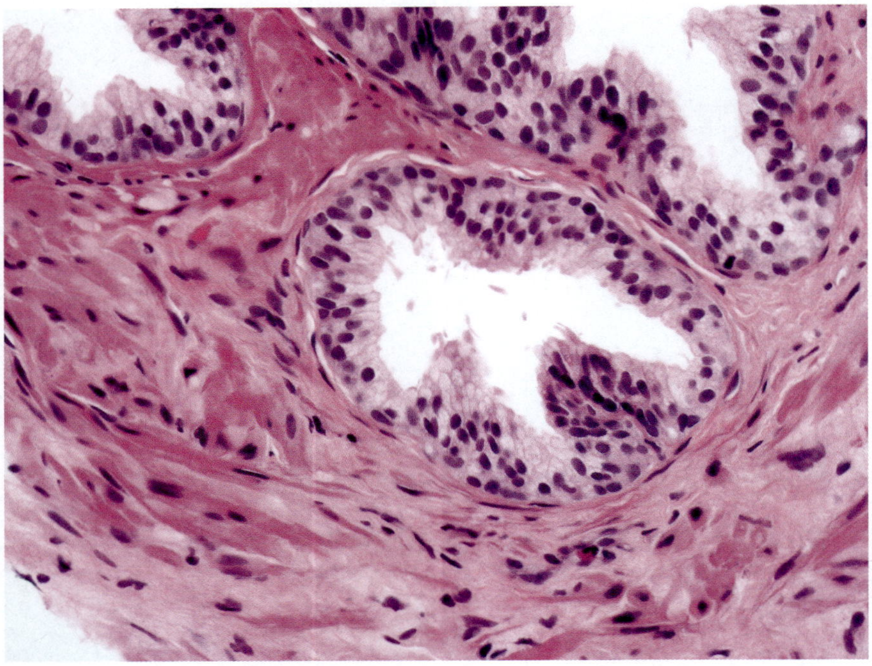

Figure 1-1.
Large benign prostatic glands composed mostly of pseudostratified secretory cells perpendicularly to the basement membrane.

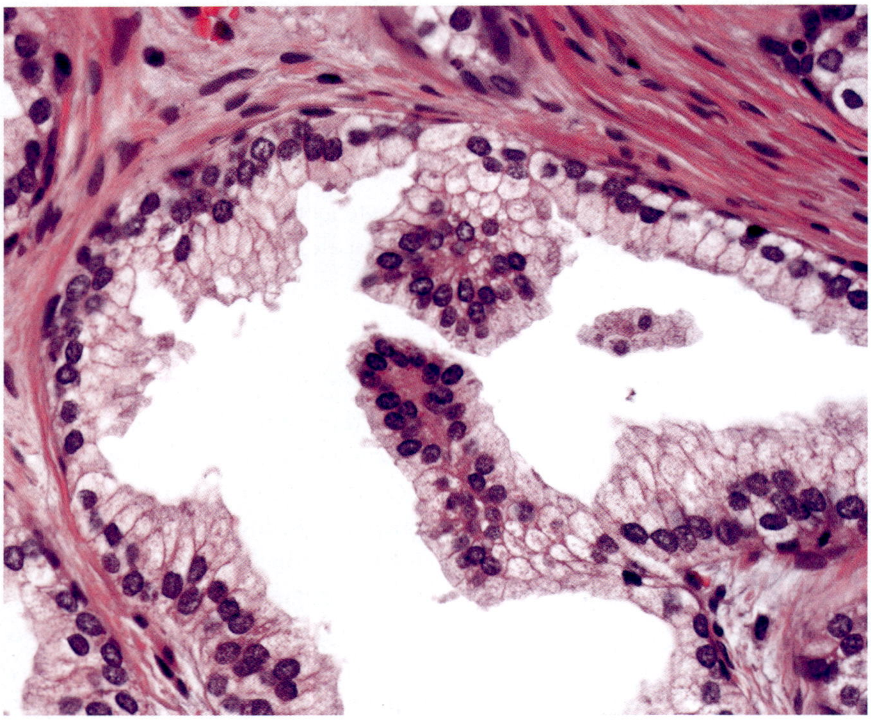

Figure 1-2.
A benign prostatic gland with infoldings consists of secretory cells demonstrating the pale to clear abundant cytoplasm. A basal cell layer can be appreciated. Prominent nucleoli are usually not seen in either secretory cells or basal cells.

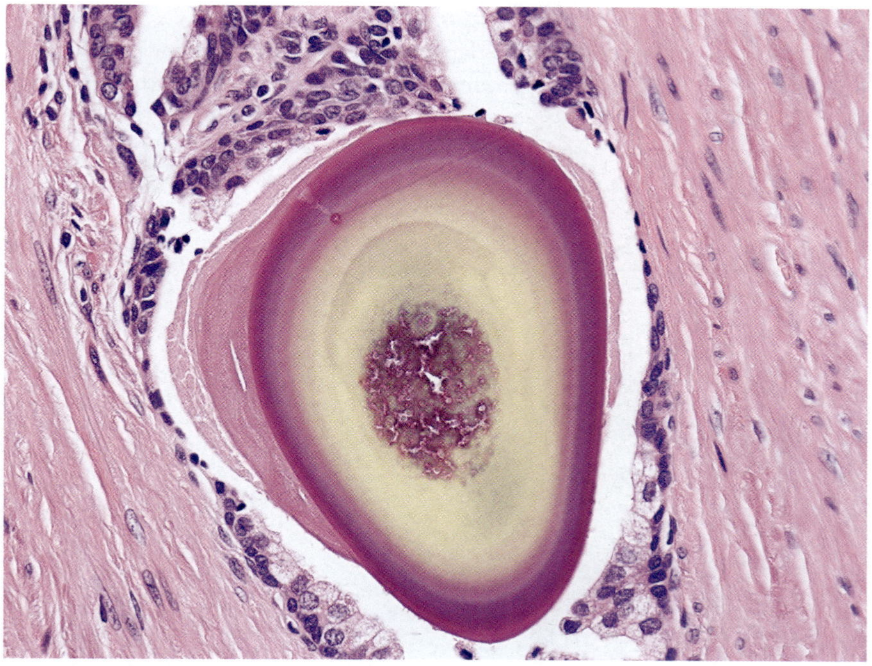

Figure 1-3.
A round corpus amylacea (amylaceum) with concentric layers is present within the lumen of a benign prostatic gland.

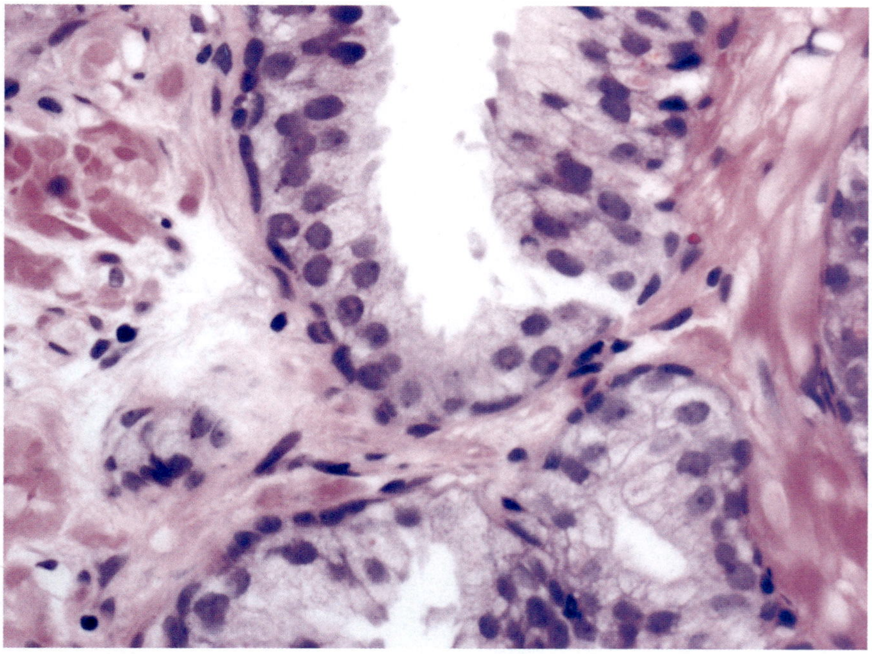

Figure 1-4.
Some special fixatives, such as zinc formalin in this case, can enhance the nuclear details. Therefore, nucleoli from benign prostatic glands can be easily appreciated much better than those fixed with buffered formalin. This case should not be diagnosed as high-grade prostatic intraepithelial neoplasia (PIN).

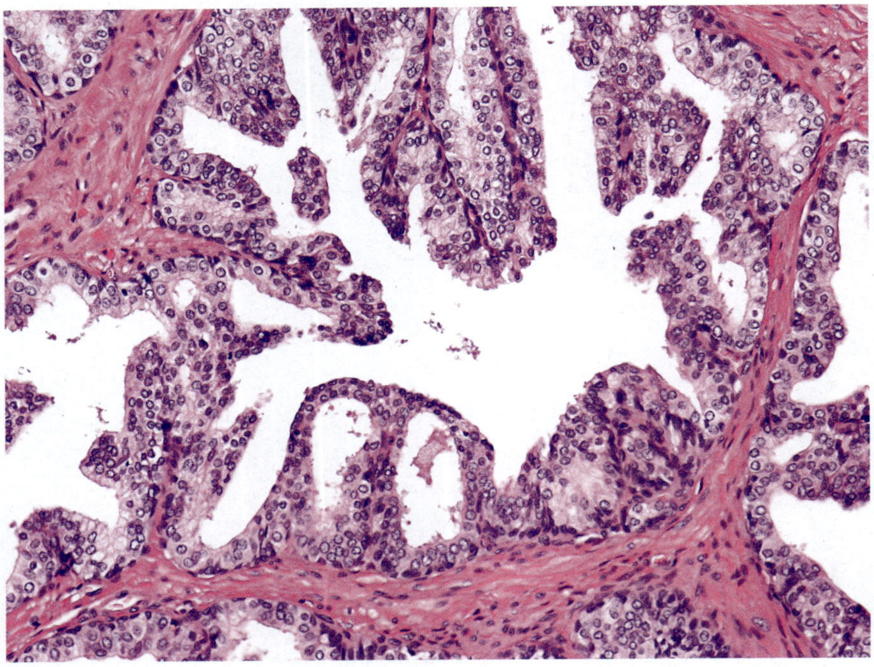

Figure 1-5.
A large benign gland located in the prostatic central zone shows the complex architecture, cribriform patterns, and "Roman bridge."

  - They secrete prostate-specific antigen (PSA) and have androgen receptors. Secretory cells may contain lipofuscin pigment, which tends to be purple, dark brown instead of golden brown
  - Prostatic adenocarcinoma typically has the immunophenotype of a secretory cell
- Basal cells
  - Located in the basilar compartment, underneath secretory cells, just above basement membrane (Figs. 1-2 and 1-4)
  - Basal cells with pale chromatin are elongated cells parallel to the basement membrane
  - In some fixatives, basal cells appear to have a perinuclear halo
  - They contain minimal PSA and androgen receptors, so that they are less responsive to hormonal therapy
  - In many ways basal cells are similar to urothelial cells in nature
- Neuroendocrine (NE) cells
  - Located in basilar compartment as well
  - NE cells cannot be distinguished from basal cells in hematoxylin and eosin (H&E)-stained sections unless they contain special NE granules
  - NE cells can be highlighted by NE markers such as neuron-specific enolase (NSE), synaptophysin, or chromogranin (Fig. 1-6)
  - They are columnar, triangular, or starry shaped, sometimes with long cell processes demonstrated by immunostaining
  - NE differentiation can be seen in prostatic adenocarcinoma
- Stem cells
  - They are primitive cells with potential to differentiate to mature cells
  - They may also be responsible for development of carcinoma or other malignant tumors of the prostate
  - They are believed to be located in the basilar component, and cannot be distinguished from basal cells in H&E sections
  - Although some stem cell markers have been studied in the prostate, the definition of the stem cells in the prostate is uncertain
- Fibromuscular stroma separating the prostatic glands. The smooth muscle can contract

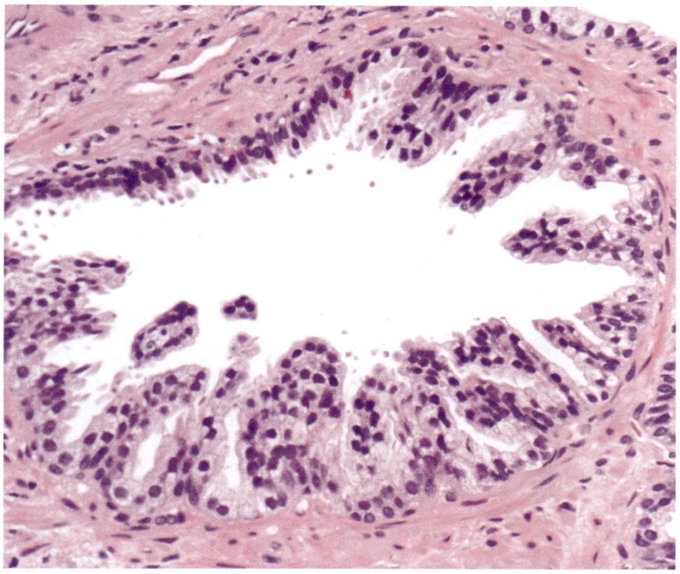

a

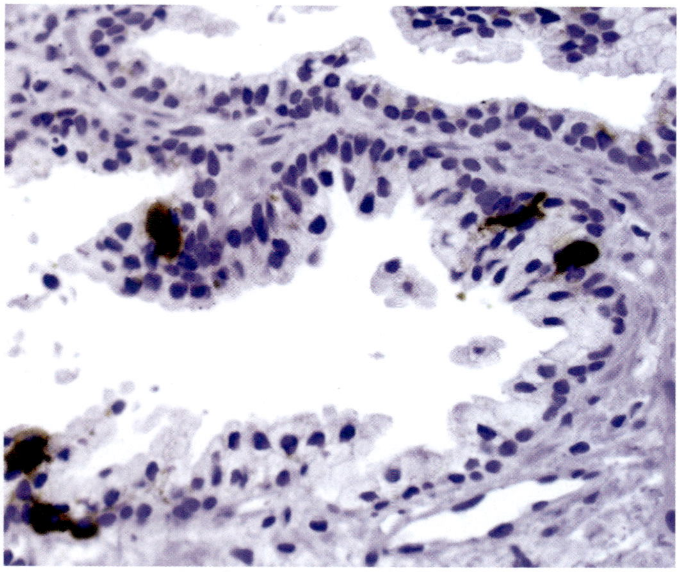

b

Figure 1-6.
Neuroendocrine cells not seen on H&E (*a*) staining, but they can be appreciated with chromogranin staining (*b*).

PROSTATIC URETHRA

- A portion of urethra within the prostate, lined by urothelium (Fig. 1-7)
- Urothelial lesions including urothelial carcinoma, nephrogenic adenoma can also develop in prostatic urethra

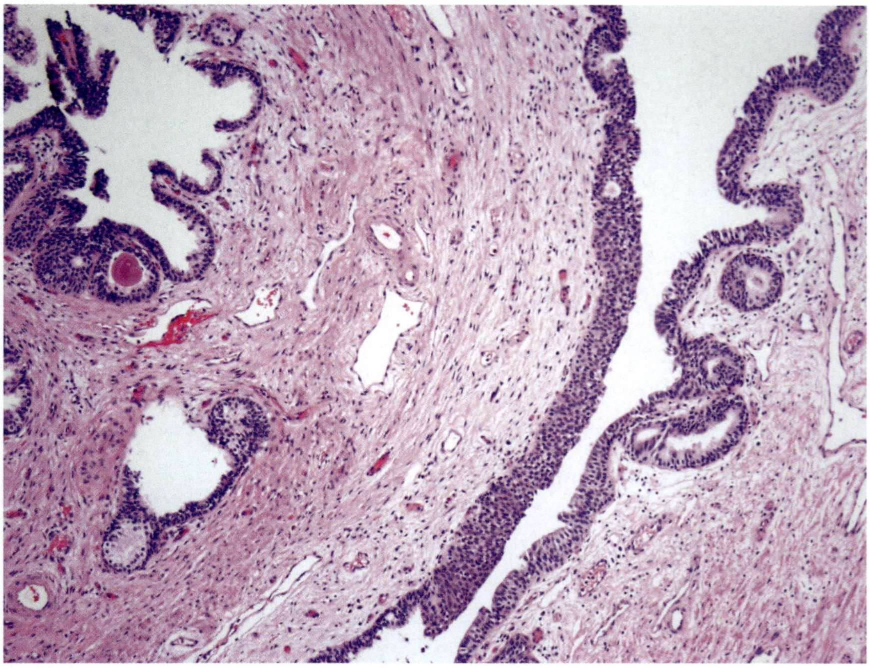

Figure 1-7.
Prostatic urethra is lined by urothelium, which is essentially the same epithelium seen in the renal pelvis, bladder, and prostatic urethra. Prostatic glands can be seen underneath the urothelium (left).

VERUMONTANUM

- A glandular structure located in the central portion of the prostatic urethra
- Next to the opening of two ejaculatory ducts on the prostatic urethra
- Cluster of closed packed small glands underneath the urothelium (Figs. 1-8 and 1-9)
- Dense secretion (corpus amylacea) within the lumen (Fig. 1-9)
- Lipofuscin may be occasionally present
- It can be confused with prostatic adenocarcinoma

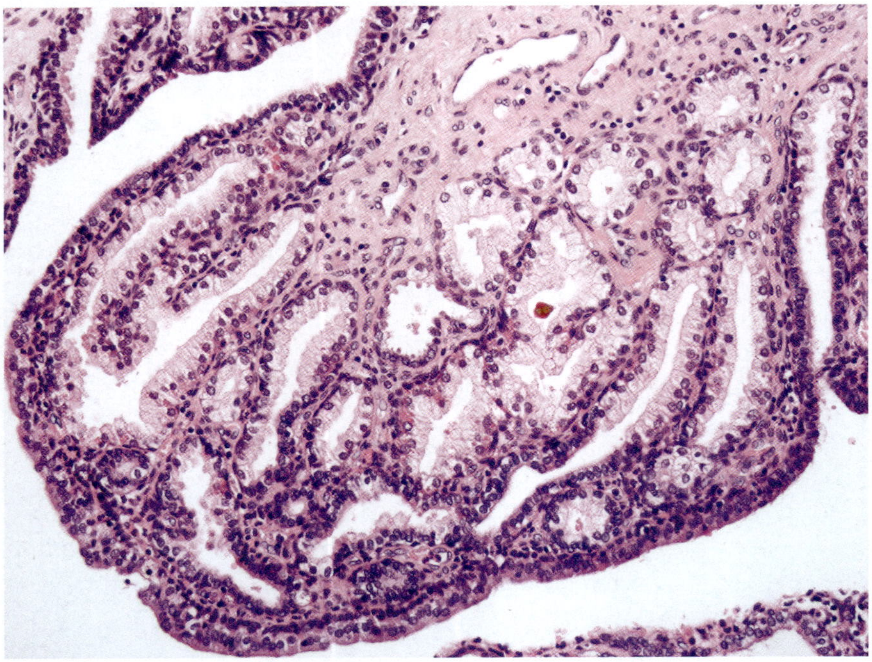

Figure 1-8.
Verumontanum is a small papillary projection composed of crowded glands.

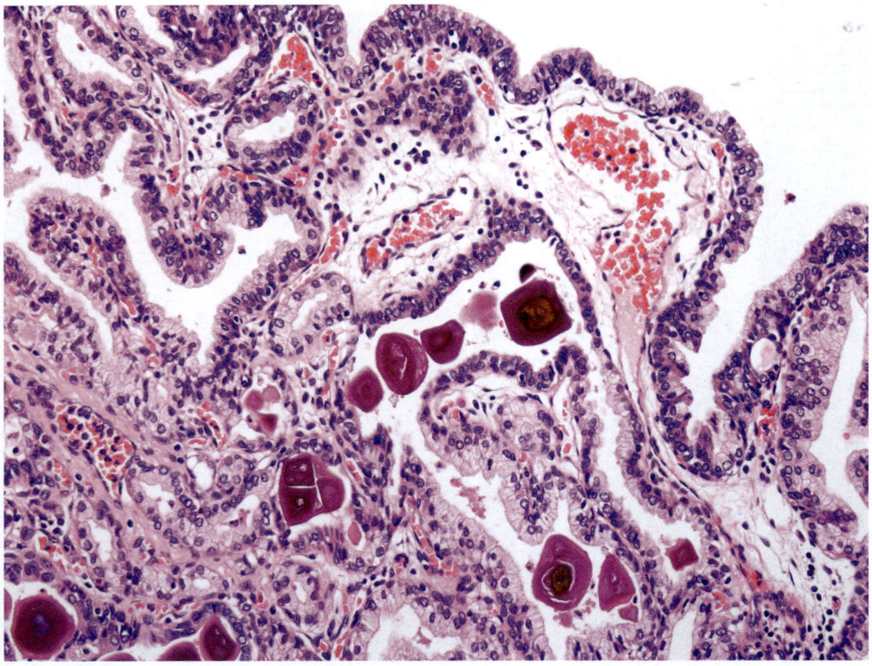

Figure 1-9.
Verumontanum located underneath the prostatic urothelium, containing dense corpora amylacea in the lumens.

SEMINAL VESICLES AND EJACULATORY DUCTS

Location

- Seminal vesicles (SVs): a pair of "rabbit ear" like glandular structures located posterior and superior to the prostate
- Ejaculatory ducts are the continuation of SVs, histologically almost identical to SVs but located within the prostate

Measurement and weight

- SVs measure 5 to 8 cm in length and weigh 4 to 5 g
- SVs insert into prostate as ejaculatory ducts, their secretion along with that of ejaculatory ducts becomes a part of the semen
- Although seminal vesicles are very similar to the prostate in morphology and development, neoplasms rarely develop in the seminal vesicles

Histology

- A seminal vesicle is composed of a large central lumen surrounded by clusters of small glands (Fig. 1-10)
- Golden brown pigment (lipofuscin) usually present in the cytoplasm (Figs. 1-11 and 1-12)
- The lining epithelium show degenerative atypia (Fig. 1-12)
- No mitosis seen
- SVs as well as ejaculatory duct glands are positive for MUC6, while prostatic glands are negative for MUC6 (Fig. 1-13)

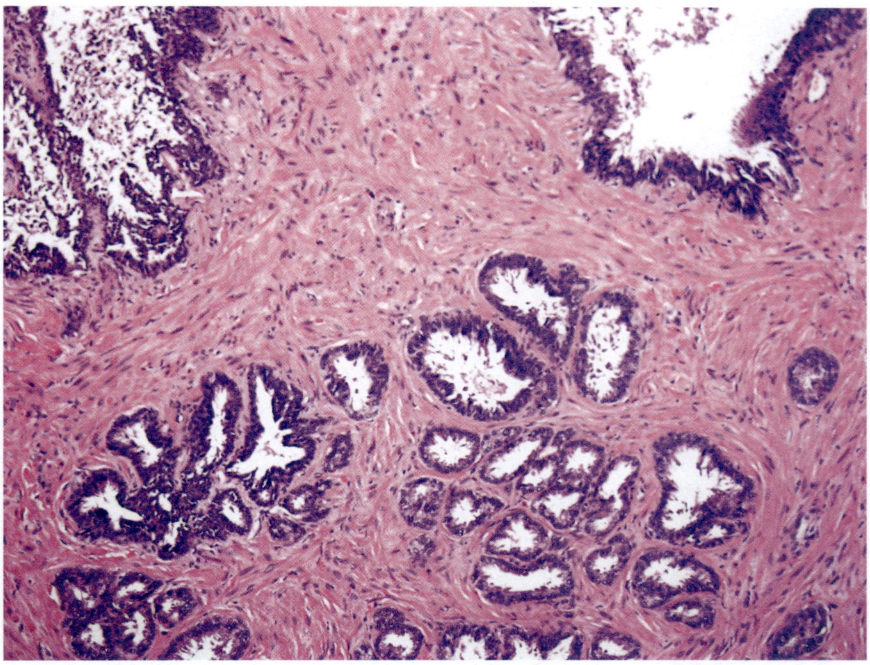

Figure 1-10.
Seminal vesicle is composed of small outpouching glands.

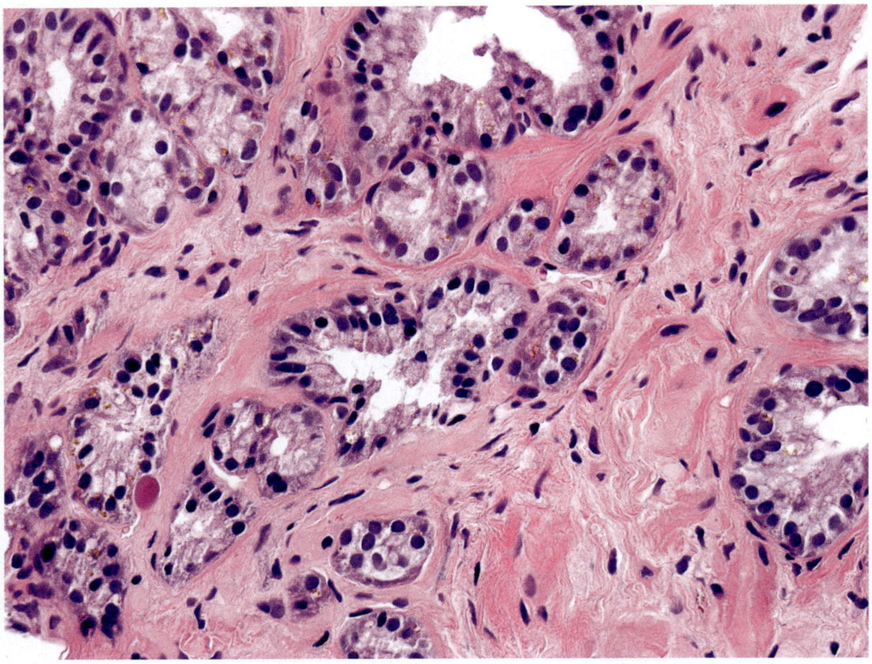

Figure 1-11.
The seminal vesicle glands contain golden yellow pigment (lipofuscin).

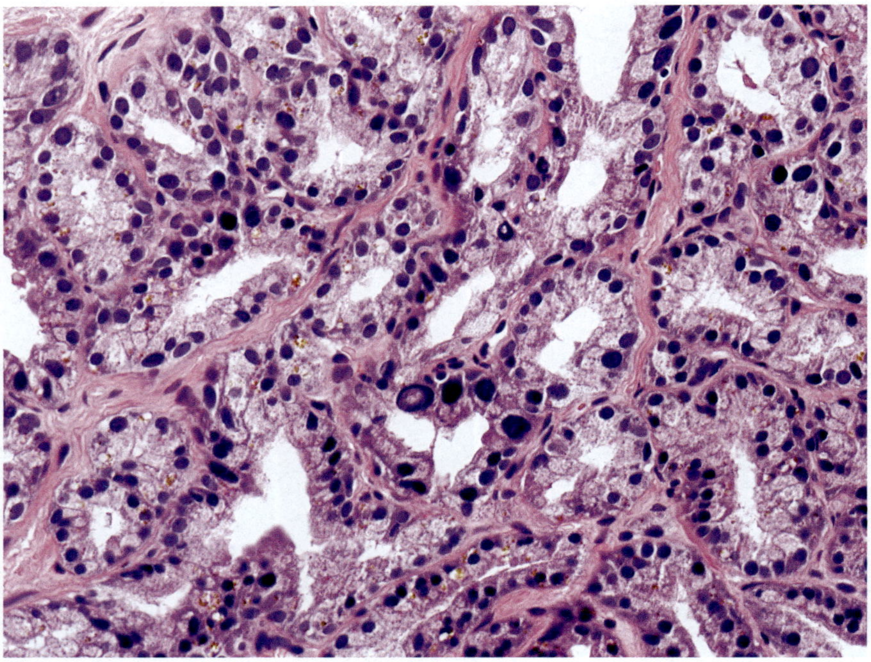

Figure 1-12.
At a high magnification, the degenerative cytological atypia can be seen.

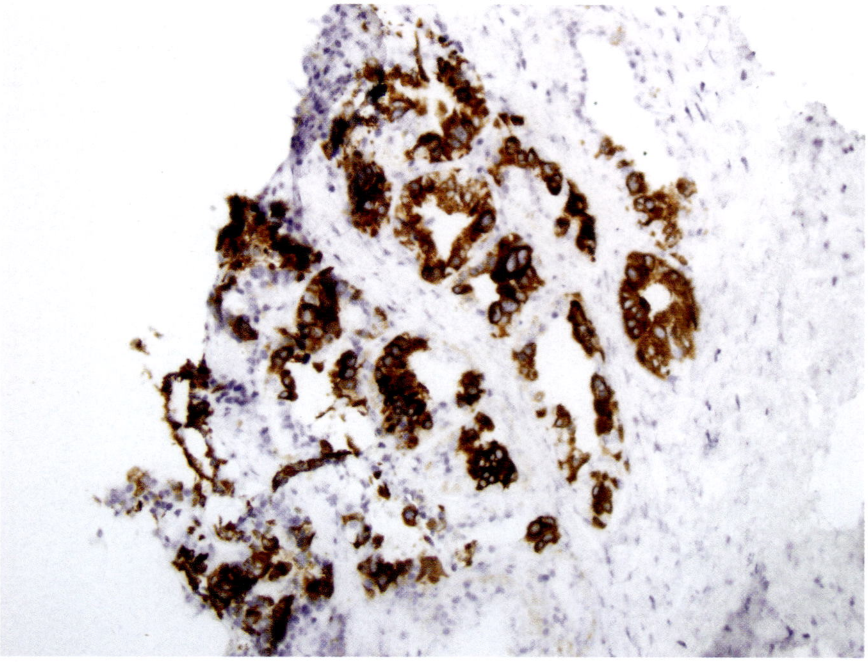

Figure 1-13.
Seminal vesicle is positive for Muc6, while the prostatic glands should be negative for Muc6.

- Ejaculatory ducts, by definition, are located within the prostate, although microscopically they are almost identical to the seminal vesicles (Figs. 1-14 and 1-15)
- When present in needle core biopsy or cytology specimens (Fig. 1-16), seminal vesicles or ejaculatory ducts can be confused with adenocarcinoma
- When involved by prostatic adenocarcinoma, the patients will have a poor prognosis
- In biopsy specimens, it is difficult or impossible to distinguish SV from ejaculatory ducts, so that the diagnosis of SV invasion by adenocarcinoma should be made with caution, and is best avoided in the biopsy diagnosis. We often use the diagnosis "prostatic adenocarcinoma adjacent to seminal vesicle/ejaculatory duct type of tissue"

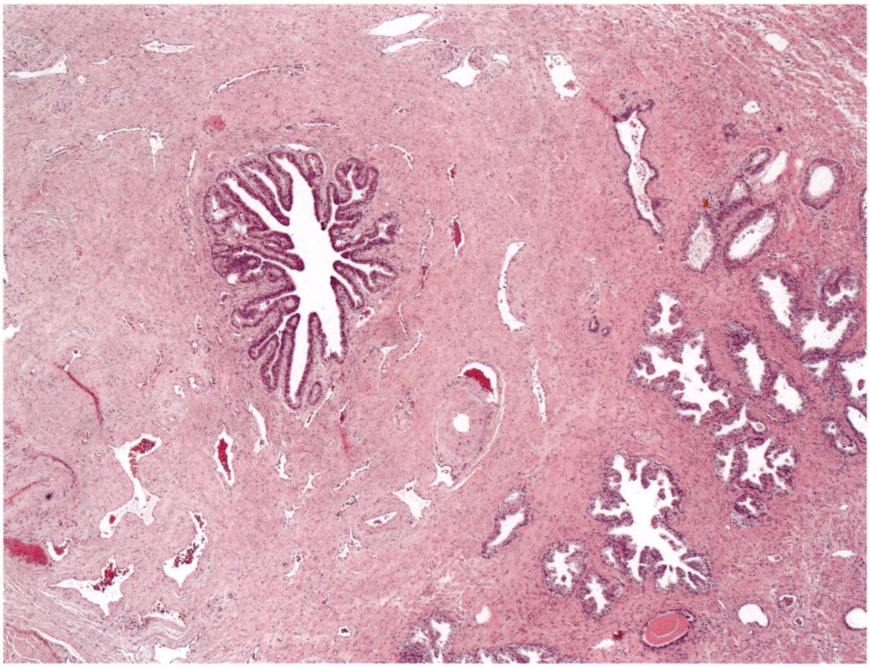

Figure 1-14.
Ejaculatory duct is present at the level of prostatic glands.

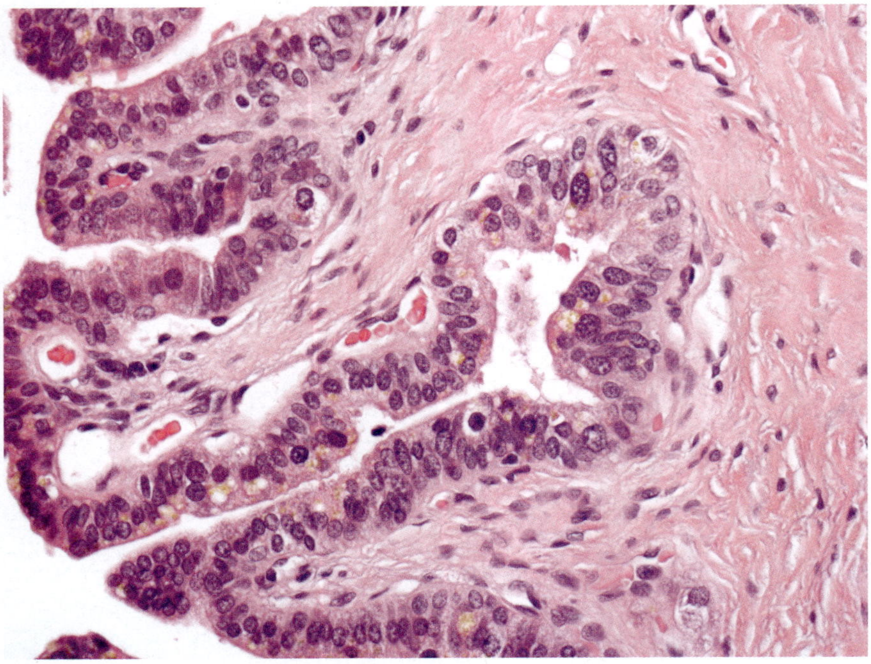

Figure 1-15.
At a higher magnification, the ejaculatory duct lining epithelium is similar to the one of seminal vesicle. There are also two types of epithelial cells and secretory cells that contain golden yellow pigment.

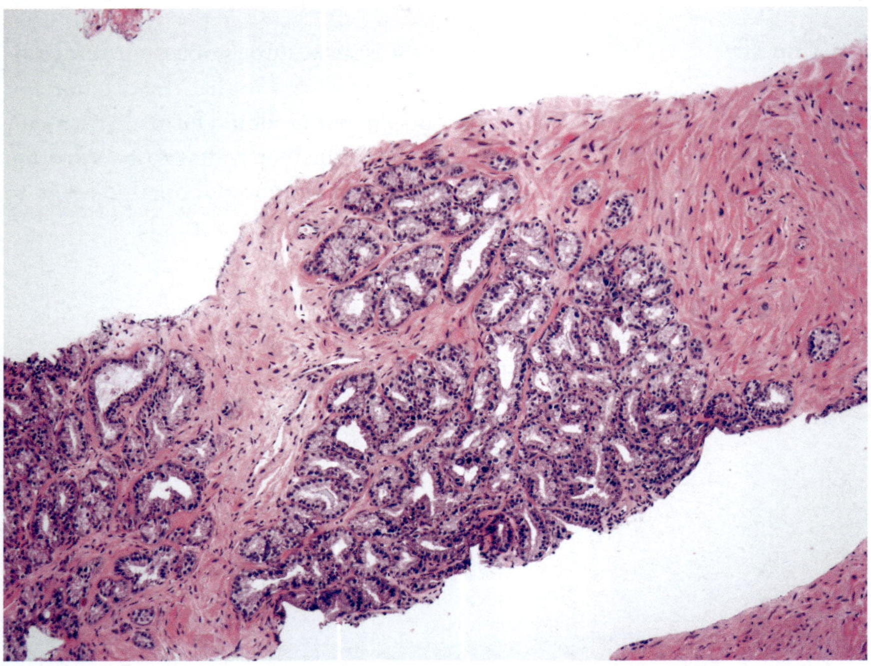

Figure 1-16.
This structure on a needle core biopsy could be either seminal vesicle or ejaculatory duct.

SEMINAL VESICLE AMYLOIDOSIS

Definition

- Amyloid deposits present in the seminal vesicle
- It is mostly localized rather than systemic involvement, therefore, no clinical significance
- Amyloidosis is seen in 5% to 10% normal men or in prostatectomy specimens harboring prostate cancer
- It is a condition related to aging because the incidence increases with age
- Histologically, the homogenous amyloid deposit is located underneath the seminal vesicle epithelium (Fig. 1-17)
- Congo red staining positive with amyloid deposit showing apple green birefringence under polarization (Fig. 1-18)

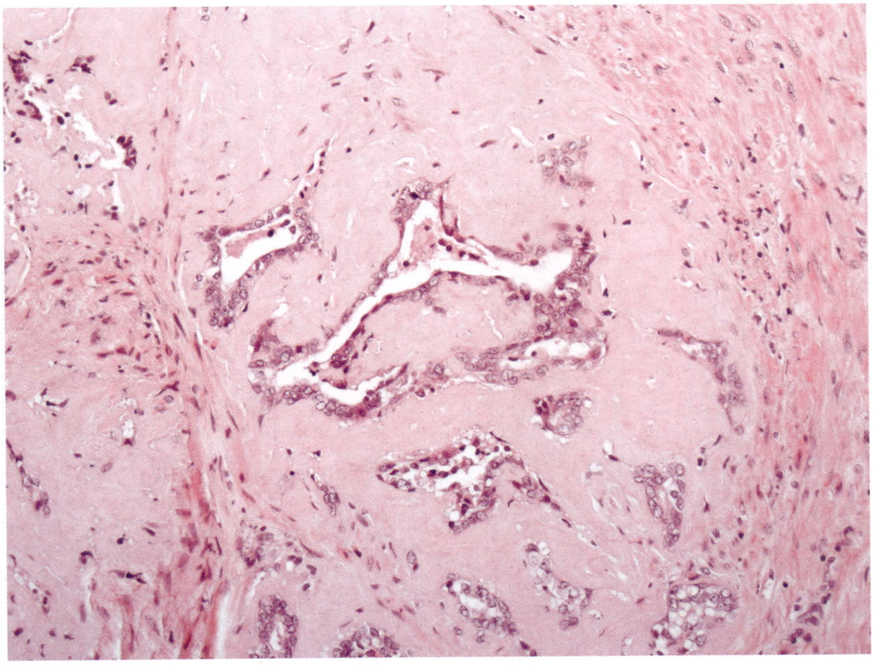

Figure 1-17.
Amyloidosis of the seminal vesicles is a common finding, which is not associated with systemic disease.

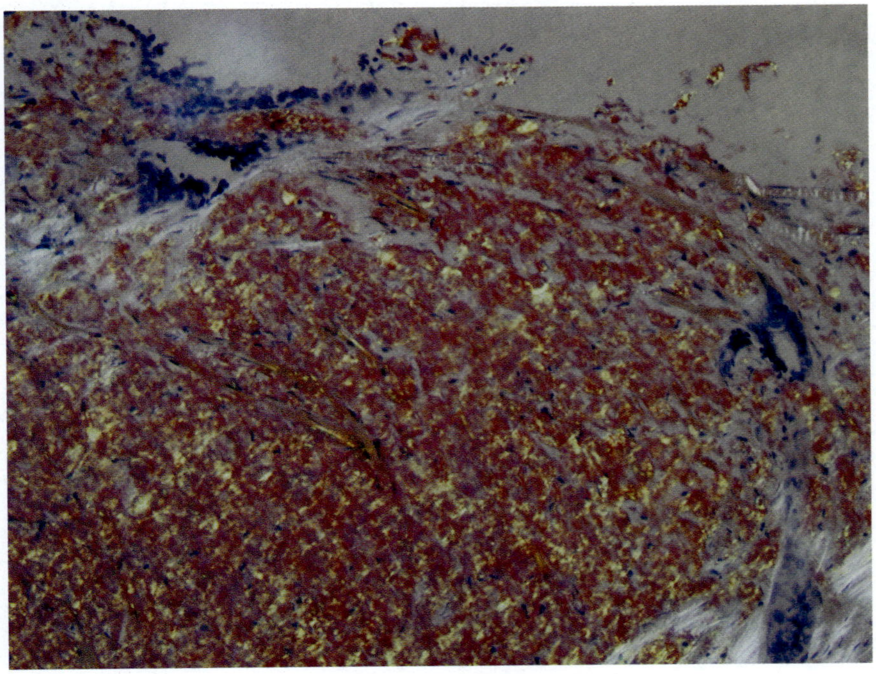

Figure 1-18.
Congo red staining demonstrates positive "apple green" amyloid material in seminal vesicle.

COWPER'S GLANDS

- Also known as bulbourethral glands, located outside (distal to) the prostate
- Surrounded by the periurethral skeletal muscle inferior to the prostate apex
- Histologically, Cowper's gland (Fig. 1-19) is composed of
  - Mucinous acini, palely stained glandular structures on H&E sections
  - Ductal structures, darker stained glandular structures on H&E sections
- It is a benign mimicker of prostate cancer, since it can be seen in prostate needle core biopsy

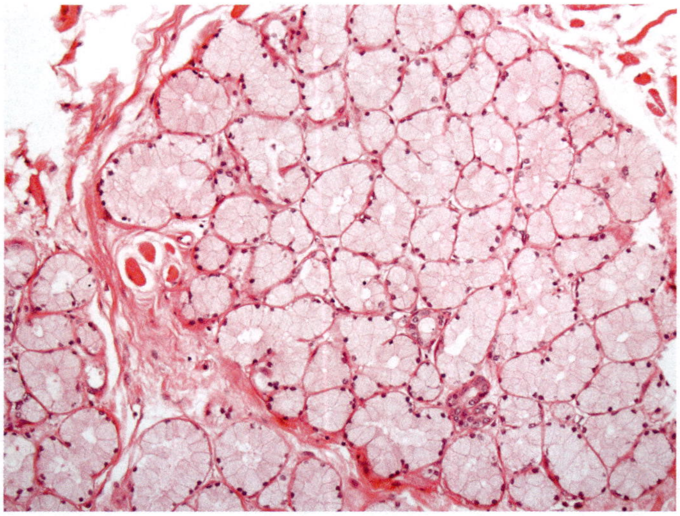

a

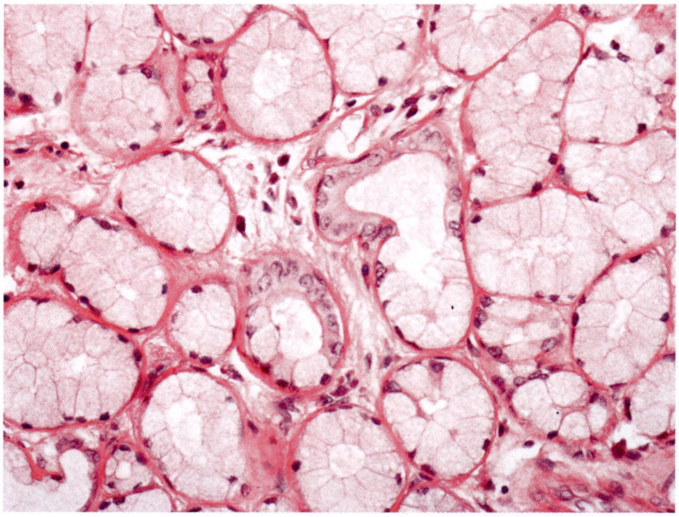

b

Figure 1-19.
Cowper's gland consists of well-organized small acini surrounded by skeletal muscle (*a*). High magnification shows the benign mucinous acini and darker ductal structures (*b*).

PARAGANGLION

Definition

- Normal nerve structure can be seen within the prostate or periprostatic tissue
- Incidental findings
- Most cases seen in prostatectomy specimens
- Rare to see on needle core biopsy

Gross pathology

- Not identifiable grossly

Histology

- Small cluster of cells without capsule but well circumscribed, mean size 1 mm (Fig. 1-20)
- Within prostatic parenchyma or periprostatic tissue
- Paraganglion is composed of uniform NE cells with either clear (Fig. 1-21*a*) or amphophilic cytoplasm (Fig. 1-20)
- "Salt and pepper chromatin" can be seen
- May be associated with nerves

Immunohistochemistry

- NSE, synaptophysin, or chromogranin positive (Fig. 1-21)
- Basal cell markers and keratin markers negative (Fig. 1-21)
- AMACR negative
- S100 negative in paraganglia but positive in associated nerve bundles

Clinical relevance

- Benign, no treatment needed
- Can be confused with high-grade adenocarcinoma

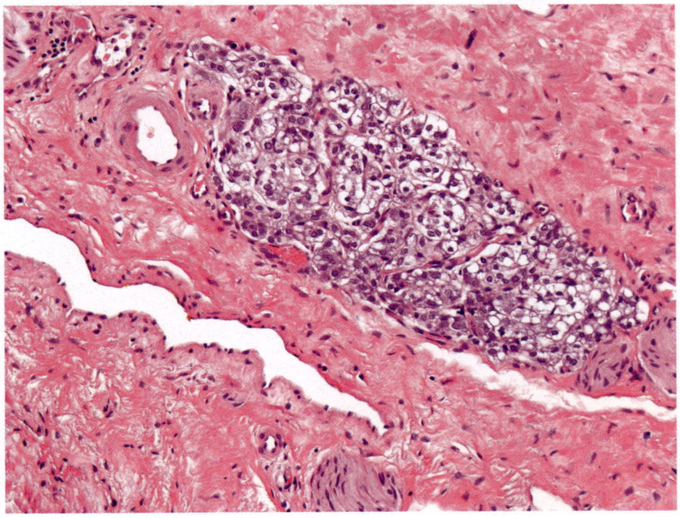

a

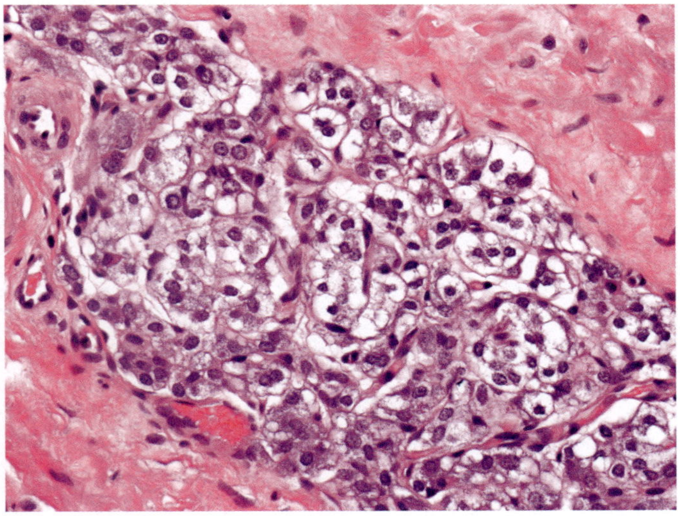

b

Figure 1-20.
Cluster of solid paraganglion cells present within the prostate (*a*). Higher magnification shows the neuroendocrine features of paraganglial cells without luminal formation (*b*), which can be confused with high-grade adenocarcinoma.

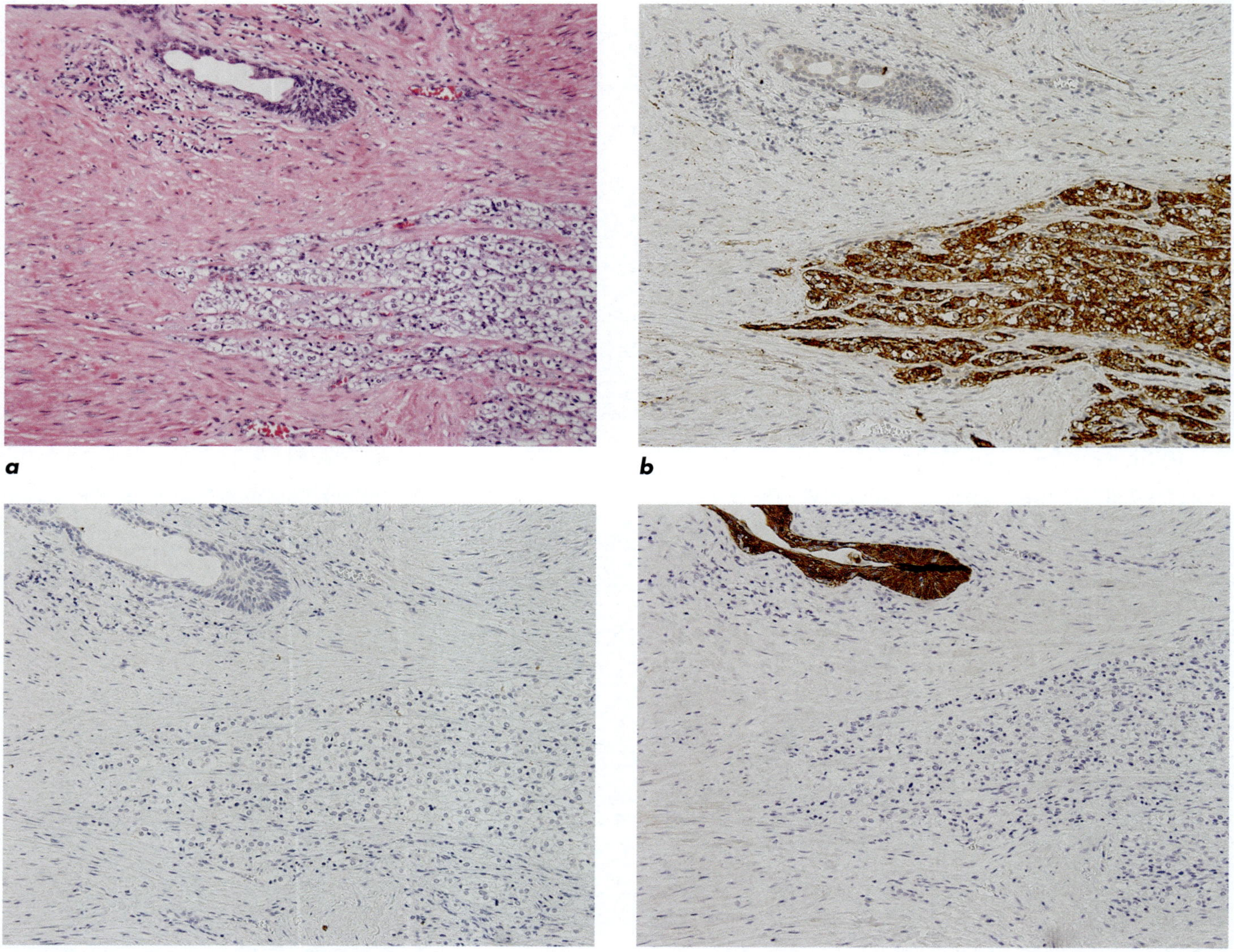

a *b* *c* *d*

Figure 1-21.
The paraganglion cells have clear cytoplasm and bland cytology on H&E (*a*). By immunohistochemistry, these cells are positive for synaptophysin (*b*), and negative for PSA (*c*) and triple stain (*d*).

CHAPTER 2

Immunohistochemical Markers of the Prostate

INTRODUCTION

- Immunohistochemistry (IHC) has been a powerful tool for pathologists to make diagnosis of prostate lesions
- Several steps need to be taken to interpret IHC results
- The diagnosis should be primarily based on the findings on hematoxylin and eosin (H&E)-stained sections
- Pre-IHC evaluation
  - Obtain clinical information, particularly the previous diagnosis
  - If necessary, talk with clinical colleagues who are more familiar with the patient situation and history
  - Carefully examine H&E-stained slides
  - Examine all the levels, and order deeper sections if tissue exposed by sectioning is not sufficient
  - Generate a list of differential diagnoses
- Selection of a panel of antibodies
  - Expected positive staining
  - Expected negative staining
  - Best to have an internal control
- Post-IHC evaluation
  - Confirm the controls
  - Examine the staining patterns
  - Document staining intensity and percentage of positive cells
  - Interpretation of positive or negative staining
  - Draw a conclusion
  - If a definitive diagnosis cannot be reached, a descriptive diagnosis may be provided
  - If necessary, discuss with your clinical colleagues if this diagnosis may have a major impact on the patient

TRIPLE STAIN

- Triple stain containing AMACR, p63, and HMWCK is one of the most commonly used immunostaining marker panels in pathology
- Using two-color chromogens to differentiate prostatic adenocarcinoma (red) from benign prostatic glands (brown) (Figs. 2-1 to 2-6)
- The major advantage is that only one slide is needed for three markers, which creates a better interpretation of the small lesion
- Using this triple staining properly, a pathologist may improve the diagnostic accuracy (Fig. 2-4)
- The advantages and disadvantages for prostate biopsy specimens are summarized in Table 2-1

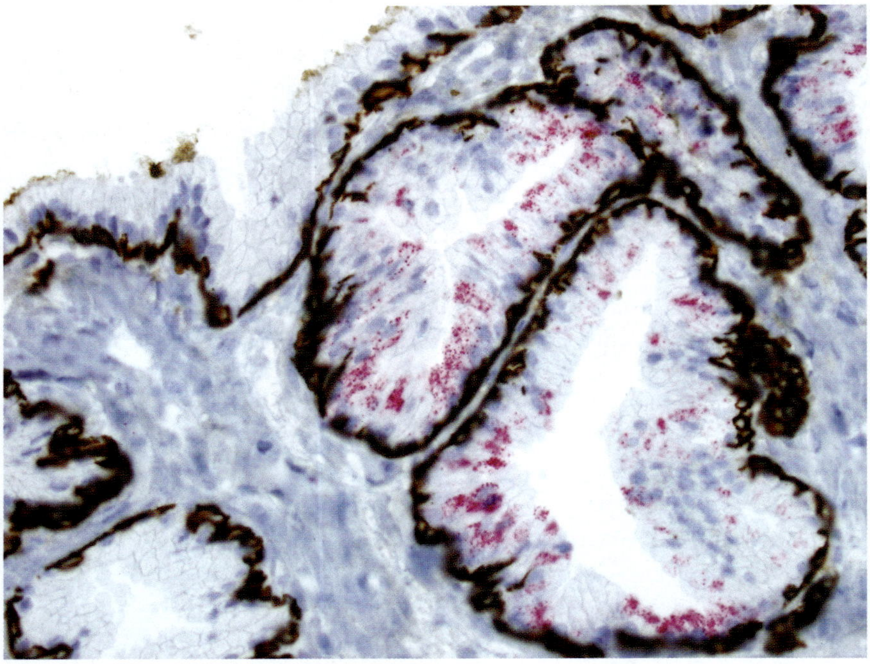

Figure 2-1.
Triple staining (AMACR, p63, and HMWC) in benign glands, which show both nuclear (p63) and cytoplasmic (HMWCK) staining in basal cells (brown). The secretory cells contain fine red granules as weak AMACR staining.

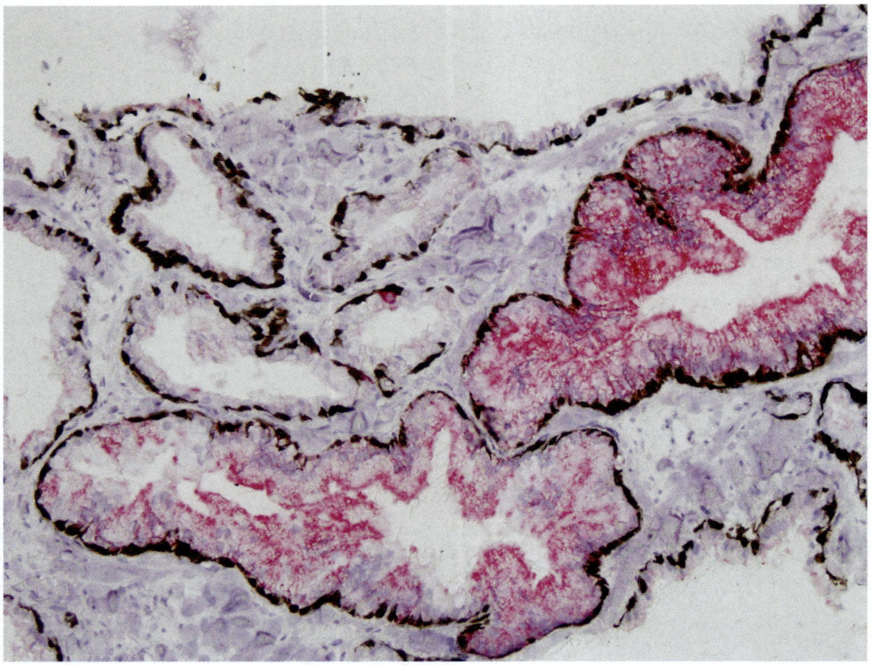

Figure 2-2.
A high-grade PIN gland with triple staining shows the presence of both basal cell staining (brown) and strong AMACR staining (red).

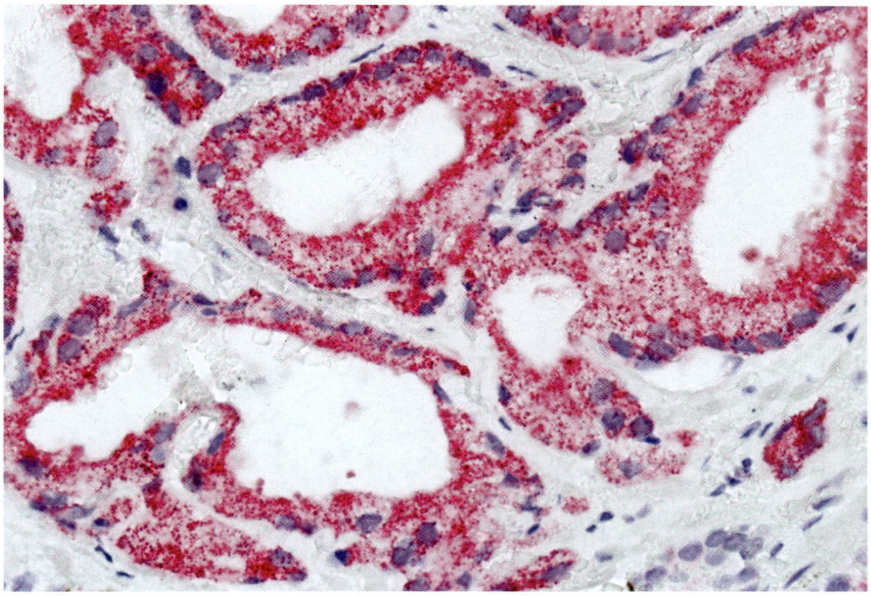

Figure 2-3.
Adenocarcinoma contains coarse red AMACR granules in the cytoplasm (strong AMACR staining) but without basal cell staining (p63 and HMWCK).

Figure 2-4.
On a prostate needle core biopsy with triple stain, a cluster of atypical glands (*a*) shows strong AMACR staining (red) and lack of basal cell staining (*b*), confirming the diagnosis of prostatic adenocarcinoma.

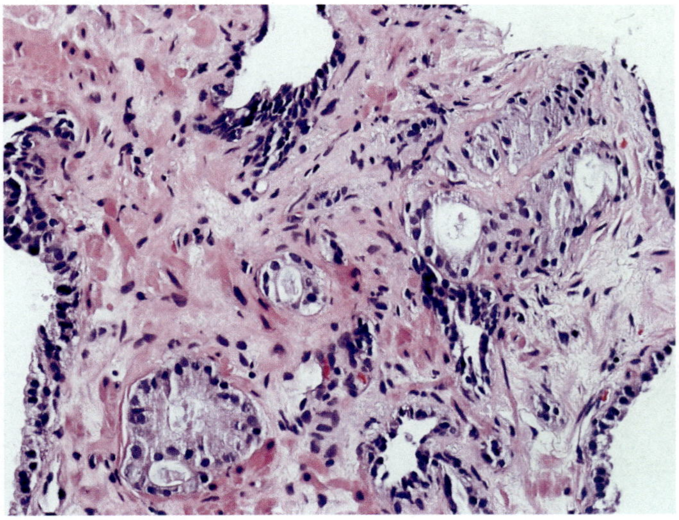

a

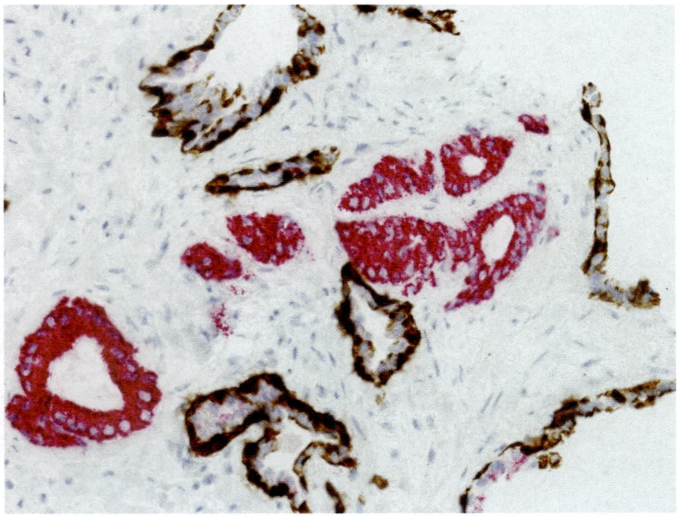

b

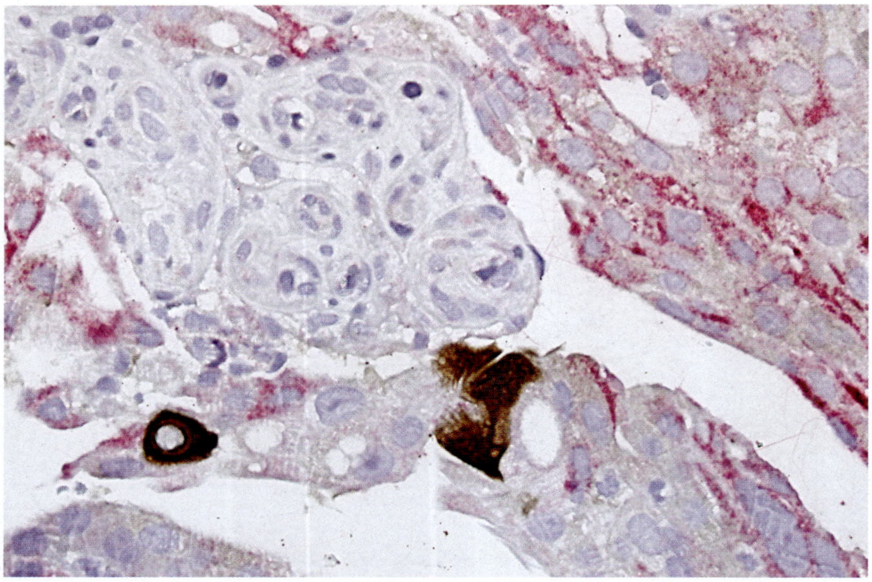

Figure 2-5.
In case of adenocarcinoma with triple staining, rare tumor cells staining positive for basal cell markers (brown), compared to the other tumor cells staining for AMACR.

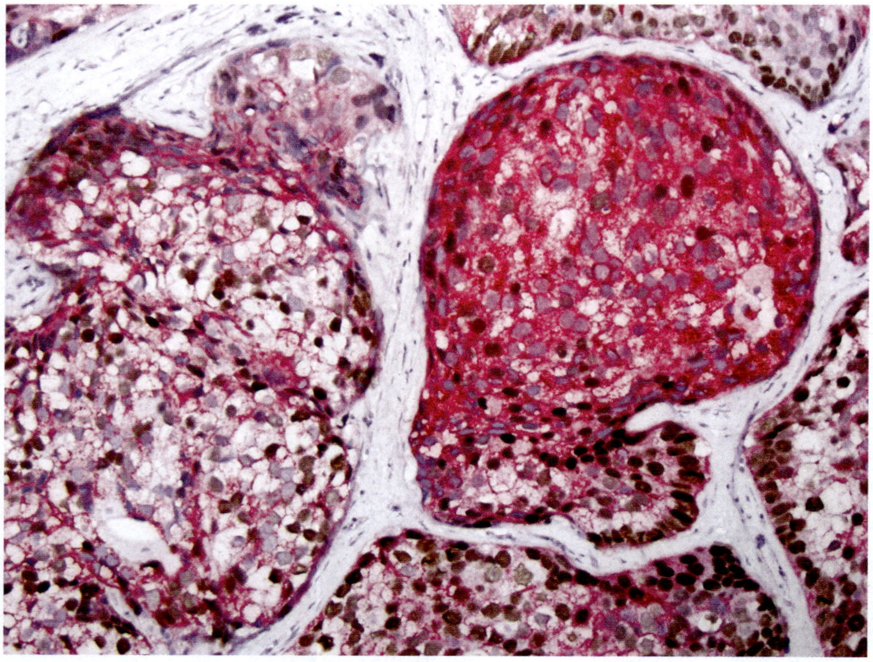

Figure 2-6.
A rare case of p63-positive prostatic adenocarcinoma with triple staining shows the presence of strong AMACR immunoreactivity and p63 immunoreactivity (nuclear staining) without HMWCK (cytoplasmic) staining in tumor cells.

Table 2-1. Advantages and Disadvantages of Triple Stain

Advantages	Only one slide needed
	No matching slides needed. A small lesion shows staining patterns for three markers together
	Colorful and easy to recognize
	Two distinct colors
Disadvantages	Technically more difficult, the red chromogen staining is particularly difficult to control
	Technical billing issue
	AMACR overstaining may lead to the wrong diagnosis

AMACR (α-METHYLACYL-CoA RACEMASE)

- Other names: p504s, racemase
- This enzyme is normally present in the liver and kidney
- It is localized in peroxisomes and mitochondria
- AMACR is related to branched fatty acid metabolism
- In the prostate, adenocarcinoma contains significantly higher levels of AMACR than benign prostatic glands or stroma
- It may be used alone or as a component of triple stain
- If staining is done properly, AMACR immunoreactivity can be seen in more than 90% of prostatic adenocarcinoma, regardless of the grades
- Typically in adenocarcinoma, AMACR staining shows larger coarse granules (Figs. 2-3 and 2-4*b*)
- In some treated prostatic adenocarcinomas, AMACR may be decreased
- AMACR can be seen in the malignant tumors from other organs, noticeably colon adenocarcinoma and papillary renal cell carcinoma, all have more than 90% positive rates
- So that AMACR may not be very specific in determining the origin of a metastatic tumor
- In high-grade PIN, the precursor lesion of prostatic adenocarcinoma, the AMACR level is also higher. However, it can be only seen in 50% of high-grade PIN cases (Fig. 2-2)
- Rare benign lesions, particularly nephrogenic adenoma can be positive for AMACR
- AMACR immunoreactivity in some conditions is summarized in Table 2-2

Table 2-2. AMACR Immunoreactivity in Prostatic Conditions and Other Lesions

	AMACR immunoreactivity
Prostatic adenocarcinoma	80% to 95%
Hormonal treated prostatic adenocarcinoma	<30%
Metastatic prostatic adenocarcinoma	70% to 80%
Irradiated prostatic adenocarcinoma	>80%
High-grade prostatic intraepithelial neoplasia	50%
Prostatic adenosis	10% to 17.5%
Nephrogenic adenoma	50%
Colonic adenocarcinoma	>90%
Papillary renal cell carcinoma	100%

P63

- P63 is a member of the p53gene family
- P63 typically shows nuclear staining
- P63 is a marker for prostatic basal cells (Figs. 2-1, 2-2, and 2-5) in a benign gland and high-grade PIN
- P63 is also a marker for benign and malignant urothelial cells
- P63 is positive in the vast majority of squamous cell carcinoma, and a small percentage of adenocarcinomas in other organs
- The marker is used to determine the origin of the tumor
- Rare cases of prostatic adenocarcinoma show focal or diffuse p63 immunoreactivity (Fig. 2-6)

HMWCK (HIGH MOLECULAR CYTOKERATINS)

- Also known as K903 or 34βE12
- Labels basal cells of the prostate (Figs. 2-1, 2-2, and 2-4*b*), urothelial cells, and squamous cells similar to p63
- Cytoplasmic staining
- In rare cases of prostatic adenocarcinoma, HWMCK can be positive in scattered distribution (Fig. 2-6)

PSA (PROSTATIC-SPECIFIC ANTIGEN)

- A protease whose function is to keep semen in liquid phase
- One of the most used markers in medicine
- It is relatively specific for prostatic secretory cells, either benign (Fig. 2-7) or malignant (Fig. 2-8)
- Benign prostatic glands produce more PSA than the malignant ones, but more PSA leaking to the circulation in adenocarcinoma, which may be related to tumor invasion
- It is uncommonly used in prostate needle core biopsy since both benign glands and adenocarcinoma will be positive
- It is mostly used in a metastatic lesion to determine whether it originated from the prostate
- In high-grade prostatic adenocarcinoma, particularly in hormonal refractile cases, the PSA immunoreactivity can be low and focal (Fig. 2-9)

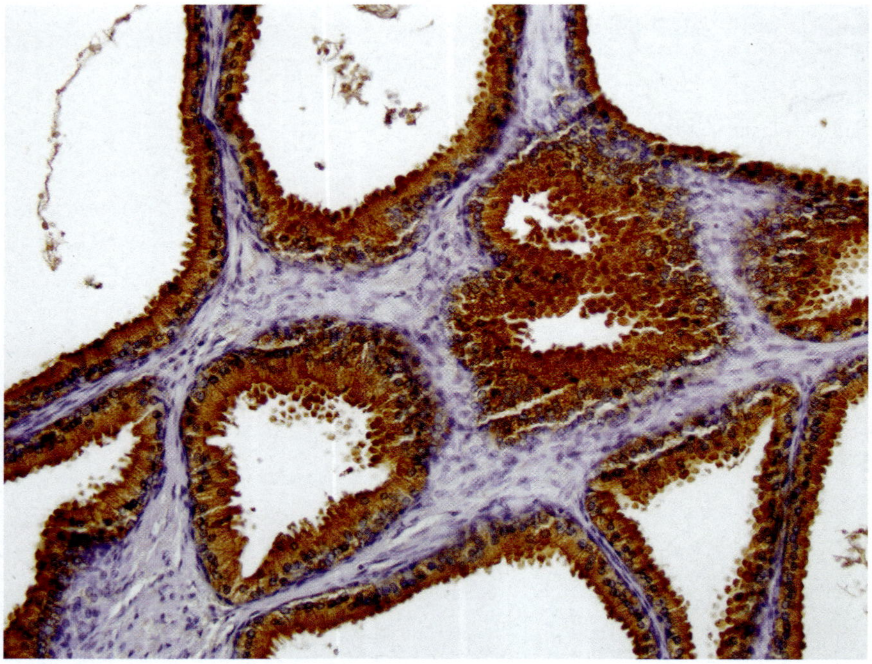

Figure 2-7.
Benign prostatic glands are diffusely positive for PSA.

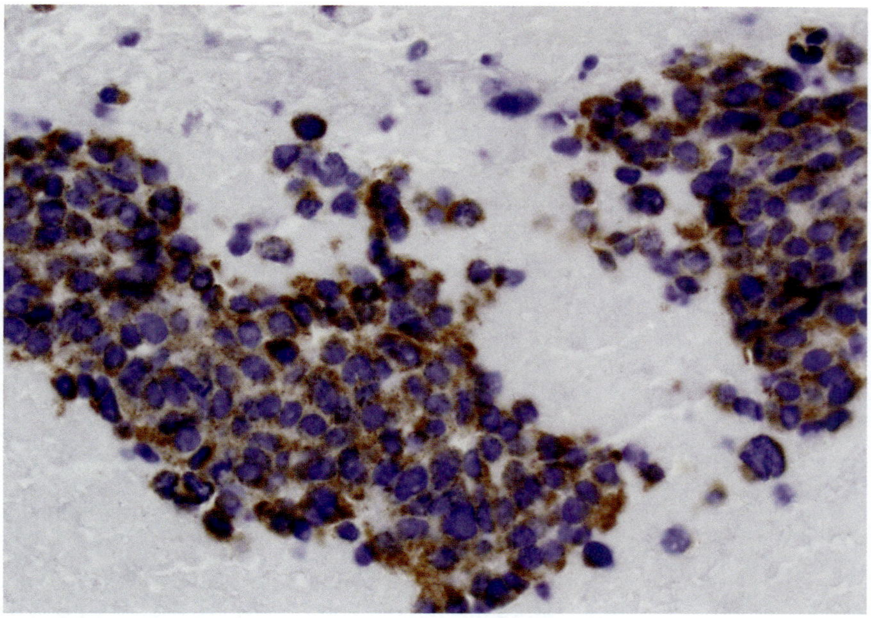

Figure 2-8.
High-grade prostatic adenocarcinoma shows diffuse PSA positivity.

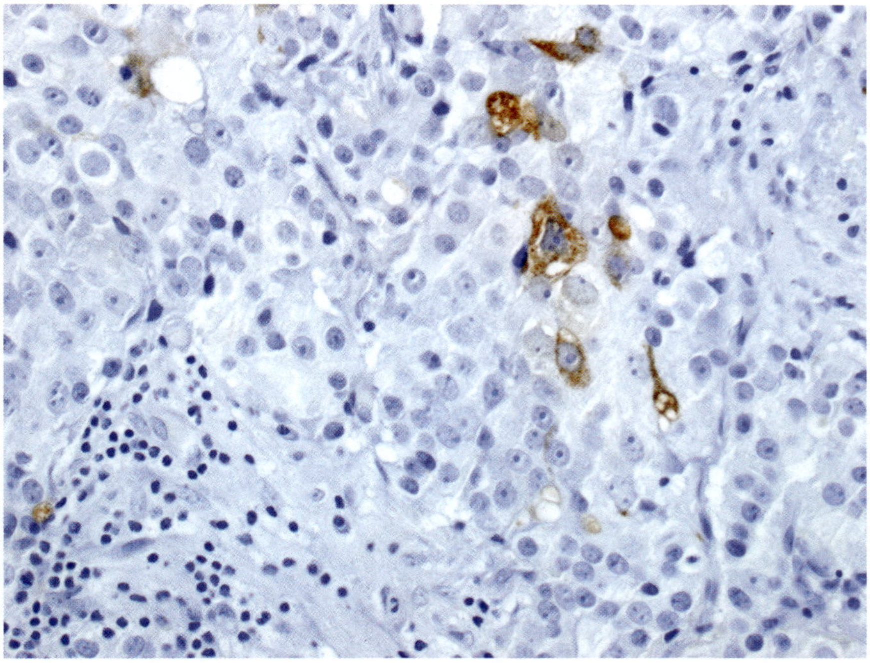

Figure 2-9.
High-grade prostatic adenocarcinoma shows rare tumor cells positive for PSA.

PSAP (PROSTATE-SPECIFIC ALKALINE PHOSPHATASE)

- Positive for both benign secretory cells and adenocarcinoma
- Similar to PSA, but less specific
- Not used frequently

PSMA (PROSTATE-SPECIFIC MEMBRANE ANTIGEN)

- Positive in both benign glands and adenocarcinoma
- However, PSMA is stronger in adenocarcinoma than in normal prostatic glands
- It is useful in identifying metastatic adenocarcinoma of the prostate in IHC or in clinical setting
- PSMA has also been seen in the vasculature within other adenocarcinoma such as gastric carcinoma

ERG (ETS-RELATED GENE)

- TMPRSS2-ERG fusion gene leads to overexpression of ERG
- ERG overexpression may contribute to development of androgen-independent prostate cancer by disruption of androgen receptor signaling
- ERG immunostaining is nuclear staining (Fig. 2-10)
- ERG is present in the normal endothelial cells as an internal positive control (Fig. 2-10*a*)
- ERG is detected by IHC in 50% of prostatic adenocarcinoma (Fig. 2-10*b*)
- There is no sufficient evidence that level of ERG is related to prognosis of prostate cancer
- ERG typically is not present in any types of carcinomas from other organs
- So that ERG is highly specific but not very sensitive marker
- The commonly used markers for prostatic cells are compared in Table 2-3

Figure 2-10.
ERG immunostaining highlights the endothelial cells, but not the benign prostatic glands (*a*). Prostatic adenocarcinoma cells exhibit positive nuclear staining (*b*).

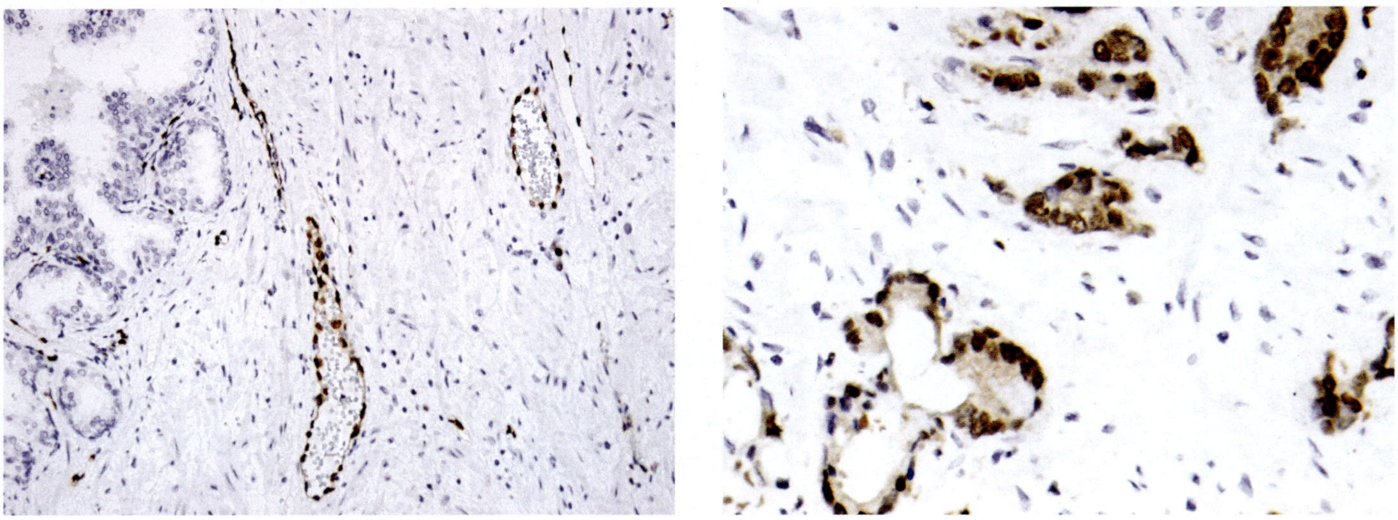

a *b*

Table 2-3. Summary of Markers Commonly Used for Prostate Pathology

Marker	*Benign secretory cell*	*Benign basal cell*	*Adenocarcinoma*
HMWCK	Negative	Positive	Negative
P63	Negative	Positive	Negative
AMACR	Negative or weakly positive	Negative	Positive (90%)
PSA	Positive	Negative	Positive
PSAP	Positive	Negative	Positive
PSMA	Positive (weak)	Negative	Positive (strong)
P501S	Positive	Negative	Positive
ERG	Negative (endothelial cells positive)	Negative	Positive (50%)

AMACR, α-methylacyl-CoA racemase; HMWCK, high molecular cytokeratins; PSA, prostatic-specific antigen; PSAP, prostate-specific alkaline phosphatase; PSMA, prostate specific membrance antigen; ERG, ETS-related gene.

CHAPTER 3 Inflammatory Lesions of the Prostate

ACUTE INFLAMMATION

Definition

- Acute inflammation of the prostate is characterized by the presence of neutrophil accumulation in the glandular structures

Other terms

- Acute prostatitis
- Typically, *focal acute inflammation* instead of *acute prostatitis* is used in the pathology diagnosis because the patient may not have any symptoms or signs

Pathogenesis

- Acute inflammation may be caused by infection or obstruction

Clinical features

- Fever, chills, and tender prostate if inflammation is extensive
- The serum PSA may be mildly increased
- The patient may not have any symptoms if inflammation is focal

Gross pathology

- No obvious change if inflammation is focal
- Microabscesses may be seen

Histology

- Accumulation of neutrophils in the lumen of prostatic glands (ducts or acini) forming microabscesses (Figs. 3-1 to 3-3)
- The glandular structures may be extended and dilated (Fig. 3-3)
- Neutrophil infiltrates may be present in the stroma as well
- Other inflammatory cells may also be present so that both acute and chronic inflammations are coexisting
- If there is tissue destruction, foamy macrophages can be seen (Fig. 3-3)
- The presence of acute inflammation should be included in the pathology report of a needle core biopsy, since it may be responsible for PSA elevation

Immunohistochemistry

- Not necessary

Clinical relevance (prognosis and treatment options)

- May or may not be associated with any symptom
- A patient with systemic symptoms of acute infection may need antibiotic treatment

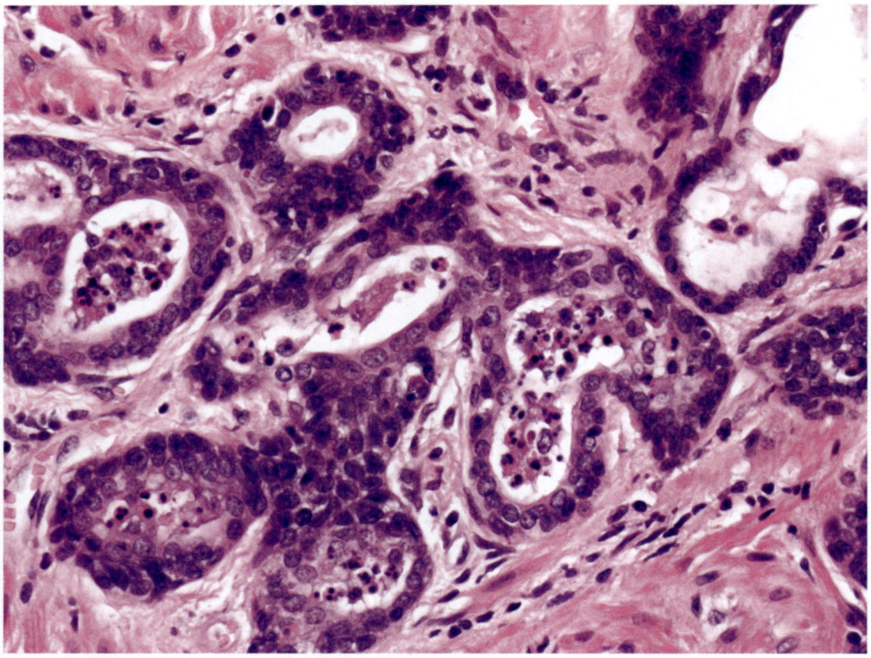

Figure 3-1.
Acute inflammation is present in multiple prostatic glands which show some reactive epithelial changes.

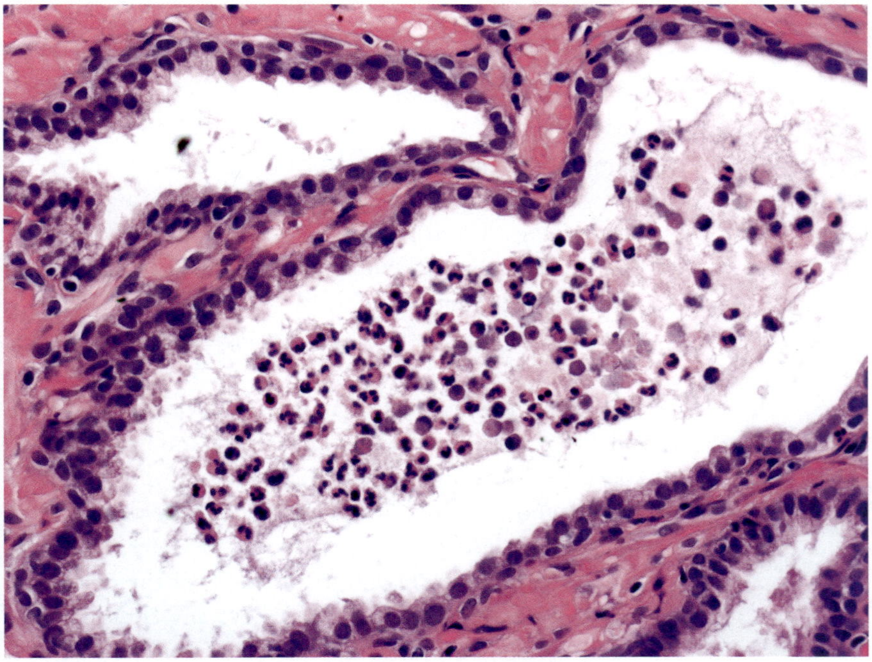

Figure 3-2.
Acute inflammation present in a dilated gland showing predominantly neutrophils and some macrophages in the lumen.

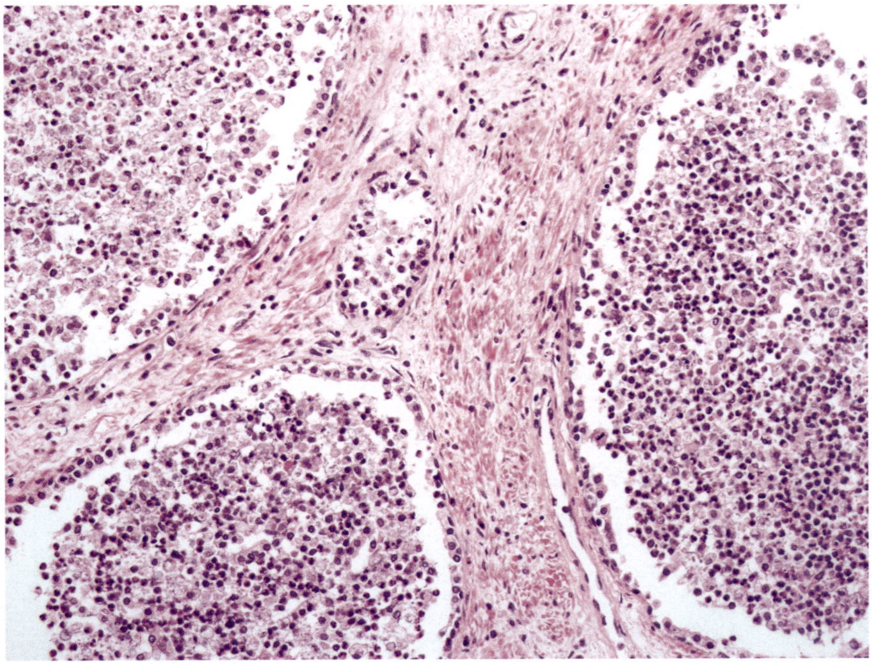

Figure 3-3.
Severe acute prostatitis from a patient with symptoms of infection. The dilated glands are all filled with neutrophils and cell debris as microabscesses.

CHRONIC INFLAMMATION

Definition

- Presence of chronic inflammatory cell infiltrates in the prostatic glands or stroma

Other terms

- Chronic prostatitis
- We typically do not use the term *chronic prostatitis* in the pathology report unless there are clinical symptoms and signs

Pathogenesis

- Many factors may contribute to the chronic inflammation
- Bacterial infection with or without benign prostatic hyperplasia (BPH) is a common cause

Clinical features

- Chronic inflammation is a very common finding in the prostate, the majority of the patients do not have any symptoms
- A dull lower back pain
- Urine positive culture for bacteria
- Mild elevation of serum PSA may be observed

Gross pathology

- No specific findings

Histology

- Chronic inflammatory cells including mostly lymphocytes and occasionally plasma cells, eosinophils, and macrophages (Figs. 3-4 to 3-6)
- The inflammation is centered around the glandular structures (Figs. 3-4 and 3-5)
- Architectural distortion and cytological atypia may be present (Fig. 3-7)
- Chronic inflammation is not associated with the increased risk for carcinoma; however, chronic inflammation may be coexisting with adenocarcinoma (Fig. 3-8)
- The diagnosis should be *chronic inflammation* rather than *chronic prostatitis* since the latter may be interpreted as a clinical entity even though the majority of the cases with focal chronic inflammation don't have any clinical symptoms and signs and there is no need for treatment

Immunohistochemistry

- Mostly not necessary
- Occasionally, AMACR and basal cell markers to rule out malignancy (Fig. 3-7*b*)
- Most chronic inflammatory cells are T cells (CD3 positive/CD20 negative)

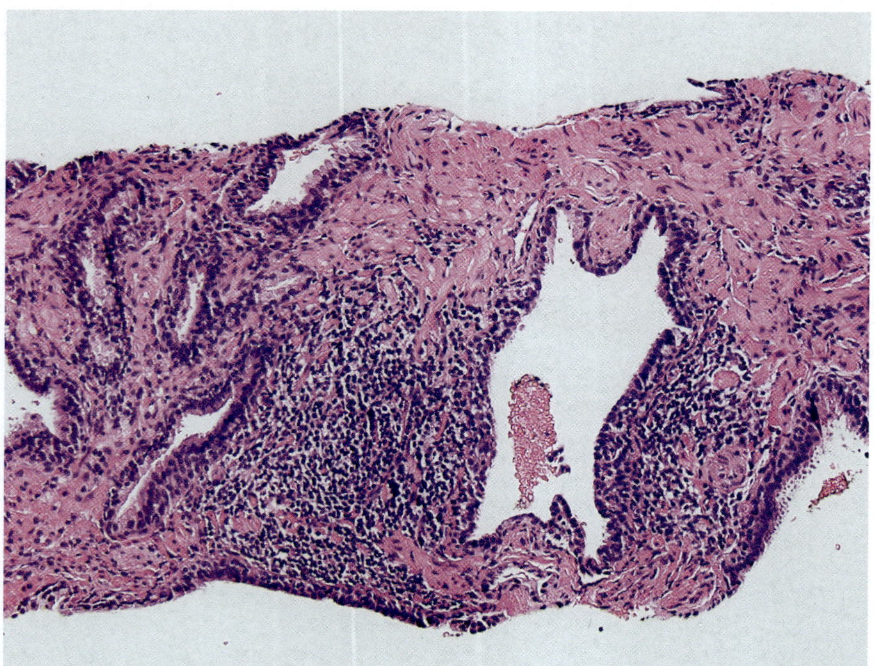

Figure 3-4.
Chronic inflammatory cells mostly lymphocytes associated with prostatic glands.

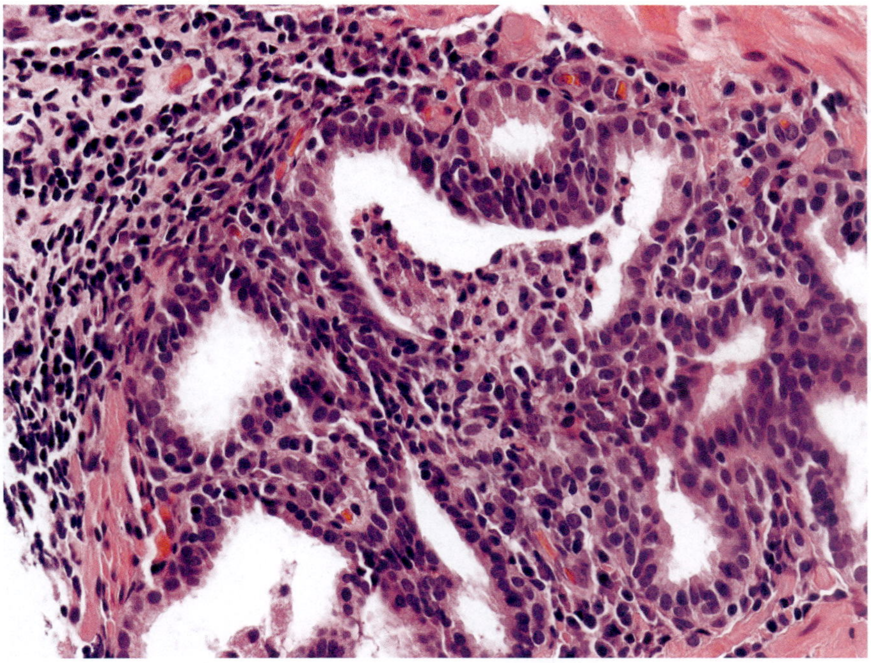

Figure 3-5.
The glandular distortion associated with chronic inflammation.

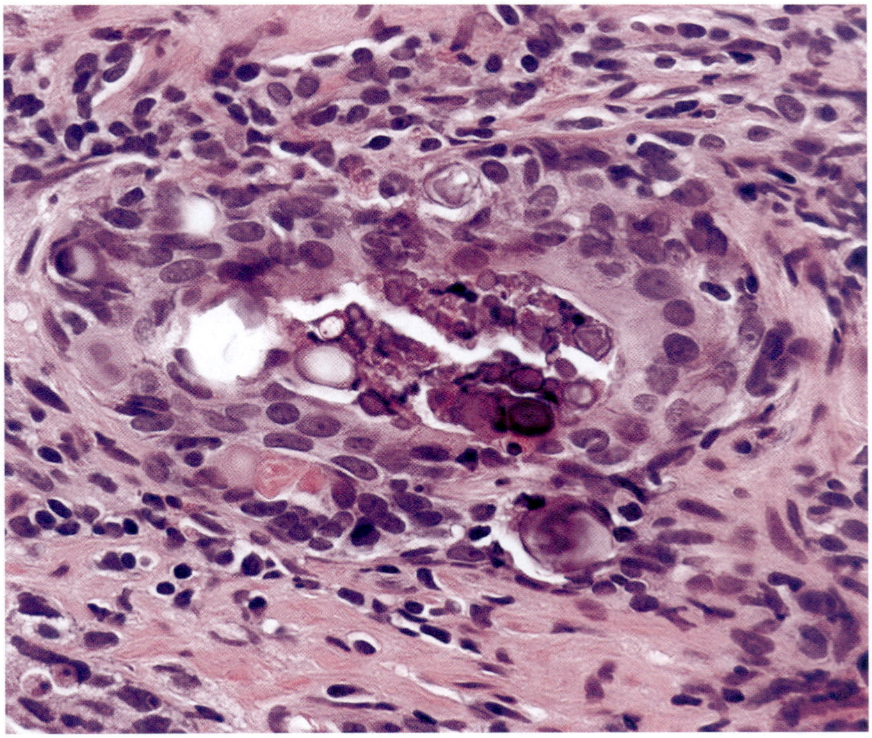

Figure 3-6.
Microcalcification associated with chronic inflammation.

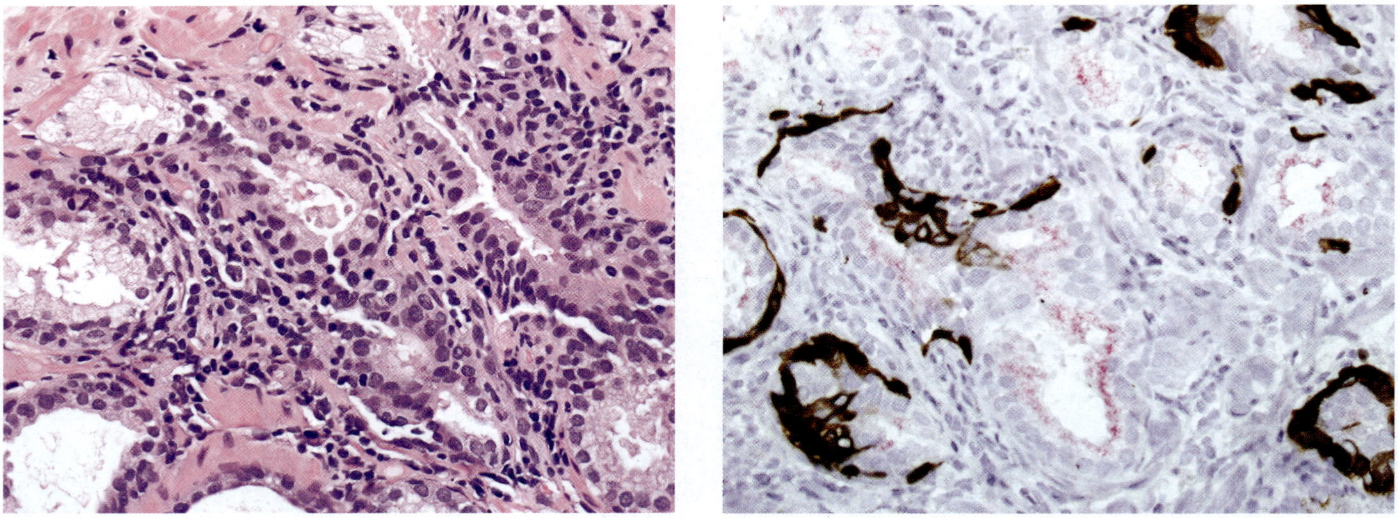

a b

Figure 3-7.
Reactive cytological atypia showing prominent nucleoli is associated with chronic inflammation (*a*). Triple immunostaining (*b*) shows the presence of patchy basal cells and weak AMACR staining in the reactive epithelial cells.

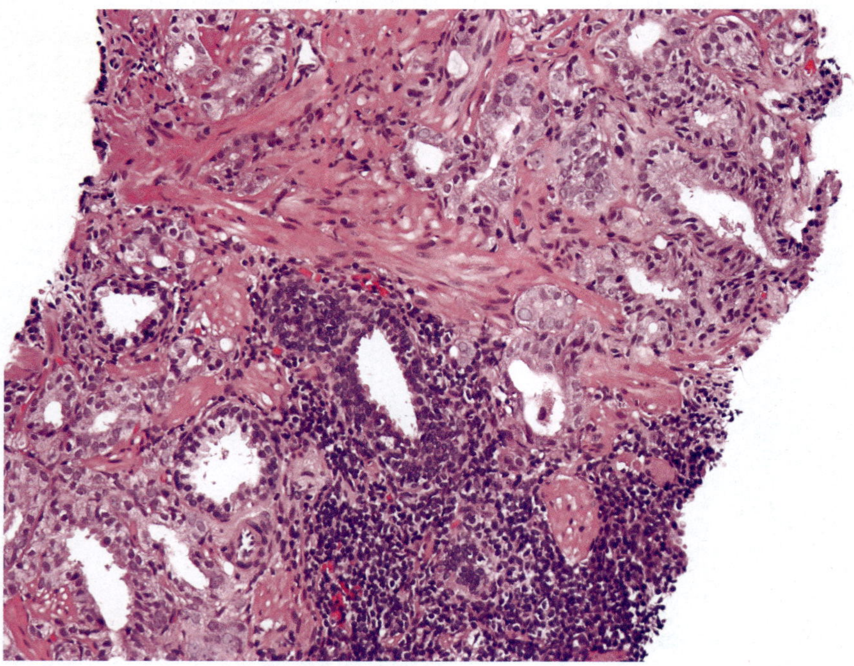

Figure 3-8.
Chronic inflammation of the prostate coexisting with prostatic adenocarcinoma.

Differential diagnosis

- Small lymphocytic lymphoma (chronic lymphocytic leukemia lymphoma) (SLL/CLL): lymphocytes are not centered around the glandular structures, and composed of monotonous B cells (CD20 positive/CD3 negative) without plasma cells and other inflammatory cells

Clinical relevance (prognosis and treatment options)

- Chronic inflammation is a very common finding seen in the majority of the prostatectomies and 20% to 30% of biopsy specimens
- We only report chronic inflammation when it is relatively extensive
- Extensive chronic prostatitis may be associated with elevated PSA

NONSPECIFIC GRANULOMATOUS PROSTATITIS

Definition

- Inflammation of the prostate with the presence of granulomas not associated with specific causes such as bacillus Calmette–Guerin (BCG) or biopsy

Clinical features

- Elevation of serum PSA up to two digits (10 to 15 μg/mL)
- Hard and nodular prostate on palpation
- Clinically suspicious for prostate cancer

Pathogenesis and epidemiology

- Nonspecific granulomatous prostatitis (NSGP) is most likely caused by the blockage of prostatic ducts, which results in epithelial disruption and the leaking cellular debris, prostatic secretions into the stroma. The leaked material induces granulomatous inflammatory response, centered around the damaged ducts or acini
- NSGP accounts for the majority of granulomatous prostatitis (50% to 70%)

Histology

- In the early phase, acute inflammation or microabscesses are centered around the ducts or acini (Fig. 3-9)
- The inflammatory process is often more diffuse (Fig. 3-10)
- Rupture and damage of the glandular epithelium can be observed (Fig. 3-10)
- Granulomas are typically poorly defined and noncaseating (Figs. 3-9 and 3-10)
- Giant cells are occasionally seen (Fig. 3-10*b*)
- In later stage, fibrosis and chronic inflammation become prominent
- When foamy macrophages are present in NSGP, it can be considered xanthogranulomatous prostatitis
- Cytologic atypia can be seen in the reactive glandular cells

Immunohistochemistry

- Basal cells can be detected
- AMACR should not be elevated in the epithelial cells with reactive atypia
- CD68 and other histiocytic markers are positive in granulomas

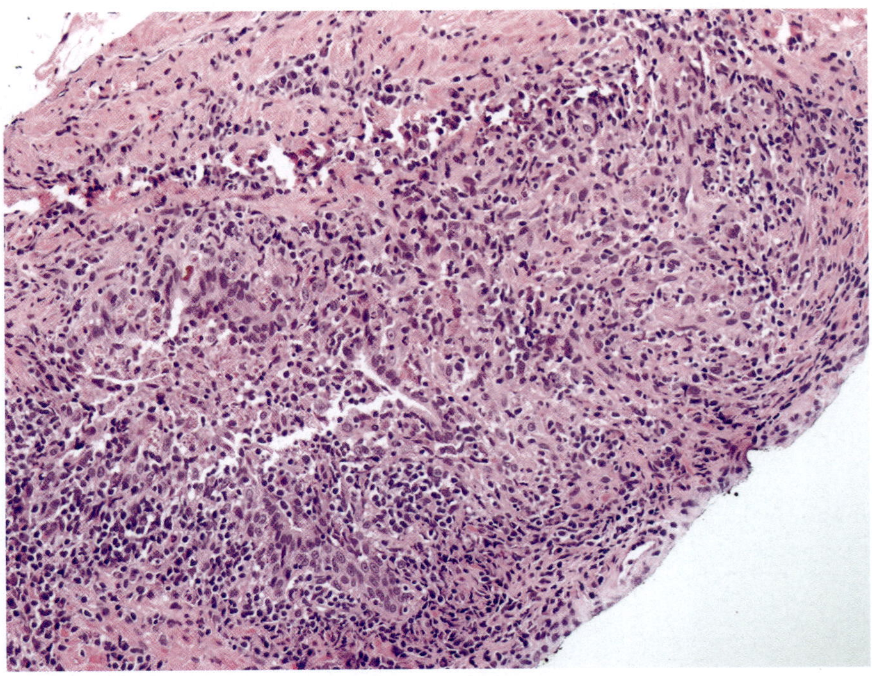

Figure 3-9.
Nonspecific granulomatous prostatitis (NSGP) with chronic inflammatory cells infiltrating around prostatic glandular structures and forming poorly defined granulomas.

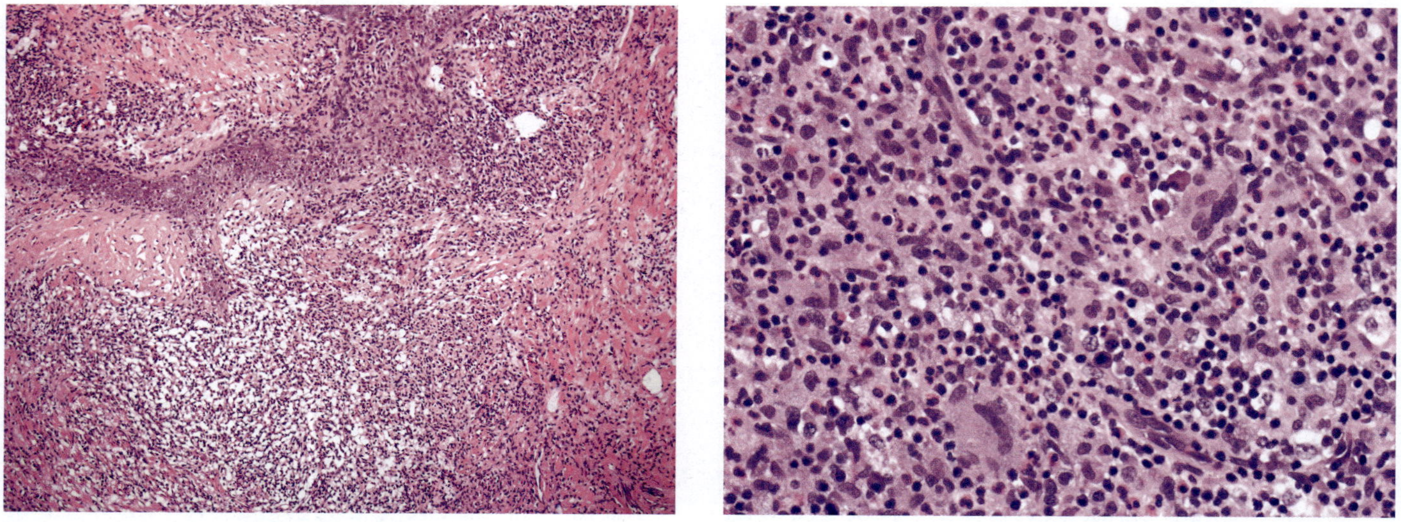

Figure 3-10.
NSGP shows extensive inflammation centered around disrupted prostatic ducts (*a*). Higher magnification (*b*) shows mixed inflammatory cells with occasional multinucleated giant cells in the granuloma.

Differential diagnosis

- In contrast, specific granulomatous prostatitis includes postbiopsy granulomas, systemic granulomatous prostatitis (such as sarcoidosis), infectious granulomatous prostatitis (such as fungi), and mycobacterial prostatitis (TB or BCG induced)
- Other granulomatous inflammations can be seen in Table 3-1

Clinical relevance (prognosis and treatment options)

- Clinical signs are highly suspicious for cancer prostatic adenocarcinoma
- A small focus of carcinoma may be masked by the heavy inflammation
- In the cases with atypia, rebiopsy may be necessary when acute inflammation subsides

Table 3-1. Differential Diagnosis of Prostatic Granulomas

	NSGP	*BCG granuloma*	*Postbiopsy granuloma*
History	Elevated PSA	History of bladder cancer with intravesical BCG administration	History of transurethral resection of bladder tumor or prostate
Symptoms	Hard prostate by palpation	Hematuria	BPH or other prostate disease
Epicenter	Disrupted ducts or acini	Not defined	Prostatic urethra
Type of necrosis	Noncaseating	Caseating necrosis	Fibrinoid necrosis, geographic necrosis
Necrosis distribution	No	Diffuse and random	Edge of resection
Acute inflammation	Yes	No	No
Key features	Granuloma associated with ruptured ducts	Granuloma with caseating necrosis and Langerhans giant cells	Granuloma with geographic fibrinoid necrotic center

BCG, bacillus Calmette–Guerin; BPH, benign prostatic hyperplasia; NSGP, Nonspecific granulomatous prostatitis; PSA, prostate-specific antigen.

POSTBIOPSY GRANULOMA AND NEEDLE TRACK

Definition

- Granulomatous reactive changes to focal tissue damage after transurethral resection of prostate (TURP) or needle core biopsy

Other terms

- Post-TURP granuloma, needle track granuloma

Pathogenesis

- TURP and needle core biopsy are invasive procedures leading to focal tissue loss and damage
- As a repair process, the body responds to this damage by granulomatous and inflammatory reactions
- Typically 12 needles cores are taken during biopsy. Therefore, it is possible to see the area of needle tracks from needle core biopsy in prostatectomy specimens

Clinical features

- History of TURP (mostly for the treatment of BPH or advanced obstructive prostate cancer) or needle core biopsy
- Some patients may develop hematospermia or hematuria after biopsy
- If complicated with infection, there will be fever, chills, pain, and tenderness of the prostate area

Gross pathology

- Prostatic urethra may show mucosal ulceration or erosion
- In some cases, the prostates are enlarged due to the presence of benign prostatic hyperplasia

Histology

- Postbiopsy granulomas are characterized by the presence of
  - A granuloma contains a large area of central necrosis surrounded by histiocytes, occasional foreign body giant cell reaction, and other chronic inflammatory cells (Fig. 3-11*a*)
  - The characteristic fibrinoid necrosis is typically irregular with a "geographic" appearance, and located in the center of the granuloma (Fig. 3-11*b*)
  - Similar postbiopsy granuloma can be also seen in the bladder after transurethral resection of bladder tumor (TURBT) (see Chapter 47)
- Needle track
  - Small well-circumscribed areas of granulomatous reaction
  - 1 to 2 mm in diameter
  - With central necrosis and histiocytic reaction, chronic inflammatory cells, with or without foreign body giant cells (Fig. 3-12)
  - Eventually the scar and fibrosis replace the granulomatous reaction

Figure 3-11.
The postbiopsy (TURP) granuloma with the center of granuloma containing the fibrinoid necrosis (*a*), surrounded by histiocytes and chronic inflammatory infiltrates (*b*).

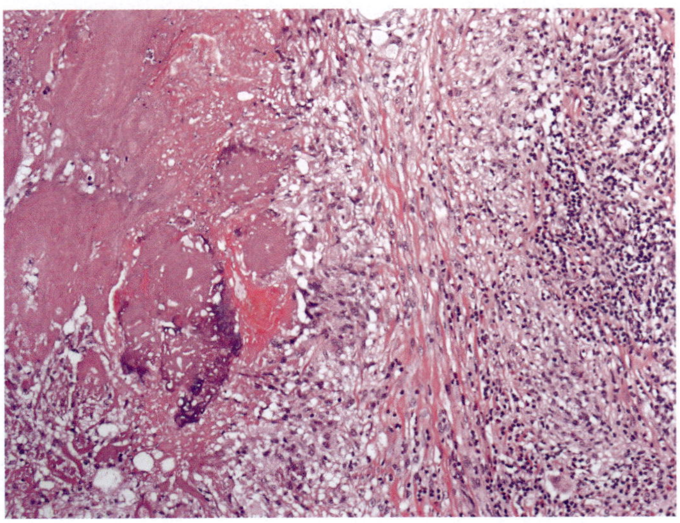

a

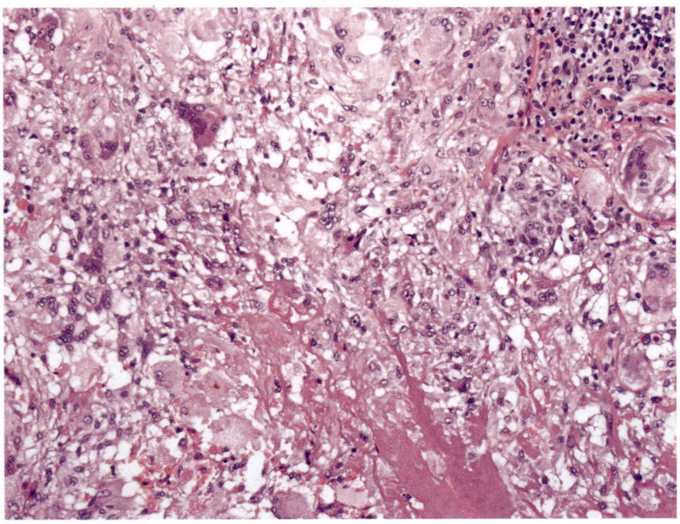

b

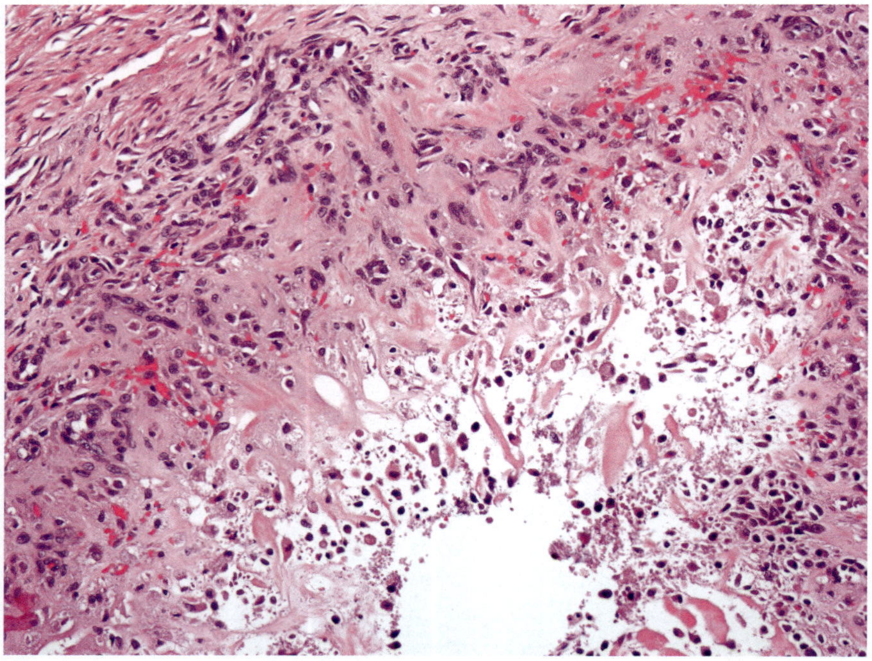

Figure 3-12.
A small needle track consists of a tissue defect caused by previous needle core biopsy and the presence of a ring of histiocytes along with lymphocytes and fibrosis.

Immunohistochemistry

- CD68 (histiocytes marker) positive. Keratin markers negative

Clinical relevance (prognosis and treatment option)

- It is a self-limiting condition
- It should not be confused with BCG or other infectious granulomatous inflammation
- Acid fast bacilli (AFB) or Grocott methenamine silver stain (GMS) stains are negative, although they are rarely necessary

BCG (INDUCED) GRANULOMA

Definition

- Granulomatous inflammation in the prostate caused by BCG therapy

Pathogenesis

- Live BCG suspension is injected intravesically into a patient with superficial bladder cancer to induce granulomatous reaction, which leads to eradication of the tumor cells in the bladder
- BCG may infect the prostate and induce granulomatous inflammation of the prostate and other organs

Clinical features

- All the patients had a history of intravesical BCG installation
- No specific symptoms except mild irritations

Histology

- Caseating or noncaseating granulomas seen in the prostate parenchyma (Fig. 3-13)
- The granuloma is composed of epithelioid histiocytes and multinucleated "horseshoe" like Langerhans giant cells (Figs. 3-13 and 3-14), morphologically identical to a TB granuloma

Immunohistochemistry and histochemistry

- AFB stain may confirm the presence of mycobacteria, but it is rarely necessary for diagnosis

Differential diagnosis (see Table 3-1)

- NSGP and postbiopsy granuloma

Clinical relevance

- No treatment necessary, unless it becomes systemic

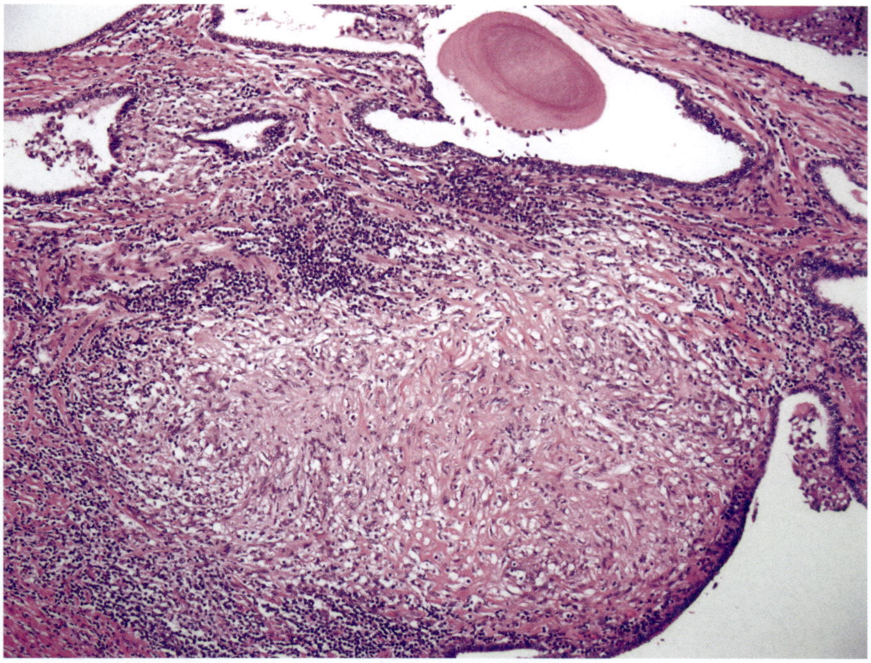

Figure 3-13.
BCG granuloma. A noncaseating granuloma is seen in a patient who received intravesical BCG treatment. No obvious necrosis is seen.

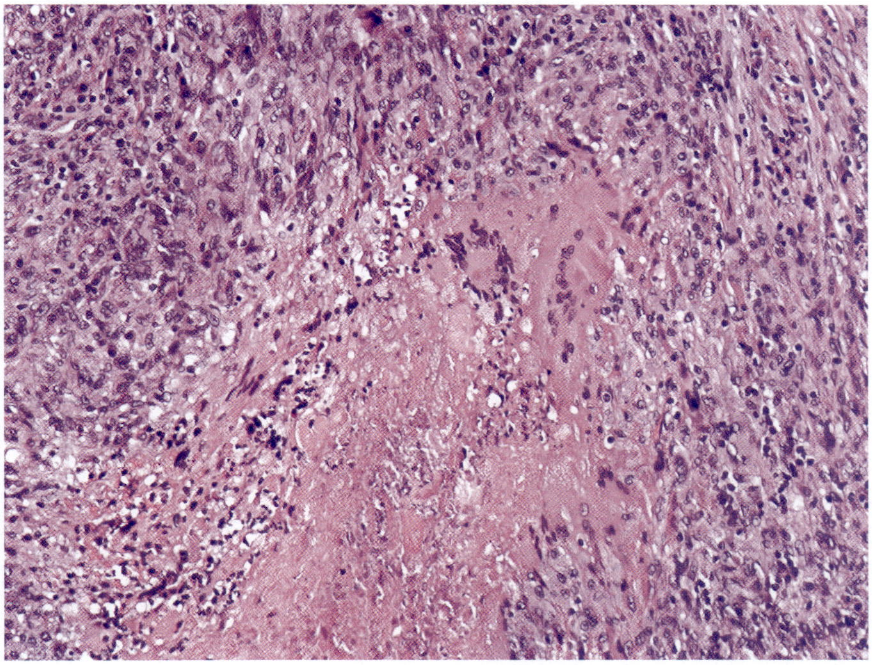

Figure 3-14.
A caseating granuloma in a patient with prior BCG treatment. Many histiocytes and occasional multinucleated giant cells with horseshoe-shaped nuclei (Langerhans cells) are seen next to caseating necrosis.

CHAPTER 4

Other Reactive Conditions of the Prostate

SIMPLE ATROPHY

Definition

- Benign atrophic lesion characteristic of small glands in lobular patterns

Other terms

- Atrophy, classic atrophy, sclerotic atrophy

Pathogenesis and epidemiology

- Increasing prevalence and extent with age
- Often mixed with benign prostatic hyperplasia (BPH)
- A frequent finding; based on our own experience, it is present in almost all prostatectomy cases and up to 40% to 50% of prostate needle core biopsies. Generally, we do not include simple atrophy in the diagnosis unless there is a special circumstance

Clinical features

- Incidental findings, with no specific clinical or imaging characteristics

Gross pathology

- The prostate size is not necessarily small unless the atrophic changes are extensive

Histology

- Lobular patterns in a low magnification (Figs. 4-1 and 4-2)
- Normally prostatic ducts and acini cannot be distinguished based on morphological features. However, in atrophy, a dilated duct is surrounded by acini (Fig. 4-1)
- Because of the atrophic stroma, the glands are closely packed. However, unlike the infiltrating patterns in adenocarcinoma, the atrophic acini are uniformly spaced (Fig. 4-3)
- The glands appear to be darker because of the scant cytoplasm. Of the attenuated secretory cells (Fig. 4-3), basal cells are prominent (Fig. 4-2*b*)
- No significant cytological atypia in either secretory cells or basal cells
- Atrophy is often focal, with or without mixing with BPH
- Atrophy can be associated with chronic inflammation (Fig. 4-2). The causative relationship, however, is difficult to prove
- Atrophy is also weak proliferative processes
- It can be confused with adenocarcinoma

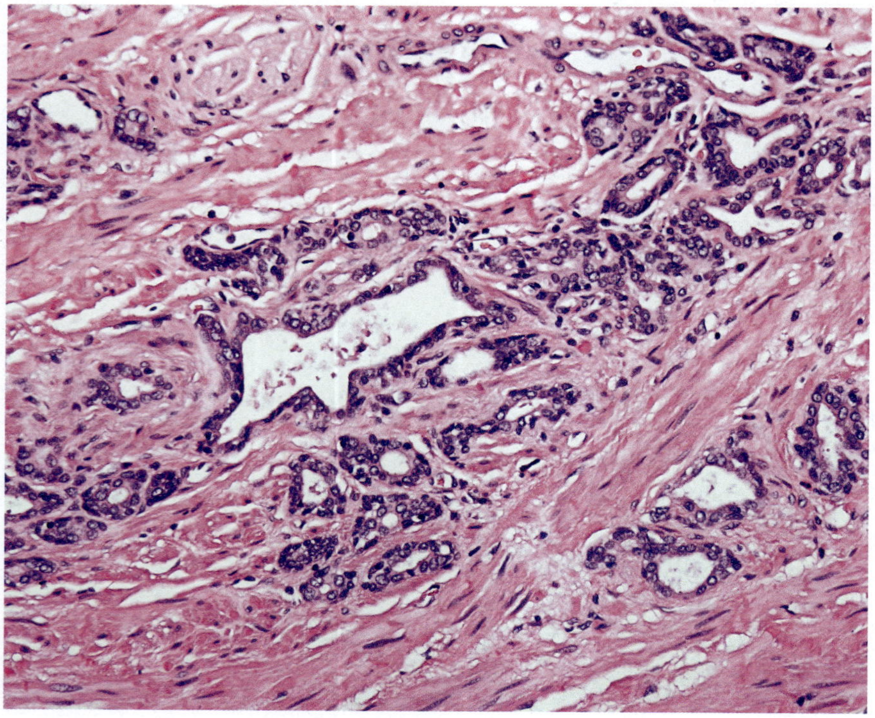

Figure 4-1.
Simple atrophy with a dilated duct in the middle, surrounded by small atrophic acini.

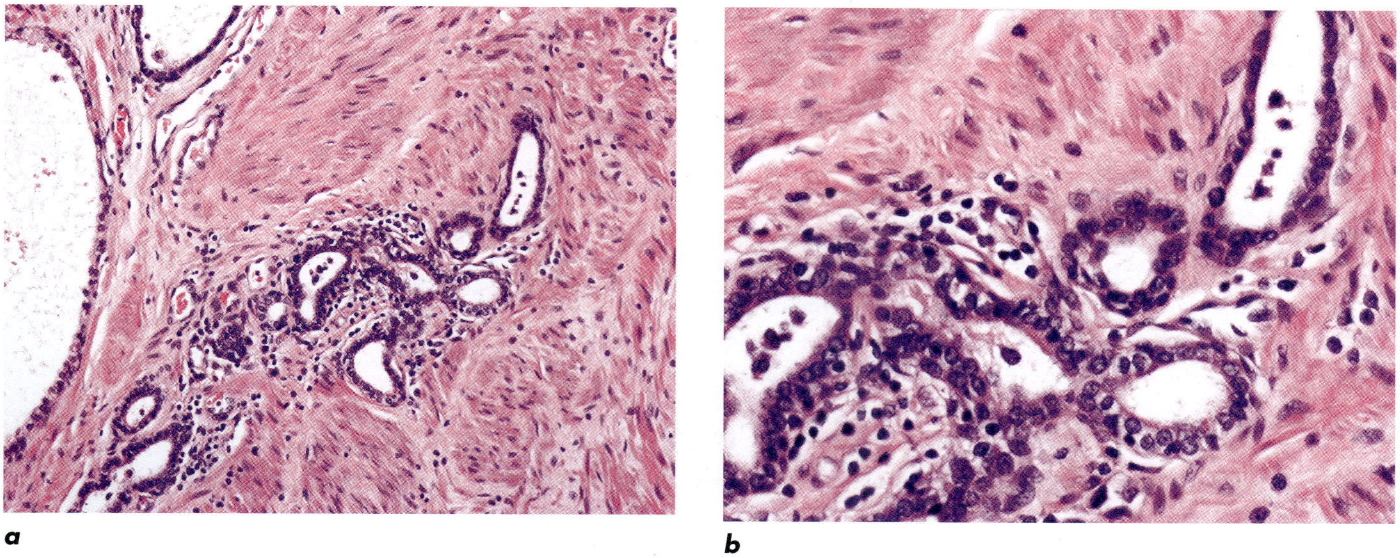

Figure 4-2.
A cluster of small glands in simple atrophy is associated with mild chronic inflammation (*a*). High magnification (*b*) shows prominent basal cells with no cytological atypia in the atrophic glandular cells.

Immunohistochemistry

- Basal cell markers positive
- AMACR negative or weakly positive
- Low Ki67 proliferative activity

Clinical relevance (prognosis and treatment options)

- Atrophy of prostatic acini and ducts in a pathology report does not correlate with the prostate size or weight
- This is a common benign condition, but it can be a mimic of adenocarcinoma

Figure 4-3.
Atrophic glands may appear to be infiltrative, but the distance between each gland (*a*) is even. At high magnification, there is no nuclear atypia (*b*).

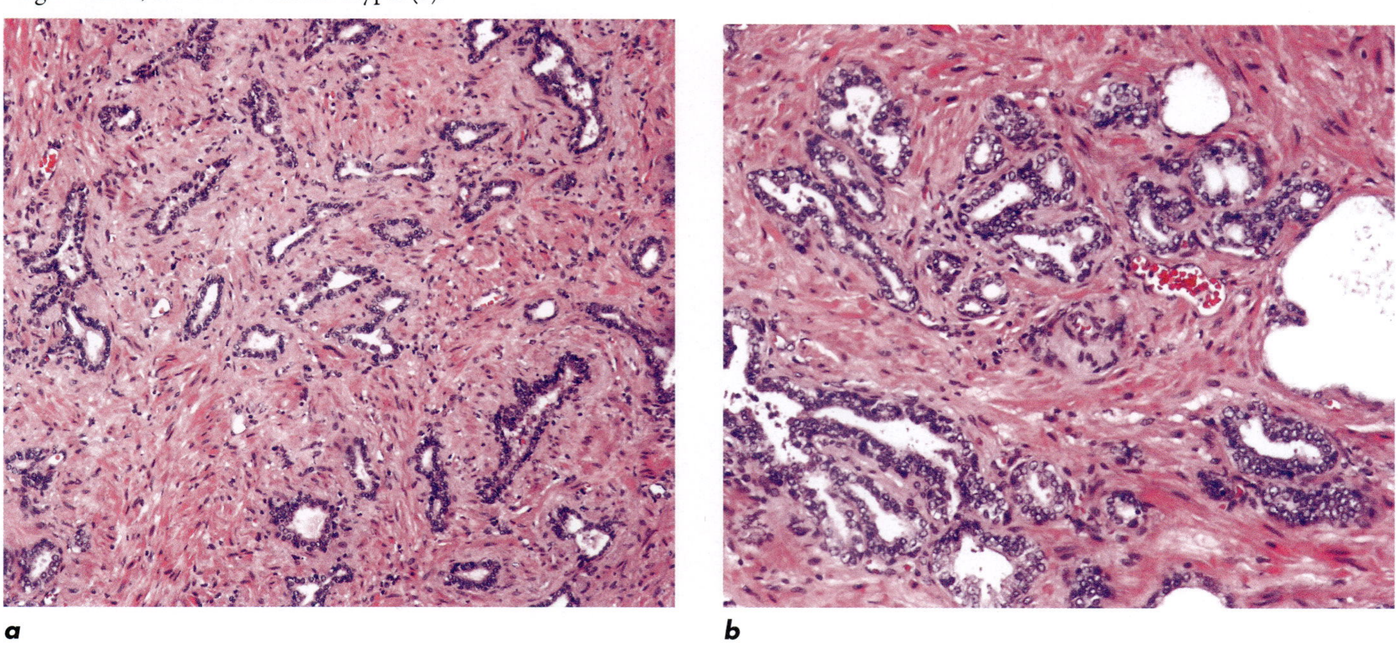

CYSTIC ATROPHY

Definition

- Benign atrophic lesion characterized by the presence of cystically dilated atrophic glands

Pathogenesis

- A form of benign atrophy
- Very common finding in the prostatectomy specimen

Clinical features

- No specific features

Gross pathology

- No specific findings

Histology

- Lobular patterns similar to simple atrophy
- Dilated glands with atrophic flat glandular cells (Fig. 4-4)
- Glandular cells with scant cytoplasm without cytological atypia

Immunohistochemistry

- Basal cell markers showing attenuated basal cells
- AMACR negative

Clinical relevance (prognosis and treatment options)

- Benign, no treatment

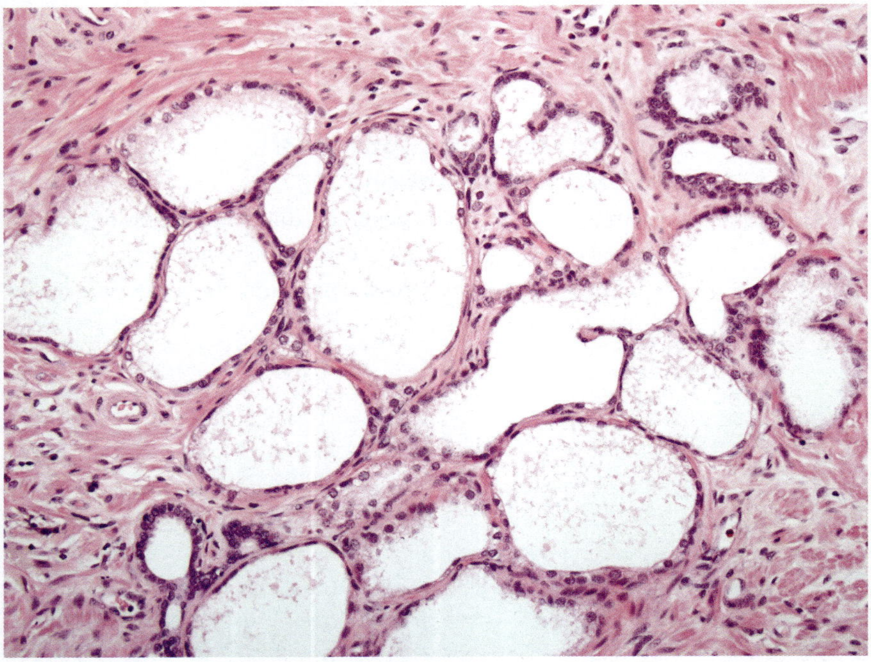

Figure 4-4.
A cluster of cystically dilated prostatic glands in a lobular pattern with attenuated epithelial cells without cytological atypia.

PARTIAL ATROPHY

Definition

- A benign atrophic lesion of the prostate characterized by angulated atrophic glands, moderate cytoplasm, and bland cytology

Pathogenesis

- Not known

Clinical features

- Relatively common in the prostate biopsy
- No specific symptoms, not known to be related to elevated PSA
- One of the most common benign conditions misdiagnosed as cancer

Gross pathology

- No specific findings

Histology

- The lesion is composed of angulated small atrophic glands (Fig. 4-5)
- Most cases showing lobular patterns (Fig. 4-6)
- Some cases may appear infiltrative
- Clusters of glandular cells with clear or pale cytoplasm and poorly recognizable lumens
- Patchy basal cells may be identified

Immunohistochemistry

- HMWCK or p63 positive, although two of three cases show patchy or minimal basal cells (Fig. 4-6*c*)
- Approximately, one of three partial atrophy cases may show positive AMACR, typically weak staining, not much higher than adjacent normal benign glands (Fig. 4-6*c*)

Differential diagnosis

- Most important is the differential diagnosis from adenocarcinoma (see Table 4-1)

Clinical relevance (prognosis and treatment options)

- Not associated with increased risk for adenocarcinoma
- It may be misdiagnosed as adenocarcinoma if one is unfamiliar with this entity
- The suspicious diagnosis, such as ASAP (see Chapter 6), should not be made on partial atrophy unless it has additional cytological atypia

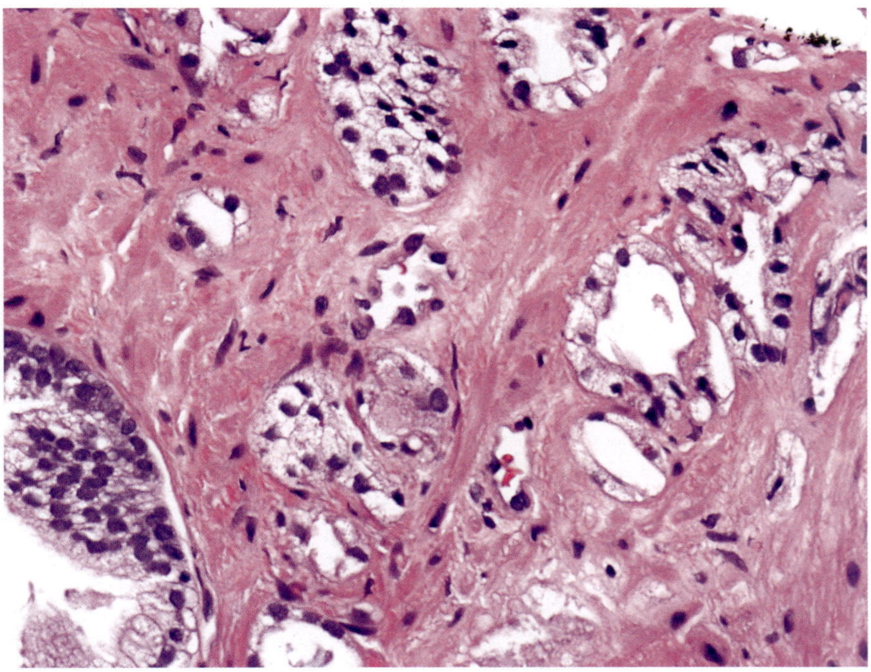

Figure 4-5.
Partial atrophy shows angulated smaller glands with scant to moderate clear cytoplasm. However, there are no prominent nucleoli in these glands.

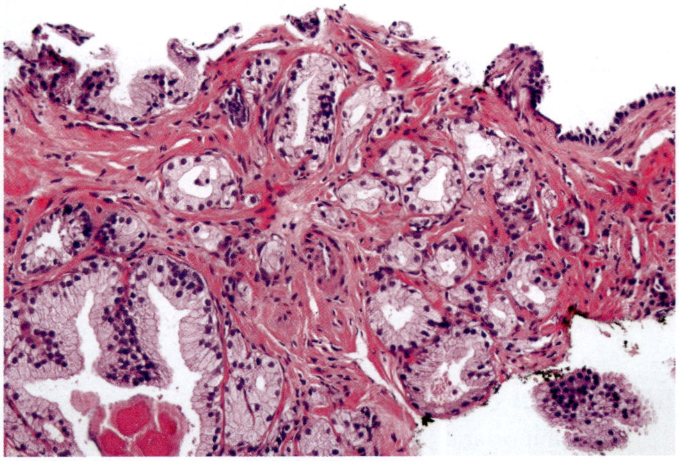

a

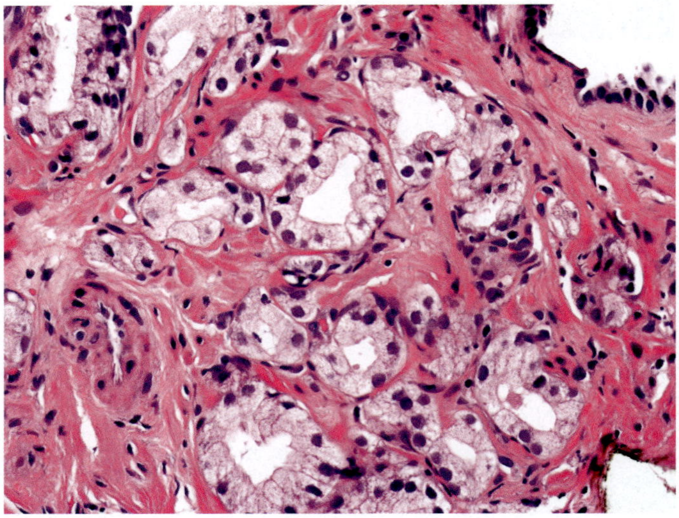

b

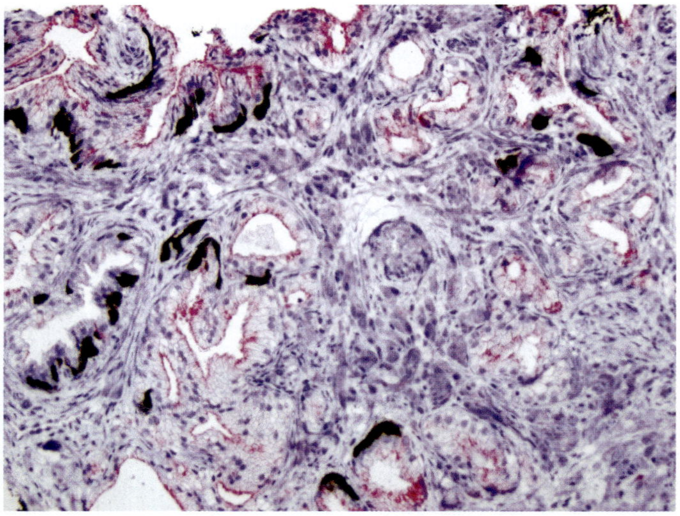

c

Figure 4-6.
(*a*) Another case of partial atrophy composed of small crowded glands with clear cytoplasm. (*b*) High magnification showing glands with angulated edges, which may appear to be single cells. No prominent nucleoli seen. (*c*) By triple immunostaining, there are patchy basal cells present in this focus. AMACR staining is weak. These features are typical for partial atrophy.

Table 4-1. Comparison of Partial Atrophy with Adenocarcinoma

	Partial atrophy	*Adenocarcinoma*
Patterns	Small crowded glands	Small crowded glands
Infiltrating	No	Yes
Nuclear atypia	No	Yes
Cytoplasm	Pale	Amphophilic or pale
AMACR	Weak, similar to benign glands	Strong, granular
Basal cell markers	Patchy basal cells in the focus	No basal cells
	Some glands may not contain basal cells	

POSTATROPHIC HYPERPLASIA

Definition

- Benign atrophic lesions with proliferative nature

Other terms

- Morphologically, there is significant overlap with simple atrophy

Pathogenesis

- Increased proliferation in benign atrophic glands as measured by Ki67 immunostaining, compared to normal prostatic glands

Clinical features

- No specific features

Gross pathology

- No specific findings

Histology

- Small crowded glands in a lobular pattern
- Secretory cells with slightly more cytoplasm (Fig. 4-7)
- Minimal cytological atypia (Fig. 4-8)
- Sometimes central dilated ducts surrounded by atrophic acini can be appreciated

Immunohistochemistry

- Basal cell markers showing presence of basal cells (Fig. 4-8*b*)
- AMACR negative
- Ki67 slightly increased compared to normal prostatic glands

Clinical relevance (prognosis and treatment options)

- Benign. Many atrophic lesions of the prostate can be proliferative

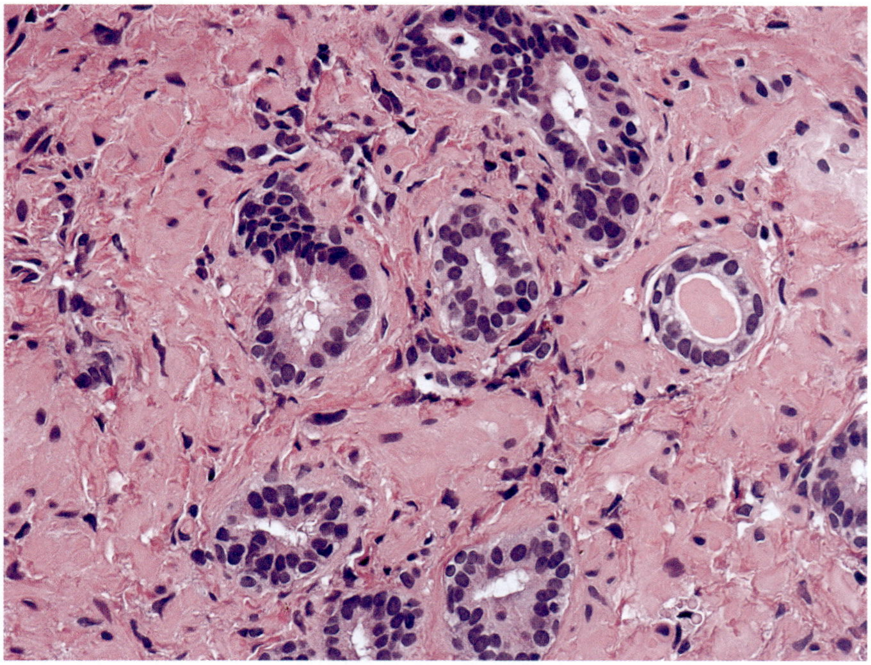

Figure 4-7.
Postatrophic hyperplasia with cluster of small glands with moderate amount cytoplasm. Mild cytological atypia is present.

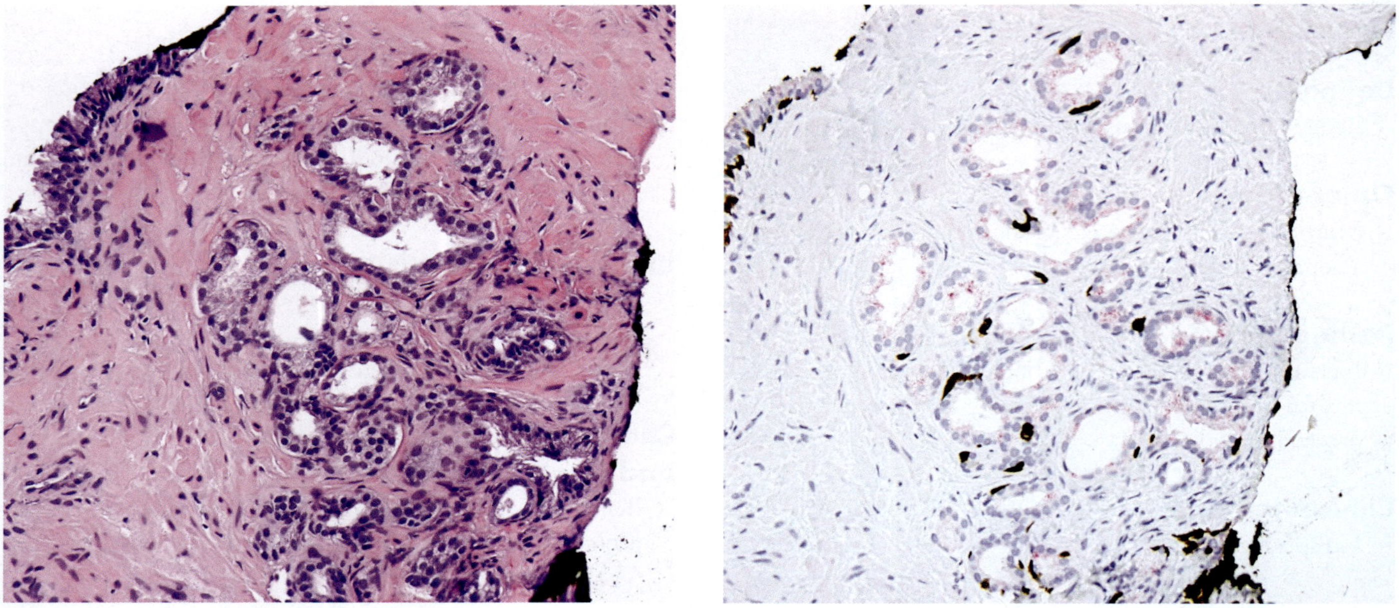

a b

Figure 4-8.
(*a*) A cluster of small atrophic glands with a lobular pattern. The glandular cells have more cytoplasm than simple atrophy. (*b*) Triple stains show the patchy basal cells and lack of significant AMACR reactivity, which confirms the diagnosis of benign atrophic glands.

OTHER BENIGN ATROPHIC LESIONS

Definition

- Any benign prostatic lesions with atrophic changes

Other terms

- Proliferative inflammatory atrophy
- Postsclerotic hyperplasia
- Sclerotic atrophy

Summary

- There are many other terms to describe benign atrophic lesions, which have the following common features:
  - These atrophic conditions are all benign
  - Like simple atrophy, some of these lesions may be proliferative in nature
  - They do not have strong association with prostate cancer, therefore, lack of clinical significance
  - The only significance is that these benign atrophic lesions may be confused with adenocarcinoma
  - There is significant overlap between them; therefore, it is difficult to reproducibly make a diagnosis using these terminologies
- We believe that understanding the morphology of these entities is more important than using the terms in clinical practice. We typically use *benign prostatic tissue* to cover most of the atrophic lesions

Proliferative inflammatory atrophy

- When there is chronic inflammation in the prostate, the glandular epithelium may appear to be reactive and proliferative (Fig. 4-9)
- It may or may not have prominent atrophic changes. It has significant overlapping with postatrophic hyperplasia
- The pathology diagnosis of this lesion is difficult without using Ki67 immunostain to demonstrate its proliferative nature
- Because of the involvement of inflammatory, this lesion has been considered to be the linker of inflammation and prostate cancer
- However, there is no evidence that inflammation and atrophy are related
- This term has never been accepted by many pathologists as a true entity. Now this term has lost its popularity and disappeared from most pathology textbooks

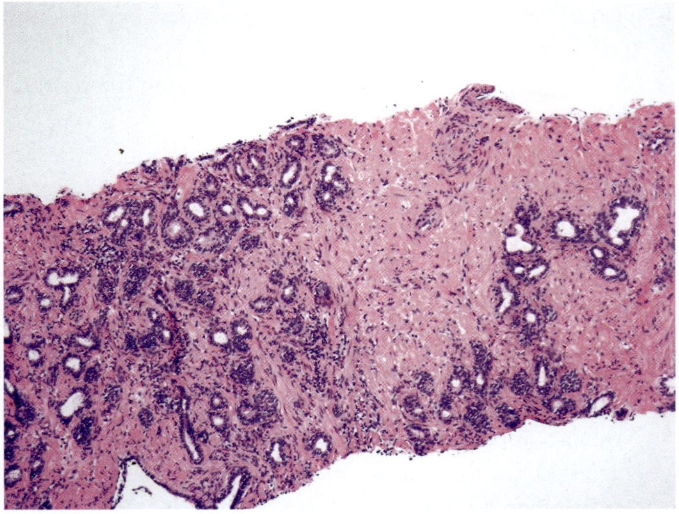

a

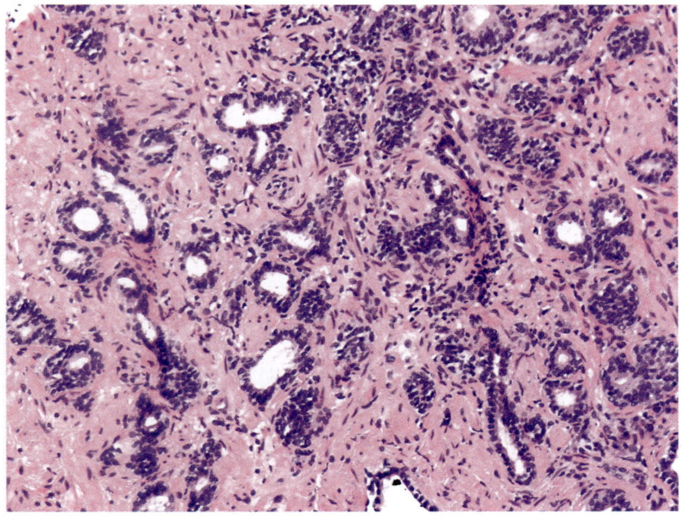

b

Figure 4-9.
Benign atrophy on needle biopsy with numerous small glands in lobular patterns (*a*). High magnification (*b*) demonstrates lack of cytological atypia and presence of chronic inflammation. This case can be considered simple atrophy, postatrophic hyperplasia, or postinflammatory hyperplasia.

Sclerotic atrophy

- An atrophic lesion that shows prominent sclerotic stromal atrophy (Fig. 4-10)

Postsclerotic hyperplasia

- Atrophic lesions with sclerotic stroma and glandular epithelium showing hyperplastic changes
- Overlaps with many atrophic or benign conditions, and the diagnosis is not easily reproducible

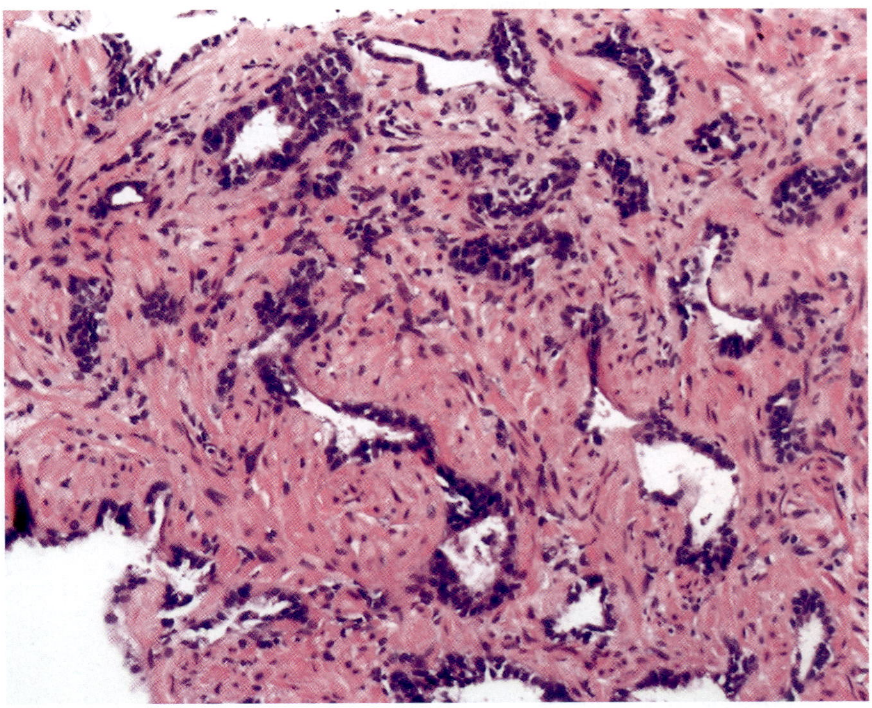

Figure 4-10.
Sclerotic atrophy with atrophic prostatic glands and sclerotic stroma.

BENIGN PROSTATIC HYPERPLASIA (BPH)

Definition

- Benign prostatic enlargement caused by increased stromal and glandular cells in a nodular fashion

Other terms

- Benign prostatic hypertrophy (incorrect term often used clinically). In pathology, hypertrophy means an increase of cell size, which is not the case for BPH
- Benign nodular hyperplasia
- Benign stromal and/or glandular hyperplasia

Pathogenesis

- The precise etiology is unknown
- More common in aging men
- The process is related to the accumulation of dihydrotestosterone (DHT), which is a more potent androgen, converted from testosterone by the enzymatic action of 5-α reductase

Clinical features

- Enlargement of prostate by palpation or imaging studies
- Urinary obstructive symptoms such as difficulty in urination, weak and discontinuous urine stream, urgency and dribbling, high residual urine volume in the bladder
- Urinary obstruction may lead to bladder hypertrophy and/or hydronephrosis in severe cases
- Clinical diagnosis will be made by measuring the residual bladder volume
- Mild increase of PSA
- Patients with BPH may develop obstruction associated infections of the prostate

Gross pathology

- Large prostate, weighing from 40 to 100 g. In the extreme cases, the prostate can reach the weight of more than 500 g
- Nodular appearance in cut surface resembling tumors (Fig. 4-11) in the central portion of the prostate (mostly transition zone)
- Prostatic urethra becomes slit-like due to compression

Histology

- Low magnification shows multiple nodules ranging from 0.1 to 10 mm in size (Fig. 4-12), mostly in the transition zone (central portion)
- Hyperplastic nodules are well circumscribed without a capsule (Figs. 4-12 and 4-13)
- A hyperplastic nodule is composed of both stromal and glandular components at different ratios (Figs. 4-12, 4-14, and 4-15)
- The glands show variables size and shapes, often with convoluted contours

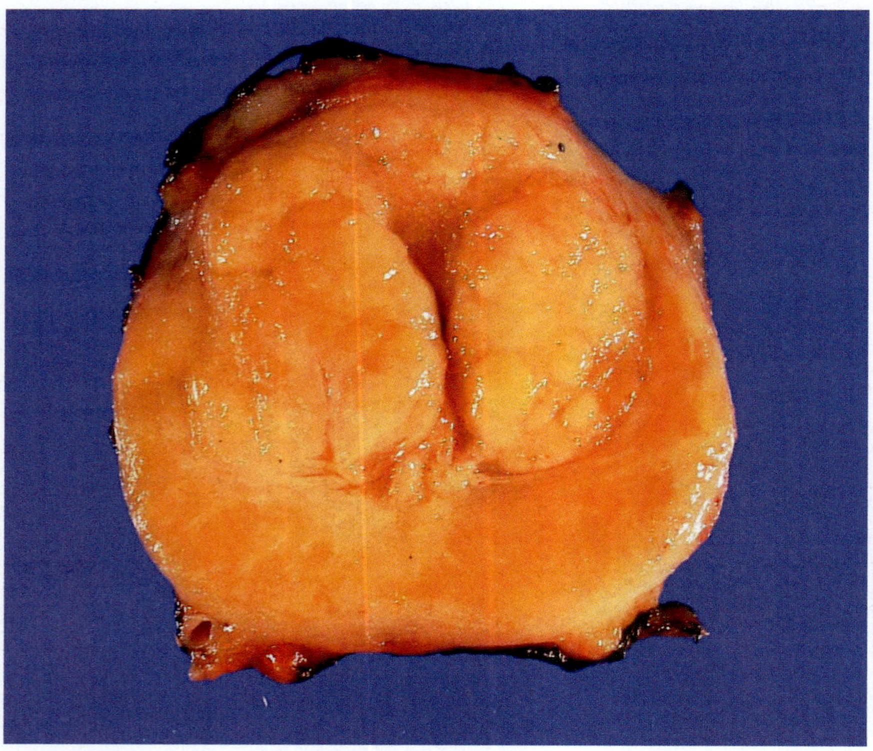

Figure 4-11.
Gross photo of a prostate with benign prostatic hyperplasia showing large BPH nodules in the central portion of the prostate compressing the prostatic urethra.

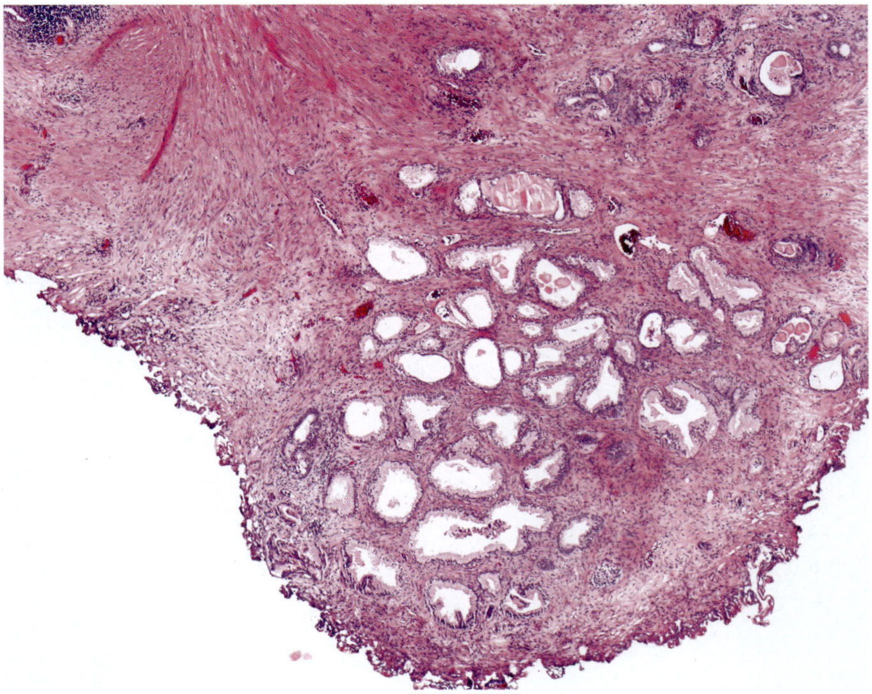

Figure 4-12.
A BPH nodule contains both components of glandular and stromal hyperplasia within the nodule.

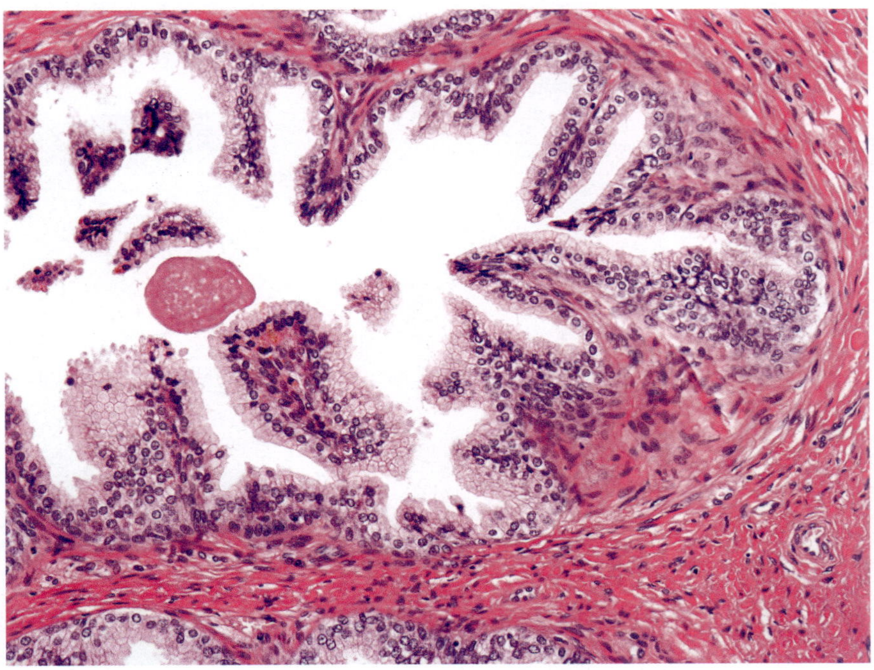

Figure 4-13.
A glandular structure within a BPH nodule shows the large convoluted lumen. The presence of secretory and basal cells can be appreciated. It is impossible to tell whether this gland is from a BPH patient or a patient without BPH at this magnification.

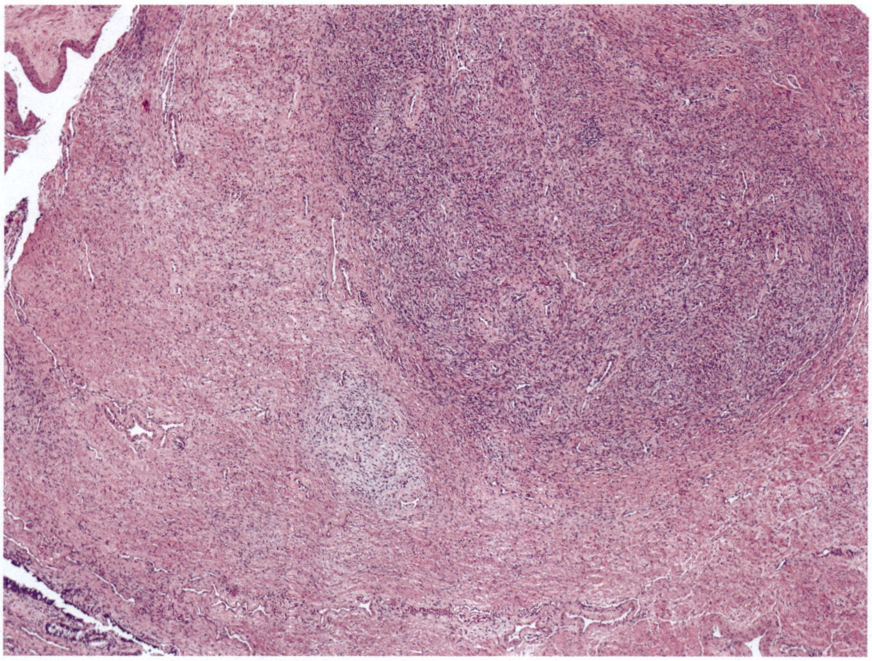

Figure 4-14.
A BPH nodule composed entirely of stromal component.

Figure 4-15.
A BPH nodule is surrounded by compressed and elongated glands (*a*). High magnification shows hyperplastic and cystically dilated glands, surrounded by a compressed elongated gland (*b*).

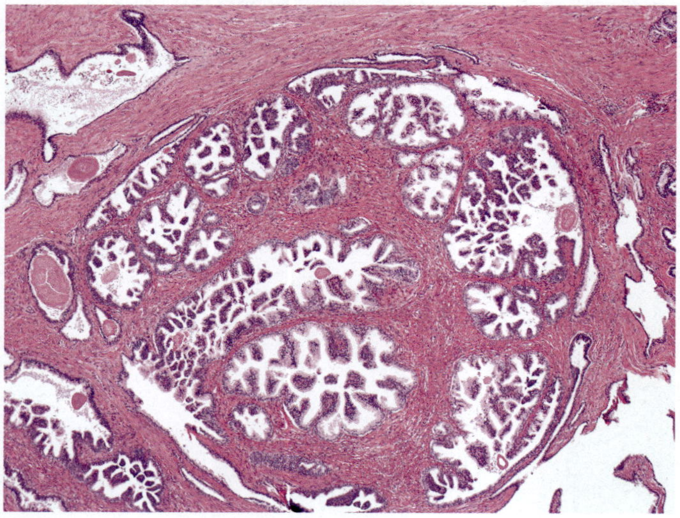

a

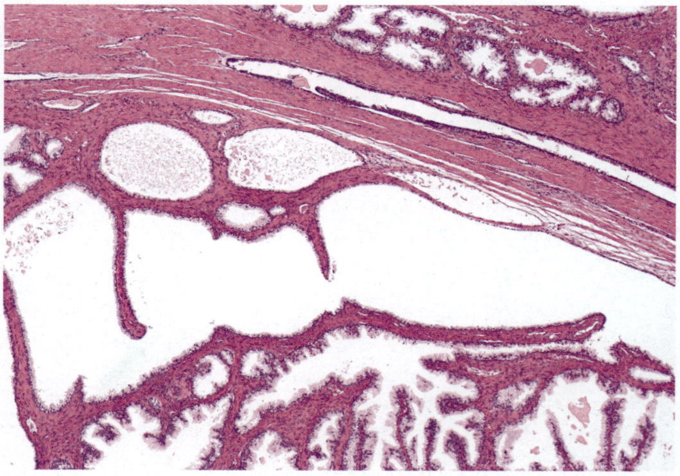

b

- The hyperplastic glands range from small to large in size, sometimes with hyperplastic basal cells
- The glandular cells show abundant pale cytoplasm without nuclear atypia (Fig. 4-13)
- Individual BPH glands can be difficult to distinguish from normal glands at higher magnification
- There may only be one dominant hyperplastic component either stromal (Fig. 4-14) or glandular
- BPH may be associated with acute or chronic inflammation; in the majority of cases, the inflammation is focal (Fig. 4-16)
- Focal infarct and microcalcifications may also be present
- In the TURP specimens, there are often several cauterization effects on the prostate, which may cause challenges to distinguish from incidental adenocarcinoma
- In needle core biopsy specimen, only hyperplastic stroma can be recognized microscopically (Fig. 4-17) but not glandular components. Therefore, the diagnosis of BPH cannot and should not be made on needle core biopsy specimens

Immunohistochemistry

- Triple stains to rule out carcinoma or high-grade prostatic intraepithelial neoplasia (PIN)

Molecular analysis

- Not contributory to pathology diagnosis

Clinical relevance (prognosis and treatment options)

- BPH is a significant medical condition
- However, pathology diagnosis is not essential, clinical diagnosis can be established with accuracy
- In fact, the pathology diagnosis of BPH should not be made from needle core biopsy material
- Medical treatment including α-blockers or finasteride (5-α-reductase inhibitors) are effective in the majority of cases
- TURP is currently used only in BPH cases refractory to medical treatment. Open prostatectomy occasionally used for severe cases

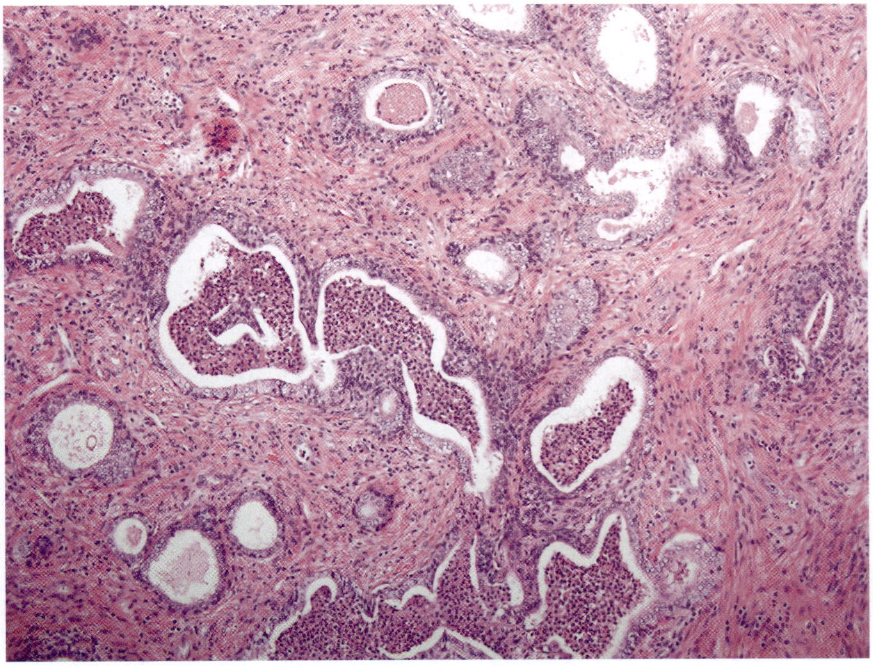

Figure 4-16.
Acute inflammation present within the BPH nodule.

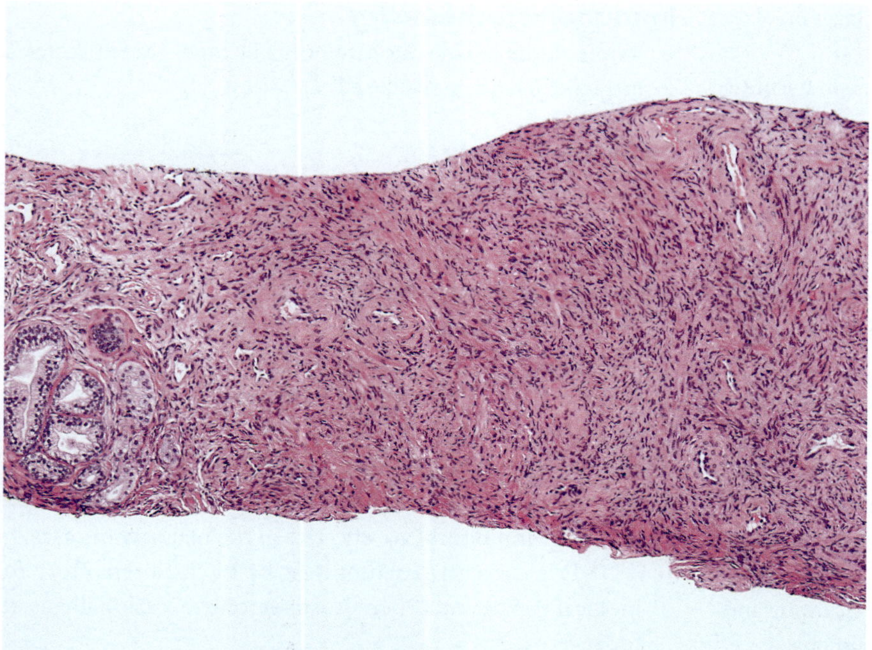

Figure 4-17.
Stromal hyperplasia seen on a needle core biopsy.

BASAL CELL HYPERPLASIA (BCH)

Definition

- Benign proliferation of basal cells of the prostate

Other terms

- Atypical basal cell hyperplasia (name not recommended)
- Florid BCH
- Basal cell adenoma

Pathogenesis

- In most cases, it appears to be a variant of BPH

Clinical features

- Enlarged prostate
- Urinary obstruction symptoms as seen in patients with BPH
- Mild to moderate elevation of serum PSA as seen in BPH patients

Gross pathology

- Variable sizes of nodules mostly in the transition zone

Histology

- Well-defined small nodules ranging from 0.1 to 2 mm (Fig. 4-18)
- The nodule is composed of clusters of basal cells (Figs. 4-19 and 4-20)
- The hallmark of BCH is the presence of multilayered cells (Fig. 4-19)
- The basal cells nuclei exhibit disorganized orientation
- The basal cells may show nuclear grooving, occasional mitoses, and rare cytological atypia (Fig. 4-21)
- In some cases of extensive basal cell nests, we use the term florid BCH (Fig. 4-18)
- Occasionally, basal cell nests may appear to be infiltrating
- In rare cases, a basal cell nodule may get large enough to be recognizable grossly, which may be referred to as *basal cell adenoma*
- The presence of focal cytological atypia may be seen, which was referred to as *atypical BCH*. Neither of these conditions have any clinical significance. Therefore, we believe that *atypical BCH* and *basal cell adenoma* are in the spectrum of BCH

Immunohistochemistry

- HMWCK and p63 positive
- AMACR negative and PSA negative

Differential diagnosis

- *Basaloid cell carcinoma*, has a more infiltrative growth pattern, diffuse cytological atypia, and extensive cribriform patterns, which resemble adenoid cystic carcinoma. Extraprostatic invasion and invasion into adjacent organs may be seen. A high proliferative rate with Ki67 and positivity for BCL1 are supportive of the diagnosis

Clinical relevance (prognosis and treatment options)

- Benign condition
- Treatment similar to BPH

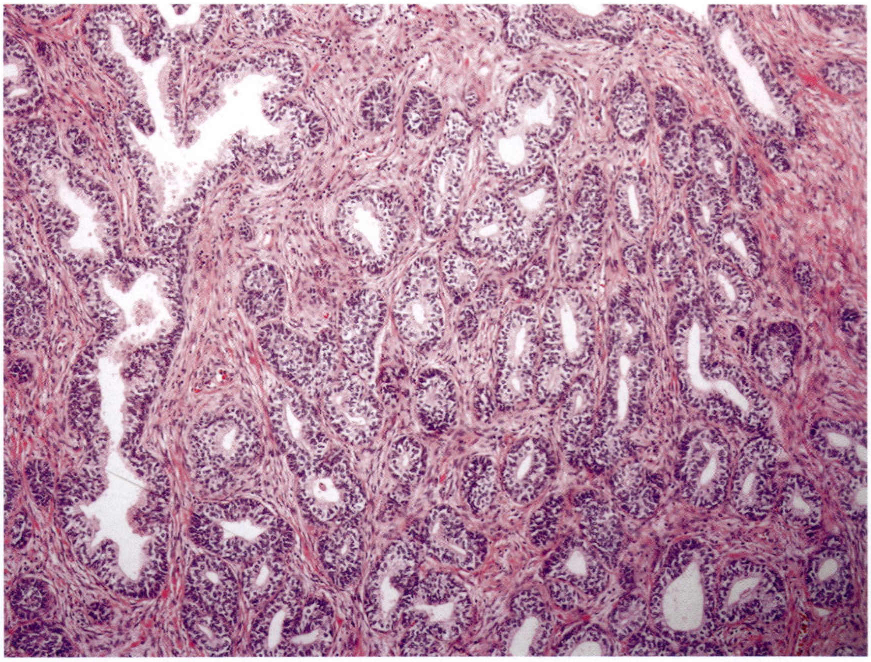

Figure 4-18.
Basal cell hyperplasia (BCH) with a lobular appearance resembling BPH, except the BCH glands are smaller.

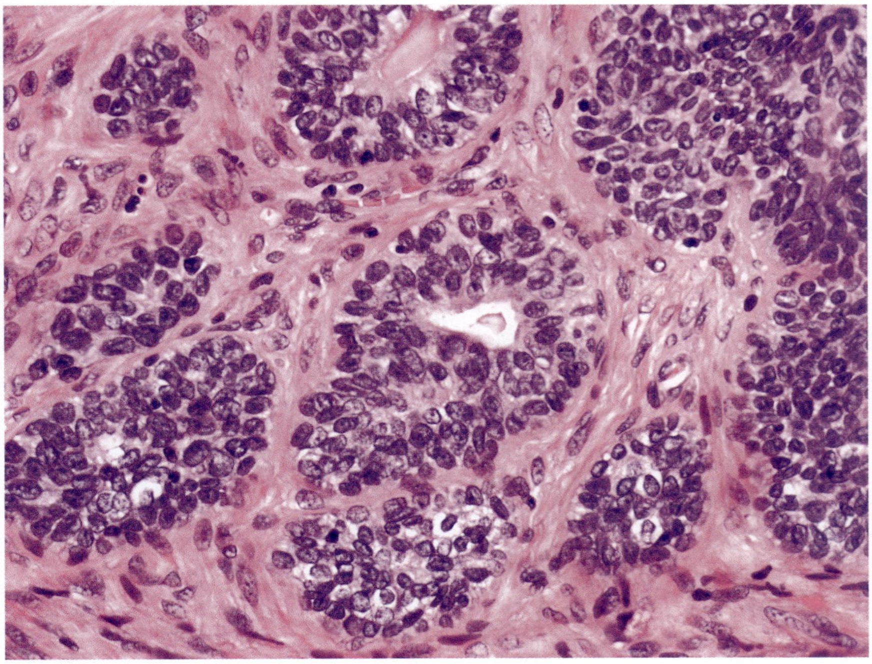

Figure 4-19.
High magnification shows the hallmark of BCH: multilayered cells. Nuclear grooves can be seen in some cells.

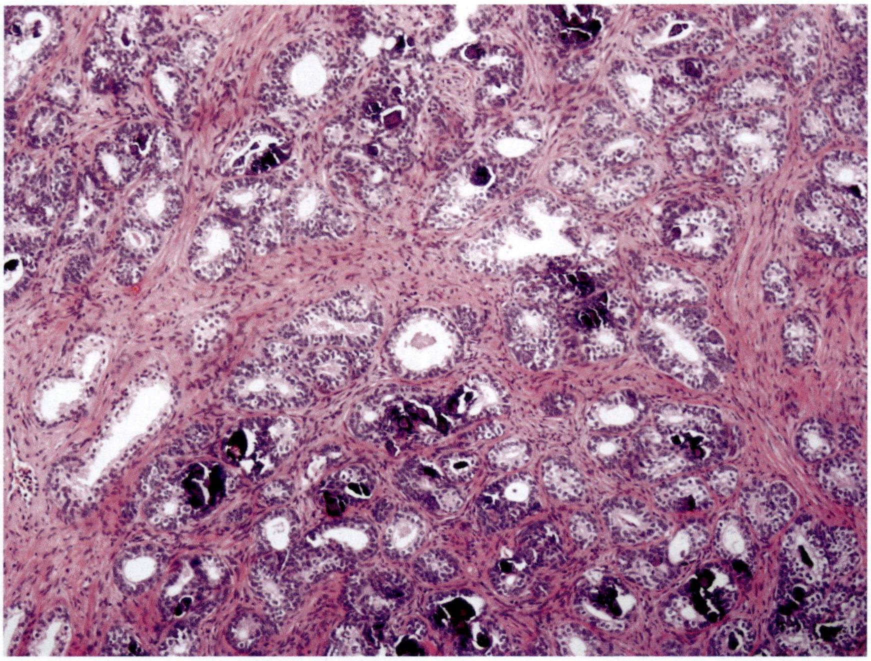

Figure 4-20.
A basal cell hyperplastic nodule contains microcalcifications.

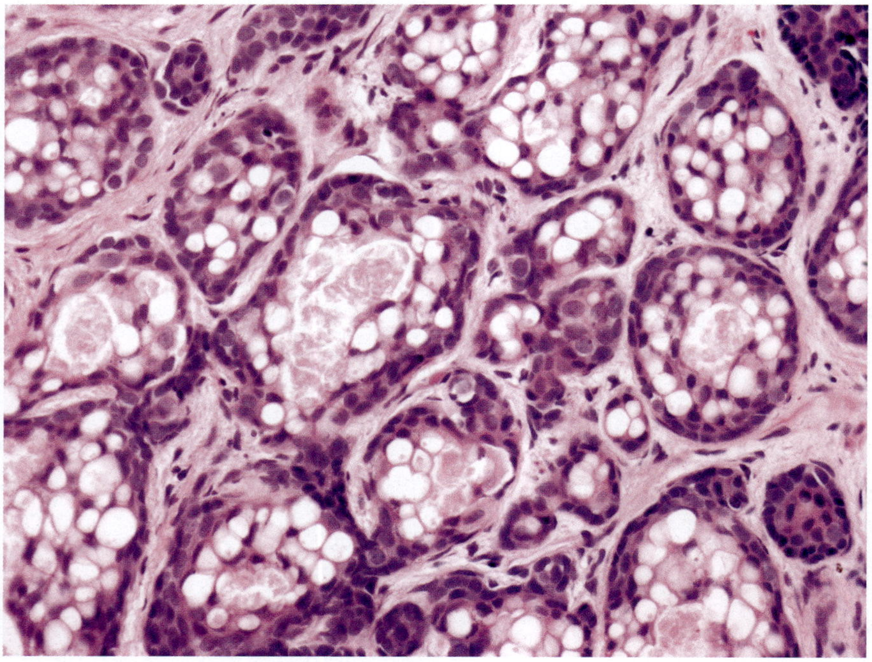

Figure 4-21.
BCH with signet ring appearance, although no significant cytological atypia present.

CLEAR CELL CRIBRIFORM HYPERPLASIA

Definition

- Benign hyperplastic lesions with cribriform patterns and composed of glandular cells with clear cytoplasm

Pathogenesis

- Most often as a part of BPH

Clinical features

- Enlargement of prostate with BPH symptoms

Gross pathology

- Large prostate with nodules similar to BPH
- Incidental finding in transurethral resection (TUR) or prostatectomy specimens, because clear cell cribriform hyperplasia (CCCH) itself cannot be recognized grossly

Histology

- Large glands with cribriform patterns (Fig. 4-22)
- These glands (ducts or acini) are noninfiltrating, confined to BPH nodules
- Glands are composed of secretory cells with abundant clear cytoplasm without cytological atypia (Fig. 4-23)
- Basal cells clusters can be seen in the periphery of the glands as crescents (Fig. 4-23*b*)

Immunohistochemistry

- Basal cells markers positive for basal cells
- AMACR negative or weakly positive

Differential diagnosis

- *Foamy gland carcinoma:* foamy cytoplasm, no basal cells
- *Pseudohyperplastic adenocarcinoma:* prominent cytological atypia, no basal cells
- *High-grade PIN:* prominent nucleoli in a large gland, patchy but not clustered basal cells

Clinical relevance (prognosis and treatment options)

- Benign
- Treatment same as BPH

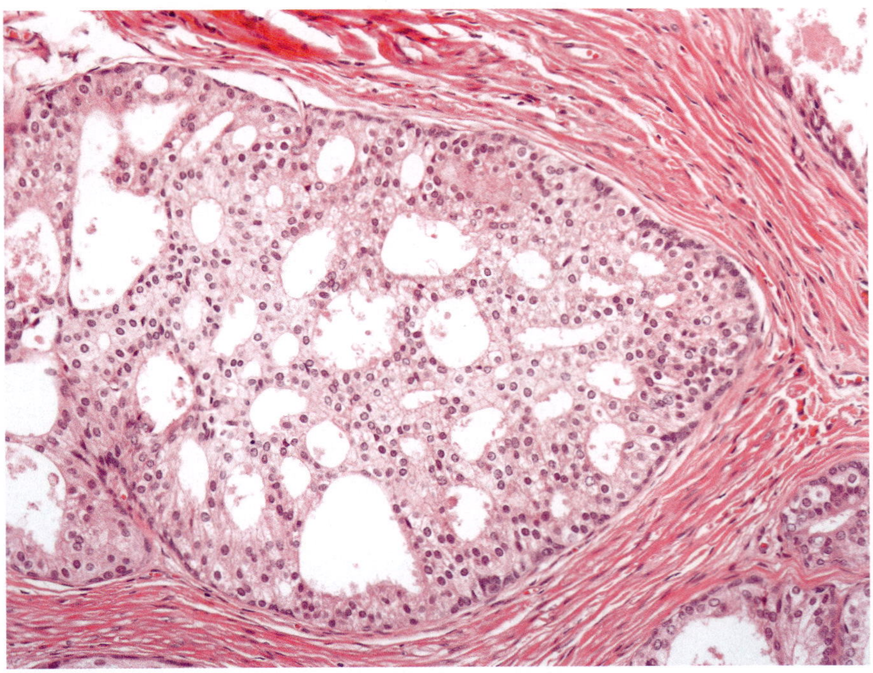

Figure 4-22.
Clear cell cribriform hyperplasia (CCCH) is composed of large complex well-circumscribed glands comprising cells with clear cytoplasm.

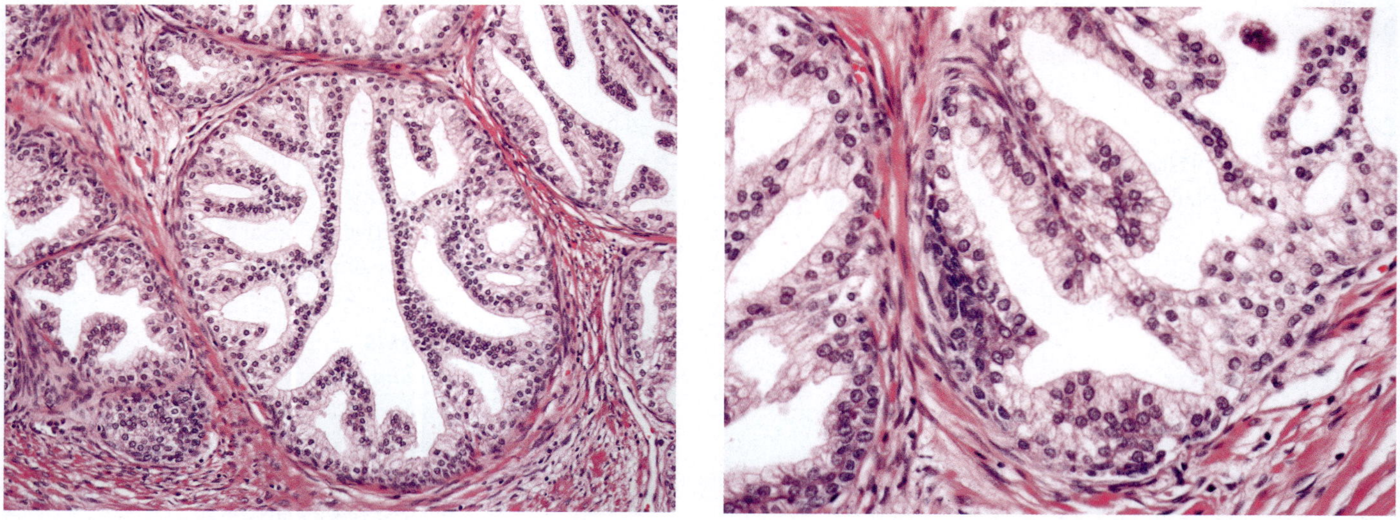

a b

Figure 4-23.
CCCH within large glands displaying a smooth contour, cribriform pattern, and "Roman bridge." No cytological atypia is seen (*a*). A cluster of basal cells can be seen in the basal layer of one end of a large gland (*b*).

SCLEROSING ADENOSIS

Definition

- Benign lesion of the prostate characterized by a lobular proliferation of small crowded glands and spindle cell stroma

Pathogenesis

- Unclear
- May be present as a histologic variant of BPH

Clinical features

- Rarely seen in prostate needle core biopsies, but more commonly seen in TUR or prostatectomy specimens
- Mostly incidental findings
- Occasionally PSA is mildly increased or there are other symptoms related to BPH

Gross pathology

- Mostly located in the transition zone as a part of BPH
- No other specific findings grossly

Histology

- Lobular patterns similar to adenosis (Fig. 4-24), with confined noninfiltrating borders
- Glandular structures are crowded, but have well-formed compressed lumens without glandular fusion (Fig. 4-24*b*)
- Glandular epithelium may show nuclear atypia including nuclear enlargement and sometimes prominent nucleoli (Fig. 4-25)
- Prominent spindle cells are present between glands. The cells have features of myofibroblasts. The cellularity ranges from mild to moderate without apparent cytological atypia (Figs. 4-24 and 4-25)
- *This is the most atypical looking benign lesion in the prostate* based on morphology alone
- Thickened basement membrane (hyaline sheets) can be seen sometimes
- The key features are noninfiltrating pattern, atypical glandular cells with cellular but bland spindle cells

Immunohistochemistry

- Glandular cells are similar to adenosis, positive for basal cell markers (patchy)
- We have seen a couple of cases of sclerosing adenosis with minimal basal cell staining
- Spindle cells, resemble myofibroblasts, are positive for S100, muscle specific actin
- AMACR negative

Differential diagnosis

- High-grade adenocarcinoma (see Table 4-2)

Clinical relevance (prognosis and treatment options)

- Benign condition, despite its deceivingly atypical appearance
- Can be easily confused with cancer histologically, especially on needle core biopsy

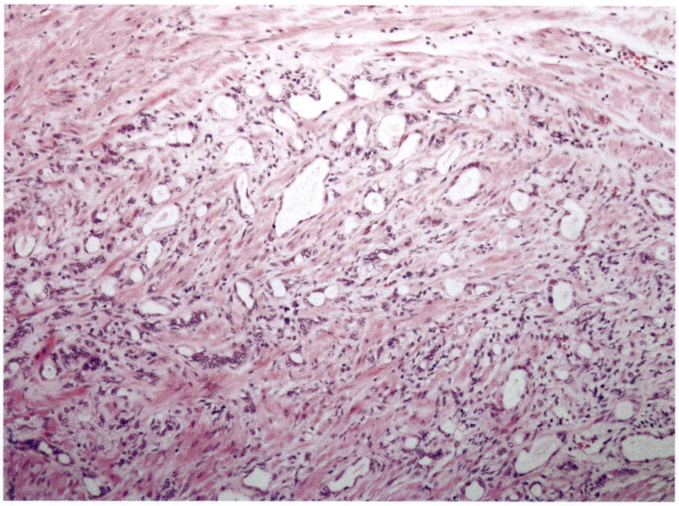

a

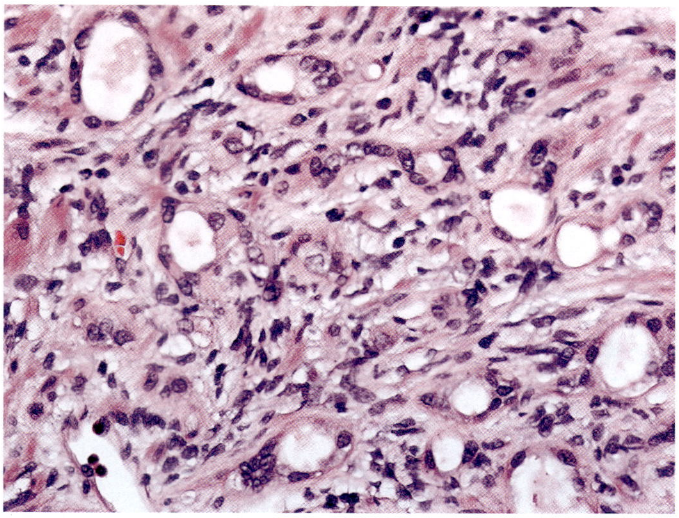

b

Figure 4-24.
Sclerosing adenosis displays a lobular pattern with a noninfiltrating border (*a*). High magnification shows minimal cytological atypia in the glandular cells and spindle cells (*b*).

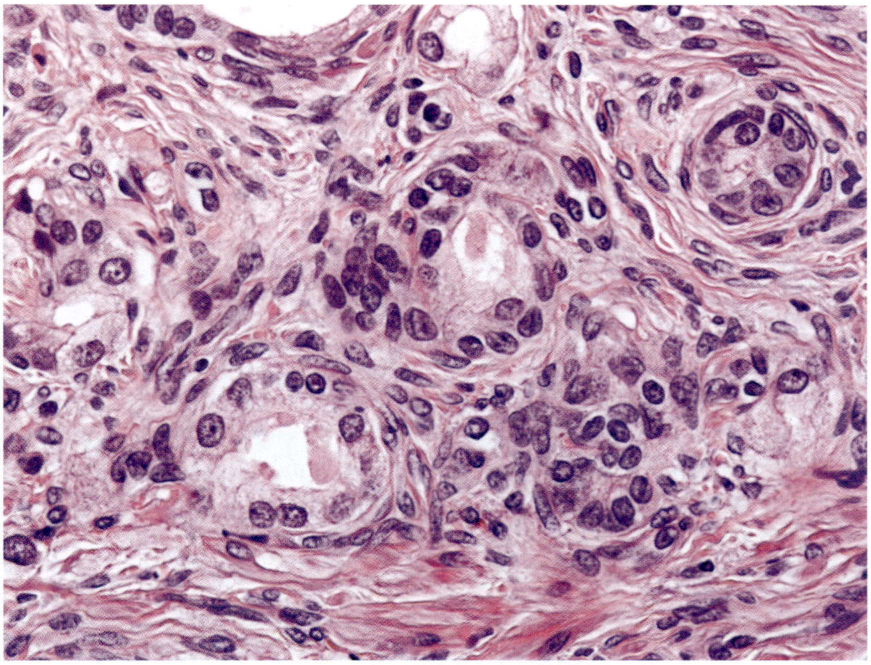

Figure 4-25.
Sclerosing adenosis showing high cellularity of the stroma, which consists of spindled myofibroblastic cells with mild to moderate cytological atypia.

Table 4-2. Comparison of Sclerosing Adenosis and Adenocarcinoma

	Sclerosing adenosis	*High-grade adenocarcinoma*
Lobular pattern	Yes	No
Infiltrating border	No	Yes, extensive
Glandular component	Compressed glands	Incompletely formed glands
Lumen	Complete, nonfused	Fused
Prominent nucleoli	Present	Present
Cell-cell variation	Little or no	Yes
Stroma	Bland spindle cells, moderate to high cellularity	Desmoplastic reaction No cellular stromal component
Hyaline sheet	May be present	Absent
P63, HMWCK	Mostly positive	Negative
S100, MSA	Positive in the stroma	Negative
AMACR	Negative	Positive

VERUMONTANUM HYPERPLASIA

Definition

- Benign glandular hyperplastic change of the verumontanum

Other terms

- Verumontanum mucosal gland hyperplasia (VMGH)

Pathogenesis

- Verumontanum is a normal papillary structure located in the prostatic urethra, composed of the small crowded glands
- VMGH was reported in 14% of prostatectomy specimens ranging from 6 glands to more than 50 glands
- Therefore, so-called verumontanum hyperplasia is either a reactive change or normal variation of the verumontanum in which there are varying numbers of glandular structures in each case

Clinical features

- Located in the prostatic urethra between the two openings of ejaculatory ducts
- No other clinical symptoms or signs

Gross pathology

- A small papillary projection in the mid prostatic urethra

Histology

- Normally, the verumontanum is composed of a small cluster of two to three layers of the small crowded glands containing dense corpora amylacea
- In verumontanum hyperplasia (Fig. 4-26), there are increased numbers of small crowded glands, giving an impression of high cellularity (no definition how many glands are necessary for verumontanum hyperplasia
- Sometimes it appears to be a papillary lesion
- Degenerative cytological atypia may be present
- Basal cells present

Immunohistochemistry

- Basal cells markers positive and AMACR negative or weakly positive

Clinical relevance (prognosis and treatment options)

- Benign, no treatment necessary

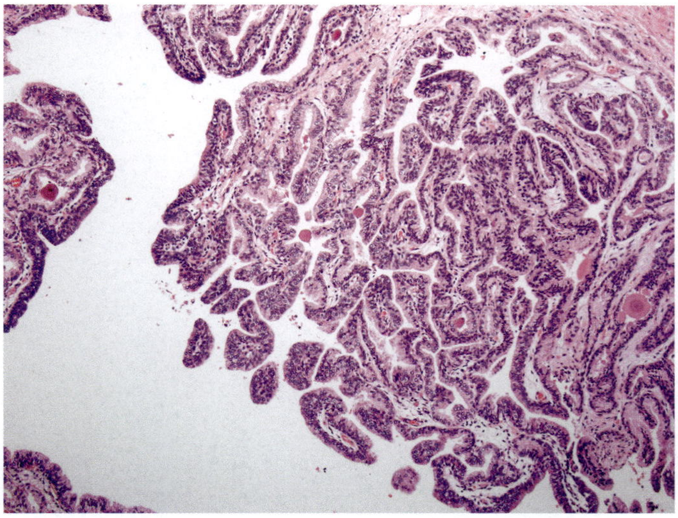

a

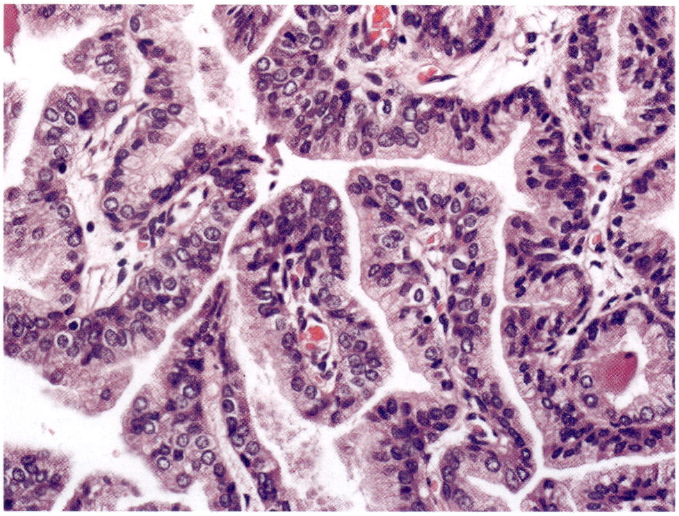

b

Figure 4-26.
Verumontanum hyperplasia contains small packed glands (*a*). Dense corpora amylacea can be seen in the lumen. High magnification shows that the glands consist of pseudostratified columnar cells without nuclear atypia or prominent nucleoli (*b*).

INFARCT

Definition

- Ischemia results in the infarction of the prostate

Pathogenesis

- Infection directly associated with BPH or BPH subsequently compromises the blood circulation in the prostate and leads to the development of infarction
- Ischemic infarcts develop in a single or multiple locations in the prostate
- Infarcted (necrotic) glandular epithelium and stroma contributes to the elevated serum PSA levels
- On the periphery of the infarct, squamous metaplasia is prominent as a repair process

Clinical features

- Large and firm prostate due to the presence of BPH
- Elevated serum PSA, which can be up to 100 ng/mL
- *This is one of the very few benign prostatic lesions, which can be associated with significantly elevated serum PSA levels*

Gross pathology

- Large prostate with BPH
- Areas of discoloration and necrosis may be seen

Histology

- Single or multiple areas of necrosis (Fig. 4-27)
- Necrotic center with ghost cells
- Prominent squamous metaplasia in the periphery of the infarct (Fig. 4-27*b*)
- Sometimes, prostatic glands are severely dilated and filled and with necrotic material
- Mitosis and cytological atypia are commonly seen in the metaplastic cells in a newly developed infarct (Fig. 4-27*b*)
- BPH present in the background
- Hemorrhage (Fig. 4-28), and acute and chronic inflammation are common in areas adjacent to infarct

Clinical relevance

- Benign condition, but prostatectomy may be a consideration
- BPH needs treatment

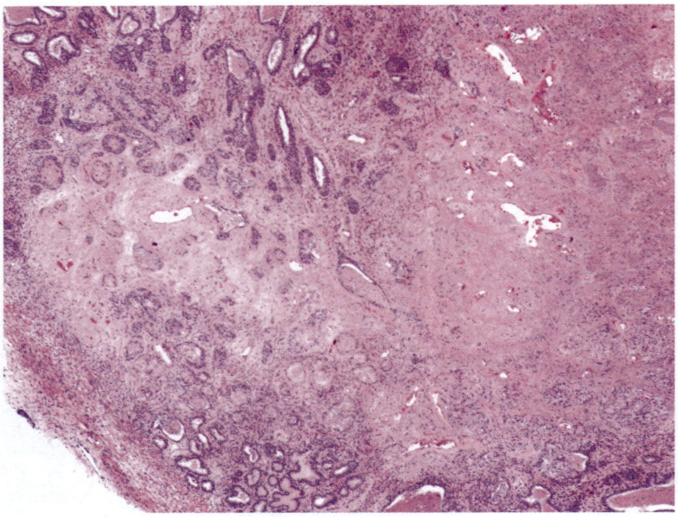

a

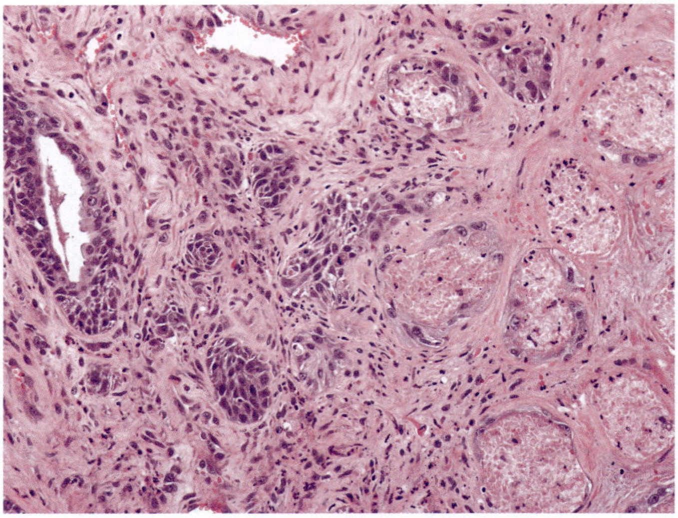

b

Figure 4-27.
A large area of infarct can be seen on the right side of photo (*a*) from a patient with PSA of 108 ng/mL. Higher magnification shows the infarct is surrounded by reactive prostatic glands undergoing squamous metaplasia (*b*).

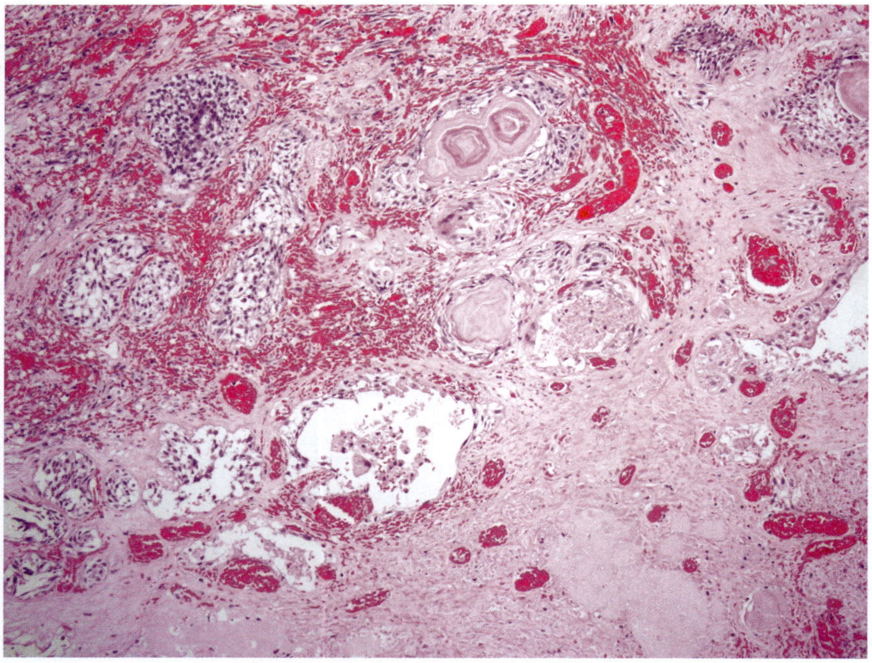

Figure 4-28.
In the periphery of an infarcted area, prostatic glands are undergoing metaplastic changes.

SQUAMOUS METAPLASIA

Definition

- Metaplastic changes from prostatic glandular epithelium to squamous epithelium

Pathogenesis

- Both benign cells and malignant epithelial cells (carcinoma) can undergo transformation to squamous cells
- In benign condition, squamous metaplasia is seen with other conditions, particularly as a repair process for infarct

Clinical features

- Nonspecific
- Possible similar symptoms as in chronic inflammation

Gross pathology

- Areas of infarct may be seen
- Squamous metaplasia is not identified grossly

Histology

- Prostatic glands are replaced by squamous epithelium (Fig. 4-29)
- Lobular patterns may be retained
- Squamous metaplasia may be seen in the periphery of the infarct
- May be associated with chronic inflammation
- Reactive atypia with mitoses may be seen as a regenerative process (Fig. 4-30)
- Squamous metaplasia may be seen without infarct (Fig. 4-31)
- Squamous metaplasia occurs frequently after estrogen treatment for prostate cancer patients

Immunohistochemistry

- P63 positive and p53 negative

Differential diagnosis

- Squamous cell carcinoma, with infiltrating patterns and significant cytological atypia

Clinical relevance (prognosis and treatment options)

- Benign

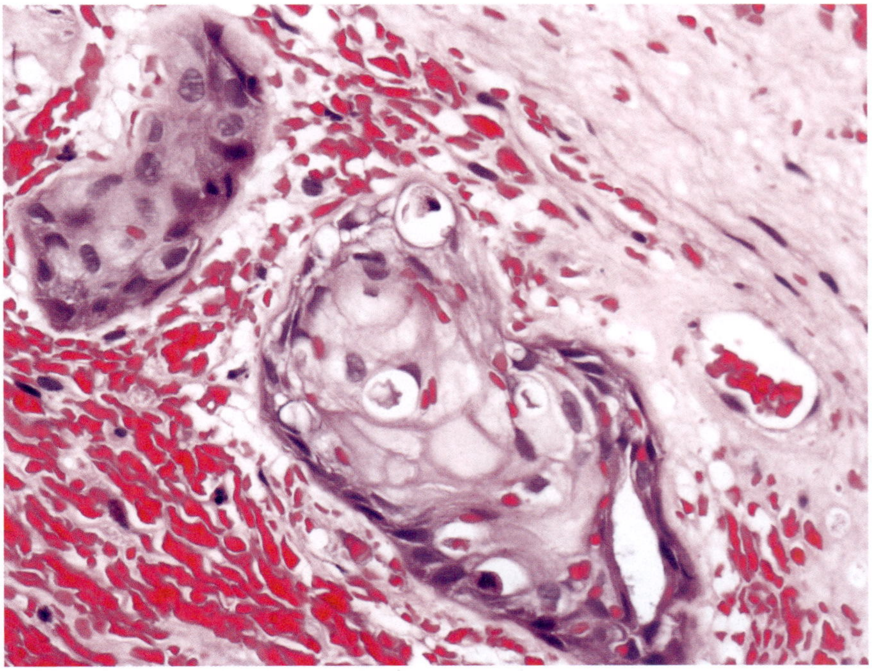

Figure 4-29.
Metaplastic squamous cells show reactive atypia adjacent to infarct.

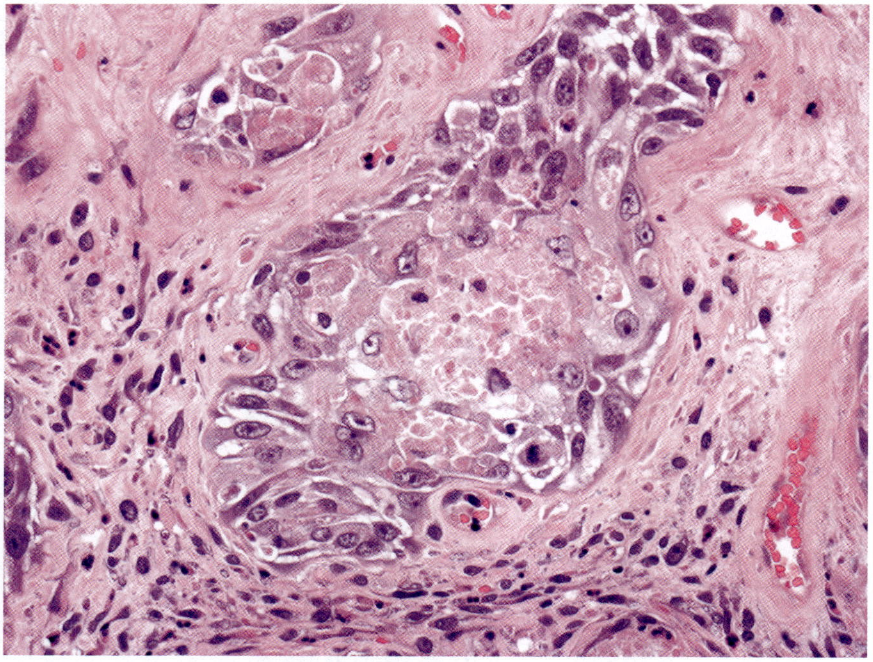

Figure 4-30.
Metaplastic squamous cells display reactive atypia with mitoses.

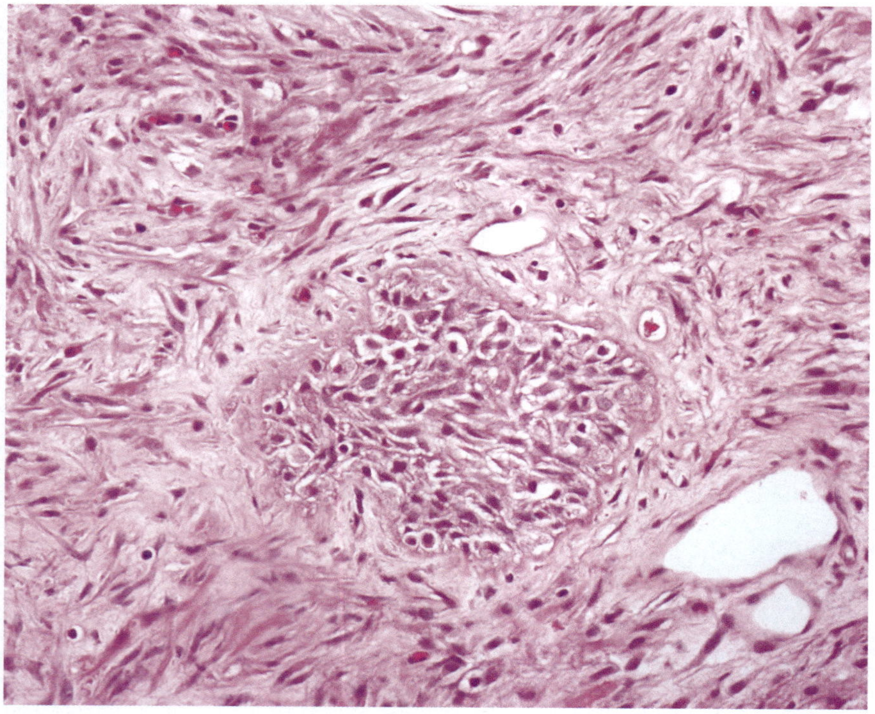

Figure 4-31.
Squamous metaplasia present without infarct.

UROTHELIAL METAPLASIA

Definition

- Benign metaplastic changes from prostatic epithelium to urothelium

Other terms

- Transitional cell metaplasia

Pathogenesis

- Proliferation of basal cells (which have the similar morphological and biochemical features as urothelium) leading to the replacement of prostatic glandular cells with urothelial like cells
- Often seen in chronic inflammatory conditions

Clinical features

- Nonspecific

Gross pathology

- Not identified grossly

Histology

- Presence of multilayered cells replacing or undermining the surface columnar secretory cells of the prostate (Figs. 4-32 to 4-34)
- Common findings in needle core biopsy or TURP specimens
- Nuclear grooving (Fig. 4-32) and prominent nucleoli (Fig. 4-33) can be seen
- The nuclei are slightly different from those of the prostatic secretory cells with small nucleoli without significant cytological atypia (Fig. 4-33)

Immunohistochemistry

- Basal markers (p63 and HMWCK) positive (Fig. 4-34)

Differential diagnosis

- *High-grade PIN:* has significant cytological atypia with patchy basal cells, which can be confirmed by basal cell staining

Clinical relevance (prognosis and treatment options)

- May be confused with urothelial lesions or high-grade PIN
- No other clinical significance

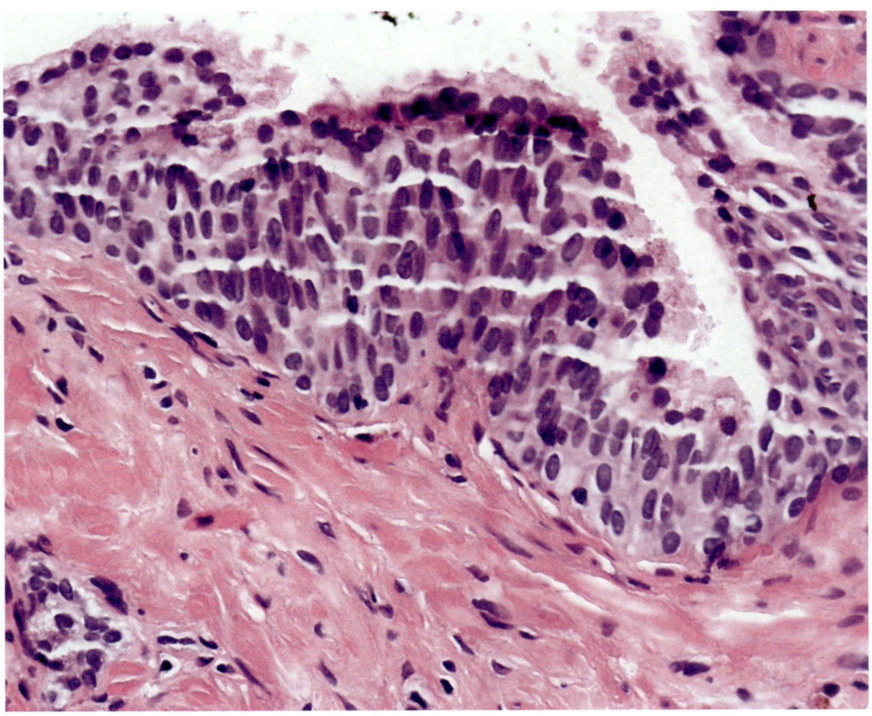

Figure 4-32.
Urothelial metaplasia shows multilayered cell proliferation underneath the prostatic secretory cells. Some metaplastic cells have nuclear grooves.

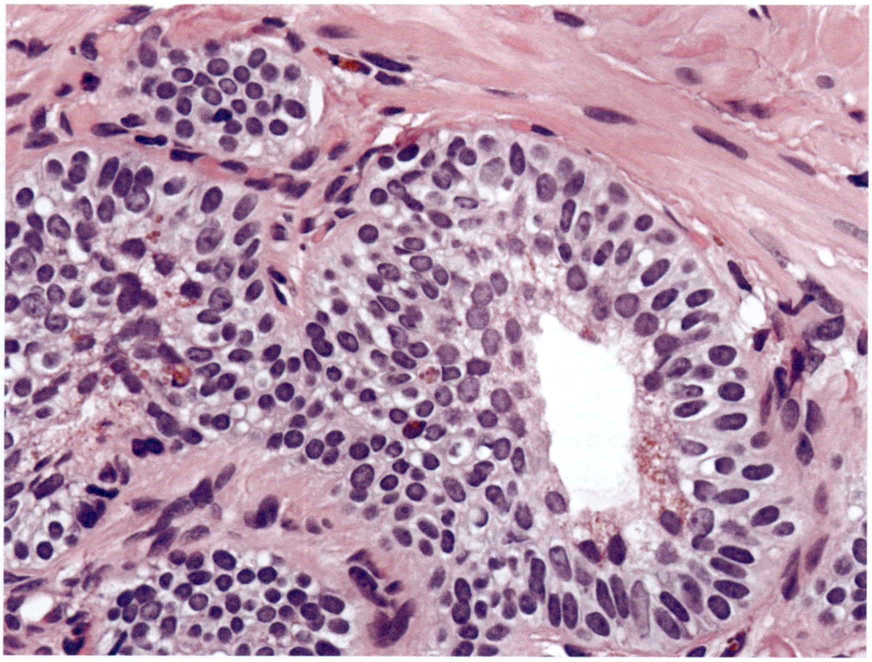

Figure 4-33.
Occasionally, urothelial metaplastic cells may show small but distinct nucleoli.

Figure 4-34.
(*a*) Multilayered urothelial metaplastic cells underneath the secretory cells. (*b*) The basal cell stains (p63 and HMWCK) are positive in metaplastic urothelial cells.

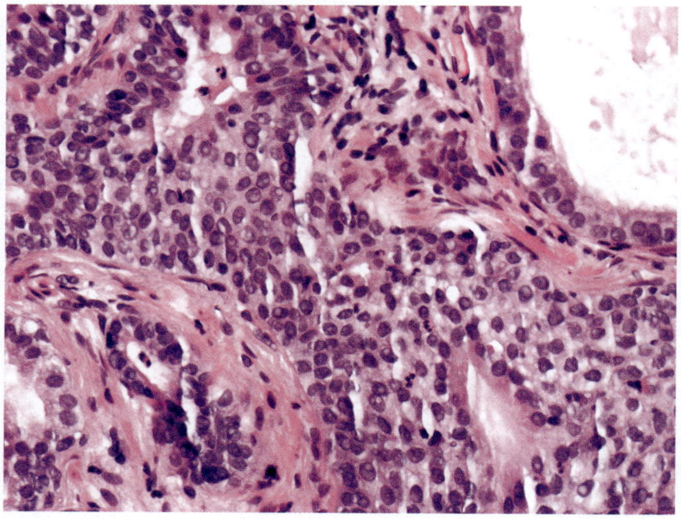

a

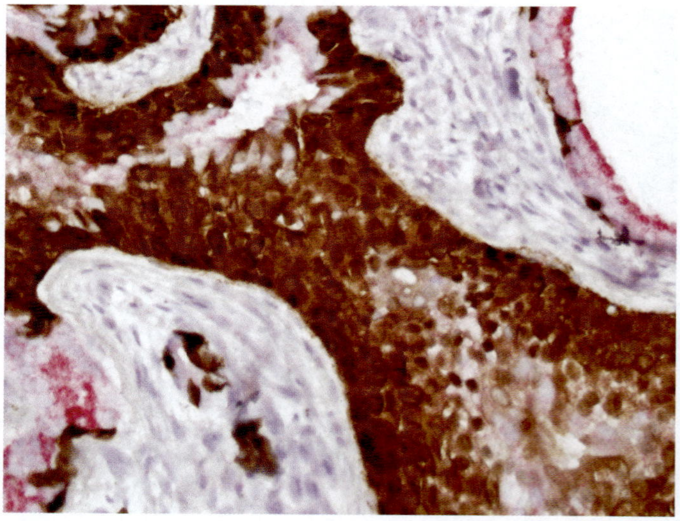

b

MUCINOUS METAPLASIA

Definition

- Benign metaplastic changes from prostatic glandular cells to mucinous glands

Other terms

- Colonic metaplasia, intestinal metaplasia

Pathogenesis

- Reactive changes to chronic stimulus

Clinical features

- Not specific

Gross pathology

- A microscopic finding, not identified grossly

Histology

- Mucinous metaplasia is present as individual cells in a gland (Fig. 4-35) or in a cluster of glands (Fig. 4-36)
- Prostatic secretory cells are replaced by goblet cells (Fig. 4-37)
- The metaplastic goblet cells have abundant blue or pale mucinous cytoplasm
- Nucleoli may be prominent, but no significant cytological atypia or infiltrating patterns are seen
- Adenocarcinoma cells can also undergo mucinous differentiation

Immunohistochemistry

- Mucicarmine positive, PSA positive in the adjacent secretory cells
- Basal cell markers positive in prostatic basal cells

Clinical relevance (prognosis and treatment options)

- No other clinical consequence, but it may mimic mucinous adenocarcinoma

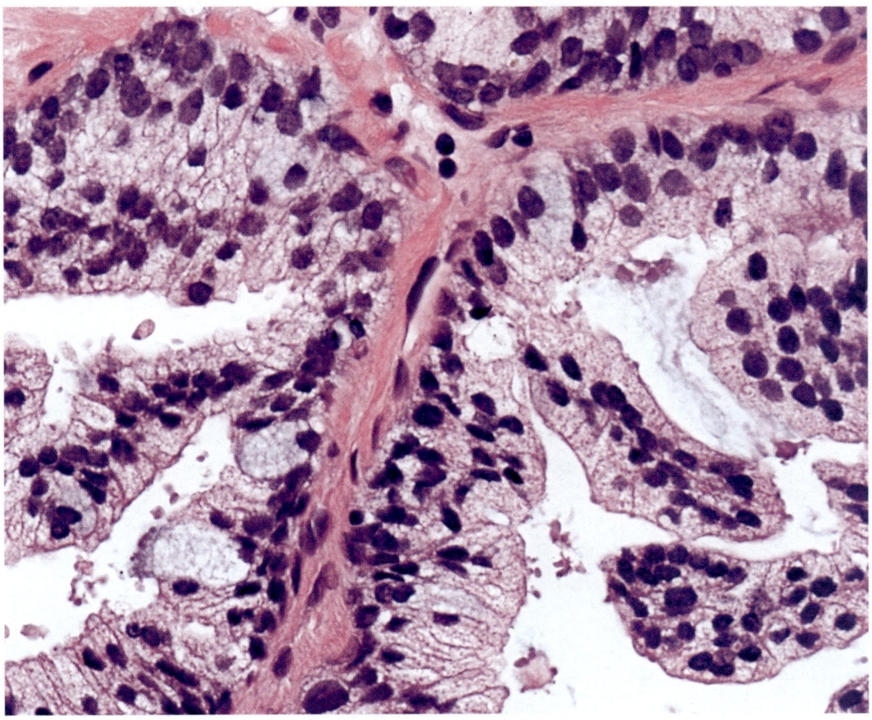

Figure 4-35.
Occasional goblet cells present in a benign prostatic gland.

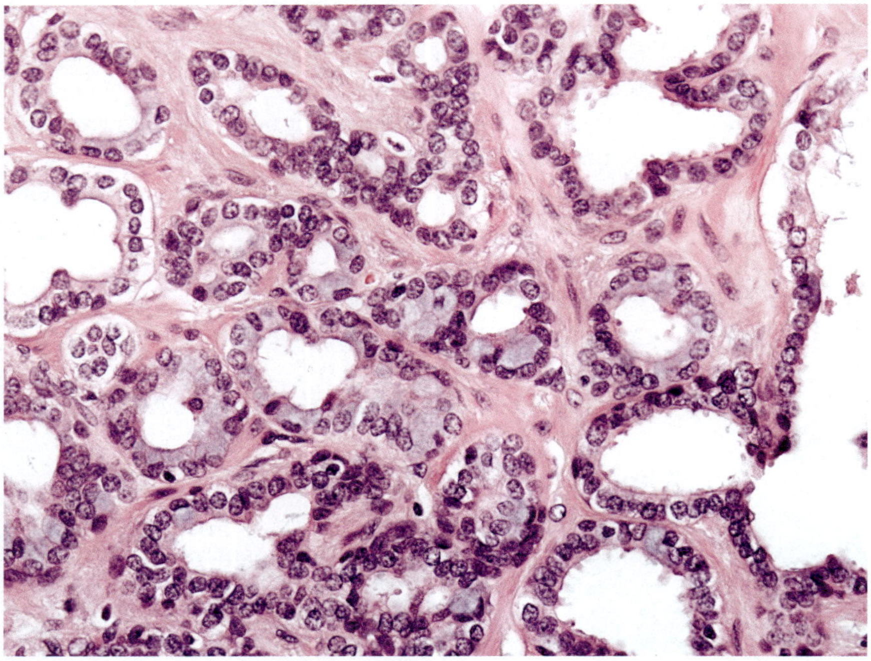

Figure 4-36.
Multiple atrophic prostatic glands with mucinous metaplasia.

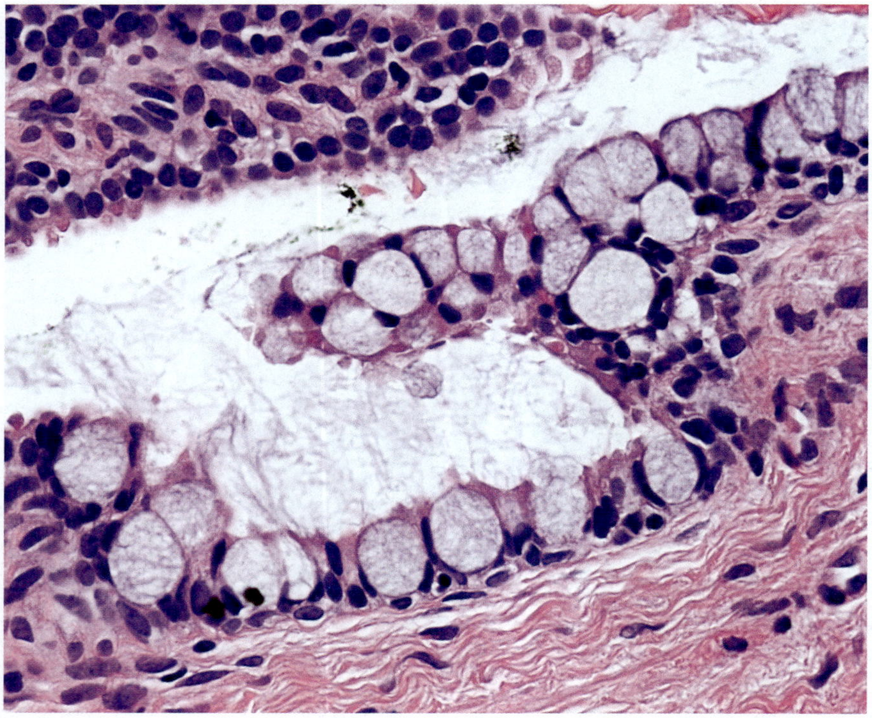

Figure 4-37.
A portion of the prostatic gland is replaced by metaplastic glandular cells (intestinal metaplasia).

MESONEPHRIC REMNANTS

Definition

- Benign tubular or acinar proliferation resembling mesonephric remnants

Other terms

- Mesonephric remnant hyperplasia

Pathogenesis

- Glandular structures resembling mesonephric remnants, it may be a metaplastic process at least in some cases
- It may resemble atrophic prostatic glands composed predominantly of basal cells or nephrogenic adenoma

Clinical features

- Incidental finding in TUR or prostatectomy specimens
- Rare condition
- No clinical symptoms or signs

Gross pathology

- Nonspecific

Histology

- Mostly located in the base or bladder neck regions
- Lobular patterns or infiltrating appearance (Fig. 4-38)
- Crowded small glands with single layer of cuboidal cells (Fig. 4-39)
  - Atrophic tubules containing colloid-like material
  - Atrophic tubules with micropapillary projections
- No significant cytological atypia and no additional basal cell layers

Immunohistochemistry

- Basal cell markers (p63 and HMWCK) positive
- Negative for PSA, PSAP, or AMACR

Clinical relevance (prognosis and treatment options)

- Benign, no treatment needed. It can be confused with adenocarcinoma

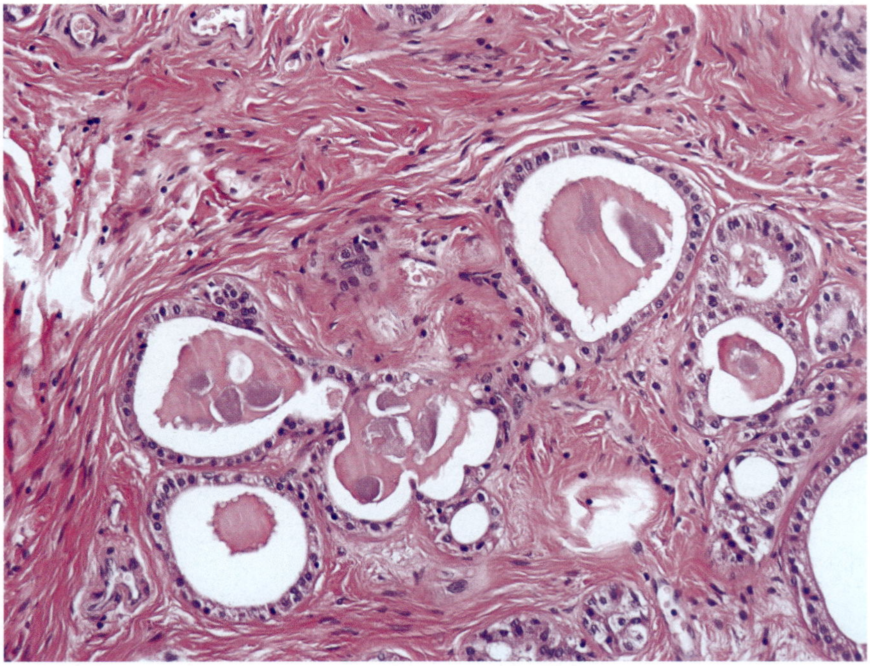

Figure 4-38.
Mesonephric remnants are composed of small glands in a lobular pattern. Some of the glands contain pink secretions.

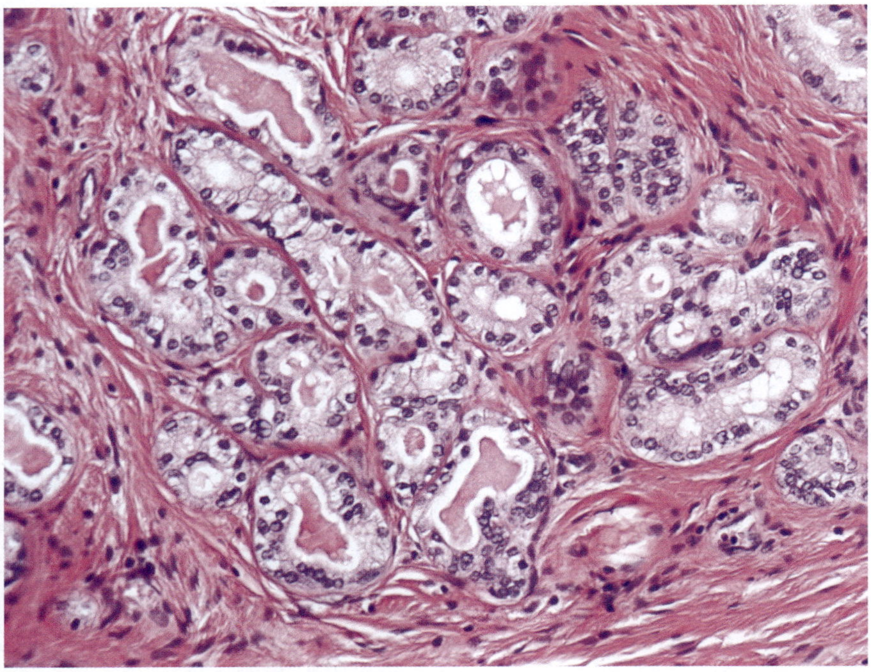

Figure 4-39.
At higher magnification, the glands are lined by a single layer of cells without cytologic atypia.

MICROCALCIFICATIONS IN THE PROSTATE

Definition

- Presence of small foci of calcifications in the prostatic parenchyma, which can only be detected by imaging studies or microscopic examination

Other terms

- Microlithiasis of the prostate

Pathogenesis

- The common causes of microcalcifications in the prostate are precipitations of prostatic secretion, chronic inflammation, or minor tissue damage
- They are very common histological findings in the prostatectomy specimens (50% to 80%)
- They are also frequently seen in seminal vesicles and ejaculatory ducts

Clinical features

- Asymptomatic, detected by imaging studies clinically or incidentally on microscopic examination

Gross pathology

- No specific gross findings if microscopic
- If calculus present, it may feel crunchy when cutting the prostate

Histology

- Microcalcifications are mostly seen within the benign prostatic glands (Fig. 4-40) or sometimes in the benign stroma
- Microcalcifications can be also seen in benign seminal vesicles, ejaculatory ducts, or prostatic urethra (Fig. 4-41)
- Only occasionally, microcalcifications can be seen within prostatic adenocarcinoma (Fig. 4-42)
- There is no major difference in the distribution of microcalcifications in different zones of the prostate

Immunohistochemistry and molecular analysis

- Not indicated

Clinical relevance (prognosis and treatment options)

- Unlike microcalcifications in the breast, which are mostly associated with breast cancer, microcalcifications in the prostate are most commonly associated with benign prostatic conditions

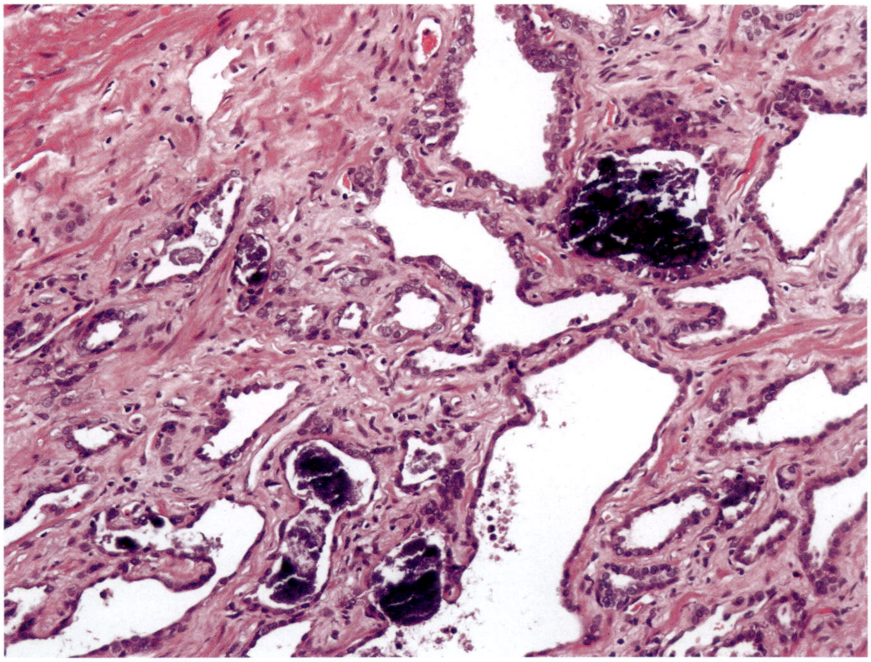

Figure 4-40.
Microcalcifications are present within the lumens of benign glands.

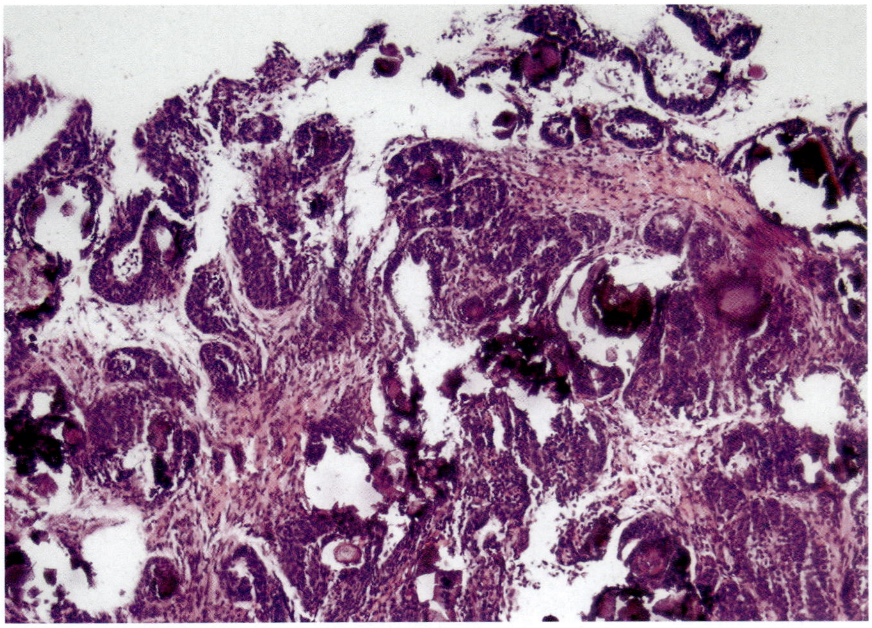

Figure 4-41.
Microcalcifications present in von Brunn's nests in the prostatic urethra.

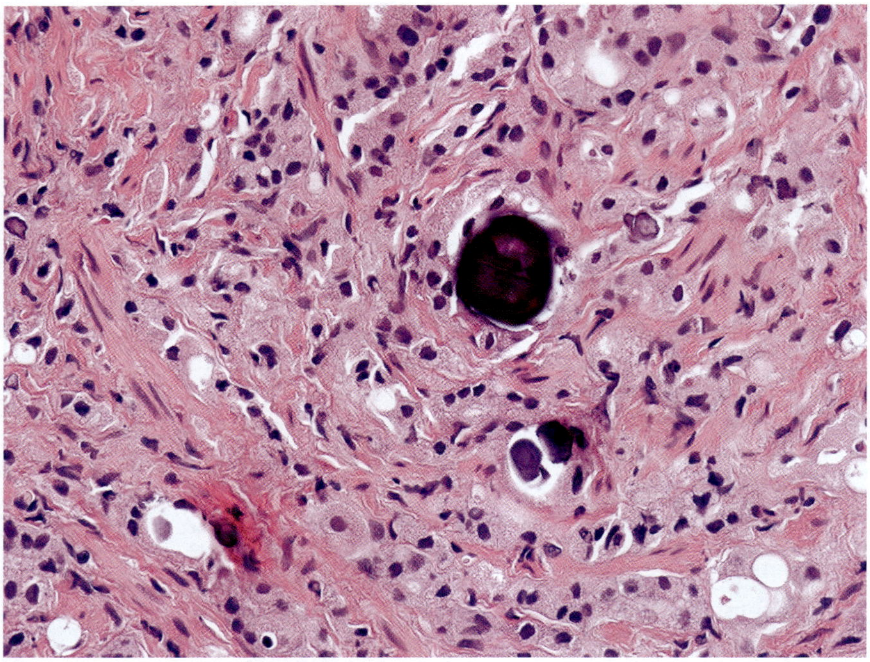

Figure 4-42.
Microcalcifications can rarely be seen within a prostatic adenocarcinoma.

POLYPOID URETHRITIS OF THE PROSTATIC URETHRA

Definition

- Inflammation of prostatic urethra with polypoid appearance

Other terms

- Polypoid prostatic urethritis
- Papillary urethritis

Pathogenesis

- Uncertain etiology
- May be related to infectious etiology or mechanical stimulus

Clinical features

- Pain and difficulty in urination
- Some discharge if infected by bacteria
- Polypoid growth in urethral mucosa

Gross pathology

- Edematous polypoid or papillary growth often close to the verumontanum

Histology

- Polypoid structures with edematous stroma (Fig. 4-43*a*)
- Chronic inflammatory infiltrates with lining urothelium showing reactive cytological atypia (Fig. 4-43*b*)

Immunohistochemistry

- Usually not necessary. P53 negative, and CK20 negative or focally positive

Differential diagnosis

- Papillary urothelial carcinoma: significant cytological atypia and branching papilla

Clinical relevance (prognosis and treatment options)

- Benign condition, may resolve spontaneously. If resected, it will not recur

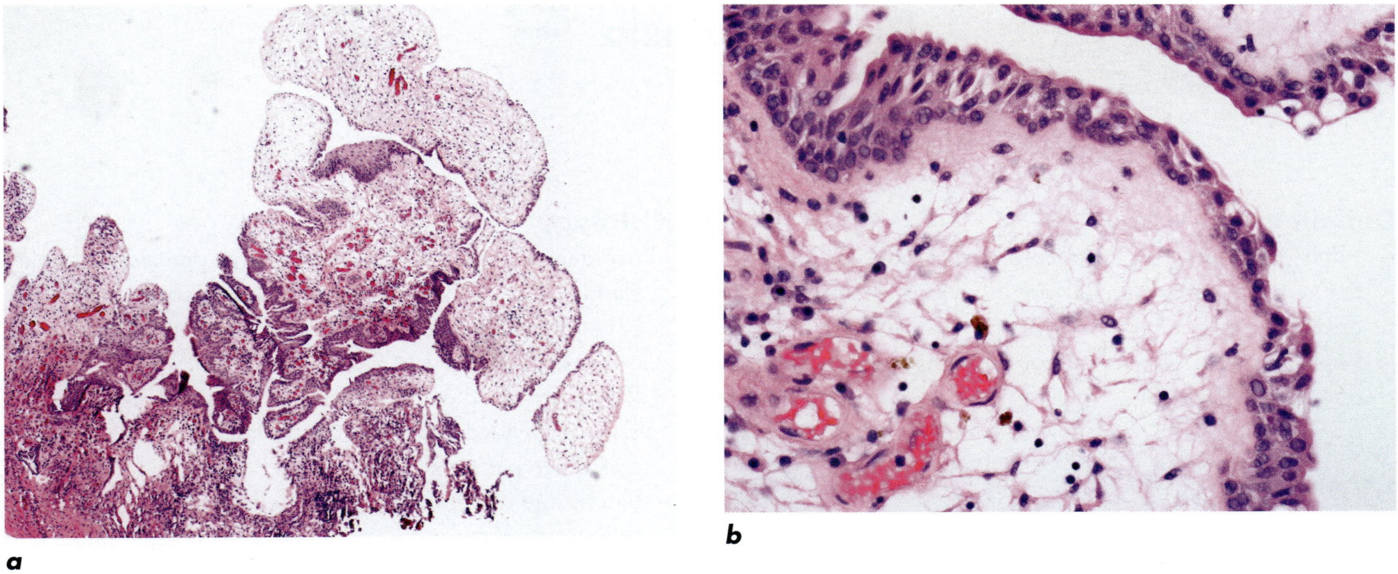

Figure 4-43.
Polypoid urethritis exhibits a polypoid appearance with an edematous stroma (*a*). Higher magnification shows a reactive urothelium (*b*).

CHAPTER 5

High-Grade Prostatic Intraepithelial Neoplasia

Definition

- High-grade prostatic intraepithelial neoplasia (PIN) is defined as neoplastic cells growing within the preexisting ducts or acini
- High-grade PIN is a microscopic finding that can be made only by pathologists

Other terms

- High-grade dysplasia, carcinoma in situ (both not used anymore)

Pathogenesis

- High-grade PIN is the precursor lesion of the prostatic adenocarcinoma

Clinical features

- No or minimal increase of serum prostate-specific antigen (PSA) levels. No specific symptoms or signs or abnormal imaging findings

Gross pathology

- Not identified grossly

Histology

- Proliferation of epithelial cells in large preexisting benign glands (ducts or acini). At low magnification, high-grade PIN glands appear to be darker because of increased cellularity (Figs. 5-1 to 5-3)
- Pseudostratified epithelium (Figs. 5-2 and 5-4)
- Can be divided into flat, micropapillary (Fig. 5-4*a*), or cribriform patterns
- Patchy and discontinuous basal cells present (Fig. 5-2*b*)
- Low-grade PIN: without identifiable nucleoli under 20× magnification
- High-grade PIN: with prominent nucleoli under 20× magnification (Fig. 5-4*b*)
- Individual cells are very similar to adenocarcinoma although high-grade PIN cells are confined within basement membrane

Immunohistochemistry

- Patchy basal cells can be confirmed by HMWCK and p63 (Fig. 5-3*b*)
- 50% high-grade PIN are AMACR positive, typically weak staining (Fig. 5-3*b*)
- Many markers, which are positive in prostatic adenocarcinoma, will be positive in high-grade PIN

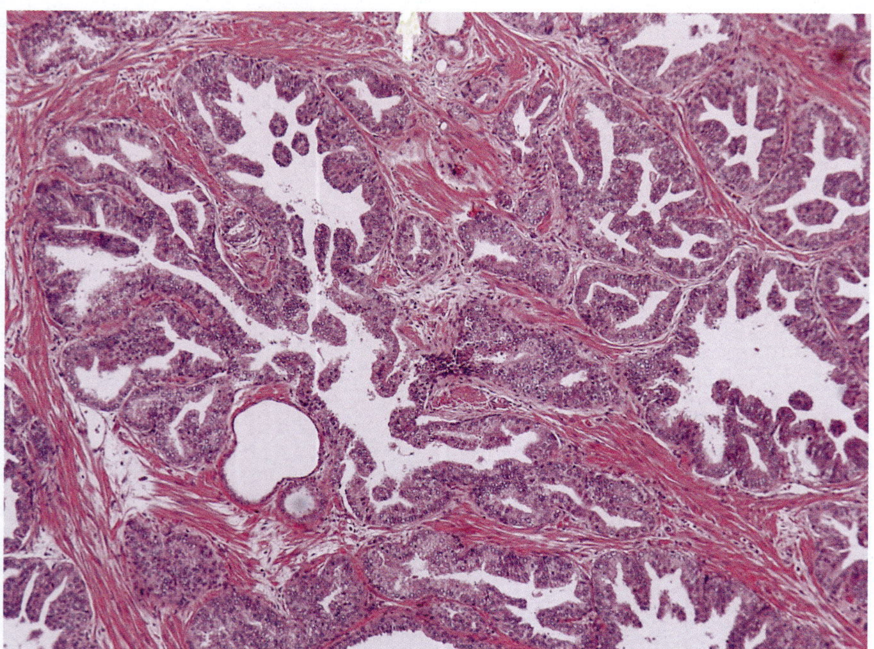

Figure 5-1.
There is increased cell proliferation in a couple of glands with high-grade PIN. The luminal spaces become smaller and more convoluted with a slit-like appearance.

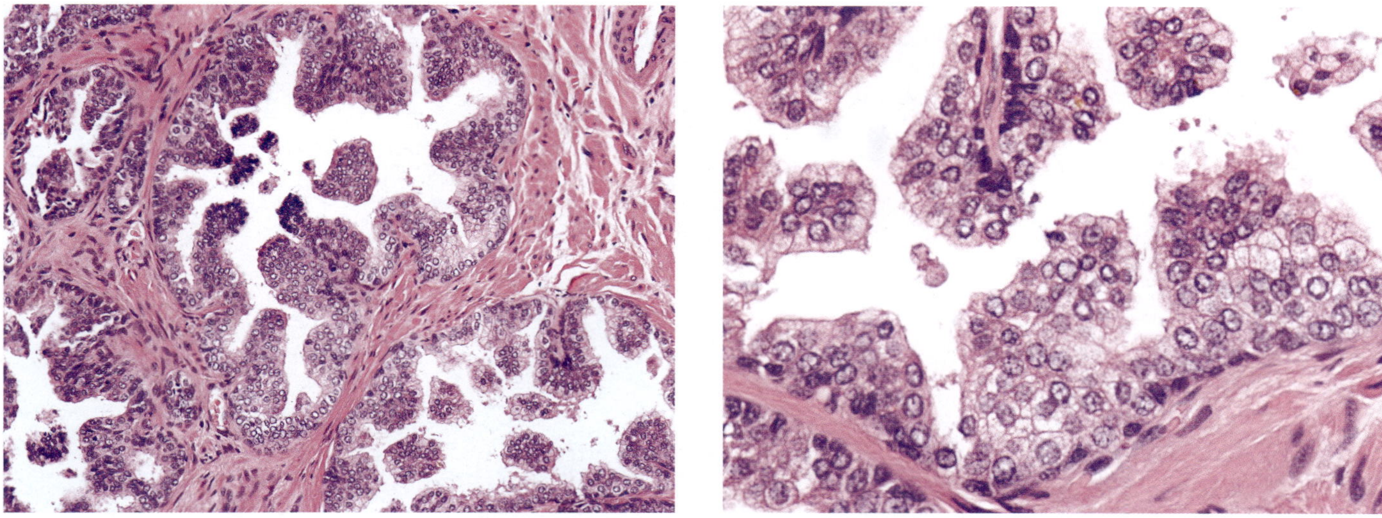

a b

Figure 5-2.
Several glands are involved by high-grade PIN (*a*). High magnification (*b*) shows pseudostratified columnar cells with prominent nucleoli. Patchy basal cells can be seen in the basal portion of the gland.

Figure 5-3.
A high-grade PIN gland shows nuclear atypia (*a*) and it is positive for both AMACR and basal cell markers (*b*).

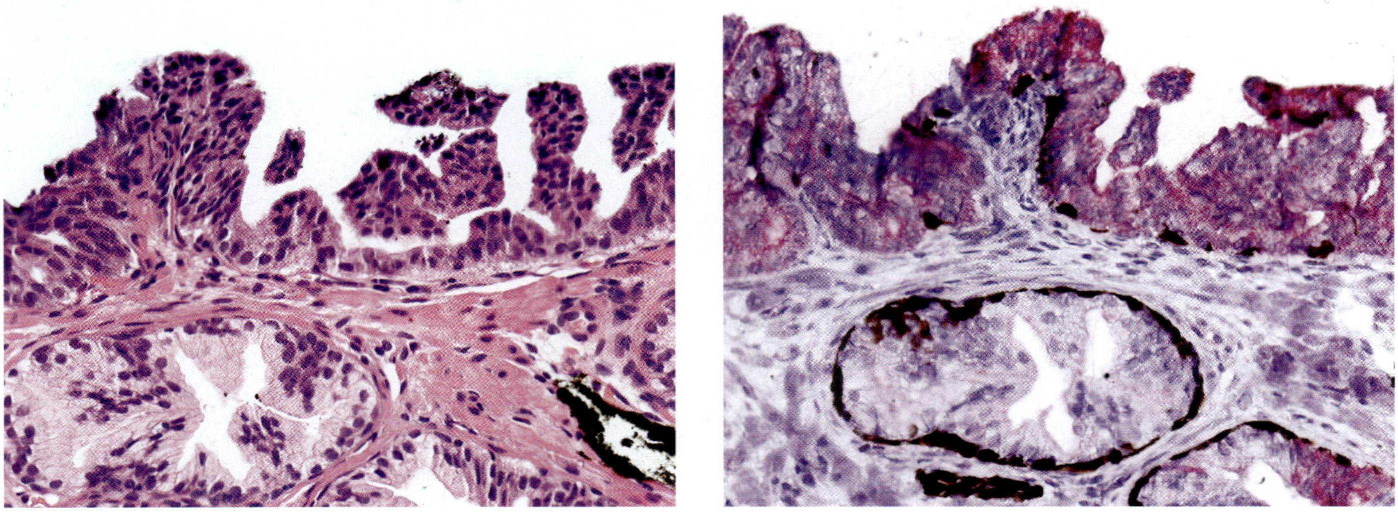

a b

Clinical relevance (prognosis and treatment options)

- Originally, the presence of isolated high-grade PIN on biopsy (without cancer) would indicate a rebiopsy
- However, the risk of finding cancer in the rebiopsy of the patients with isolated high-grade PIN is not much higher than those with a benign biopsy. Therefore, a recent recommendation by some experts is that there is no need of rebiopsy for the patients with a diagnosis of an isolated high-grade PIN in the first year
- A rebiopsy is indicated when there is clinical suspicion such as elevated PSA and high PSA velocity
- There is also suggestion that rebiopsy should be necessary if there are multiple foci of high-grade PIN detected initially, which might have a slightly higher risk for cancer
- During biopsy, taking more cores (or saturated biopsy) may help increase the cancer detection rate from the location with high-grade PIN. However, all the six or 12 (including lateral) areas should be sampled

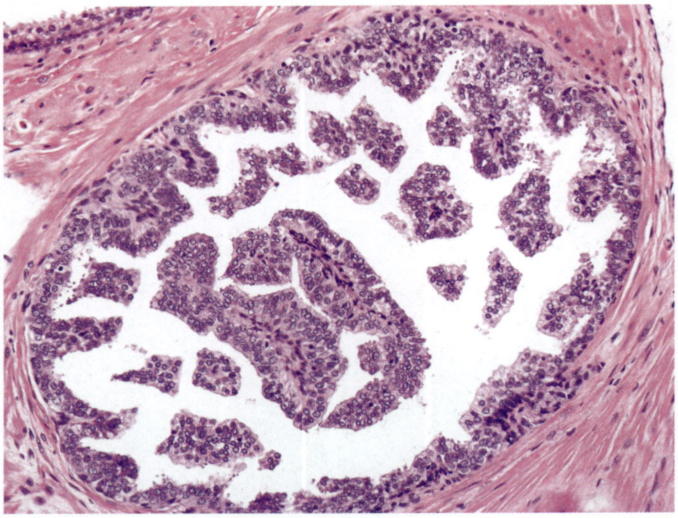

a

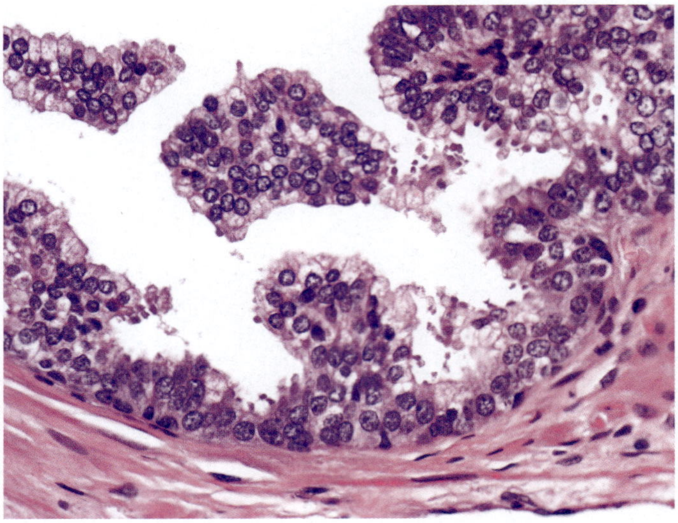

b

Figure 5-4.
A high-grade PIN gland with micropapillary configuration (*a*) and high magnification showing prominent nucleoli (*b*).

CHAPTER 6

Other Atypical Lesions of the Prostate

ADENOSIS

Definition

- Small glandular proliferation in a lobular pattern and the proliferating cells lacking cytological atypia
- Typically seen in the transitional zone
- A well-known mimic of prostatic adenocarcinoma

Other terms

- Atypical adenomatous hyperplasia (AAH), atypical adenosis (should not be used)

Clinical features

- Typically asymptomatic. It is often seen in the patients with BPH, which is associated with urinary obstruction symptoms

Gross pathology

- Not possible to identify adenosis grossly

Histology

- Small crowded glands in a well-circumscribed lobule. At low power, it is difficult to distinguish from Gleason pattern 2 of prostatic adenocarcinoma (Figs. 6-1 and 6-2)
- Patchy basal cells can be recognized (Fig. 6-1*b*)
- Lack of significant cytological atypia (Fig. 6-1*b*). Prominent and enlarged nucleoli seen in adenocarcinoma should not be present. If they are present, they are more likely to be adenocarcinoma than adenosis
- Crystalloid can been seen in the lumen occasionally (Fig. 6-3)
- In the old literature, some cases were called *atypical adenosis*. By today's standards and application of immunostaining, these cases are low-grade adenocarcinomas

Immunohistochemistry

- Presence of patchy basal cells confirmed by positive 34βE12 and/or p63 staining (Figs. 6-2*b* and 6-3*b*)
- Most adenosis cases are negative for AMACR (Fig. 6-2*b*). Only a small subset (5% to 10%) of adenosis can be positive for AMACR (Fig. 6-3*b*)

Figure 6-1.
Adenosis is composed of small crowded glands in a lobular pattern. At a lower power, it is difficult to distinguish adenosis from low-grade adenocarcinoma (*a*). High magnification shows lack of cytological atypia and occasional basal cells present (*b*, arrows).

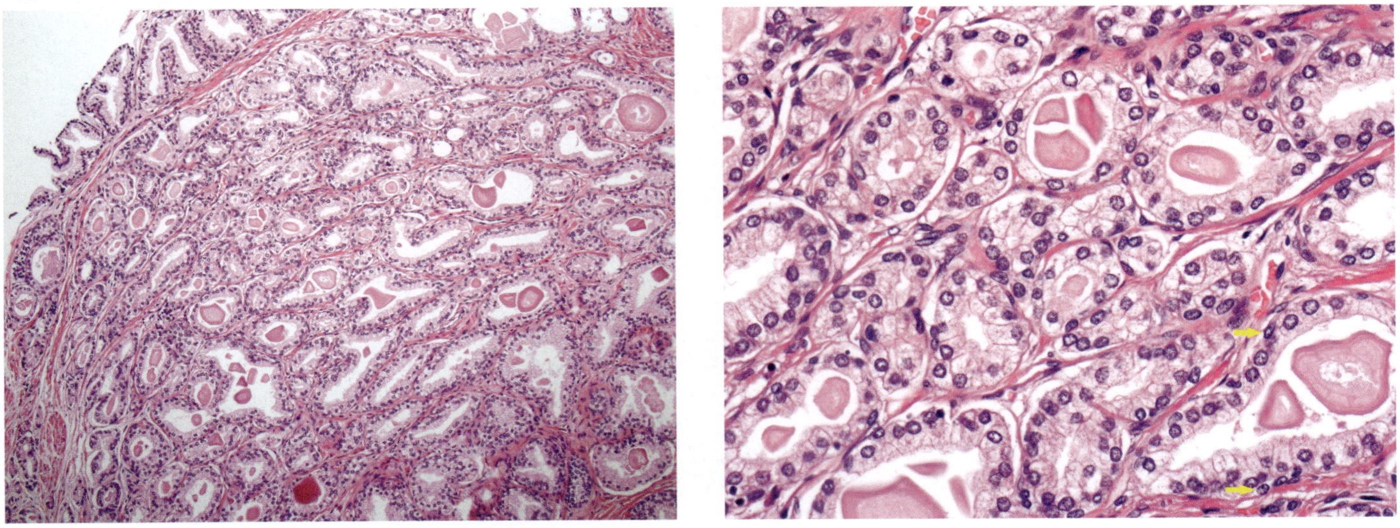

a *b*

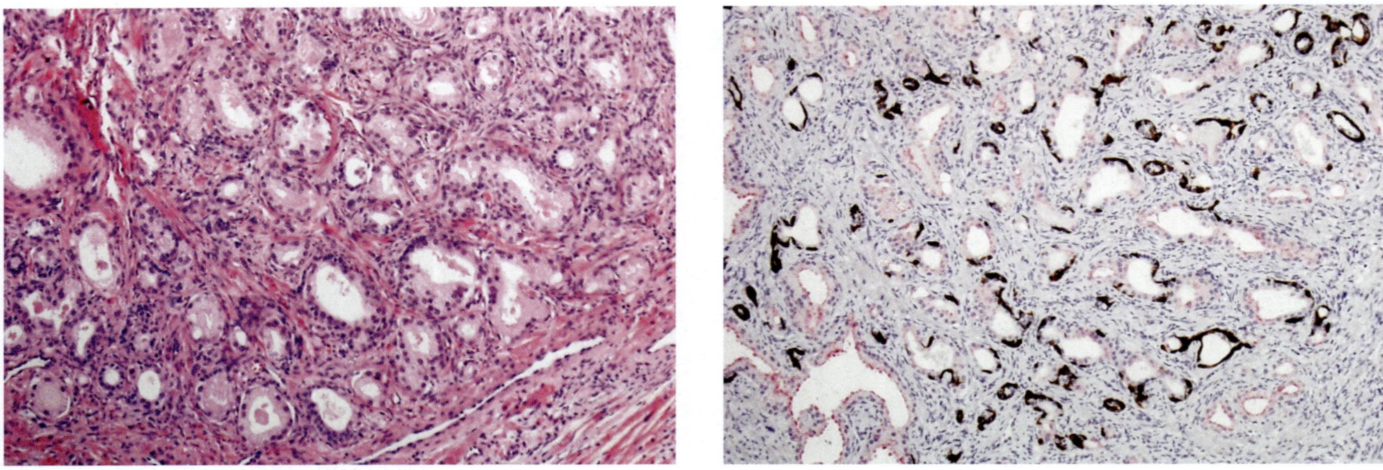

a *b*

Figure 6-2.
Adenosis (H&E, *a*) with corresponding triple staining (*b*) shows discontinuous basal cells (brown stain). AMACR (red stain) is weakly positive in adenosis, similar to that in benign glands.

Figure 6-3.
Another case of adenosis (*a*) with matching triple staining (*b*) shows unusual AMACR positivity while patchy basal cells are present. Some glands do not have basal cells but with AMACR immunoreactivity similar to that of adenocarcinoma. However, the focus should be reviewed as a whole.

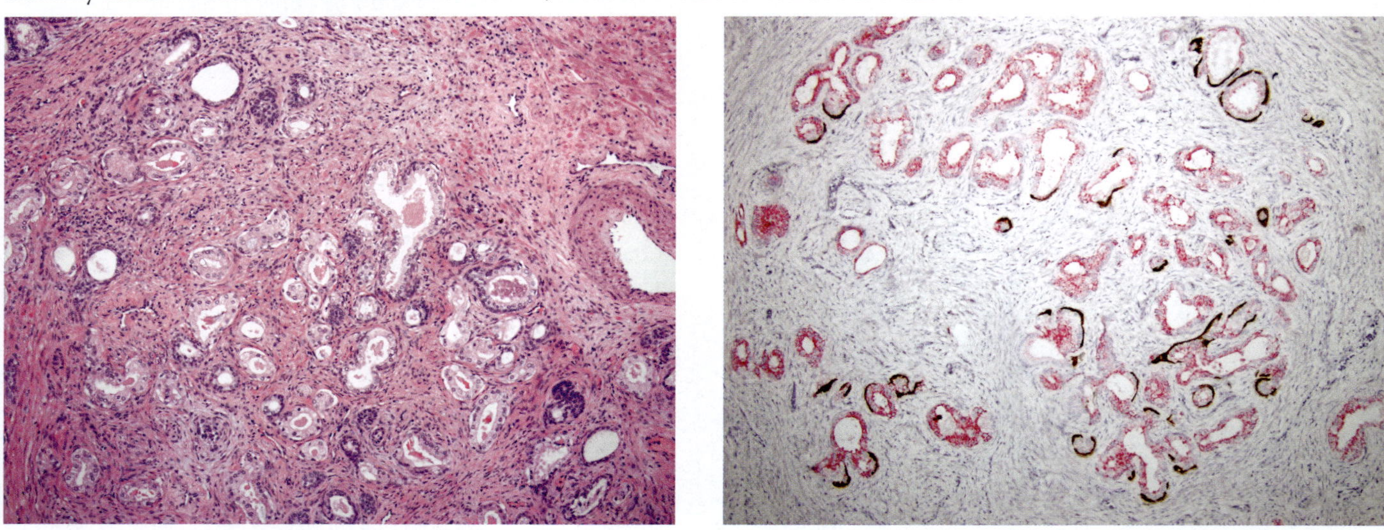

a *b*

Differential diagnosis

- Adenocarcinoma: two major features distinguish adenocarcinoma from adenosis: (1) adenocarcinoma with significant cytological atypia including prominent nucleoli, while adenosis does not and (2) adenocarcinoma does not have basal cells, while adenosis contains patchy basal cells
- High-grade PIN: two key features present in high-grade PIN but not in adenosis: cytological atypia (prominent nucleoli) and presence of large glands (see Table 6-1)

Molecular analysis

- Not established for diagnosis

Clinical relevance (prognosis and treatment options)

- Mostly benign, probably a histological variant of benign prostatic hyperplasia, although a small subset of adenosis may be related to adenocarcinoma development
- A repeat biopsy is not indicated immediately unless there is other clinical indication
- Clinical follow-up may be necessary

Table 6-1. Comparison of High-Grade PIN and Adenosis

	High-grade PIN	*Adenosis*
Architecture	Benign (preexisting benign glands)	Atypical (crowded small glands)
Cytology	Atypical (similar to adenocarcinoma)	Benign (similar to BPH)
Basal cells	Present, patchy	Present, patchy
Lobular pattern	No	Yes
Infiltrating pattern	No	No
Precursor for adenocarcinoma	Yes	Not conclusive Possibly a small subset
34be12/p63	Positive	Positive
AMACR	Positive 50% Usually weaker that in carcinoma	Mostly negative 5% to 10% positive
Repeat biopsy	Not necessary in the year	Not necessary unless clinically indicated

AMACR, α-methylacyl-CoA racemase; BPH, benign prostatic hyperplasia; PIN, prostatic intraepithelial neoplasia.

SMALL ATYPICAL GLANDS SUSPICIOUS FOR ADENOCARCINOMA (ATYPICAL SMALL ACINAR PROLIFERATION)

Definition

- A diagnostic term used in an uncertain situation when histological features suspicious for cancer are present, but fall short of a definitive malignant diagnosis

Other terms

- Also known as ASAP (atypical small acinar proliferation), atypical hyperplasia (this old term should be avoided)

Pathogenesis

- This is not a clinicopathological entity but rather a description of suspicious situations

Clinical features

- No specific features, but similar to prostate cancer patients with elevated PSA and undergoing needle core biopsy

Gross pathology

- No specific gross appearance

Histology

- Small focus of glands showing mild to moderate cytological atypia (one cannot really tell if it is a duct or acinus in a normal prostate), which are clearly different from the adjacent benign glands (Figs. 6-4 and 6-5)
- Atypical glands are small in number, typical two to five. Some experts suggest this diagnosis when there are less than three atypical glands
- Usually no basal cells can be seen (Figs. 6-4*b* and 6-5*b*)
- The diagnostic criteria for this condition is very subjective

Immunohistochemistry

- Triple stain has been used for ASAP cases and proven to be helpful in reducing uncertainty and establishing a definitive diagnosis
- AMACR typically weak (Figs. 6-4*b* and 6-5*b*), or negative
- HMWCK and p63 may or may not be detectable in a small focus of atypical glands (Figs. 6-4*b* and 6-5*b*)

Clinical relevance (prognosis and treatment options)

- There is an increased risk in finding cancer in a repeat biopsy of a patient with ASAP diagnosis. Therefore, a rebiopsy is recommended within 6 months
- More than 50% of patients with ASAP diagnoses will be found to have prostatic adenocarcinoma by repeat biopsies
- Do not use ASAP in the case of high-grade PIN

Figure 6-4.

Two small atypical glands found on needle core biopsy, which are significantly different from benign glands (*a*), both of them show negative basal cell staining and AMACR reactivity (*b*). This finding is highly suspicious for adenocarcinoma.

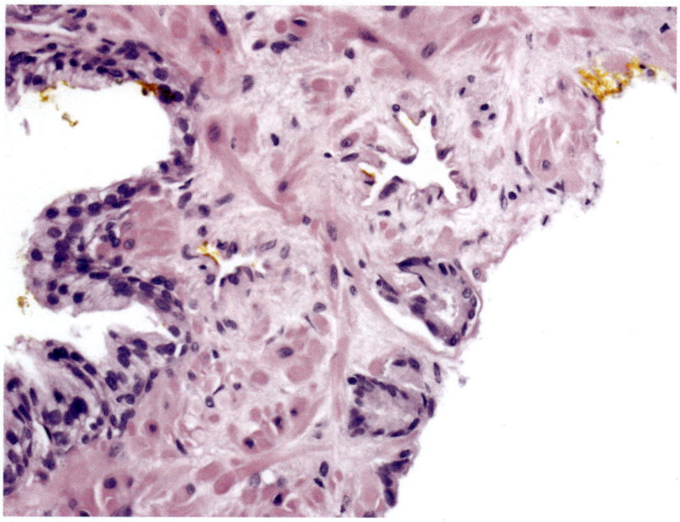

a

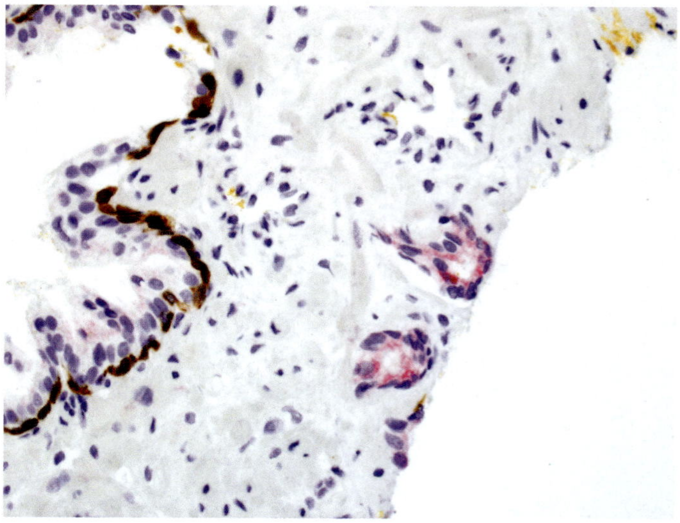

b

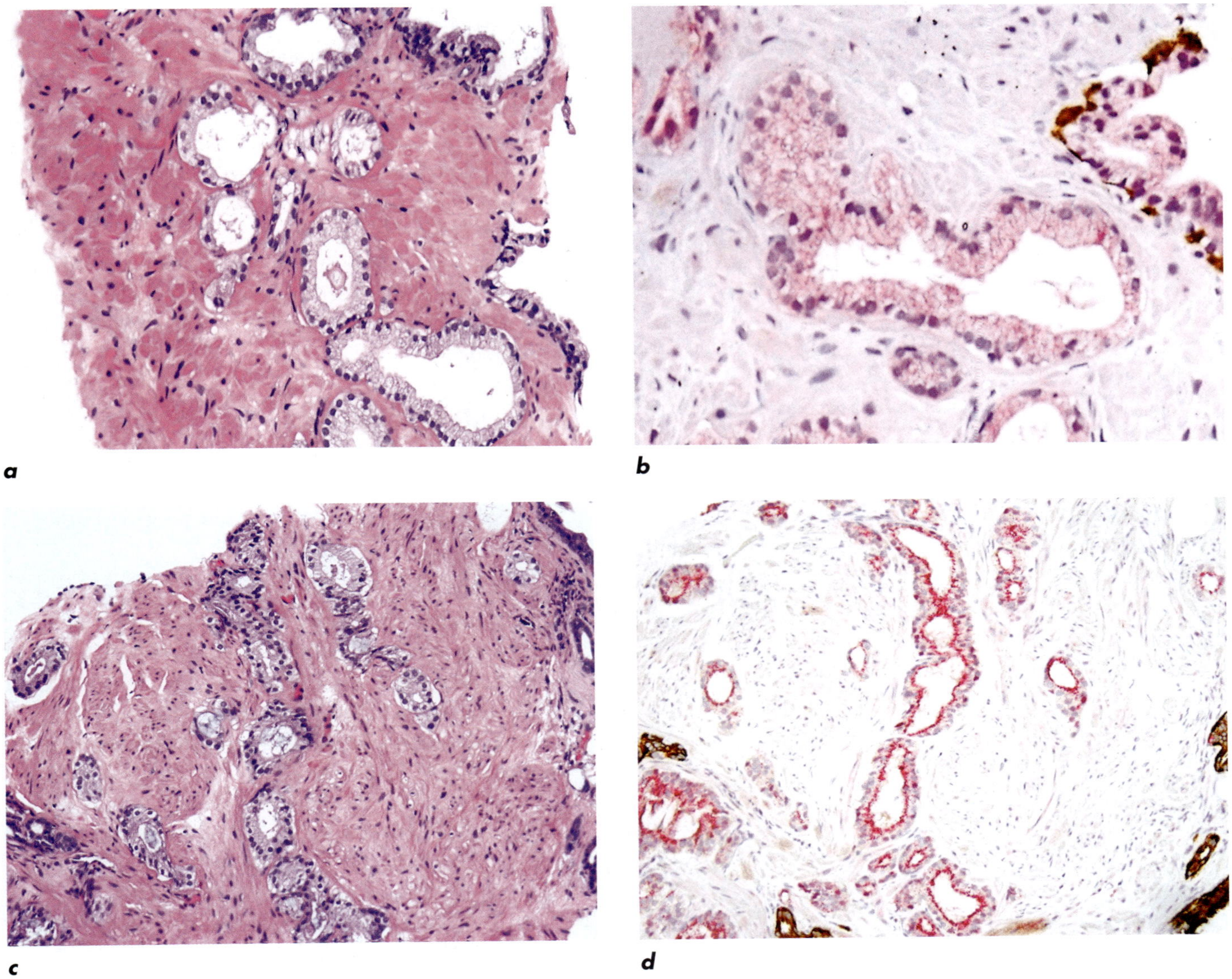

Figure 6-5.
ASAP followed by a repeat biopsy positive for cancer. These small atypical glands do not have prominent nucleoli although they appear to be infiltrative (*a*). By immunostaining the atypical glands are negative for basal cells and weakly positive for AMACR (*b*). The findings are suspicious but not diagnostic of cancer. Repeat biopsy a few months later shows sufficient evidence to make a definitive diagnosis of adenocarcinoma (*c*), confirmed by the triple immunostaining (*d*).

HIGH-GRADE PROSTATIC INTRAEPITHELIAL NEOPLASIA WITH ADJACENT SMALL ATYPICAL GLANDS

Definition

- Presence of high-grade prostatic intraepithelial neoplasia (PIN) and adjacent small focus of atypical glands suspicious but not diagnostic of prostatic adenocarcinoma

Other terms

- High-grade PIN with atypia (PINATYP), high-grade PIN with atypical small acinar proliferation (PIN+ASAP)

Pathogenesis

- High-grade PIN is a precursor lesion of adenocarcinoma. It can develop into an adenocarcinoma when small clusters of neoplastic cells budding off the large PIN glands. During the process, the small abnormal glands are losing basal cells and becoming invasive adenocarcinoma
- This condition is somewhere in the middle between high-grade PIN and carcinoma, which may represent early adenocarcinoma
- It is not a true pathologic entity as high-grade PIN, but represents an uncertain condition that needs special attention

Clinical features

- No specific clinical symptoms
- Typically, a man with elevated PSA undergoing prostatic needle core biopsy

Gross pathology

- Biopsy situation, gross pathology does not apply

Histology

- The lesion is composed of both high-grade PIN and a cluster of small atypical glands (Fig. 6-6)
- Nuclear atypia is present (Fig. 6-6) and similar to the adjacent high-grade PIN
- The PIN glands and small atypical glands are similar in cytological features. There should not be a sharp contrast in morphology between small atypical glands and adjacent high-grade PIN

Immunohistochemistry

- AMACR positive or negative, similar to high-grade PIN (Fig. 6-6*c*)
- Basal cell markers negative or patchily positive (Fig. 6-6*c*)

Clinical relevance (prognosis and treatment options)

- If the transition from high-grade PIN with small atypical glands is detected in a prostate needle core biopsy, it could be difficult to determine if it is still a high-grade PIN or if it is already an early adenocarcinoma. In this situation, we use PINATYP diagnosis
- It also may represent the tangential sectioning of a focus of high-grade PIN or small focus of adenocarcinoma next to high-grade PIN
- Rebiopsy is indicated as in the case of ASAP
- No radical treatment such as surgery or radiation is indicated, but clinical follow-up is necessary
- Some of the atypical prostatic lesions are summarized in Table 6-2

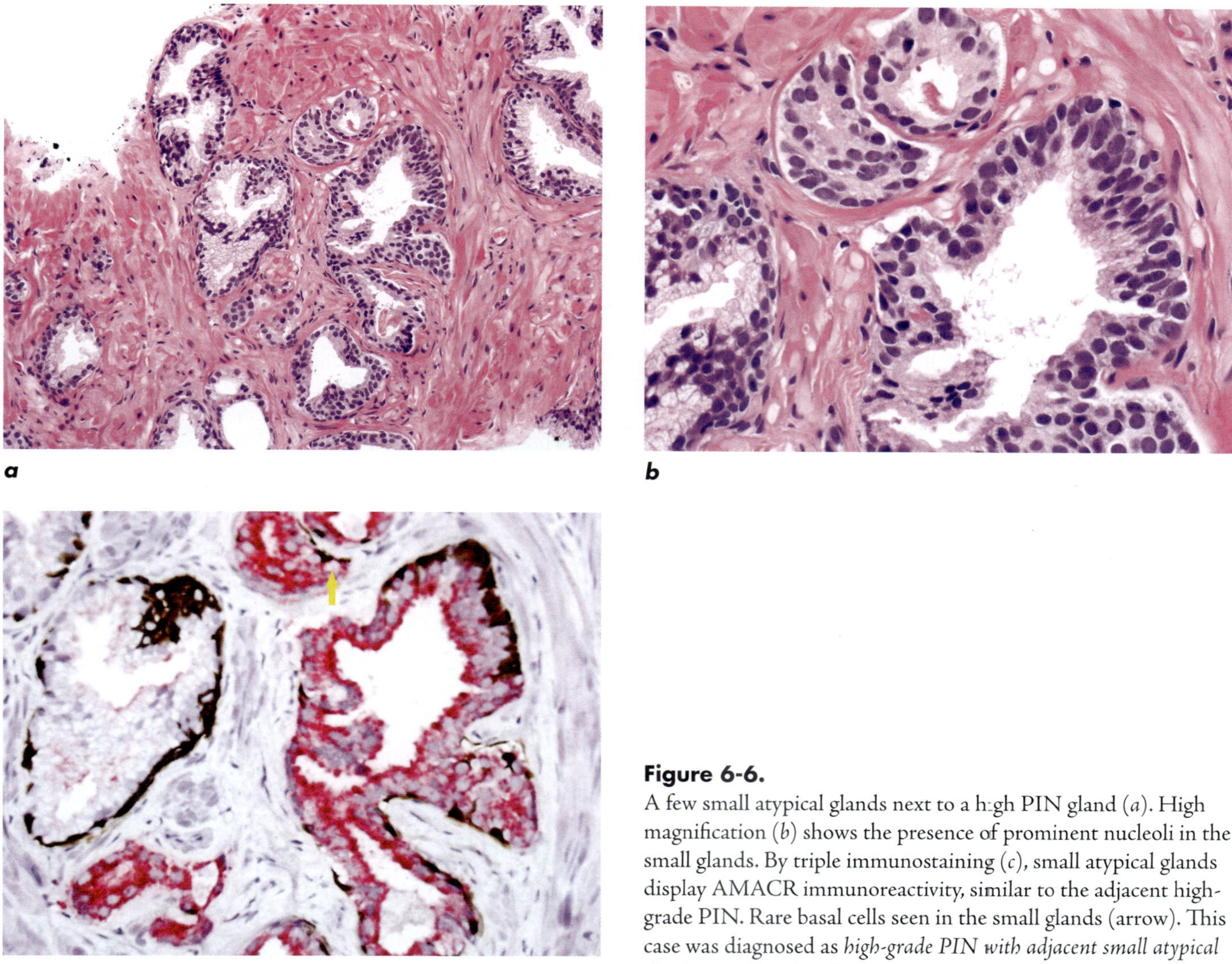

Figure 6-6.
A few small atypical glands next to a high PIN gland (*a*). High magnification (*b*) shows the presence of prominent nucleoli in the small glands. By triple immunostaining (*c*), small atypical glands display AMACR immunoreactivity, similar to the adjacent high-grade PIN. Rare basal cells seen in the small glands (arrow). This case was diagnosed as *high-grade PIN with adjacent small atypical gland suspicious for adenocarcinoma.*

Table 6-2. Atypical Conditions of the Prostate and Their Clinical Relevance

Condition on initial biopsy	*Risk finding cancer on rebiopsy*	*Indication for rebiopsy*
Adenocarcinoma on active surveillance	Almost 100%	Yes, yearly
ASAP	50%	Yes, immediately
High-grade PIN with atypia	50%	Yes, immediately
High-grade PIN	20% to 25%	Not immediately in 1 year
Adenosis*	<20%	No
Atrophy*	<20%	No
Benign prostate*	<20%	No
*Anyone with clinically suspicious factors	Not sure	Yes

ASAP, atypical small acinar proliferation; PIN, prostatic intraepithelial neoplasia.

CHAPTER 7 Diagnostic Features of Prostatic Adenocarcinoma

Definition

- Histological features commonly seen in prostatic adenocarcinoma
- These features are not highly specific, because they may be seen in benign conditions. Therefore, it requires a combination of multiple diagnostic features to establish a diagnosis of adenocarcinoma

Common histological features

- Adenocarcinoma accounts for more than 95% of malignancies of the prostate, which is the focus of this chapter
- Other types of cancers including urothelial cell carcinoma, carcinosarcoma, basal cell carcinoma, lymphomas, or stromal sarcomas do occur within the prostate
- No single feature is sensitive and specific enough to establish diagnosis of prostatic adenocarcinoma in all the cases. Although the most common known histological feature for prostatic adenocarcinoma is *small infiltrating glands with big nucleoli*, this feature can be seen in the majority of the prostatic adenocarcinoma cases but does not sufficiently cover all the cases
- The diagnosis of prostatic adenocarcinoma, particularly on limited material from needle core biopsy, is based on a constellation of architectural, cytological, and other features (listed on Table 7-1). Some of the diagnostic features should be included in the pathology report for their clinical relevance (Table 7-2)

Architectural patterns

- Small glands
  - Malignant glands are usually smaller in diameter than normal prostatic glands (acini or ducts) (Figs. 7-1 and 7-2)
- Infiltrating patterns
  - Malignant glands, unless in a low-grade tumor, do not form a lobular pattern as normal glands do
  - They infiltrate the stroma tissue in a haphazard manner, which refers to the irregular distribution and angulation of the malignant glands (Fig. 7-3)
- Straight luminal borders
  - The malignant glands have smaller lumens, less convoluted than larger benign glands (Fig. 7-3)
  - A large malignant gland has straight luminal border (Fig. 7-4) or it may have papillary projections (Fig. 7-5)
  - The malignant glands may be complex and cribriform forming "Roman bridges"
- Poorly formed glands
  - In less differentiated tumors, the glandular pattern is irregular, less organized, fused (Fig. 7-6)
- Solid patterns
  - In a very high-grade tumor, the tumor cells lost the glandular formation, they tend to grow in cords, nests, or sheets of solid cells
- Glomus-like blood vessel proliferation
  - It has been observed that the smooth muscle cells in small arteries within the areas of prostatic adenocarcinoma may exhibit proliferative change (Fig. 7-7)
  - There are increased layers of small muscles in a small artery. It resembles the appearance of a glomus tumor or the appearance of an onion skin
- Invading muscle
  - Tumor cells may invade smooth or skeletal muscles of the prostatic stroma, splitting or eroding into muscle fibers (Figs. 7-8, arrow, and 7-9)
- Invading nerve and adipose tissue
  - The tumor cells may also invade nerve bundles (perineural invasion) or ganglion, or adipose tissue (extraprostatic extension). These features will be discussed in the next chapters
- Desmoplastic reaction
  - Low-grade and intermediate-grade tumors do not induce desmoplastic reaction. However, some higher grade tumors (Gleason 7 or above) may cause desmoplastic or fibrotic reaction of the prostatic stroma (Fig. 7-10)
- Retraction artifact
  - This retraction feature is seen more commonly in malignant glands than benign glands, mostly seen in prostatectomy specimens, rarely seen in needle core specimens (Fig. 7-11)
  - But, it is not a good diagnostic feature for needle core biopsy. Furthermore, it is also seen associated with high-grade PIN (Fig. 7-12) or benign glands (Fig. 7-13)

Cytological features

- Prominent nucleoli
  - This is the single most important diagnostic feature, well known for prostate cancer cells
  - Typically the diameter of the nucleolus of a malignant cell is bigger than 3 μm (half of a lymphocyte) in diameter, with "cherry red" color on H&E stained slides (Figs. 7-14 and 7-15, arrow)
  - High-grade PIN or basal cells may display prominent nucleoli

Table 7-1. List of Histological Diagnostic Features of Prostate Cancer

Architectural patterns	Small glands
	Infiltrating patterns
	Straight luminal borders
	Poorly formed glands or solid patterns
	Glomus-like artery proliferation
	Invading muscle
	Invading nerve and adipose tissue
	Desmoplastic reaction
	Retraction artifact
Cytological features	Prominent nucleoli
	Lack of basal cells
	Nuclear hyperchromasia
	Nuclear enlargement
	Amphophilic cytoplasm
	Multiple nucleoli
	Marginated nucleoli
	N/C ratio
Extracellular material	Blue mucin
	Pink secretion
	Crystalloids
	Intraluminal collagen fragments
Pathognomonic features	Perineural invasion
	Collagenous micronodules
	Glomeruloid structure

N/C ratio, nuclear/cytoplasmic ratio.

Table 7-2. Diagnostic Items to Be Included in Pathology Report of Prostate Needle Core Biopsy

When adenocarcinoma present	*When adenocarcinoma absent*
Gleason score (3 + 3, 3 + 4, 4 + 5 ...)	Presence of high-grade PIN
Volume (involving % of tissue core or tumor mm in length)	Presence of acute inflammation
Side (right or left)	Presence of marked chronic inflammation
Number of positive cores	Presence of granuloma
Location (right apex, left, mid ...)	Presence of infarct (coagulative necrosis)
Presence of perineural invasion	Presence of treatment effect
Presence of extraprostatic extension (fat)	
Presence of special type of carcinoma, such as • Ductal • Foamy gland • Small cell type • Intraductal	Diagnosis should be avoided in biopsy: • Low-grade PIN • Benign prostatic hyperplasia • Atrophy • Normal colonic mucosa
Options but may not be required: • High-grade PIN • Granulomatous or prominent inflammation	
Tumor involving seminal vesicle/ejaculatory ducts if specified biopsy	

PIN, prostatic intraepithelial neoplasia.

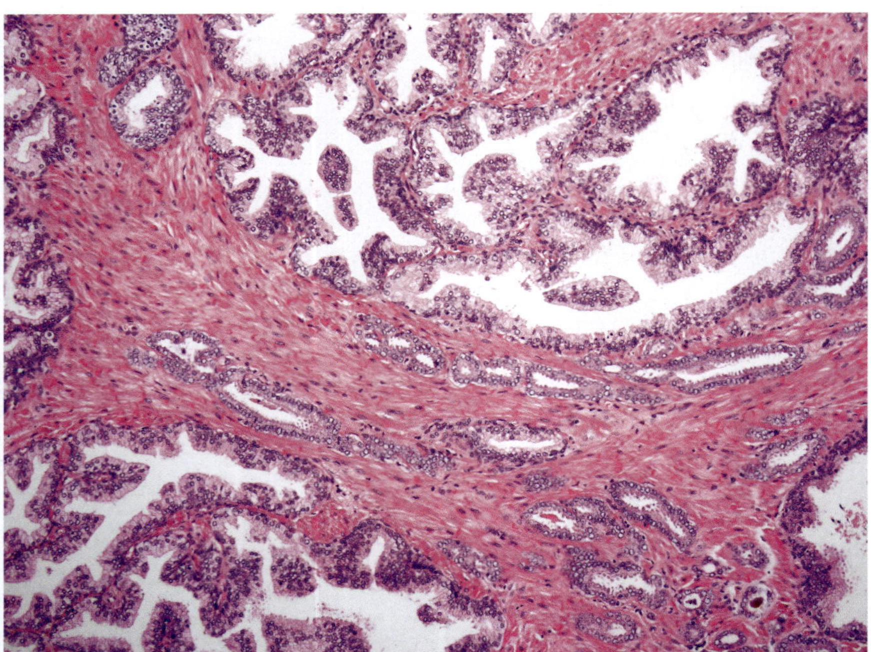

Figure 7-1.
Several small glands infiltrate between two groups of large benign glands. The cytoplasm of the malignant glands is darker than those of benign glands.

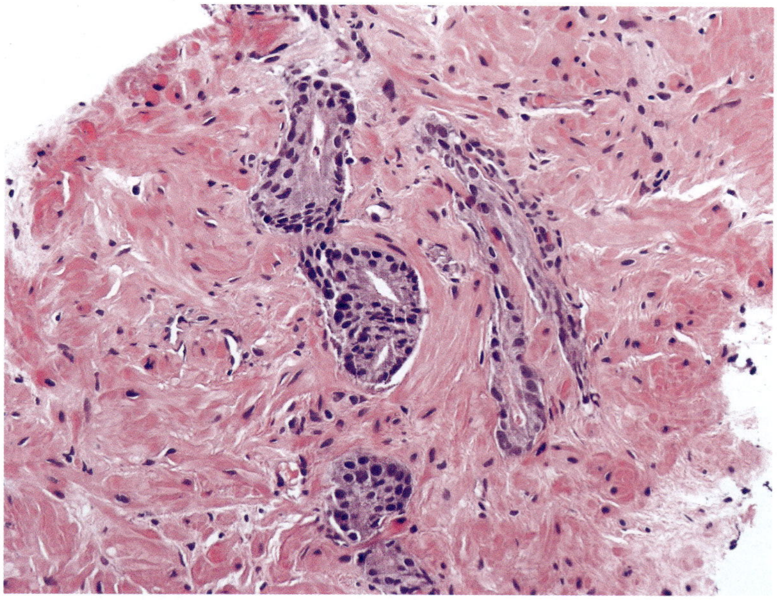

Figure 7-2.
A cluster of malignant glands on the right side are severely elongated and infiltrating. The pattern is rarely seen in benign glands.

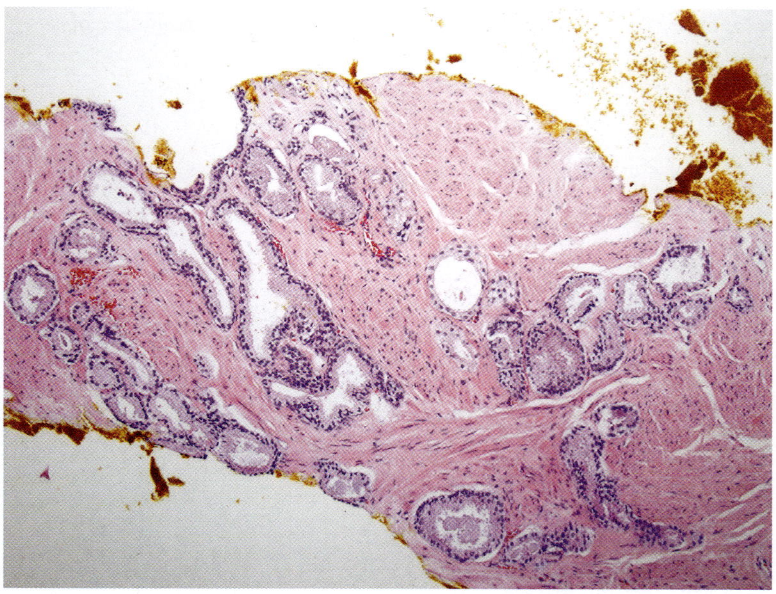

Figure 7-3.
Several adenocarcinoma glands show a haphazard infiltrating pattern without forming a lobule.

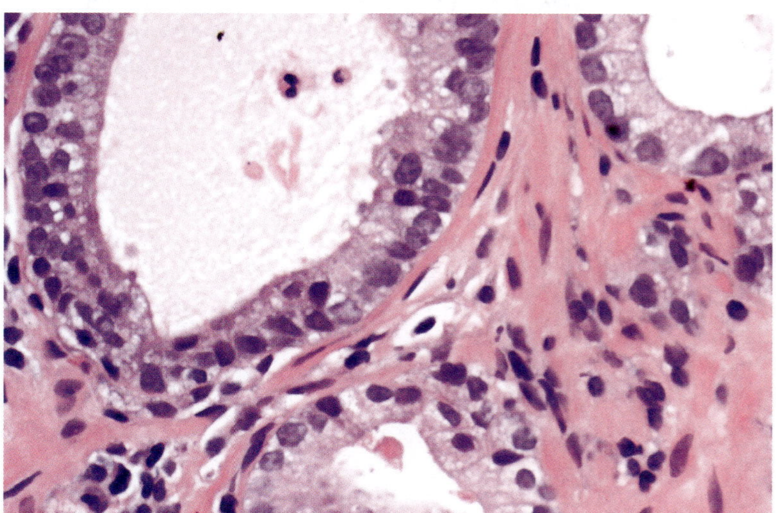

Figure 7-4.
Adenocarcinoma glands with straight luminal borders and nuclear atypia.

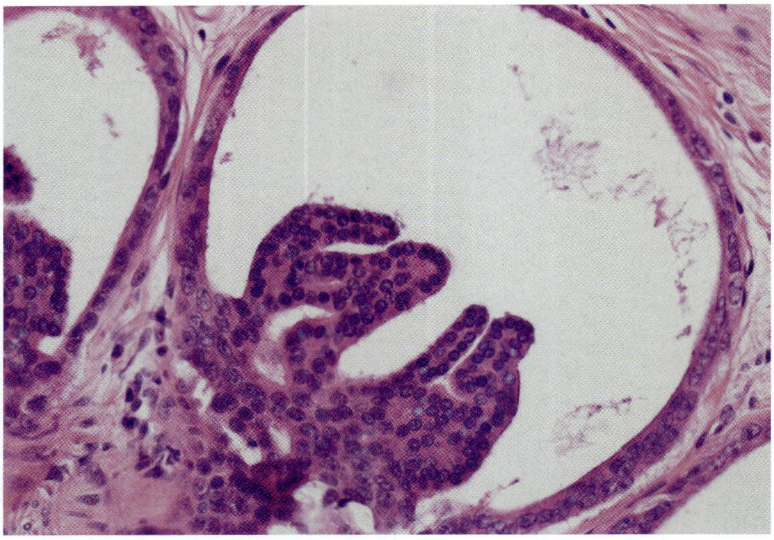

Figure 7-5.
A large dilated malignant gland with very rigid and straight luminal border and finger-like projections into the lumen.

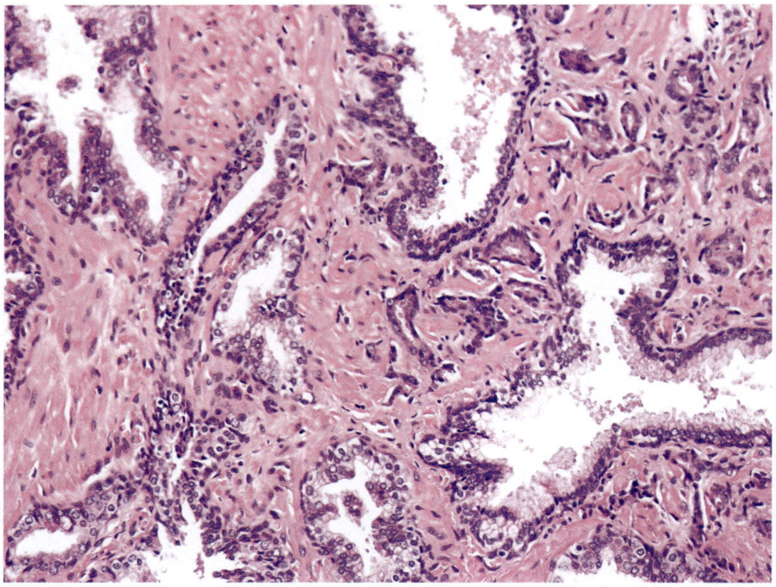

Figure 7-6.
Several poorly formed small glands infiltrating between large benign glands. These features are diagnostic of adenocarcinoma.

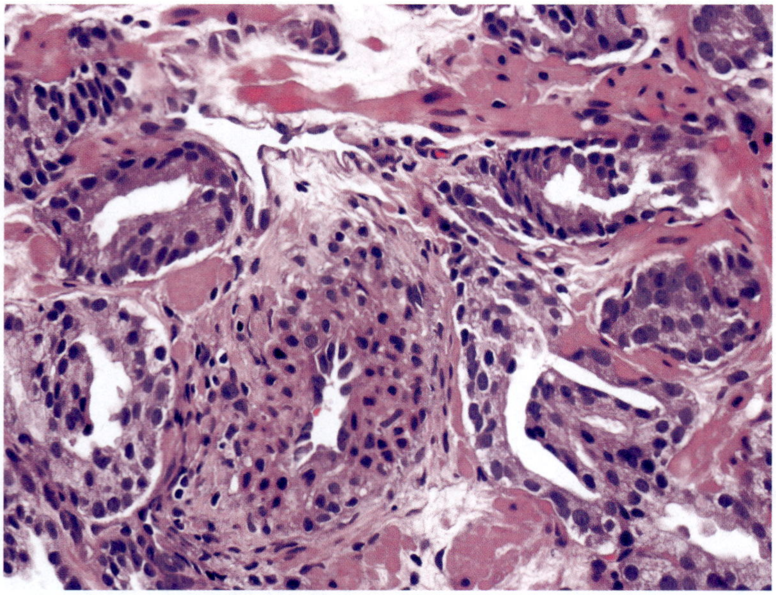

Figure 7-7.
A small artery located within an area of infiltrating adenocarcinoma shows marked proliferation of smooth muscle cells, giving the appearance of "onion skin" or "glomus tumor."

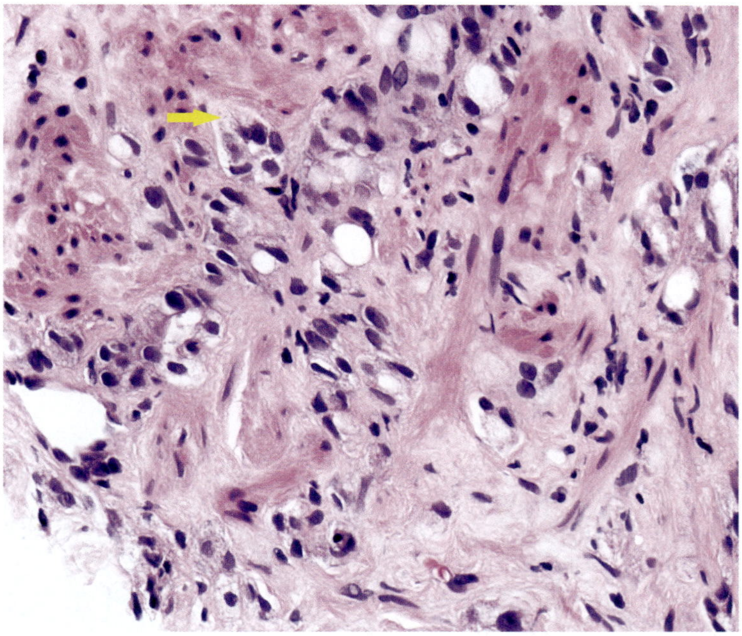

Figure 7-8.
Malignant glandular cells split and erode muscle fibers (arrow).

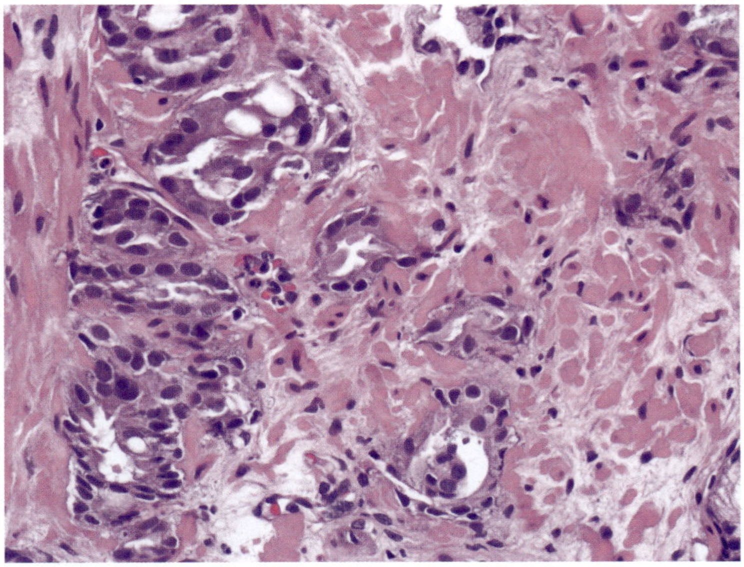

Figure 7-9.
Adenocarcinoma cells invading muscle fibers.

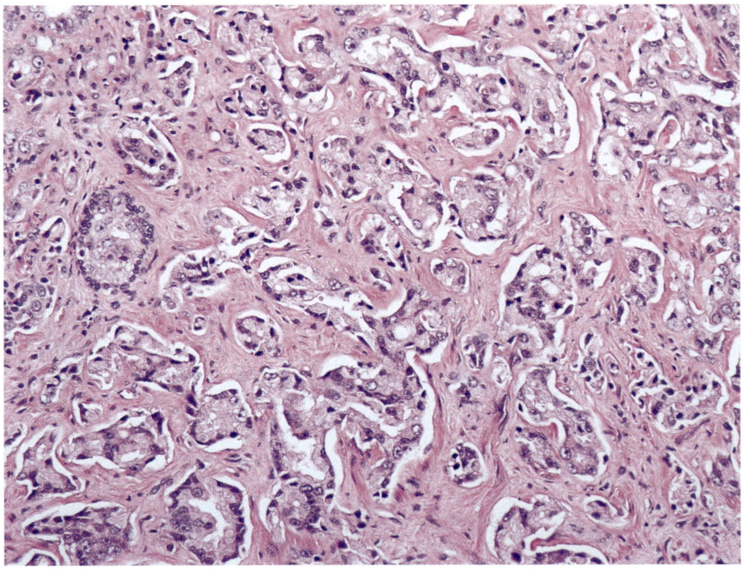

Figure 7-10.
Prominent fibrotic stroma reaction induced by (Gleason pattern 4) adenocarcinoma.

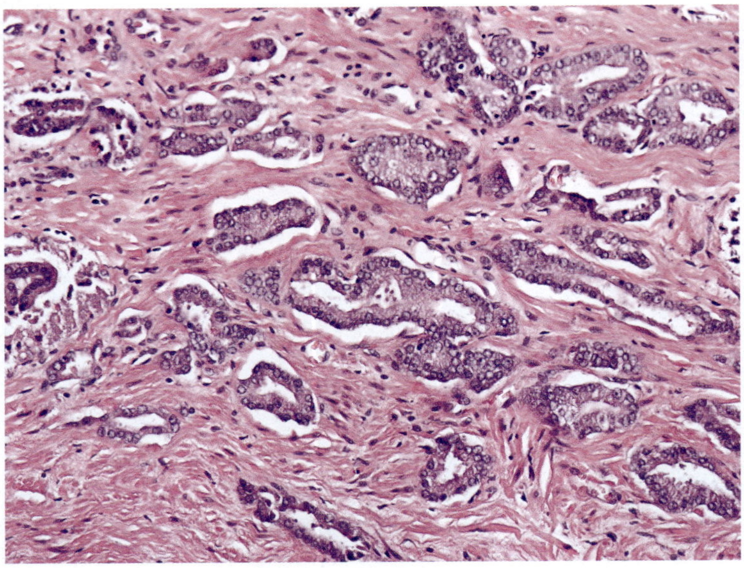

Figure 7-11.
Adenocarcinoma with retraction artifacts (clefts) around malignant glands.

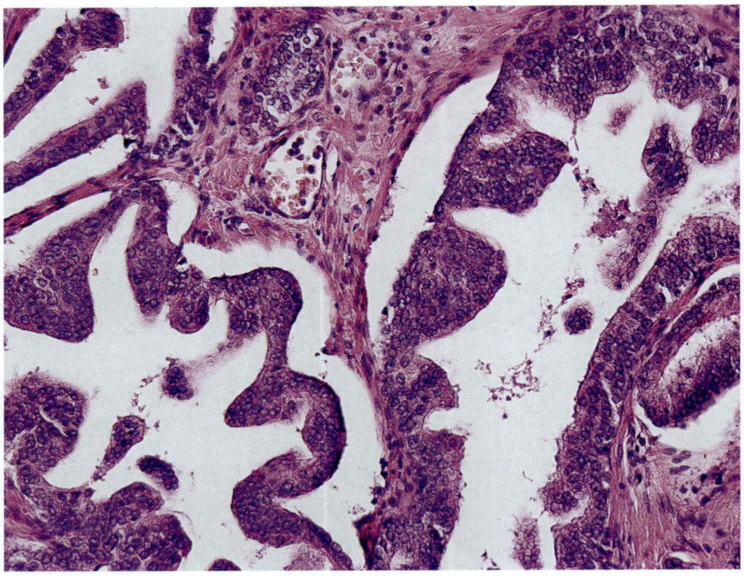

Figure 7-12.
High-grade PIN with retraction artifacts.

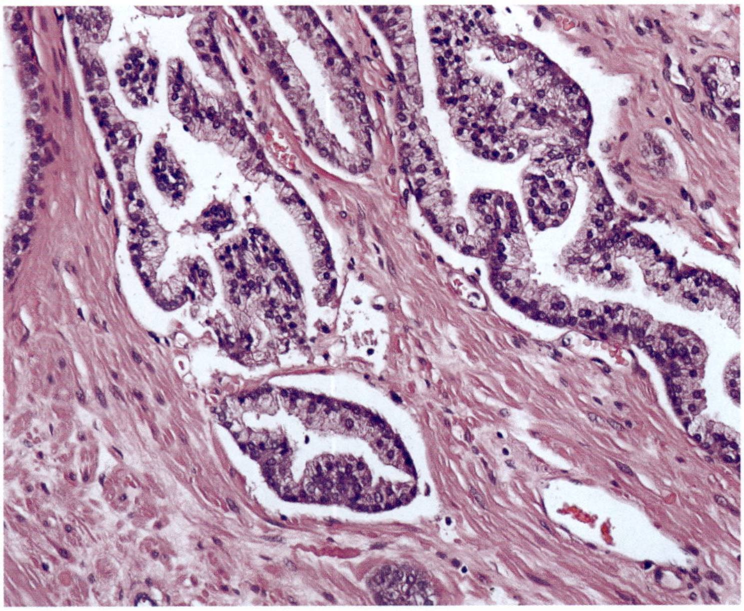

Figure 7-13.
Benign glands with retraction artifacts.

- Lack of basal cells
  - Typically adenocarcinoma of the prostate lack basal cells (Figs. 7-14 and 7-16), they have the phenotype of prostatic secretory cells
  - The lack of basal cells can be confirmed by the negative staining of basal cell markers such as p63 and HMWCK
- Nuclear hyperchromasia
  - Tumor cells show increased (darker) chromatin compared to benign glandular cells (Fig. 7-16)
- Nuclear enlargement (nucleomegaly)
  - Malignant glandular cells have larger and more irregular nuclei than normal glandular cells (Fig. 7-17)
- Amphophilic cytoplasm
  - Tumor cells have purple or darker cytoplasm than a benign gland (Fig. 7-16)
- Multiple nucleoli
  - Multiple nucleoli are common in malignant cells (Fig. 7-15). This feature is uncommon in a benign gland, but can be seen in high-grade PIN and other lesions

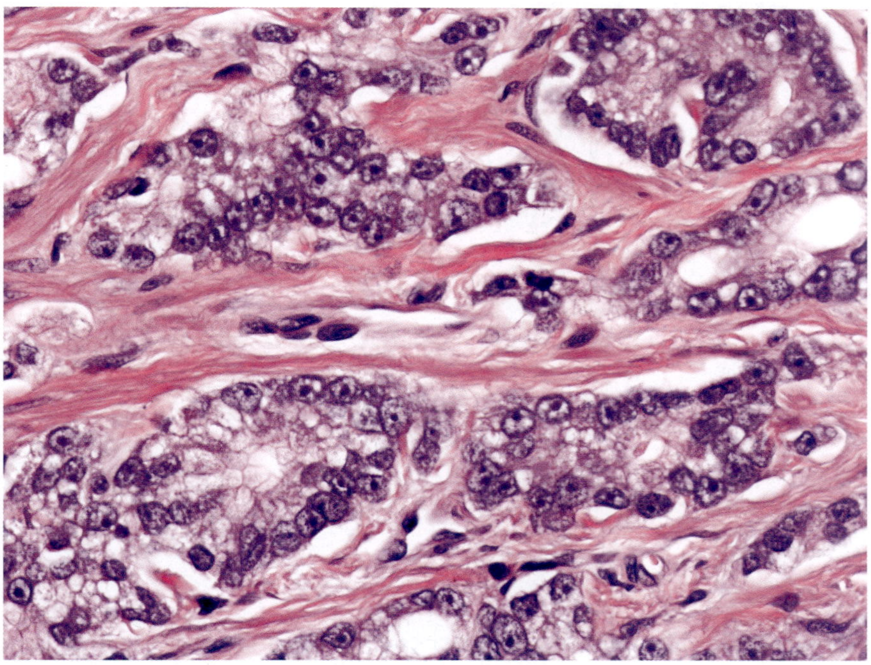

Figure 7-14.
Adenocarcinoma cells with prominent nucleoli, most are singular and occasionally two nucleoli.

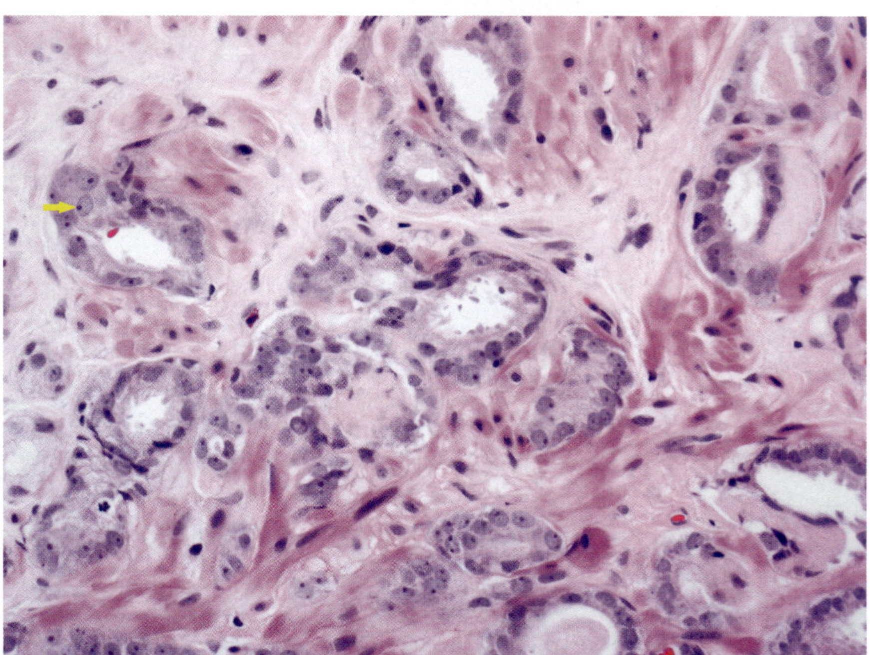

Figure 7-15.
Adenocarcinoma cells, relatively uniform in size and shape, contain one or multiple prominent "cherry red" nucleolus, greater than 3 μm in diameter, centrally located. Marginated nucleoli (arrow) and mitoses can be seen.

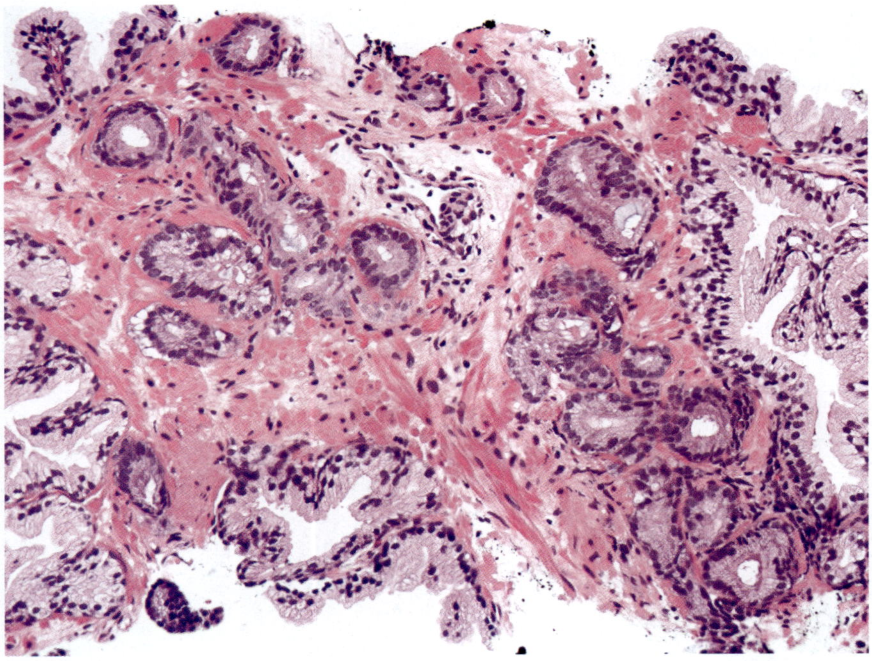

Figure 7-16.
Adenocarcinoma infiltrating between benign glands. The tumor cells do not contain basal cells and they have a higher N/C ratio than the adjacent benign glandular cells.

- Marginated nucleoli
  - Nucleoli are closer to nuclear membrane of the tumor cell (Fig. 7-15, arrow), which can hardly be used as diagnostic criteria because it may require a special fixative to show nuclear detail
- Nuclear/cytoplasmic (N/C) ratio
  - Tumor cells may display higher nucleus to cytoplasm ratio (Fig. 7-16)
  - However, this feature is not reliable or consistent in prostatic adenocarcinoma

Special extracellular material

There are several types of extracellular material often seen in the lumen of a malignant gland, but can be occasionally seen in a benign condition.

- Blue mucin
  - blue-tinged mucinous secretions, typically small amount (Figs. 7-17 and 7-18)
- Crystalloids
  - Cystalloids are more commonly seen in well-differentiated malignant glands (Figs. 7-19 and 7-20)
  - Crystalloids are typically seen in carcinoma of Gleason pattern 2 or 3, rarely in a high-grade one
  - But they can also been seen in benign conditions such as adenosis and occasionally seen in benign atrophic glands
- Pink amorphous secretion
  - Intraluminal amorphous eosinophilic secretions more commonly in malignant glands than in benign glands (Figs. 7-21 to 7-23)
  - On the other hand, corpora amylacea are more commonly seen in a benign gland
- Intraluminal collagen fragments
  - Related to collagenous micronodules, the fragmented collagen fibers may be released to the lumen of a malignant gland, confirmed by ultrastructural studies in the past
  - These fibers are eosinophilic and highly refractile (Fig. 7-24)

Comparison and contrast of adenocarcinoma with benign glands

- *One of the most important methods* to diagnose prostate cancer is to compare and contrast benign and malignant glands (Figs. 7-25 and 7-26)
- The difference can be obvious or subtle
- A benign gland, which is almost always present in the prostate needle core biopsy, can be used as a reference for such a comparison (Figs. 7-26 and 7-27)
- The different sizes of the glands (Figs. 7-25 and 7-26)
- The different shapes of the glands (Figs. 7-25 and 7-26)
- The luminal borders of the glands (Fig. 7-28)
- The colors of the cytoplasm (Figs. 7-25 and 7-28)
- The nuclear sizes (Fig. 7-27)
- The nucleolus sizes (Figs. 7-25 and 7-28)
- Finally, the differences between malignant and benign glands can be highlighted by using immunostains (Fig. 7-28*b*)

The major differences between adenocarcinoma and benign glands are listed in Table 7-3.

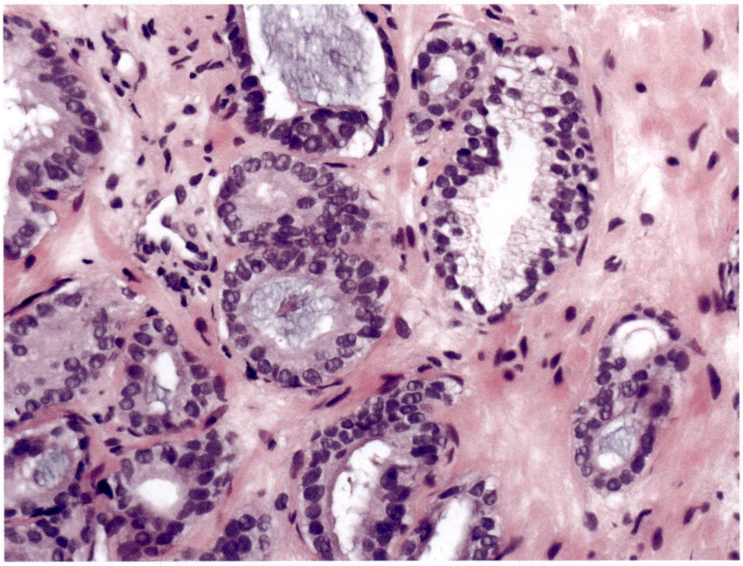

Figure 7-17.
Adenocarcinoma. Small amount of blue mucin present in the malignant glands but not in the benign prostatic glands (right).

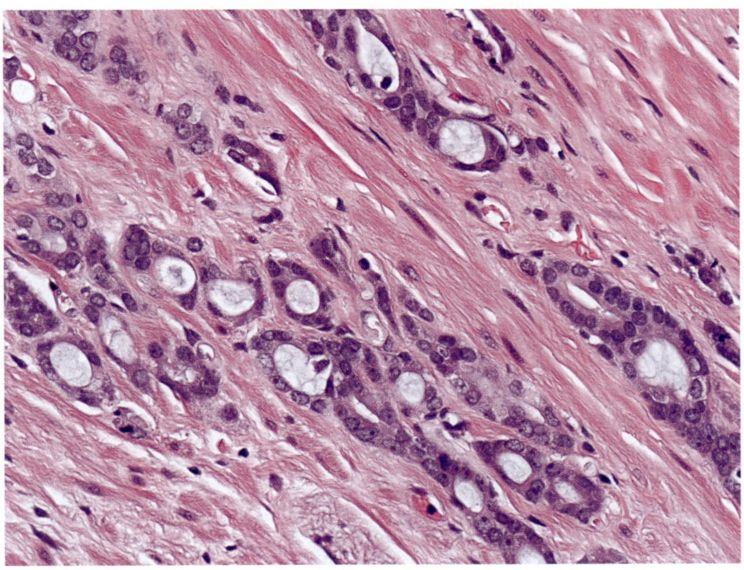

Figure 7-18.
Adenocarcinoma with blue-tinged mucin.

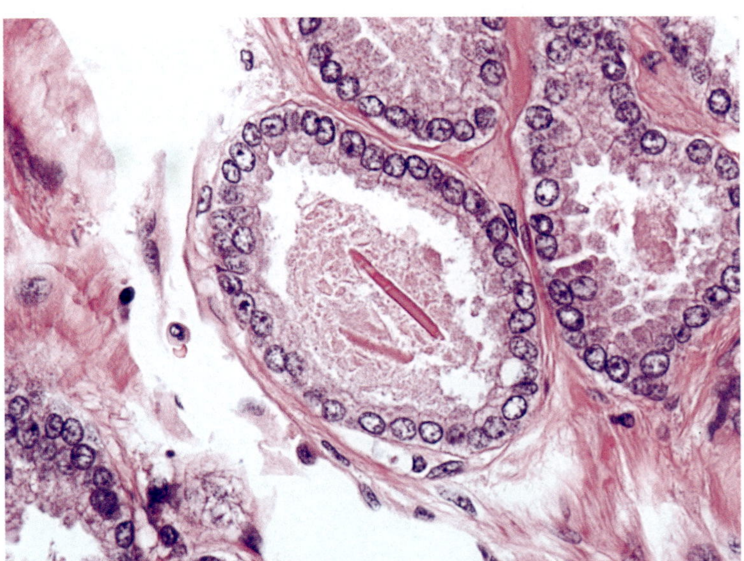

Figure 7-19.
Adenocarcinoma with crystalloids.

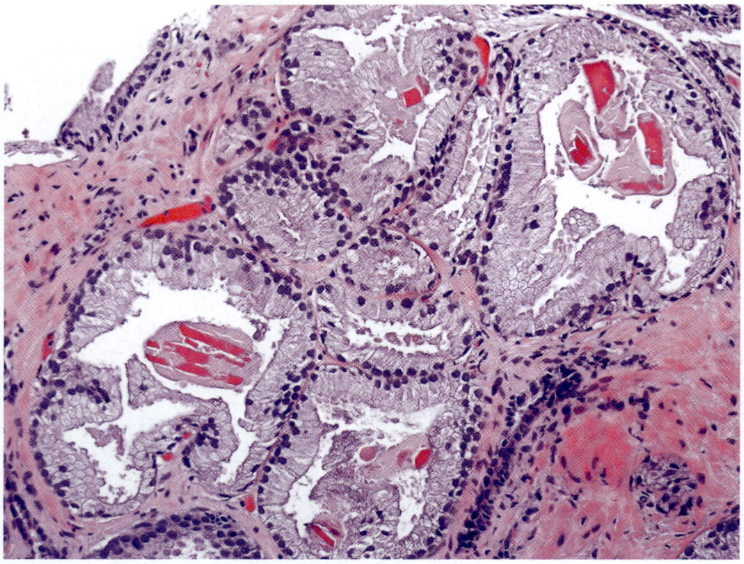

Figure 7-20.
Adenocarcinoma. Crystalloids present in multiple malignant glands although they have deceiving benign appearance.

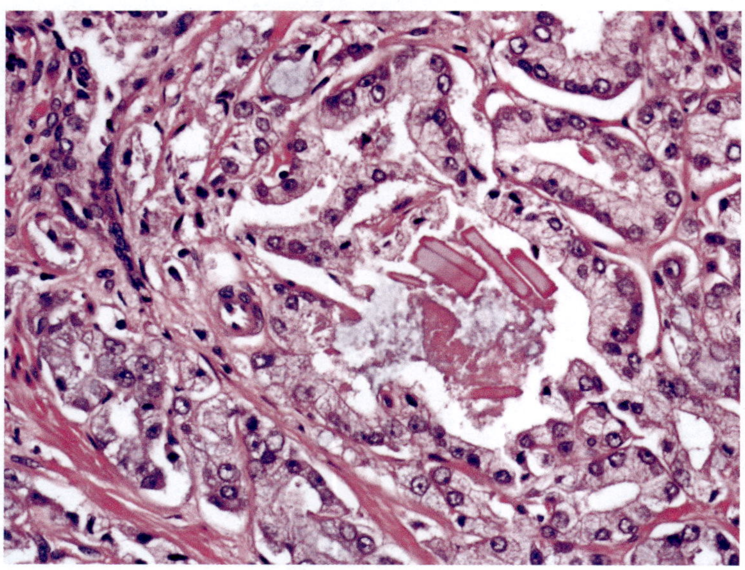

Figure 7-21.
Adenocarcinoma containing both crystalloids and blue mucin.

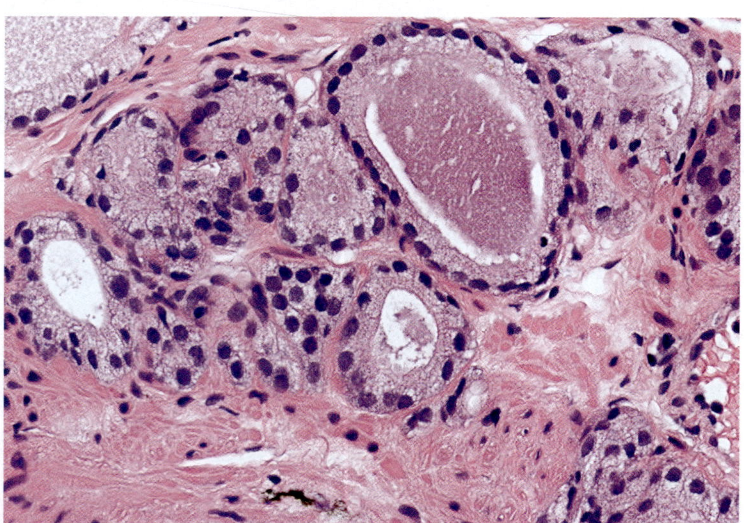

Figure 7-22.
Adenocarcinoma. Pink amorphous secretion is seen in several malignant glands.

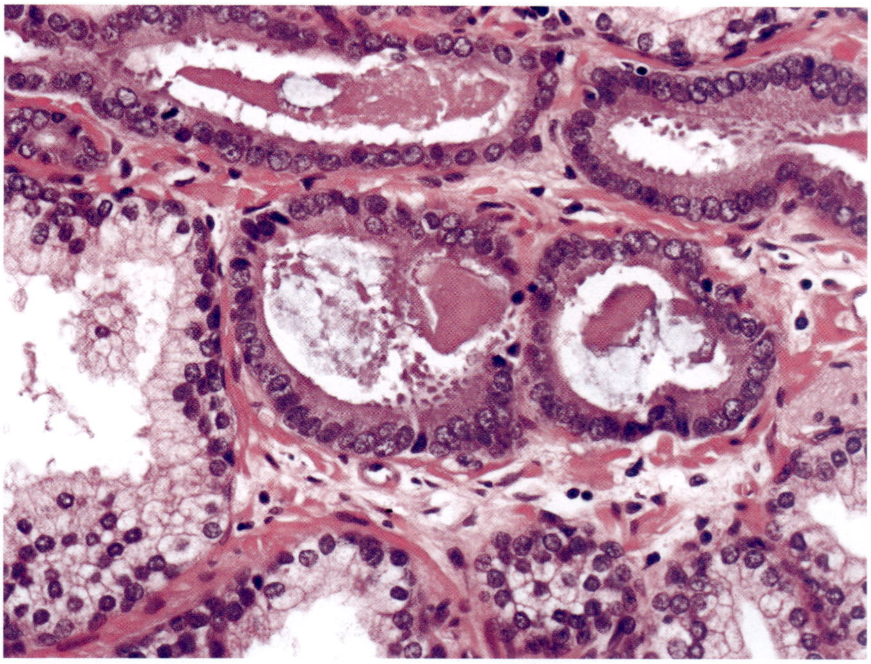

Figure 7-23.
Adenocarcinoma with pink secretion and small amount of blue mucin.

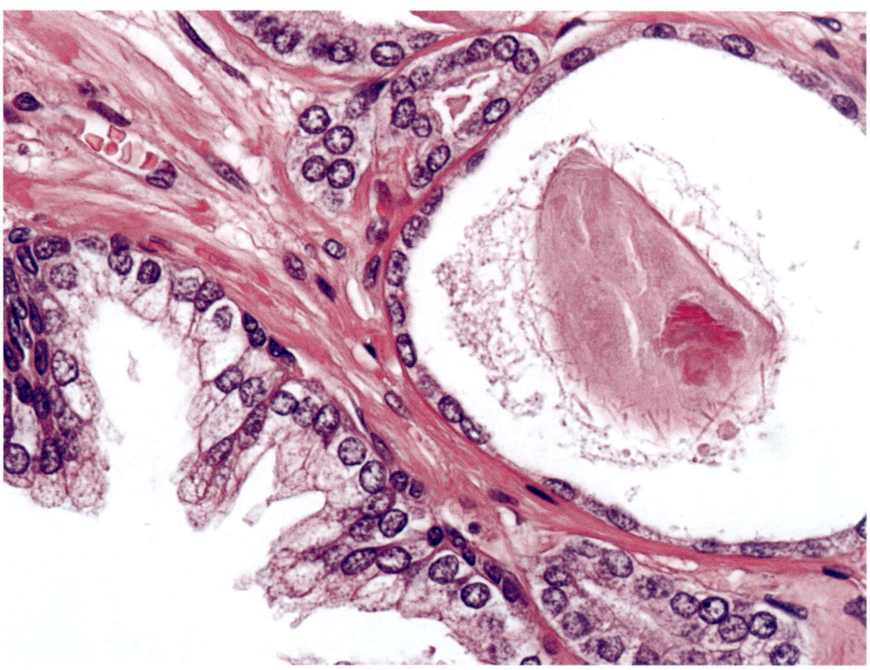

Figure 7-24.
Fragmented collagen fibers are seen in the lumen of a malignant gland.

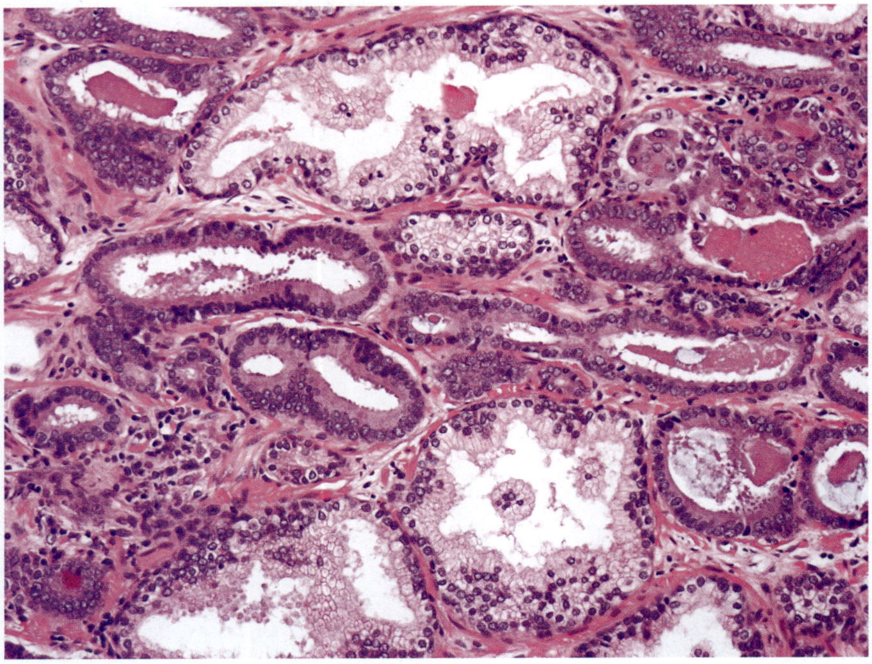

Figure 7-25.
Adenocarcinoma. A group of small malignant glands are infiltrating between large benign glands.

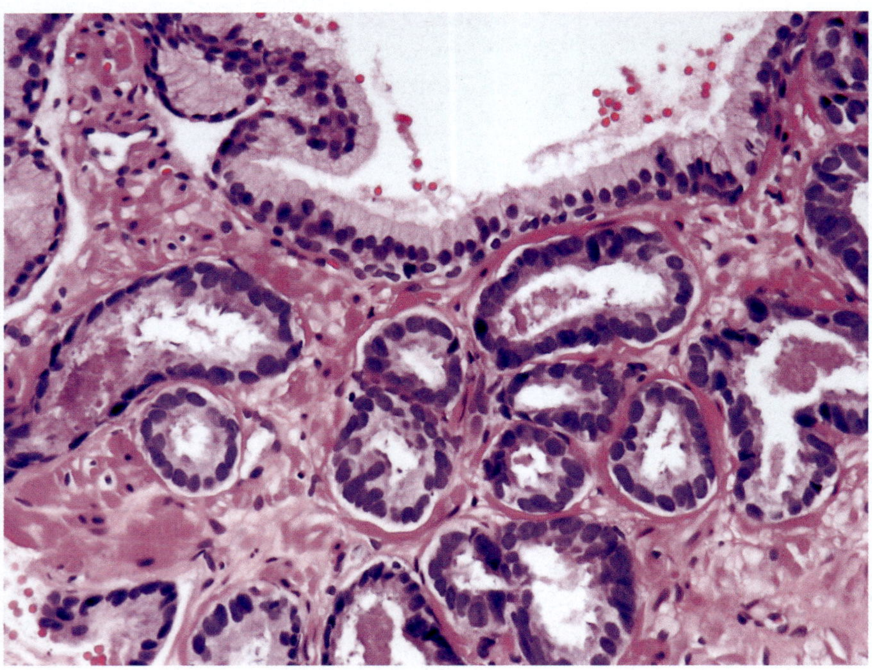

Figure 7-26.
Adenocarcinoma. A large benign gland, with a basal cell layer, is adjacent to a cluster of small malignant glands with no basal cells. Nuclei are larger in the malignant glands than in the benign one, although the prominent nucleoli are not easily seen in the malignant glands.

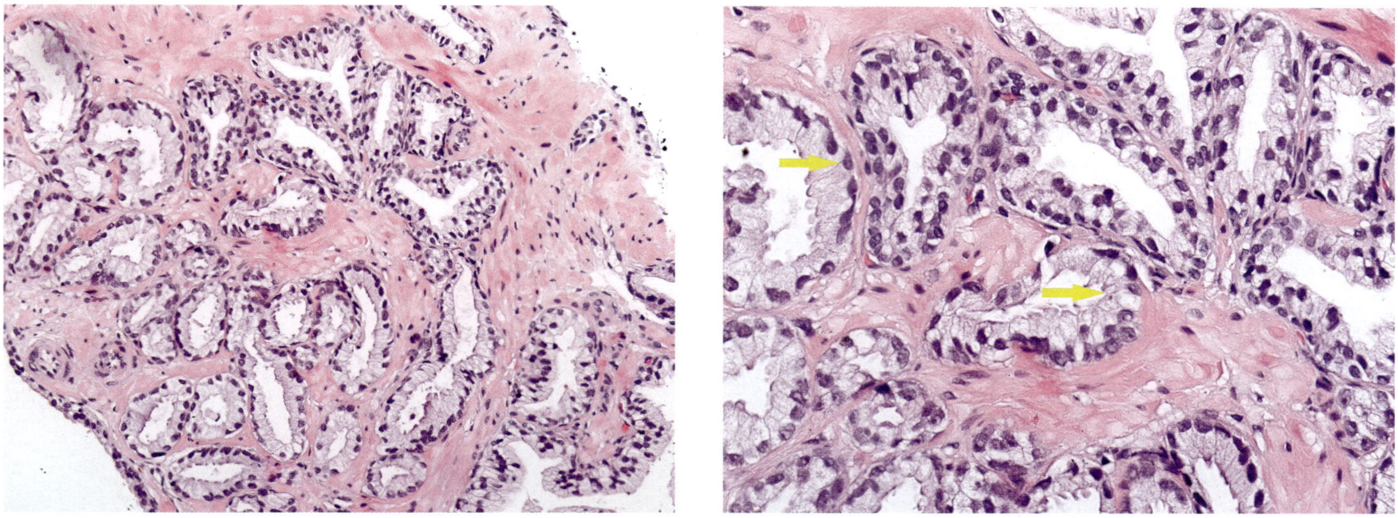

a b

Figure 7-27.
Adenocarcinoma showing a subtle difference between malignant glands (left) and benign glands (right) at low magnification (*a*). At high magnification, the presence of nuclear enlargement, prominent nucleoli, and lack of basal cells in the malignant glands (*b*, arrows) can be seen.

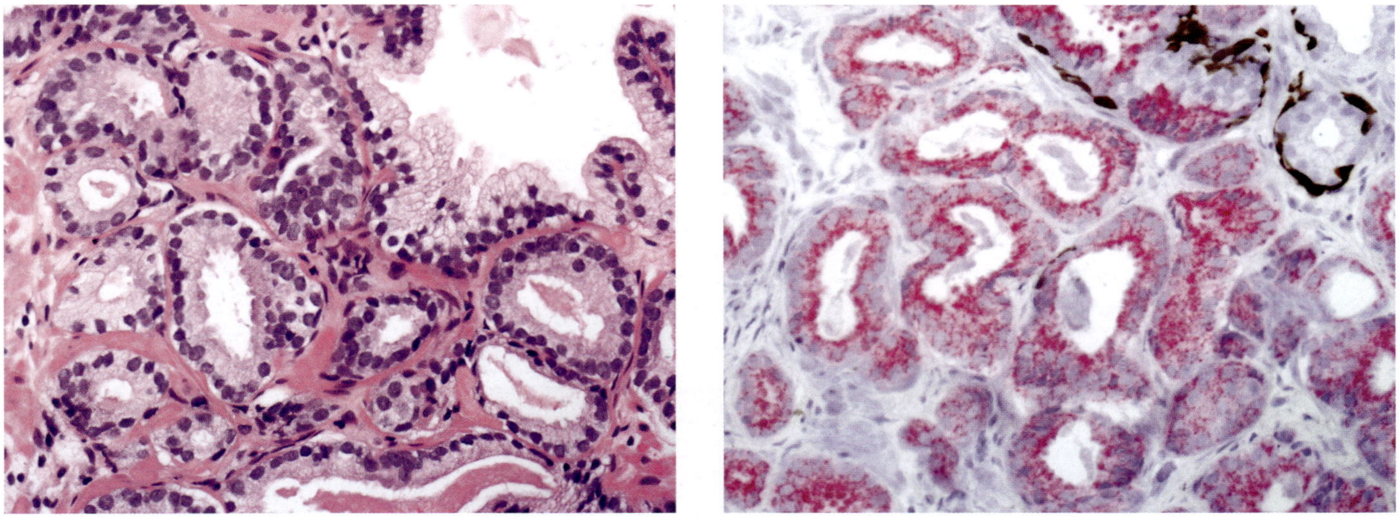

a b

Figure 7-28.
Adenocarcinoma (*a*). Application of immunohistochemistry (triple stain, *b*) enhances the differences between adenocarcinoma and benign glands, which demonstrates malignant glands with strong AMACR (red) reactivity and lack of basal cells (negative p63/HMWCK), and benign glands with basal cells (brown) and negative for AMACR staining.

Table 7-3. Major Histological Differences Between Prostatic Carcinoma and Benign Glands

	Gland size	*Lumen border*	*Nuclear size*	*Cytoplasm*	*Nucleoli*	*Pink secretion*
Carcinoma	Small	Straight	Larger	Dark	Prominent	Present
Benign	Large	Convoluted	Smaller	Pale	Not prominent	Absent

Pathognomonic features of prostatic adenocarcinoma

- Several histological features, highly specific for prostatic adenocarcinoma and not seen in any benign conditions, are considered to be *pathognomonic* features of prostatic adenocarcinoma
- These features include perineural invasion, collagenous micronodule, and glomeruloid structure (which are summarized in Table 7-4)
- Although their presence is a strong indicator for diagnosis of prostatic adenocarcinoma, several structures in the benign conditions mimic their appearance
- These pathognomonic features are not very sensitive markers for diagnosis of prostatic adenocarcinoma since they can be seen only in a small subset of needle core biopsy cases positive for cancer

Perineural invasion by adenocarcinoma

- This is a common finding associated with prostatic adenocarcinoma
- It is characterized by adenocarcinoma cells grow around the nerve up to 70% to 100% of the perineural spaces (Figs. 7-29 to 7-31). It is not lymphatic invasion because the spaces around the nerve do not have endothelial lining
- When tumor cells get into the perineural spaces, it is easier for them to extend to outside the prostate
- The presence of perineural invasion (PNI) in the biopsy (Fig. 7-31) or prostatectomy specimens is associated with high volume disease and a high risk of extraprostatic extension based on our experience and studies from other investigators, although the results from other studies are variable. We include the presence of PNI in our pathology reports
- The quantitative measure of PNI is unnecessary although some studies suggested a relation between the numbers of PNI and tumor prognosis
- It is a common sense that the more tumor cells present (high volume), the more PNI will be identified
- Perineural indentation by benign glands can be occasionally seen, typical less than 50% of the peripheral spaces of the nerve (Fig. 7-32). Only in rare cases, perineural indentation can be up to 70% of periphery a nerve

Collagenous micronodules

- Also known as mucinous fibroplasia
- Collagenous micronodules (CMNs) is an uncommon finding associated with prostatic adenocarcinoma, present in 2% to 10% of prostatic specimens with cancer
- It is characterized by the presence of eosinophilic extracellular material next to carcinoma cells (Figs. 7-33 to 7-35)
- These nodules are eosinophilic and homogenous measuring 10 to 100 μm (Fig. 7-33)
- In the early phase of development, they often form a dome-shaped structure underneath the malignant glands (Fig. 7-34)
- The epithelial cells associated with the CMN typically exhibit darker amphophilic cytoplasm, probably because of the increased protein synthesis in the tumor cells including the production of collagenases (it functions to digest and degrade the stroma)

Table 7-4. Summary of Pathognomonic Features of Prostatic Adenocarcinoma

	Description	*Meaning*	*Pitfall*
Perineural invasion	Tumor cells next to nerve or wrap around the nerve >75%	Tumor cells involving the perineural spaces, higher risk for extraprostatic invasion	Perineural indentation by benign gland
Glomerulation	Tumor cells form a structure resembling glomerulus	Tumor cells overgrowing in a gland cell overgrowth	High-grade PIN can show similar pattern
Collagenous micronodules	Eosinophilic material accumulated adjacent to malignant glandular cells	Formed by fragmented collagen fibers, results from the collagenase released by tumor cells; indication of invasion	

PIN, prostatic intraepithelial neoplasia.

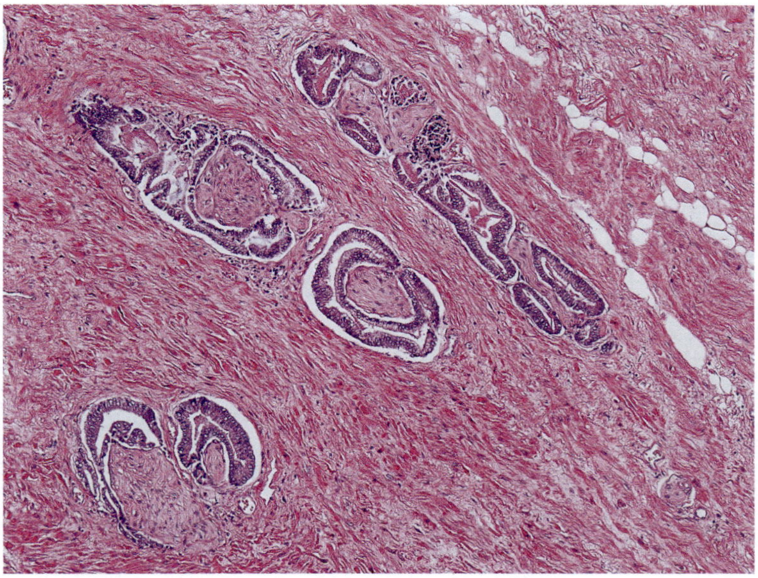

Figure 7-29.
Adenocarcinoma. Several malignant glands show perineural invasion.

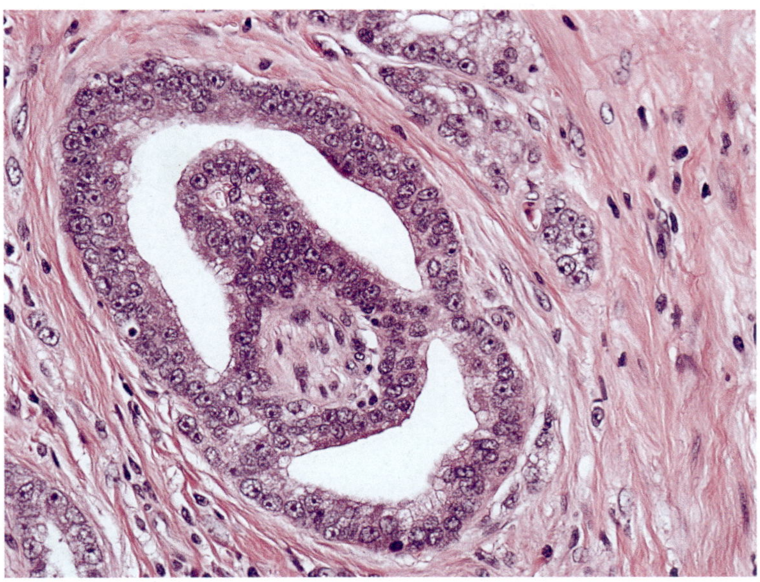

Figure 7-30.
Adenocarcinoma. A large malignant gland entirely surrounds a nerve bundle.

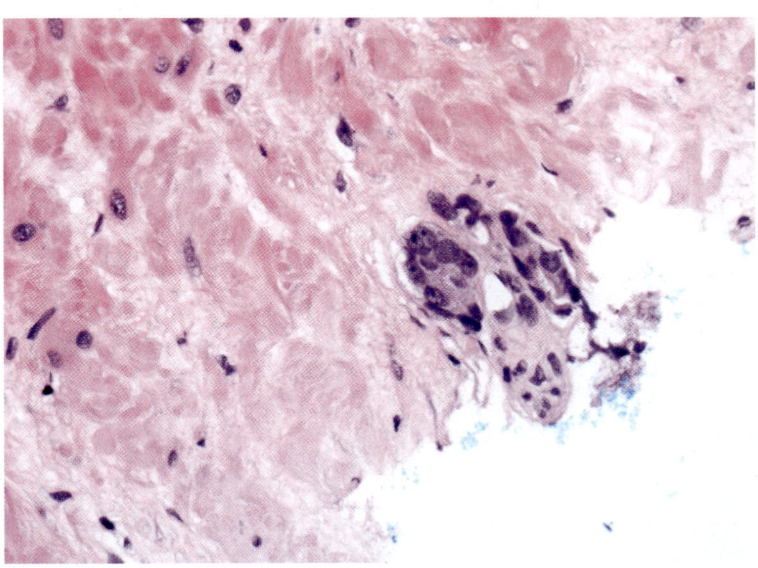

Figure 7-31.
Small focus of adenocarcinoma with perineural invasion on needle core biopsy.

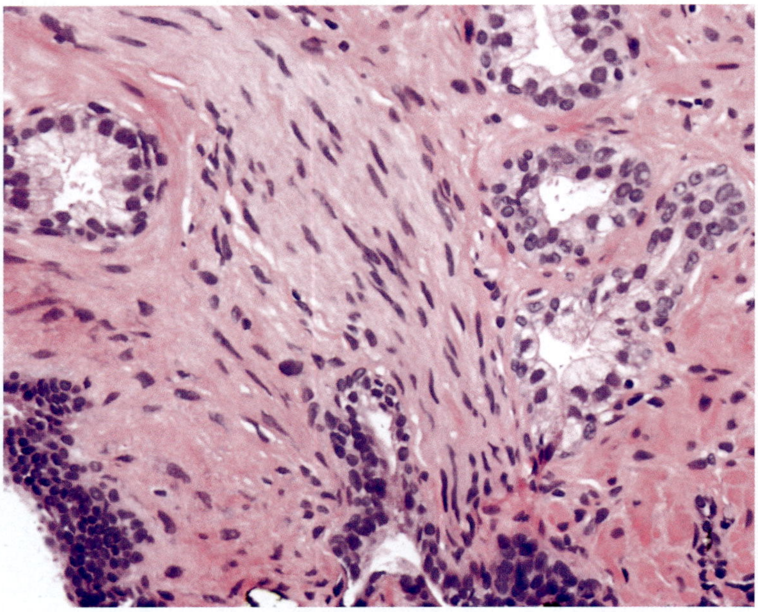

Figure 7-32.
Benign glands with perineural indentation. A nerve bundle is indented by several benign glands, mimicking perineural invasion.

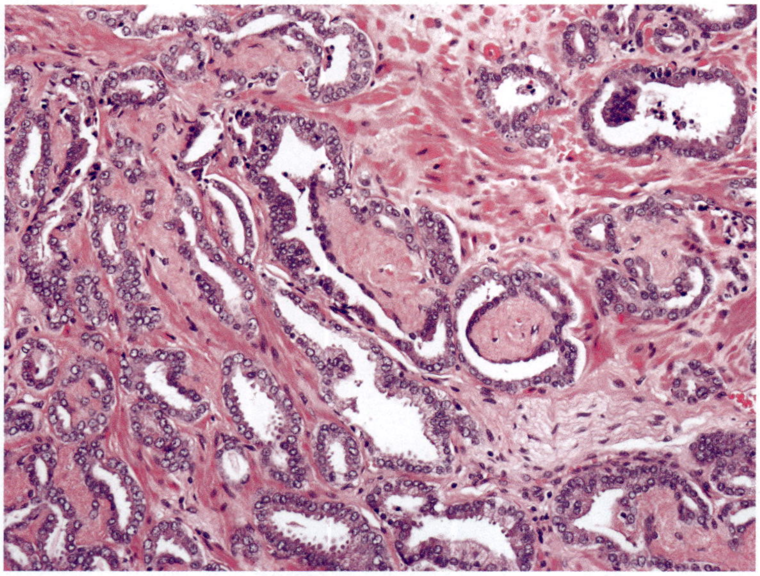

Figure 7-33.
Adenocarcinoma with several collagenous micronodules (CMNs).

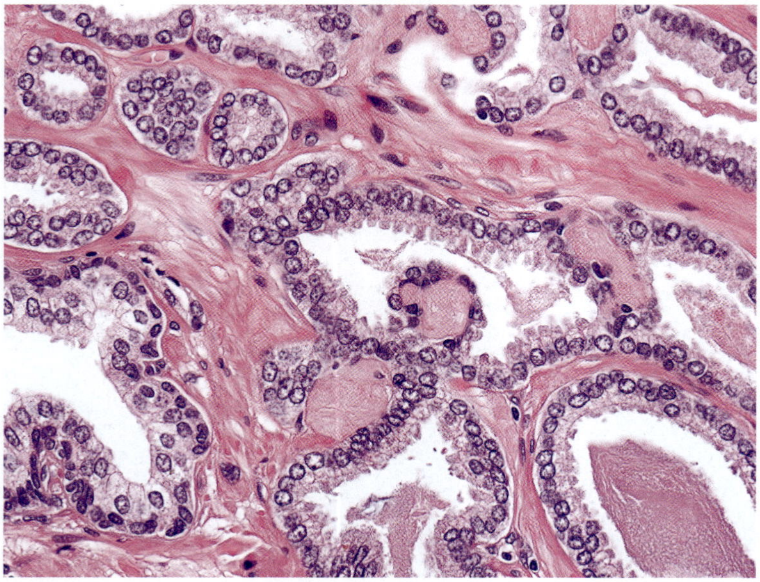

Figure 7-34.
Adenocarcinoma with distinct dome-shaped pink CMNs underneath tumor cells.

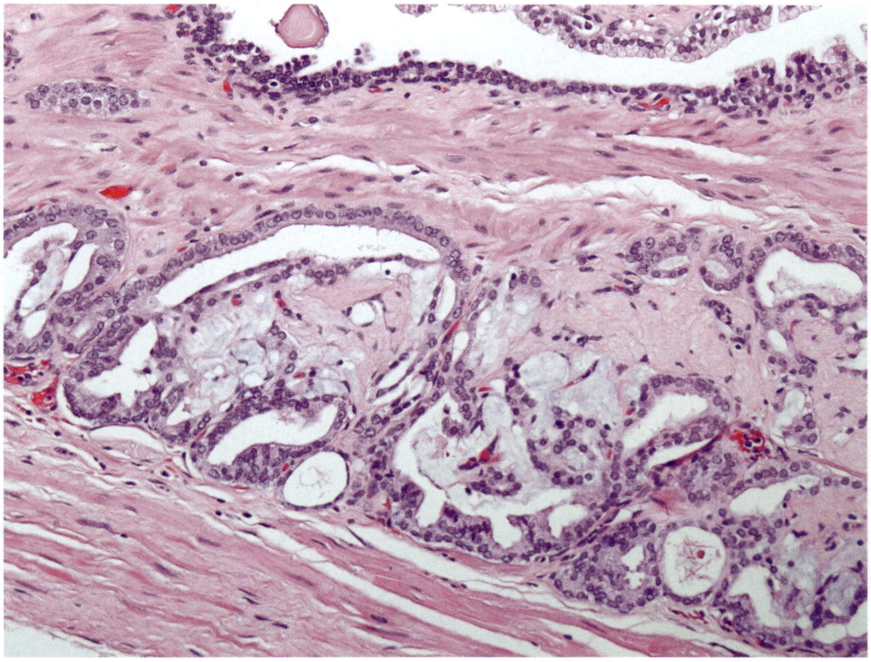

Figure 7-35.
Adenocarcinoma. Occasionally, CMN can be seen with mucin-producing malignant glands.

- It is highly specific for cancer because it is probably related to the invasive nature of prostatic adenocarcinoma
- Based on our studies, CMN is composed of fragmented collagen fibers, which are believed to be the production by the action of collagenases secreted by carcinoma cells (such as MMP-9)
- CMN may be seen in mucin-producing adenocarcinoma cells (Fig. 7-35), but most cases do not have mucin production
- Normal prostatic epithelium lacks the production of sufficient amount of collagenase so that they cannot invade the prostatic stroma as tumor cells do
- Reactive benign glands may trap stromal cells mimicking CMN (Fig. 7-36)
- CMN is not associated with a poor prognosis
- CMN may be calcified

Glomeruloid structures

- Also known as *glomerulation* or *glomeruloid bodies* of malignant prostatic glands
- Glomeruloid structure is an uncommon finding associated with prostatic adenocarcinoma, only seen in less than 5% of prostatic adenocarcinoma cases
- It is characterized by the presence of a cluster of cells within a gland, which resemble the structure of glomerulus (Figs. 7-37 and 7-38)
- Both lining cells and centrally located cluster of cells are all malignant, which typically contain prominent nucleoli and other typical features of adenocarcinoma (Figs. 7-39 and 7-40)
- It may be present in singular or multiple glands (Fig. 7-37)
- Basal cells are absent in this structure, which can be demonstrated by negative basal cell marker staining
- Occasionally high-grade PIN may mimic glomeruloid structures, because they do contain basal cells in the glandular structures
- IDC of the prostate may show similar features to glomeruloid structures except the presence of basal cells in IDC (Fig. 7-41)
- Glomeruloid structures are still graded as Gleason pattern 3
- It is not associated with a poor prognosis

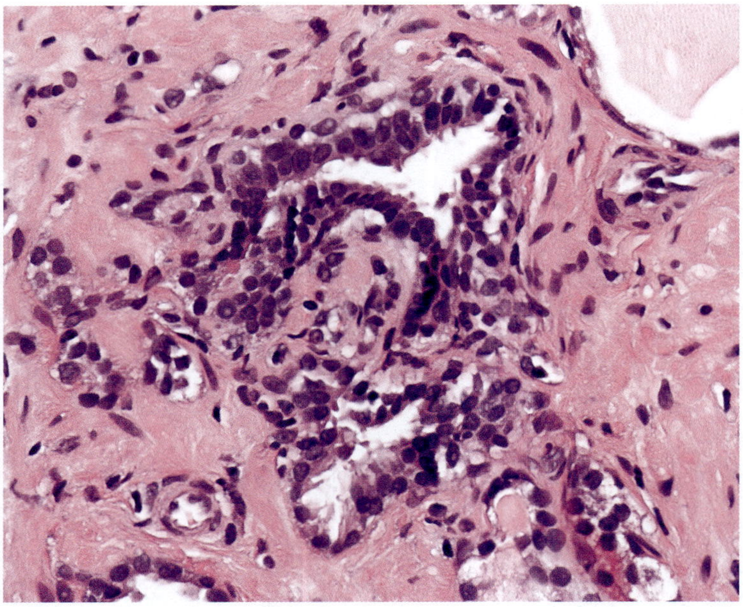

Figure 7-36.
A benign gland associated with chronic inflammation shows glandular distortion, mimicking CMN.

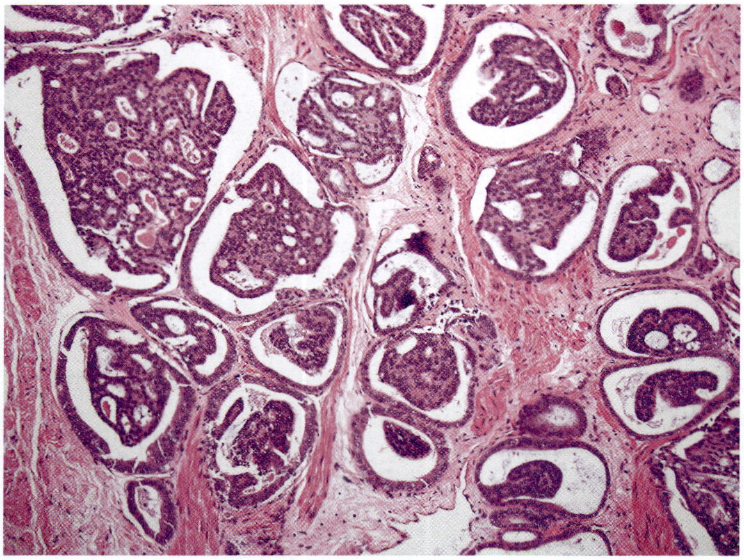

Figure 7-37.
Adenocarcinoma with glomeruloid structures.

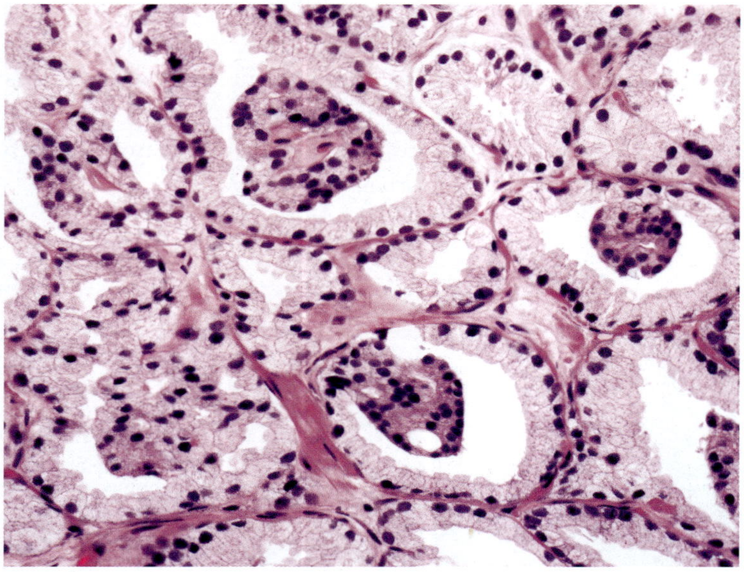

Figure 7-38.
Adenocarcinoma. A number of malignant glands contain glomeruloid structures, clusters of tumor cells growing in the lumen.

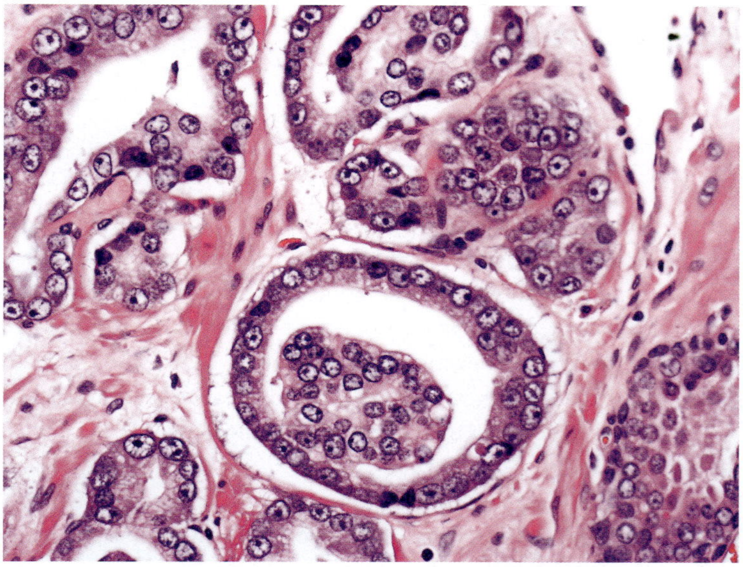

Figure 7-39.
Adenocarcinoma with glomeruloid structures.

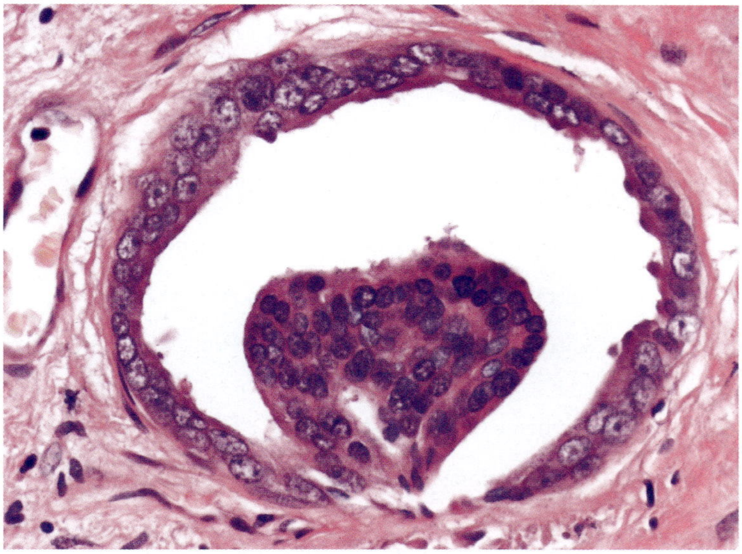

Figure 7-40.
Adenocarcinoma. One malignant gland displays a glomeruloid structure.

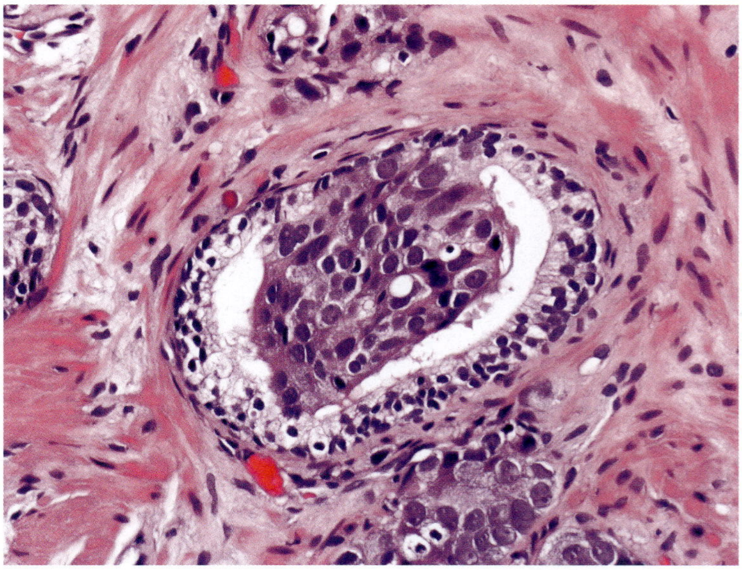

Figure 7-41.
Intraductal carcinoma of the prostate with a glomeruloid formation containing malignant cells in the center and benign glandular cells in the periphery.

CHAPTER 8

Grading of Prostatic Adenocarcinoma

GLEASON GRADING SYSTEM

- The Gleason grading system is based on the architectural features of prostatic adenocarcinoma
- There are five grades or patterns from 1 (least aggressive) to 5 (most aggressive). Their characteristics are summarized in Table 8-1
- Other old grading systems such as nuclear grading system have been replaced by the Gleason grading system
- The Gleason grading system is one of the best histological grading systems for cancers
- It has been widely used in the world, more than any other cancer grading system, because it is simple and correlates well with clinical outcomes
- The Gleason score is the combination of the most dominant pattern and second-most prevalent pattern (original)
- The recently proposed modified Gleason score is the combination of the most dominant pattern and the highest pattern with, particularly in biopsy. Because of limited application, whether this modified Gleason grading system can outperform the original one is unknown
- Grade 1
    - The least common pattern. Some of the old cases with Gleason 1 pattern have been determined as adenosis with contemporary immunostaining
    - Lobular pattern
    - Composed of packed malignant glands in similar size and shape (Fig. 8-1)
    - Nuclear atypia present and no basal cells

Table 8-1. Summary of Gleason Patterns

Grade (pattern)	*Lobular pattern*	*Infiltrating*	*Gland shape*	*Location*	*Frequency*	*Prognosis*
1	Yes	No	Packed regular	Central zone	Rare	Almost benign
2	Yes	May be on periphery	Packed slightly irregular	Central zone	Less common	Probably indolent
3	No	Yes	Donut shaped	Peripheral zone	Most common	Potentially aggressive
4	No	Yes	Fused gland	Peripheral zone	Common	Aggressive
5	No	Yes	No luminal formation	Peripheral zone	Less common	Very aggressive

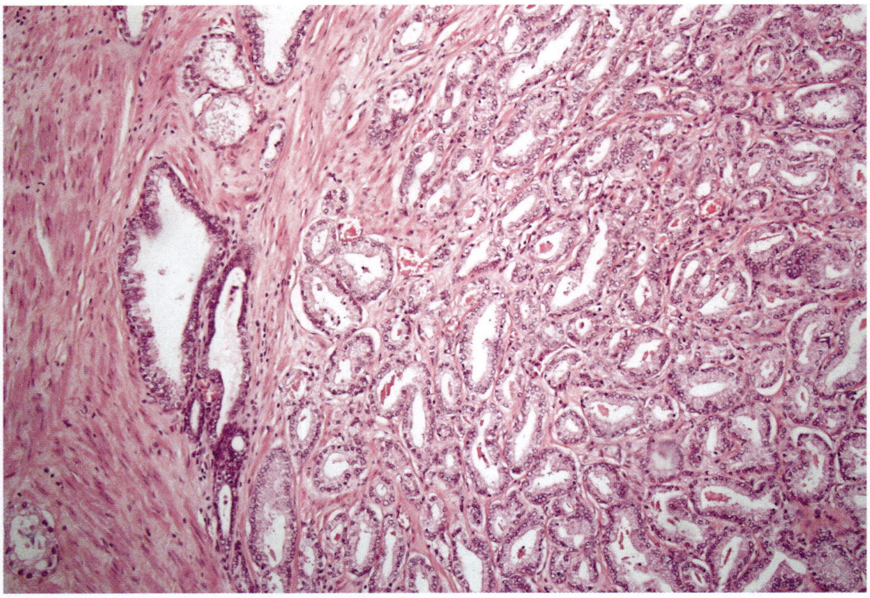

Figure 8-1.
Gleason pattern 1 adenocarcinoma is composed of regular-shaped glands back-to-back packed in a well-defined lobule. No infiltrating pattern is seen.

- Grade 2
  - Lobular pattern in transition zone
  - Composed of packed malignant glands in a confined nodule, with a slight variation of size and shape (Figs. 8-2 and 8-3)
  - Minimal invasion
  - Nuclear atypia present and no basal cells (Fig. 8-4)
- Grade 3
  - This is the most common pattern of prostate cancer
  - Malignant glands are well-formed glands, as small donuts in shape, with smooth round contours (Figs. 8-5 and 8-6)
  - Infiltrating but no desmoplastic stromal reaction
  - Nuclear atypia present and no basal cells (Figs. 8-6 and 8-7)

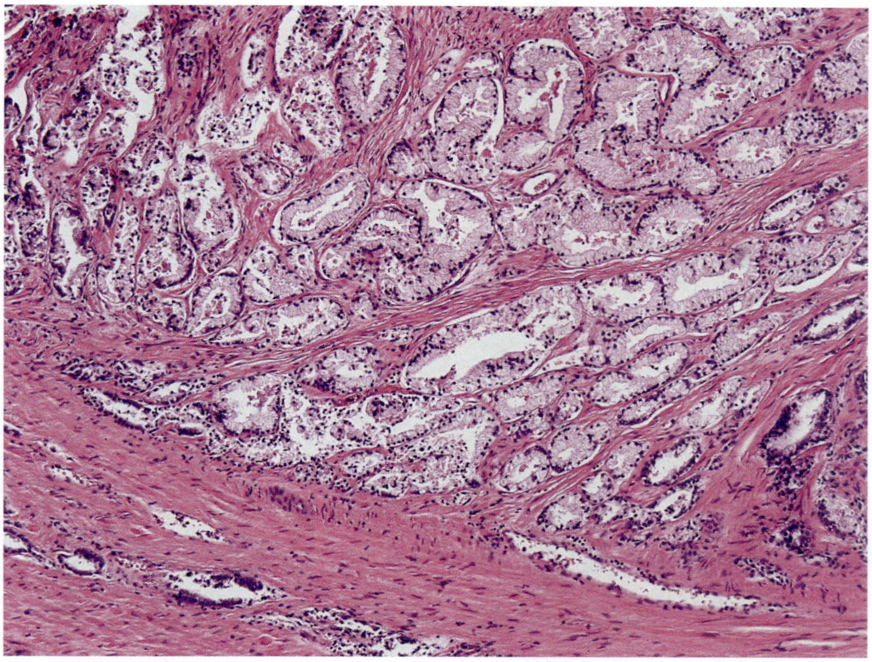

Figure 8-2.
Gleason pattern 2 adenocarcinoma composed of slightly irregularly shaped glands in a defined lobule.

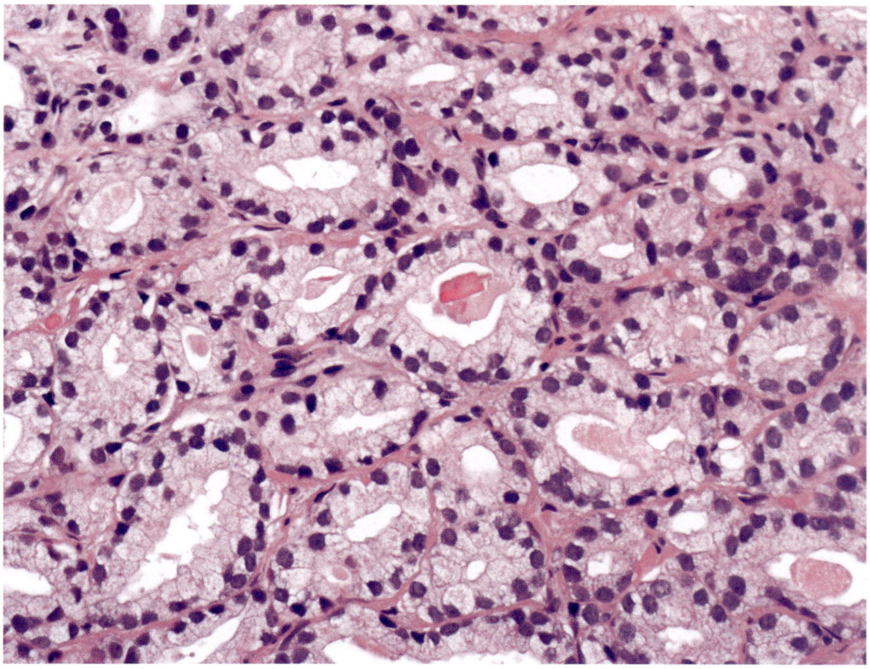

Figure 8-3.
Higher magnification of a Gleason pattern 2 adenocarcinoma shows the back-to-back malignant glands with moderate cytological atypia including occasional prominent nucleoli.

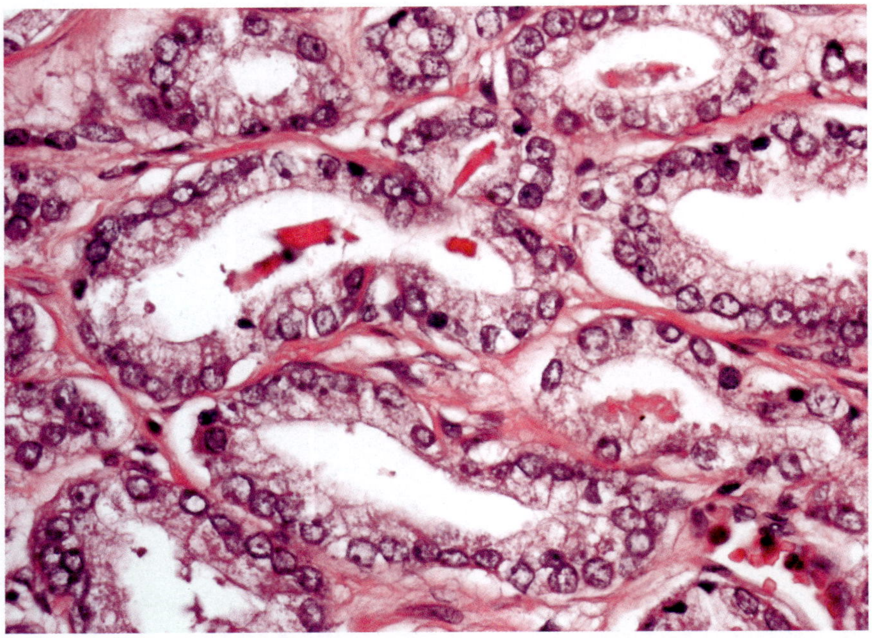

Figure 8-4.
Gleason pattern 2 adenocarcinoma shows the presence of cytological atypia including prominent nucleoli in the malignant cells.

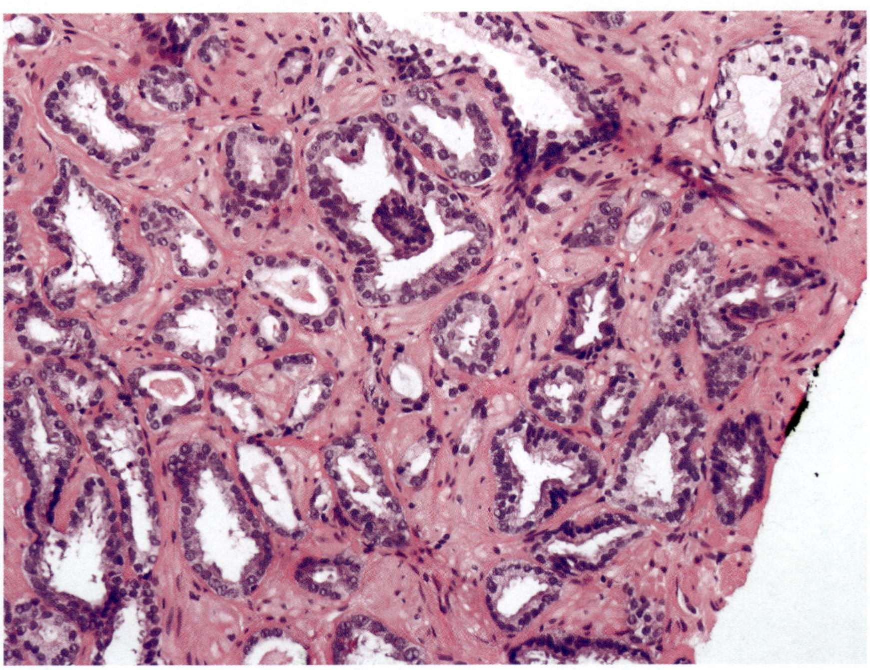

Figure 8-5.
Gleason pattern 3 adenocarcinoma is characterized by small glands with well-formed lumens, resembling the shape of a donut.

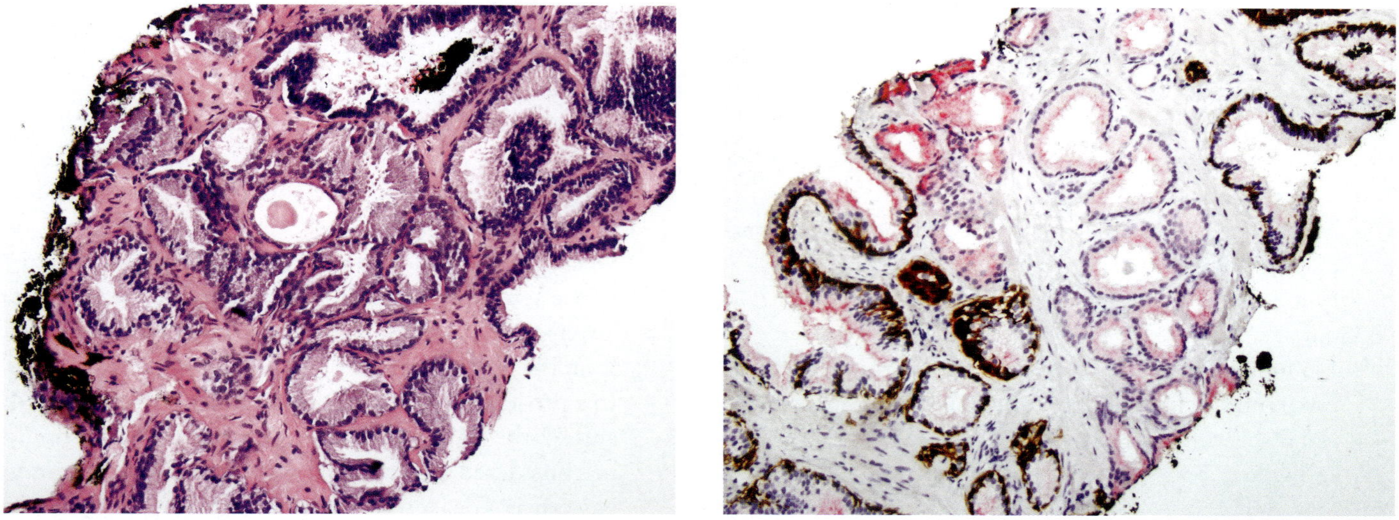

a b

Figure 8-6.
A small focus of Gleason pattern 3 adenocarcinoma on needle core biopsy displaying well-formed lumens (*a*). By triple immunostaining, the presence of adenocarcinoma is confirmed with no basal cells and moderate AMACR immunoreactivity (*b*).

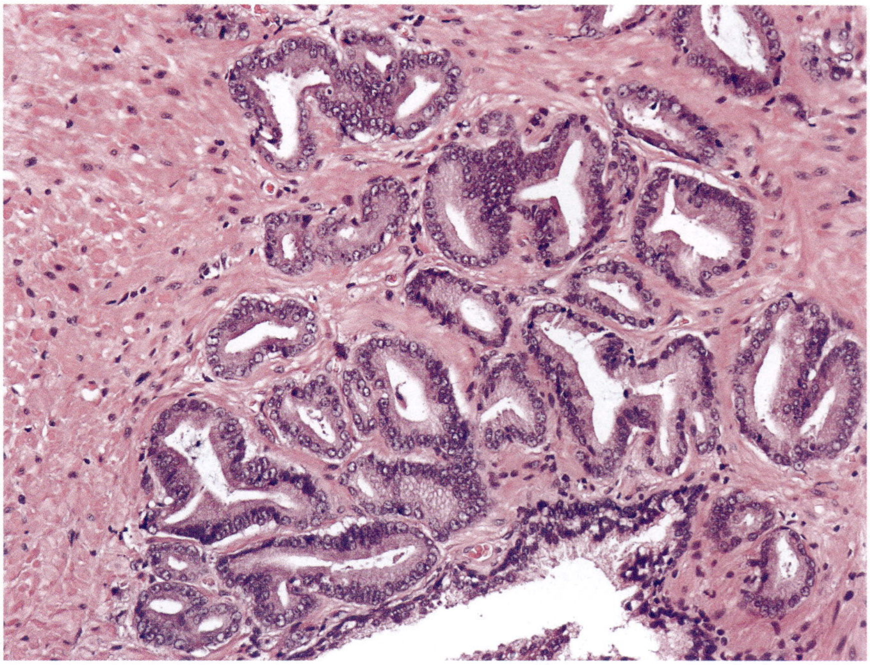

Figure 8-7.
A focus of small glands with some branching, form Y- and T-shaped glands. This is still considered to be Gleason pattern 3.

- Grade 4
  - Malignant glands with glandular fusion and irregular contours (Figs. 8-8 to 8-10)
  - Cribriform patterns (Fig. 8-9)
  - Clear cell (hypernephroid) (Fig. 8-11), mucinous or foamy glands mostly fall into this pattern
  - Infiltrating tumor cells often with desmoplastic stromal reaction (Fig. 8-10)
  - Nuclear atypia present and no basal cells
- Grade 5
  - No luminal formation, can be mistaken this high-grade carcinoma for lymphoma or other high-grade malignancy
  - Solid sheets (Figs. 8-12 and 8-13)
  - Individual cells (Fig. 8-14) or Indian filing patterns (Fig. 8-15)
  - Comedo necrosis in a malignant cribriform gland (Fig. 8-16)
  - Gleason pattern 5 may displace greater degree of cytological pleomorphism
- Several modifications and interpretations of original Gleason grading have been proposed and applied in daily practice:
  - Gleason score 2 to 4 should be used rarely in needle core biopsy
  - Most cribriform adenocarcinoma should be graded as Gleason pattern 4
  - Ductal adenocarcinoma can be graded as Gleason pattern 4
  - In the setting of dominant high grade adenocarcinoma, lower grade patterns (if less than 5%) may be obmited from the report
  - In a prostatectomy case with 3 Gleason patterns (3, 4, and 5), the least common pattern less than 5% should be considered a tertiary pattern; if the least common pattern is Gleason 5 but greater than 5%, it should be included in the Gleason score as the secondary pattern

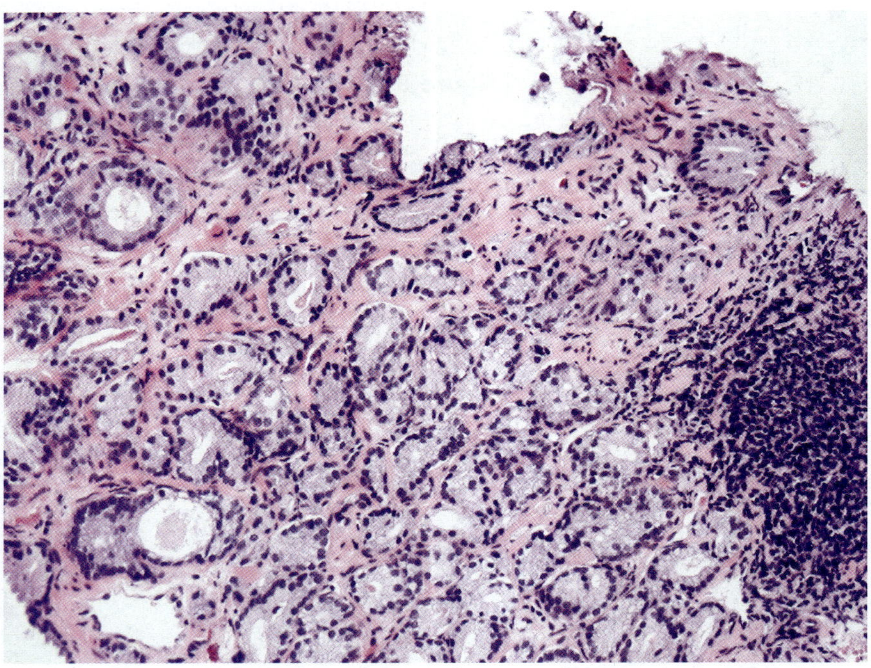

Figure 8-8.
Gleason 3 adenocarcinoma with both well-formed glands (Gleason 3 on the left) and some fused glands (Gleason 4 on the right). The diagnosis is prostatic adenocarcinoma, Gleason score 3 + 4 = 7.

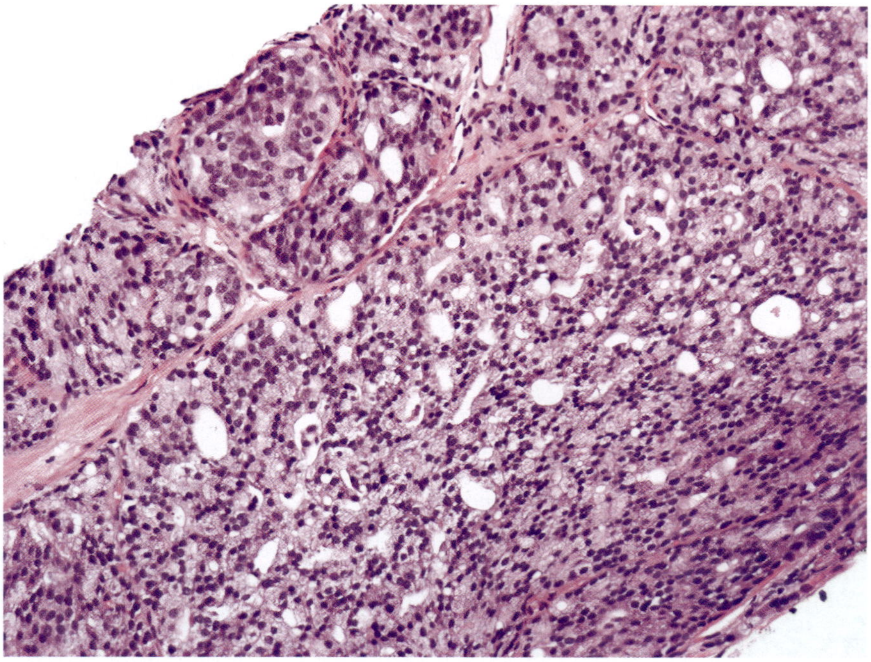

Figure 8-9.
Gleason pattern 4 adenocarcinoma. A needle core biopsy contains adenocarcinoma with prominent cribriform patterns, which is considered to be Gleason pattern 4.

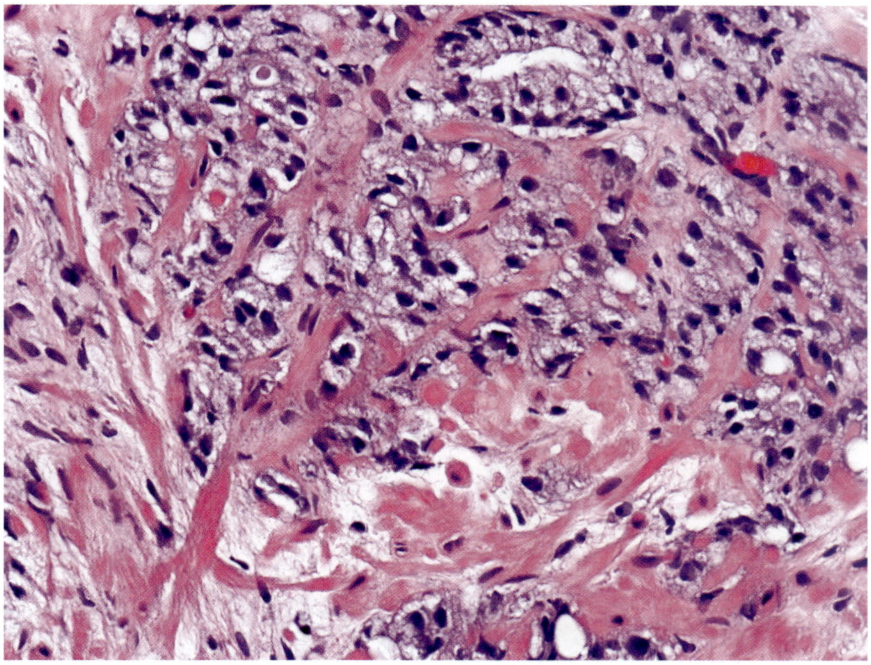

Figure 8-10.
Gleason pattern 4 adenocarcinoma with prominent glandular fusion.

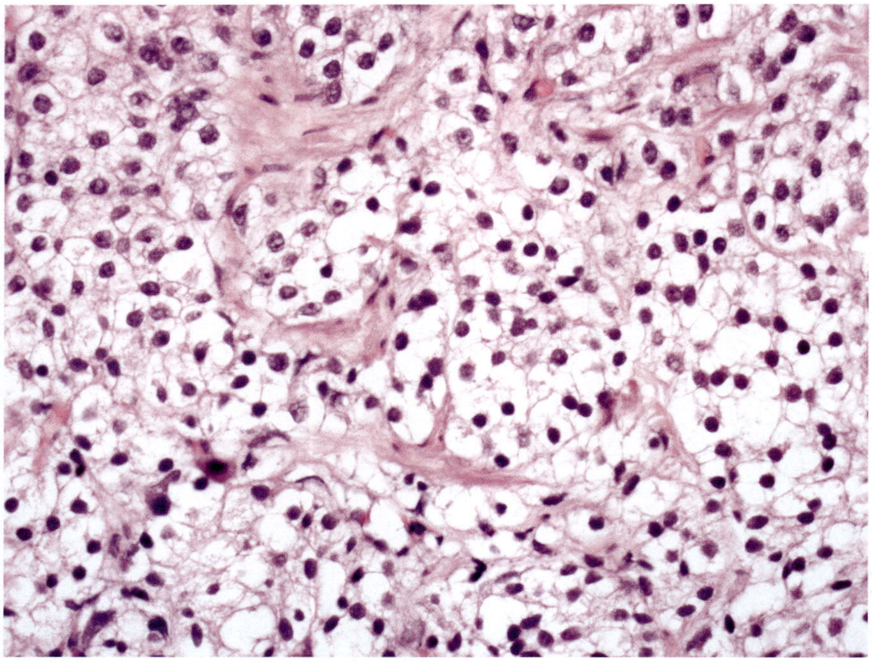

Figure 8-11.
Gleason 4 hypernephroid adenocarcinoma with prominent clear cytoplasm, resembling clear cell renal cell carcinoma (RCC).

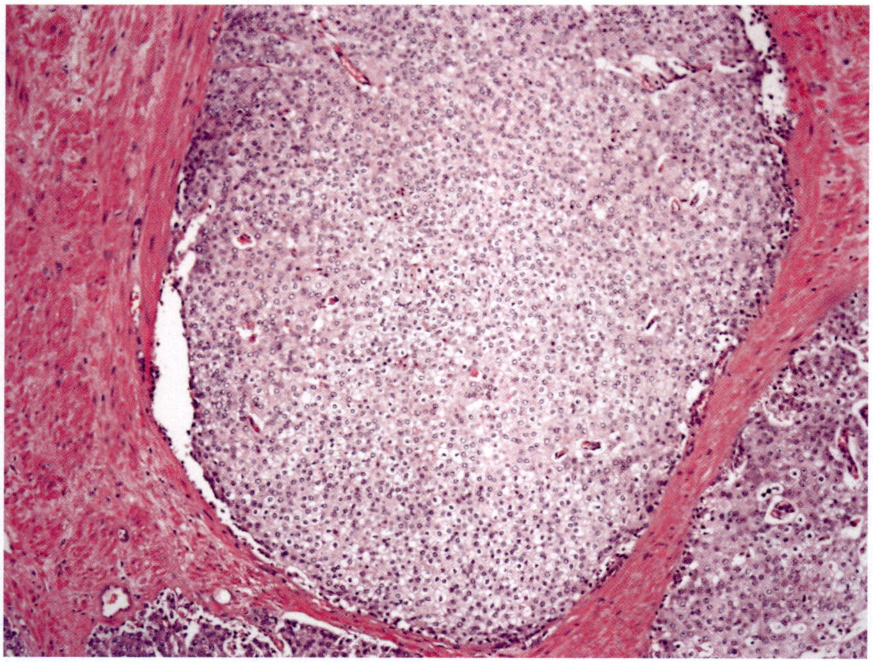

Figure 8-12.
Gleason pattern 5 adenocarcinoma is defined as tumor without luminal formation. In this case, adenocarcinoma cells form solid sheets without luminal formation.

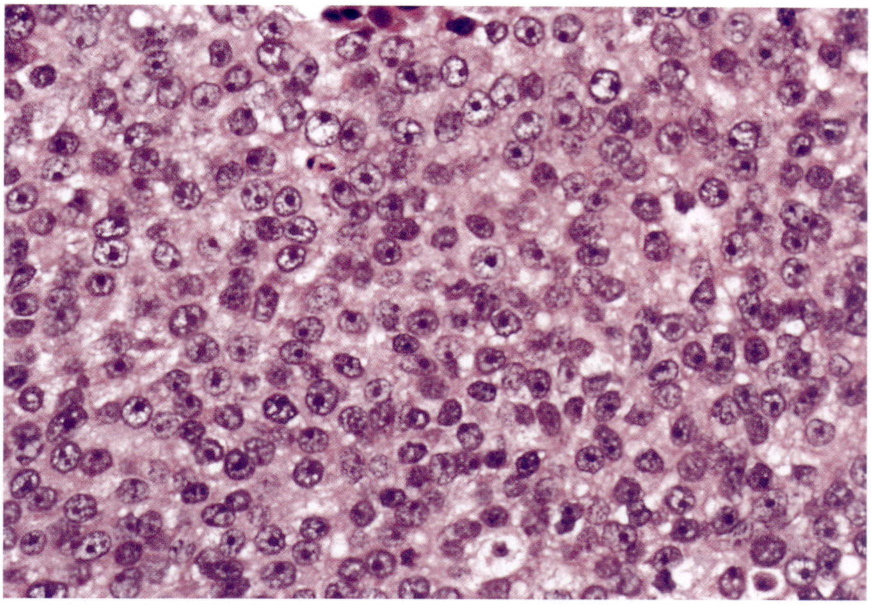

Figure 8-13.
A Gleason pattern 5 adenocarcinoma, composed of solid sheets of tumor cells.

Figure 8-14.
Gleason pattern 5 adenocarcinoma with diffusely infiltrating small carcinoma cells, resembling chronic inflammatory cells at low magnification (*a*). Higher magnification shows carcinoma cells with cytological atypia and subtle nesting patterns (*b*).

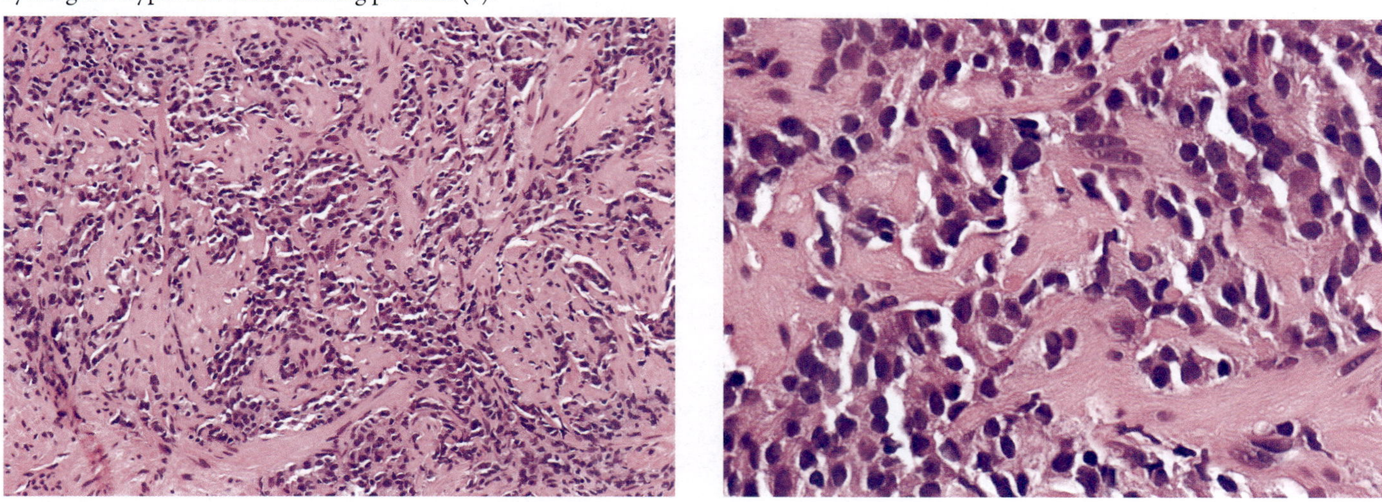

a **b**

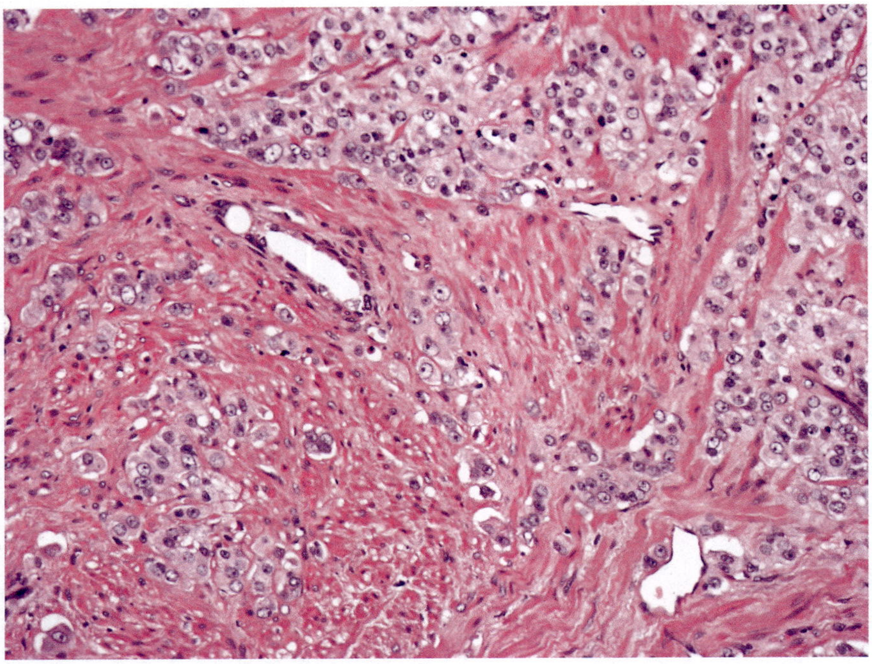

Figure 8-15.
Gleason pattern 5 adenocarcinoma cells extensively infiltrate the prostatic stroma in single-cell "Indian-file" pattern.

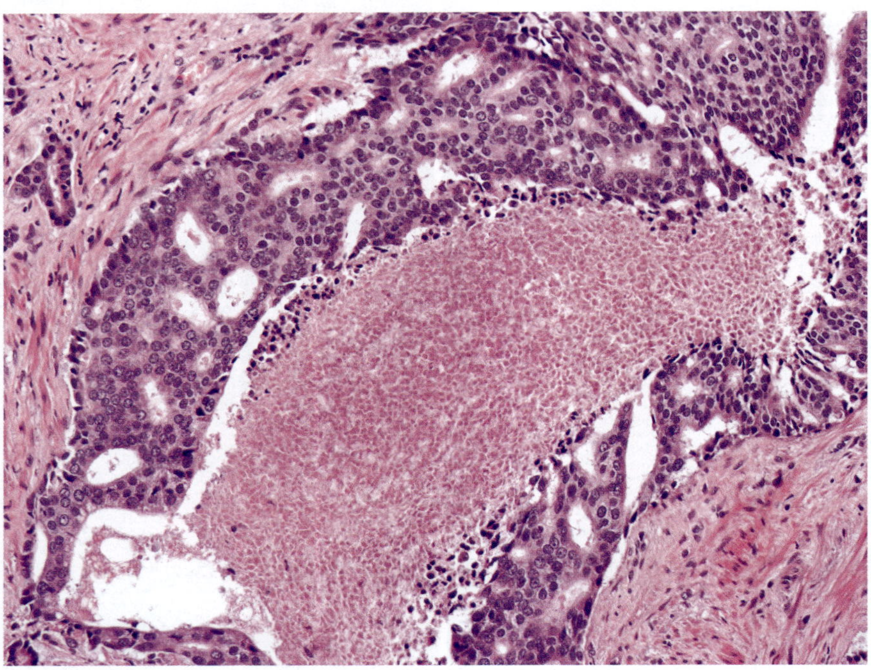

Figure 8-16.
A cribriform malignant gland with central comedo necrosis, which is defined as a Gleason 5 pattern.

CHAPTER 9

Evaluation and Staging of Prostatic Adenocarcinoma

STAGE T1A PROSTATIC ADENOCARCINOMA

Definition

- In a transurethral resection (TUR) specimen, the presence of prostatic adenocarcinoma in less than or equal to 5% of tissue chips and less than or equal to Gleason score 6 (T1A)

Pathogenesis

- T1A mostly representing transition zone low-grade carcinoma

Clinical features

- Symptoms of benign prostatic hyperplasia with serum PSA levels mildly elevated within the limit for benign prostatic hyperplasia (BPH)
- TUR performed as treatment for BPH

Gross pathology

- Prostatic tissue chips, not specific finding

Histology

- Incidental finding of limited cancer on TUR specimens. Severe cauterization may cause difficulty to detect an adenocarcinoma focus
- Typically low-grade adenocarcinoma with Gleason score 4 to 6 (Figs. 9-1 and 9-2)
- The percentage of chips involved by cancer (positive chips/total chips) will be reported. If only a small portion of the chip is involved, combining a few positive chips as one positive chip may be necessary
- If greater than 5% of tissue chips or greater than Gleason score 6 (T1B)
- In a prostate needle core biopsy, the presence of prostatic adenocarcinoma (T1C)

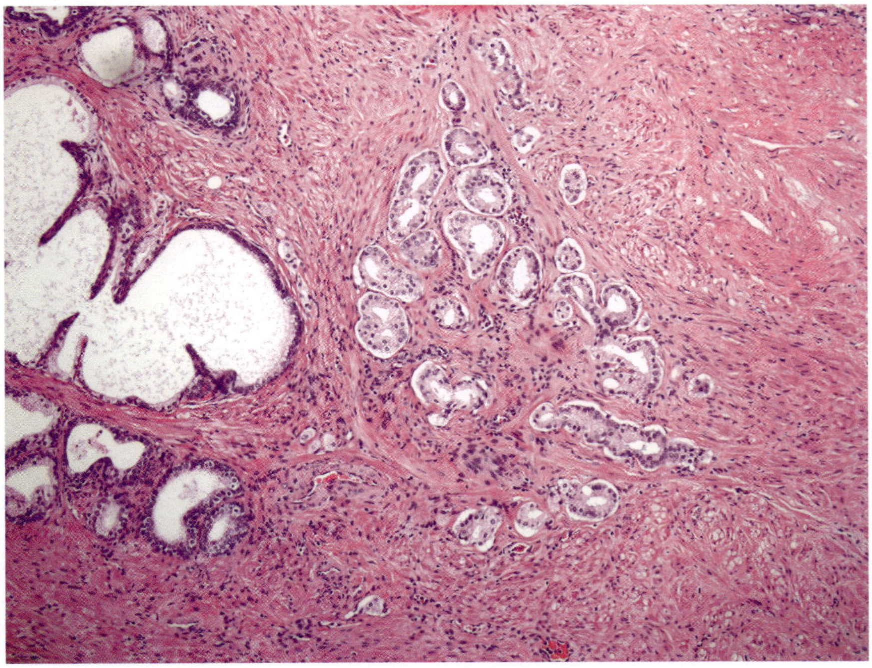

Figure 9-1.
T1A prostate cancer is defined as adenocarcinoma, Gleason score 6 or less, with a volume less than or equal to 5% of TURP chips. This case contains only one small focus of adenocarcinoma, Gleason score 2 + 2.

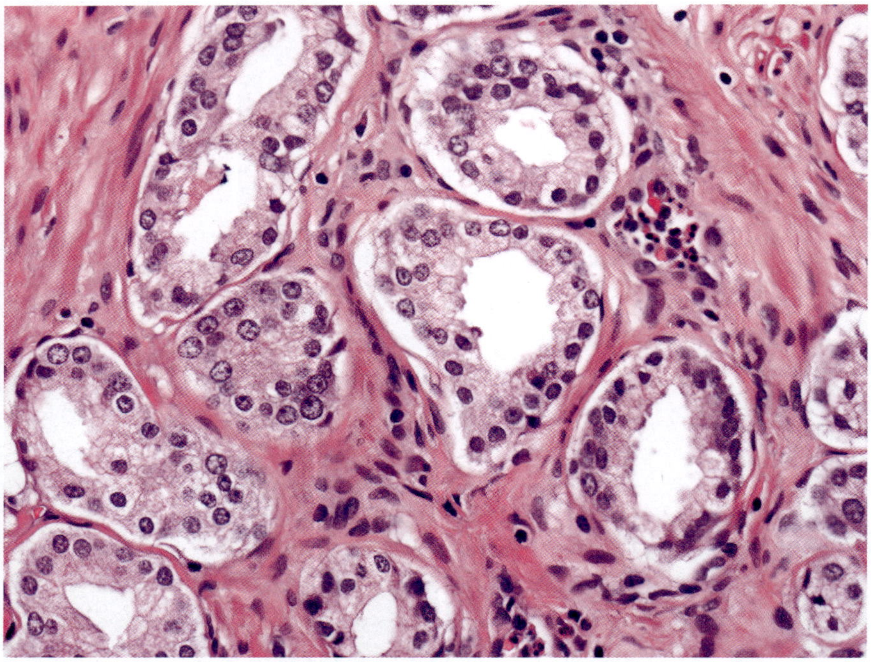

Figure 9-2.
High magnification of the T1A cancer focus showing nuclear atypia of the tumor cells.

Immunohistochemistry

- If needed, triple stain including AMACR, p63, and HMWCK can be applied

Clinical relevance (prognosis and treatment options)

- Typically T1A prostatic adenocarcinoma does not need treatment for the patient
- The tumor (T), node (N), and metastasis (M) pathology stage of prostate cancer is used for determination of the extent of prostate cancer
  - Low stages of prostatic adenocarcinoma
    - T1A: incidental carcinoma present in less than or equal to 5% of chips *and* Gleason score 2 to 6
    - T1B: incidental carcinoma present in 5% or more of the chips *or* Gleason score 7 or greater in TURP specimens
    - T1C: prostate needle core positive for carcinoma
    - T2A: (prostatectomy) with tumor confined to one lobe but less than 50% of the lobe, which is very rare
    - T2B: (prostatectomy) with tumor confined to one lobe but greater than 50% of volume of the lobe
    - T2C: (prostatectomy) with tumor involving both right and left lobes
    - T1B and T1C need further treatment including surgery, radiation, hormonal therapy, or active surveillance

EXTRAPROSTATIC EXTENSION BY ADENOCARCINOMA (STAGE T3A)

Definition

- Extraprostatic extension (EPE) is defined as prostatic adenocarcinoma that extends outside the prostate capsule into extraprostatic tissue
- Focal EPE: single microscopic foci of carcinoma cells outside the prostate capsule
- Established EPE: two or more separate microscopic foci of carcinoma cells outside the prostate capsule

Other terms

- Capsule penetration or capsule perforation (no longer used)

Pathogenesis

- The nature of a malignant epithelial neoplasm is its ability to invade outside the prostate into adjacent tissues. The prostate capsule, as we discussed in Chapter 1, is a thin layer of condensed fibrous tissue rather than a true capsule

Clinical features

- No specific clinical symptoms

Gross pathology

- Areas of large poorly defined masses bulging out of the capsule

Histology

- Adenocarcinoma cells are found outside the prostatic capsule, mostly in the adipose tissue (Fig. 9-3)
- On biopsy, if there is adipose tissue at the tip of the needle core, that is mostly likely extraprostatic tissue (Fig. 9-4). Although adipose tissue is reportedly found within the prostate, I have not seen true adipose tissue within the prostatic capsule. Some of the reported findings of fat within the prostate were caused by architectural distortion or vacuoles
- In evaluating the prostatectomy specimen, drawing a line (either imaginary or by using a marker pen on the glass slide) can be helpful in determining the presence of EPE

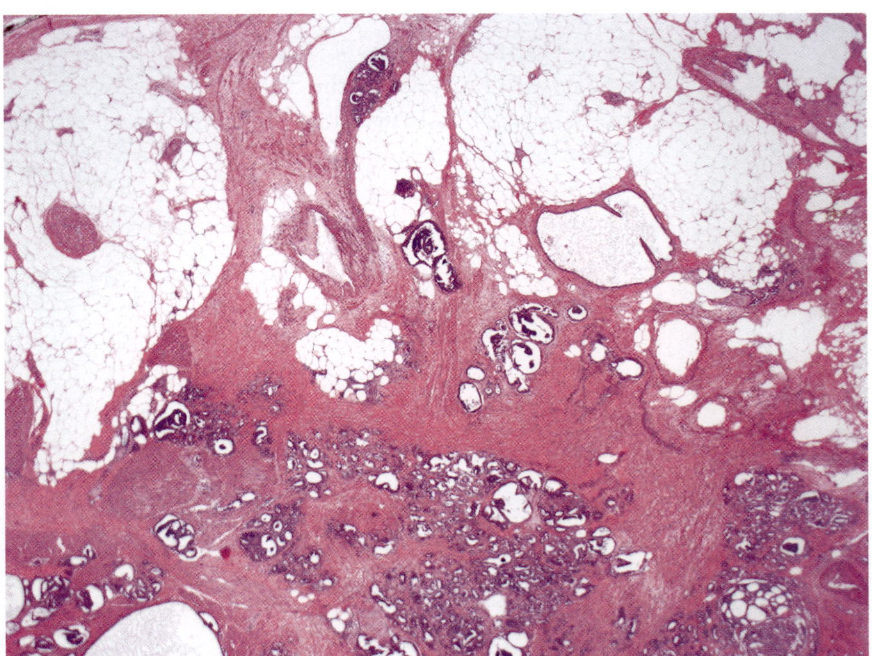

Figure 9-3.
A prostatectomy specimen shows the tumor cells extending into periprostatic adipose tissue.

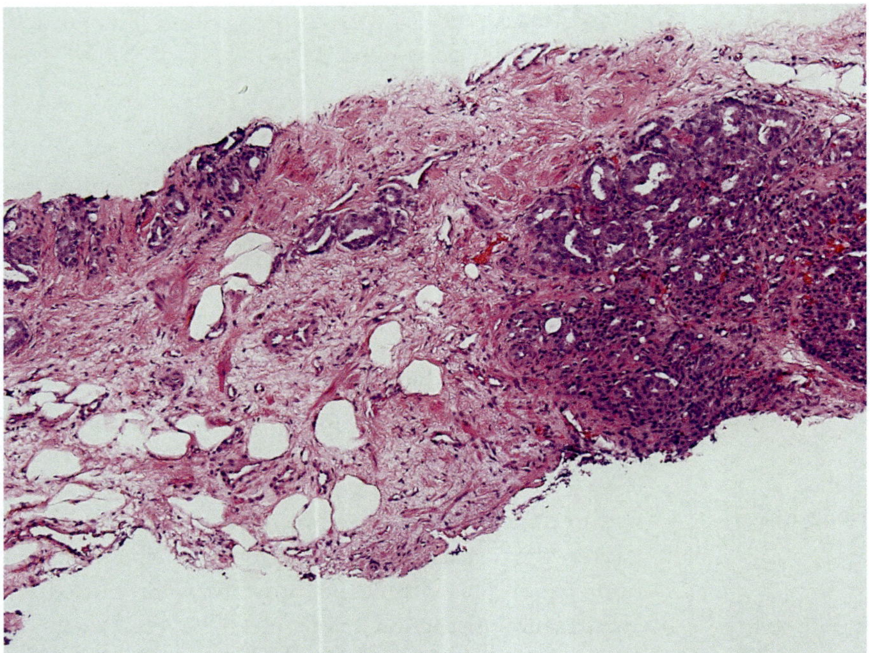

Figure 9-4.
A needle core biopsy specimen shows clearly a focus of high-grade adenocarcinoma within the adipose tissue (typically at the end of a needle core), representing extraprostatic extension.

Clinical relevance (prognosis and treatment options)

- T3A: extraprostatic extension; T3B: seminal vesicle involvement
- Needle biopsy with EPE indicates potential positive surgical margins
- The finding of EPE on needle biopsy is associated with high-volume or high-grade disease, which may lead to a change of strategy in treatment options
- Nerve sparing may not be possible because the nerve bundles can be involved in the cases of EPE (Fig. 9-5)
- External beam radiation may be better than seeding (brachytherapy) for cases with EPE

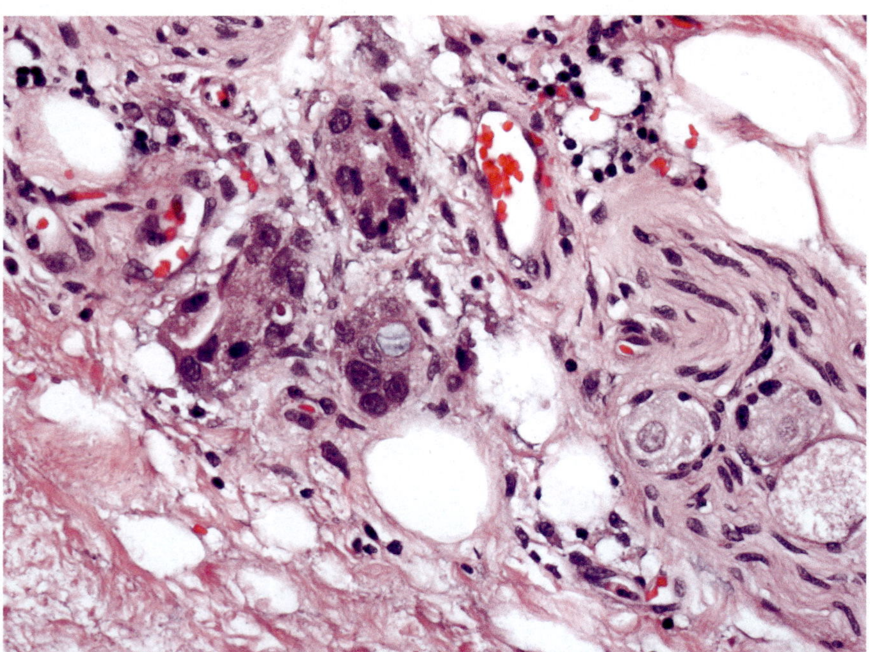

Figure 9-5.
Adenocarcinoma with extraprostatic extension and ganglion cell involvement.

SEMINAL VESICLE INVASION (STAGE T3B)

Definition

- Prostatic adenocarcinoma involves one or both seminal vesicles

Pathogenesis

- Tumor cells involve the seminal vesicle mostly by direct extension, or by lymphovascular spreading

Clinical features

- High serum PSA levels
- Typically high-grade and high-volume disease

Gross pathology

- No specific finding
- Occasionally, a large tumor mass involving a portion of the seminal vesicle may be seen

Histology

- Tumor cells are found in the muscular wall of the seminal vesicle (Figs. 9-6 and 9-7), not in the adipose tissue outside the seminal vesicle
- Tumor cells in a section containing both seminal vesicle–like structure and benign prostatic glands should not be considered seminal vesicle invasion because it most likely represents a portion of ejaculatory duct (Fig. 9-7)
- The seminal vesicle–like tissue with the prostate glands should be defined as the ejaculatory duct
- Unless the seminal vesicle is specifically targeted during biopsy, it is not possible to distinguish seminal vesicle from ejaculatory ducts on needle core biopsy material (Fig. 9-8). In this situation, we typically use the statement, "Tumor cells involve seminal vesicle/ejaculatory duct tissue. Clinical correlation is necessary"

Immunohistochemistry

- Generally not necessary, occasionally, triple stain is needed to confirm the presence of adenocarcinoma
- MUC 6 can be used for confirming the presence of seminal vesicles or ejaculatory ducts

Clinical relevance (prognosis and treatment options)

- Adenocarcinoma with seminal vesicle involvement is Stage 3B disease
- Associated with poor prognosis

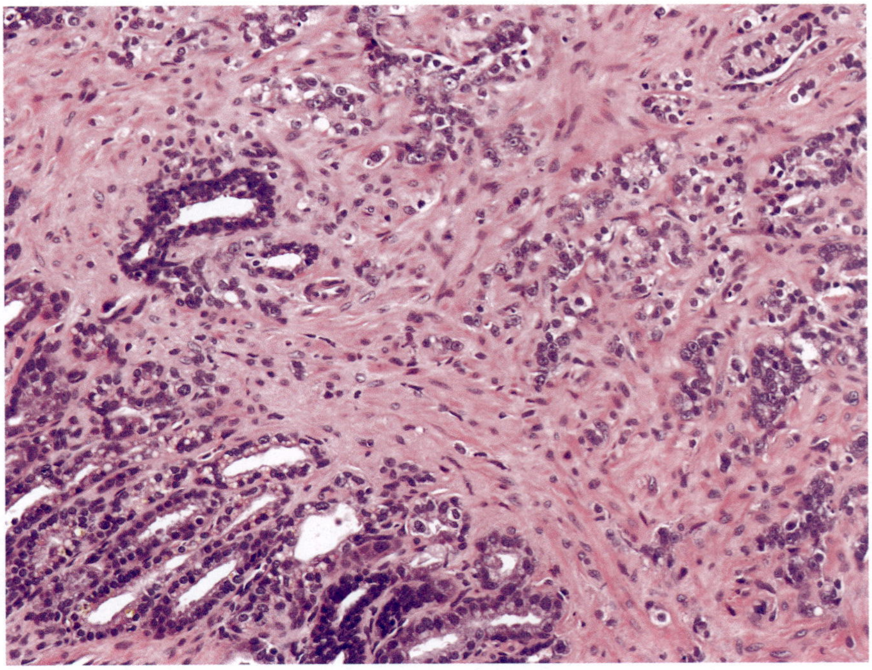

Figure 9-6.
High-grade (Gleason 4 + 5) adenocarcinoma invading into the wall of the seminal vesicle.

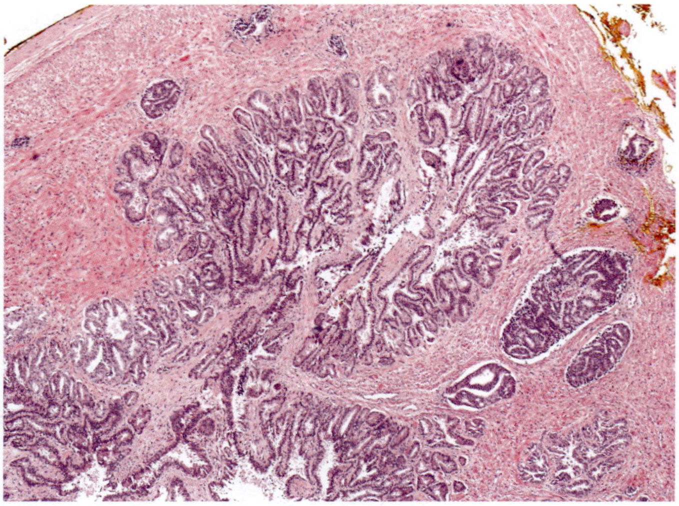

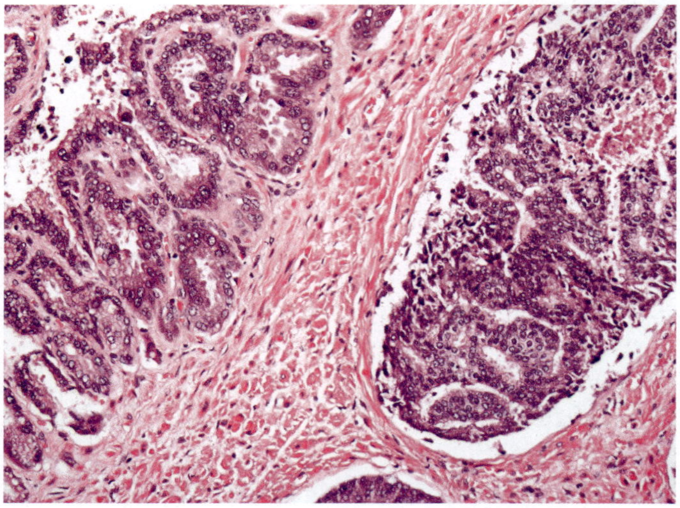

a *b*

Figure 9-7.
A seminal vesicle is invaded by adenocarcinoma (*a*). High magnification shows that the seminal vesicle cells on the left containing pigment, while tumor cells on the right do not (*b*).

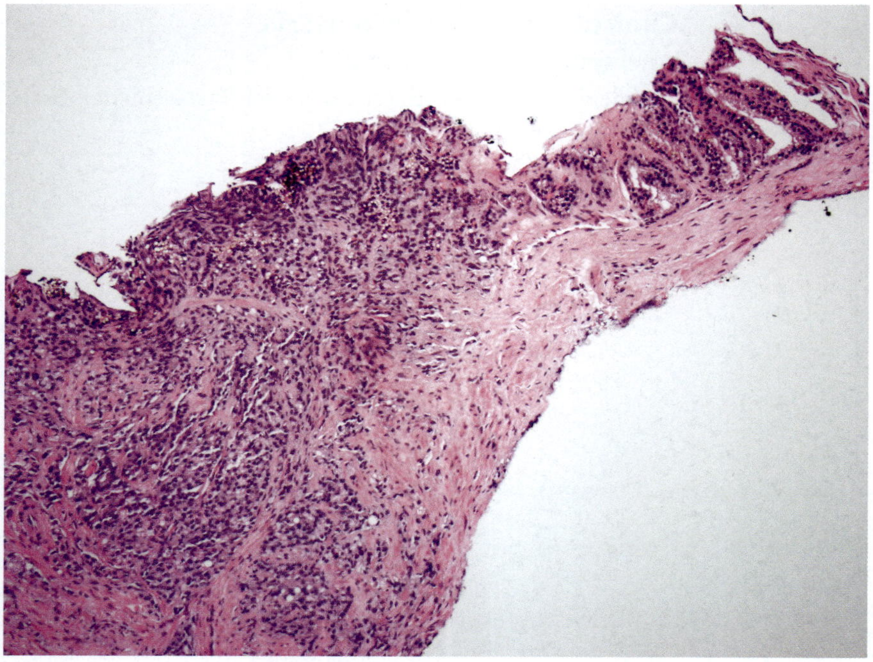

Figure 9-8.
A prostate needle core specimen is mostly involved by high-grade adenocarcinoma. The seminal vesicle type tissue can be appreciated; however, this may be a part of ejaculatory duct, not seminal vesicle.

POSITIVE SURGICAL MARGIN

Definition

- Tumor cells extend to the inked surgical margins
- Positive margin status does not change the stage of prostate cancer but it is associated with a significant risk of recurrence. It is most commonly seen in T3 cases

Pathogenesis

- Two possible situations for positive margins
  - Tumor cells invade extraprostatic tissue and complete surgical removal by prostatectomy is not possible
  - The surgeon cut into the prostate parenchyma and the result is "capsule incision" with benign (not positive margin) or malignant tissue (positive margin) present at the inked margins

Gross pathology

- The shape, surface, and integrity of the prostate should be evaluated
- If the prostate from a radical prostatectomy specimen is arriving disrupted or in pieces, it will be difficult to determine the surgical margin status, and this must be carefully described in the gross description. This could be a concern in robotic prostatectomy when the prostate is pulled out from a small hole in the abdominal wall
- The prostate should be inked before cutting with left and right side in different colored inks
- Avoid overinking, which will run over to the cut surface to create false-positive margins
- The cut surface may show the yellow-white firm and solid areas, which may present carcinoma. Its relationship to the capsule or surface of the prostate can be carefully evaluated

Histology

- The ink has to be over the tumor cells to be considered to be a positive margin (Fig. 9-9). Even one layer of fibrous tissue is sufficient for a negative margin (Fig. 9-10)
- Sometimes, the tumor cells are cauterized at the margins, which should be considered to be a positive margin
- The grading of the margins has not been well accepted, but it may provide some quantitative measures of the extent of the disease
  - Grade 1. Apical positive margin with Gleason 3 pattern tumor in one or two small foci (reportedly related to a good prognosis)
  - Grade 2. Focal positive margins elsewhere in the prostate (most positive margins fall into this category, the prognosis is variable)
  - Grade 3. Extensive positive margins (≥3 foci) with high-grade adenocarcinoma are generally considered to be associated with a poor prognosis

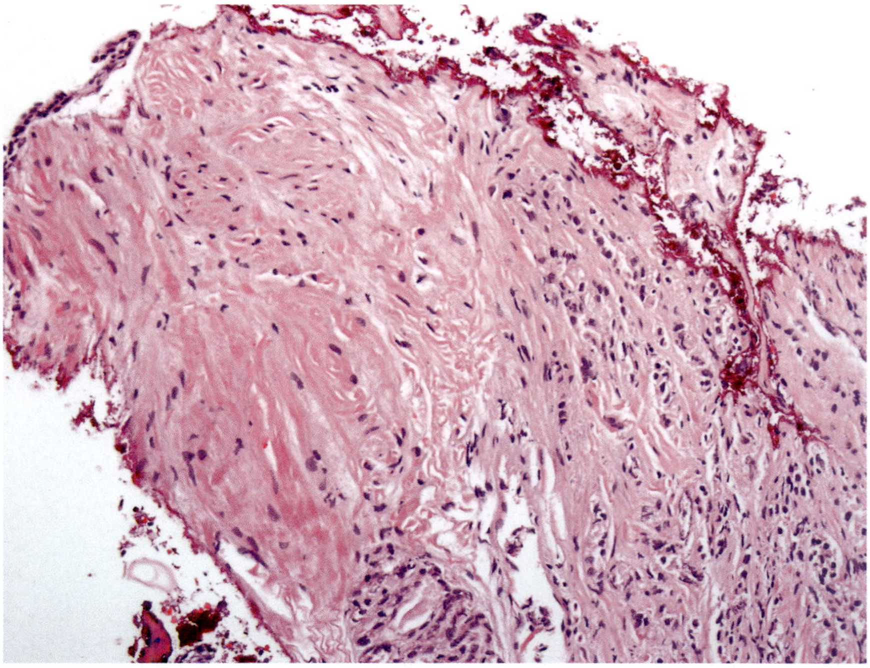

Figure 9-9.
Apical margin is involved by tumor cells that have to be on the inked surface.

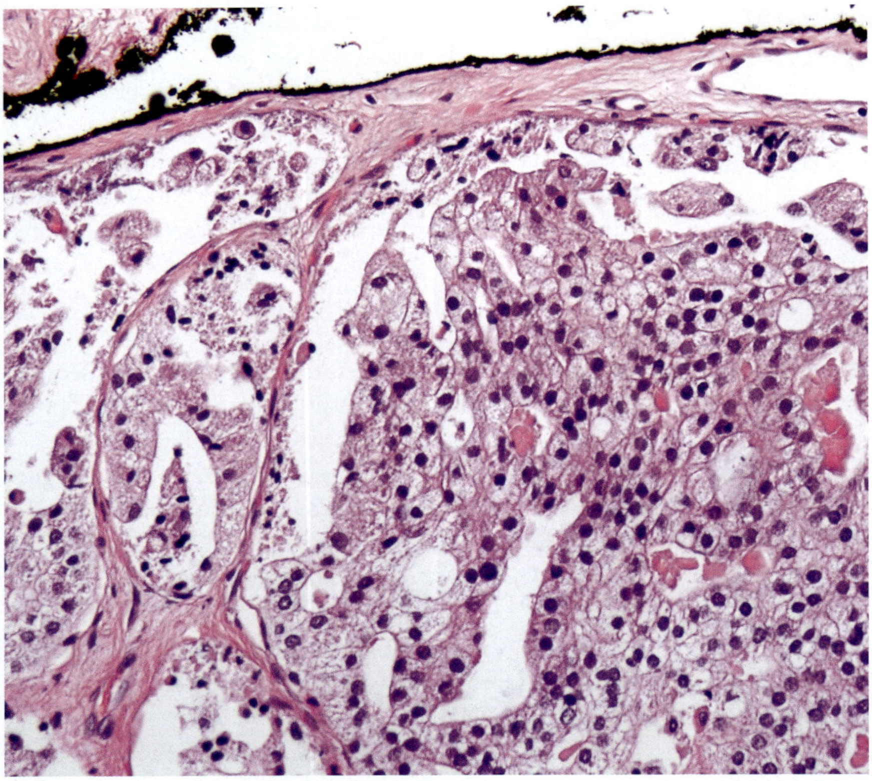

Figure 9-10.
Adenocarcinoma is close to the inked margin but separated by a thin layer of fibrous tissue, which is not considered to be a positive margin.

Clinical relevance (prognosis and treatment options)

- Positive surgical margin is one of the most common predictive factors for recurrence
- A good prostatectomy is typically associated with a positive margin rate less than 10%, although it may heavily depend on the selection of patients

LYMPHOVASCULAR INVASION

- Lymphovascular invasion is one of the malignant features of prostatic adenocarcinoma
- Although the presence of lymphovascular invasion does not change the tumor stage, it is the prelude of metastases to the lymph nodes and distal organs
- Lymphovascular invasion is more commonly seen in high-grade and high-volume diseases (Fig. 9-11)
- The identification of lymphovascular invasion is best done in an area away from the bulk of the tumor since a vessel with endothelium can be appreciated better (Fig. 9-12)
- When there is any doubt, the application of CD31 or CD34 immunohistochemistry can be helpful to confirm the presence of endothelial cells

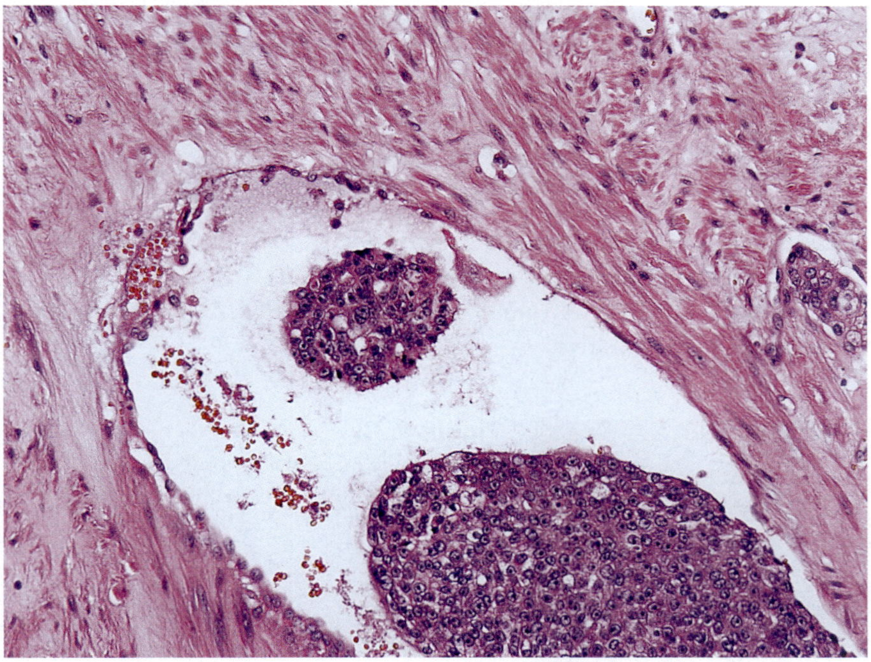

Figure 9-11.
Vascular invasion: Adenocarcinoma tumor thrombi are present in a large vascular space, which may represent a small vein.

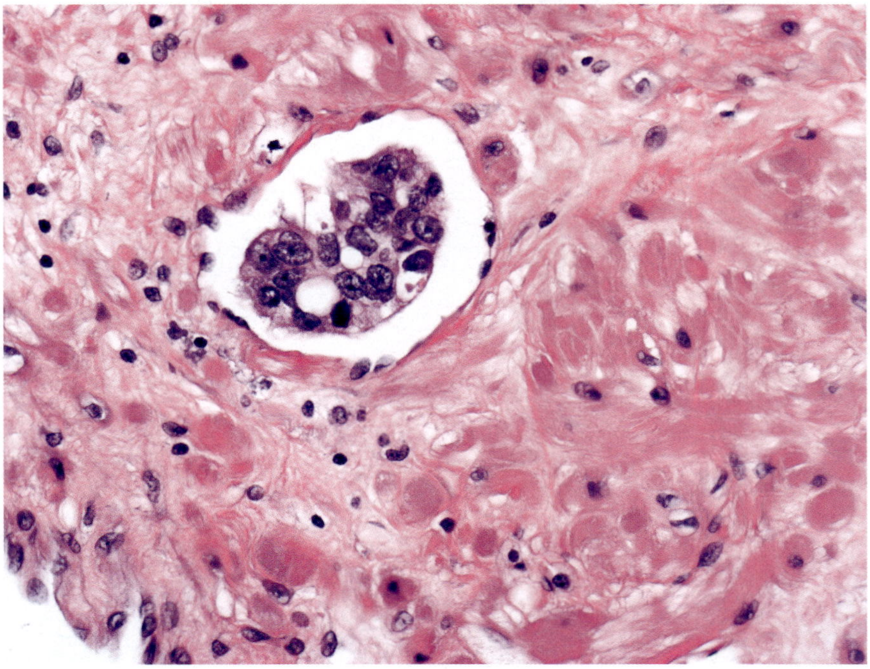

Figure 9-12.
Lymphovascular invasion seen in a prostatectomy specimen.

PROSTATIC ADENOCARCINOMA METASTATIC TO LYMPH NODES (STAGE N1 OR M1A)

Definition

- Metastatic prostatic adenocarcinoma in a regional lymph node (N1) or nonregional lymph node (M1A)
- No metastasis in lymph node(s) = pN0, lymph node not examined = pNx

Pathogenesis

- Tumor cells in the prostate invade into the lymphatics, migrate to and develop colonies in the draining lymph nodes

Clinical features

- High-grade and high-volume primary prostatic adenocarcinoma
- High PSA levels
- No symptoms directly related to the pelvic LN metastasis

Gross pathology

- In many cases, it is not possible to identify a node positive for metastatic prostate cancer based on the size. Only occasionally, a positive node can be grossly identified. Microscopic examination is essential

Histology

- Small or large clusters of tumor cells in the lymph node (Fig. 9-13)
- Tumor cells show prominent nucleoli, relatively mild pleomorphism. The most common patterns are cribriform patterns (Gleason pattern 4) (Fig. 9-14)
- Long-standing hormonal retractile tumors can be very pleomorphic histologically

Immunohistochemistry

- PSA positive (can be focal)
- PSMA (more specific) and/or AMACR (less specific) positive

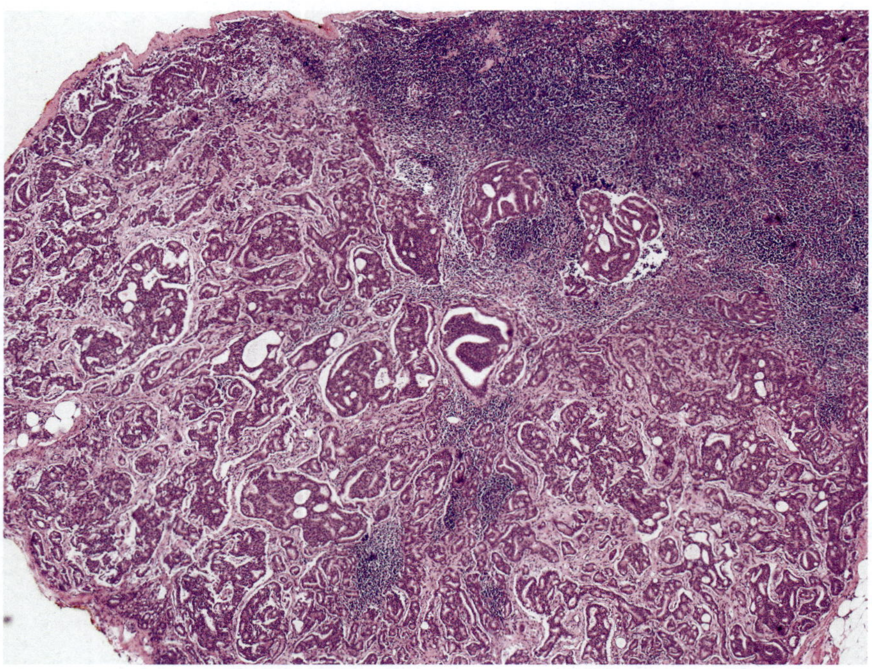

Figure 9-13.
Lymph node metastasis of prostatic adenocarcinoma with prominent cribriform patterns.

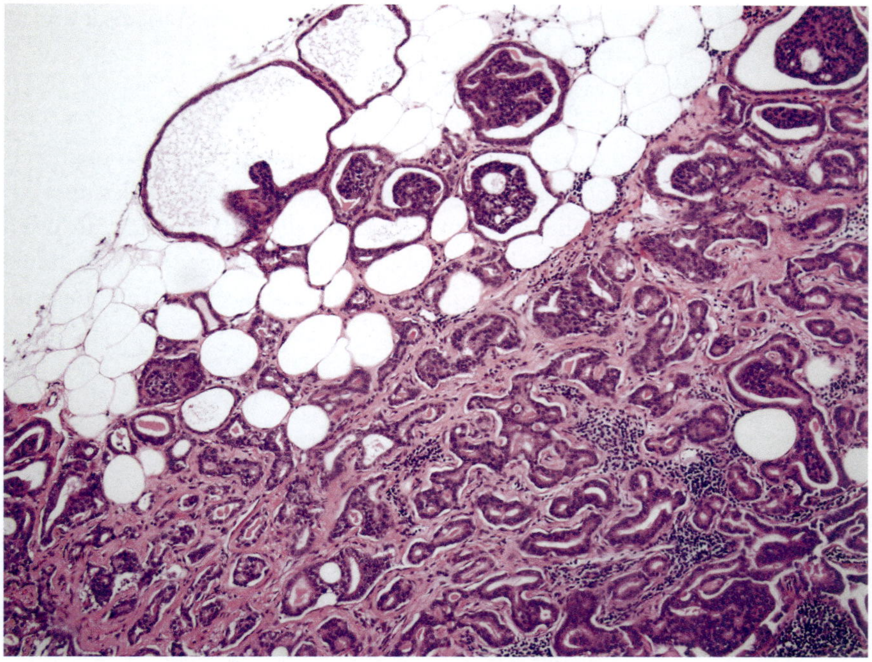

Figure 9-14.
Lymph node metastasis of a case of prostatic adenocarcinoma exhibits glandular, cribriform patterns and cystically dilated glands. Tumor cells also extend into the adipose tissue (extranodal extension).

Molecular analysis

- Not indicated

Clinical relevance (prognosis and treatment options)

- In most situations, finding a positive pelvic lymph node intraoperatively will probably result in aborted radical prostatectomy
- Removal of a prostate harboring cancer in a patient with lymph node metastasis may be considered *debulking*. But its benefit has not been proven
- The presence of positive lymph nodes in the radical prostatectomy patient population in our practice is very low (<0.5%)
- The frozen section diagnosis of pelvic lymph nodes (Fig. 9-15) may carry a significant high false-negative rate for detecting metastatic prostate cancer
- Therefore, it is not recommended to perform routine frozen section examination of all the pelvic lymph nodes from a patient undergoing radical prostatectomy unless there is a significant risk
- Some surgeons routinely remove prostates regardless of the status of the pelvic lymph nodes for metastasis

Figure 9-15.
A frozen section (*a*) of a pelvic lymph node shows the presence of small cluster of glands. Permanent section (*b*) confirms the presence of metastatic adenocarcinoma in the node.

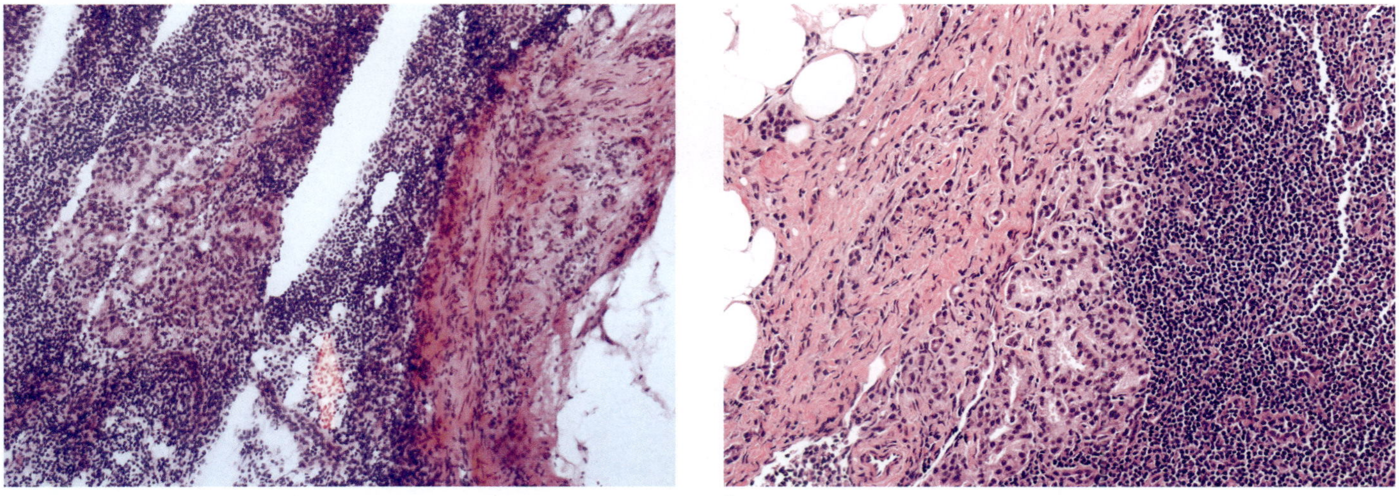

a **b**

METASTATIC PROSTATIC ADENOCARCINOMA IN THE BONE (STAGE M1B)

Definition

- Establishment of colonies of prostatic adenocarcinoma in the bone

Other terms

- None

Pathogenesis

- Prostatic adenocarcinoma appears to have a certain degree of affinity to migrate to bone and establish metastatic foci
- It is not clear whether it is mostly related to the environment of the bone or the intrinsic feature of the prostatic adenocarcinoma cells

Clinical features

- History of prostate cancer
- It is important to know the history and grade of the prostatic adenocarcinoma. A typical small focus of Gleason 3 + 3 tumor is very unlikely to develop metastasis if undersampling is not an issue
- Elevated serum PSA
- Positive PET scan (metabolically active cells)
- Imaging studies show an osteoblastic lesion (most metastatic tumors from other origins are osteolytic lesions)
- This phenomenon is relatively specific for metastatic prostate cancer, it is probably because prostatic adenocarcinoma cells produce or induce some factors stimulating the osteoid production

Gross pathology

- Not usually seen

Histology

- The presence of adenocarcinoma cells in clusters (Fig. 9-16) in the bone
- Evidence of prominent new bone formation in addition to the presence of adenocarcinoma includes thick hyperplastic bone trabecular structures and osteoblastic rimming (Fig. 9-17)
- Cribriform patterns are seen in the majority of metastatic cases (Fig. 9-17)
- Prominent cherry red nucleoli may be seen

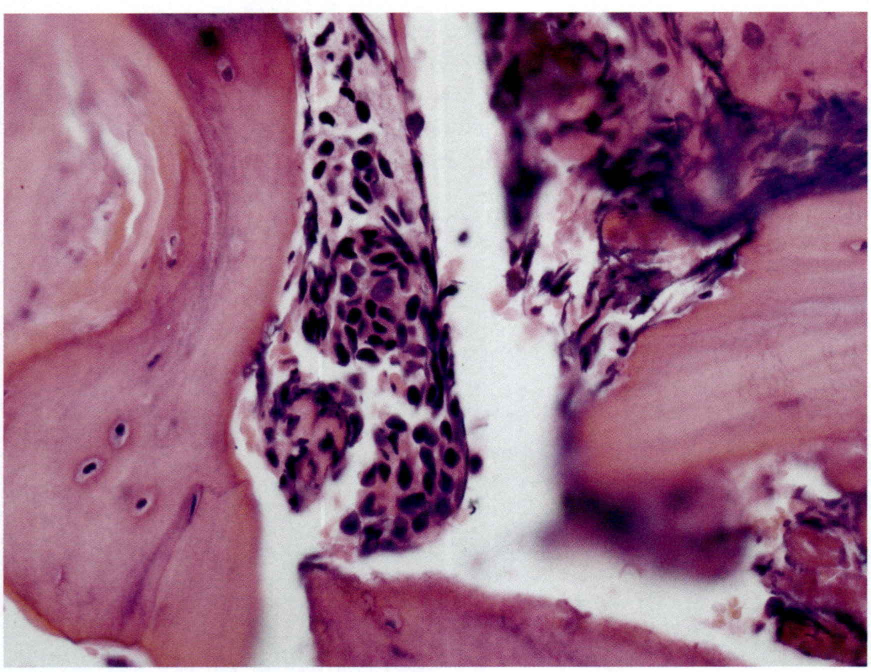

Figure 9-16.
A vertebral bone biopsy shows the presence of a cluster of prostatic adenocarcinoma cells, which can be difficult to classify.

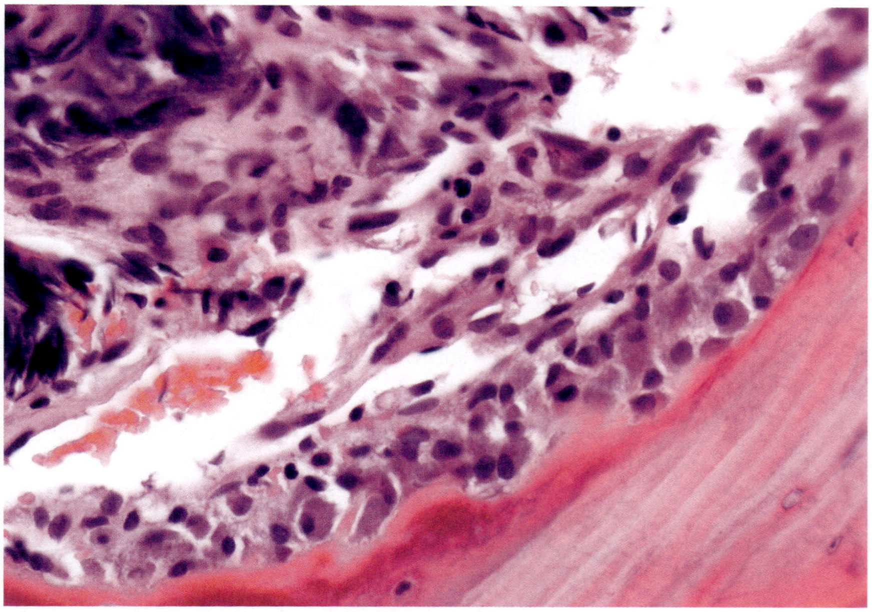

Figure 9-17.
The presence of osteoblasts in the bone suggests an osteoblastic lesion, which is characteristic of metastatic prostate cancer.

Immunohistochemistry

- It is obligatory for a pathologist to perform PSA or other immunostains to confirm the diagnosis of metastatic prostatic adenocarcinoma because of significant clinical consequences
- PSA positivity is specific (Fig. 9-18), but it can be very focal in a higher grade tumor
- AMACR positivity is less specific, because it may be positive for other cancers such as colon adenocarcinoma or papillary RCC
- PMSA positivity. High-grade prostate adenocarcinoma demonstrates a stronger staining than either low-grade tumor or benign epithelium

Clinical relevance (prognosis and treatment options)

- Metastasis in bone carries a poor prognosis
- It is a sign of systemic disease, which requires systemic treatment such as hormonal therapy or chemotherapy
- Surgical resection is usually not indicated for cure but for palliative purpose. A metastatic tumor in the bone may be resected if it causes pathologic fracture or other morbidities
- Bone metastasis of prostate cancer can also be radiated to relieve bone pain

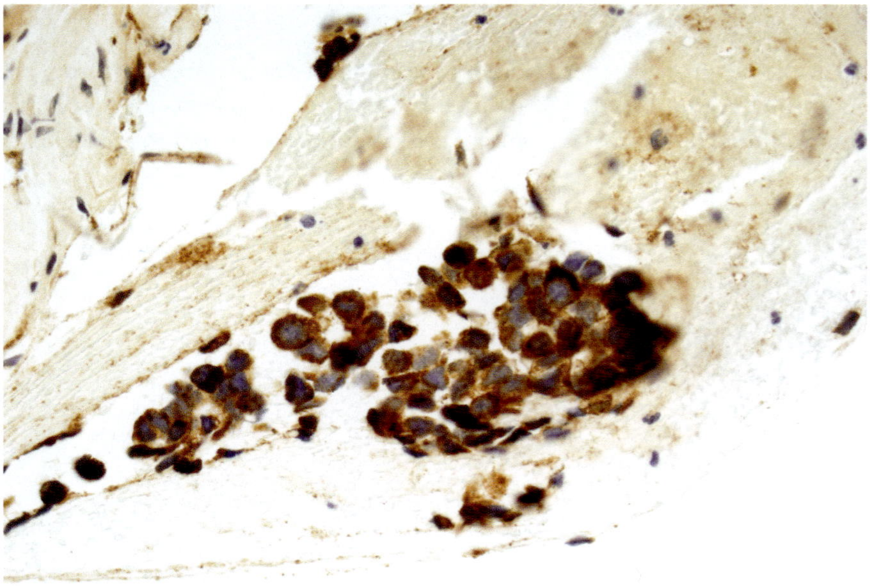

Figure 9-18.
The PSA immunostaining confirms the nature of prostatic primary.

METASTATIC PROSTATIC CANCER IN THE LUNG AND OTHER ORGANS (STAGE M1C)

Definition

- Prostatic carcinoma metastasizes to any other organ
- Stage M1 does not include seminal vesicles

Other terms

- T4 prostate cancer
- Metastatic prostate cancer

Pathogenesis

- Tumor cells invade the blood vessels, migrate through blood into other organs, and develop metastatic foci

Clinical features

- Not associated with a specific clinical symptom
- Typically high-grade and high-volume primary adenocarcinoma
- Some will be hormone refractile and some will be hormone naïve
- A small volume tumor with Gleason score $3 + 3 = 6$ is very unlikely to metastasize to other organs
- It may be detected by imaging studies showing metabolically active lesions
- ProstaScint scanning is a prostate-specific detecting system that can be used to reveal metastatic disease or localized recurrence
- The mechanism of ProstaScint is using a labeled antibody specific for PSMA, which recognizes prostatic adenocarcinoma but not other tumors. Then the radioactive Indium^{111} label will be detected in the tissue if the metastatic or recurrent tumor is present
- Because PSMA is also present in the normal prostate, ProstaScint does not help detect a primary prostate cancer

Gross pathology

- Variable size and shape of the metastatic foci
- Not specific findings

Histology

- Mostly poorly differentiated adenocarcinoma (Gleason pattern 4 or 5) (Fig. 9-19)
- Some cases will show cribriform patterns, with typically prominent nucleoli and less pleomorphic features
- Hormonal refractile (hormone treated but recurring) adenocarcinoma will show marked cytologic atypia, difficult to distinguish from a primary malignance from the other organs

Immunohistochemistry

PSA	Positive (Fig. 9-19*b* and *f*), but it can be weak or focal
AMACR	Positive (Fig. 9-19*c*)
PSMA	Positive

Molecular analysis

- Not currently available for clinical use

Clinical relevance (prognosis and treatment options)

- Metastatic prostate cancer has a poor prognosis
- However, detection of metastatic prostate cancer is important since some of these cases can still respond to hormonal therapy
- In the majority of cases of a primary carcinoma, surgical resection is useful. However, resection of metastatic prostate cancer has not been proven to improve prognosis

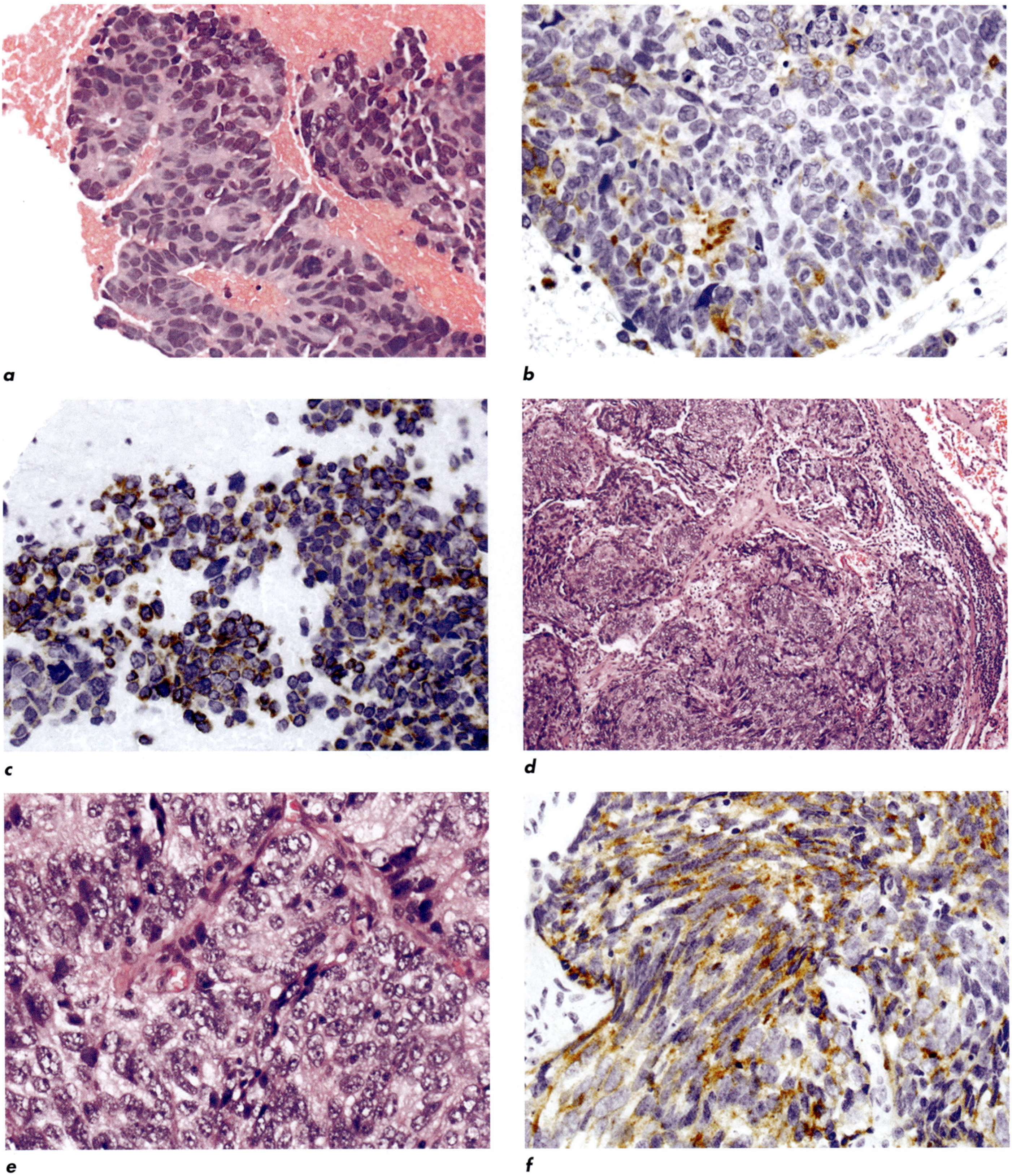

Figure 9-19

Metastatic prostatic adenocarcinoma. High-grade (Gleason 4 + 5) adenocarcinoma is present (*a*) and tumor cells are positive for PSA (*b*) and AMACR (*c*). Another case of high-grade metastatic prostatic adenocarcinoma (*d*) showing relative uniform tumor cells with prominent nucleoli typical for prostatic adenocarcinoma (*e*), also demonstrating PSA positivity (*f*).

CANCER VANISHING SYNDROME

Definition

- A situation of inability to identify residual cancer in the radical prostatectomy specimen in a man with biopsy-confirmed prostatic adenocarcinoma
- The cancer is not vanished but it cannot be detected anymore due to limitation of tissue sampling

Pathogenesis and epidemiology

- This is not a condition that the cancer disappears as the title is indicated
- It is a small focus of adenocarcinoma detected by biopsy, but not detected in the prostatectomy specimen because of sampling issues
- With extensive sampling, even a small focus of prostatic adenocarcinoma can be evaluated microscopically
- Based on our studies, this phenomena represents 0.1% to 0.3% of our several thousand of cases over more than 10 years of experience
- Strictly speaking, a wrong diagnosis on biopsy (false positive) leading to prostatectomy should not be considered *cancer vanishing syndrome*

Clinical features

- Normal or slightly increased PSA
- Small focus of adenocarcinoma on needle core biopsy
- No evidence of metastatic carcinoma

Gross pathology

- Normal appearance of the prostate with or without BPH

Histology

- Biopsy material needs to be reviewed and confirmed as prostatic adenocarcinoma
- As a routine practice, we review all the outside biopsy material before a prostatectomy is performed for prostate cancer patients in house. This provides an extra protection from litigation
- Typically the cancer on biopsy is a single small focus of carcinoma of Gleason 3 + 3 = 6
- Methods to handle this situation
  - Providing preoperative information to the patients that there is a small chance that cancer may not be detected in the prostatectomy specimens particularly for the patients with single small focus of Gleason 3 + 3 tumor
  - Reviewing the biopsy material again
  - Submitting all the remaining prostate tissue
  - Submitting all the harvested frozen tissue from tumor banking
  - Ordering deeper sections of suspicious areas
  - Occasionally flip the tissue blocks in the biopsy positive area if necessary
  - Perform triple immunostaining on the suspicious areas

Immunohistochemistry

- Triple stains are often performed to confirm the presence of prostate cancer

Molecular analysis

- Genotyping to confirm the match between the patient and the biopsy material is usually not necessary unless there is a high-grade or high-volume tumor present in needle biopsy or a high clinical suspicion that the patient does not have prostate cancer

Clinical relevance (prognosis and treatment options)

- Currently, vigorous PSA screening can lead to detection of early prostate cancer
- As consequence, it is also associated with an increasing number of cases with a very low volume of cancer detected. Therefore, there is either no residual cancer (cancer vanishing) or very little residual cancer found at radical prostatectomy
- The rising incidence of very low-volume prostate cancer detected should be considered by clinicians when discussing treatment options with patients
- The prognosis is excellent, indicating that there is no clinical significance to microscopic foci of cancer that remain undetected after complete pathologic sampling

CHAPTER 10

Special Histological Variants of Prostatic Adenocarcinoma

DUCTAL ADENOCARCINOMA

Definition

- Prostatic adenocarcinoma composed of tall columnar cells

Other terms

- Papillary carcinoma
- Endometrioid carcinoma

Pathogenesis

- Histological variant of prostatic adenocarcinoma, pathogenesis is not different from acinar adenocarcinoma

Clinical features

- Elevated PSA and a palpable mass

Gross pathology

- Most cases are associated with acinar adenocarcinoma, and located in the peripheral zone
- Only a minority of cases are located in the prostatic urethra as a polypoid lesion

Histology

- Tumor is composed of tall columnar cells with prominent nucleoli (Figs. 10-1 and 10-2)
- Morphologically, it is similar to endometrium. Therefore it was termed *endometrioid carcinoma* in the past (Figs. 10-3 and 10-4)
- Papillary structures may be seen (Figs. 10-2 and 10-5)
- Nuclear atypia is present in ductal carcinoma, including prominent nucleoli (Figs. 10-2, 10-4, and 10-5), similar to acinar type of prostatic adenocarcinoma
- Majority of cases are associated with high-grade acinar adenocarcinoma (mixed) (Fig. 10-4)
- Biologically and biochemically, ductal adenocarcinoma is similar to acinar adenocarcinoma, Gleason pattern 4
- Since it's often associated with a high-grade acinar component, ductal adenocarcinoma will typically be Gleason score 7 to 9 if graded

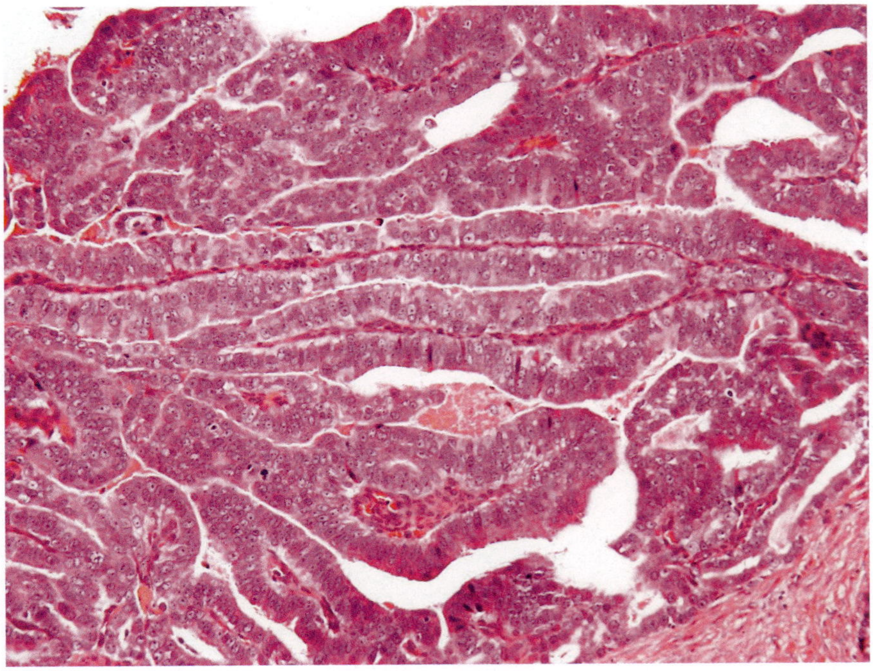

Figure 10-1.
A ductal adenocarcinoma characterized by the presence of tall columnar tumor cells.

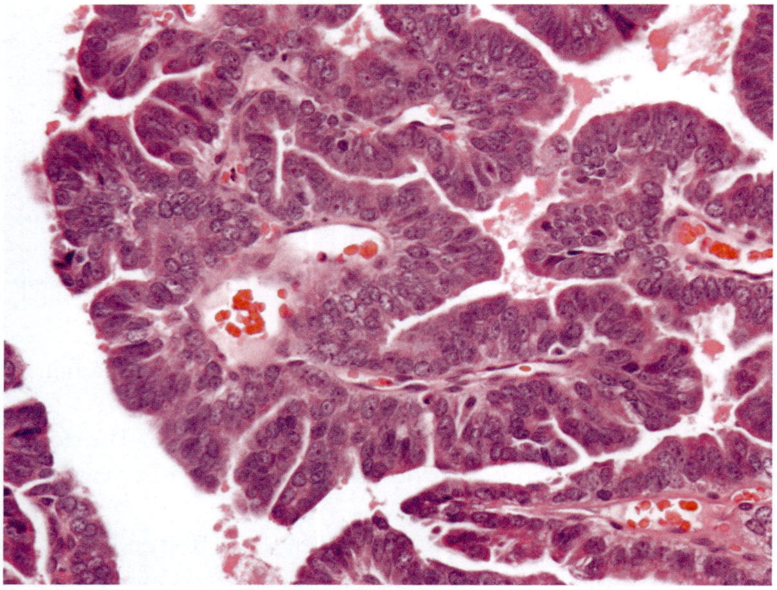

Figure 10-2.
Ductal adenocarcinoma showing papillary structures, which are lined by pseudostratified malignant columnar cells.

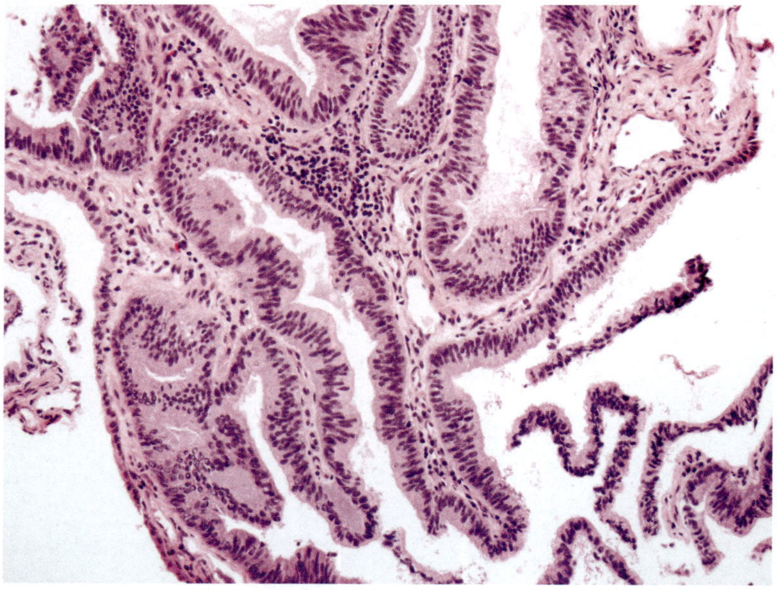

Figure 10-3.
A ductal adenocarcinoma protruding into the prostatic urethra. The presence of atypical columnar cells is characteristic.

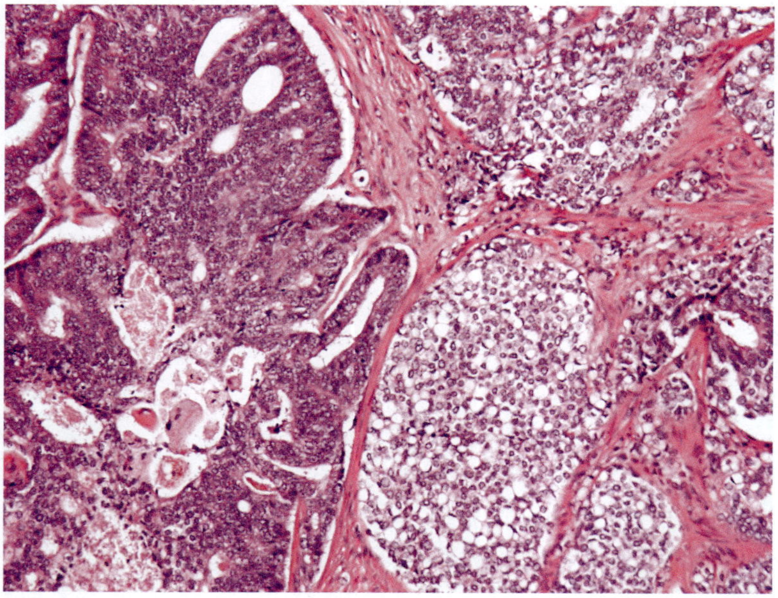

Figure 10-4.
Presence of both ductal component (left) and acinar component of adenocarcinoma.

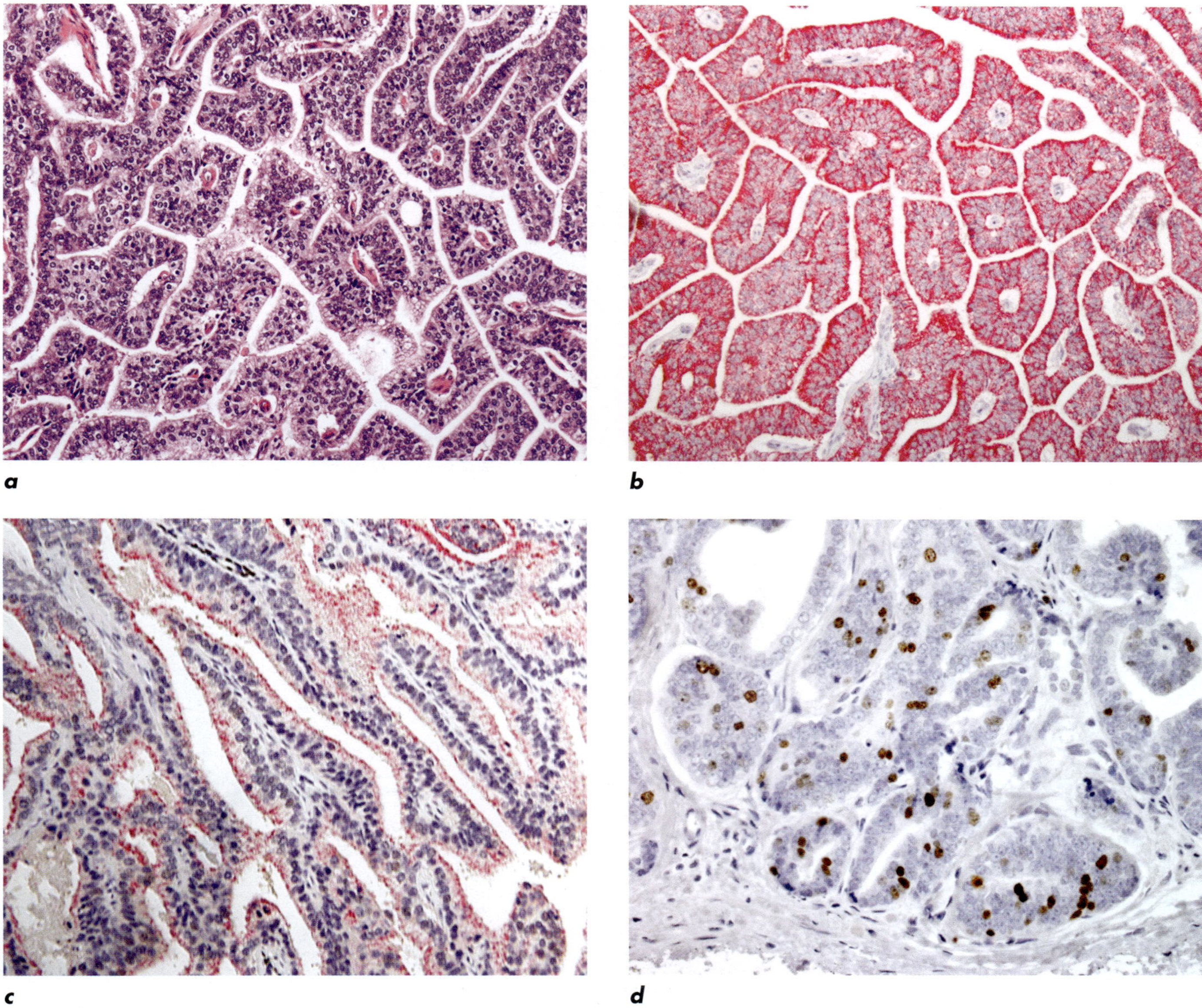

Figure 10-5.
Ductal adenocarcinoma with papilla (*a*), confirmed by positive AMACR staining and lack of basal cells (*b*). Another case of adenocarcinoma showing weak AMACR staining and negative basal cell marker staining (*c*) with relatively high Ki67 proliferative activities (*d*), similar to that of Gleason 7 or 8 acinar adenocarcinoma.

Immunohistochemistry

- AMACR strongly (Fig. 10-5*b*) to weakly (Fig. 10-5*c*) positive
- Basal cell markers are negative (Figs. 10-5*b* and 10-5*c*)
- PSA positive
- Androgen receptor positive, ER and PR negative
- Ki67 proliferative rate is high (Fig. 10-5*d*)
- When basal cells are present, the tumor is considered to be intraductal carcinoma

Differential diagnosis

- Acinar adenocarcinoma: much more common, not tall columnar cells
- Intraductal carcinoma of the prostate (see Table 10-1)

Clinical relevance (prognosis and treatment options)

- Aggressive behavior similar to Gleason 4 + 4 = 8
- Expected to be responsive to hormonal treatment since its AR positivity

Table 10-1. Comparison of Intraductal Carcinoma and High-Grade PIN of the Prostate

	IDC	*High-grade PIN*
Nature	Malignant	Premalignant
Gland size	Large	Large
Atypia	Marked	Less prominent
Mitosis	Frequent	Rare
Comedo necrosis	Common	Rare
Basal cells	Present, patchy	Present, patchy
AMACR	Strong	Weak or moderate
HMWCK/p63	Positive	Positive
Treatment	Needed	Not needed

AMACR, α-methylacyl-CoA racemase; HMWCK, high molecular cytokeratins; IDC, intraductal carcinoma of the prostate; PIN; prostatic intraepithelial neoplasia.

INTRADUCTAL CARCINOMA OF THE PROSTATE

Definition

- Malignant epithelial cells filling large acini and prostatic ducts

Pathogenesis

- It is considered to be an advanced phase of prostate cancer development, not a premalignant lesion such as high-grade PIN

Clinical features

- Same symptoms and signs as prostate cancer, such as elevated PSA

Gross pathology

- Typically associated with high-grade and high-volume cancer

Histology

- Tumor cells present in a preexisting prostatic gland
- Tumor cells form solid or dense cribriform patterns (Figs. 10-6 and 10-7)
- Loose cribriform or micropapillary pattern with marked cytologic atypia
- With preservation of basal cells
- Tumor cells may show partial involvement of a gland (Figs. 10-6 and 10-8)

Immunohistochemistry

- AMACR positive (Figs. 10-7*b* and 10-7*d*), weak to strong
- Basal cell markers positive (Figs. 10-7*b* and 10-7*d*)

Clinical relevance (prognosis and treatment options)

- IDC is typically associated with high-grade and high-volume invasive adenocarcinoma in the vast majority of cases. Therefore, it is important to make an accurate diagnosis especially on biopsy
- Treatment such as radical prostatectomy, radiation or hormonal therapy, or combination of these therapies recommended

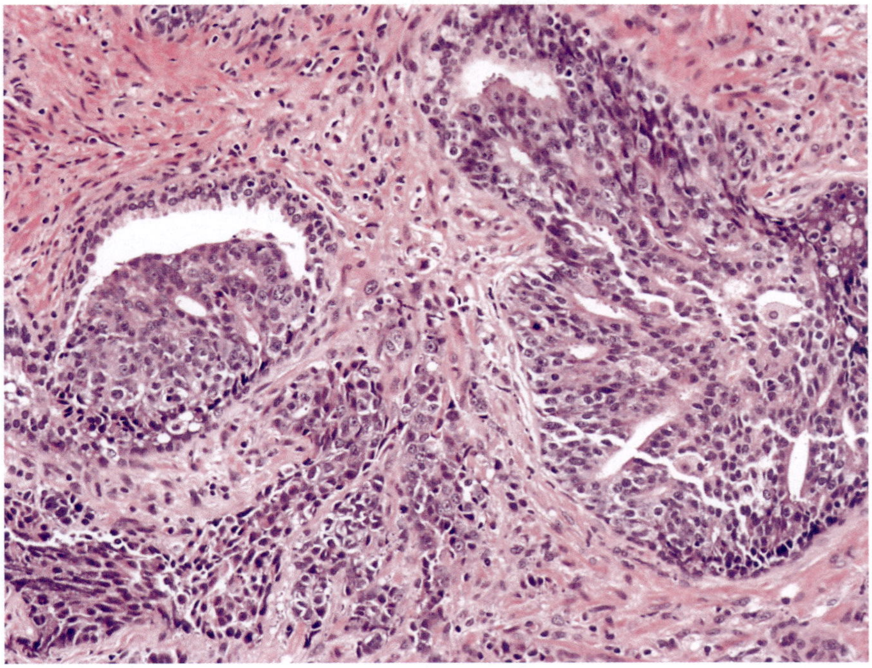

Figure 10-6.
Intraductal carcinoma (IDC) of the prostate. On the left side of the photo, a benign gland is filled with cribriform adenocarcinoma. On the right side, a large gland with florid cribriform growth in the lumen.

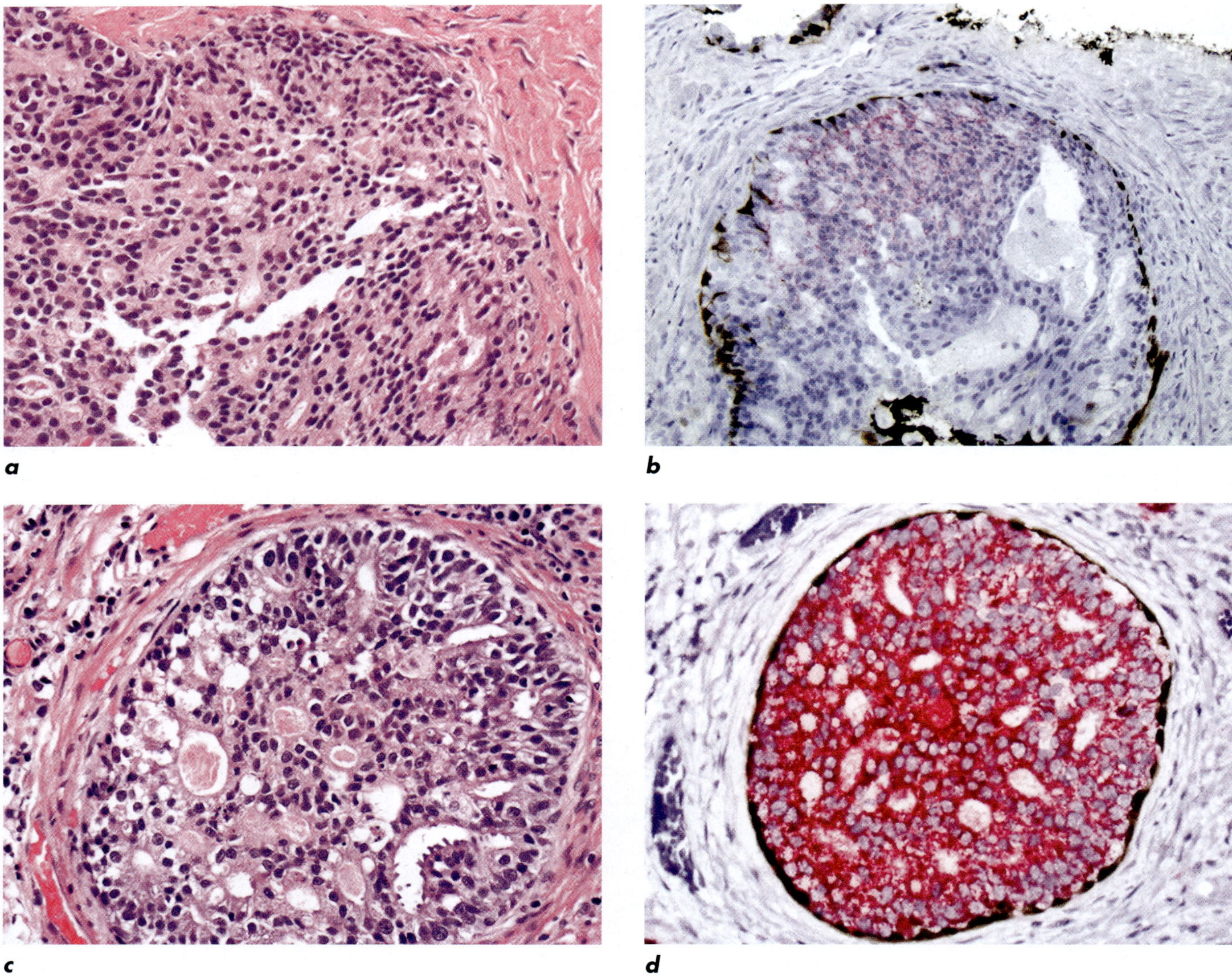

Figure 10-7.
IDC in a large gland with confluent cribriform pattern (*a*). The presence of basal cells is confirmed by positive triple staining. The tumor cells are weakly positive for AMACR (*b*). Another case of IDC with cribriform patterns (*c*), triple immunostaining showing strong AMACR staining and the presence of basal cells (*d*).

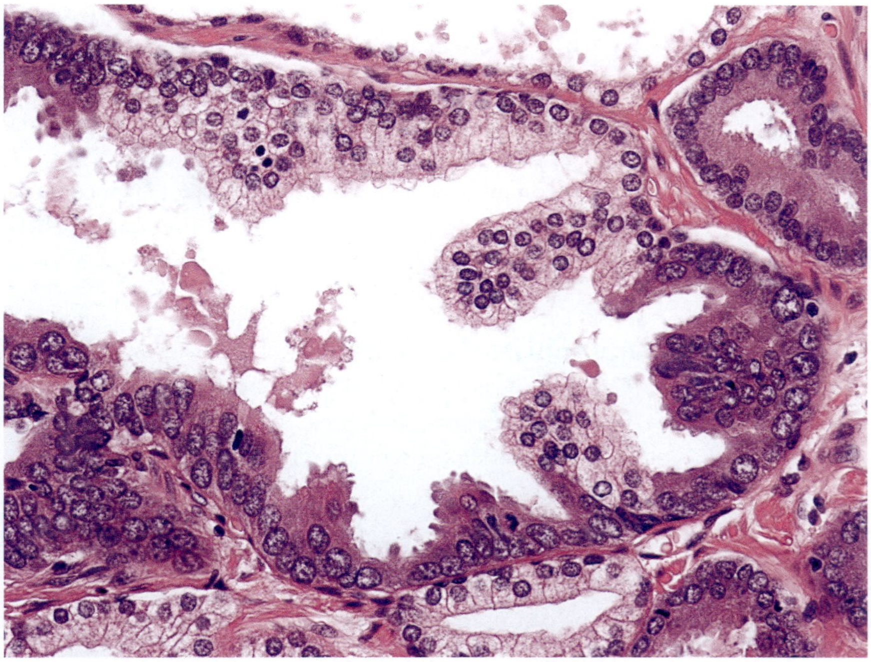

Figure 10-8.
IDC with tumor cells partially involve a large gland (lower portion), similar to invasive tumor cells arranged in small glands (right).

FOAMY GLAND ADENOCARCINOMA

Definition

- Prostatic adenocarcinoma composed of tumor cells with abundant foamy cytoplasm

Clinical features

- Typically associated with relatively aggressive behaviors as Gleason score 7 or above
- PSA elevation and palpable tumor mass

Gross pathology

- Not identifiable

Histology

- Tumor composed of large cells with abundant foamy cytoplasm (Figs. 10-9 and 10-10)
- Patterns of well-formed glands (Gleason pattern 3), fused or cribriform glands (Gleason pattern 4), or individual cells (Gleason pattern 5) can be seen (Figs. 10-9 and 10-10)
- Nuclear atypia may not be prominent (Fig. 10-11)
- Often associated conventional acinar adenocarcinoma, rarely in pure form
- By electron microscopy, the tumor cell cytoplasm contains membrane-bound vesicles similar to those seen in chromophobe renal cell carcinoma

Immunohistochemistry

- AMACR positive (Fig. 10-11*b*) but often weaker than typical acinar adenocarcinoma
- Basal cell markers absent (Fig. 10-11*b*)

Clinical relevance (prognosis and treatment options)

- Can be confused with benign glands because of the bland cytology
- However, most foamy gland adenocarcinoma cases are associated with a relatively aggressive behavior

Figure 10-9.
A group of glands with foamy cytoplasm and deceivingly benign appearance at a low magnification (*a*). At higher magnification, the tumor cells demonstrate foamy cytoplasm and nuclear atypia with occasional nucleoli (*b*).

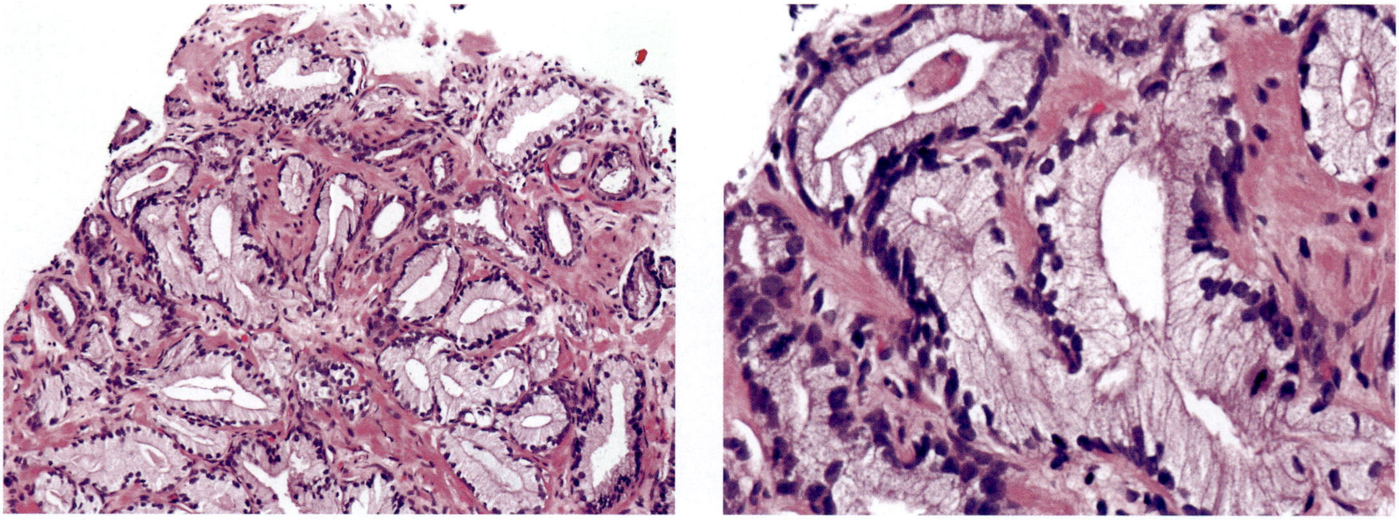

a **b**

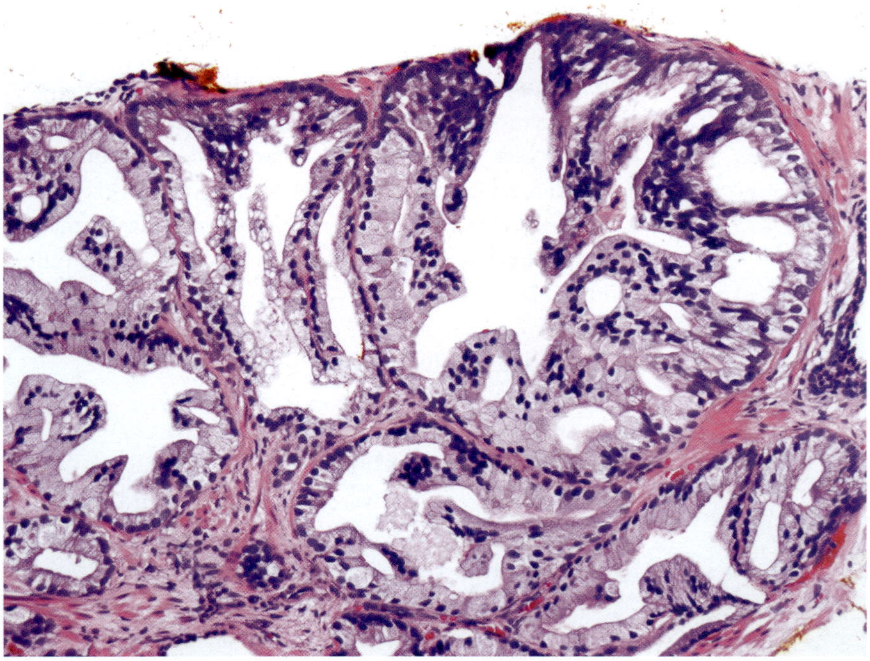

Figure 10-10.
Foamy gland adenocarcinoma: several large glands for cribriform patterns and foamy cytoplasm.

Figure 10-11.
A case of foamy gland adenocarcinoma with minimal cytological atypia and abundant foamy cytoplasm on H&E section (*a*), a diagnosis of carcinoma is made with the help of triple immunostaining showing strong AMACR reactivity and no basal cells (*b*).

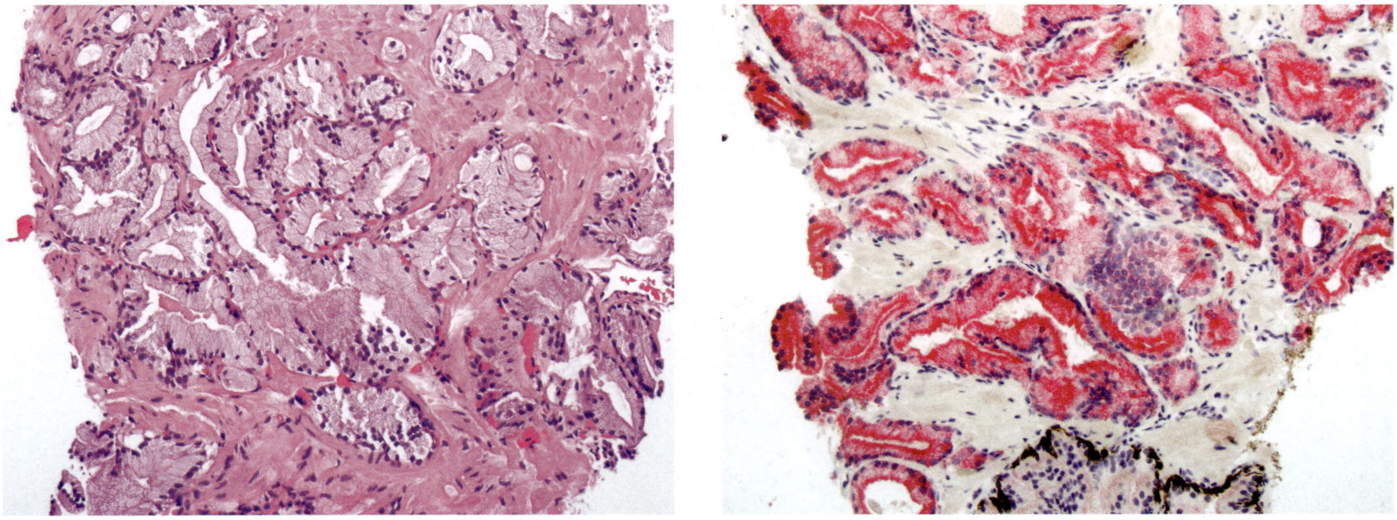

a **b**

MUCINOUS ADENOCARCINOMA

Definition

- Prostatic adenocarcinoma characterized by tumor cells producing abundant mucin

Other terms

- Colloid carcinoma

Pathogenesis

- Tumor cells producing a large amount of mucin

Clinical features

- Same as conventional adenocarcinoma

Gross pathology

- Myxoid or mucinous areas

Histology

- Abundant intracellular or extracellular mucin associated with adenocarcinoma (Figs. 10-12 and 10-13)
- Typically tumor cells show Gleason pattern 4 with glandular fusion
- Rarely a pure form, often mixed with conventional acinar adenocarcinoma (Fig. 10-13)
- In rare cases, conventional acinar adenocarcinoma may undergo focal mucinous metaplasia (Fig. 10-14)
- Collagenous micronodules (mucinous fibroplasia) may be present, but they are not exclusively associated with mucin production
- Grading of special variants of prostatic adenocarcinoma is summarized in Table 10-2

Immunohistochemistry

- AMACR weakly positive, ERG positive, and basal cell markers negative
- MUC8 may be positive

Clinical relevance (prognosis and treatment options)

- Typically behavior as Gleason pattern 4 (Gleason score 7 or above)

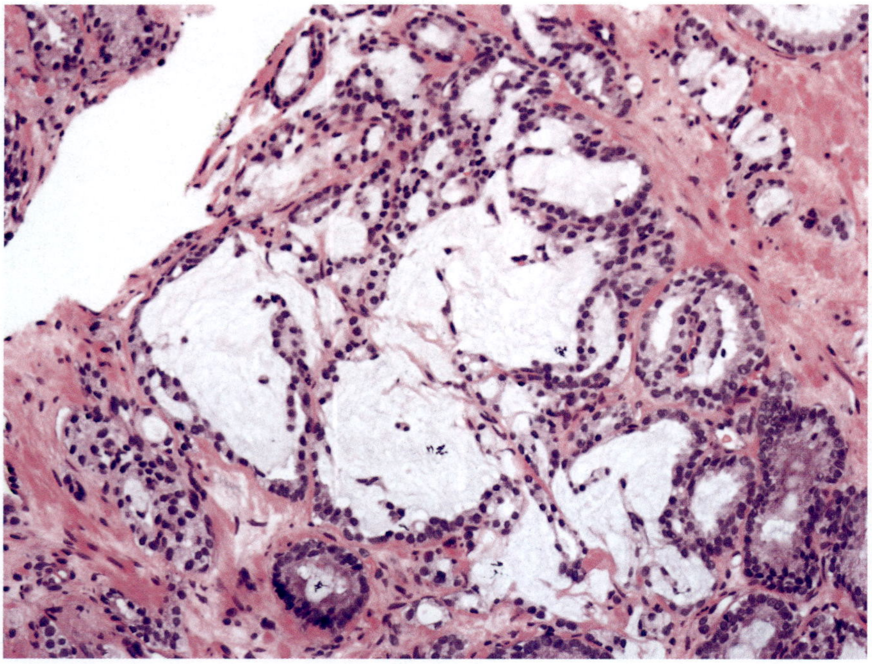

Figure 10-12. Adenocarcinoma with abundant mucin production.

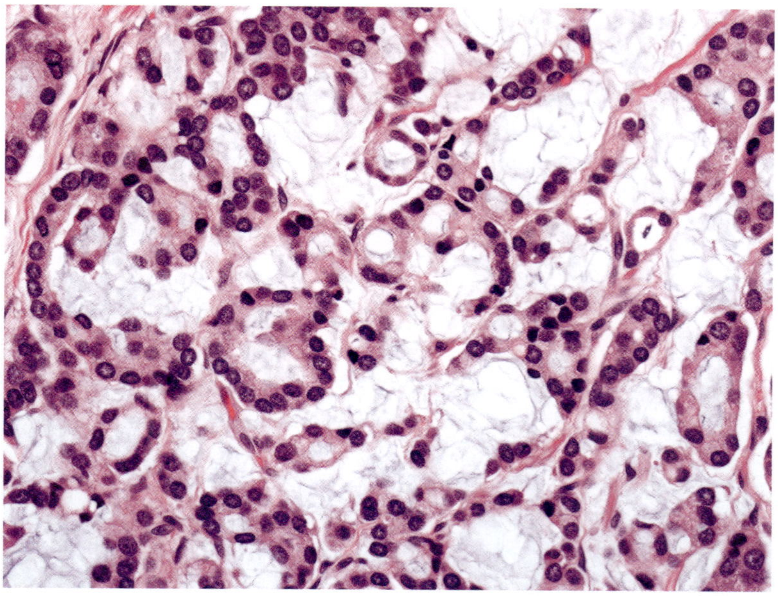

Figure 10-13.
Mucinous adenocarcinoma contains a large amount of mucin and cribriform patterns.

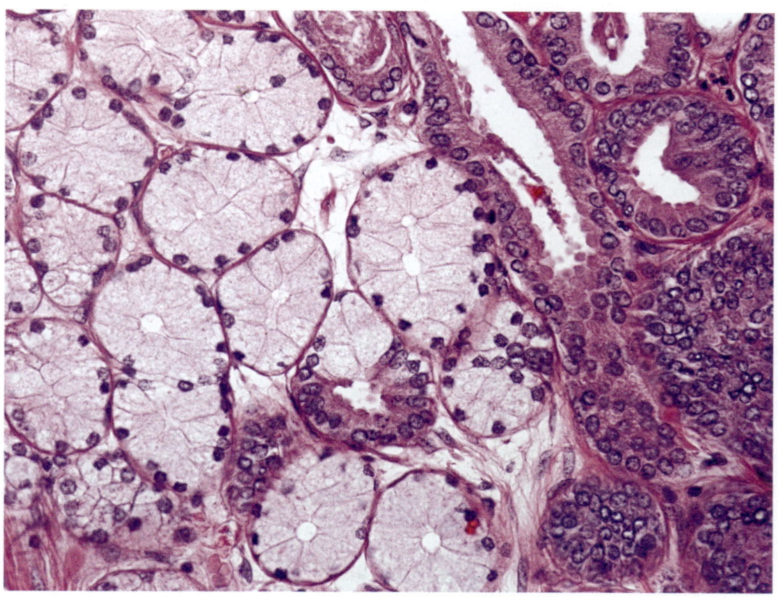

Figure 10-14.
Adenocarcinoma undergoing mucinous differentiation (left) next to typical adenocarcinoma (right).

Table 10-2. Grading Unusual Variants

Adenocarcinoma variants	*Corresponding Gleason pattern*
Mucinous (type)	4
Foamy gland (type)	4
Pseudohyperplastic type	3
Large gland type	3
Atrophic type	3
Signet ring type	4 to 5
Ductal adenocarcinoma	4

SIGNET RING CELL CARCINOMA

- Signet ring cell carcinoma is a special morphological variant of prostatic adenocarcinoma
- It is characterized by the presence of vacuoles in the tumor cells (Fig. 10-15)
- But the vacuoles may not be mucin, but intracellular lumen or dissolved fat in the cytoplasm
- The presence of intracellular lumen and microvilli has been observed using electron microscopy
- It is commonly seen in a high-grade tumor, in which conventional high-grade adenocarcinoma can also be seen. It is associated with aggressive behavior
- The tumor is graded as Gleason pattern 4 (with irregular lumen) or pattern 5 (without lumen formation by the tumor cells) (Fig. 10-16)

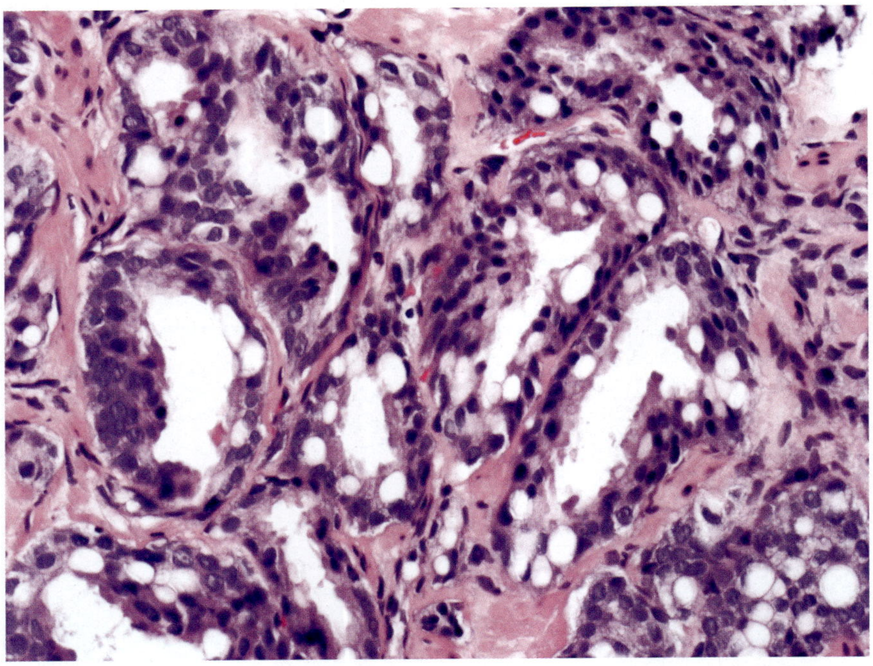

Figure 10-15.
Adenocarcinoma cells with prominent large vacuole in the cytoplasm, resembling signet rings.

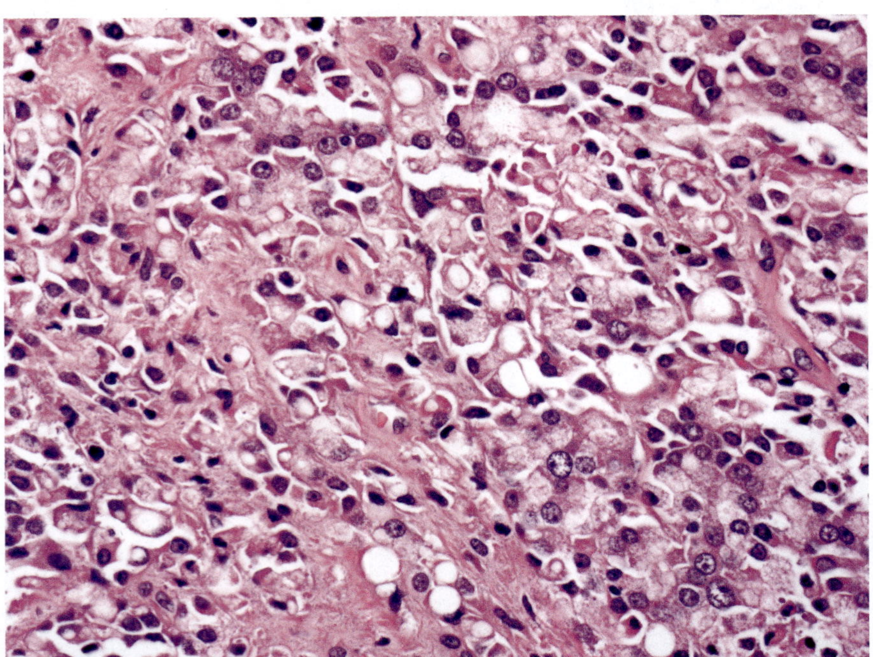

Figure 10-16.
Signet ring carcinoma. High-grade (Gleason pattern 5) adenocarcinoma with intracytoplasmic vacuoles, resembling signet rings.

PSEUDOHYPERPLASTIC ADENOCARCINOMA

- Adenocarcinoma cells forming large benign-appearing glands mimicking benign prostatic hyperplasia (Figs. 10-17 to 10-19)
- Pathogenesis is unknown, but probably similar to conventional acinar adenocarcinoma
- Nuclear atypia present but may not be obvious
- No basal cells, confirmed by immunostaining (Fig. 10-17*c*)
- AMACR can be positive either strong or weak (Figs. 10-18*b* and 10-19*b*)
- It is important to recognize this pattern particularly on needle core biopsies since it can be mimicking benign hyperplastic lesions

Figure 10-17.
Pseudohyperplastic adenocarcinoma composed of numerous large glands with deceiving benign appearance on a needle core biopsy (*a*). Higher magnification (*b*) shows the straight luminal borders with minimal cytological atypia, but lack of basal cell staining (*c*).

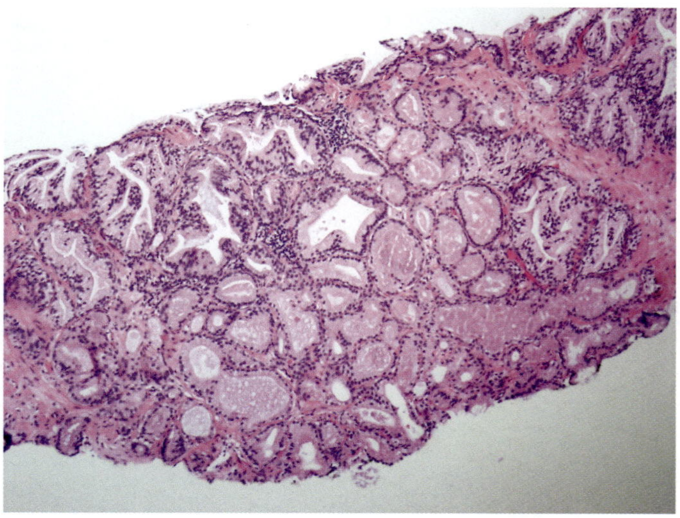

a

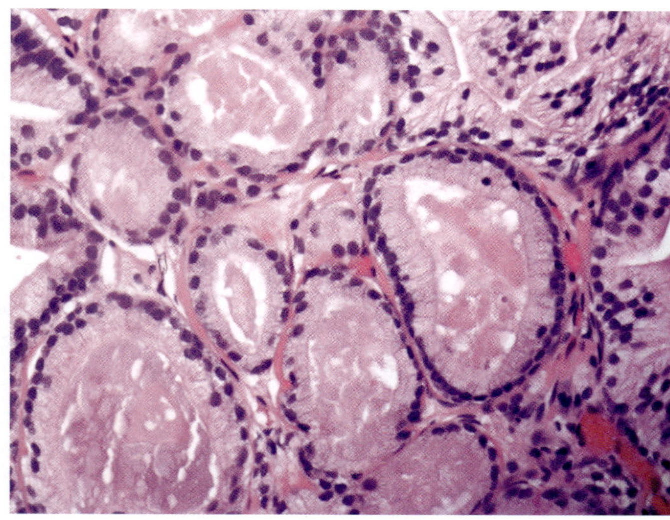

b

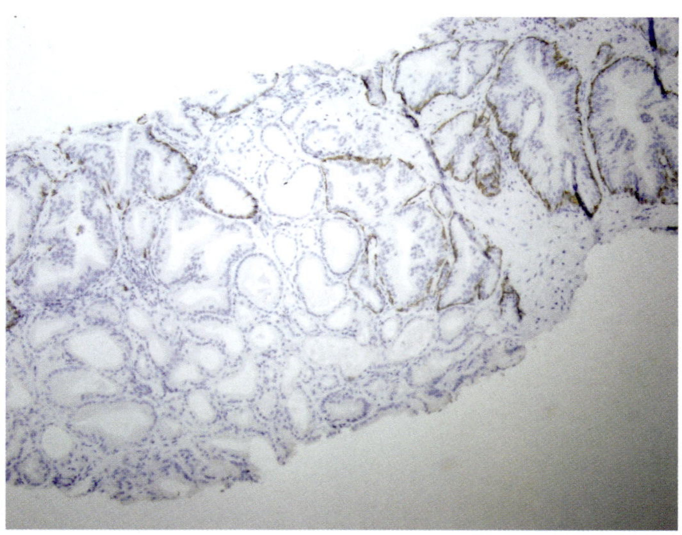

c

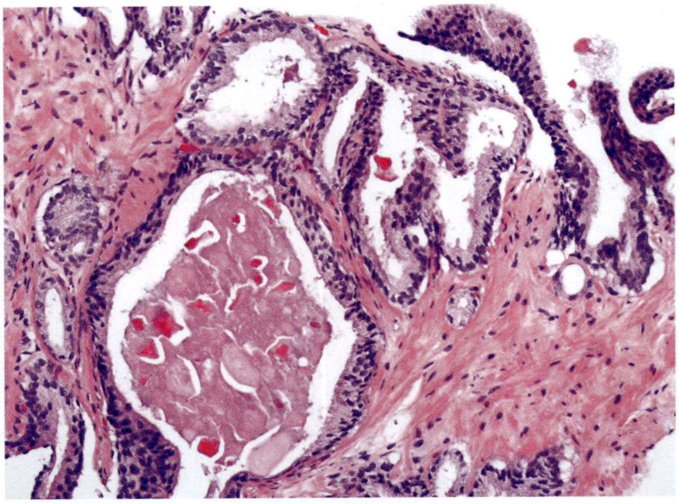

a

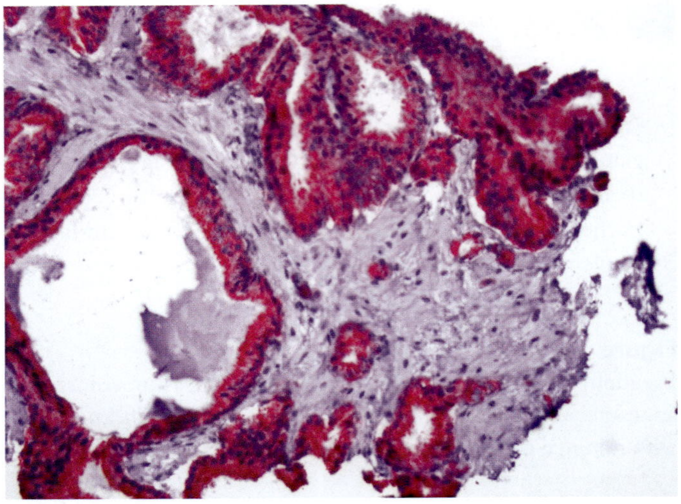

b

Figure 10-18.
Pseudohyperplastic adenocarcinoma contains a group of benign looking glands (*a*), triple staining shows the tumor cells strongly positive for AMACR and negative for basal cell staining (*b*).

Figure 10-19.
Large foamy gland carcinoma. Two large glands and several adjacent smaller glands with foamy cytoplasm on needle core biopsy; no obvious nuclear atypia can be appreciated except for the straight luminal borders (*a*). Triple immunostaining (*b*) shows the two large malignant glands (AMACR weakly positive with no basal cells).

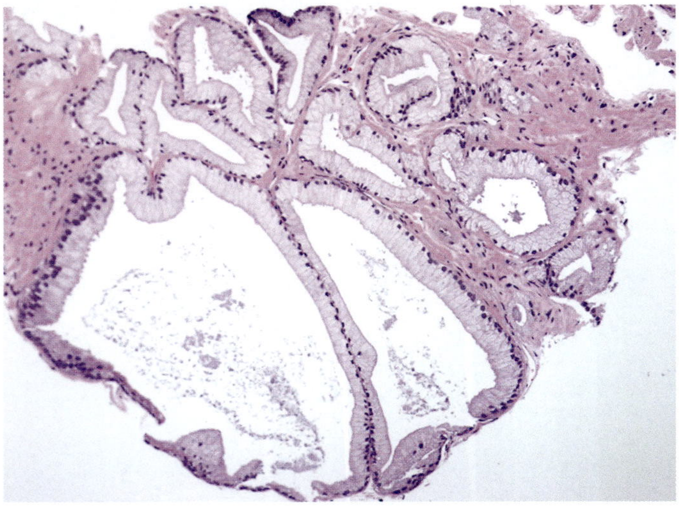

a

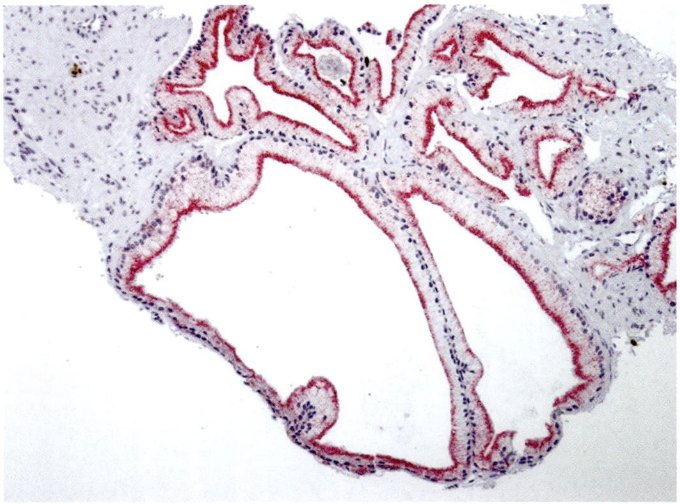

b

LARGE GLAND ADENOCARCINOMA

- Tumor cells are characterized by very large dilated glands (Figs. 10-20 and 10-21)
- Not known to be associated with aggressiveness
- The malignant large glands with straight luminal border (Fig. 10-20*a*) and prominent nucleoli present (Fig. 10-20*b*)
- AMACR positive, and no basal cells (Figs. 10-20*d*, 10-21*b*, and 10-21*c*)
- The infiltrating patterns are difficult to appreciate
- It can be misdiagnosed as cystic atrophy
- They are usually not present alone, but mixed with conventional adenocarcinoma

Figure 10-20.
Large gland carcinoma is composed of several very large dilated glands (*a*). Between the large glands, there are several small malignant glands with typical features of carcinoma (*b*). Higher magnification (*c*) shows the flat lining epithelium has small round nuclei. The triple stain (*d*) confirms the large and small glands are all malignant.

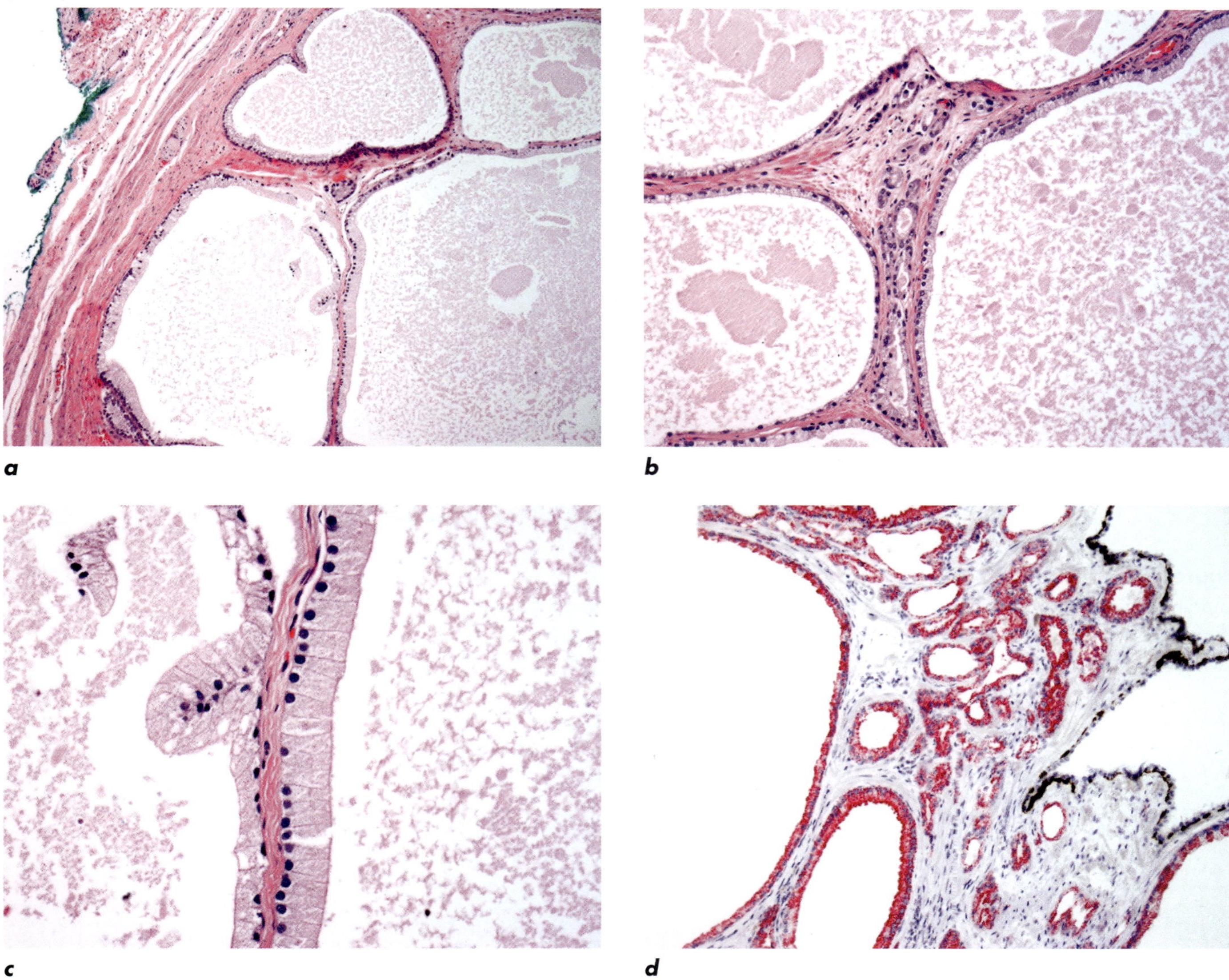

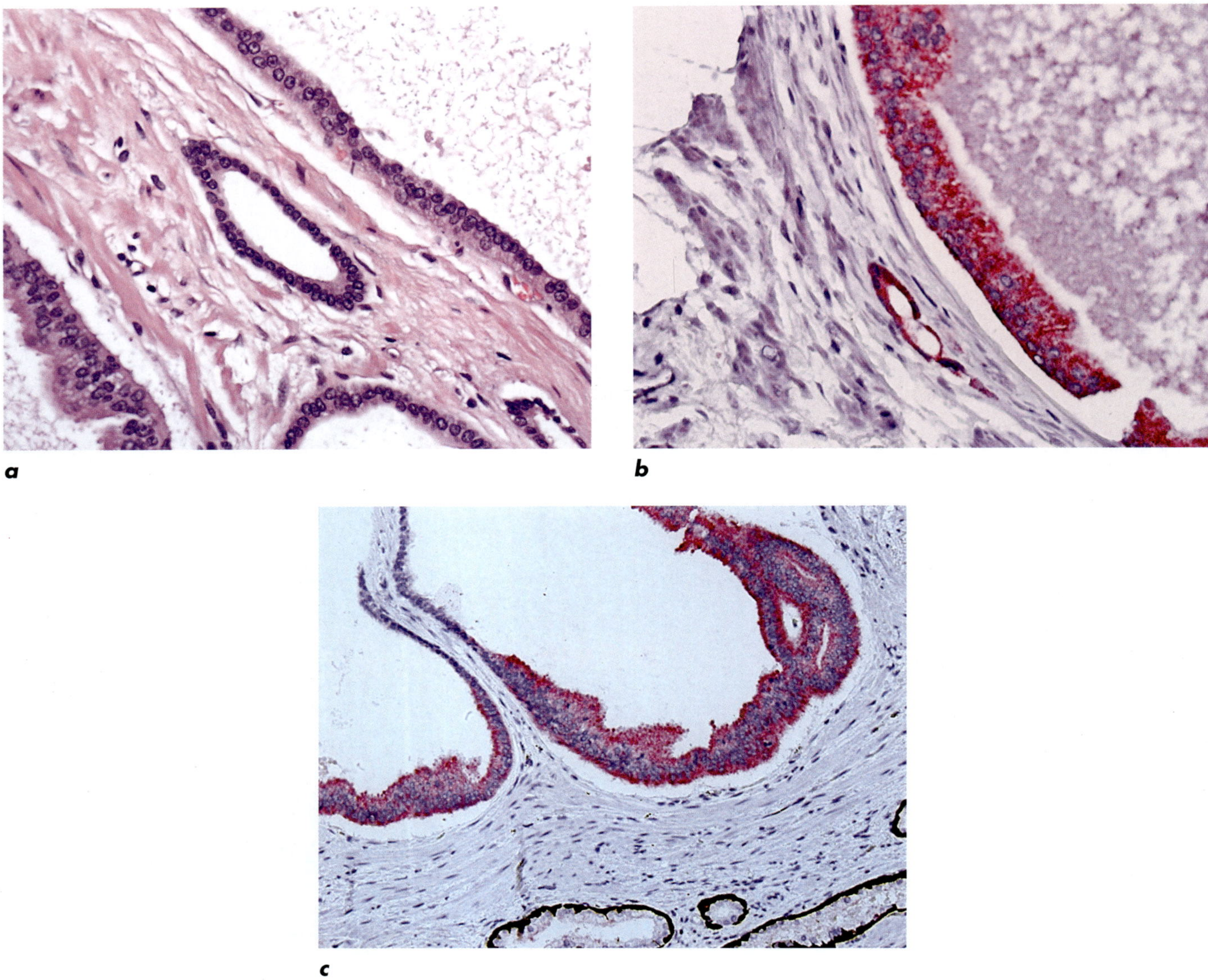

Figure 10-21.
Another large gland carcinoma with straight luminal borders and flat lining epithelium (*a*). The triple immunostain (*b, c*) confirms the malignant nature of the large glands with strong AMACR immunoreactivity.

ATROPHIC ADENOCARCINOMA

- Characteristic of tumor cells with scant cytoplasm forming atrophic glands (Figs. 10-22 and 10-23)
- Nuclear atypia is not obvious because of the compression of the nuclei by the cytoplasm (Fig. 10-23*c*)
- This type of carcinoma can be easily missed on needle core biopsy because of the subtle cytological atypia
- The key for diagnosis is its infiltrating patterns (Fig. 10-22*a*) and the coexistent typical adenocarcinoma
- Application of immunochemistry will be helpful (Figs. 10-23*b* and 10-23*d*)
- Adenocarcinoma undergoing atrophic changes after treatment will be discussed in separate chapters

Figure 10-22.

Atrophic adenocarcinoma. A cluster of small atrophic glands present between two large benign glands. The infiltrating patterns and presence of intraluminal blue mucin and crystalloids (*a*) suggest the diagnosis of carcinoma. At high magnification (*b*), the presence of subtle nuclear atypia can be seen, confirming the diagnosis of atrophic adenocarcinoma.

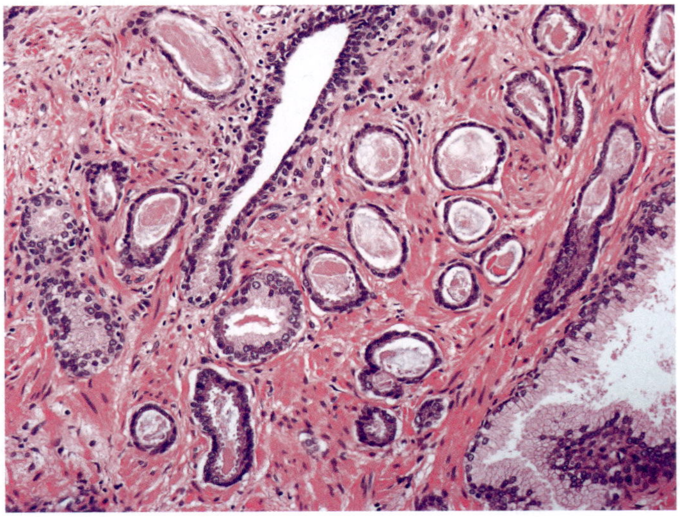

a

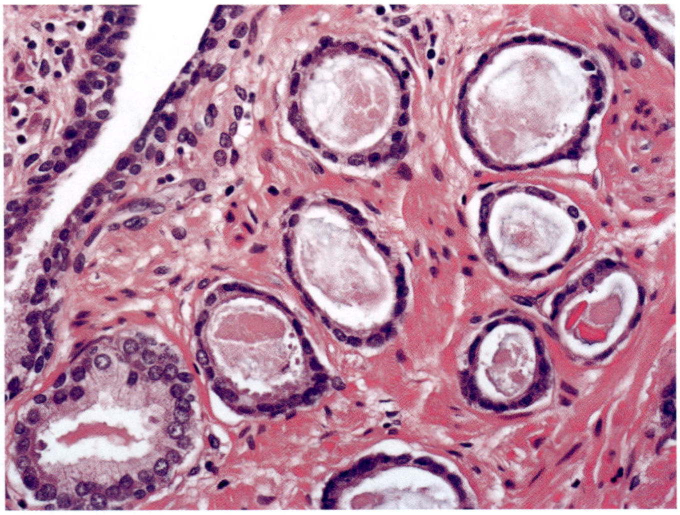

b

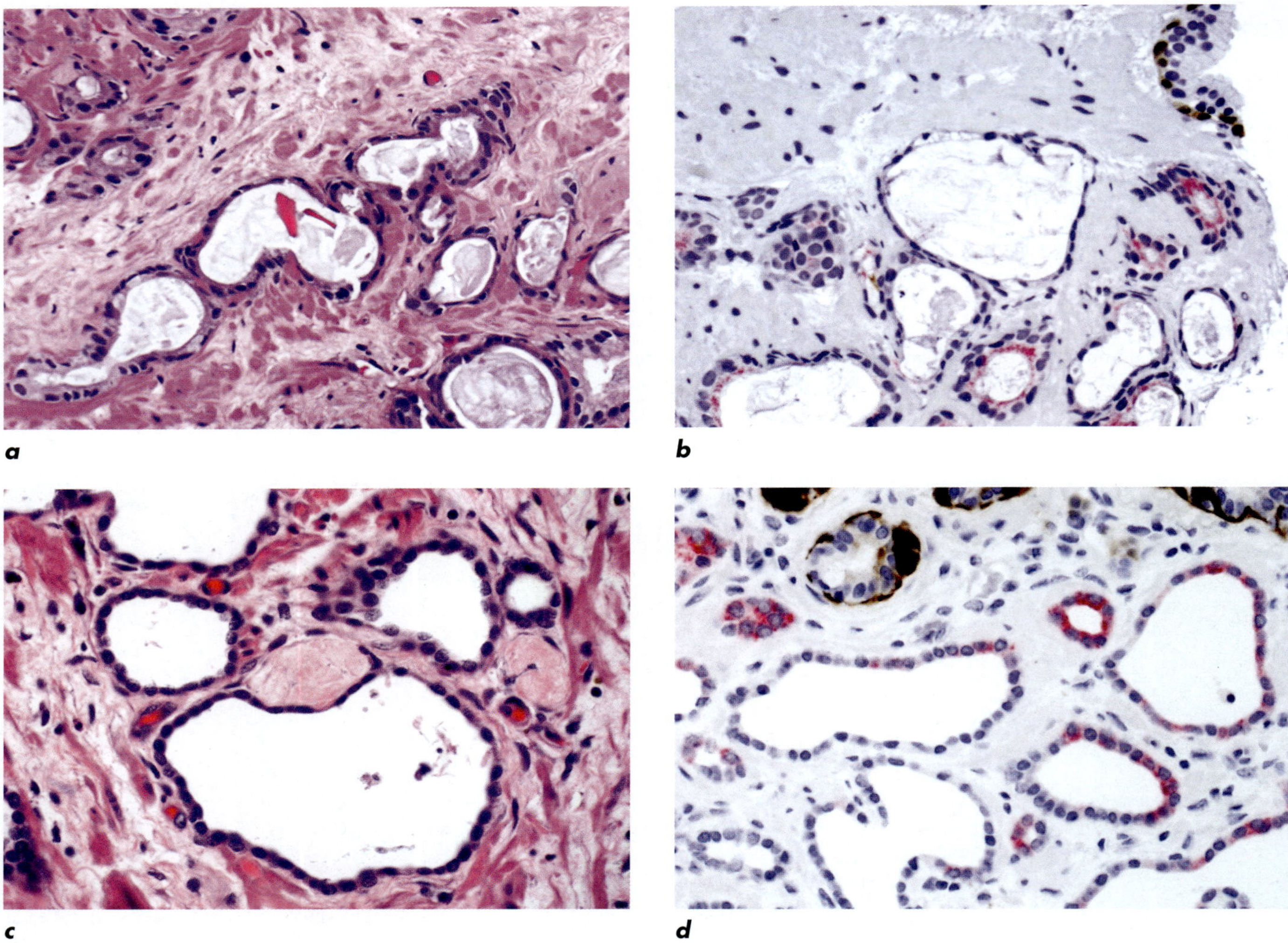

Figure 10-23.
Atrophic adenocarcinoma adjacent to typical adenocarcinoma on the left upper corner (*a*). By triple immunostaining (*b*), the nature of these malignant cells is confirmed (AMACR positive, basal cell markers negative). Another case of atrophic carcinoma composed of a few dilated glands with flat epithelial cells with minimal cytological atypia (*c*). However, two collagenous nodules are present. Triple immunostaining confirms the lack of basal cells and AMACR immunoreactivity in the atrophic malignant glands (*d*).

NEUROENDOCRINE DIFFERENTIATION OF PROSTATIC ADENOCARCINOMA

Definition

- Neuroendocrine cells are present in normal prostatic glands
- Neuroendocrine differentiation can be seen in high-grade PIN or prostatic adenocarcinoma as neoplastic components

Pathogenesis

- Neuroendocrine cells (NEC) secrete peptide hormones, which regulate cell growth and differentiation
- Neoplastic neuroendocrine cells are also secreting hormones, which may contribute to the continuous growth and aggressiveness of the tumor

Clinical features

- Normally neuroendocrine cells are present in the prostatic glandular compartments. However, the number of these cells is small, so that serum levels of neuroendocrine markers are not detectable in a man without prostate cancer
- In many cases of prostatic adenocarcinoma, there may be a small subset of malignant neuroendocrine cells scattered throughout the tumor. The clinical significance of scattered neuroendocrine cells in prostatic adenocarcinoma is unknown
- In high-grade prostatic adenocarcinoma, particularly androgen independent cancer, there is an increased number of neuroendocrine cells, which may lead to increased serum levels of neuroendocrine markers such as chromogranin

Gross pathology

- Not grossly visible

Histology

- Generally speaking, neuroendocrine cells cannot be identified in a normal or benign prostate on the H&E-stained sections
- By immunostaining specific for neuroendocrine markers, such as chromogranin, neuron specific enolase, or synaptophysin, one or two neuroendocrine cells may be highlighted in a normal prostatic gland (Fig. 10-24)
- The neuroendocrine cell hyperplasia is not a well-defined condition. We are not sure how many NEC should be present in normal glands because almost all the prostate specimens that we see in surgical pathology are not totally "normal"
- The neuroendocrine cells are located in the basal cell compartment or between secretory cells and basal cells
- By immunostaining, they are irregular in shape: columnar, oval, or triangular
- Sometimes star-like with long cytoplasmic projections (Fig. 10-24*b*)

Figure 10-24.
A benign prostatic gland with no neuroendocrine cells can be identified on H&E-stained section (*a*). Chromogranin stain (*b*) showing several neuroendocrine cells in this gland.

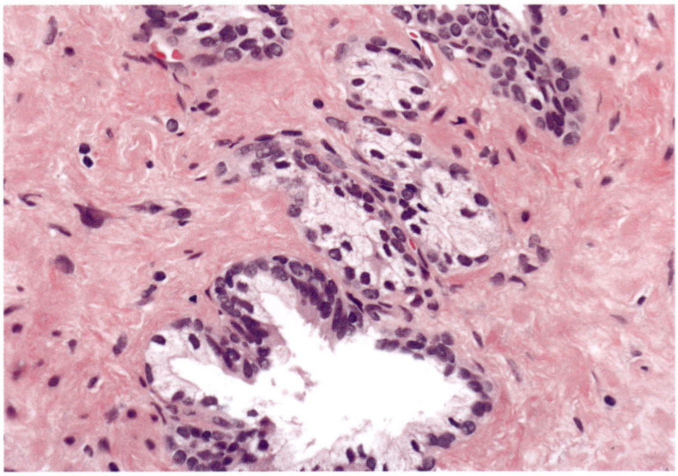

a

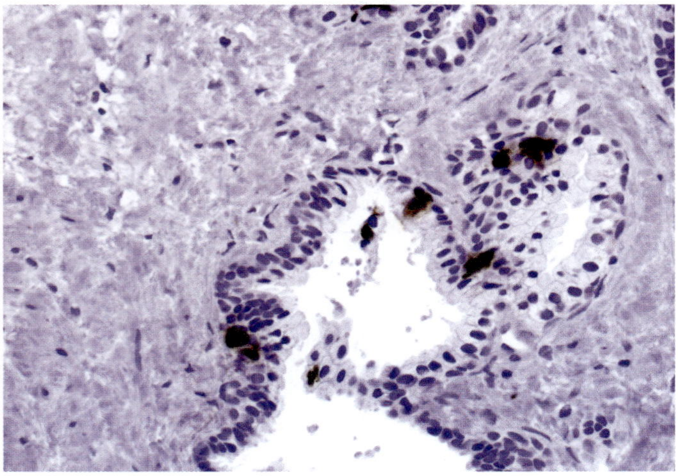

b

- Occasionally, neuroendocrine cells can be identified on H&E-stained section, when they have eosinophilic neuroendocrine secretory granules in the cytoplasm of benign or neoplastic epithelial cells of the prostate (Figs. 10-25 and 10-26). This change is also known as Paneth cell metaplasia
- In prostatic adenocarcinoma, 5% to 10% of unselected cases will show focal neuroendocrine differentiation by chromogranin immunostaining. The number of neuroendocrine cells in each case of prostatic adenocarcinoma is variable, ranging from a few to more than 50% of tumor cells positive for neuroendocrine markers (Fig. 10-27)
- In high-grade prostatic adenocarcinoma, sometimes, the presence of neuroendocrine differentiation can be appreciated when "salt-and-pepper" chromatin is present (Fig. 10-28)
- The conditions with neuroendocrine cells in the prostate are summarized in Table 10-3

Immunohistochemistry

- Chromogranin A (Figs. 10-24*b* and 10-27), synaptophysin (Fig. 10-28*b*), neuron specific enolase, and p56 are positive in neuroendocrine cells

Clinical relevance (prognosis and treatment options)

- High-grade prostatic adenocarcinoma along with small cell carcinoma with a large number of neuroendocrine cells have a poor prognosis. The patients with these tumors may need adjuvant chemotherapy for a systemic disease
- If a patient with prostate cancer has neuroendocrine differentiation and elevated serum chromogranin level, this finding may be used for monitoring the treatment effects and possible recurrent status
- Carcinoid tumor in the prostate will be similar to the one in other organs
- The clinical significance of focal neuroendocrine differentiation in adenocarcinoma is not known

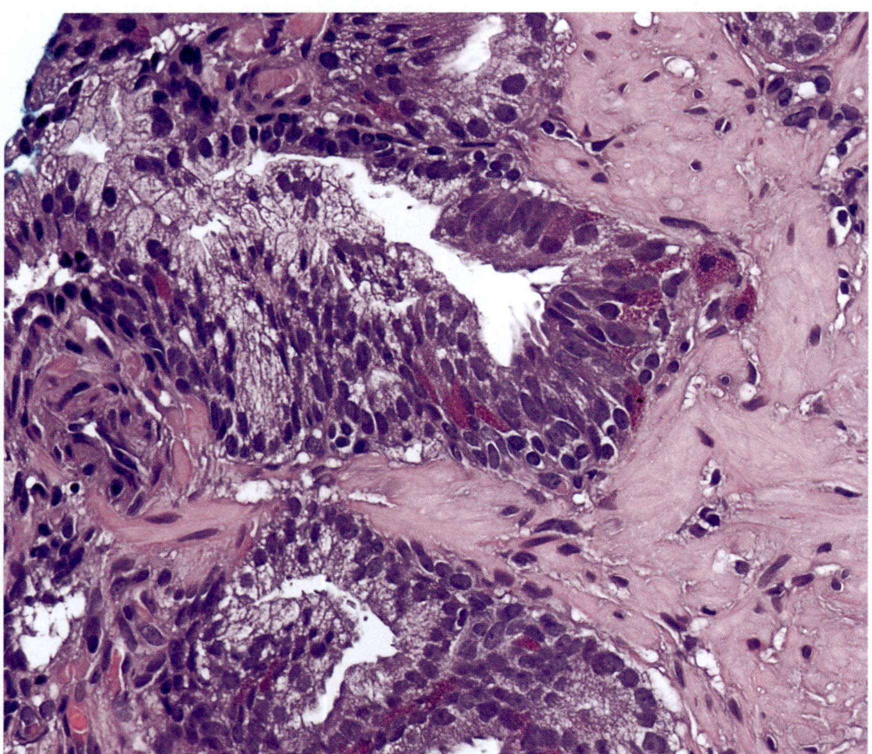

Figure 10-25.
High-grade PIN containing a few neoplastic cells with large eosinophilic granules.

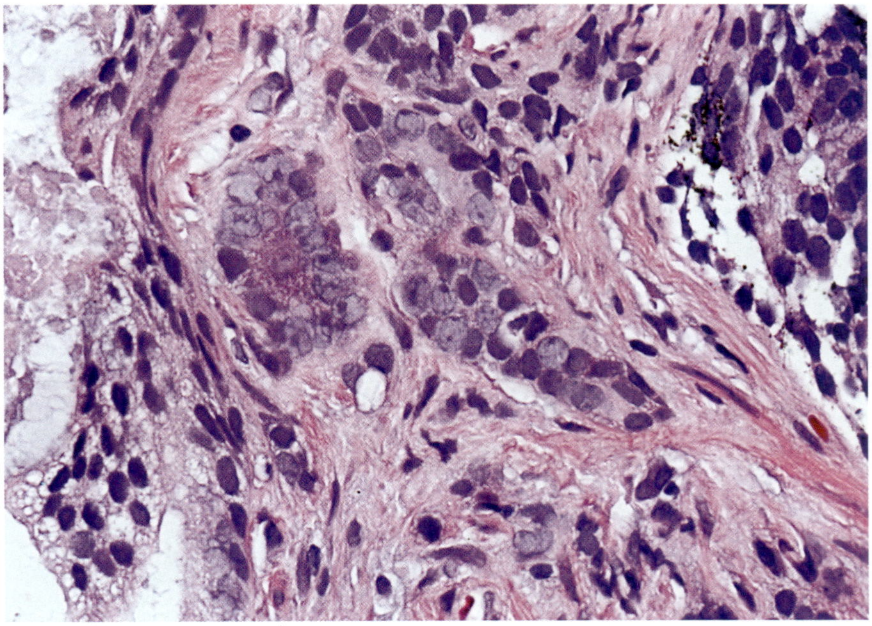

Figure 10-26.
Prostatic adenocarcinoma cells contain large eosinophilic granules in the cytoplasm.

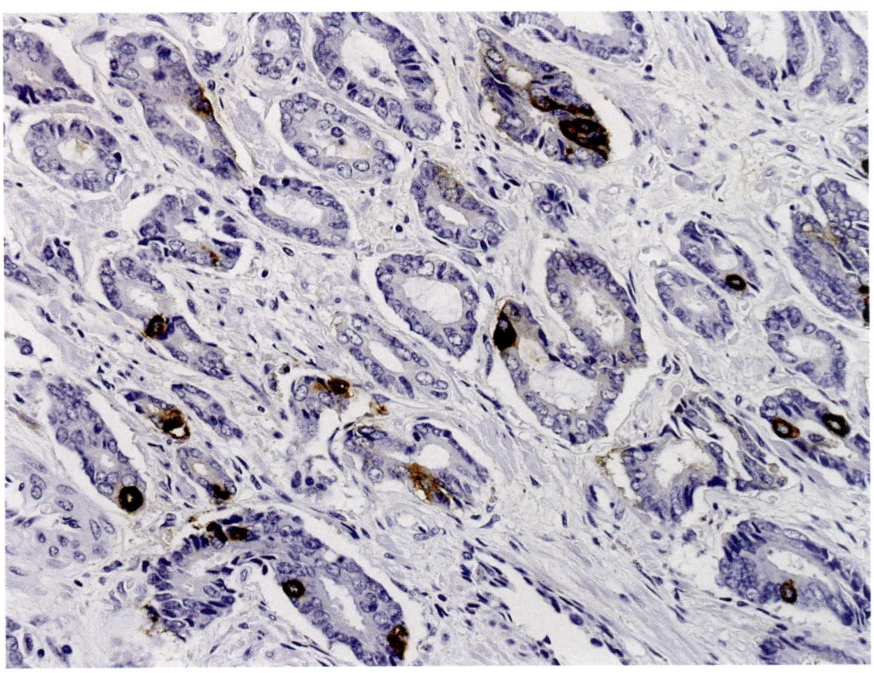

Figure 10-27.
Gleason score 3 + 3 adenocarcinoma with 10% neuroendocrine cells in well-formed glandular structures confirmed by chromogranin staining.

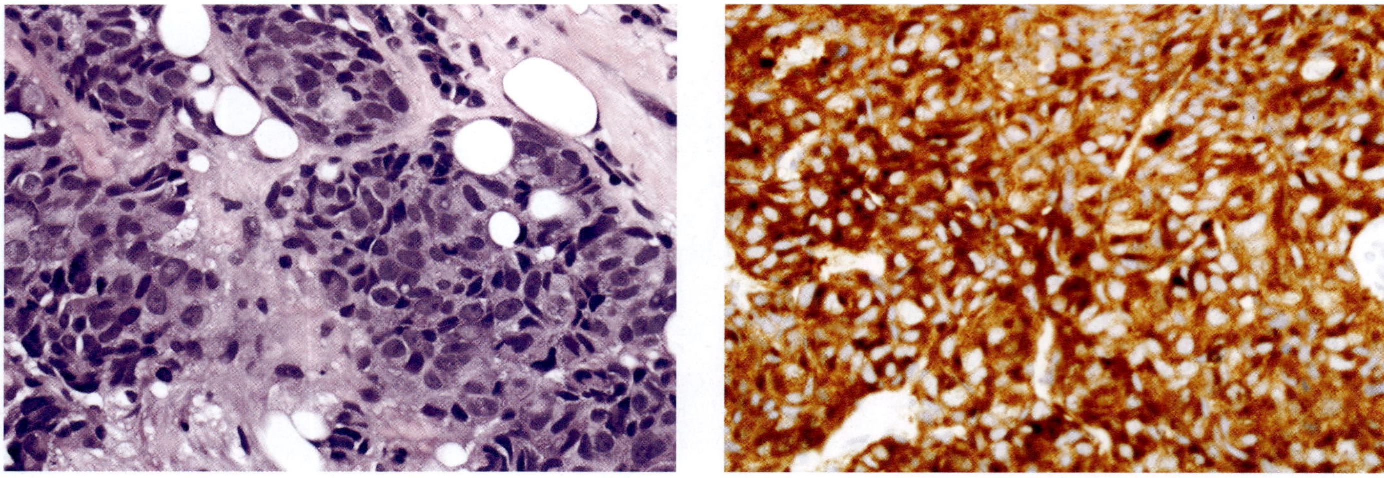

a *b*

Figure 10-28.
Gleason score 5 + 5 adenocarcinoma show extensive neuroendocrine differentiation with characteristic "salt-and-pepper" chromatin patterns (*a*). The positive synaptophysin immunostaining confirms the nature of neuroendocrine differentiation of the tumor cells (*b*).

Table 10-3. Conditions of Neuroendocrine Cells in the Prostate

Neuroendocrine cells	*H&E*	*Neuroendocrine markers*	*Clinical significance*
Normal prostate	Not visible	Scattered positive cells	No (normal)
	Intracytoplamic eosinophilic granules	Rare positive cells	No
High-grade PIN	Eosinophilic granules	Rare positive cells	Not known
Adenocarcinoma	Not visible	Focally positive cells	Not known
	Salt-and-pepper chromatin	Diffusely positive cells >50%	Systemic treatment needed
Carcinoid	Typical carcinoid features	Diffusely positive cells	Low-grade malignancy similar to carcinoid of other organs
Small cell carcinoma	Small cells with molding, salt-and-pepper chromatin, high mitotic counts	Diffusely positive	Chemotherapy candidate

H&E, hematoxylin and eosin.

CHAPTER 11 Special Treatment Effects on the Prostate

POSTRADIATION CHANGES IN BENIGN PROSTATIC GLANDS

Definition

- Histological changes in the benign prostatic tissue induced by radiation applied as treatment of prostate cancer or other pelvic neoplasms

Other terms

- Postradiation atypia in the prostate, radiation changes in the prostate

Pathogenesis

- Radiation is one of the major treatment options for patients with prostate cancer
- The prostate can also be irradiated in the radiation field when other tumors in the pelvis are being irradiated
- Radiation may induce marked changes in benign prostatic tissue in addition to changes in adenocarcinoma cells

Clinical features

- Typical scenario is that a patient with a history of prostate cancer, status postradiation now presents with an elevated serum PSA level
- Prostate needle core biopsy is performed to rule out recurrent or persistent prostate cancer
- Postradiation changes can been seen in a prostate with adenocarcinoma
- Postradiation changes are common findings in a radical salvage prostatectomy specimen from a patient with a history of pelvic radiation with or without prostate cancer

Gross pathology

- No specific changes
- Radiation will cause increased fibrotic tissue and scarring of the prostate

Histology

- Postradiation stromal changes (Fig. 11-1)
  - Dilated small vessels with prominent endothelium or hyalinization
  - Increased lymphocytic infiltrates in the stroma
  - Fibrosis may be present but it is difficult to appreciate on biopsy
- Postradiation epithelial changes (Figs. 11-1 and 11-2)
  - Irregularity of the glands
  - Nuclear enlargement two to three times the size of normal secretory cells
  - The characteristic features of degenerative atypia are no mitotic activity, smudged chromatin, with or without prominent nucleoli
  - Streaming appearance and arrangement of the atypical nuclei
  - These changes can persist years after radiation

Immunohistochemistry

- AMACR negative in the benign glands with postradiation atypia (Figs. 11-3 and 11-4)
- Basal cell markers (p63 and HMWCK) positive; most of the atypical cells are basal cells in nature (Figs. 11-3 and 11-4)

Molecular analysis

- Not indicated

Clinical relevance (prognosis and treatment options)

- Although the elevation of PSA strongly indicates the recurrence of prostate cancer in a patient with radiation, the definitive diagnosis of recurrent prostatic adenocarcinoma has to be based on histological evidence of carcinoma
- The postradiation atypia in the benign prostatic glands appears to be more pleomorphic than cancer cells, which can be mistakenly diagnosed as adenocarcinoma if one is not familiar with these histological characteristics

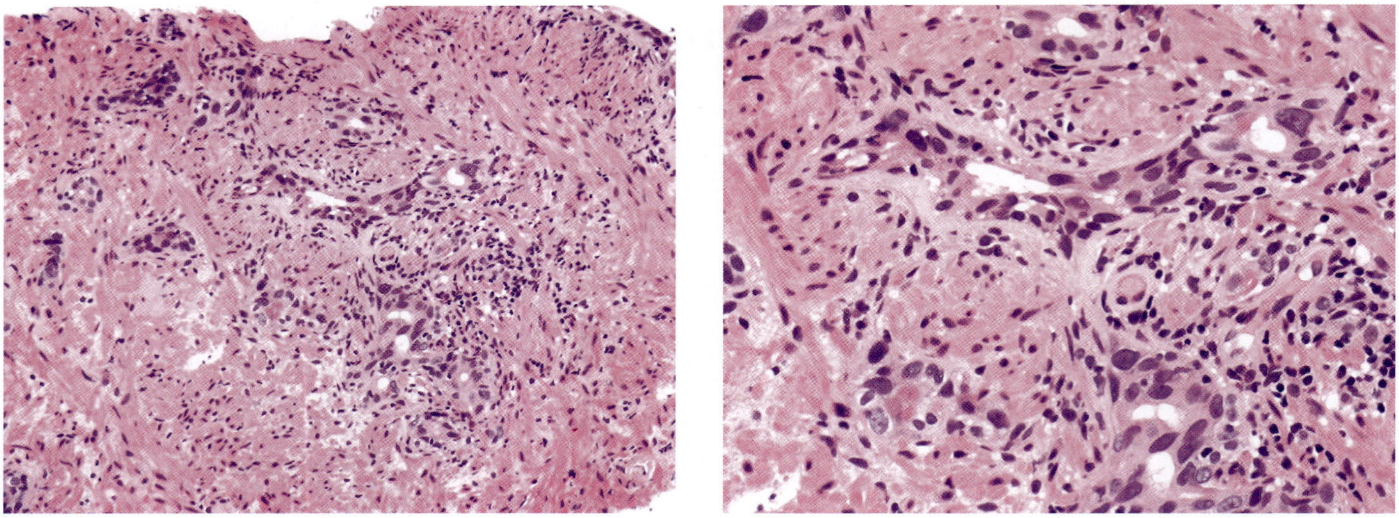

a b

Figure 11-1.
Benign glands with postradiation atypia display architectural distortion and chronic inflammation (*a*). High magnification shows the prominent cytological atypia with a "streaming" appearance where elongated epithelial nuclei are parallel to each other (*b*).

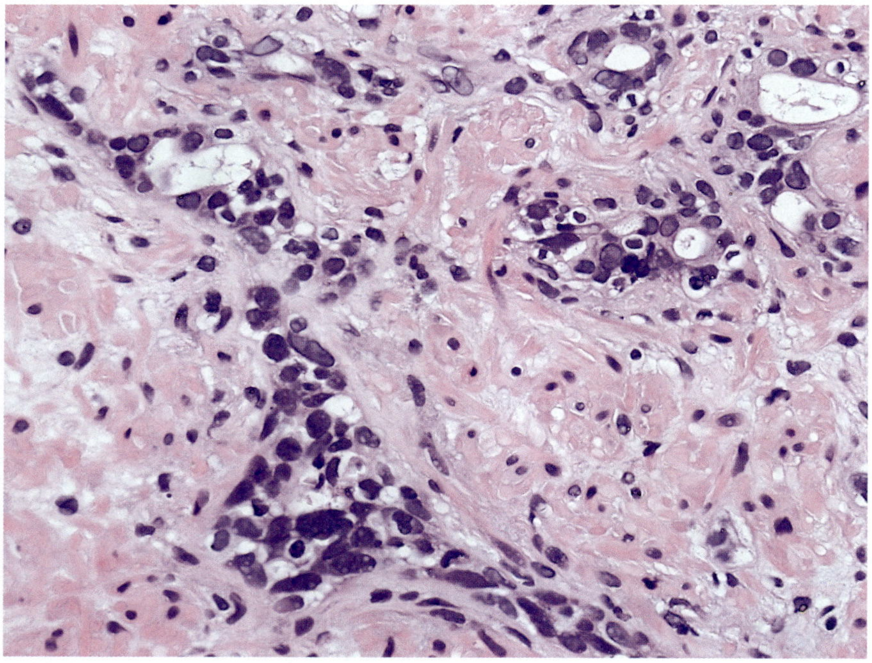

Figure 11-2.
Benign glands with postradiation changes showing degenerative atypia without mitosis. Streaming appearance is evident.

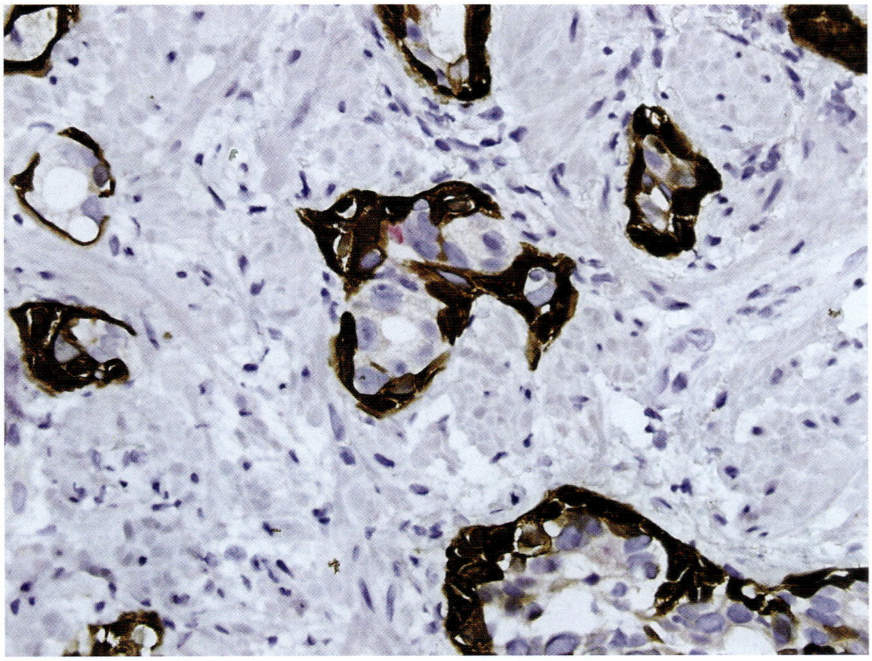

Figure 11-3.
Immunostaining confirms the presence of basal cells in the atypical irradiated benign glands without AMACR reactivity.

Figure 11-4.
A few distorted benign glands with prominent cytological atypia on H&E section (*a*); immunostaining (*b*) confirms the basal cell nature of these atypical cells (p63 and HWMCK positive).

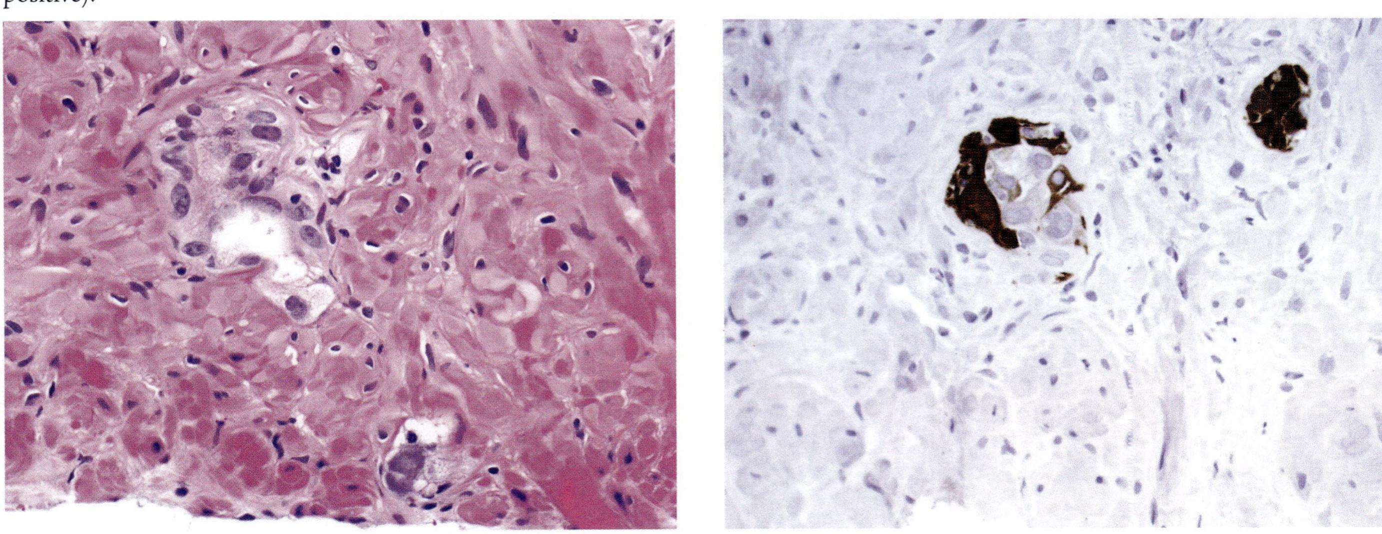

a

b

POSTRADIATION CHANGES IN PROSTATIC ADENOCARCINOMA

Definition

- Radiation induces cell death and other histological changes in prostatic adenocarcinoma
- Most morphologic changes of postradiation prostate reported in literature were obtained from the cases with external beam radiation. Brachytherapy (radioactive seeding) induces the histological changes, which are indistinguishable from those caused by external beam radiation
- Postradiation changes can also be seen in a radical salvage prostatectomy specimen from a patient with a history of pelvic radiation

Other terms

- Recurrent adenocarcinoma postradiation, persistent adenocarcinoma postradiation

Pathogenesis

- Radiation, as one of the major treatment options for the patients with prostate cancer, will induce marked changes in adenocarcinoma cells

Clinical features

- Typical scenario is that a patient with a history of prostate cancer, status postradiation now presents with an elevated serum PSA level
- Prostate needle core biopsy is performed to determine the presence of recurrent/persistent prostate cancer

Gross pathology

- No specific changes
- Radiation will cause increased fibrotic tissue and scarring of the prostate
- The presence of yellowish spots of adenocarcinoma may be identified

Histology

Several types of changes have been observed in a postradiation setting:

- Early postradiation changes a few days or weeks after radiation are rarely seen in clinical specimens. Most adenocarcinoma cells show necrosis, marked degenerative changes along with edema, and acute inflammatory infiltrates in the stroma
- Late changes in adenocarcinoma occur a few years after radiation. The tumor cells are small, in single cells or in clusters infiltrating the stroma. The tumor cells are bland with minimal cytological atypia (Fig. 11-5). Adjacent benign glands show cytological atypia as discussed previously (Fig. 11-6). The tumor cells may show poorly formed glands (Fig. 11-7). Well-formed glandular structures are not commonly seen

Figure 11-5.
Prostatic adenocarcinoma with postradiation effect. Scattered carcinoma cells (*a*, arrows) exhibit vacuolated cytoplasm with small nuclei. The infiltrating pattern of these cells indicates that they are malignant. Triple immunostaining (*b*) confirms the strong AMACR reactivity and lack of basal cells in these scattered carcinoma cells.

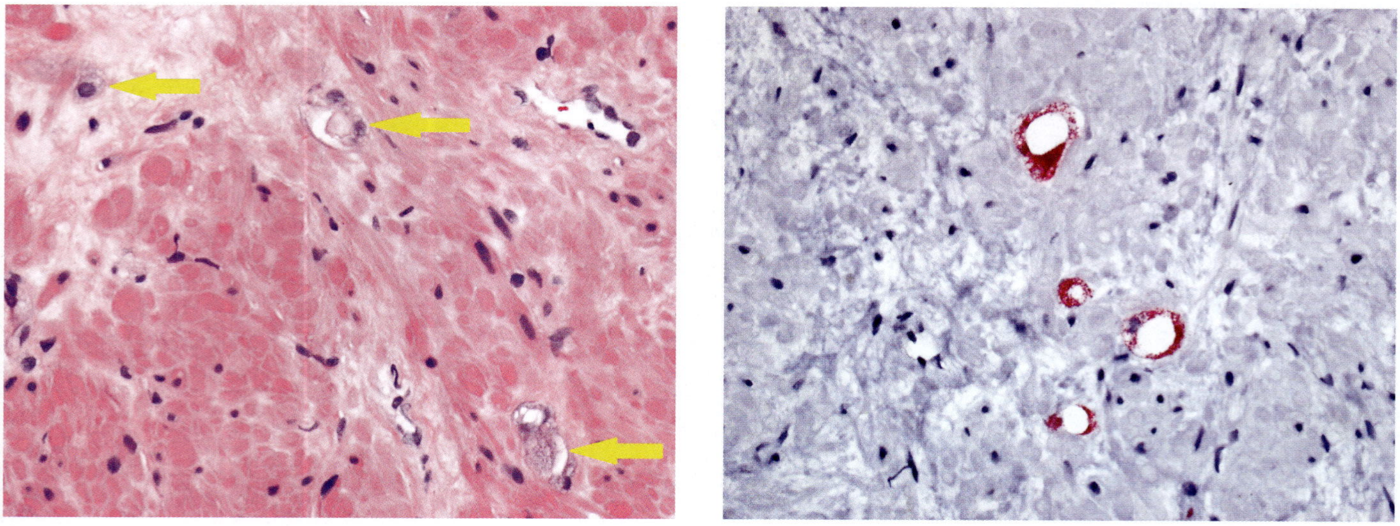

a **b**

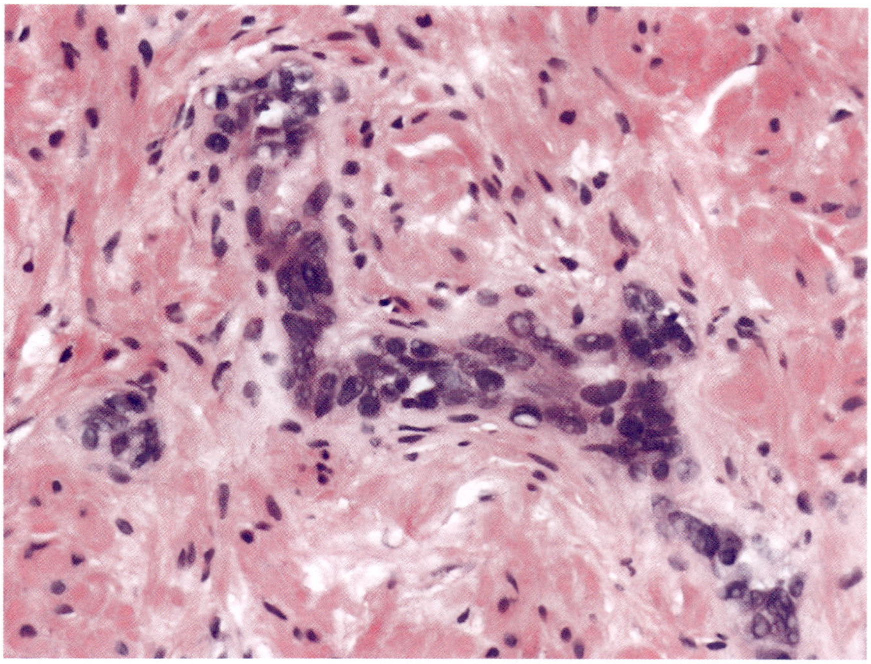

Figure 11-6.
Benign prostatic glands with postradiation atypia. In comparison to the bland malignant cells, the benign epithelial cells show marked cytological atypia.

- The diagnosis of adenocarcinoma postradiation is primarily based on the infiltrating patterns rather than the cytological appearance of the tumor cells, since benign epithelial cells often show more pleomorphic appearance (Fig. 11-6) than the malignant cells after radiation (Figs. 11-5 and 11-7)
- Some adenocarcinoma cells show no obvious or minimal cytological changes after radiation. These tumor cells may represent the population resistant to radiation
- As we previously mentioned, chronic inflammation, fibrosis, and marked cytological atypia can be seen in the benign prostatic tissue

Immunohistochemistry

- AMACR positive in postradiation prostatic adenocarcinoma (Figs. 11-5*b* and 11-7*c*)
- For some unknown reason, a single AMACR (brown) immunostain is more sensitive than the popular triple (AMACR, p63, and HWMCK) stain in highlighting the tumor cells
- Basal cell markers are negative in postradiation prostatic adenocarcinoma (Fig. 11-7*c*)
- PSA, PSMA may be positive in adenocarcinoma as well as benign glands, but the staining intensity tends to be variable

Clinical relevance (prognosis and treatment options)

- Recurrent prostatic adenocarcinoma cannot be distinguished from persistent prostatic adenocarcinoma in postradiation patients by histological features alone, so we use the term *"recurrent/persistent prostatic adenocarcinoma"* in the report
- These patients may require (salvage) radical prostatectomy although it is technically difficult because of extensive fibrosis and adhesion of the prostate to the adjacent organs after radiation
- Hormonal therapy and chemotherapy may also be an option in these cases

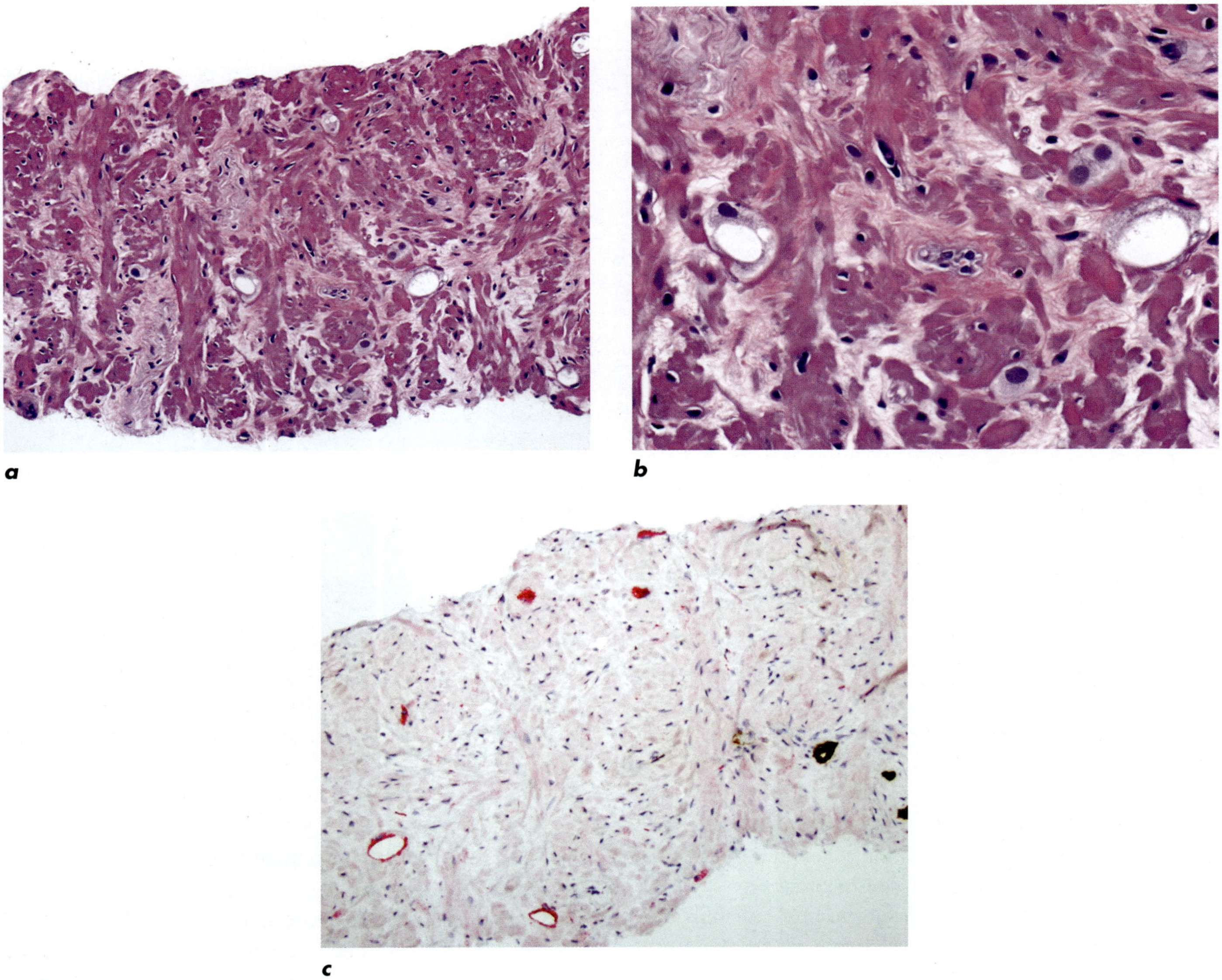

Figure 11-7.
Recurrent adenocarcinoma after radiation. Scattered cells with pale cytoplasm are found on a needle core biopsy (*a*). High magnification shows infiltrating cells with moderate cytological atypia (*b*). Immunostaining (*c*) confirms the diagnosis of adenocarcinoma (positive AMACR and negative basal cell staining) in comparison to the benign glands (on the left) with basal cell staining.

THERMAL EFFECTS ON PROSTATE TISSUE

Definition

- A variety of modalities have been used in the urological field to treat benign prostatic hyperplasia (BPH) and prostatic adenocarcinoma by causing thermal injuries to the tissue

Other terms

- These treatment modalities include cryoablation using liquid nitrogen (rapid deep freezing), microwave (heating), laser (burning), and high-intensity-focused ultrasound (HIFU)

Pathogenesis

- Although there may be some differences in treatment efficacy, these modalities essentially induce thermal injury to prostatic tissue, leading to the demise and reduction of benign, hyperplastic, or neoplastic tissue of the prostate in a nonspecific fashion

Clinical features

- These therapies have been used as initial treatment for prostate cancer although some of them, such as HIFU, are not approved or available in the United States
- They may also be used as a second line of treatment for locally recurrent prostate cancer after radiation failure

Gross pathology

- No specific findings except fibrosis and cystic degenerative changes

Histology

- Effects on benign prostatic tissue
  - Coagulative and hemorrhagic necrosis as early changes (Figs. 11-8 and 11-9)
  - Chronic inflammation and foreign body giant cell granulomatous inflammation occur later
  - Fibrosis and calcification in the areas of necrosis in long standing cases
  - Basal cell hyperplasia may be present
- Effects on prostatic adenocarcinoma
  - The tumor cells undergo coagulative necrosis (Fig. 11-9), which may be difficult to evaluate histologically
  - Chronic inflammation, hemosiderin-laden macrophages, or foreign body giant cell reaction present in the periphery of the necrotic tumor
  - Sometimes, the prostatic adenocarcinoma shows no obvious morphologic changes after thermal therapy, representing either a poor-response or improper procedures
  - Biopsy or transurethral resection of prostate (TURP) may reveal no evidence of residual adenocarcinoma

Immunohistochemistry

- AMACR is positive and p63 and HMWCK are negative in treated adenocarcinoma (Fig. 11-9*b*)

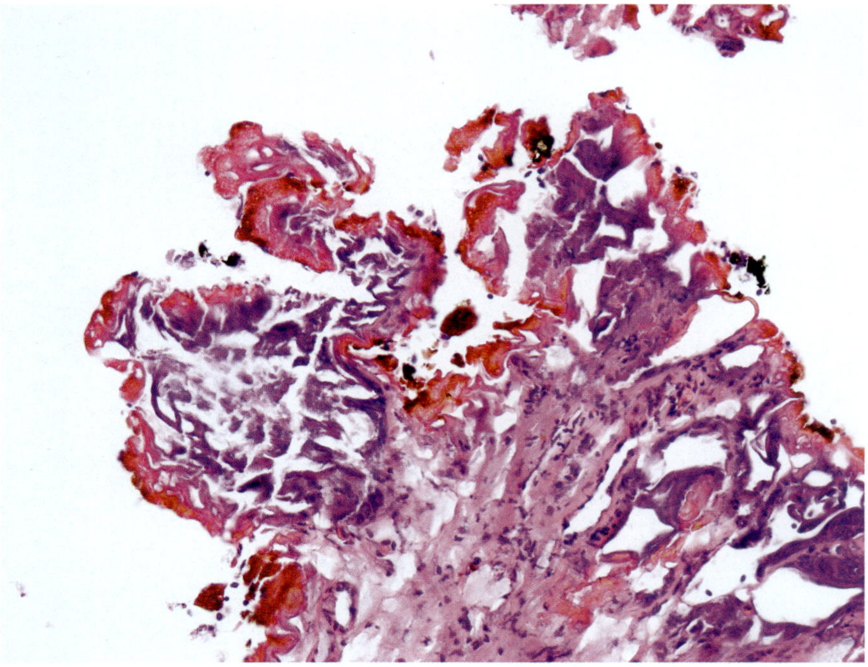

Figure 11-8.
Benign prostatic tissue with severe cauterization from a patient with benign prostatic hyperplasia (BPH) undergoing TURP.

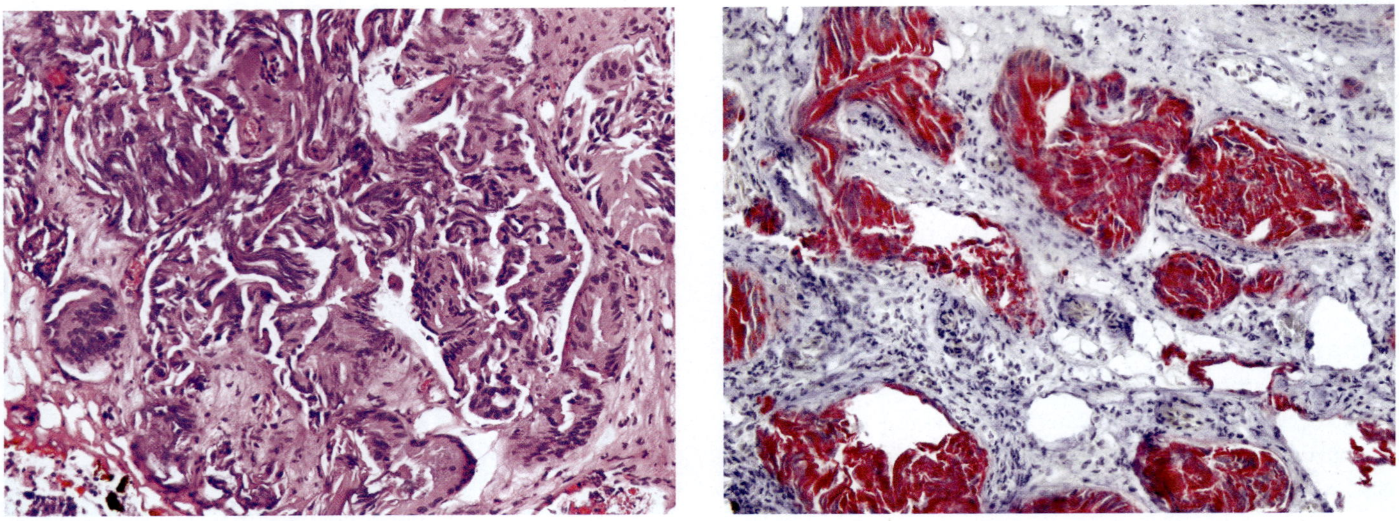

a b

Figure 11-9.
Adenocarcinoma with severe thermal effect showing distorted epithelial clusters difficult to make a diagnosis of carcinoma (*a*). A triple immunostaining (*b*), less effected by the thermal damage, demonstrating the presence of adenocarcinoma (AMACR positive and basal cell markers negative).

Clinical relevance (prognosis and treatment options)

- These therapies provide additional options for treatment of BPH or prostatic adenocarcinoma. The efficacy of these treatments is inconclusive and highly operator dependent. No strong evidence that one is better than the others
- For pathologists, it is important to be familiar with these posttherapy changes
- Sometimes, it could be difficult to determine whether there is a viable residual tumor present
- In addition, similar to radiation, these high-energy therapies are not discriminating benign or malignant, prostate, or adjacent organs. If these are not applied properly, the adjacent organs such as the rectum or bladder can be thermally damaged, even perforated, leading to serious medical problems

ANDROGEN ABLATION AND OTHER HORMONAL THERAPY–INDUCED CHANGES IN PROSTATE

Definition

- Hormonal therapy, generally referring to androgen ablation (actually antihormonal therapy), is one of the major proven therapies for prostate cancer
- In a wide sense, therapies with other hormones or manipulations of hormones can be considered hormone therapy for prostate cancer
- The other types of hormonal therapy include estrogen administration, finasteride (discussed in a separate entity), or even glucocorticoids (experimental)

Other terms

- Androgen deprivation, castration, antiandrogen therapy

Pathogenesis

- Androgenic influences are important for both the growth and malignant transformation of prostatic tissue. The testes account for more than 90% of total circulating testosterone. In the prostate, testosterone is converted into dihydrotestosterone (DHT) by the enzyme 5-α-reductase. DHT is the primary androgen that stimulates the growth of both benign and malignant prostate tissues
- Charles Higgins received the Nobel prize for his pioneering work in hormonal treatment by performing orchiectomy on prostate cancer patients
- Nowadays, in addition to orchiectomy, androgen deprivation can be achieved by chemical agents such as gonadotropin-releasing hormone antagonists (such as Lupron), androgen blockers, or estrogen

Clinical features

- Androgen ablation can be used as an initial therapy for some prostate cancer patients when surgery or radiation is not an option
- More commonly, androgen ablation is used as adjuvant therapy combining with surgery, radiation, or chemotherapy for advanced or metastatic disease
- Preoperative (neoadjuvant) hormonal ablation, not commonly used in the United States, is sometimes used for clinically localized prostate cancer to slow the tumor growth before surgery
- Adverse effects of hormonal therapy include hot flashes, loss of libido, or impotence

Gross pathology

- Prostate is reduced in size and weight

Histology

- Effects on benign prostatic tissue
  - Nonspecific histologic changes, including basal cell hyperplasia, transitional cell, and squamous cell metaplasia in benign epithelium, and chronic inflammation are present (Figs. 11-10 and 11-11)
  - These nonspecific histologic changes in benign prostatic epithelial cells (Fig. 11-10*a*) often provide a clue to the pathologist that hormonal therapy has been used
- Effects on adenocarcinoma
  - Regardless of the method of androgen ablation, the histological changes in the prostatic tissue are indistinguishable
  - The effects are most prominent on secretory epithelial cells since they express androgen receptors
  - Regression and degenerative changes, such as pyknotic nuclei, clear cytoplasm, or vacuolated cytoplasm are evident
  - The usual features of adenocarcinoma, such as cytologic atypia, are diminished or absent (Figs. 11-12 and 11-13)
  - These changes can cause difficulty in assessment of prostate biopsies, and may result in underestimation of the extent of disease if hormone therapy was administered prior to a biopsy or prostatectomy
  - Furthermore, because of the severe histological changes in tumor cells caused by prior hormonal therapy, the assignment of a Gleason score is unreliable
  - The infiltrating pattern of a prostatic adenocarcinoma is mostly retained and can be recognized (Figs. 11-12 and 11-13)
  - In particular, identification of scattered individual malignant epithelial cells in the stroma is diagnostic evidence of prostatic adenocarcinoma
  - In the case of hormonally treated adenocarcinoma, we still give a Gleason score with a note indicating that grading hormonal-treated prostate cancer may not be accurate to be used as a reliable prognostic indicator
- Estrogen effect
  - Administration of estrogen is rare in a current clinical setting; diethylstilbestrol is no longer commercially available. However, estrogens can cause severe squamous metaplasia in benign or malignant prostatic cells in addition to the atrophic changes in the prostate

Immunohistochemistry

- AMACR can be positive in hormonally treated prostatic adenocarcinoma; however, the intensity and percentage of positive cases are reduced. Only approximately 50% of hormonally treated prostate cancer cases show AMACR immunoreactivity. Interestingly, when these tumor cells become refractory to hormonal therapy, the AMACR staining returns in a high percentage of cases

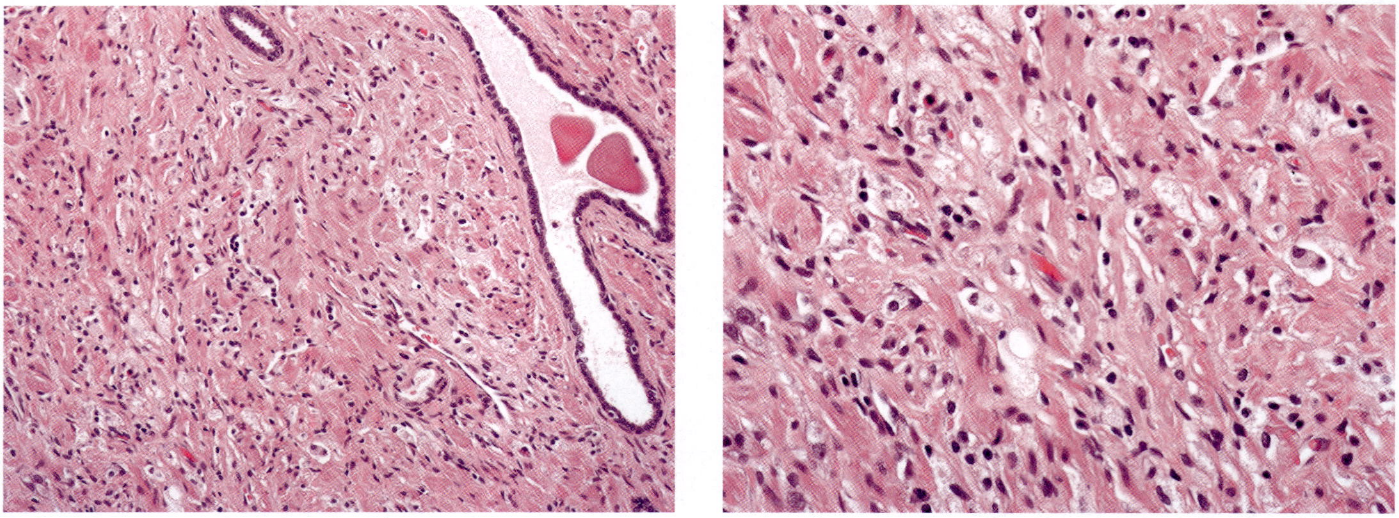

a b

Figure 11-10.
Adenocarcinoma with hormonal effects. At a low magnification, it is difficult to appreciate the presence of tumor cells (*a*, left). The benign gland on the right is showing atrophic changes. Scattered infiltrating tumor cells with pale cytoplasm can be seen at higher magnification (*b*).

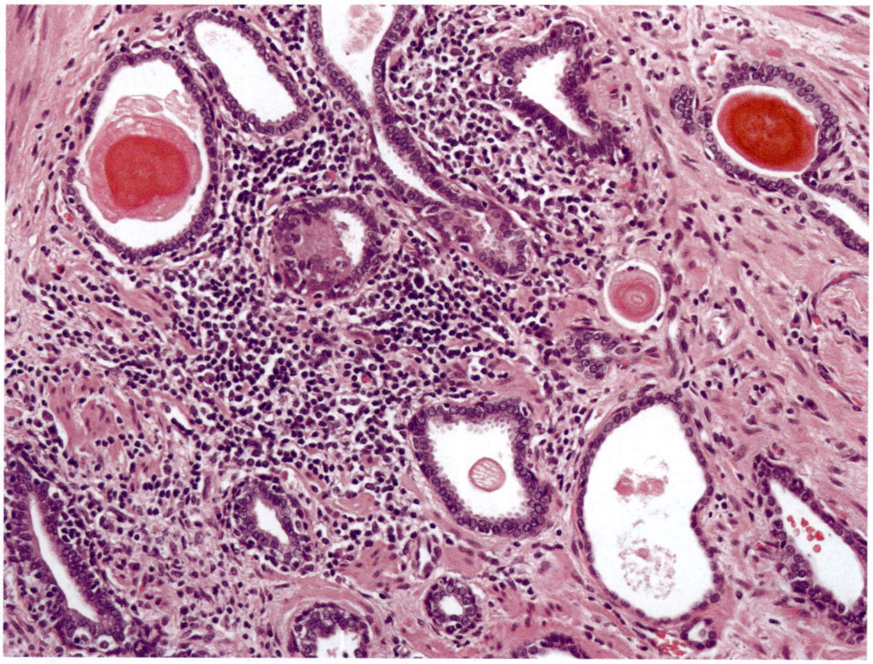

Figure 11-11.
Benign glands posthormonal therapy showing atrophic glandular changes surrounded by chronic inflammatory cells.

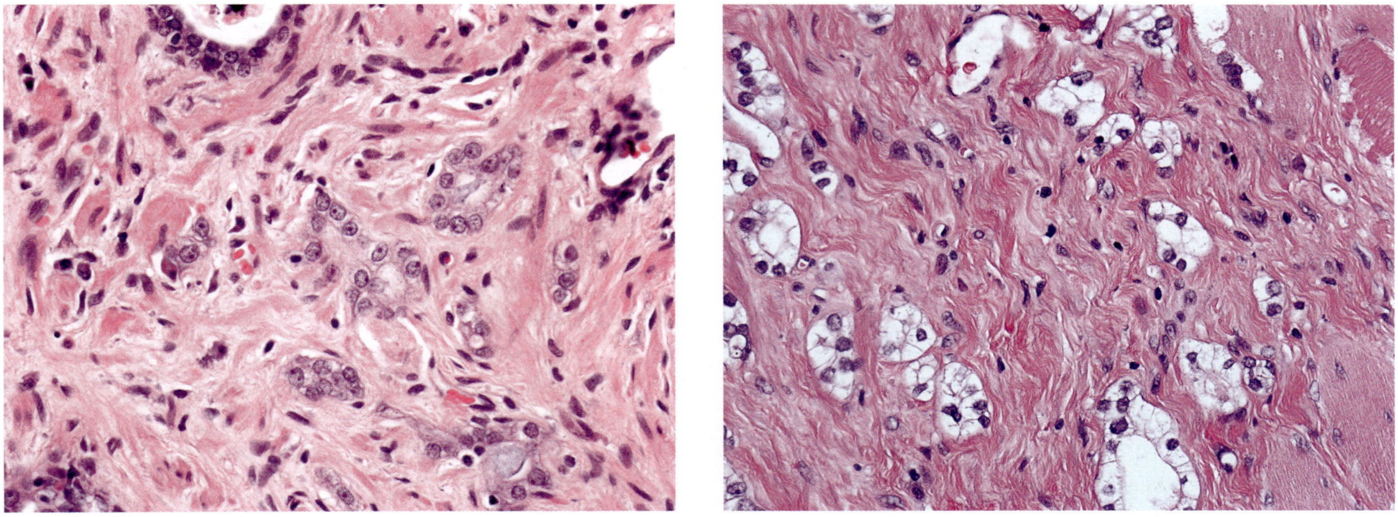

a b

Figure 11-12.
In one area of the prostate, tumor cells (*a*) do not show obvious treatment effects in morphology, while in another area from the same prostate, tumor cells show clear cell atrophic change (*b*).

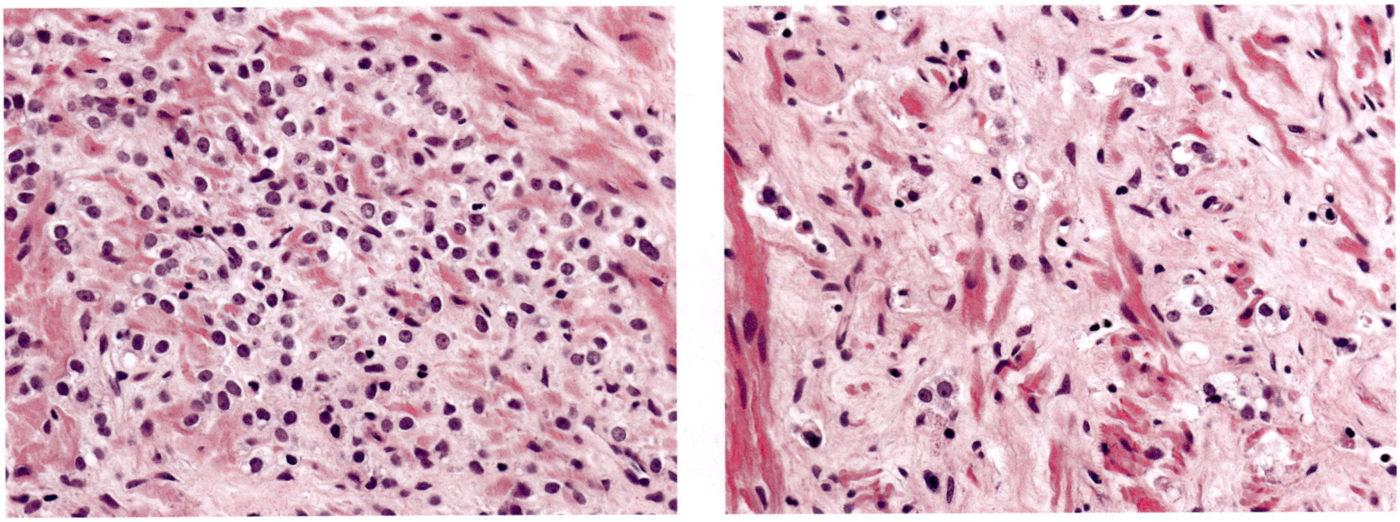

a b

Figure 11-13.
Adenocarcinoma with hormonal effects. A focus of tumor cells is arranged in a solid pattern without glandular structures (*a*). Tumor cells show prominent nucleoli and degenerative changes (*b*).

- Immunostaining for keratins or PSA may be helpful in identifying the individual tumor cells in this situation to confirm the diagnosis

Clinical relevance (prognosis and treatment options)

- Because of the marked atrophic changes of the cancer cells, preoperative (neoadjuvant) hormonal therapy may cause diagnosis of small-volume cancer difficult
- Preoperative (neoadjuvant) hormonal therapy has been proposed by some experts to reduce positive margin rate and downstage of prostate cancer. However, there is no evidence it is improving the survival rate
- Therefore, it may be artificially creating a false-negative result because of the difficulty in identifying treated cancer cells. Nevertheless, the neoadjuvant hormonal therapy is not commonly used in most U.S. institutions

5-α-REDUCTASE INHIBITORS–INDUCED CHANGES

Definition

- Morphologic changes in the prostate induced by administration of 5-α-reductase (5-aR) inhibitors, which are considered weaker antiandrogen agents

Pathogenesis

- 5-aR catalyzes the conversion of testosterone to more potent dihydrotestosterone (DHT) in the prostate. While finasteride blocks the conversion of testosterone to DHT in the prostate by inhibiting the type 2 5-aR isoenzyme, dutasteride is a dual inhibitor of both the type 1 (present in liver and skin) and type 2 isoenzymes of 5-aR (in the prostate), and may be more potent than finasteride
- The reduction of DHT leads to atrophic changes in both malignant and benign prostate tissue

Clinical features

- History of 5-aR is mostly used for treatment of BPH
- 5-aR can also be used along with other antiandrogen such Lupron for treatment of prostate cancer
- 5-aR has been used in prostate cancer chemoprevention clinical trials for patients with high-grade PIN
- Administration of either drug may complicate the clinical diagnosis of a prostate cancer because they produce a nearly 50% decrease in serum PSA concentrations during the first 3 months of therapy, which persists as long as the drug is continued

Gross pathology

- No obvious change grossly
- Possible a reduction in size and weight of the prostate after 5-aR treatment

Histology

- Finasteride can induce mild chronic inflammation (Fig. 11-14)
- It also reduces prostate volume and causes mild atrophic changes of the benign prostatic glands (Fig. 11-15)
- Both finasteride and dutasteride appear to cause mild atrophic changes of prostatic adenocarcinoma (Fig. 11-16)
- But these changes are subtle and have a limited effect on the diagnosis of prostatic adenocarcinoma based on the histological appearance on biopsy
- Whether 5-aR can induce changes of prostatic adenocarcinoma, which may appear higher grade, is not known

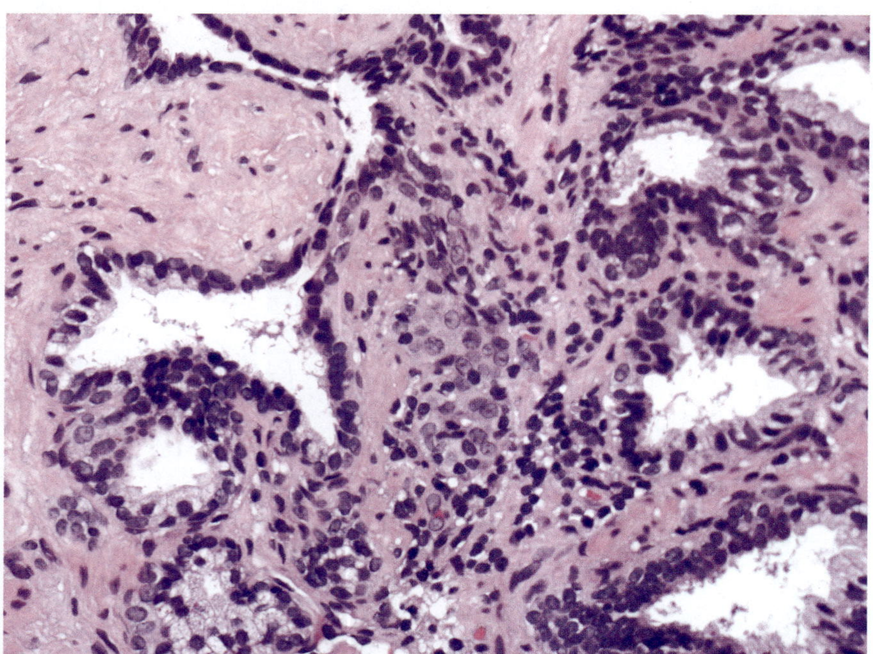

Figure 11-14. Benign glands post-5-α-reductase (5-aR) treatment with glandular atrophy, basal cell hyperplasia, and chronic inflammation are present.

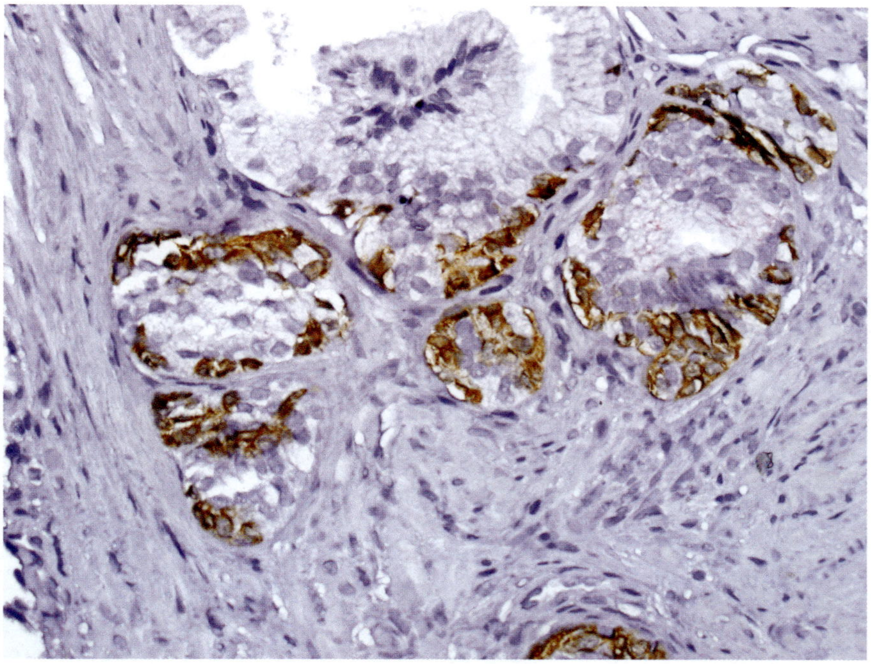

Figure 11-15.
Benign glands post-5-aR treatment with basal cell staining (HMWCK) confirms the prominent basal cells in benign glands.

Immunohistochemistry

- Basal cell markers are present in benign prostatic tissue and not in adenocarcinoma of the prostate after 5-aR treatment (Fig. 11-15)
- We have seen weak AMACR staining in prostatic adenocarcinoma cells after 5-aR treatment (Fig. 11-16*c*). Whether 5-aR can reduce PSA staining or AMACR staining intensity of most cases of prostate cancer is unknown

Clinical relevance (prognosis and treatment options)

- It has been suggested that 5-aR inhibitors have the potential to elevate the Gleason score of prostate cancers
- This suggestion was based on the findings of the Prostate Cancer Prevention trial, a placebo-controlled trial in which men treated with finasteride had fewer prostate cancers overall but significantly more tumors of Gleason score 7 to 10 as compared to those in the control group
- It is possible that the high-grade appearance of those tumors was due to the finasteride effect
- Thus, it is not clear that the "high-grade" prostate cancers that developed in the men receiving finasteride are truly more aggressive than those that arose in men not receiving finasteride
- The relationship between 5-aR inhibitors and Gleason score remains unsettled
- The effects on the prostate histology by 5-aR inhibitors and other therapeutic agents are summarized (Table 11-1)

Table 11-1. Treatment Effects on Benign Prostatic Tissue and Adenocarcinoma

Therapy	*Benign prostate*	*Adenocarcinoma*
Androgen ablation	Atrophy of secretory cells	Severe atrophic changes
	Basal cell hyperplasia	Degenerative changes
Estrogen	Squamous metaplasia	Squamous metaplasia
5-α-reductase inhibitor	Mild atrophy of secretory cells	Minimal change
	Basal cell hyperplasia	Some may show high-grade appearance
Radiation	Secretory cell atrophy	Early: necrosis
	Prominent basal cells with marked atypia (streaming)	Later: clear cell cytoplasm and atrophic change

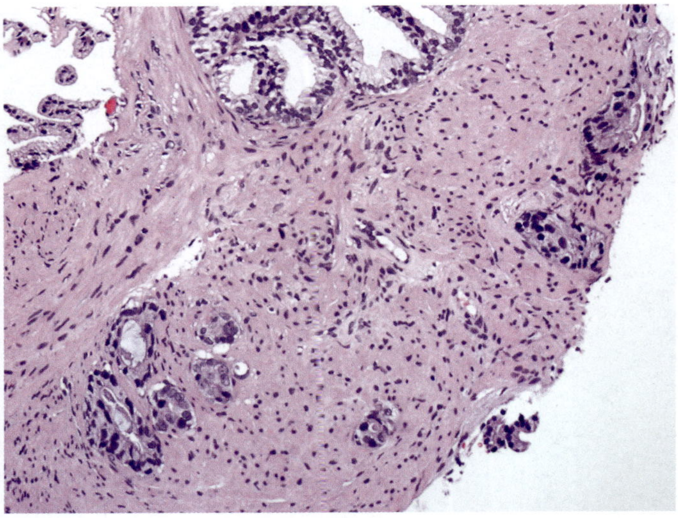

a

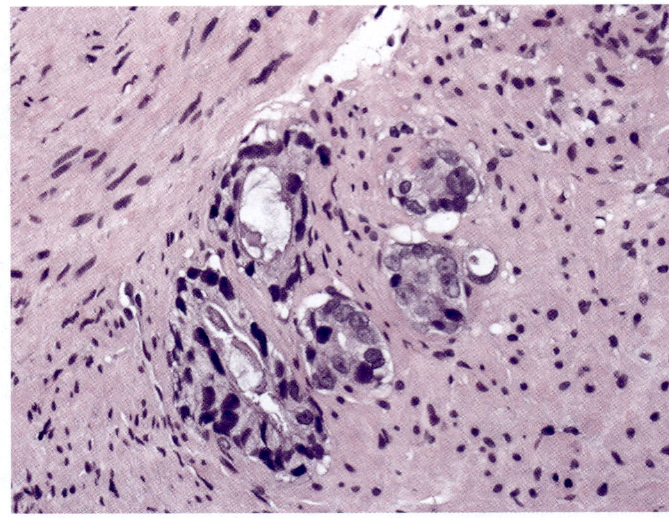

b

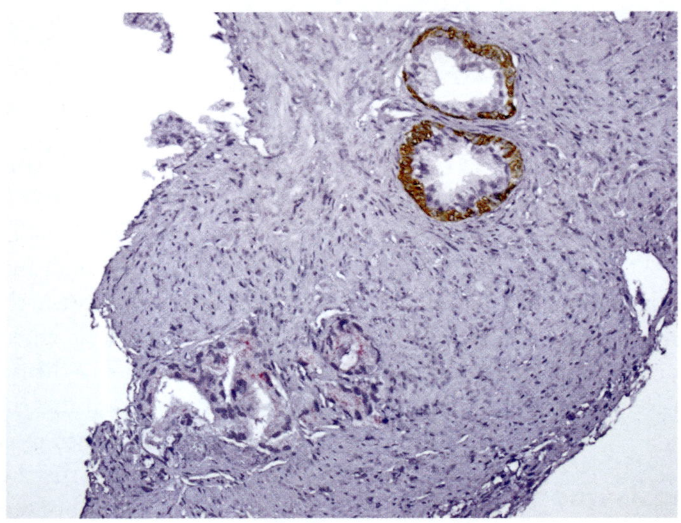

c

Figure 11-16.
Adenocarcinoma post-5-aR treatment with a small focus of adenocarcinoma displaying some glandular fusion (*a*). Higher magnification shows the presence of cytological atypia in tumor cells (*b*). Triple immunostaining shows weak AMACR staining in tumor cells (*c*).

CHAPTER 12

Other Malignant Neoplastic Lesions of the Prostate

UROTHELIAL CARCINOMA OF THE PROSTATE

Definition

- Primary urothelial carcinoma derives from urothelial cells of the prostatic urethra
- It may be invasive or in situ urothelial carcinoma
- In practice, urothelial carcinoma of the prostate may include the following conditions, which may be difficult to distinguish microscopically:
  - The prostatic primary urothelial carcinoma without the bladder involvement
  - The bladder primary urothelial carcinoma involving the prostate
  - The primary urothelial carcinoma simultaneously develops in both the prostate and the bladder

Clinical features

- Prostate enlargement
- Elevated serum PSA may be present, usually mild, depending on the degree of prostate tissue destruction

Gross pathology

- Diffuse enlargement of the prostate or poorly defined infiltrating mass in the prostate
- Indistinguishable from high-grade prostatic adenocarcinoma grossly

Histology

- Urothelial carcinoma of the prostate is usually high grade, morphologically similar to that of the bladder (Fig. 12-1)
- Urothelial carcinoma in situ is confined within the basement membrane of the urothelium or a prostatic gland without evidence of invasion (Figs. 12-2 and 12-3)
- Invasive urothelial carcinoma is characterized by the presence of stromal invasion by nests or small cords of tumor cells with desmoplastic reaction of the stroma (Fig. 12-4)
- Tumor cells are pleomorphic, often with areas of necrosis
- Cribriform patterns are uncommon in urothelial carcinoma

Immunohistochemistry

- P63 and HMWCK positive (Fig. 12-5)
- AMACR negative or weakly positive (Fig. 12-5)
- Positive for new urothelial markers such as S100P, Gata3, uroplakin, negative for PSA

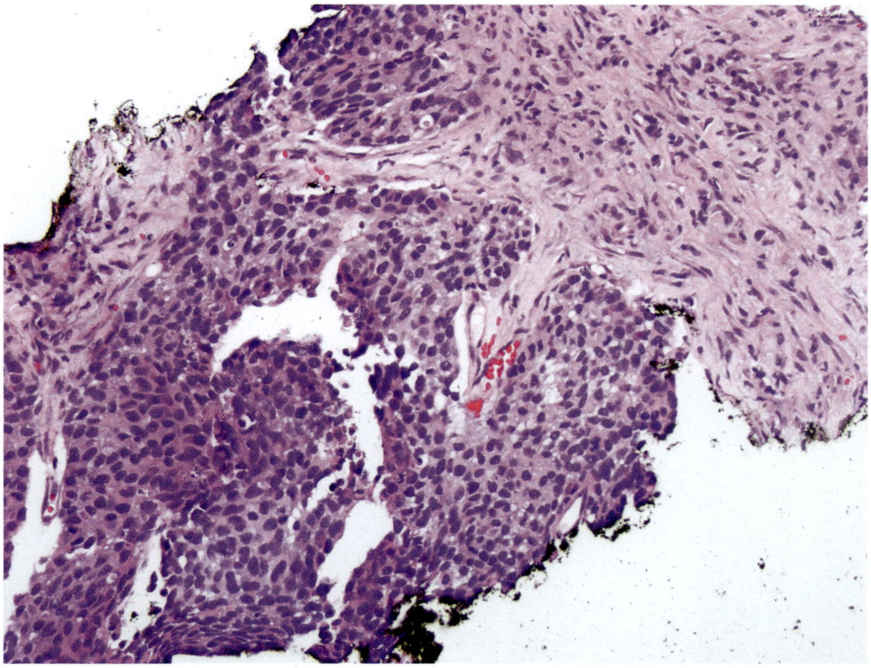

Figure 12-1.
High-grade urothelial carcinoma present on a prostate needle core biopsy, which is composed of large nests of tumor cells without any glandular differentiation.

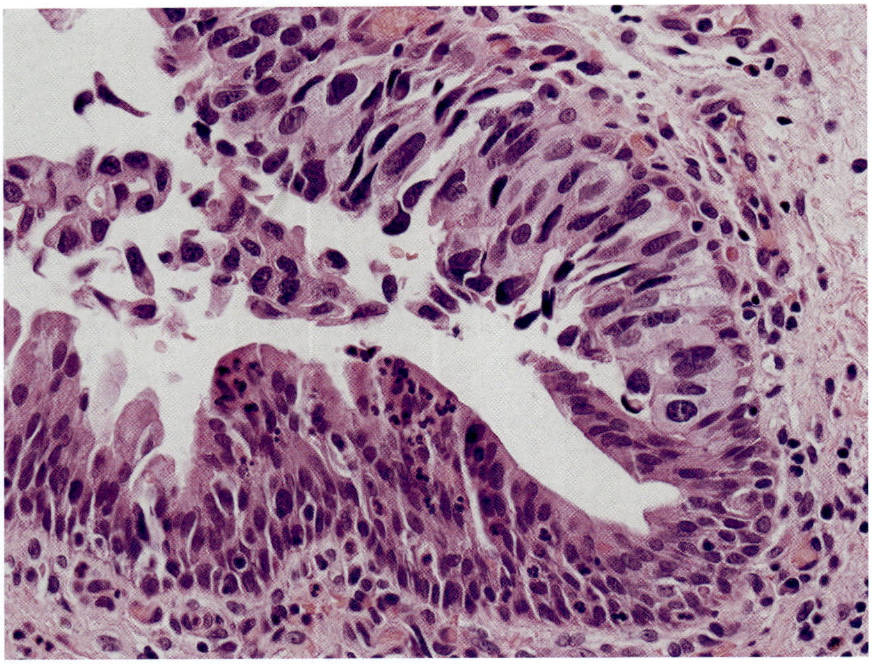

Figure 12-2.
Urothelial carcinoma in situ involving the urothelium of the prostatic urethra.

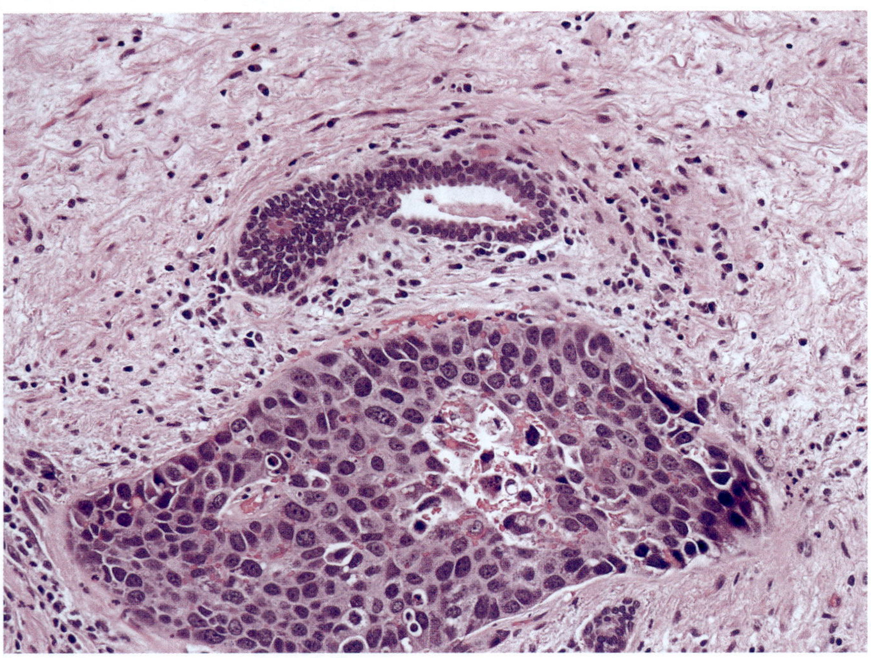

Figure 12-3.
Urothelial carcinoma in situ involving a prostatic gland, which is not considered to be invasive unless stromal invasion is present.

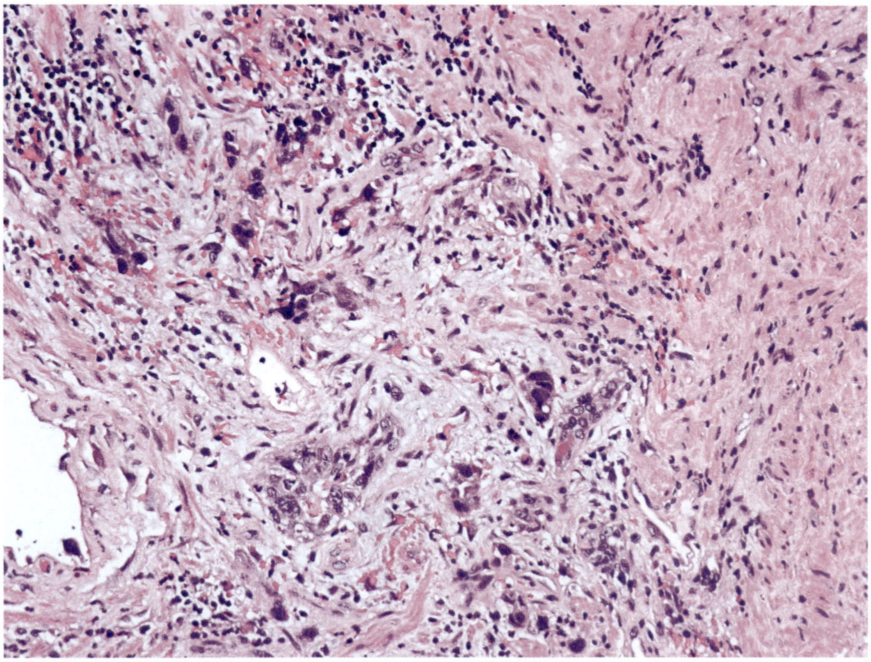

Figure 12-4.
High-grade urothelial carcinoma invading prostatic stroma with marked desmoplastic reaction.

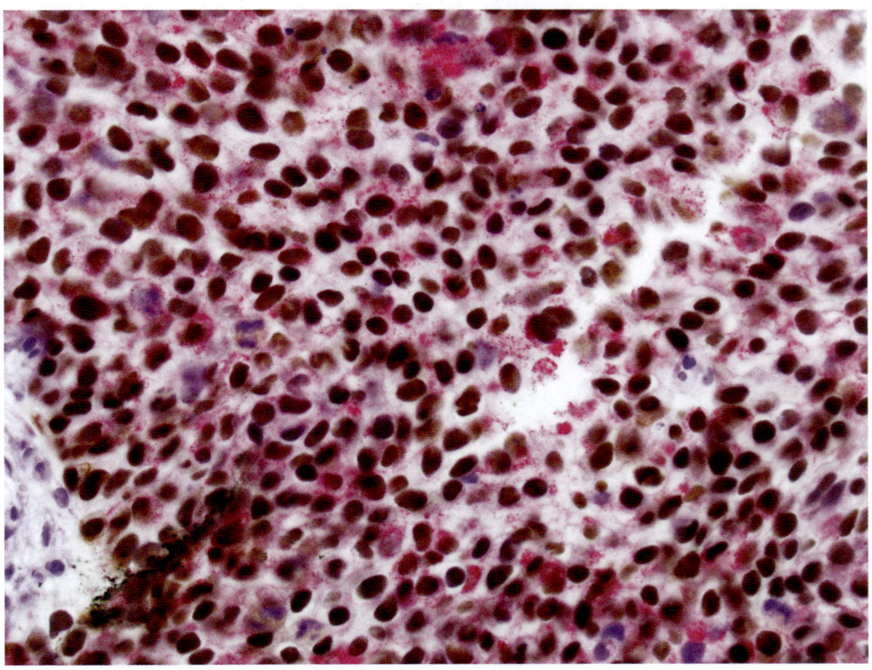

Figure 12-5.
Urothelial carcinoma cells are positive for p63 (brown, nuclear staining) and weakly positive for AMACR (red, cytoplasmic).

Differential diagnosis

- The major differential diagnosis is a high-grade prostatic adenocarcinoma, which has different treatment implications (see Table 12-1)

Clinical relevance (prognosis and treatment options)

- Primary urothelial carcinoma of the prostate is uncommon. The diagnosis requires the negative bladder examination confirmed by negative biopsy. Treatment of choice is prostatectomy
- The majority of urothelial carcinoma of the prostate is the secondary involvement by bladder urothelial carcinoma. Therefore, the cystoscopy and biopsy of bladder lesions are critical for establishing the diagnosis
- Theoretically, urothelial carcinoma may develop simultaneously in both the prostatic urethra and the bladder. On the other hand, the advanced prostatic urothelial carcinoma may secondarily involve the bladder. However, in practice, it is difficult to distinguish these two conditions in advanced stages
- The secondary urothelial carcinoma of the prostate is an advanced stage cancer with poor prognosis. The main treatment option is cystoprostatectomy with adjuvant chemotherapy

Table 12-1. Comparison of Urothelial Carcinoma and Adenocarcinoma of the Prostate

	Urothelial carcinoma	*Prostatic adenocarcinoma*
Morphology of tumor cells	More pleomorphic	Relatively uniform
Urothelial CIS	May be present	Absent
Bladder cancer	May be present	Absent
Glandular formation	Occasional	Common
Cribriform pattern	Rare	Common
Squamous differentiation	Common	Rare
Serum PSA	Normal or mildly elevated	Elevated
AMACR	Negative or weakly positive	Positive
PSA	Negative	Positive
P63/HMWCK	Positive	Negative
Gata3/S100P	Positive	Negative
Prognosis	Very poor	Good to poor depending on the grade and stage
Treatment	Surgery and chemotherapy	Surgery, hormone, and radiation therapy

AMACR, α-methylacyl-CoA racemase; HMWCK; high molecular cytokeratins; PSA, prostate-specific antigen.

BASALOID CARCINOMA OF THE PROSTATE

Definition

- Malignant epithelial neoplasm deriving from (or with features of) basal cells of the prostate

Other terms

- Basal cell carcinoma, adenoid cystic carcinoma of the prostate

Clinical features

- Wide age range
- Urinary obstruction symptoms
- PSA normal or mildly elevated (if there is destruction of prostatic tissue)

Gross pathology

- Infiltrating mass
- White to fleshy on cut surface

Histology

- Common features of basal cell carcinoma
  - The hallmark of this tumor is: infiltrating nests of basal cells
  - Nests of tumor cells with scant cytoplasm appear to be blue
  - Mild cytological atypia
- Classic basal cell type
  - Nests of cells with scant cytoplasm, the blue cells nests under at low magnifications (Fig. 12-6)
  - The tumor morphologically resemble basal cell carcinoma of the skin
- Adenoid cystic type
  - Nests of cells with cribriform patterns
  - Glandular differentiation and microcystic patterns can be seen (Fig. 12-7)
  - Perineural invasion can be observed. Morphologically resembles adenoid cystic carcinoma of the salivary glands

Immunohistochemistry

- P63 and HMWCK positive
- CK7 positive/CK20 negative (most urothelial carcinoma CK20 positive)
- PAS negative, AMACR weakly positive in a small subset of tumors, BCL2 positive
- High Ki67 proliferative index

Differential diagnosis

- Adenocarcinoma: glandular formation, prominent nucleoli, and positive PSA and AMACR
- Urothelial carcinoma: more pleomorphic, positive S100p and Gata3
- Basal cell hyperplasia: no sufficient cytological atypia and no infiltrative patterns (see Table 12-2)

Clinical relevance (prognosis and treatment options)

- Most cases are locally invasive
- Local recurrence and distant metastasis can be seen in a minority of the cases

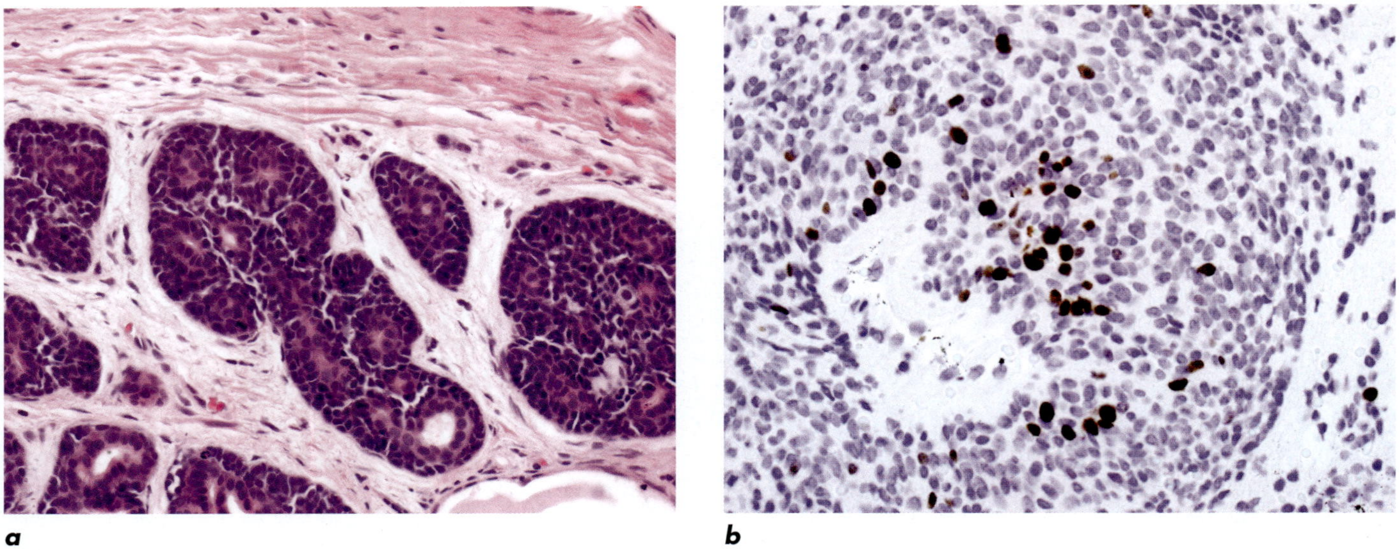

Figure 12-6.
Irregular nests of basal cells with scant cytoplasm infiltrating the prostate (*a*). The Ki67 proliferative activity of the tumor cells is high (*b*).

Figure 12-7.
Adenoid cystic type of basaloid cell carcinoma of the prostate composed of islands of tumor cells with cribriform patterns (*a*) invading the stroma. Perineural invasion can be seen (*b*).

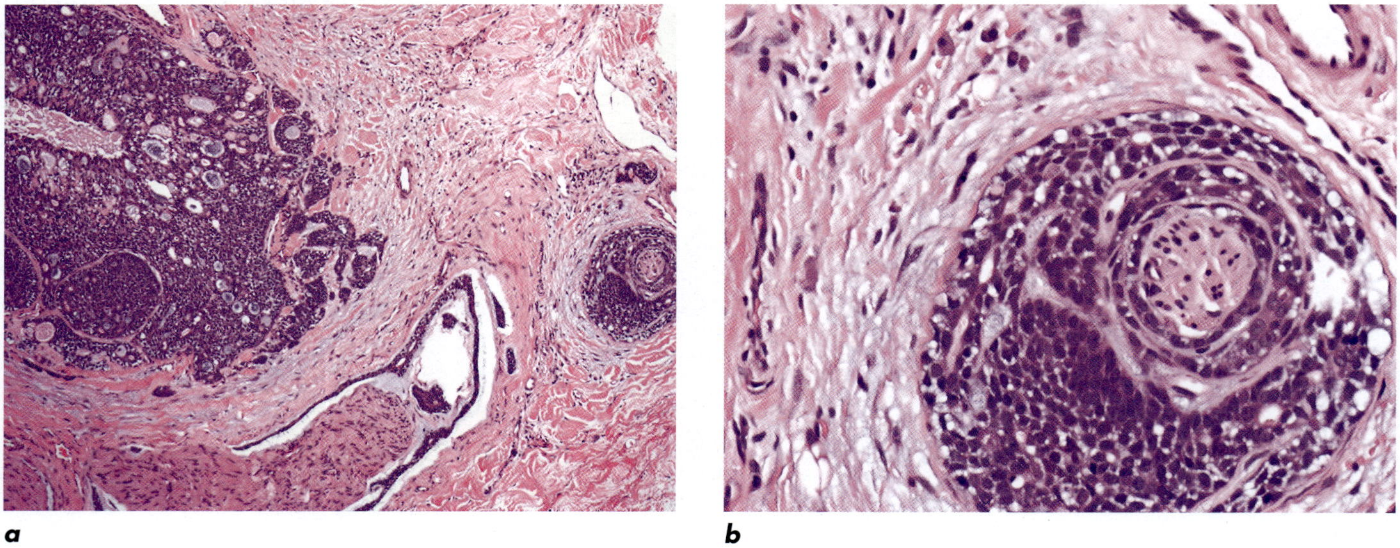

Table 12-2. Comparison of Basaloid Carcinoma with Basal Cell Hyperplasia

	Basaloid carcinoma	*Basal cell hyperplasia*
Nature	Destructive but low-grade malignant neoplasm	Benign proliferative lesion
Symptoms	Hematuria	Urinary obstruction
Prostate enlargement	Yes	Yes
Serum PSA	Possibly elevated	Mildly elevated
Gross	Poorly defined infiltrating mass	BPH-like nodules
Adenoid cystic pattern	Yes	No
Basal cell nests	Yes	No
Growth patterns	Infiltrative	Lobular
Ki67	Increased	Normal
Bcl2	Positive	Negative
Treatment	Prostatectomy	Treatment for BPH
Prognosis	Locally invasive but metastasis rare, good prognosis if resected	Benign, excellent

BPH, benign prostatic hyperplasia; PSA, prostate-specific antigen.

SQUAMOUS CELL CARCINOMA

Definition

- A malignant tumor entirely composed of squamous cell carcinoma components
- Prostatic adenocarcinoma with squamous cell differentiation is defined as the presence of both adenocarcinoma malignant squamous cell components
- Prostatic adenocarcinoma can undergo squamous differentiation with or without estrogen treatment

Clinical features

- Primary prostatic squamous cell carcinoma is very rare
- In most cases, squamous cell carcinoma is secondary, either it is extended from the adjacent organ such as anal-rectal or distant metastasis from other organs

Gross pathology

- Poorly circumscribed, destructive mass lesion
- Necrosis with keratin debris may be present

Histology

- Usually high-grade carcinoma (Figs. 12-8 and 12-9)
- Invasive with desmoplastic reaction of the stroma
- Keratinization or without keratinization present
- If both adenocarcinoma and malignant squamous carcinoma present, it will be considered adenocarcinoma with squamous differentiation (Fig. 12-10)

Immunohistochemistry

- Keratins are positive in both squamous cell carcinoma and adenocarcinoma with squamous differentiation. P63 will be positive in squamous cell carcinoma and possibly positive in the differentiated squamous components
- PSA and AMACR negative in squamous components, positive in glandular component

Clinical relevance (prognosis and treatment options)

- When a diagnosis of squamous cell carcinoma is made in the prostate, a workup is necessary to rule out another primary
- If it is considered to be a primary, prostatectomy is indicated
- Poor prognosis as either primary or secondary
- The prognosis of prostatic adenocarcinoma with squamous differentiation is not known, most likely related to the grade and stage of the glandular component

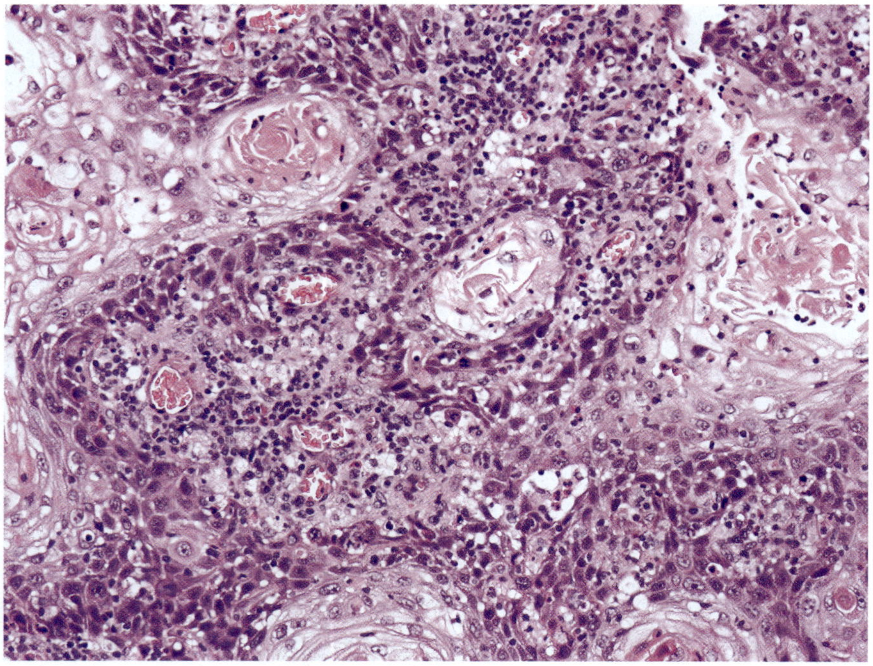

Figure 12-8.
High-grade squamous cell carcinoma of the prostate with invasive growth patterns and keratinization.

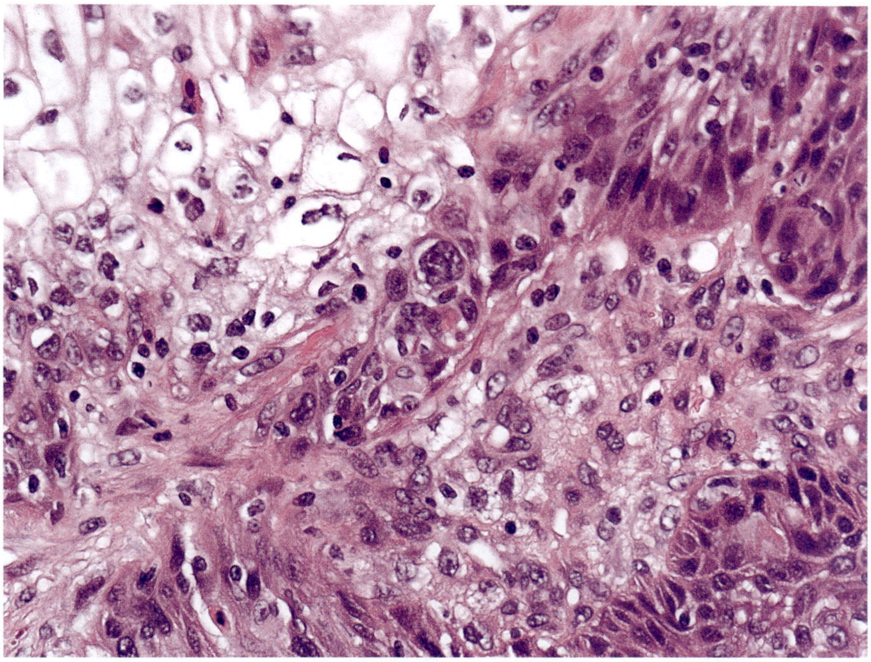

Figure 12-9.
High-grade squamous cell carcinoma displaying marked cytological atypia.

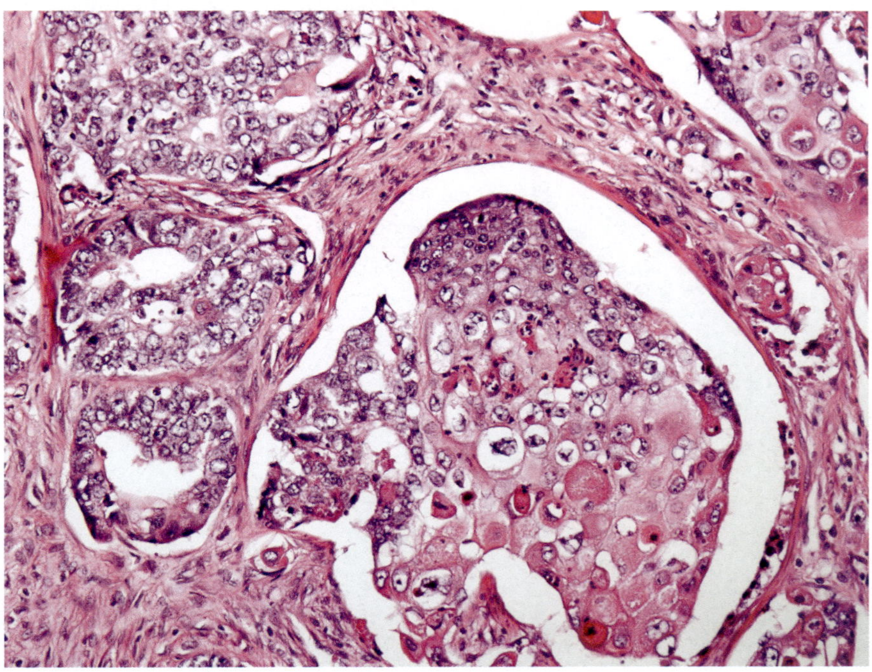

Figure 12-10.
High-grade adenocarcinoma of the prostate undergoing squamous differentiation.

SMALL CELL CARCINOMA

Definition

- Prostatic adenocarcinoma with features of small neuroendocrine cells

Pathogenesis

- Majority of small cell carcinoma of the prostate is associated with high-grade prostatic adenocarcinoma. Most likely, this is a dedifferentiation of adenocarcinoma
- Pure small cell carcinoma is very rare in the prostate

Clinical features

- Typically present as advanced stage of prostate cancer
- PSA elevation
- Serum neuroendocrine markers such as chromogranin may be elevated

Gross pathology

- Large solid areas with extensive infiltration of the prostate

Histology

- This tumor composed of sheets of small neuroendocrine cells with scant cytoplasm and salt-and-pepper chromatin, similar to small cell carcinoma of the lung (Figs. 12-11 and 12-12)
- High rates of mitosis and apoptosis
- High-grade acinar adenocarcinoma component is often present

Immunohistochemistry

- PSA and AMACR focally positive
- Keratins and neuroendocrine markers positive
- Thyroid transcription factor (TTF1) positive in less than 50% of cases (Fig. 12-13)

Clinical relevance (prognosis and treatment options)

- A very aggressive tumor with survival time of only a couple of years with treatment
- The benefit of surgery is mostly reducing symptoms but probably not associated with an increased survival
- Systemic treatment such as chemotherapy with or without radiation is necessary to prolong the survival time

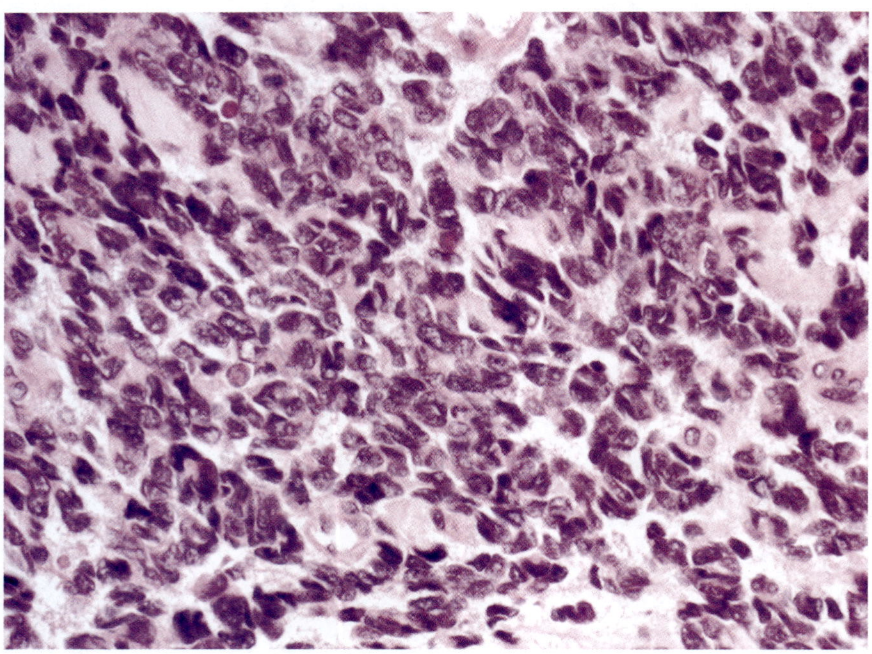

Figure 12-11.
Small cell carcinoma cells with scant cytoplasm and crowding. No glandular differentiation is seen.

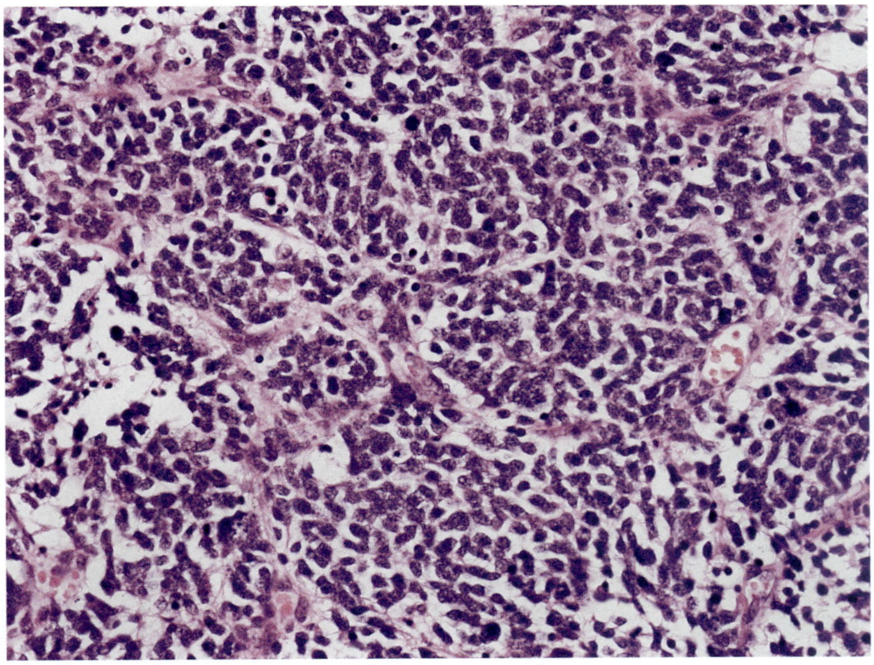

Figure 12-12.
Small cell carcinoma cells with "salt-and-pepper" chromatin. Mitosis and apoptosis are common.

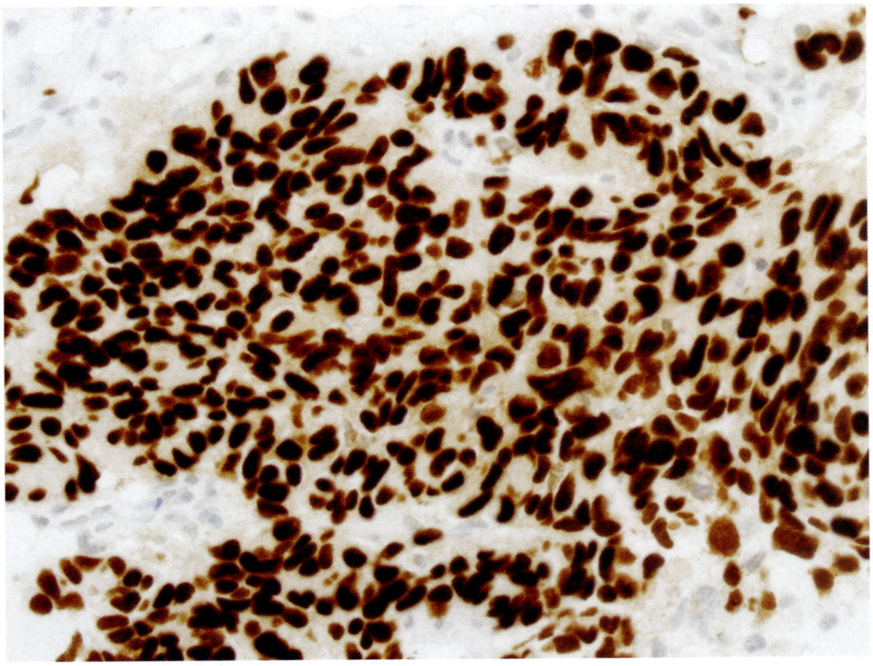

Figure 12-13.
Small cell carcinoma of the prostate showing TTF1 positivity.

SARCOMATOID CARCINOMA

Definition

- Malignant neoplasm containing both epithelial and sarcomatoid components

Other terms

- Carcinosarcoma

Pathogenesis

- In most instances, the tumor starts as an adenocarcinoma followed by dedifferentiation and development of sarcomatoid component
- It may also be derived from a stem cell that differentiates into malignant epithelial and stromal components
- We have seen cases with a small focus of prostatic adenocarcinoma, Gleason 3 + 3 = 6 initially, developing into sarcomatoid carcinoma after receiving unproven treatment, which may include cell growth stimulating factors

Clinical features

- Urinary obstruction
- Elevated serum PSA possible if the tumor is large
- Metastatic lesions are present at the time of diagnosis or after diagnosis

Gross pathology

- Large destructive mass with infiltrating borders with fleshy cut surface
- Prostate distortion, hemorrhage, and necrosis are frequent

Histology

- The diagnosis requires the presence of both carcinomatous and sarcomatoid components (Fig. 12-14*a*)
- Carcinomatous component
  - Usually high-grade carcinoma (Gleason pattern 4 or 5) can be seen (Fig. 12-14*b*)
  - In some cases, Gleason 3 and 4 patterns are present
  - Other carcinomatous components such as squamous, small cell carcinoma may be occasionally seen
- Sarcomatoid component
  - Typically undifferentiated high-grade spindle cell component (Figs. 12-14*c*)
  - Occasionally, heterologous elements such as osteosarcoma, chondrosarcoma may be seen
- Carcinomatous and sarcomatoid components are present in separate areas or mixed together
- The carcinomatous component can range from 1% to 99% of the tumor

Immunohistochemistry

- Carcinomatous components positive for PSA, AMACR, and keratin
- Sarcomatoid components positive for keratins (AE1/AE3 or Cam5.2)

Clinical relevance (prognosis and treatment options)

- Often present in an advanced stage of disease with metastasis in 30% to 50% of patients at diagnosis
- Poor prognosis with most patients dying within 1 year of diagnosis. No effective treatments have been established

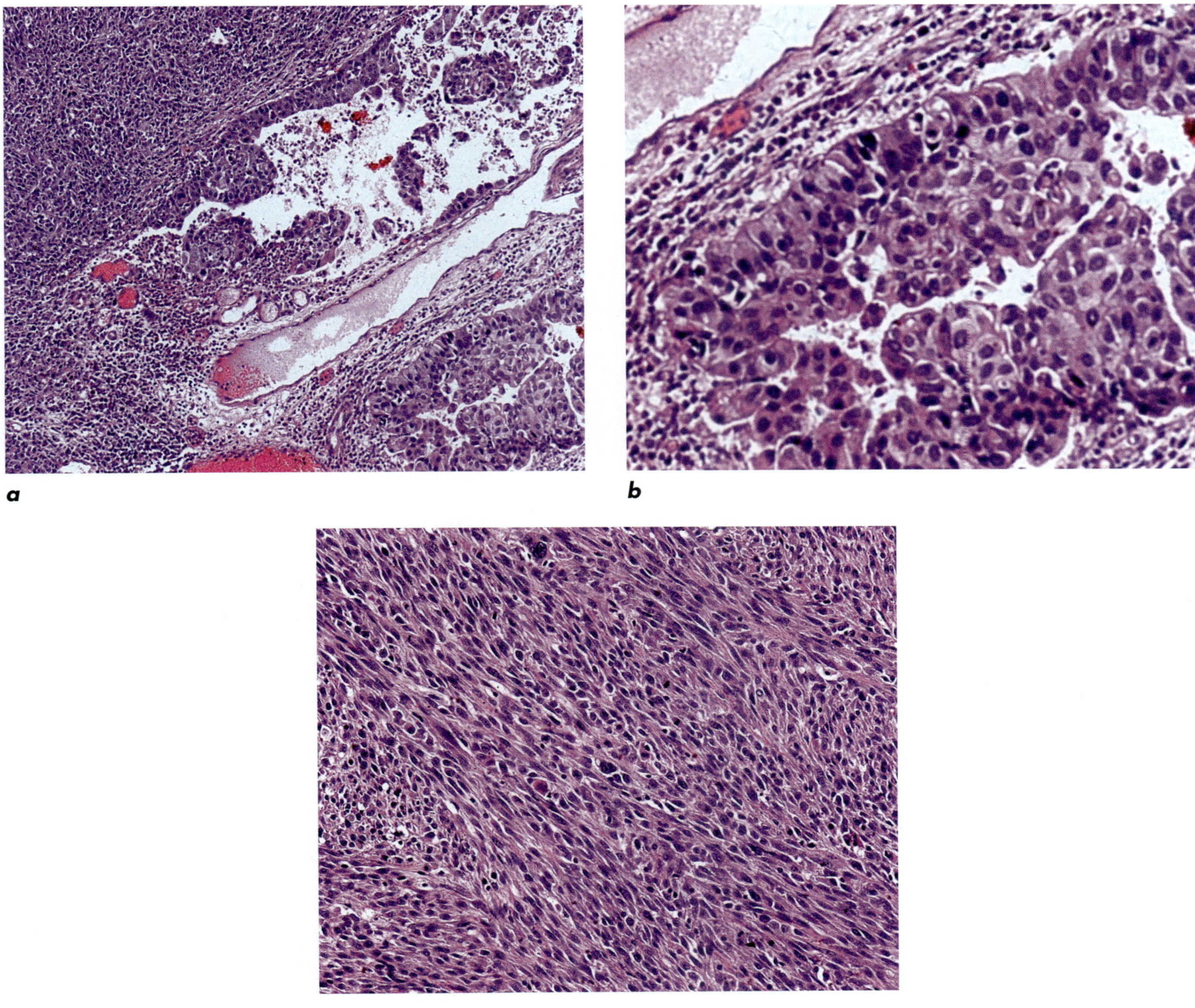

Figure 12-14.

Sarcomatoid carcinoma (*a*) of the prostate composed of both sarcomatoid (left) and carcinomatous components. High magnifications show a high-grade carcinomatous component with vague glandular appearance and marked cytological atypia (*b*) and a high-grade spindle cell component with cytological pleomorphism and brisk mitotic figures (*c*).

SARCOMAS OF THE PROSTATE

Definition

- Primary malignant mesenchymal neoplasms arising in the prostate
- Common types: leiomyosarcoma, rhabdomyosarcoma, fibrosarcoma, and synovial sarcoma

Pathogenesis

Rare conditions in the prostate, probably develops from stem cells in the prostate

Clinical features

- Enlargement of prostate, typically with urinary obstruction
- In late stage, hematuria can be seen

Gross pathology

- Large mass replacing the prostate with a flashy cut surface
- Focal hemorrhage, necrosis, and invasion outside prostatic capsule to adjacent organs are common findings

Histology

- Spindle cell proliferations with high cellularity, high mitotic activity, and pleomorphic cytology (Fig. 12-15)
- Invasive nature including, destruction of the prostatic parenchyma, invasion of the capsule and surrounding tissues
- Other features of a specific type of sarcoma

Clinical relevance (prognosis and treatment options)

- Treatment of choice is surgical removal
- The chemotherapy and radiation may be used but their efficacy is of question
- High-grade sarcoma has worse prognosis than the low-grade one

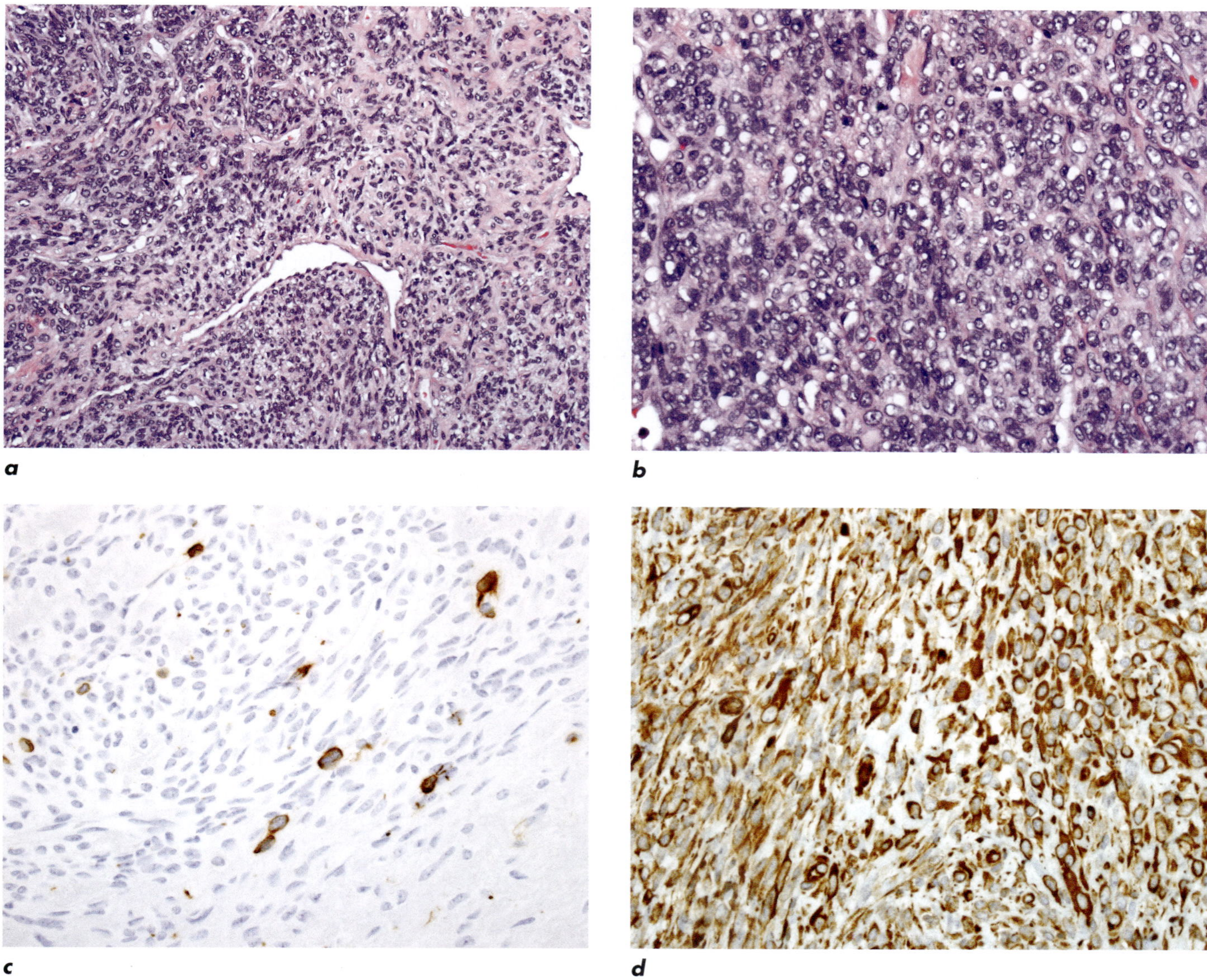

Figure 12-15.
Primary monophasic synovial sarcoma. The prostate is largely replaced by a large infiltrating mass, which is composed of cellular spindle cells around a branching vessel forming a "staghorn" appearance (*a*). The tumor is very cellular with brisk mitotic figures (*b*). By immunohistochemistry, the tumor cells are focally positive for AE1/AE3 keratins (*c*) and diffusely positive for vimentin (*d*).

PROSTATIC STROMAL TUMOR OF UNCERTAIN MALIGNANT POTENTIAL

Definition

- A neoplasm of uncertain malignant potential, arising from specialized prostatic stroma

Other terms

- Atypical spindle cell proliferation, atypical stromal hyperplasia, phyllodes tumor, or cystic epithelial stromal tumor

Clinical features

- Symptoms of lower urinary tract obstruction similar to those of BPH
- Palpable irregular mass on digital rectal examination
- Minimal PSA elevation, hematuria, or hematospermia is uncommon
- Occasionally, the patient may be asymptomatic and the lesion detected by prostate needle core biopsy

Gross pathology

- Irregularly enlarged prostate
- Poorly defined mass with cut surface showing white-tan fibroid appearance
- Hemorrhage and necrosis are uncommon

Histology

- Spindle tumor cells with scant cytoplasm surrounding the trapped glands (Fig. 12-16)
- Several patterns have been observed; however, mixed patterns are often seen in one case
- Pleomorphic pattern: hypercellular spindle cells with blizzard appearance, but degenerative nuclei (Fig. 12-17). Mitosis is common
- Eosinophilic pattern: hypercellular stromal cells with eosinophilic cytoplasm
- Phyllodes pattern: leaf-like hypercellular stroma with extended and dilated benign prostatic glandular epithelium (Fig. 12-18), resembling phyllodes tumor of the breast
- Myxoid pattern

Immunohistochemistry

- CD34 positive, PR may be positive
- Myoepithelial cell and smooth muscle markers, such as smooth muscle actin and desmin, can be positive

Clinical relevance (prognosis and treatment options)

- Surgical resection for completion is the treatment of choice
- Tumor may recur if resection is not complete
- Tumor may be locally invasive and be adherent to adjacent organs such as the rectum
- It may be associated with sarcoma as either transformation or coexisting
- Metastasis is usually absent

Figure 12-16.
Pleomorphic pattern of prostatic stromal tumor is characterized by the presence of cellular stromal cells surrounding the prostatic glands (*a*). At a higher magnification, the glandular cells are hyperplastic (*b*) and proliferating stromal cells are spindle shaped and cellular.

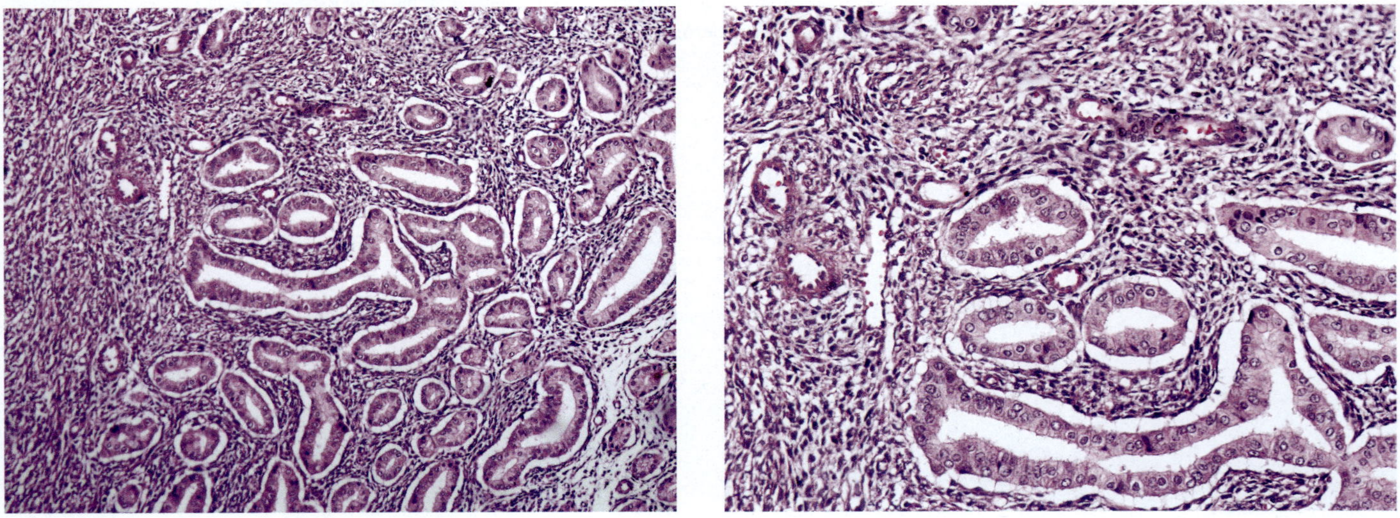

a **b**

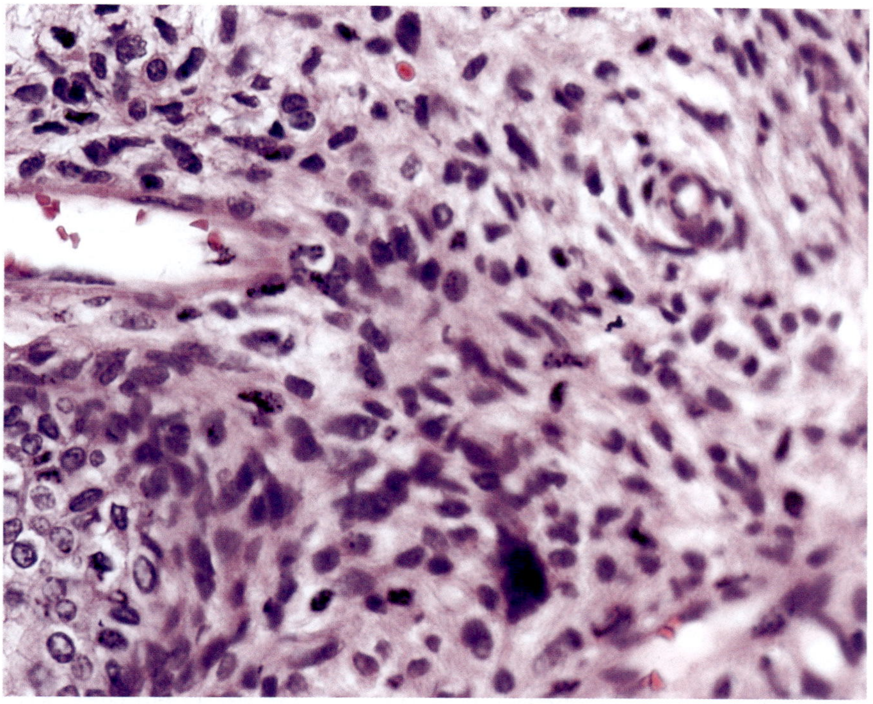

Figure 12-17.
Prostatic stromal tumor with focal degenerative atypia.

Figure 12-18.
Phyllodes tumor of the prostate with leaf-like lobular growth patterns (*a*). High magnification (*b*) shows the abnormal stromal cells covered by hyperplastic epithelium.

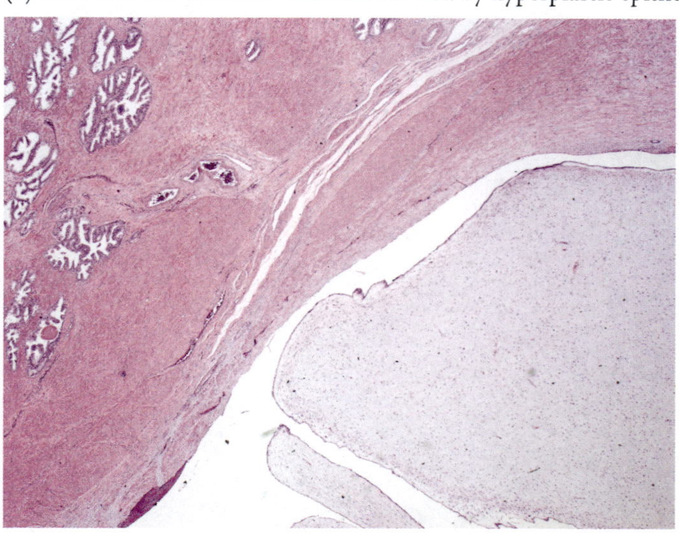

a

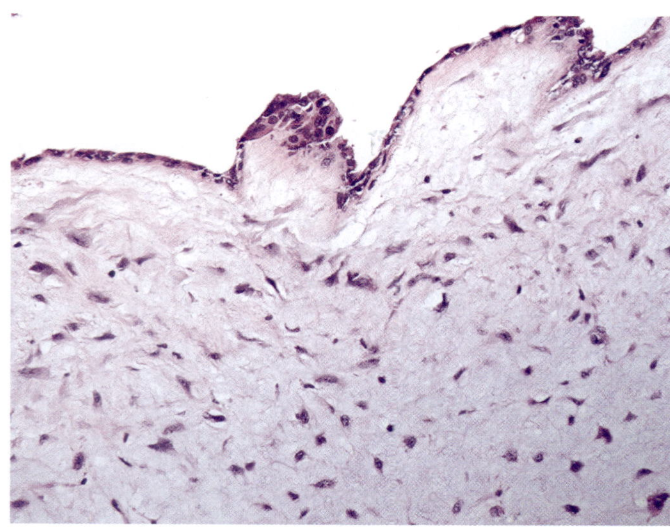

b

SECONDARY CARCINOMAS OF THE PROSTATE

Definition

- Any carcinomas from other organs secondarily involving the prostate by direct extension or metastasis

Pathogenesis and epidemiology

- Advanced carcinomas of any other organs may directly invade into or metastasize to the prostate
- The most common type is urothelial carcinoma, which has been discussed as a separate entity earlier in the chapter
- The secondary carcinoma involving the prostate is much less common than prostatic adenocarcinoma involving other organs

Clinical features

- A history of a primary carcinoma in other organs, with or without treatment
- Typically found as workup of the primary carcinoma
- Occasionally identified as the initial presentation
- Imaging studies can confirm the diagnosis

Gross pathology

- Mass lesion, single or multiple, well defined except urothelial carcinoma in the prostate
- Involvement of the prostate capsule if by direct extension

Histology

- High-grade carcinoma (Fig. 12-19), which does not have the typical morphological features of a prostatic adenocarcinoma

Immunohistochemistry

- Depending on the primary tumor, organ-specific markers such as lung TTF1, colon CDX2 can be helpful
- Prostate markers negative

Clinical relevance (prognosis and treatment options)

- In a patient with a known history of a high-grade carcinoma elsewhere, the secondary carcinoma in the prostate should be considered when its history is not typical for prostate cancer
- Sometimes, primary and secondary urothelial carcinoma in the prostate cannot be distinguished easily, but cystoprostatectomy will be the treatment of choice

Figure 12-19.
Metastatic colonic adenocarcinoma in the prostate, diffusely infiltrating the prostate (*a*).
High magnification shows the presence of sheets of mucin-containing signet ring cells (*b*).

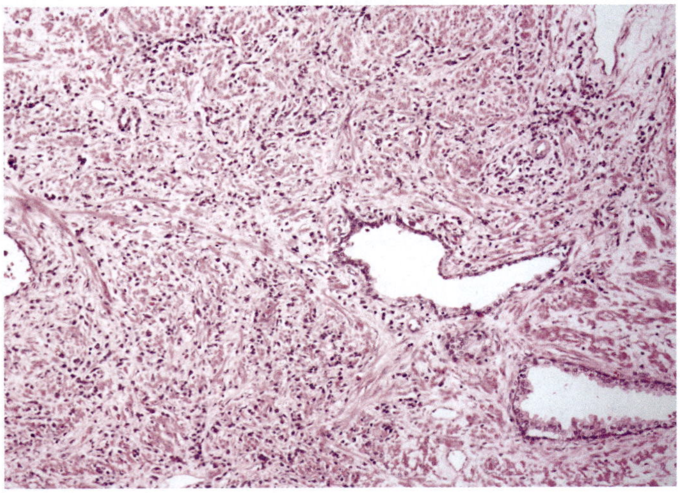

a

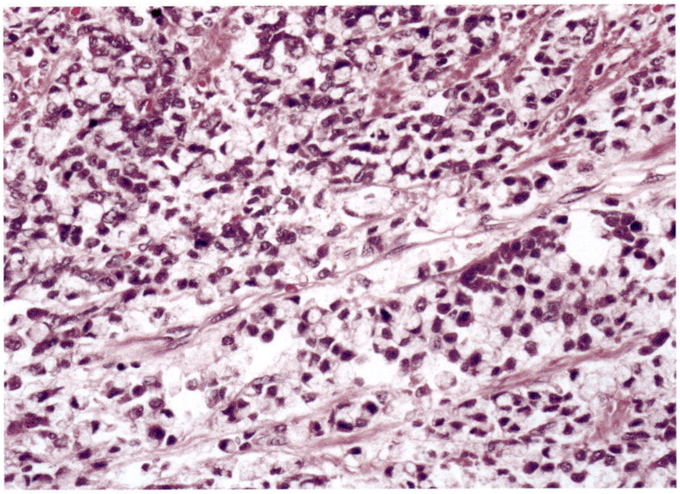

b

CHRONIC LYMPHOCYTIC LEUKEMIA IN THE PROSTATE

Definition

- Chronic lymphocytic leukemia (CLL) in the prostate is characterized by an accumulation of monoclonal small (mature) B lymphocytes in the prostate

Other terms

- Small lymphocytic lymphoma (SLL) or B-cell CLL involving the prostate

Pathogenesis

- Typically CLL/SLL involves the prostate as a part of systemic disease
- Isolated CLL in the prostate is very rare
- Other lymphomas such as large B-cell lymphoma can also involve the prostate

Clinical features

- Most cases may be asymptomatic
- Constitutional symptoms such as fever, night sweat, weight loss, or enlarged lymph nodes may be seen
- Occasionally, urinary obstruction is the presenting symptom
- Blood analysis shows an increase of mature lymphocytes

Gross pathology

- Prostate is diffusedly enlarged, no defined mass lesions

Histology

- Heavy lymphocytic infiltrates, which are not centered around the prostatic glandular structures (Fig. 12-20)
- A homogenous or monotonous population of mature-appearing lymphocytes, with minimal cytological atypia (Fig. 12-20*b*)
- No plasma cells or other inflammatory cells present, which are usually present in inflammatory processes
- Intraepithelial lymphocytes are uncommon
- Destruction of glandular structures usually not present
- Sometimes, CLL/SLL may coexist with prostatic adenocarcinoma

Immunohistochemistry

- B-cell markers; CD5, CD19, CD20, CD23 positive

Clinical relevance (prognosis and treatment options)

- In the men with prostate biopsy material showing heavy lymphocytic infiltrates, which is away from the glands and with no other inflammatory cells, the diagnosis of CLL in the prostate should be considered or suggested
- However, a definitive diagnosis of CLL in the prostate can hardly be based on morphologic evidence alone. Such a diagnosis is mostly depending on the clinical history, immunohistochemistry, and other ancillary studies
- Confirmation with blood tests to demonstrate increased lymphocytes in the blood is relatively easy
- Because of the slow and progressive nature of the disease, patients are clinically monitored with no treatment
- However, recent studies have shown some effectiveness of chemotherapeutic regiments for this condition
- Therefore, the establishment of CLL in the prostate may have some therapeutic value

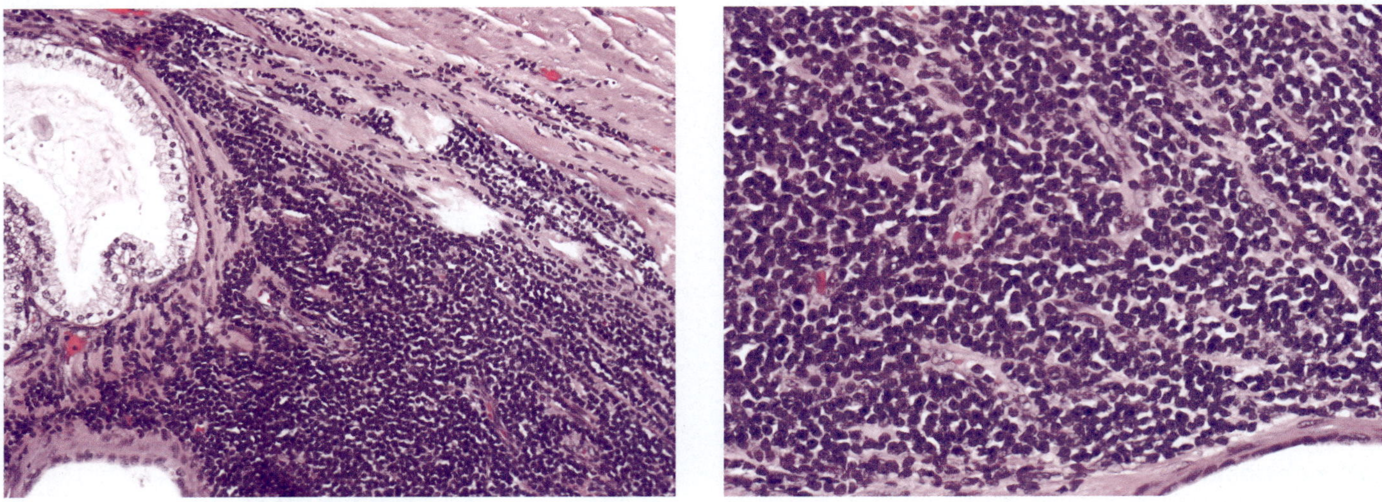

a b

Figure 12-20.

Chronic lymphocytic lymphoma (CLL) involving the prostate. The prostatic glands are surrounded by the heavy lymphocytic infiltrates. The infiltrates may be close to or away from the glandular structures (*a*). High magnification shows monotonous small lymphocytes (*b*) without other inflammatory cells and plasma cells.

SECTION 2
The Testis

CHAPTER 13 Normal Histology of Testis and Paratesticular Tissue

TESTIS

Anatomy

- A pair of testes are hanging organs connected by spermatic cords and located within the scrotum
- Each testis weighs approximately 20 g with volume of 15 to 25 mL
- The testis is confined by a thick fibrotic membrane called tunica albuginea and segmented by septa into small lobes

Histology

- The major components of the testis are seminiferous tubules (Fig. 13-1), each measures 150 to 200 μm in diameter and 30 to 80 cm in length
- The combined length of seminiferous tubules runs 0.5 to 1 km long, which provides a sufficient space and environment the production of millions of sperm
- There are three major populations of specific cells in the testis
- Germ cells
  - Undergoing maturation within seminiferous tubules
  - Each cycle of spermatogenesis will take 1 to 2 months
  - The most primitive germ cells are spermatogonia, located close to the basement membrane of the tubules, which will eventually transform into spermatozoa (sperm)
  - The germ cells are listed below starting from the most primitive ones (Fig. 13-1*b*): Spermatogonia → Primary spermatocytes → Secondary spermatocytes → Spermatids → Spermatozoa
  - The different types of immature germ cells (spermatogonia and spermatocytes) are difficult to distinguish in routine surgical pathology specimens
  - But spermatids can be recognized by their small nuclei, and spermatozoa can be recognized by their tadpole-shaped heads
- Sertoli cells
  - Columnar cells within seminiferous tubules with indistinguishable pale cytoplasm
  - Sertoli cells have abundant cytoplasm in which germ cells are inserted. Sertoli cells are "nurse" cells that provide an environment for spermatogenesis
  - Sertoli cells have oval nuclei, pale chromatin, and prominent centrally located nucleolus (Fig. 13-2)
  - They also produce a large number of factors and hormones such as GnRH-like factor, estrogen, TGF-α, inhibin, Mullerian duct inhibitory factor
  - Sertoli cells are positive for inhibin, but negative for calretinin
- Leydig cells
  - Polygonal cells are present in clusters between seminiferous tubules (Fig. 13-3)
  - Leydig cells have abundant eosinophilic cytoplasm in which crystal of Reinke (Fig. 13-4) may be seen in normal, hyperplastic, or neoplastic Leydig cells
  - Leydig cells are the major producers of androgen, and they also produce b-endorphin and other factors
  - They are positive for inhibin and calretinin

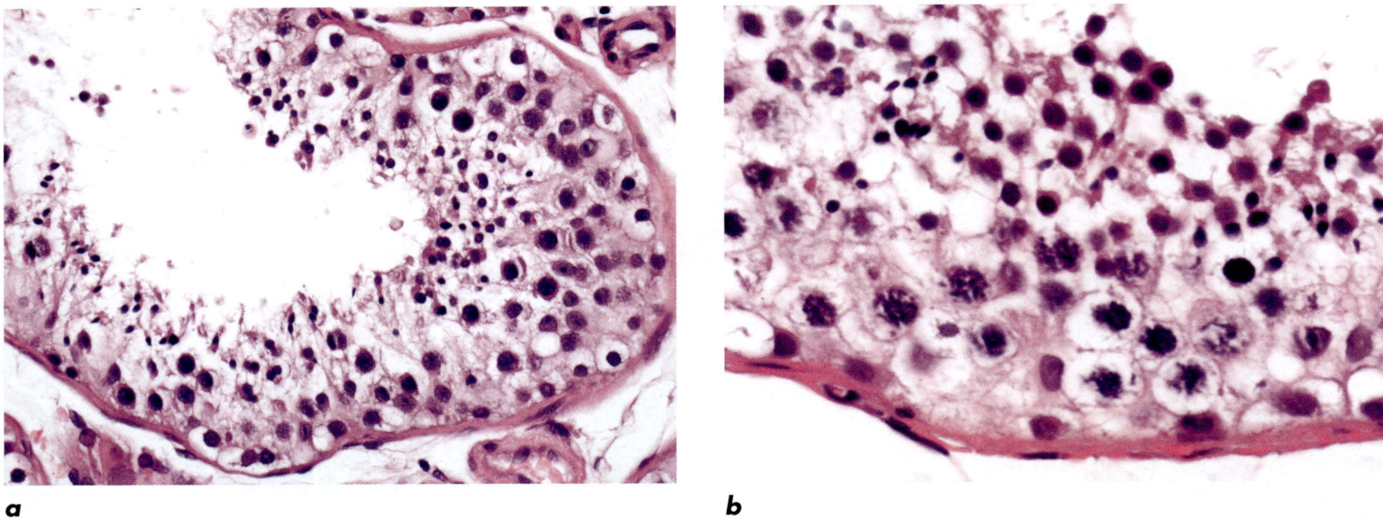

Figure 13-1.
An adult testis. A seminiferous tubule is filled with immature and developing germ cells as well as mature spermatozoa (*a*). High magnification (*b*) shows immature germ cells (spermatogonia and spermatocyte) are located in the base of the tubule, spermatids (intermediate cells with dense nuclei), and spermatozoa (tadpole-like blue dots) are located at the luminal side. Occasional Sertoli cell nuclei can be seen.

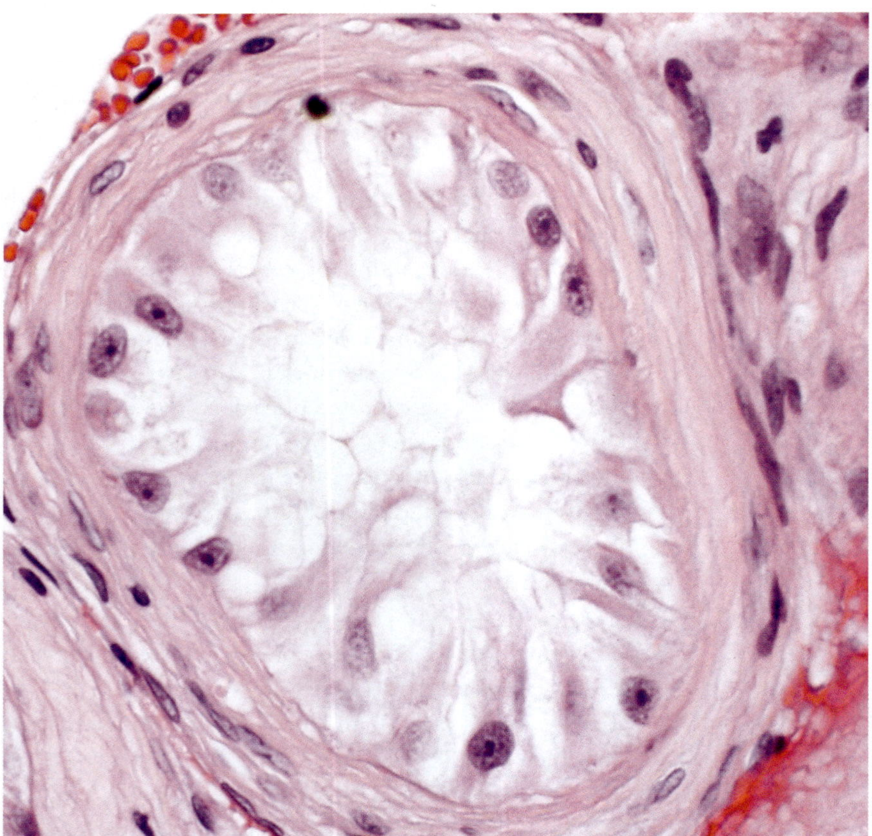

Figure 13-2.
Sertoli cells (Sertoli only pattern) are the only cell population in this seminiferous tubule with abundant pale cytoplasm and an oval-shaped nucleus with a prominent nucleolus.

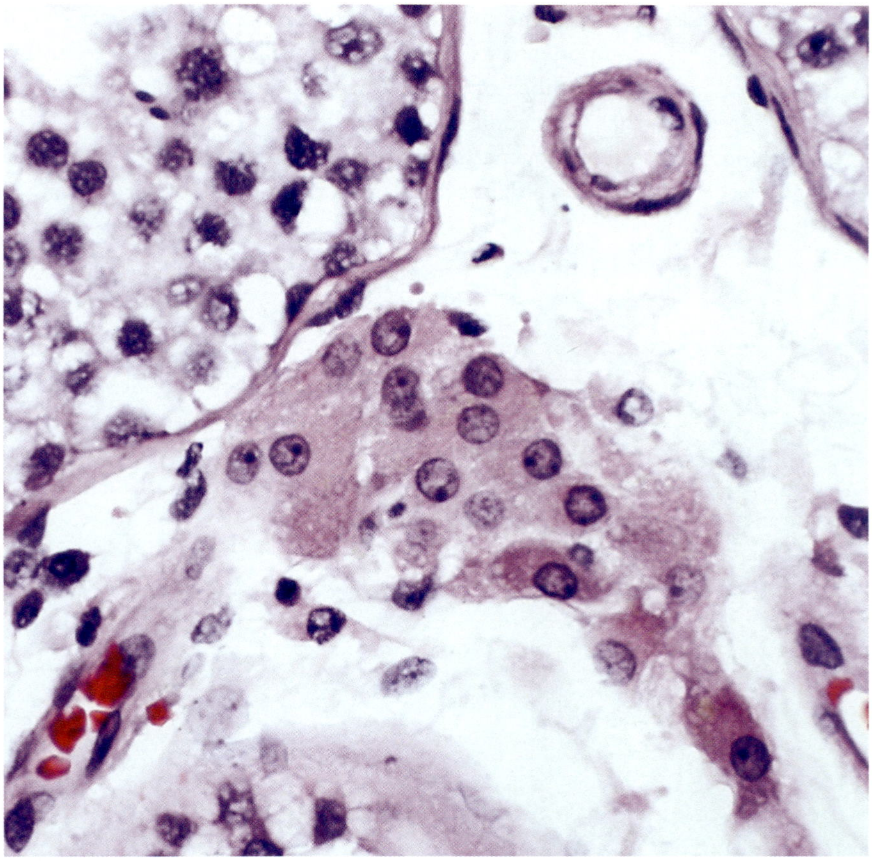

Figure 13-3.
A cluster of Leydig cells present between seminiferous tubules displaying abundant eosinophilc cytoplasm and round nuclei, and containing lipofuscin.

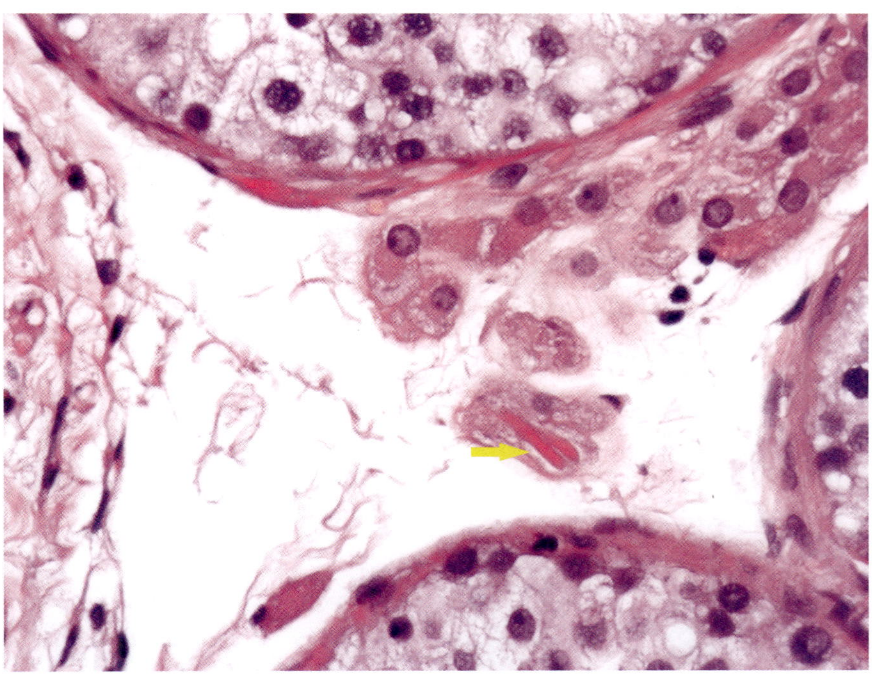

Figure 13-4.
Reinke crystals (arrow) in a Leydig cell.

Development of the testis

- A fetal testis contains seminiferous tubules with mostly immature Sertoli cells and occasional immature germ cells. Leydig cells are rarely seen (Fig. 13-5)
- A testis in preadolescent boy contains an increasing number of germ cells in the seminiferous tubules. But no spermatozoa can be identified. Leydig cells can be seen occasionally (Fig. 13-6)
- A testis in an adolescent contains all the germ cell components, as well as Sertoli cells and Leydig cells. But the number of spermatozoa is smaller (Fig. 13-7) than that in an adult
- Spermatogenesis can be seen in the testis of men over 70 years old, but decrease in the number of germ cells

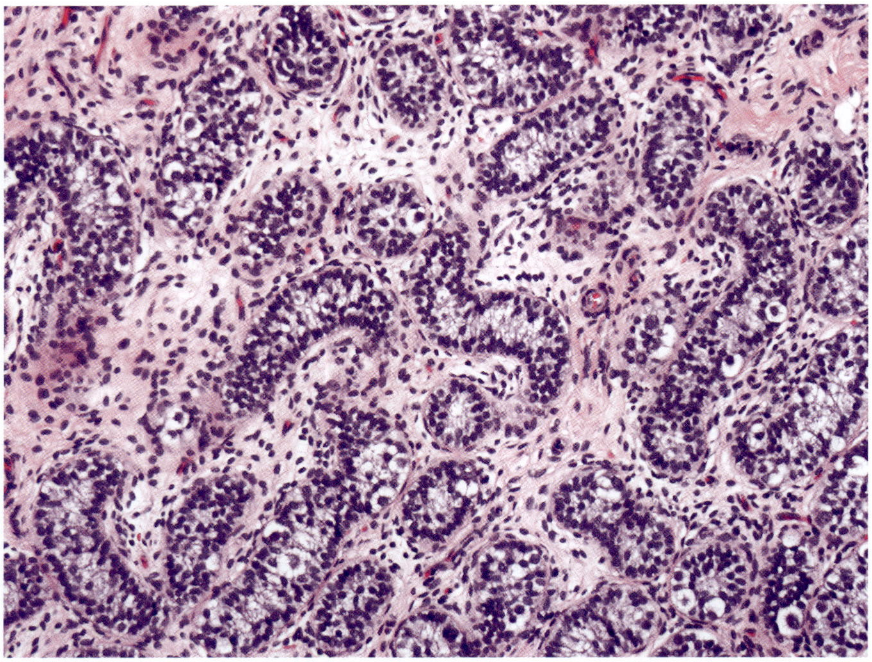

Figure 13-5.
A fetal testis with seminiferous tubules containing mostly immature Sertoli cells and occasional immature germ cells with a perinuclear halo.

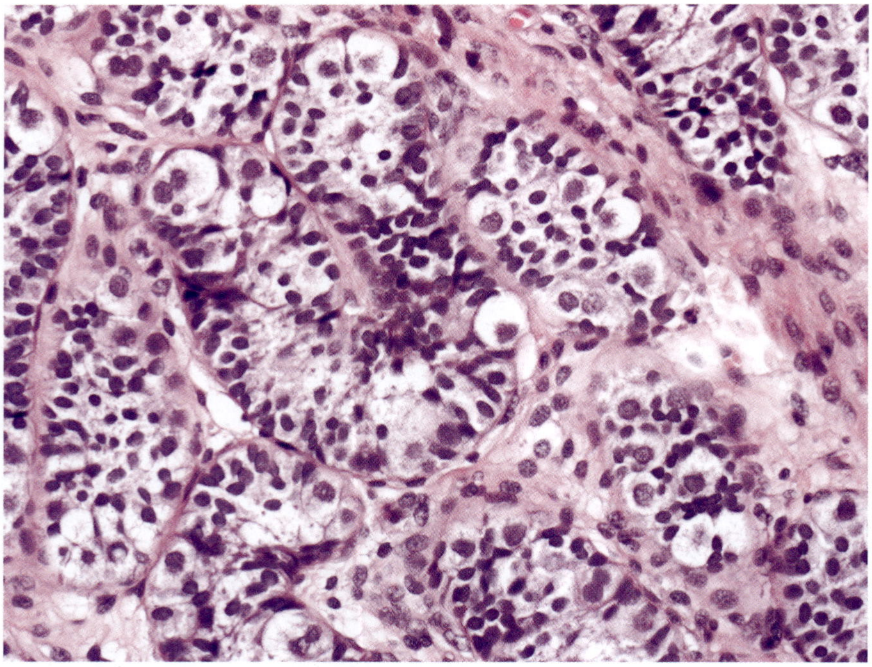

Figure 13-6.
A preadolescent testis showing increased number of germ cells within seminiferous tubules.

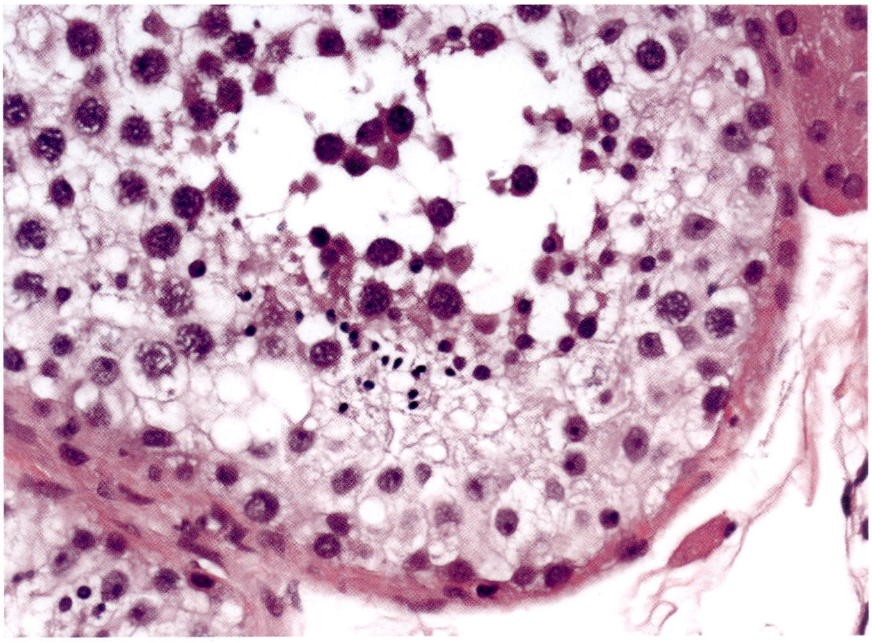

Figure 13-7.
An adolescent testis showing the presence of a small number of spermatids and spermatozoa.

RETE TESTIS AND EFFERENT DUCTS

Rete testis

- Located in the hilar region of the testis
- Composed of a network of anastomosing channels (Fig. 13-8*a*)
- The lining cells of the rete channels are flat or cuboidal cells with occasionally columnar cells (Fig. 13-8*b*)
- The rete testis connects to seminiferous tubules proximally and the efferent ducts distally
- The sperm will be transferred from the seminiferous tubules → rete testis → efferent ducts → epididymis → vas deferens

Efferent ducts

- Composed of convoluted tubular structures lined by ciliated pseudostratified columnar epithelium connecting between the rete testis and epididymis
- Different from the epididymis, the efferent ducts are smaller in diameter, with epithelial infoldings (projections) and more irregular nuclear location without the luminal clearing zone of the epididymis (Fig. 13-9)
- Both the rete testis and efferent ducts are the Wolffian (mesonephric) duct derivatives along with other male reproductive structures such as epididymis, seminal vesicles, and ejaculatory ducts (Table 13-1). All these structures are positive for PAX8

Figure 13-8.
The rete testis composed of dilated tubules separated by thick fibrous septa (*a*). The lining cells are flat or cuboidal epithelium (*b*).

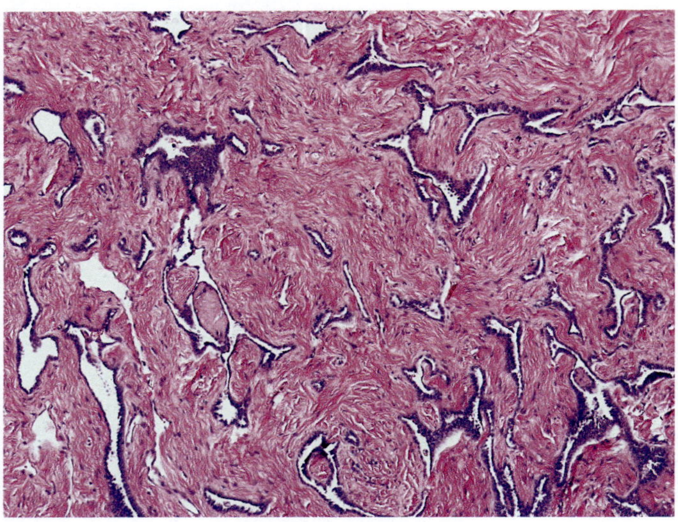

a

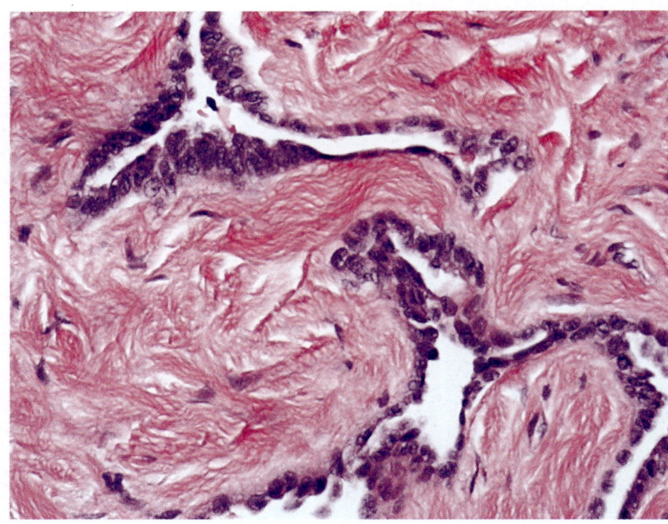

b

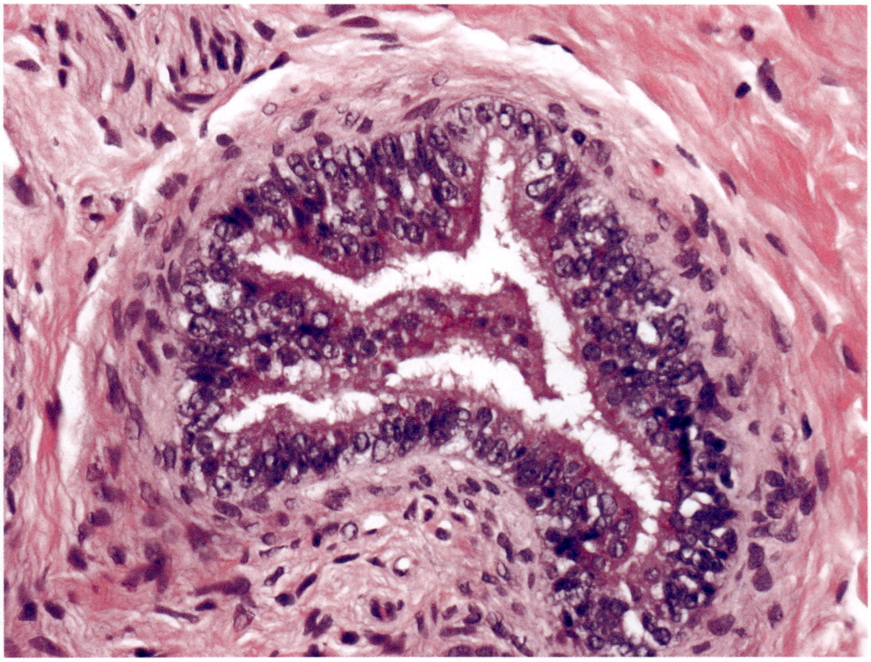

Figure 13-9.
The efferent duct is lined by pseudostratified columnar epithelium.

Table 13-1. Derivatives for the Woffian Duct and Mullerian Duct

	Male	*Female*
Wolffian duct (pair)	Seminal vesicles	(Regression)
	Ejaculatory ducts	Gartner ducts
	Vas deferens	
	Epididymis	
	Efferent ducts	
	Rete testis	
Mullerian duct (pair)	(Regression)	Fallopian tubes
	Appendix testis	Uterus
		Cervix
		Upper vagina

EPIDIDYMIS

- A pair of duct structures attached to each testis
- It can be divided into the head (connecting to testis), body, and tail (connecting to vas deferens)
- Consisting of highly coiled tubules with regularly round lumens (Fig. 13-10)
- Each tubule is lined by tall pseudostratified columnar epithelial cells, which have immobile cilia called sterocilia (Fig. 13-11)
- The epithelial nuclei are located in the basal half of the epithelium so that the luminal half of the epithelium is clear of nuclei, creating a luminal clearing zone (Fig. 13-11)

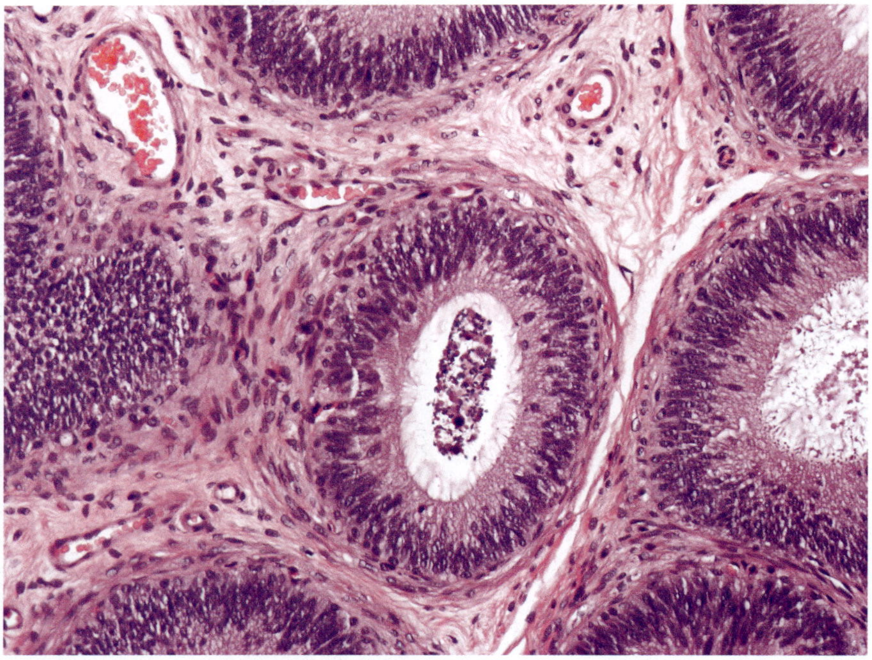

Figure 13-10.
The epididymis consists of packed large tubules lined by tall columnar cells with regularly round lumens, lined by columnar epithelium cells with a luminal clearing zone.

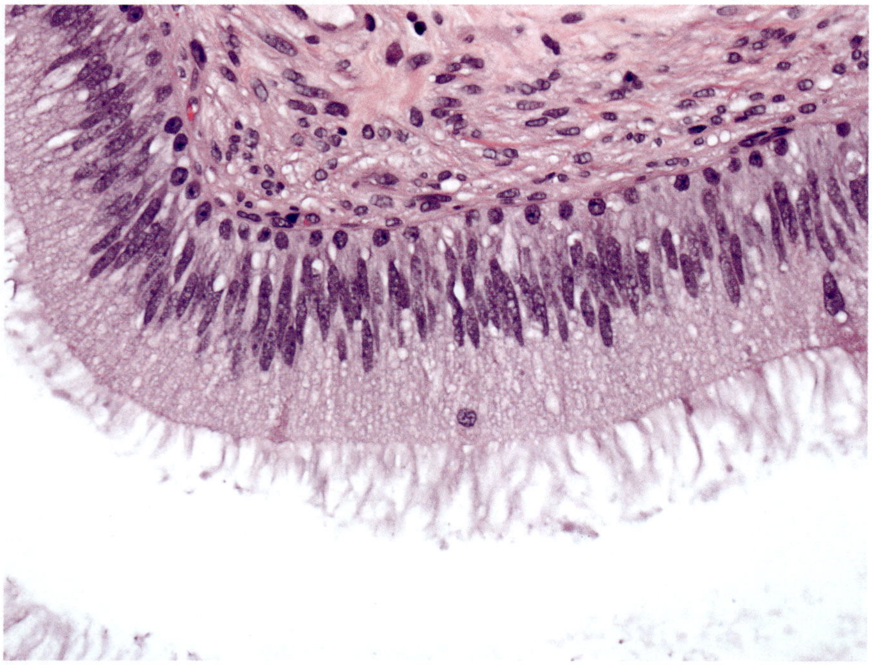

Figure 13-11.
An epididymis tubule display regularity of columnar cells with basally located cigar-shaped nuclei and long sterocilia.

VAS DEFERENS

- A pair of long muscular tubular structures with a small lumen, lined by pseudostratified columnar epithelium with sterocillia (Fig. 13-12*a*)
- Vas deferens has a thick muscular wall with inner longitudinal layer, middle circular layer, and outer longitudinal layer (Fig. 13-12*b*)
- In a vasectomy specimen, complete cross sections of the lumen of a vas deferens need to be confirmed by histological examination

SPERMATIC CORDS

- A pair of structures including vas deferens and surrounding tissues located mostly in inguinal canal, connecting the testis and abdomen
- In addition to the vas deferens (Fig. 13-12*c*), the spermatic cord specimen contains both arteries and veins, lymphatic vessels, nerve plexus, skeletal muscle, fibroadipose tissue, and tunica vaginalis, sometimes even lymph nodes (Fig. 13-12*d*)
- The spermatic cord margins are important for evaluation of a orchiectomy specimen of a patient with a germ cell tumor

Figure 13-12.
Vas deferens has a very thick smooth muscle wall and small caliber lumen (*a*). The pseudostratified columnar epithelium forms an irregularly shaped lumen (*b*). Spermatic cord contains vas deferens (*c*), skeletal muscle, a lymph node and vessels, as well fibroadipose tissue (*d*).

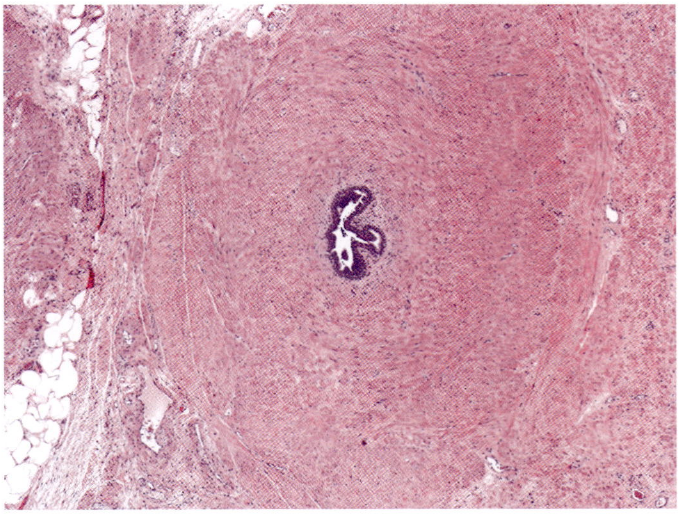
a

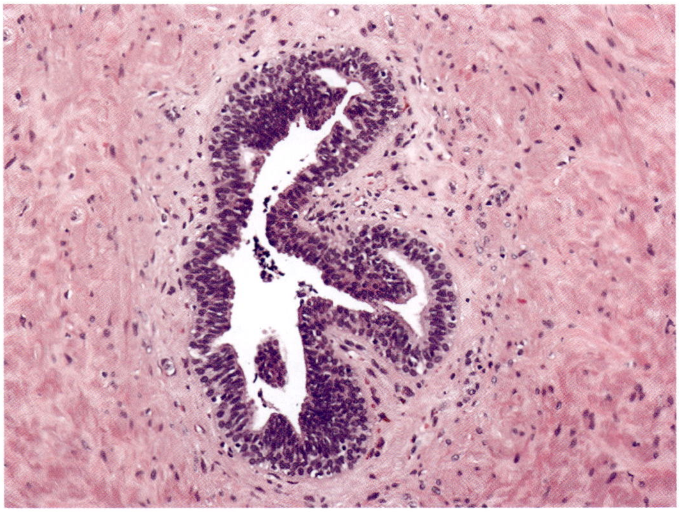
b

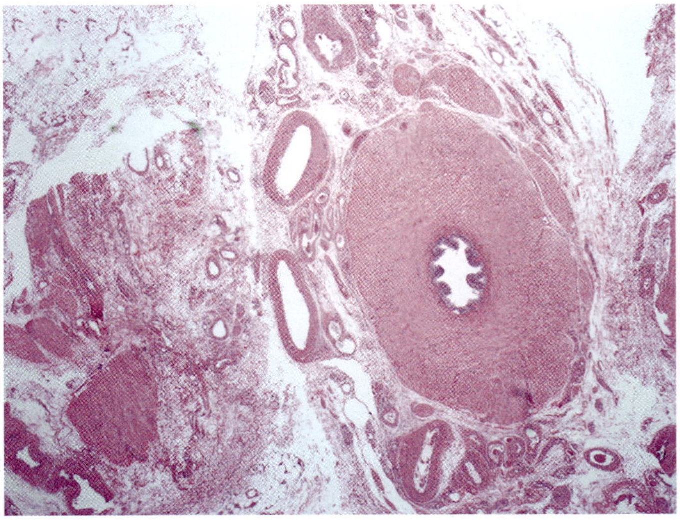
c

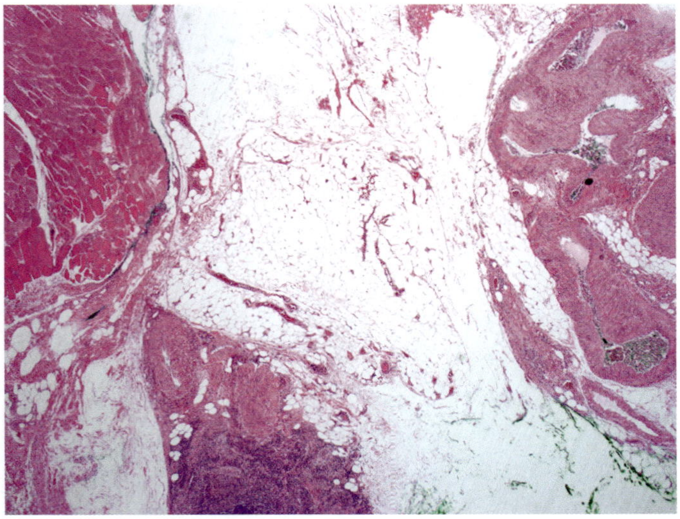
d

CHAPTER 14

Immunohistochemical Markers for Testicular Cells

Ximing J. Yang, Sean K. Wang

LACTATE DEHYDROGENASE

- Lactate dehydrogenase (LDH) is an enzyme present in many types of cells
- Serum marker to measure the tumor load
- Not specific for any tumor type; besides germ cell tumors, metastatic carcinomas or lymphomas can also cause elevated LDH

PLACENTAL ALKALINE PHOSPHATASE

- Placental alkaline phosphatase (PLAP) is an enzyme normally present in the placenta
- Tissue marker with cytoplasmic staining (Fig. 14-1)

Figure 14-1.
PLAP staining. Intratubular germ cell neoplasia, unclassified (ITGCNU) with H&E staining (*a*) and PLAP staining (*b*) showing scattered neoplastic germ cells within a tubule are positive for PLAP. PLAP positive staining in seminoma (*c*) and embryonal carcinoma (*d*).

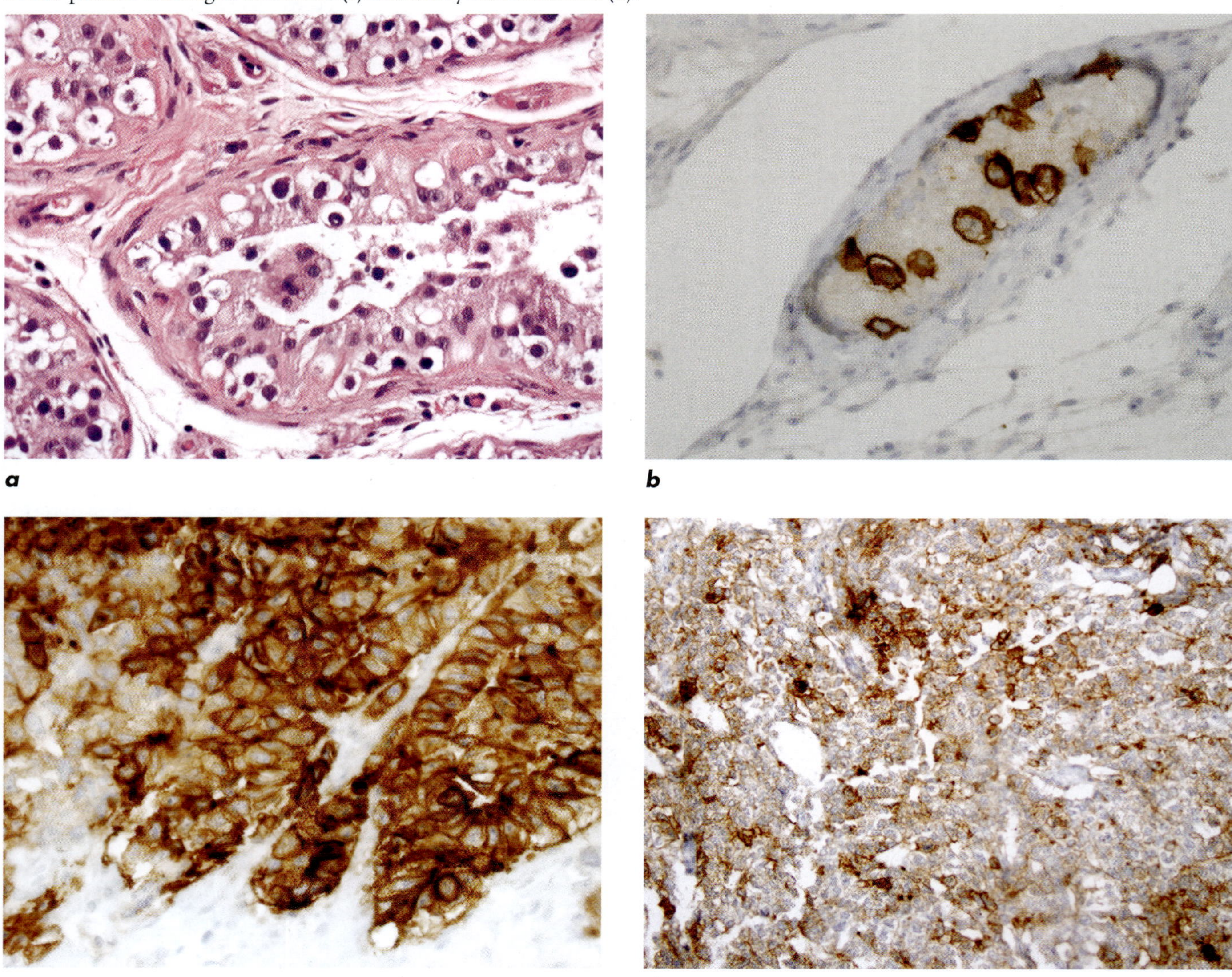

- Present in intratubular germ cell neoplasias, unclassified (ITGCNU) (Fig. 14-1*b*) and all subtypes of germ cell tumors of the testis including seminomas (Fig. 14-1*c*), embryonal cell carcinomas (Fig. 14-1*d*), yolk sac tumors, and immature teratomas
- Positive in ovarian germ cell tumors
- Useful for diagnosis but not subtyping of germ cell tumors

CD117

- CD117 (C-kit protein) is a receptor tyrosine kinase related to cell growth and differentiation
- Tissue marker with predominantly membrane and some cytoplasmic staining
- Positive in ITGCNUs (Fig. 14-2*a*) and seminomas (Fig. 14-2*b*)
- Potential therapeutic target since inhibitors for this tyrosine kinase are available

Figure 14-2.
C-kit staining (mostly membranous) in neoplastic germ cells in ITGCNU (*a*) and a classic seminoma (*b*). OCT-4 positivity (nuclear staining) in scattered neoplastic cells of ITGCNU (*c*) and seminoma cells (*d*).

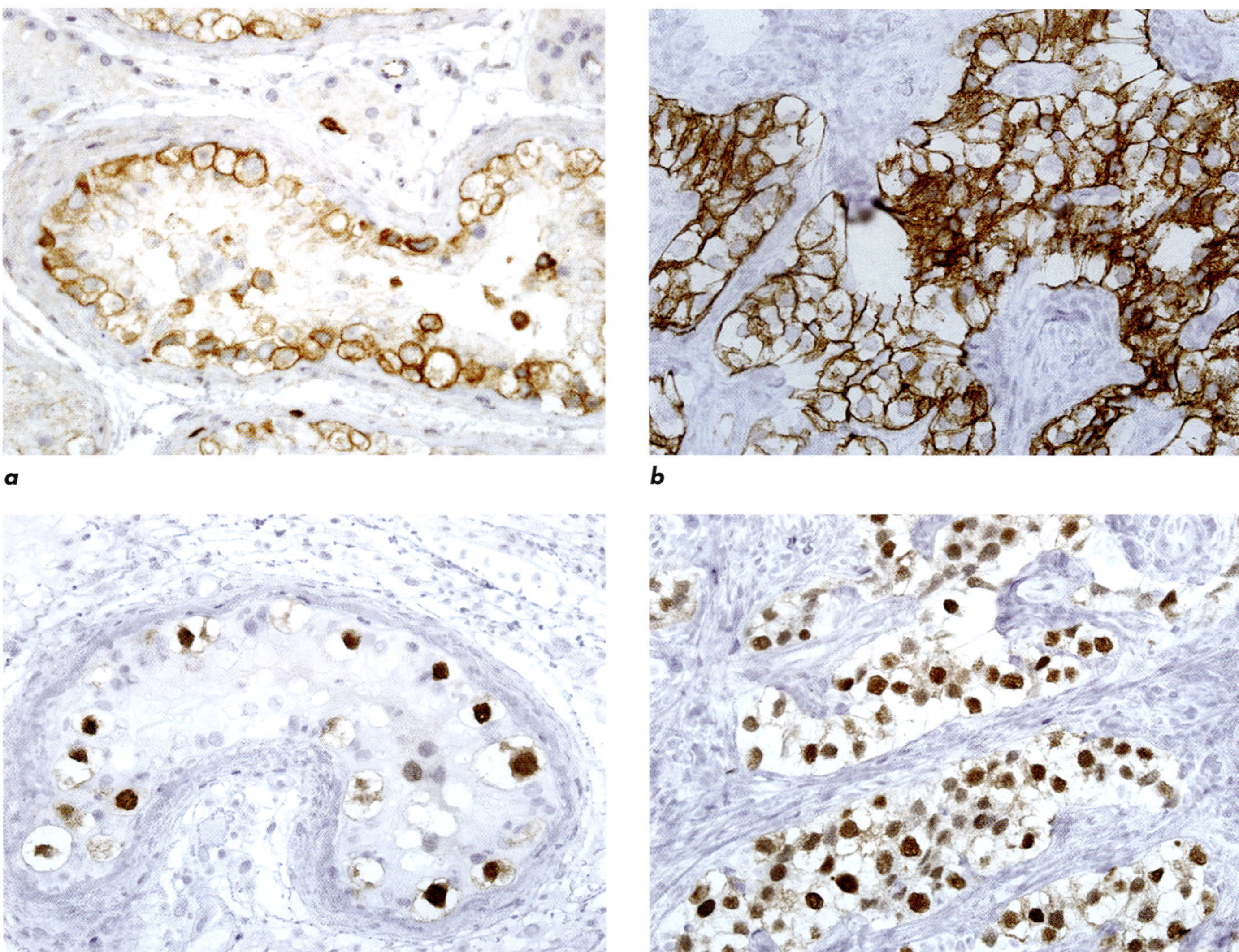

a **b** **c** **d**

OCTAMER-BINDING TRANSCRIPTION FACTOR 4

- Octamer-binding transcription factor 4 (OCT-4) is a transcription factor related to self-renewal of undifferentiated embryonic stem cells
- Tissue marker with nuclear staining
- Positive in ITGCNUs (Fig. 14-2*c*), seminomas (Fig. 14-2*d*), and embryonal carcinomas (Fig. 14-3)
- Reliable marker for these subtypes
- Negative in normal germ cells, yolk sac tumors, and sex cord stromal tumors

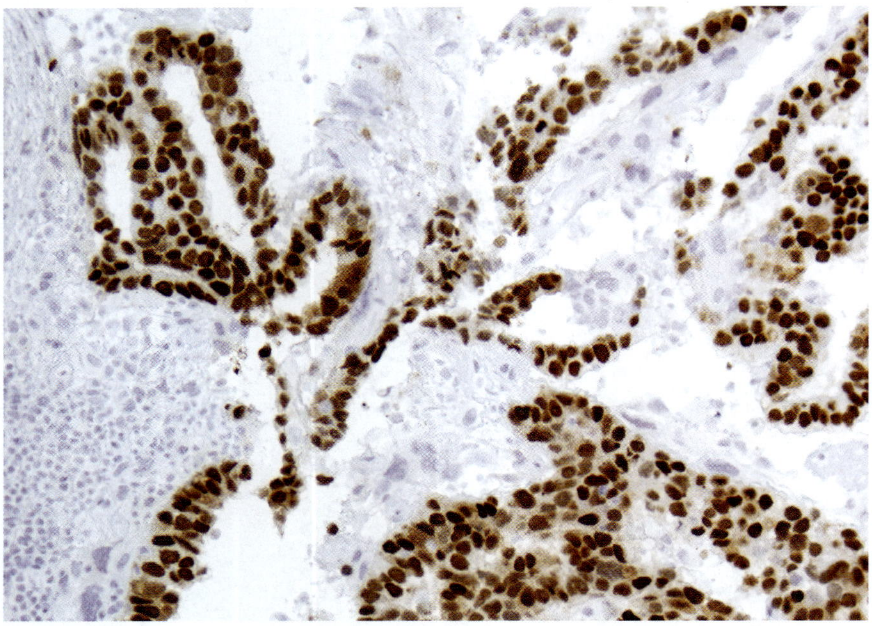

Figure 14-3.
OCT-4 positive nuclear staining in embryonal carcinoma cells, which form nests or glandular structures.

CD30

- CD30 is a cell membrane protein belonging to the tumor necrosis factor receptor family
- Positive in embryonal carcinomas with cytoplasmic staining (Fig. 14-4), although not very sensitive, and the staining may be focal
- Can be positive in some lymphomas

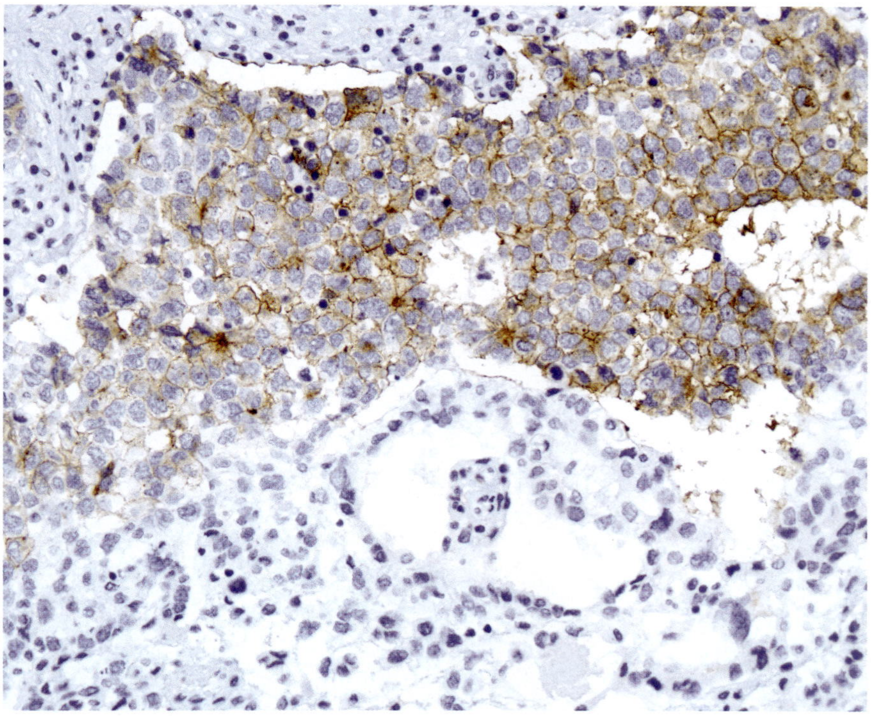

Figure 14-4.
CD30 positivity in an embryonal carcinoma.

GLYPICAN 3

- Glypican 3 is a fetoprotein normally produced by fetal tissue, which may play a role in the regulation of cell growth and proliferation
- Tissue marker with cytoplasmic staining and possible serum marker
- Positive in yolk sac tumors (Fig. 14-5*c*) and choriocarcinomas (Fig. 14-5*d*)
- Positive in hepatocellular carcinomas as well as hepatoblastomas and nephroblastomas (Wilms tumor) in children
- More sensitive than AFP

α-FETOPROTEIN

- α-Fetoprotein (AFP) is normally produced by fetal tissue
- Tissue marker with cytoplasmic staining and serum marker
- Positive in yolk sac tumors (Fig. 14-5*e*) and hepatocellular carcinomas
- Not very sensitive, staining may be focal

Figure 14-5.
Yolk sac tumor (*a*) and choriocarcinoma with H&E staining (*b*). Both yolk sac tumor (*c*) and choriocarcinoma (*d*) show glypican 3 (GPC3) immunoreactivity. Yolk sac tumor is also positive for AFP (*e*) and choriocarcinoma is positive for β-HCG (*f*).

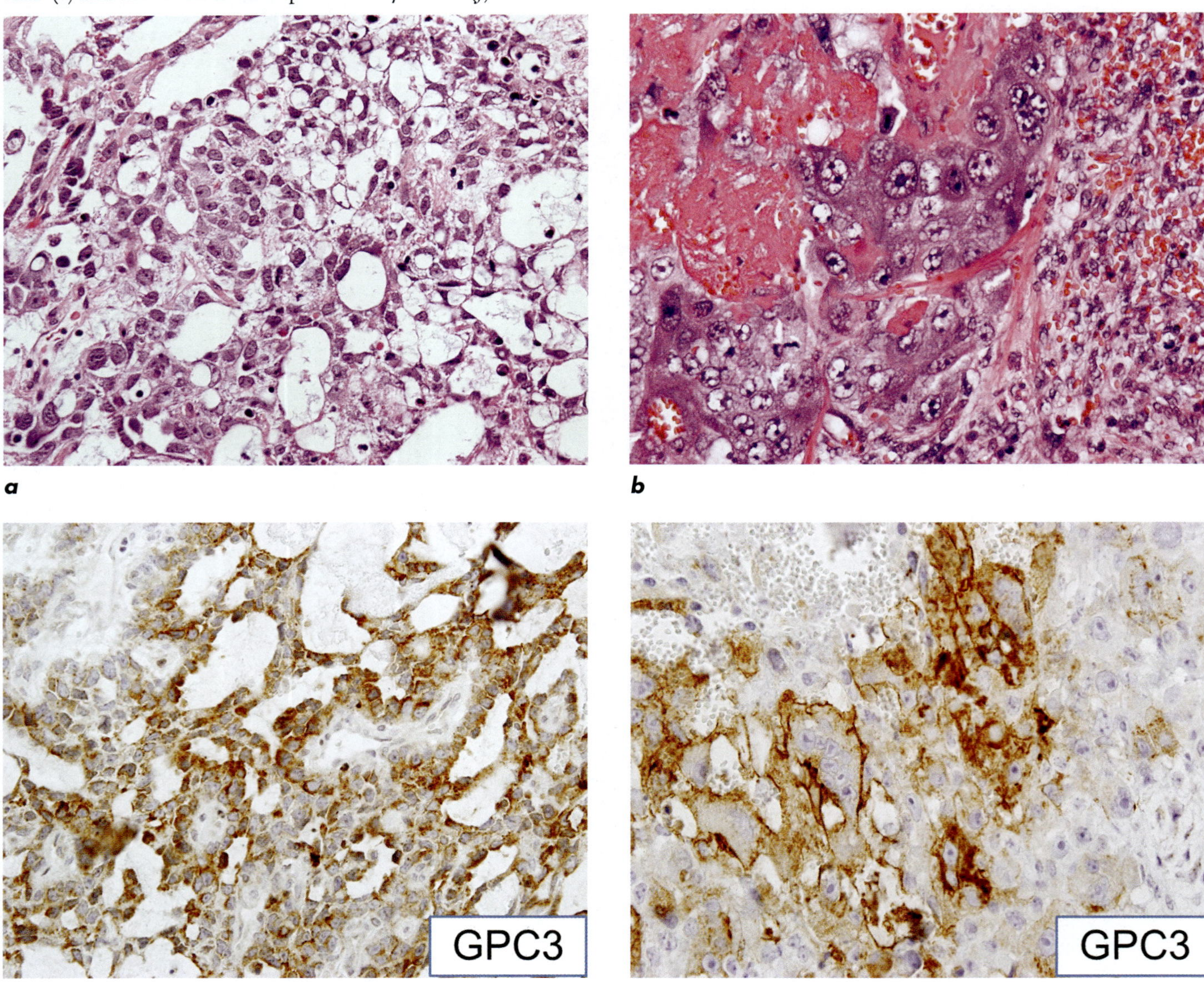

a b c d

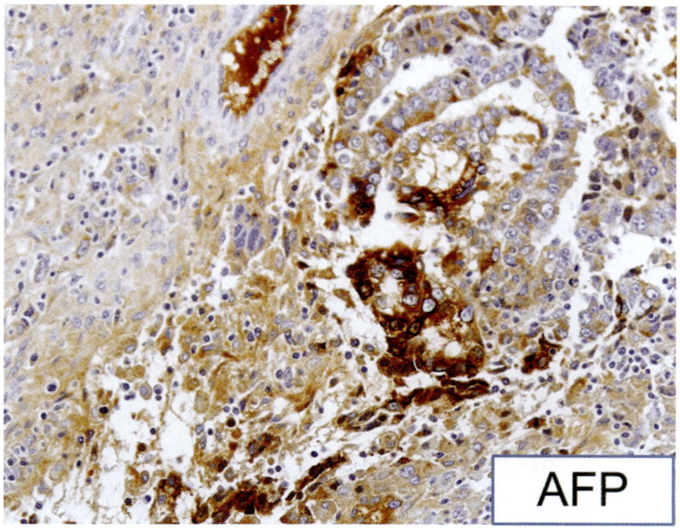

e

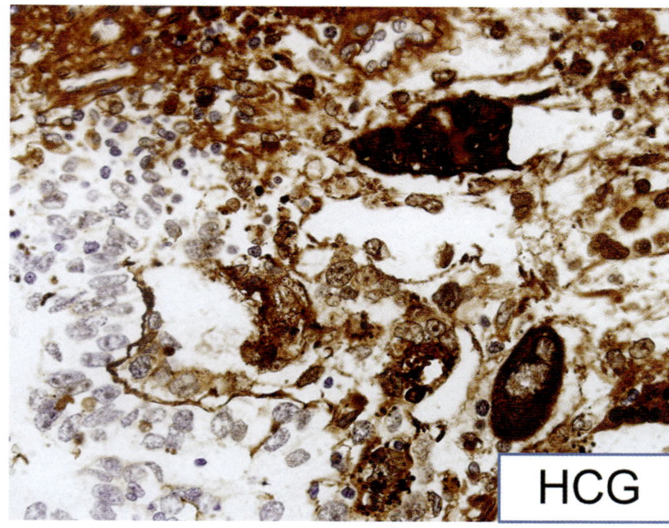

f

Figure 14-5.
(*Continued*)

BETA UNIT OF HUMAN CHORIONIC GONADOTROPIN

- Beta unit of human chorionic gonadotropin (β-HCG) is produced by syncytiotrophoblasts and normally present in the placenta
- Tissue marker with cytoplasmic staining and serum marker
- Positive in choriocarcinomas (Fig. 14-5*f*)
- Occasionally low levels of HCG can be detected in patients with seminomas, which contain a small number of neoplastic syncytiotrophoblasts
- High background in tissue sections if serum HCG level is high
- The immunohistochemical markers for classification of germ cell neoplasms are summarized in Table 14-1

Table 14-1. Immunohistochemistry Markers in Different Types of Testicular Germ Cell Neoplasms

Markers	*ITGCNU*	*Seminoma*	*Embryonal carcinoma*	*Yolk sac tumor*	*Choriocarcinoma*
PLAP	Positive	Positive	Positive	Positive	Positive
CD117	Positive	Positive	Negative	Negative	Negative
OCT-4	Positive	Positive	Positive	Negative	Negative
CD30	Negative	Negative	Positive	Negative	Negative
AFP[a]	Negative	Negative	Negative	Positive	Negative
Glypican 3	Negative	Negative	Negative	Positive	Positive
β-HCG[a]	Negative	Negative	Negative	Negative	Positive

AFP, α-fetoprotein; β-HCG, beta unit of human chorionic gonadotropin; OCT-4, octamer-binding transcription factor 4; PLAP, placental alkaline phosphatase.

[a]Used as tissue marker and serum marker.
Negative: less than 1% cases positive.

INHIBIN

- Inhibin is produced by Sertoli cells. Androgens stimulate inhibin production, which regulates spermatogenesis
- Inhibin downregulates follicle-stimulating hormone (FSH) synthesis and inhibits FSH secretion
- Can be detected in sex cord stromal cells including Sertoli cells and Leydig cells (Fig. 14-6) and their neoplasms
- Can also be found in adrenal cortical cells and ovarian sex cord stroma cells

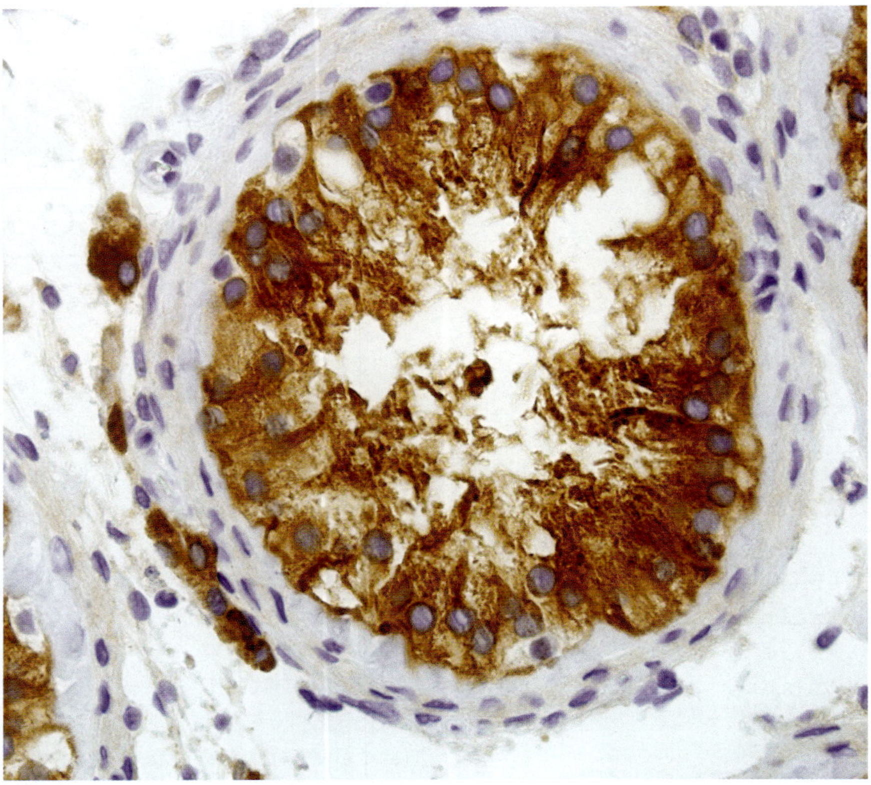

Figure 14-6.
Inhibin positivity in Sertoli cells in the seminiferous tubules and Leydig cells between tubules.

DOUBLE STAINING WITH C-KIT AND INHIBIN

- We have developed the C-kit/inhibin double immunostaining, which is commercially available
- C-kit reactivity is demonstrated with a red chromogen
  - Neoplastic cells (red) in ITGCNU (Fig. 14-7)
  - Seminomas (red)
  - Benign germ cells: negative for both C-kit and inhibin
  - Mast cells (red)
  - GI stromal tumors, renal oncocytomas, and chromophobe RCCs (red)
- Inhibin reactivity is demonstrated with a brown chromogen
  - Sertoli cells and Leydig cells (brown)
  - Sertoli adenomas and other Sertoli and Leydig cell tumors (brown)
  - Adrenal cortical cells and tumors (brown)
- Useful in subtyping testicular germ cell tumors with seminomas positive for C-kit (Fig. 14-8)
- Useful to confirm the nature of Sertoli cells and Leydig cells (Fig. 14-8)
- Useful in studying infertility cases

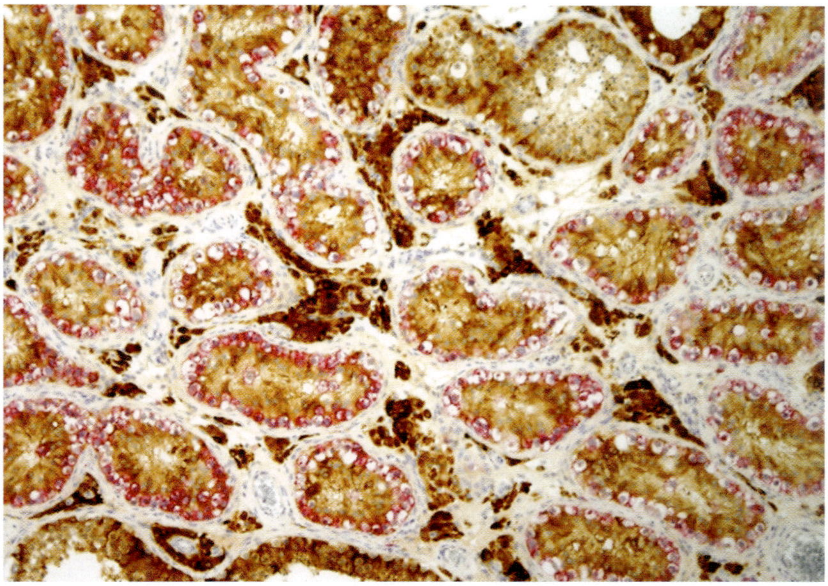

Figure 14-7.
Double immunostaining with C-kit and inhibin in ITGCNU. Within seminiferous tubules, ITGCNU neoplastic cells are stained red and Sertoli cells are stained light brown; outside tubules, Leydig cells are stained darker brown.

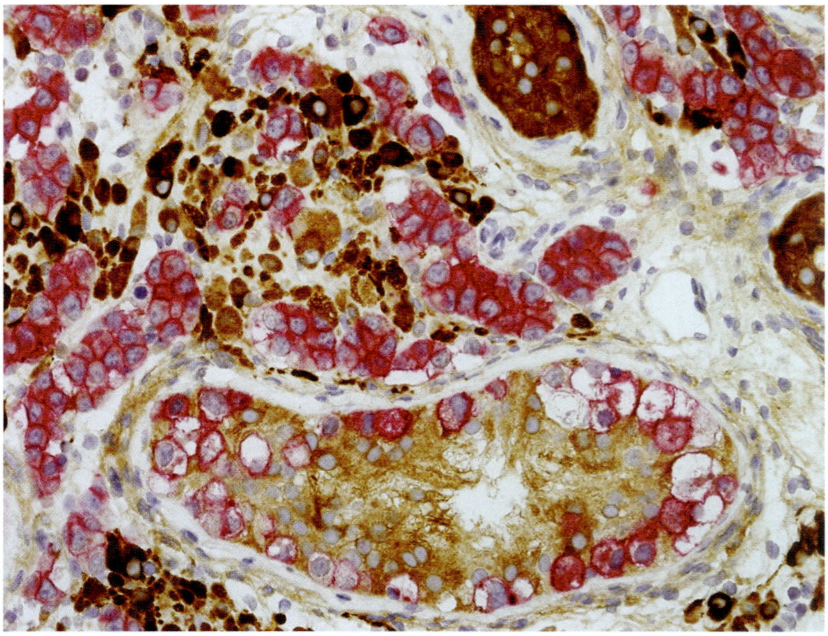

Figure 14-8.
Double immunostaining with C-kit and inhibin in ITGCNU and seminoma. Within seminiferous tubules, ITGCNU cells are stained red and Sertoli cells are stained light brown; outside tubules, seminoma cells are stained red and Leydig cells are stained darker brown.

ISOCHROMOSOME 12P

- Isochromosome 12p [I(12p)]
- Seen in all subtypes of testicular germ cell tumors
- Also seen in germ cell tumors from other organs
- This molecular genetic change can be detected using fluorescence in situ hybridization (FISH) or other molecular analysis
- Sensitivity of detecting I(12p) is only 50% for germ cell tumors

CHAPTER 15 Inflammatory Lesions of the Testis and Paratesticular Tissues

INFECTIOUS GRANULOMATOUS ORCHITIS

Definition

- Granulomatous inflammation of the testis by infectious etiology

Pathogenesis

- Most infectious causes are tuberculosis or fungi

Clinical features

- Localized form presents as a testicular mass
- Imaging studies can confirm the presence of a testicular mass
- If systemic disease, typically associated with lung or other organ involvement
- Patients may have symptoms such as fever or fatigue

Gross pathology

- Poorly defined mass lesions, single or multiple
- When the testis is bisected, focal or extensive cheesy necrotic material may be present in the center of caseating granulomas (Fig. 15-1)

Histology

- Caseating granulomas (necrotizing granulomas) are characterized by the presence of caseating (caseous) necrosis, which contains soft, white to yellow proteinaceous dead material resembling cheese grossly (Fig. 15-2)
- A granuloma is composed of histiocytes and Langerhans giant cells with central necrosis (Fig. 15-2)
- Granulomas caused by bacteria and infectious agents may contain neutrophils in addition to histiocytes, which may be called pseudotuberculous granulomas
- Granulomas caused by syphilis are called gummas, which contain central vessels with coagulative necrosis, and numerous plasma cells in the periphery
- Sarcoidosis, a disease of noninfectious etiology, is composed of granulomas that cannot be distinguished from infectious granulomas. Diagnosis is based on exclusion
- In practice, morphological features in a granuloma alone are often not specific for identifying infectious etiology. Special stains and more importantly microbiology studies including culture, biochemical, and molecular tests are more accurate
- Scar tissue and hyalinization are present in chronic cases. Residual seminiferous tubules show normal or reduced spermatogenesis

Immunohistochemistry

- AFB, GMS stains may demonstrate organisms
- Microbiology studies may be needed for confirmation of organisms

Clinical relevance (prognosis and treatment options)

- Specific antibacterial or antifungal infection is effective for systemic disease
- Generally, the etiology of a granuloma cannot be identified by a surgical pathologist unless with positive staining for organisms. Therefore, granulomatous inflammation is typically reported with AFB/GMS staining results. Clinical correlation, workup, and microbiology studies are necessary to further determine the etiology
- Surgical resection for localized lesions if suspicious for a neoplasm or removal of necrotic tissue

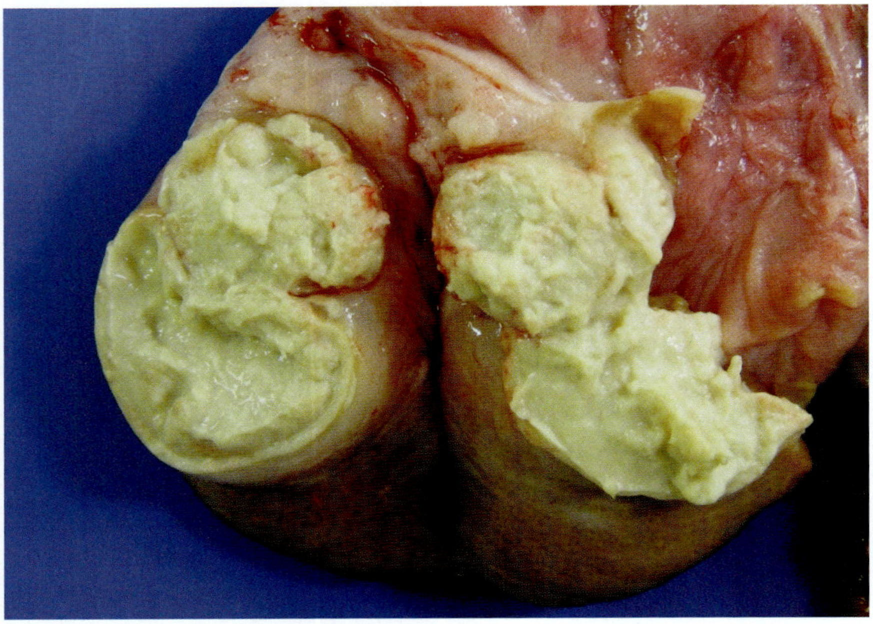

Figure 15-1.
An orchiectomy specimen with caseating granulomas from a patient with tuberculosis, showing abundant cheesy material in the center.

Figure 15-2.
A typical tuberculosis granuloma (*a*) is composed of caseating necrosis in the center surrounded by epithelioid histiocytes, and lymphocytic infiltrate. Higher magnification (*b*) shows a Langerhans' giant cell containing horseshoe-arranged nuclei along with other inflammatory cells.

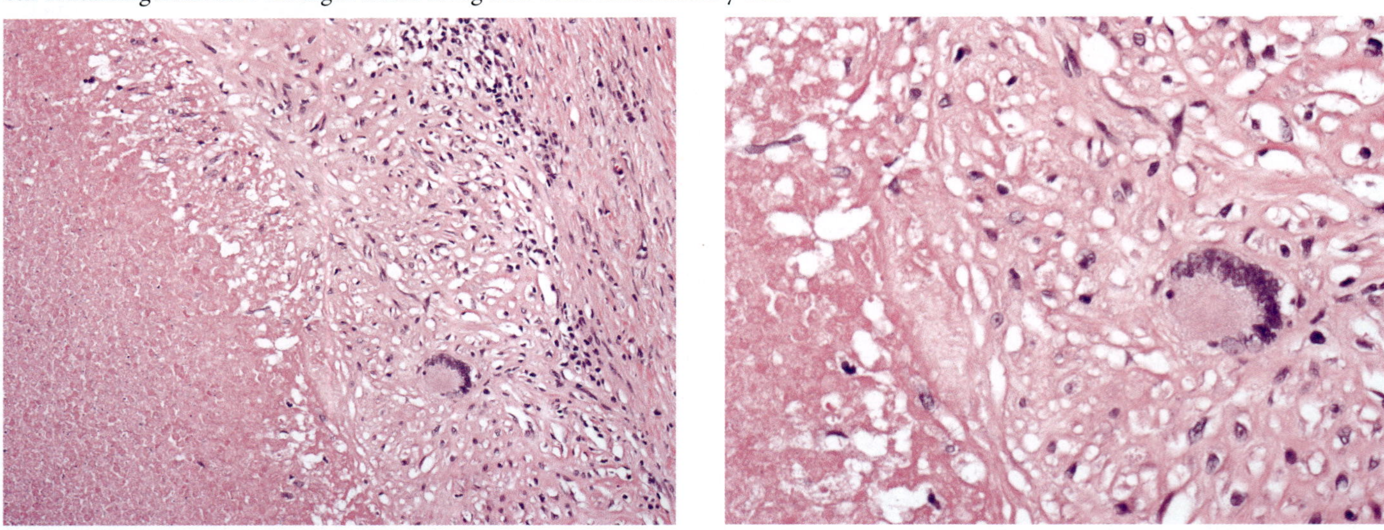

a **b**

NONSPECIFIC GRANULOMA ORCHITIS

Definition

- Chronic granulomatous inflammation of the testis with unknown etiology

Pathogenesis

- Causes of this condition are unknown and may be associated with autoimmune, infection, or trauma
- Inflammation may start from the seminiferous tubules and over time diffusely involve the entire testis

Clinical features

- Patients with nonspecific granulomatous orchitis (NSGO) may have flu-like symptoms such as fever, headache, sneeze, and cough
- Enlargement of the testis, firm but not palpable nodules, typically unilateral
- Hydrocele or inguinal hernia may be associated

Gross pathology

- Testis is diffusely enlarged without obvious nodules, different from other types of granulomatous orchitis in which nodules with caseating necrosis are typically seen
- Homogenous cut surface of an enlarged testis (Fig. 15-3)
- Epididymis may be involved

Histology

- Extensive chronic granulomatous inflammation containing histiocytes, lymphocytes, and multinuclear giant cells (Figs. 15-4 and 15-5)
- Inflammation may be centered around seminiferous tubules initially with the presence of intratubular histiocytes and sloughed germ cells (Fig. 15-6)
- Severely damaged residual tubular structures with germ cells and Sertoli cells surrounded by inflammatory cells may be seen (Fig. 15-7)
- Caseating necrosis is absent and fibrosis is prominent in the late stage

Immunohistochemistry

- CD68 positive for histiocytes, GMS and AFB should be negative

Clinical relevance (prognosis and treatment options)

- Although benign, this condition may cause extensive destruction of the testis; no effective medical treatment is available because of unknown etiology. Anti-inflammatory treatment could relieve symptoms
- Orchiectomy is the treatment of choice if medical treatment fails

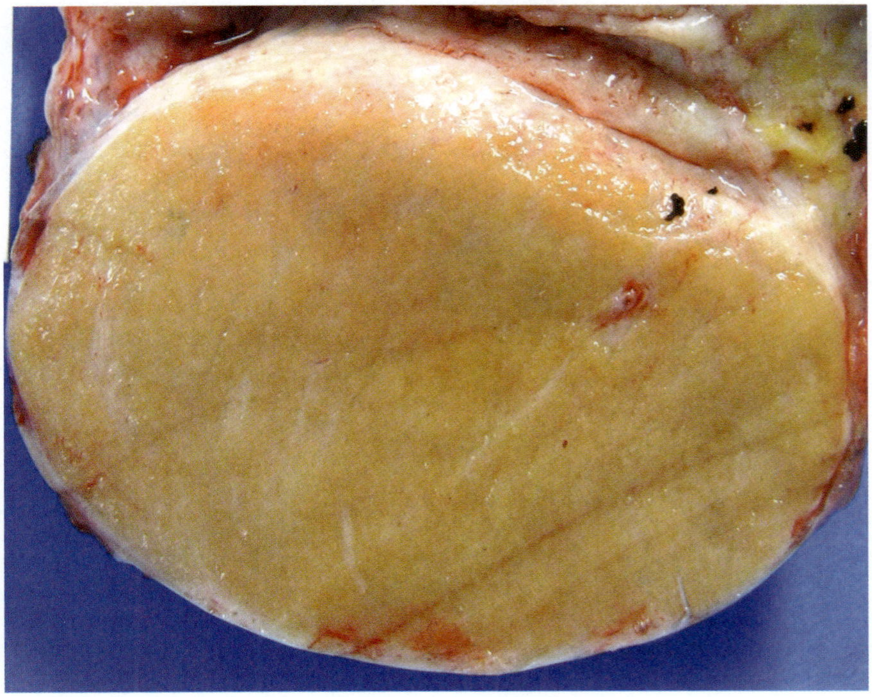

Figure 15-3.
Nonspecific granulomatous orchitis (NSGO) in an orchiectomy specimen shows diffuse enlargement of the testis, which is solid, firm with homogenous cut surface.

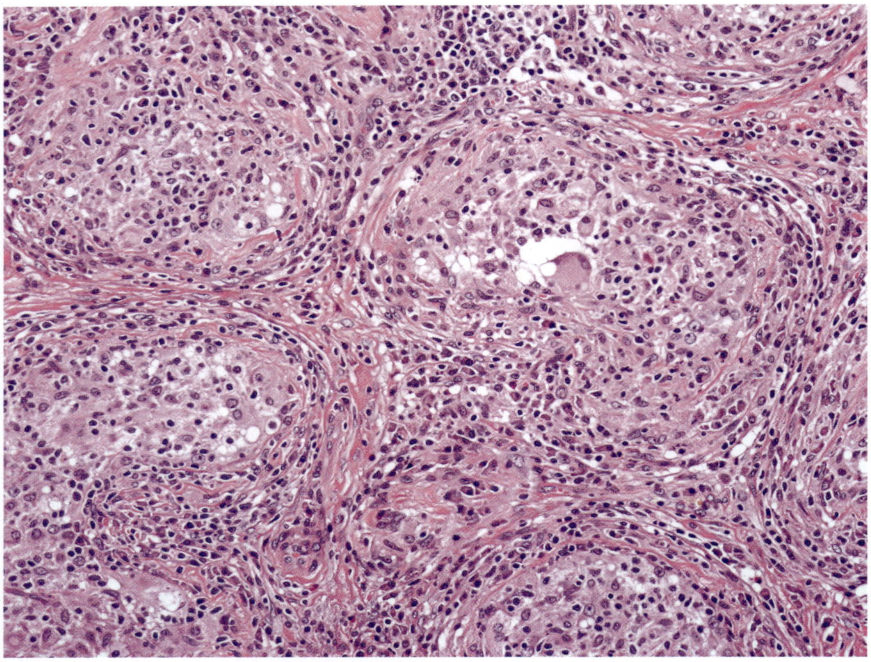

Figure 15-4.
Nonspecific granulomatous orchitis (NSGO) shows numerous granulomas replacing the entire testis.

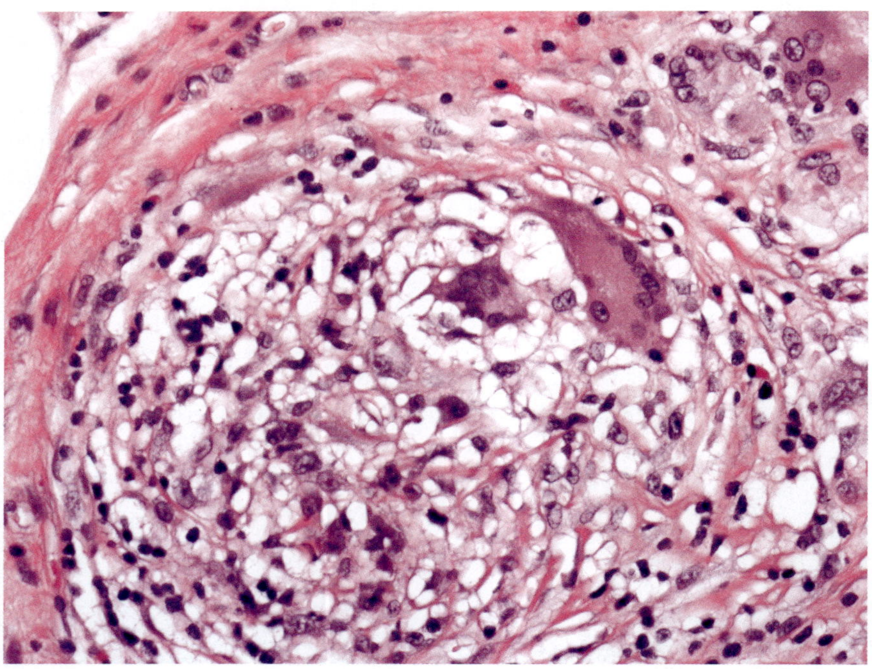

Figure 15-5.
A granuloma in NSGO consists of mostly epithelioid histiocytes, some lymphocytes and multinuclear giant cells without necrosis.

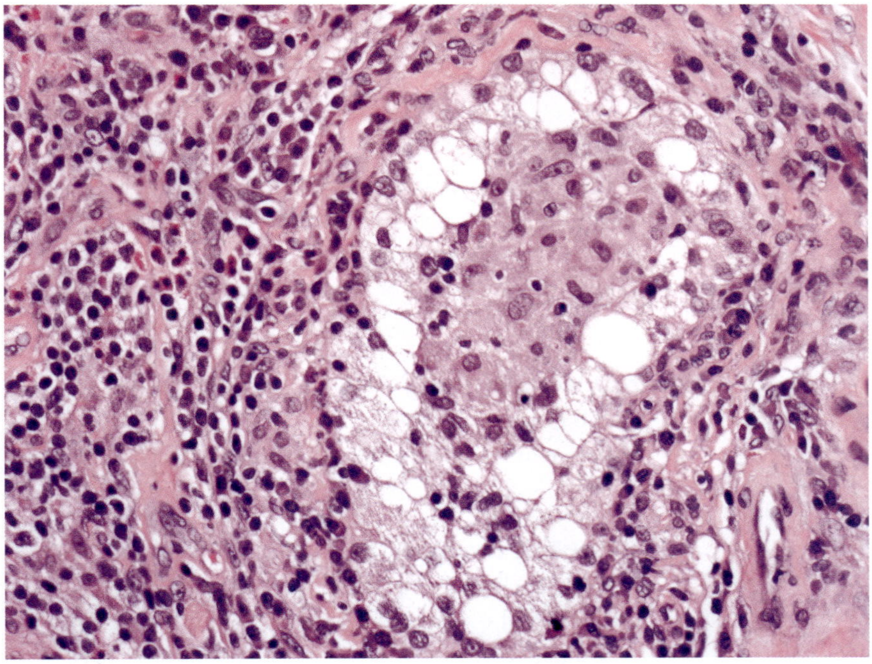

Figure 15-6.
A granuloma is forming within the residual tubule in NSGO.

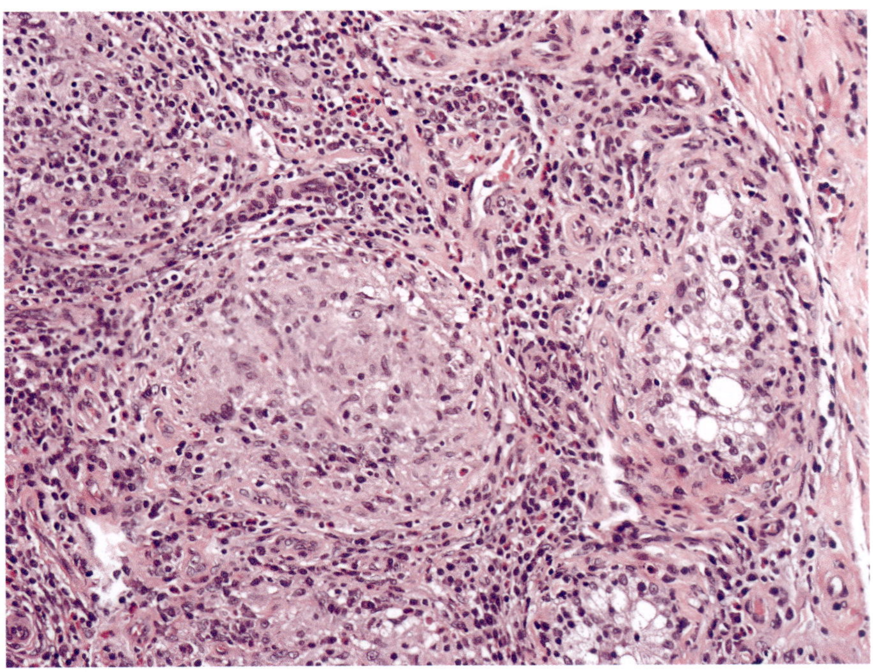

Figure 15-7.
A granuloma is present adjacent to seminiferous tubules in NSGO.

XANTHOGRANULOMA OF THE TESTIS

Definition

- Xanthogranuloma is a granulomatous inflammation with collection and lipid-laden macrophages

Other terms

- Xanthoma, xanthogranulomatous orchitis

Pathogenesis

- Xanthogranuloma (xanthoma = yellow tumor) is not a neoplasm, but a reactive granulomatous process
- Most likely caused by focal tissue damages. Destruction of cells releases abundant cholesterol, which is ingested by numerous macrophages
- Hyperlipidemia can be a risk factor

Clinical features

- May have a history of injury
- Localized mass lesion in the testis, often incidental finding by imaging studies

Gross pathology

- Can be well-defined mass or poorly circumscribed lesion
- Lesion appears bright yellow in cut surface because of its high lipid content, mostly cholesterol (Fig. 15-8)
- Focal hemorrhage, necrosis, and cystic changes may be present

Histology

- Numerous lipid-laden macrophages (Fig. 15-9)
- Granulomatous reaction includes mixed inflammatory cells and foreign body giant cells
- Cholesterol clefts can be seen

Immunohistochemistry

- CD68 positive
- Negative for keratins and other tumor markers

Differential diagnosis

- Metastatic clear cell renal cell carcinoma
  - Composed of sheets of clear cells with a "chicken-wire" vascular pattern
- Other granulomatous inflammations
  - Not predominantly composed of foamy histiocytes

Clinical relevance (prognosis and treatment options)

- Benign condition

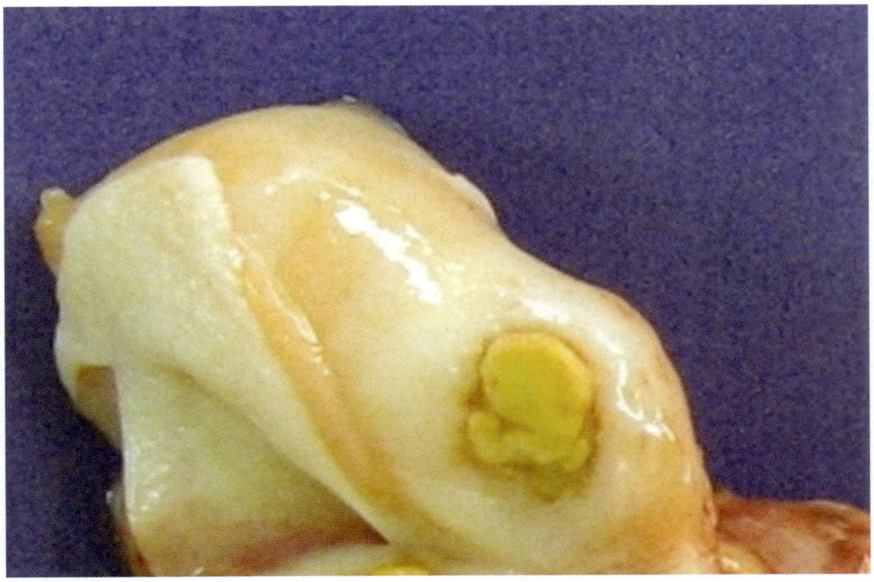

Figure 15-8.
Xanthogranuloma of the testis is a well-circumscribed yellow mass lesion, surrounded by scaring tissue.

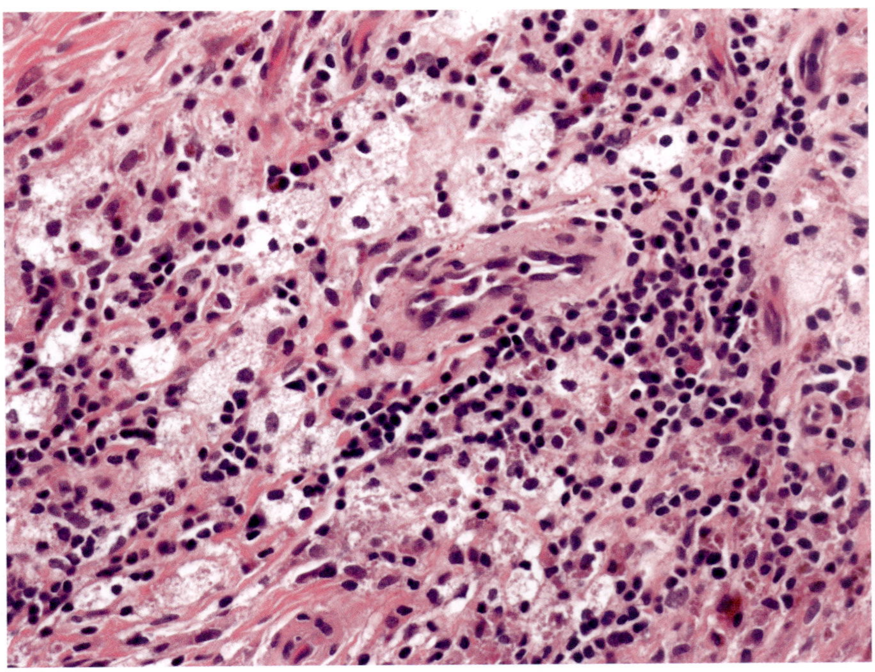

Figure 15-9.
Xanthogranuloma is composed of foamy macrophage and chronic inflammatory cell infiltrate, mostly lymphocytes.

EPIDIDYMITIS

Definition

- Inflammation of the epididymis

Pathogenesis

- Often associated with orchitis or trauma
- Inflammation can be acute or chronic
- Causes include bacterial (often acute), chlamydial (chronic), fungal, or viral infections

Clinical features

- Acute epididymitis presents with fever, pain, and pyuria
- Symptoms of chronic epididymitis are mild
- In young men, chlamydia or gonorrhea is a common cause
- In older men, *E coli* and pseudomonas infections are common
- Can coexist with testicular torsion in trauma cases

Gross pathology

- Testis with acute epididymis is swollen with or without abscesses
- In chronic phase, fibrosis and adhesion may be more prominent, causing tissue distortion

Histology

- Acute inflammation is characteristic of neutrophil infiltrates and microabscess formation. Tissue destruction is prominent (Fig. 15-10). Microabscesses are typically centered around glandular epithelium
- Chronic inflammation with or without granulomas, marked fibrosis may be present in the late stage

Immunohistochemistry and cytohistochemistry

- GMS, AFB may be necessary for granulomatous cases
- Cytomegalovirus (CMV) or other immunostains for viral infections

Microbiology studies

- Pathological features are often not specific enough for a definitive diagnosis of etiology. Therefore, microbiology studies are essential

Clinical relevance (prognosis and treatment options)

- Conservative anti-inflammatory therapy
- If an infectious agent is detected, specific therapies such as antibiotics can be applied
- Needs to be distinguished from testicular torsion or an infarct clinically, since the latter is a medical emergency that requires surgery

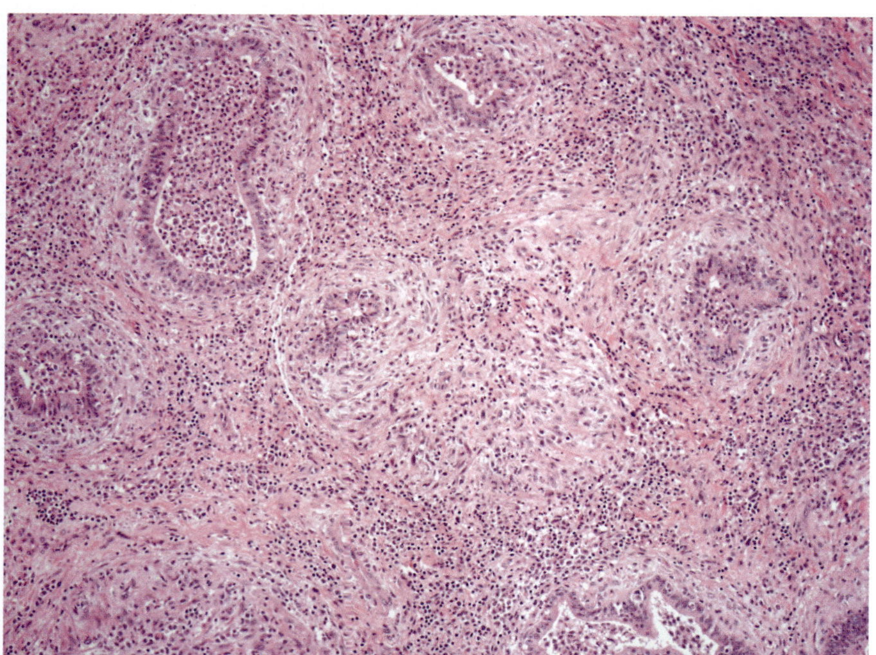

Figure 15-10.
Acute epididymitis shows the epididymis is almost entirely replaced by acute inflammatory cells. Multiple microabscesses are present inside or outside the tubules.

VASITIS NODOSA

Definition

- Benign proliferation of regenerating epithelium of the vas deferens

Pathogenesis

- Reactive process of the vas deferens after vasectomy

Clinical features

- Male patients with a history of vasectomy
- Tender small nodule at vasectomy site on the scrotum

Gross pathology

- Small nodular lesion subcutaneous in the scrotum

Histology

- Segment of the vas deferens with distortion (Fig. 15-11*a*) and obstructed sperm in the lumen (Fig. 15-11*b*)
- Small glandular structures infiltrating deeply into the muscular wall of vas (Fig. 15-11*c*)
- Epithelial cells show no obvious atypia (Fig. 15-11*d*)
- Fibrosis is common, which can be mistaken for desmoplastic reaction (Fig. 15-11*c*)
- Granulomatous reactions to leaking sperm (sperm granulomas) are commonly seen

Differential diagnosis

- Invasive adenocarcinoma exhibits significant cytological atypia and contains no spermatozoa

Clinical relevance

- In many cases, this condition will be resolved or becomes inactive without surgery. Surgical removal if symptomatic

Immunohistochemistry

- Rarely needed and epithelial markers are positive

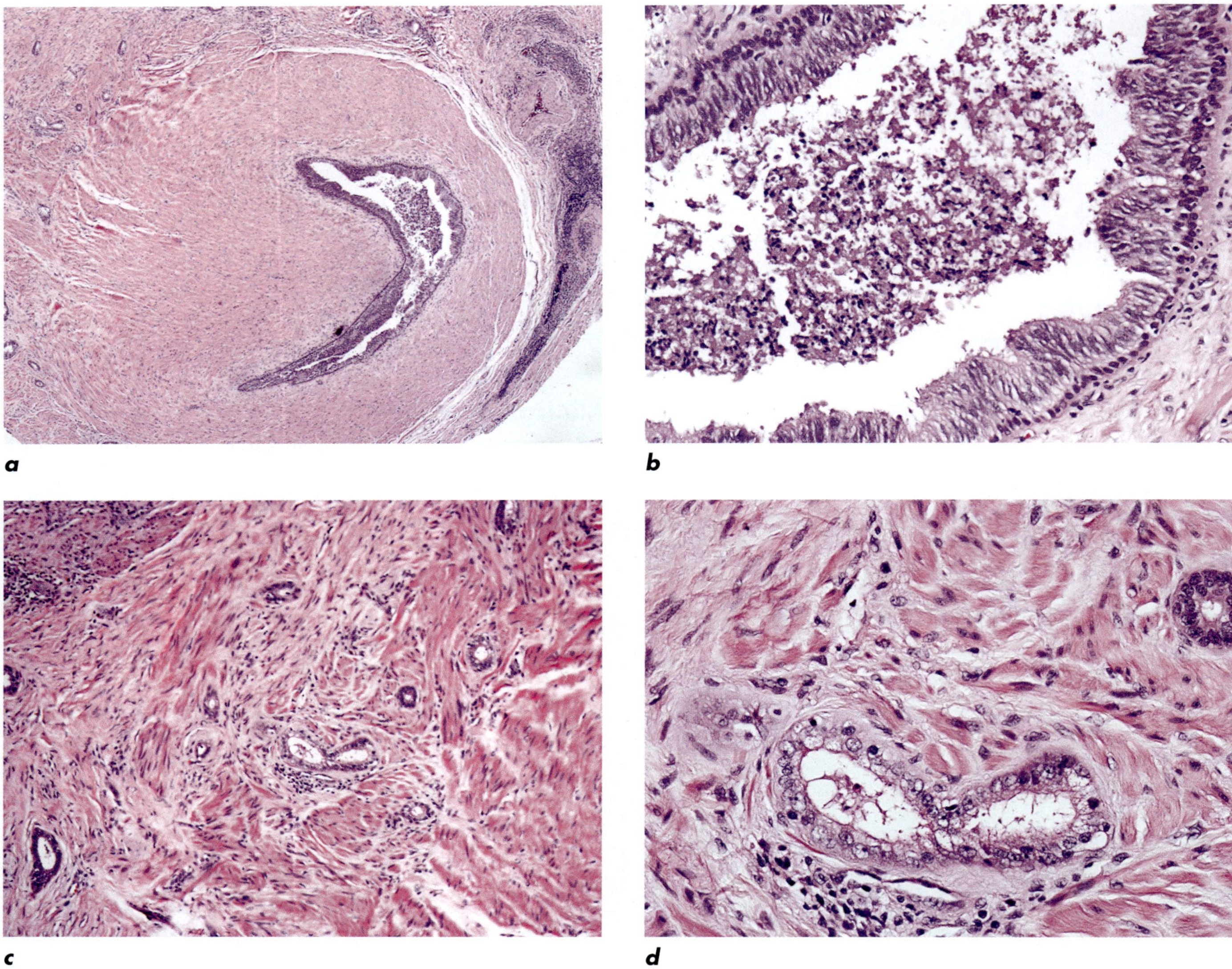

Figure 15-11.
Histologic features of vasitis nodosa. Vasitis nodosa is present in a distorted van deferens with small regenerative tubular structures infiltrating the muscular wall on the left side of the photo (*a*). In the lumen of dilated vas deferens, there are a large number of spermatozoa (*b*). The muscular wall of the vas is infiltrated by small proliferating tubules, associated with chronic inflammation and stromal reaction (*c*). The infiltrating tubular structures are well formed without significant cytological atypia (*d*).

SPERM GRANULOMA

Definition

- Granulomatous inflammation induced by extravasated sperm

Pathogenesis

- Tissue damage to the testis, epididymis, vas deferens, or any site of the sperm transport route results in spermatozoa (sperm) leaking out and inducing foreign body reactions

Clinical features

- Occurs in the reproductive age
- History of trauma, inflammation, or vasectomy
- Small painful nodules in the early phase or painless firm nodule in the late phase

Gross pathology

- Small white or tan nodules, single or multiple. May be associated fibrosis and tissue distortion

Histology

- Areas of tissue damage (liquefied necrosis) (Fig. 15-12) and granulomatous reaction with histiocytes and occasional foreign body giant cells
- Identification of pools of spermatozoa (tadpole-like blue dots) in the granuloma is key for diagnosis (Figs. 15-12 and 15-13)
- Other inflammatory cells may be present

Immunohistochemistry

- Usually not indicated
- Regenerative epithelial cells are positive for keratins
- CD68 can be used to confirm the presence of histiocytes

Clinical relevance (prognosis and treatment options)

- Benign, can be self-limiting if sperm leaking is stopped
- Surgical removal when symptomatic, associated with other lesions or suspicious for neoplasm

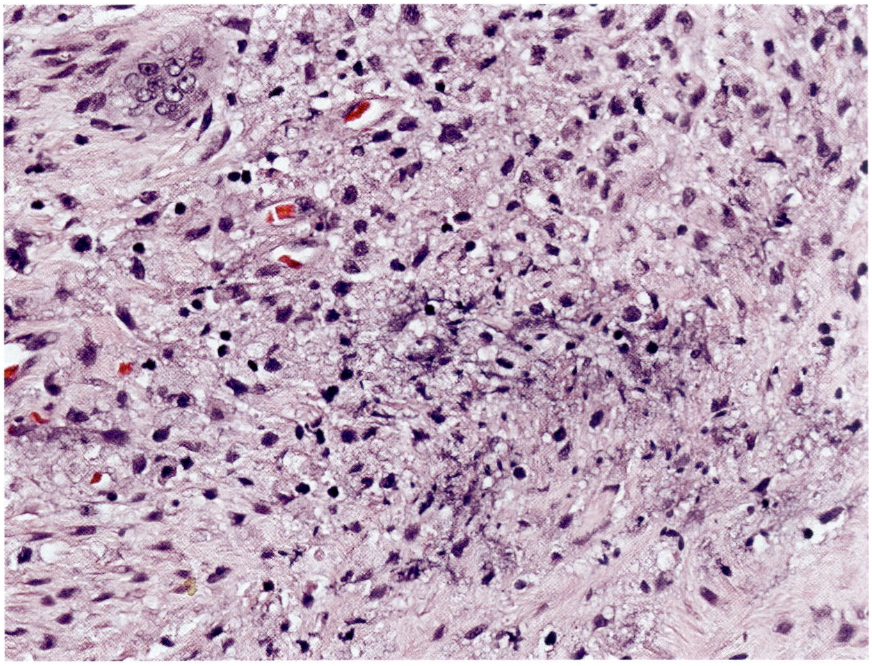

Figure 15-12.
Sperm granuloma contains numerous histiocytes, and spermatozoa can be seen mixed with histiocytes.

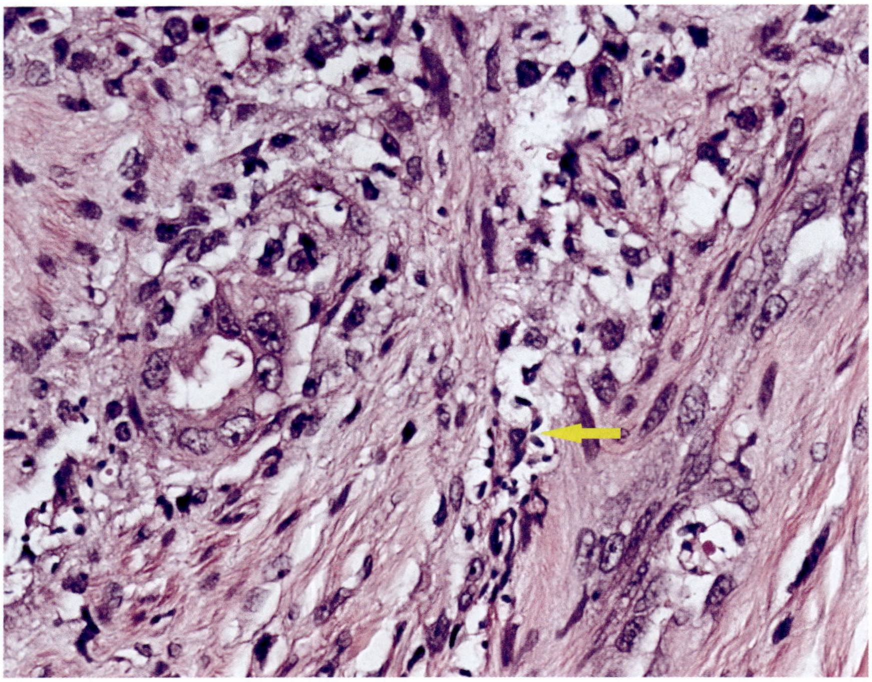

Figure 15-13.
A cluster of spermatozoa (arrow) leaking out of the regenerative tubules induce granulomatous reaction.

CHAPTER 16

Testicular Lesions Related to Infertility

HYPOSPERMATOGENESIS

Definition

- Decreased production of spermatozoa (mature germ cells or sperm)

Pathogenesis

- Many factors can contribute to decreased production of sperm
- One of the most common pathological findings of testicular biopsies for infertility patients
- Many causes cannot be determined from histological findings by a pathologist

Clinical features

- Infertility with azoospermia (no sperm) or oligospermia (low sperm count)

Gross pathology

- Normal or smaller testes

Histology

- The overall number of mature and immature germ cell is reduced. The diameters of the seminiferous tubule are smaller than normal (Fig. 16-1)
- Occasional spermatids or spermatozoa present (Fig. 16-1)

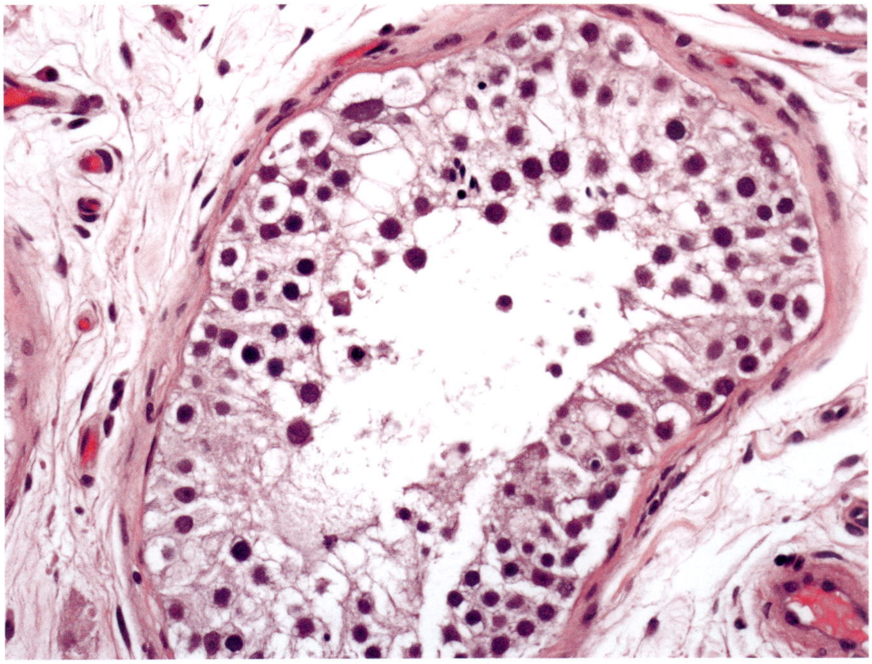

Figure 16-1. Hypospermatogenesis. A seminiferous tubule showing the decreased number of germ cells with only a few spermatozoa and spermatids seen at the luminal side.

- Tubules with hypospermatogenesis can be mixed with tubules of Sertoli-cell-only patterns (Fig. 16-2) or hyalinization (Fig. 16-3)
- The relative ratio of germ cells to Sertoli cells will decrease (normally 10-15:1 in men of reproductive age)

Immunohistochemistry

- Inhibin can be used to highlight Sertoli cells to evaluate the germ cell/Sertoli cell ratio

Molecular analysis

- May be necessary to detect genetic diseases

Clinical relevance (prognosis and treatment options)

- Correct the cause of hypospermatogenesis if possible
- Sperm retrieval may be necessary

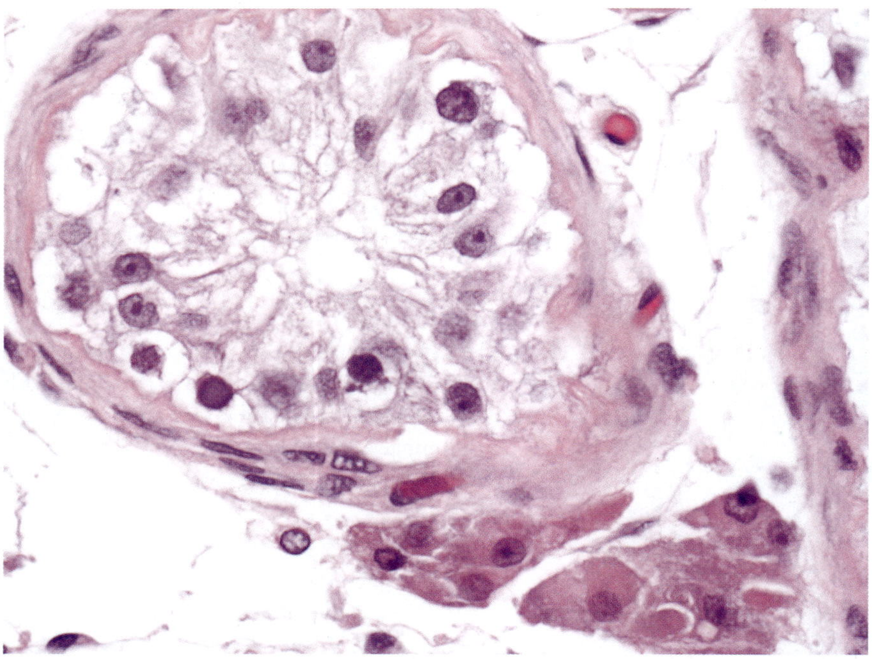

Figure 16-2.
Hypospermatogenesis with Sertoli-cell-only patterns in the tubule and a cluster of Leydig cells containing crystals of Reinke in the cytoplasm.

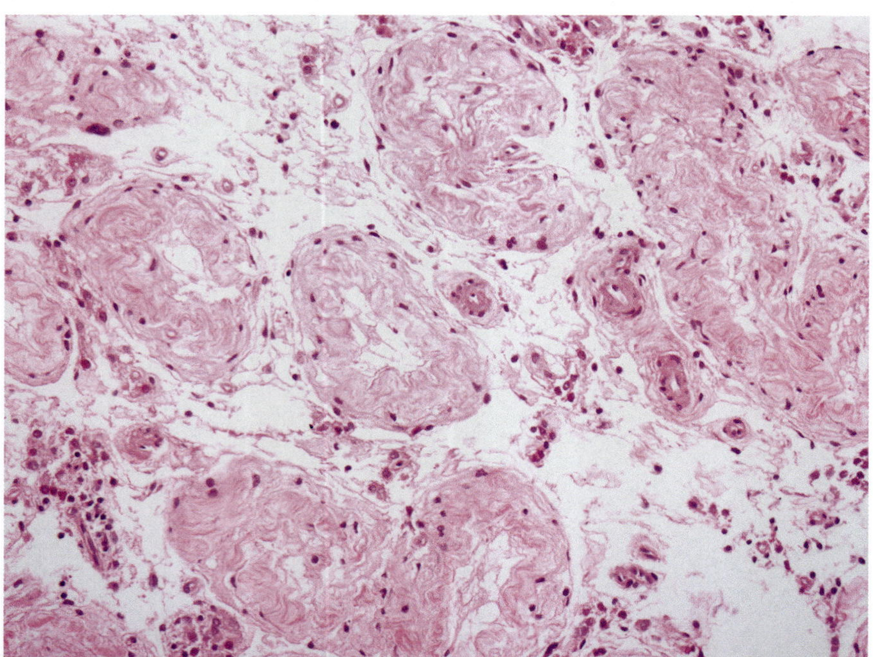

Figure 16-3.
Hypospermatogenesis with an area of all hyalinized tubules with any germ cells.

SERTOLI-CELL-ONLY SYNDROME (PATTERN)

Definition

- Seminiferous tubules contain only Sertoli cells without any germ cells

Pathogenesis

- Not a specific disease; rather it is a pathological finding that can be caused by many conditions such as infective, neoplastic, therapy related, or unknown etiology
- One of common findings in end stage testicular disease, which lacks germ cell production

Clinical features

- Infertility and associated with azoospermia
- Typically normal appearing males if onset in adult age
- Modern chemotherapy and radiation are common causes

Gross pathology

- Small or normal sized testis, typical bilateral

Histology

- All seminiferous tubules are lined by Sertoli cells only (Figs. 16-4 and 16-5)
- Classification based on Sertoli cell morphology has not been shown to relate to any clinical presentation or outcomes
- No mature or immature germ cells can be found in the tubules (Fig. 16-6)
- Leydig cell hyperplasia may be present between the tubules (Fig. 16-4)
- Hyalinized tubules, which can be derived from Sertoli-cell-only patterns (Fig. 16-6)
- *Sertoli-cell-only pattern* means the area examined contains seminiferous tubules with only Sertoli cells, which is different from Sertoli-cell-only syndrome in which there is no evidence of spermatogenesis in the entire testis. Other areas of the same testis may contain spermatogenesis in a case with Sertoli-cell-only pattern on the biopsy

Immunohistochemistry

- Inhibin positive in Sertoli cells (Fig. 16-7)
- Germ cell neoplastic markers (C-kit, OCT-4) negative

Clinical relevance (prognosis and treatment options)

- No effective treatment available to reverse this condition

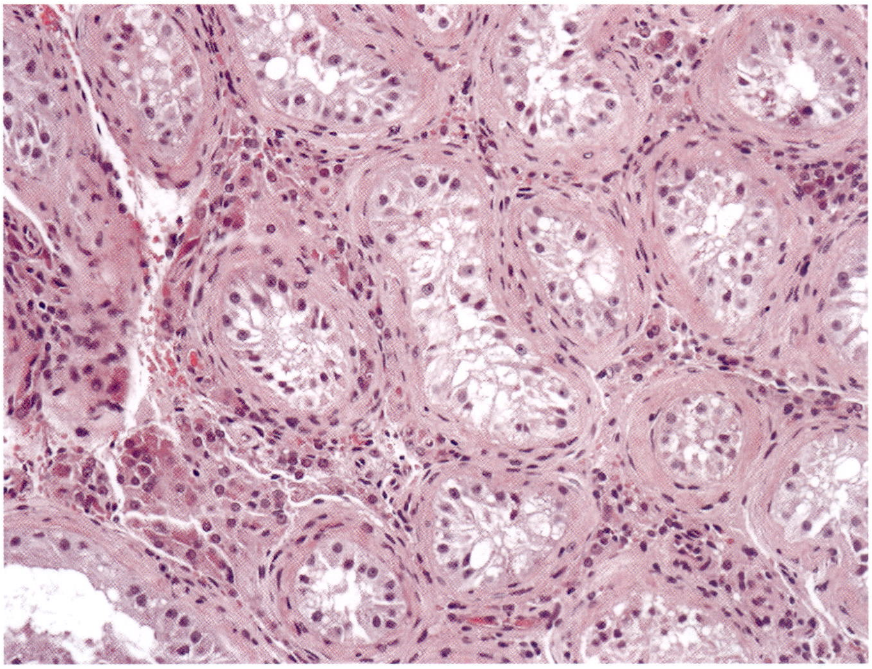

Figure 16-4.
Sertoli-cell-only pattern present in all the tubules in this photo.

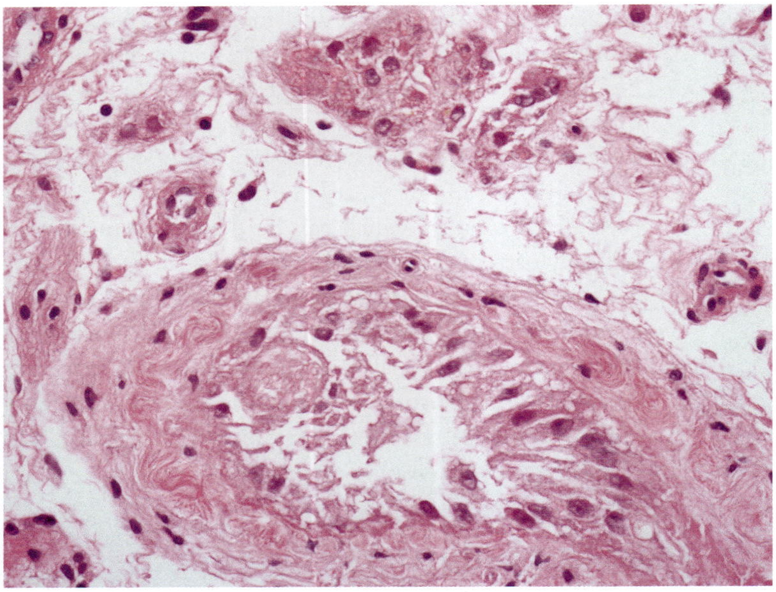

Figure 16-5.
Sertoli-cell-only pattern. A tubule contains only Sertoli cells with oval shape nuclei without any germ cells. Leydig cells can be seen outside the tubules.

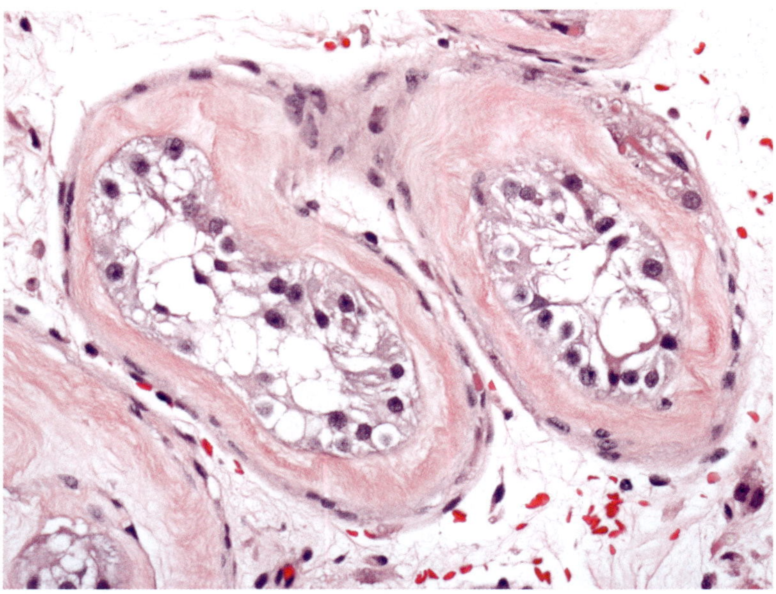

Figure 16-6.
Sertoli-cell-only pattern. Several tubules showing Sertoli-cell-only patterns as well significantly increased basement membranes.

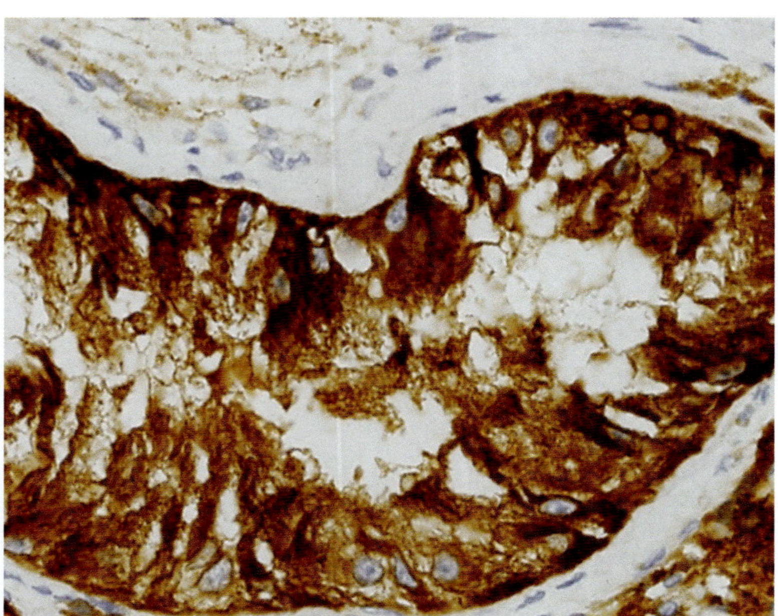

Figure 16-7.
Sertoli-cell-only pattern. Immunostaining for inhibin confirms the all the cells present in this tubule are Sertoli cells.

HYALINIZED SEMINIFEROUS TUBULES

Definition

- Germ cells and Sertoli cells in seminiferous tubules are completely replaced by hyalinized fibrotic tissue

Other terms

- End stage testicular disease, totally fibrotic testis

Pathogenesis

- Any injuries, infection, genetic, traumatic, or idiopathic can lead to this condition

Clinical features

- Testicular failure

Gross pathology

- Small and firm testis

Histology

- Germ cells and Sertoli cells absent in seminiferous tubules (Fig. 16-8), which are replaced by hyalinized tubular-shaped fibrotic tissue (Fig. 16-9)
- Hyalinized tubules can be diffuse or focal as seen in many conditions
- Leydig cells are present

Clinical relevance (prognosis and treatment options)

- Essentially irreversible, non-reproductive condition, if it is diffuse

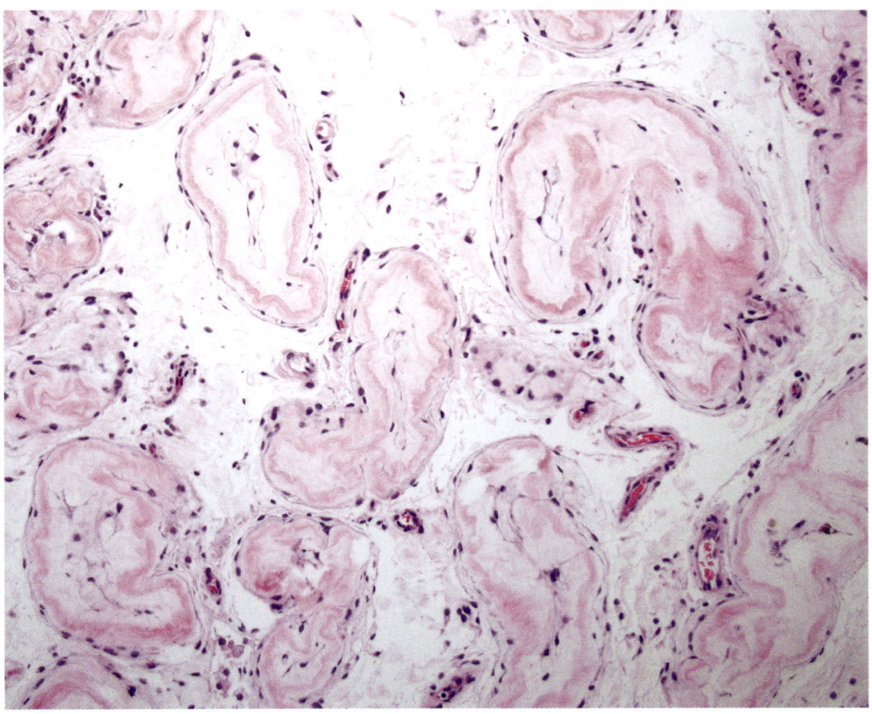

Figure 16-8.
Hyalinized seminiferous tubules. The testis is diffusely replaced by hyalinized tubules.

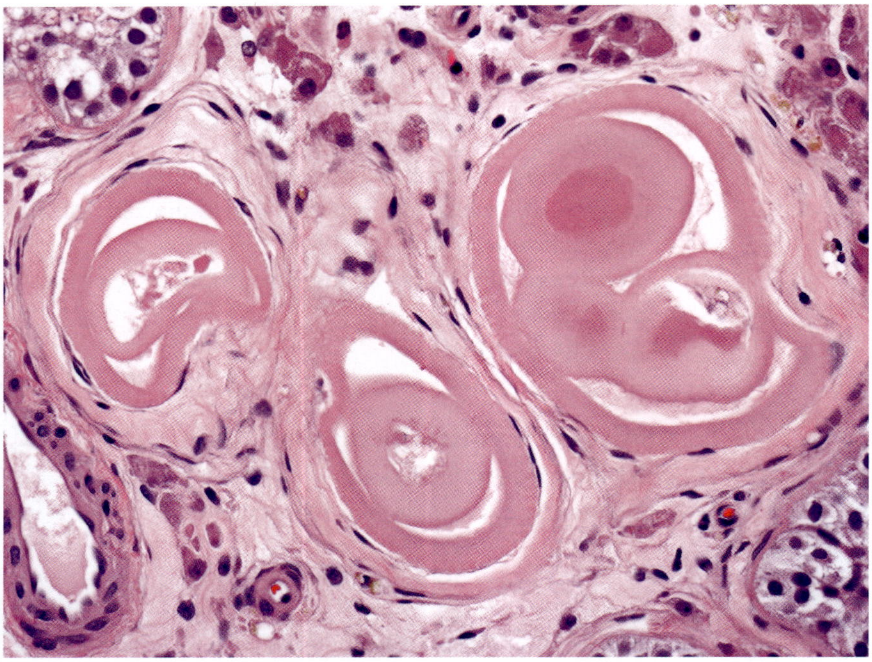

Figure 16-9.
Hyalinized seminiferous tubules. Several tubules are obliterated by hyalinized fibrosis. No germ cells or Sertoli cells are present. Occasionally Leydig cells outside the tubules are seen.

GERM CELL SLOUGHING

Definition

- A pathological condition characterized by immature germ cells separating from the base of the seminiferous tubule and falling into the lumen

Other terms

- Obstruction (not accurate, should be avoided since sloughing is not equal to obstruction)
- Sloughing is a pathological change that may be caused by obstruction or other causes
- A pathologist cannot make a diagnosis of "obstruction," although the finding of germ cell sloughing may be suggestive of duct obstruction or other causes

Pathogenesis

- Normally developing germ cells are inserted into the cytoplasm of Sertoli cells, which are attached to the basement of the seminiferous tubules
- When obstruction or other injury occurs, germ cells slough from Sertoli cells to the lumen of the tubules
- Production and maturation of germ cells may be normal, but transportation is compromised
- Finding of sloughing is most often associated with extratesticular or intratesticular obstruction, which cannot be confirmed by histological examination
- Other conditions such as inflammation, fever, or thermal injury can also cause damage to germ cells and Sertoli cells, leading them to slough off the wall of the tubules

Clinical features

- Normal testis size with azoospermia or hypospermia
- Evidence of obstruction, anatomically or surgically created such as a history of vasectomy may present

Gross pathology

- No obvious specific abnormality

Histology

- Spermatogenesis production is normal with sufficient number of immature and mature germ cells in tubules (Fig. 16-10)
- Mature and immature germ cells slough of the wall of seminiferous tubules into the lumen (Figs. 16-10 and 16-11), sometimes forming a cellular cast (Fig. 16-10)
- Germ cells are severely disorganized in the tubules with spermatids in the peripheral while spermatogonia found in the middle of the cast or tubules (Fig. 16-11)

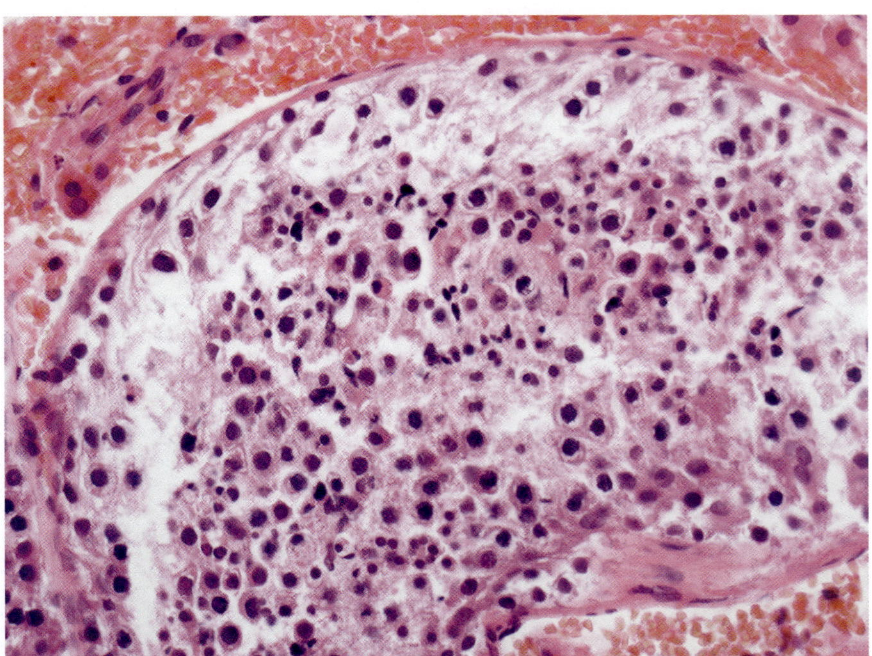

Figure 16-10.
Germ cell sloughing shows germ cell sloughing off, while Sertoli cells are still attached to the tubular wall.

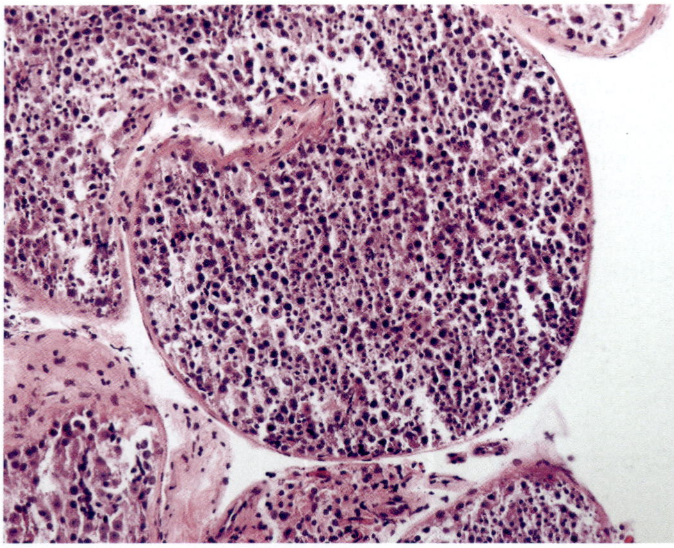

a

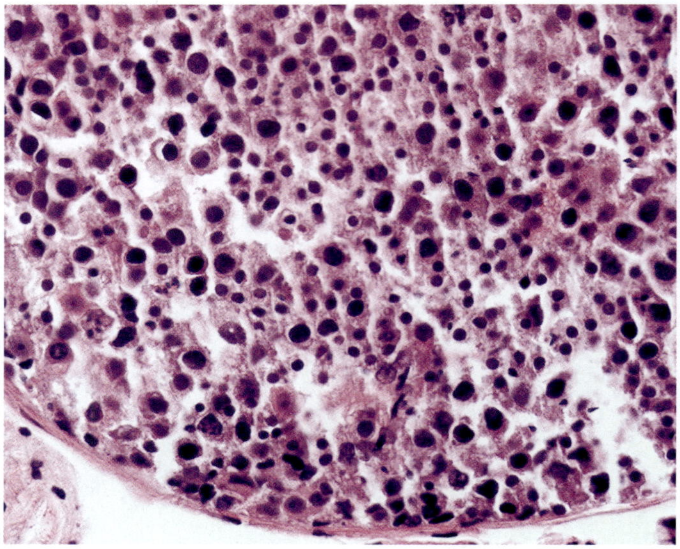

b

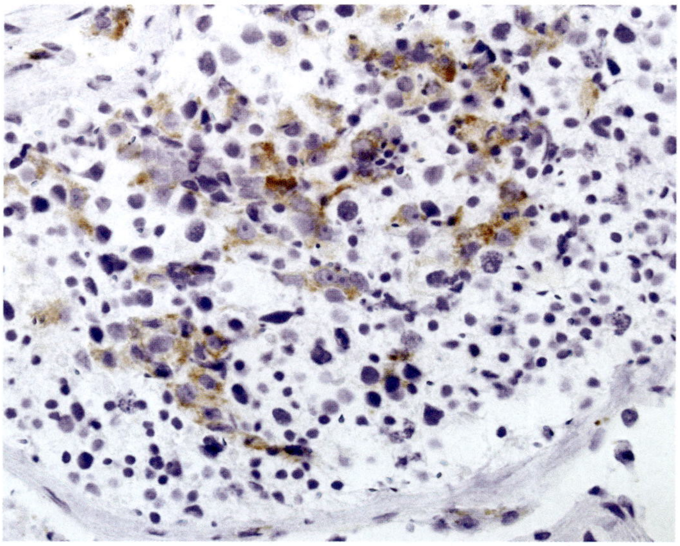

c

Figure 16-11.
Germ cell sloughing with extended seminiferous tubules that are filled with disorganized germ cells (*a*). High magnification shows disorganized mature and immature germ cells (*b*). Notice that the spermatozoa abnormally present closely to the basement membrane. The presence of macrophages is highlighted by CD68 immunostaining (*c*) along with the sloughed germ cells in the lumen.

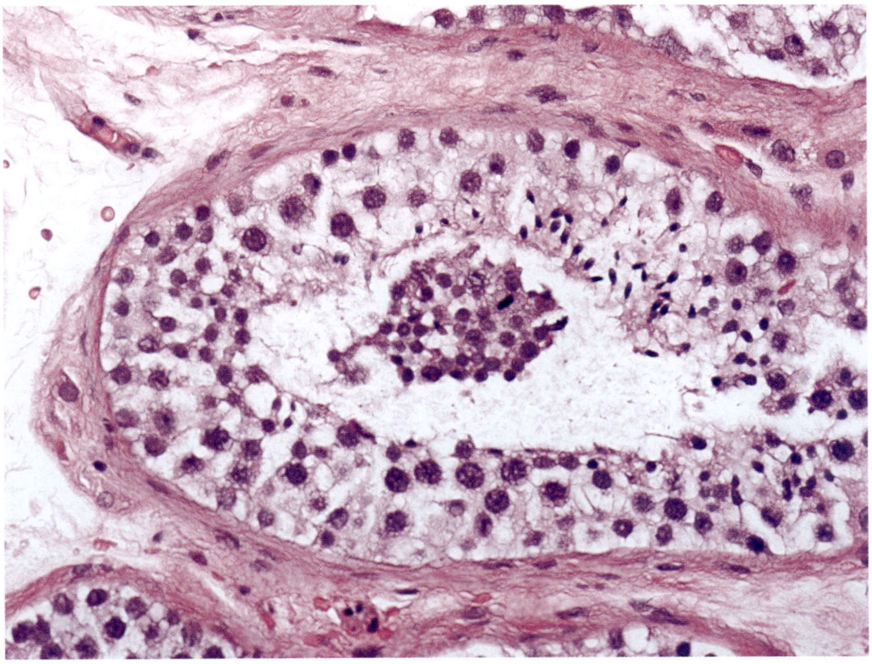

Figure 16-12.
Pseudosloughing. Although there are a few detached germ cells in the lumen, the germ cell maturation is still retained with spermatozoa present in the luminal side.

- Pseudosloughing or "plugging" is a phenomenon that there are some germ cells present in the lumen (Fig. 16-12). However, the germ cells are organized and attached to the wall of seminiferous tubules. The phenomena of pseudosloughing may be an artifact similar to the telescope event in the endometrium

Immunohistochemistry

- Presence of macrophages within a tubule can be confirmed by CD163 or CD68 immunostains in some cases (Fig. 16-11*c*)

Clinical relevance (prognosis and treatment options)

- Prognosis is mostly depending on the cause
- Extratesticular obstruction can be done in some cases if necessary, such as vasectomy
- Other obstruction or causes can be identified and removed if possible
- Sperm retrieval can be an option for some cases

MATURATION ARREST

Definition

- Failure of germ cells to mature in the seminiferous tubules
- Early maturation arrest: immature germ cells fail to progress to mature germ cells
- Late maturation arrest: failure of production of spermatozoa (sperm) although other maturing germ cells (such as spermatids) are present

Pathogenesis

- Typically, a germ cell will undergo maturation and meiosis to eventually become a spermatid and sperm (mature germ cell). In some conditions, the germ cells stop at immature stages without becoming mature spermatozoa (sperm)

Clinical features

- Azospermia (no sperm) in complete maturation arrest cases; or oligospermia (low sperm count) in incomplete maturation arrest cases

Gross pathology

- No abnormality

Histology

- Complete form: all the germ cells in the tubules are large and immature (spermatogonia and spermatocytes) without maturing germ cells, which have elongated nuclei and dense chromatin (spermatids) or spermatozoa (sperm)
- Incomplete form: spermatids are present focally but are markedly reduced in number compared to the immature germ cells. This is a very difficult situation to make a definitive diagnosis
- Early maturation arrest: only immature germ cells (spermatogonia and spermatocytes) present, without maturing germ cells (spermatids or spermatozoa) (Fig. 16-13)
- Late maturation arrest: immature germ cells present, spermatids are also present, but mature spermatozoa are absent or significantly reduced in number (Fig. 16-14)

Figure 16-13.
Early maturation arrest. Presence of only immature germ cells without spermatids and spermatozoa (*a*). The inhibin immunostaining confirms the presence of immature germ cells (negative staining) in the background of positively stained Sertoli cells (*b*).

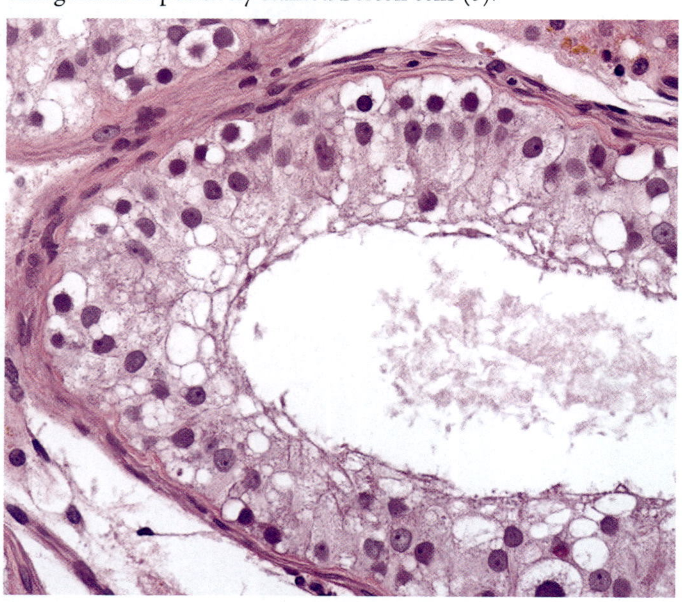

a

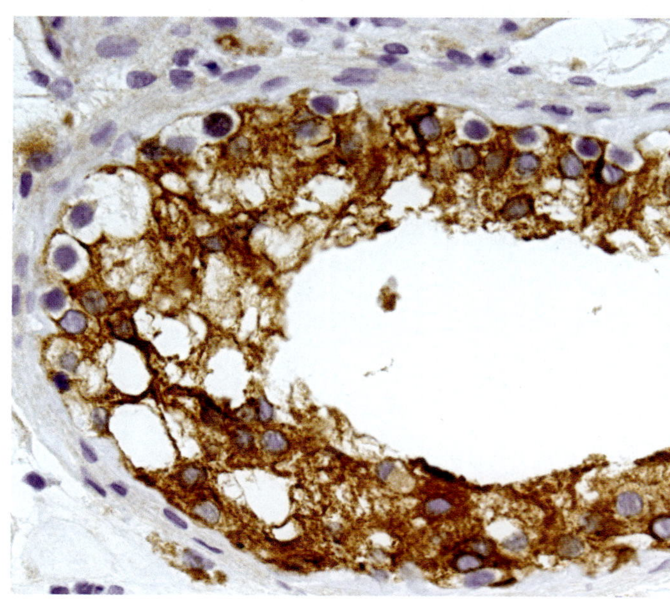

b

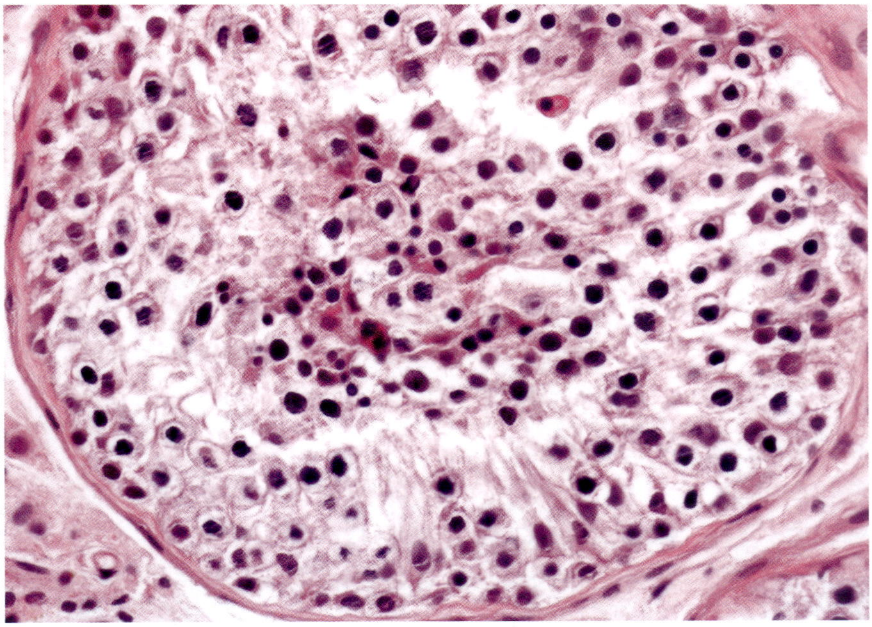

Figure 16-14.
Late maturation arrest with significant reduction of spermatozoa (sperm) although spermatids and immature germ cells are present in a normal number.

Immunohistochemistry

- Inhibin negative staining cells in the tubules are germ cells (Fig. 16-13*b*)

Differential diagnosis

- Testicular conditions associated with infertility are summarized in Table 16-1

Clinical relevance (prognosis and treatment options)

- Medical treatment and sperm retrieval

Table 16-1. Comparison of Infertility-Related Pathological Findings

Conditions	*Causes*	*Histology*	*Germ cells*	*Sperm count*
Tubular hyalinization	End stage	Hyalinized tubules	No germ cells	No[a]
Sertoli cells only	Many factors	Sertoli cells only in the tubules	No germ cells	No[a]
Sloughing	Obstruction and others	Germ cells fall to the tubular lumen	Present, detached cast in lumen	No or low
Maturation arrest	Many	Immature germ cells present	Mature germ cells low or absent	No or low
Hypospermatogenesis	Many	Reduced number of germ cells	Present but small in number	Low

[a]No sperm production from the particular groups of diseased tubules. However, these pathological changes can be focal. The sperm count is from total collection of all seminiferous tubules.

CRYPTORCHIDISM

Definition

- Failure of one or both testes descending to the scrotum

Other terms

- Undescended testis, intra-abdominal testis, or inguinal testis

Pathogenesis

- During fetal development, the testes, originally located inside the abdominal cavity, will descend into the scrotum by ninth month before birth
- Many infants have an open inguinal canal so that the testis moves up and down between the abdominal cavity and the scrotum
- The majority of cases of undescended testes in infants will descend into scrotum in the first year of life
- True cryptorchidism refers to boys or men with persistent undescended testes after the first year of infancy
- Temperature for an undescended intra-abdominal testis is higher than that of a normal testis in the scrotum, which will lead to the failure or decrease of germ cell development and the increase of the risk for development of germ cell tumors

Clinical features

- Absence of one or both testes in the scrotum
- Infertility in adulthood if bilateral
- Most undescended testes are located within abdominal cavity, some in the inguinal canal
- Imaging studies are helpful to identify where the testis is located outside the scrotum

Gross pathology

- Affected testis or testes are grossly normal or smaller (Fig. 16-15)
- Scar for fibrosis may be present (Fig. 16-16)

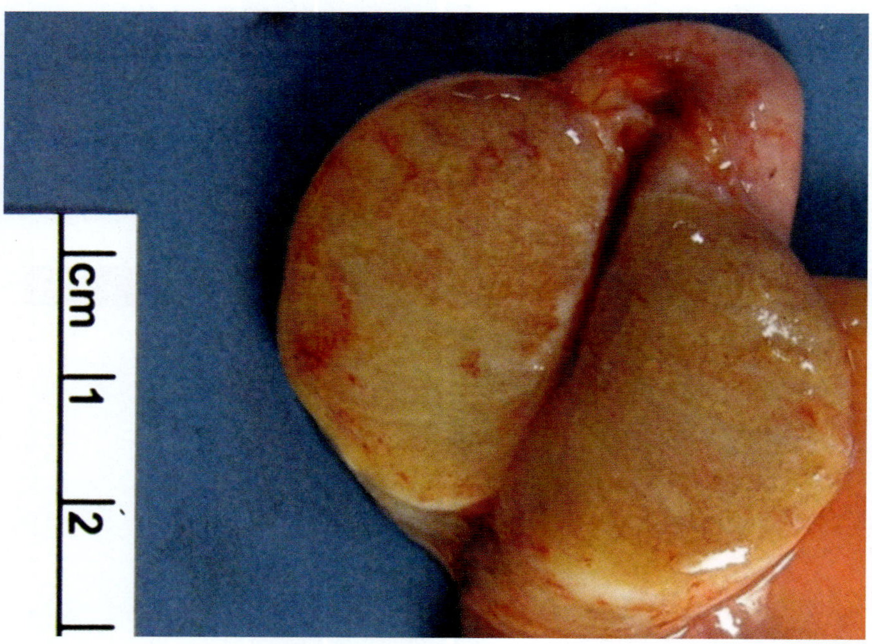

Figure 16-15.
An undescended testis (cryptorchidism) from a young adult is bivalved to reveal significant reduction in size (less than 3 cm) and more solid appearance in the testicular parenchyma.

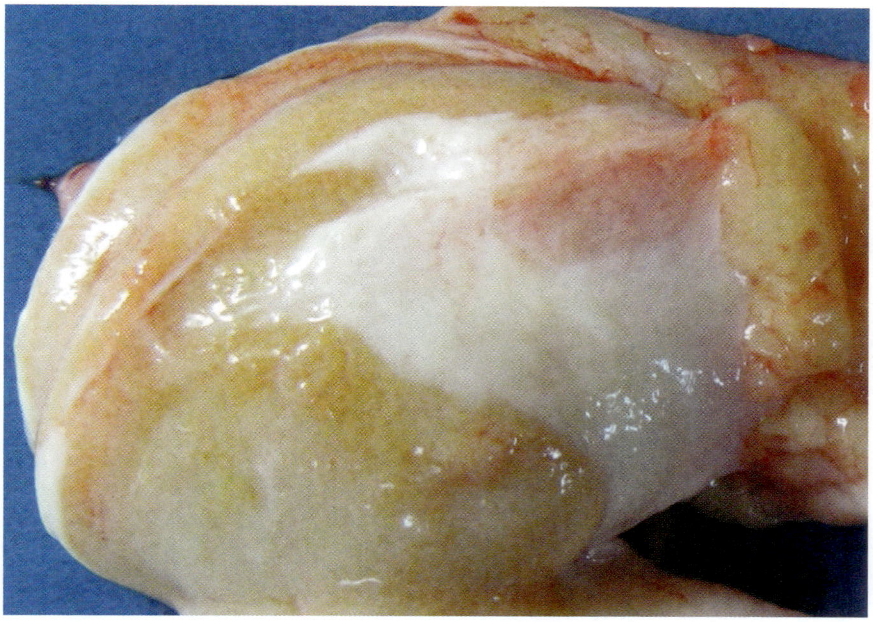

Figure 16-16.
Cryptorchidism shows a scar replacing almost a half of the testis.

Histology

- Different degrees of hypospermatogenesis present (Figs. 16-17 and 16-18)
- Sertoli-cell-only patterns are commonly seen (Fig. 16-19)
- Leydig cell hyperplasia present (Fig. 16-19*a*)
- In long-standing cases, areas of testis may show hyalinization of tubules (Fig. 16-19*b*)
- Presence of atypical germ cells with halos may be seen within tubules, which is intratubular germ cell neoplasia, unclassified (discussed in Chapter 18)

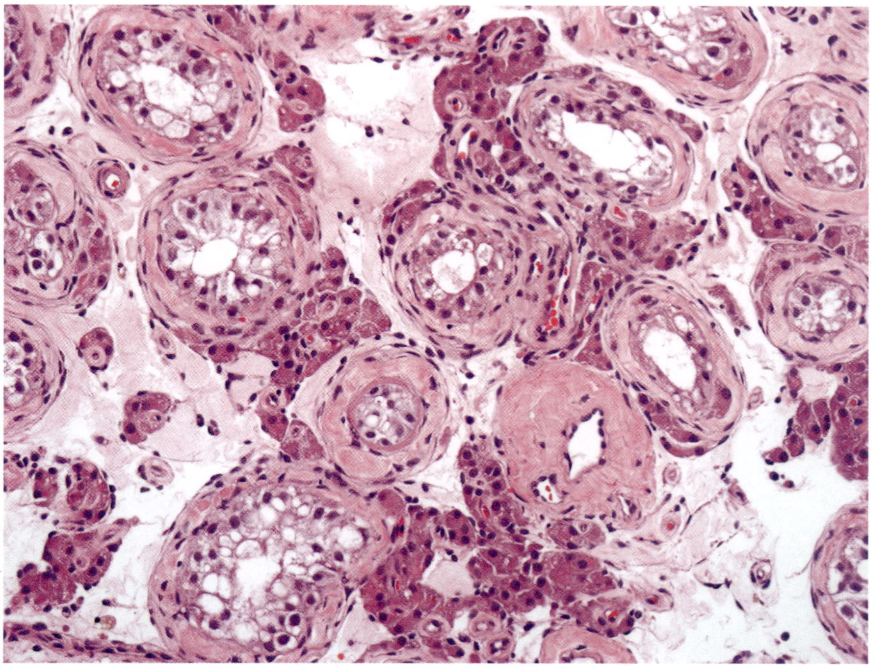

Figure 16-17.
Cryptorchidism. Most of tubules demonstrate Sertoli-cell-only patterns and occasional hyalinized tubules. Leydig cell hyperplasia is seen.

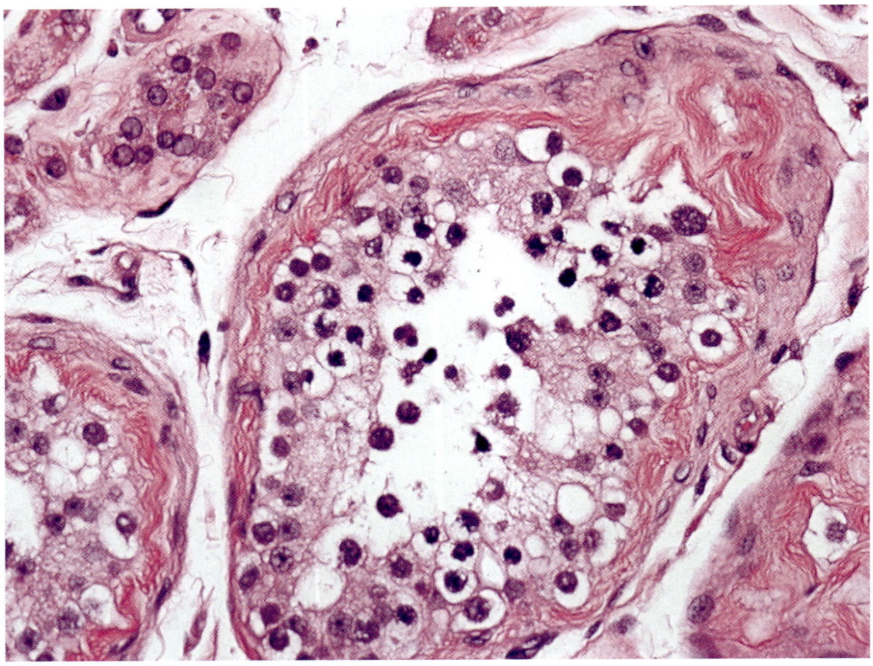

Figure 16-18.
A seminiferous tubule from a man with cryptorchidism showing hypospermatogenesis including reduced number of germ cells in all stages and no mature spermatozoa.

Clinical relevance (prognosis and treatment options)

- Because of the increased risk for testicular cancer, early detection and early orchiopexy in childhood are important for fertility
- Early orchiopexy, which may promote spermatogenesis, does not seem to decrease the risk for developing germ cell tumors
- Close clinical follow-up needed on patients with cryptorchidism even after the testis is brought down into the scrotum after orchiopexy AMACR, α-methylacyl-CoA racemase; HMWCK, high molecular cytokeratins; PSA, prostatic-specific antigen; PSAP, prostate-specific alkaline phosphatase.

Figure 16-19.
Cryptorchidism. Nodular Leydig cell hyperplasia (*a*), Sertoli-cell-only pattern and severe hyalinization of seminiferous tubules can be seen in this case (*b*).

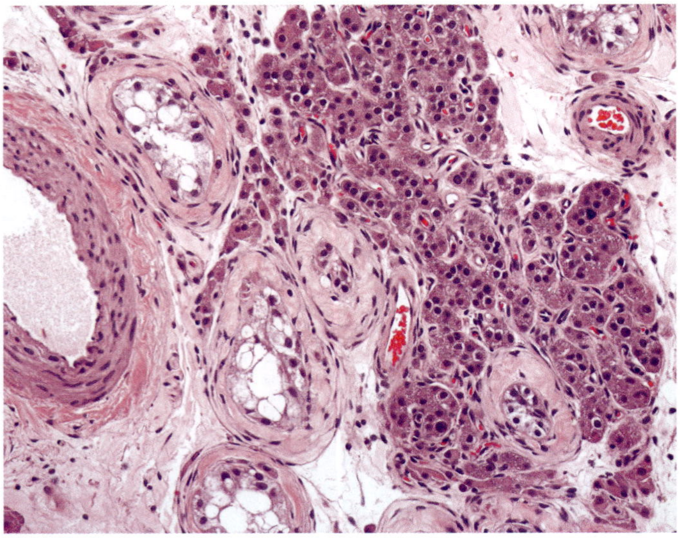

a

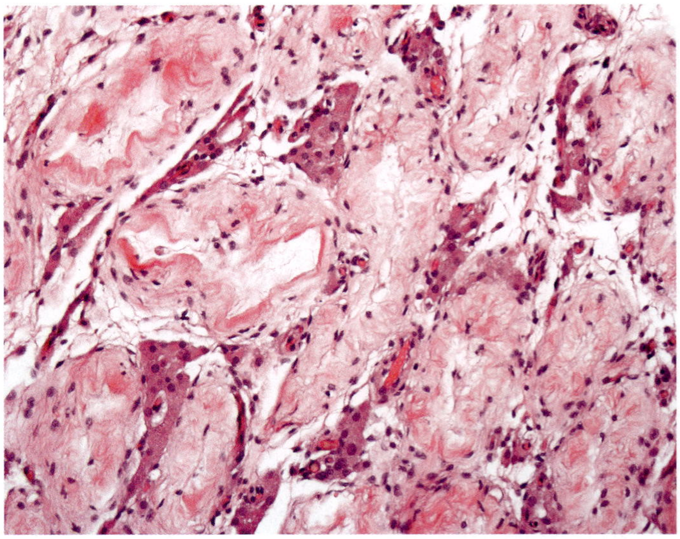

b

CHAPTER 17

Other Benign Lesions of the Testis and Paratesticular Tissue

APPENDIX TESTIS AND APPENDIX EPIDIDYMIS

Definition

- A small benign cystic lesion in the testis or epididymis
- Appendix testis: a remnant of Mullerian duct, located in the surface of upper pole of the testis
- Appendix epididymis: a remnant of Wolffian duct, located in the head of the epididymis

Other terms

- Hydatid of Morgagni (appendix testis)

Clinical features

- Very common in normal individuals, mostly asymptomatic as an incidental finding
- A solitary small cystic lesion filled with clear fluid

Gross pathology

- A small bud-like structure on the surface of testis or epididymis

Histology

- Simple columnar or cuboidal epithelial lining
- Histologically appendix testis (Fig. 17-1) and appendix epididymis (Fig. 17-2) are difficult to be distinguished since their lining cells are similar. Clinical finding of the location is the key for diagnosis

Clinical relevance (prognosis and treatment options)

- No treatment is necessary if asymptomatic. Surgical removal if symptomatic or there is a suspicion for a neoplasm

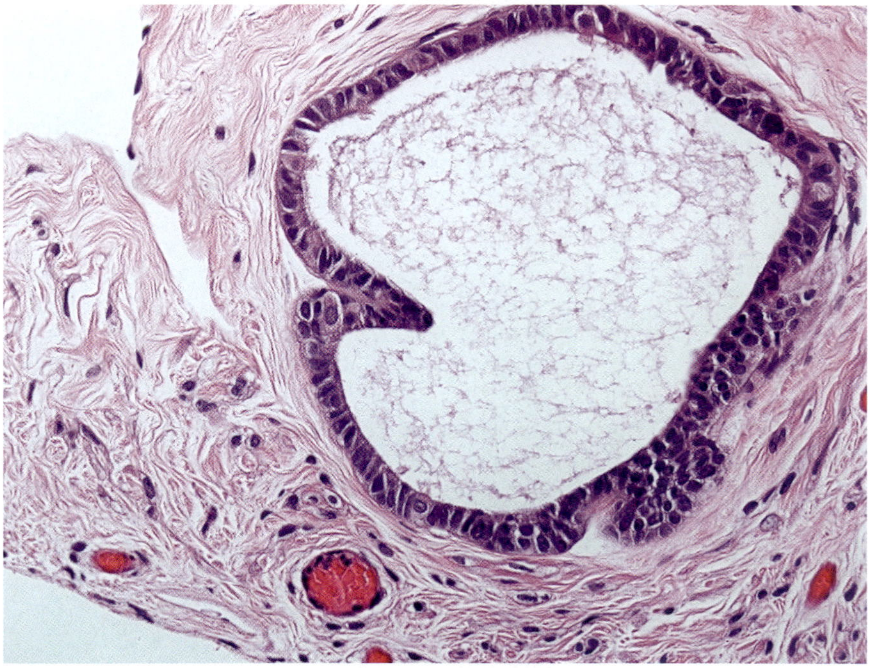

Figure 17-1.
Appendix testis is lined by cuboidal cells with cilia.

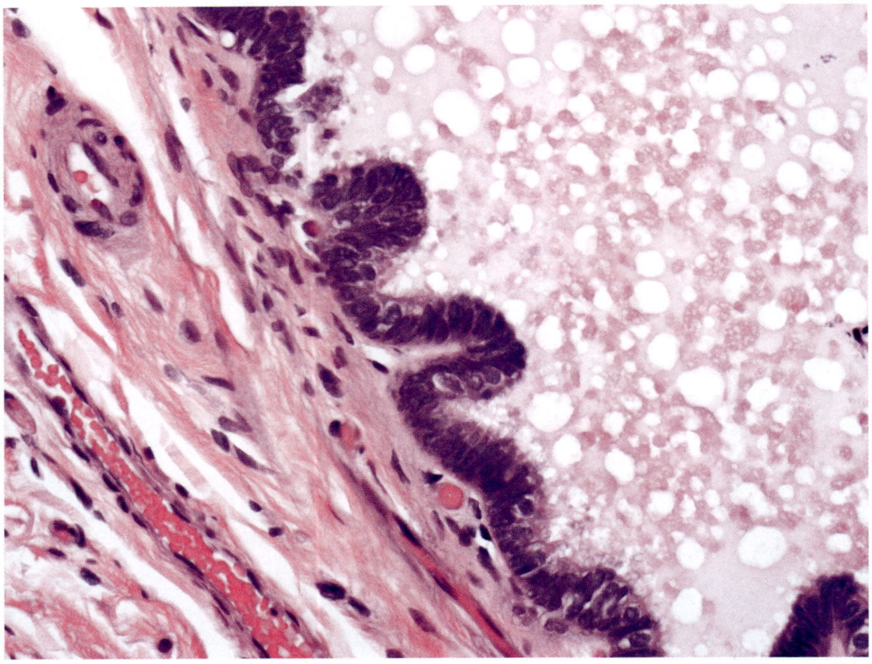

Figure 17-2.
Appendix epididymis is lined by taller columnar cells with cilia.

HYDROCELE AND HEMATOCELE

Definition

- Hydro = water; cele = space
- In a broad sense, hydrocele refers to a pathology accumulation of serous fluid in a body cavity, which may also happen in spermatic cord or the canal of Nuck in females
- Strictly speaking, a hydrocele is the accumulation of fluid around the testis. More precisely, accumulated fluid present between parietal and visceral layers of tunica vaginalis
- Hematocele: accumulation of blood or bloody fluid between parietal and visceral layers of tunica vaginalis, typically caused by trauma

Pathogenesis

- The cause of hydrocele is the patent inguinal canal where the testes descend from the abdominal cavity
- If the canel is not closed as it should be in an adult, the fluid of abdominal cavity will drain to the lower point, which is the space between the parietal (scrotum) and visceral of tunica vaginalis of the testis

Clinical features

- Hydroceles are common in newborn infants; most of them will disappear during the first year of life when the canal closes
- In adults, the typical presentation is painless swollen testis/scrotum
- Hydrocele, as a soft mass like a water balloon, can be unilateral or bilateral
- Hydrocele may be associated with inguinal hernia
- Positive transillumination test by shining a flashlight through the swollen part of the scrotum, which will light up because of the presence of clear fluid

Gross pathology

- Thin wall cyst filled with clear fluid with the testis suspended (Fig.17-3)
- Similarly, a thin-walled cyst filled with bloody fluid is called hematocele (Fig. 17-4)

Histology

- Hydrocele sac is lined by a single layer of mesothelium (Fig. 17-5)
- Sometimes, reactive mesothelium (Fig. 17-6) or associated inflammation may be present
- In hematocele, red blood cells can be seen in the space

Clinical relevance (prognosis and treatment options)

- May resolve spontaneously. A large hydrocele may compress the testis and compromise its function
- Needle drainage may be used in a large lesion or a symptomatic patient
- A hydrocele with an inguinal hernia should be fixed with surgery as quickly as possible
- Surgical repair is a simple procedure with excellent outcome

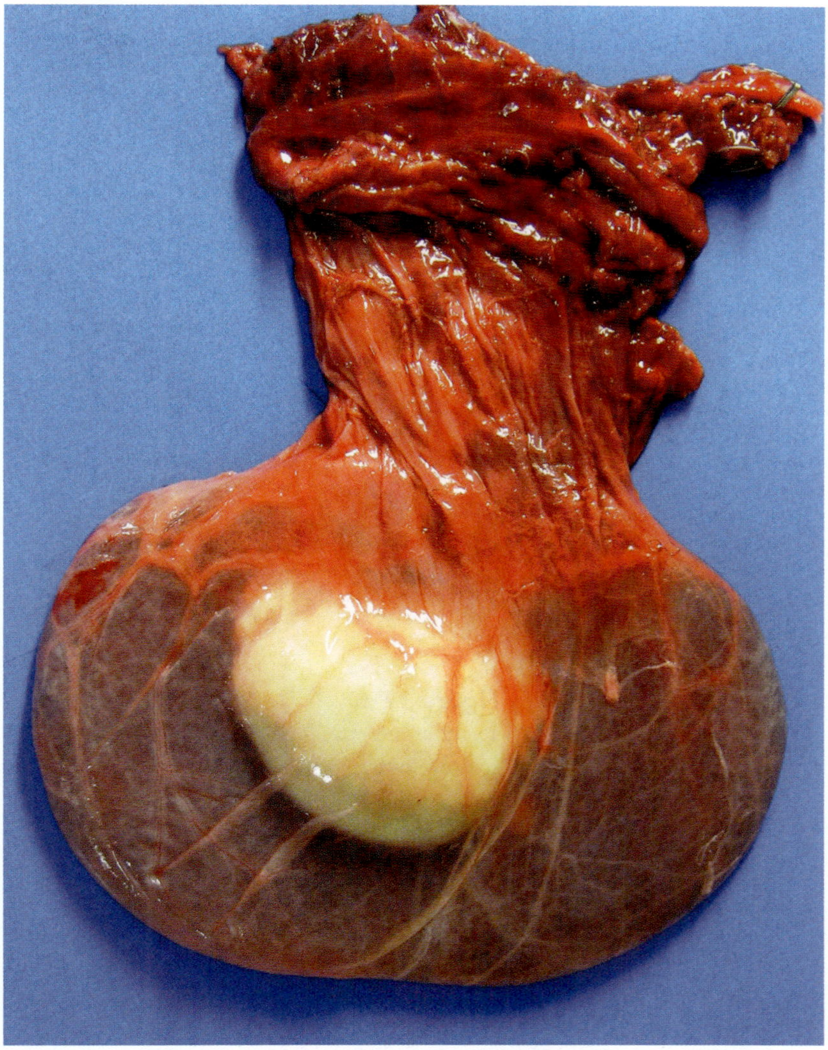

Figure 17-3.
Hydrocele with an atrophic testis suspended in a fluid-filled cystic space.

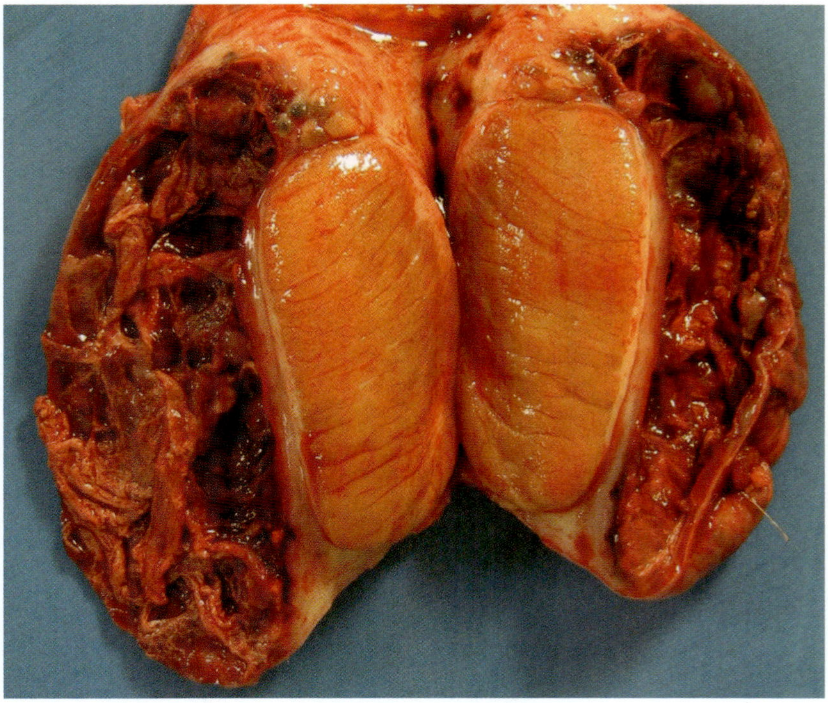

Figure 17-4.
Hematocele with clotted blood in the space between parietal and visceral layers of tunica vaginalis.

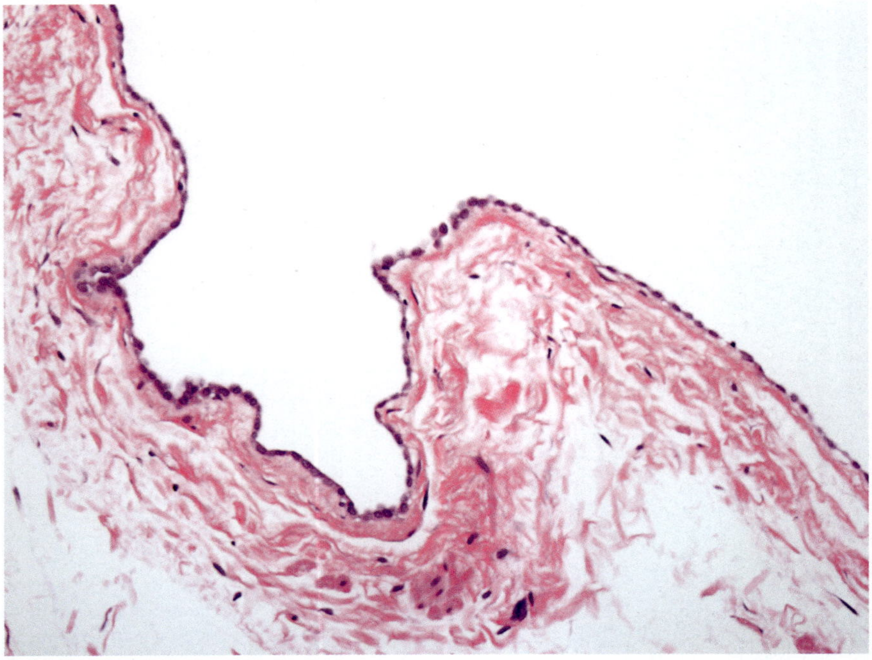

Figure 17-5.
Hydrocele with a flat mesothelial lining.

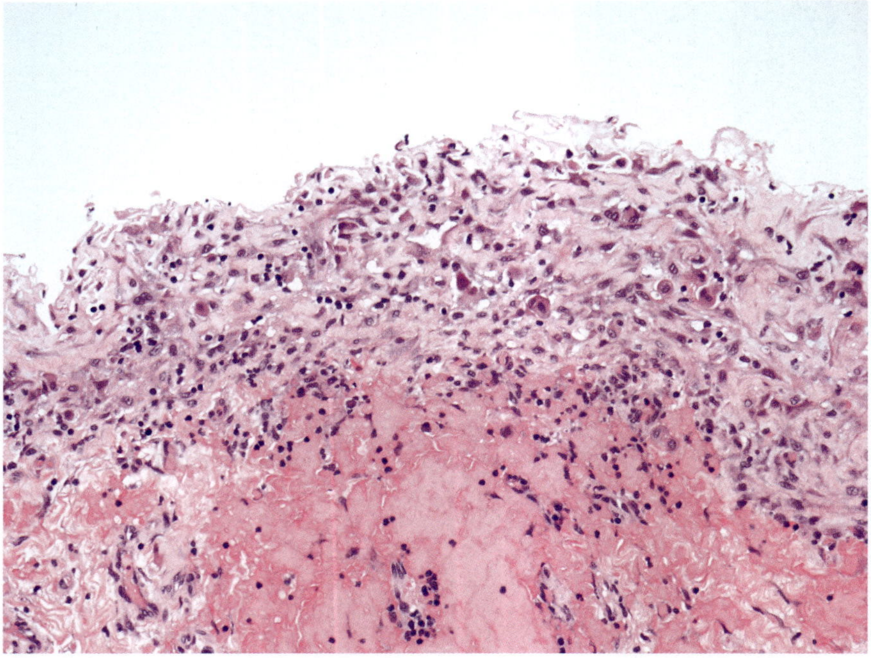

Figure 17-6.
Reactive mesothelium on the inner surface of a hydrocele.

SPERMATOCELE

Definition

- Different from hydrocele, spermatocele is the cystic dilatation of an efferent duct, proximal rete testis, or epididymis, and accumulation of fluid containing spermatozoa (sperm)

Clinical features

- Swelling testis or mass lesion, with or without pain
- Torsion may happen because of increasing weight of testis or paratesticular tissue

Gross pathology

- Thin-walled cyst with clear serous fluid

Histology

- Cystic lesion is lined by benign columnar or cuboidal epithelium (Fig. 17-7*a*), smooth muscles may be seen in the wall
- Presence of tadpole-like spermatozoa (sperms) in the cystic fluid (Fig. 17-7*b*) is another key difference from hydrocele

Clinical relevance (prognosis and treatment options)

- Surgical removal because of the risk of torsion

Figure 17-7.
Spermatocele with a cystic space lined by cuboidal epithelium (*a*). High magnification shows the presence of spermatozoa in the lumen (*b*).

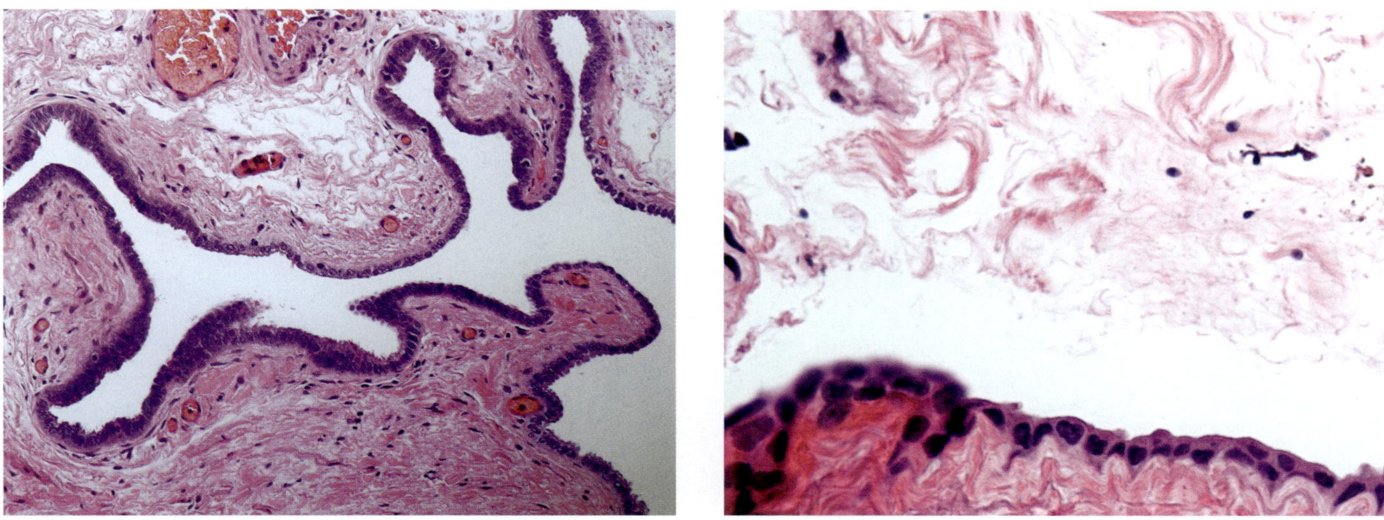

a ***b***

TORSION AND INFARCT OF TESTIS

Definition

- Torsion is the twisting of the spermatic cord
- Infarct is testicular necrosis caused by lack of blood supply due to complete torsion

Clinical features

- Typically occurs in young men with acute onset of unilateral scrotal pain
- Torsion lasting more than 24 hours will lead to testicular infarct
- Orchiectomy for cases if there is evidence of infarct

Gross pathology

- Dark red appearance of the testicular surface and cut surface (Figs. 17-8 and 17- 9)

Histology

- In partial infarct or early infarct, the seminiferous tubules are filled with sloughed cells with nuclear debris and other degenerative changes (Fig. 17-10)
- Extensive necrosis with ghost cells and hemorrhage (Fig. 17-11)
- Inflammatory cells and organizing granulation tissue may be seen in a few days
- Eventually fibrosis and scar will develop testis if untreated

Immunohistochemistry

- Not indicated

Differential diagnosis

Acute orchitis: characterized by acute inflammation without large areas of necrosis, and the hemorrhage is minimal

Clinical relevance (prognosis and treatment options)

- Timing is critical in clinical management. Torsion will be nonreversible in 6 hours once the irreversible ischemic damages to the germ cells are done
- If torsion lasts more than 24 hours, infarct will develop
- Orchiectomy is treatment of choice if infarct is present. Orchiopexy is possible if torsion is early and the testis is viable

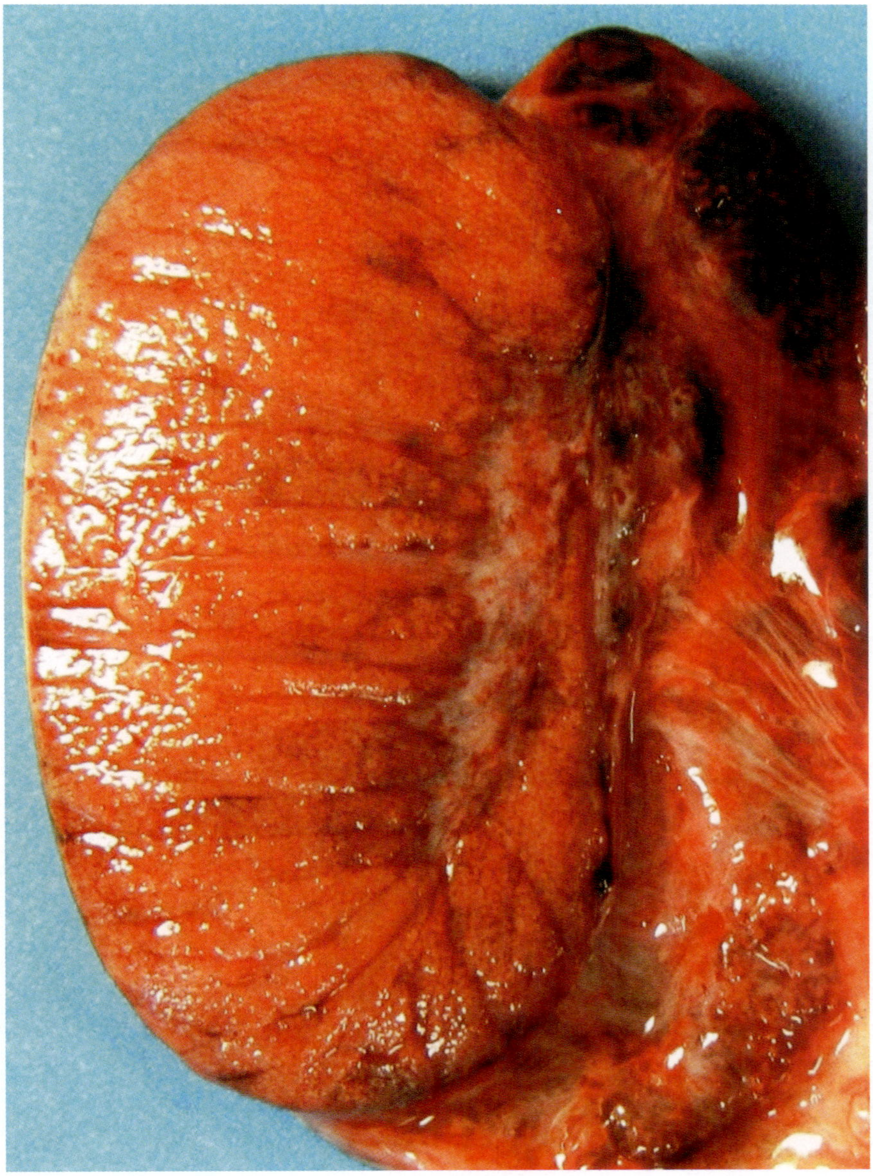

Figure 17-8.
Testicular torsion with early infarct. The cut surface of the infarcted testis shows focal hemorrhage and discoloration but the testicular architectures are retained.

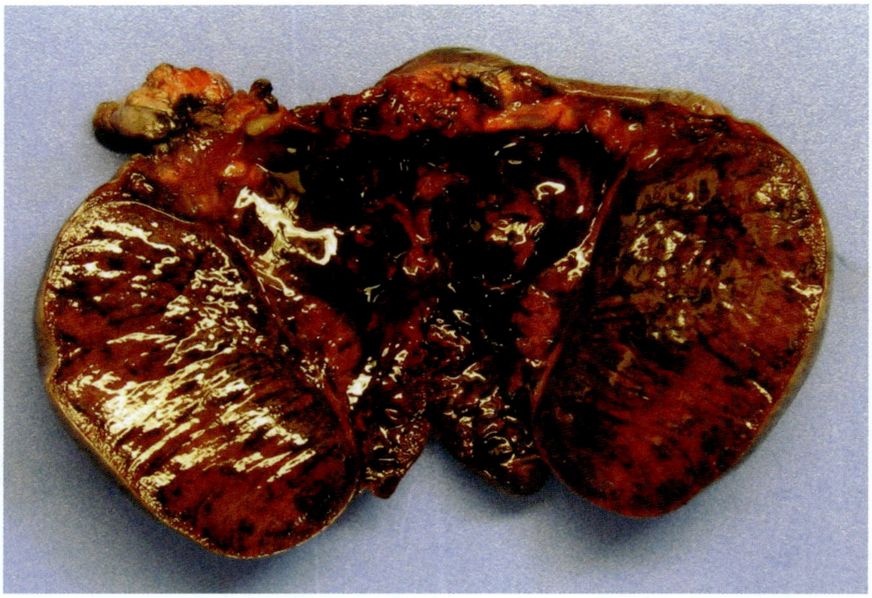

Figure 17-9.
Late stage testicular infarct by torsion showing severe hemorrhage and necrosis leading to a loss of granular appearance of the normal testicular parenchyma.

Figure 17-10.
Infarcted testis with some tubules showing early necrosis (*a*, right). High magnification shows degenerative changes, sloughing, and germ cell necrosis in the tubules (*b*).

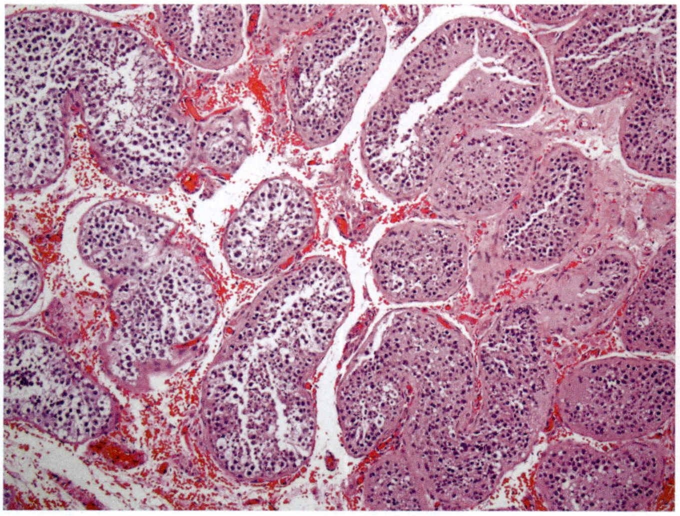

a

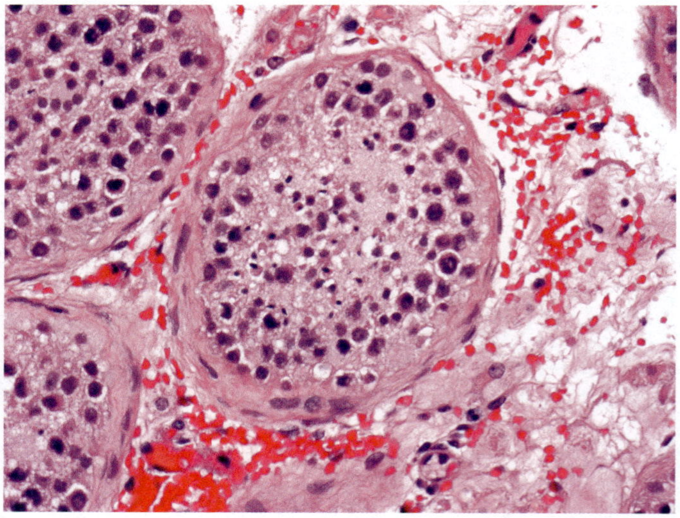

b

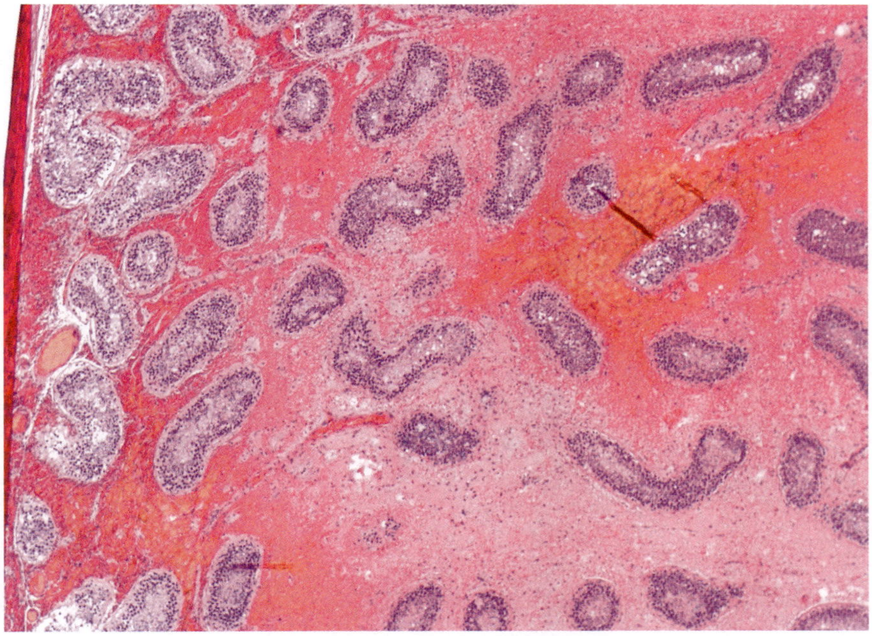

Figure 17-11.
Late hemorrhagic infarct showing the majority of seminiferous tubules with necrosis and extensive hemorrhage, although the tubular contour can be recognized.

TESTICULAR MICROLITHIASIS

Definition

- Presence of microcalcifications in the testis, either within or outside the seminiferous tubules
- Can be seen in benign or malignant conditions of the testis

Other term

- Microcalcification

Pathogenesis and epidemiology

- Testicular microlithiasis (TML), found in between 1.5% and 5% of normal testes, is a relatively frequent condition
- More common in individuals with infertility or germ cell tumors (up to 20%)
- Cause is unknown but probably related to injuries and fibrosis of seminiferous tubules, which are commonly seen in cryptorchism or infertility patients
- Classic TML is defined as five or more echogenic (calcification) foci per view. Limited TML is defined as >1 but <5 foci per view by radiological studies

Clinical features

- Condition is usually incidentally identified on testicular ultrasound scan
- By ultrasound or other imaging studies, calcified foci can be seen throughout the testis
- Bilateral involvement in 80% of cases

Gross pathology

- No specific abnormality can be seen, but the testis may contain a tumor or benign nonneoplastic conditions

Histology

- Microscopically, TML is recognized as a small focus of microcalcification, mostly round or oval in shape, 50 to 300 μm in diameter (Fig. 17-12)
- Calcifications can be present in the tubules (Fig. 17-12) or in the stroma (Fig. 17-13), which does not indicate tubular obstruction as the name implies
- Microcalcifications can be seen within malignant germ cell tumors (Fig. 17-14), or they may be present within atrophic seminiferous tubules of benign testicular conditions such as cryptorchidism

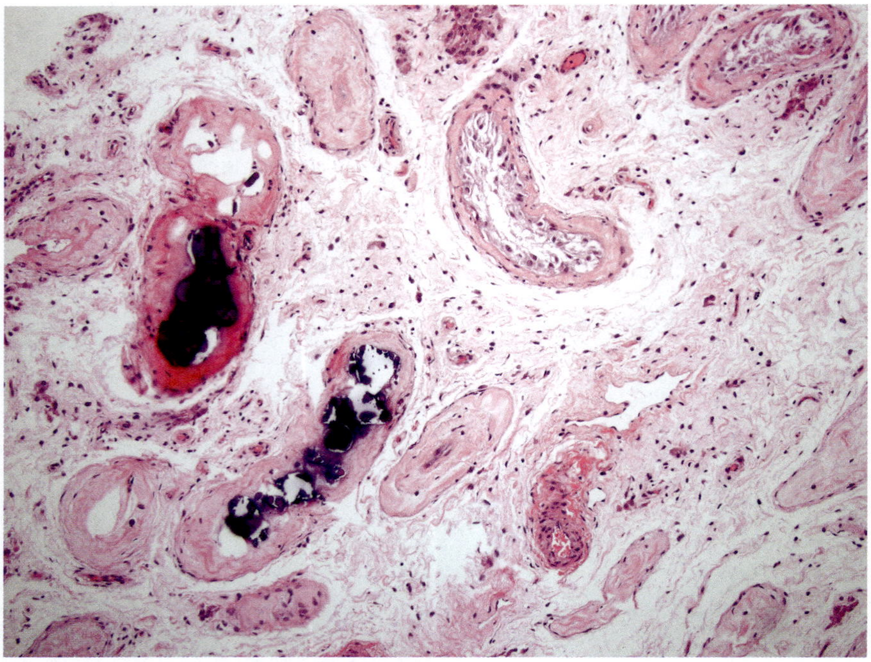

Figure 17-12.
Microcalcification (microlithiasis) present within two benign hyalinized tubules.

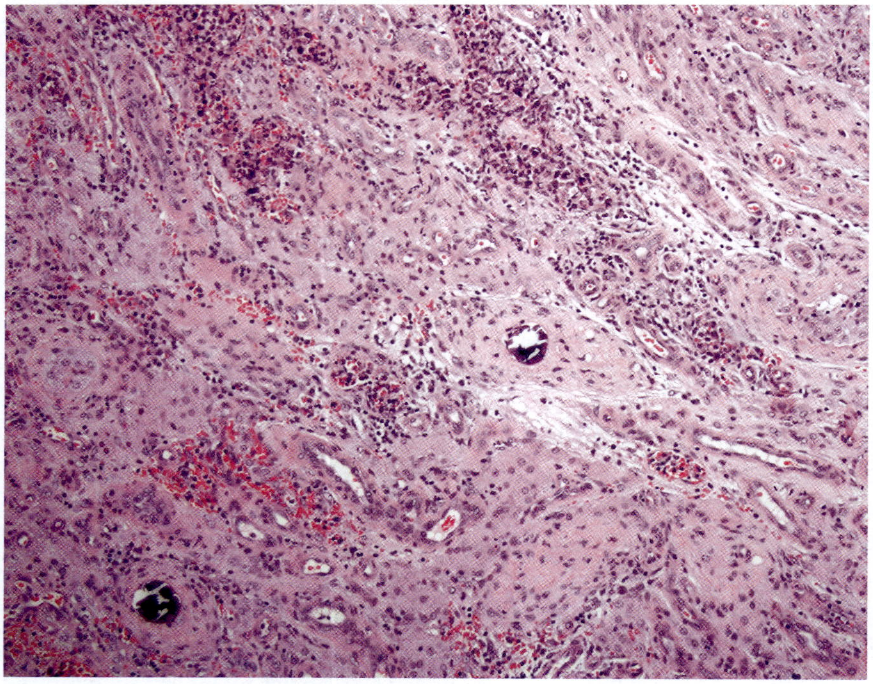

Figure 17-13.
Microlithiasis in the benign testicular tissue.

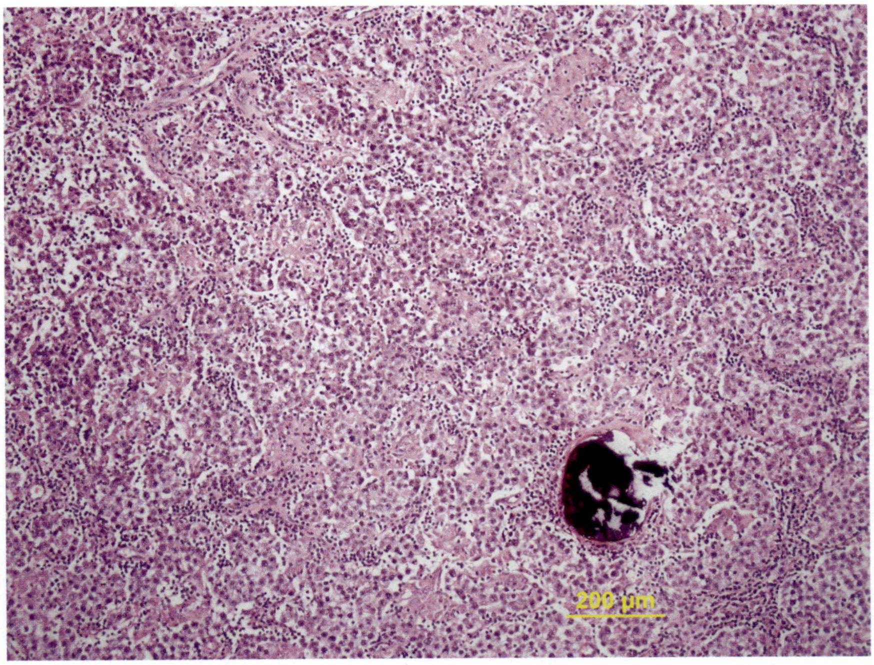

Figure 17-14.
Microcalcification (measuring 200 μm in diameter) present within a seminoma.

Clinical relevance (prognosis and treatment options)

- Asymptomatic, nonprogressive condition
- There is a controversy on whether TML is associated with testicular germ cell tumor
- TML is not associated with an increased risk of testicular cancer in asymptomatic individuals with no other risk factors for testicular germ cell tumor
- However, in men with microlithiasis and risk factors for testicular germ cell tumor, the presence of germ cell tumor or ITGCNU is increased eight- to tenfold. These men should be followed by imaging studies and serum marker measurement
- Some experts suggest that these men should undergo testicular biopsy to exclude the presence of intratubular germ cell neoplasia of unclassified type. But this practice is not accepted in the United States

OVOTETIS

Definition

- A gonad with both testicular and ovarian components in human

Other terms

- Hermaphroditic gland, gonad of true hermaphroditism, gonad of intersex

Pathogenesis

- Both testicular and ovarian components developing in one person is an abnormal genetic condition (both these sex organs can be seen in some other animals as a normal phenomenon)
- Genetically, these individuals have 47XXY, 46XX/46XY, or 46XX/47XXY, and various degrees of mosaicism

Clinical features

- Ambiguous external genitalita
- Almost all the patients are infertile, with only a few reported cases with fertility
- Both male and female hormones can be measured

Gross pathology

- Oval-shaped gonad

Histology

- Presence of both normal testicular tissue and ovarian tissues in one gonad (Fig. 17-15)
  - Testicular tissue: seminiferous tubules with Sertoli cells and a small number of germ cells depending on the age (Fig. 17-16)
  - Ovarian tissue: oocytes and ovarian stromal cells can be seen (Fig. 17-17)

Immunohistochemistry

- May be necessary to rule out germ cell neoplasia

Molecular analysis

- Cytogenetic studies are necessary to determine the genotype

Clinical relevance (prognosis and treatment options)

- Condition may be associated with many social issues of sexual preference
- Ovotestis may be detected as a suspicious mass lesion
- Surgery may be performed because of the increased risk for germ cell tumor

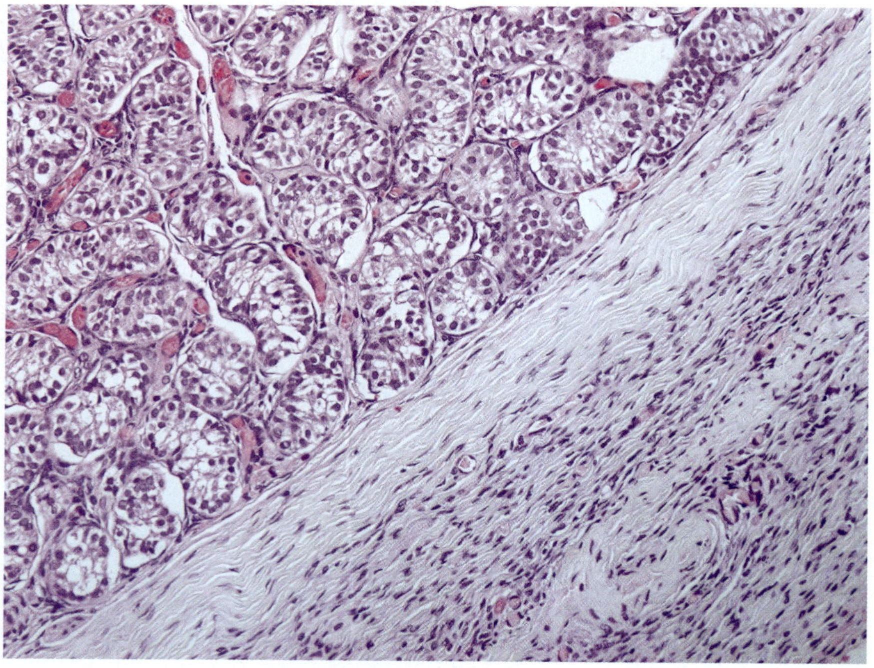

Figure 17-15.
The interface between testicular component (upper left) and dense ovarian stromal component (lower right) in an ovotestis from a young child.

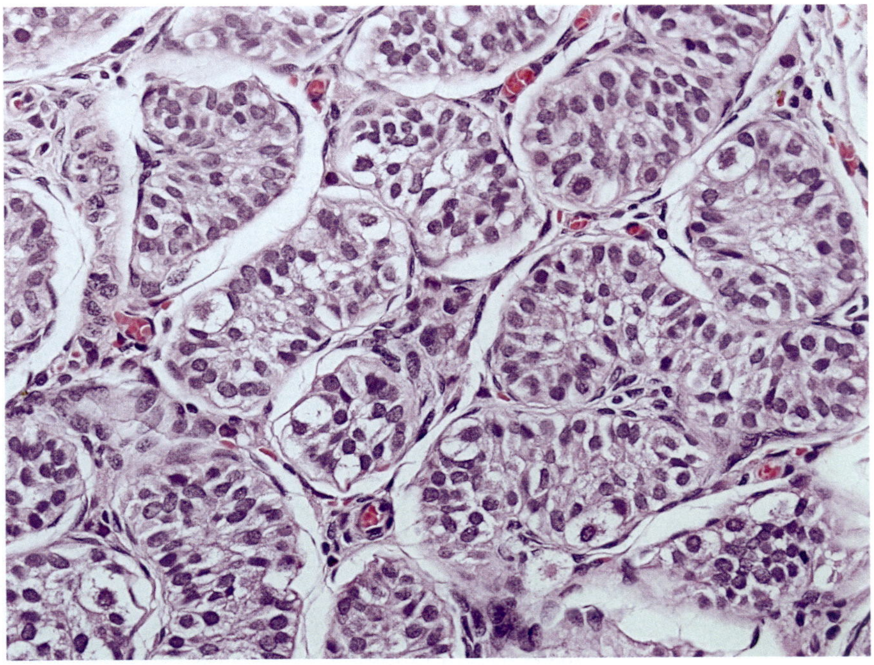

Figure 17-16.
The testicular component is composed of infantile seminiferous tubules with occasional germ cells.

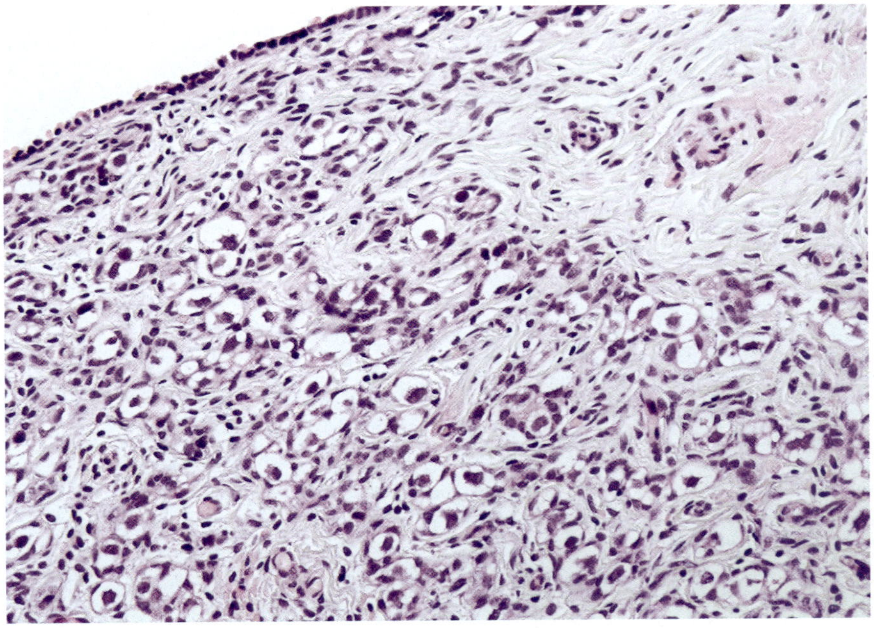

Figure 17-17.
The ovarian component is composed of ovarian tissue consisting of many round primitive oocytes and spindle-shaped stromal cells.

ANDROGEN INSENSITIVE SYNDROME

Definition

- A genetic male with inability to respond to androgen, resulting from a mutation of the androgen receptor

Other terms

- Testicular feminization syndrome

Pathogenesis

- Androgen receptor mutation leads to a male patient to have female appearance, because of the lack of androgen effect during early development

Clinical features

- Androgen insensitive syndrome (AIS) can be divided into complete and incomplete forms
- Patients with a complete form (unfunctional androgen receptors) exhibits female appearance after adolescence
- Typically, the AIS patients are tall, with well-developed breasts, sparse axillary and pubic hair
- No uterus, only a pouch-like "vagina"
- Inguinal testes or intra-abdominal testes
- Increase risk for malignant germ cell tumor at 3% to 5% at the age of 25 years, and 30% to 50% at the age of 50 years

Gross pathology

- Underdeveloped gonads (immature testes)
- Mass lesions in the gonad mostly are germ cell tumors

Histology

- Immature testis (fetal type) with minimal or no spermatogenesis (Fig. 17-18)
- Diffuse or nodular Leydig cells hyperplasia (Fig. 17-19)
- Seminoma or mixed germ cell tumor may be present when the person reaching adulthood (Fig. 17-20)

Immunohistochemistry

- Rarely required
- May be applicable to subtype germ cell tumors if present

Molecular genetics

- Cytogenetic studies show 46XY
- Androgen receptor mutation can be confirmed by molecular analysis

Clinical relevance (treatment option and prognosis)

- Removal of testes at younger age to prevent development of germ cell tumors
- If germ cell tumors develop, surgery with or without adjuvant therapies

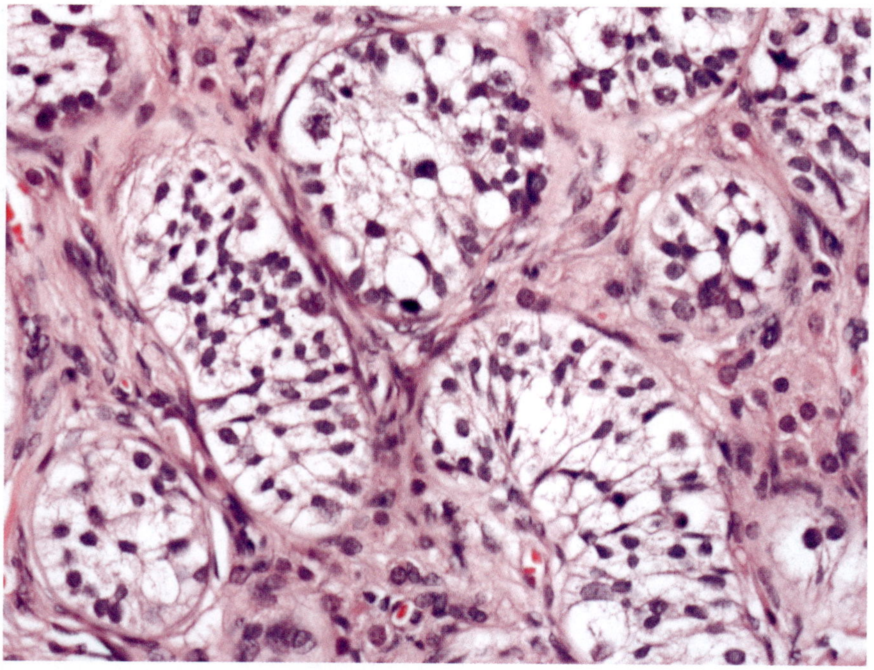

Figure 17-18.
Androgen insensitive syndrome (AIS). Testis from a 30-year-old man contains fetal seminiferous tubules with no active spermatogenesis.

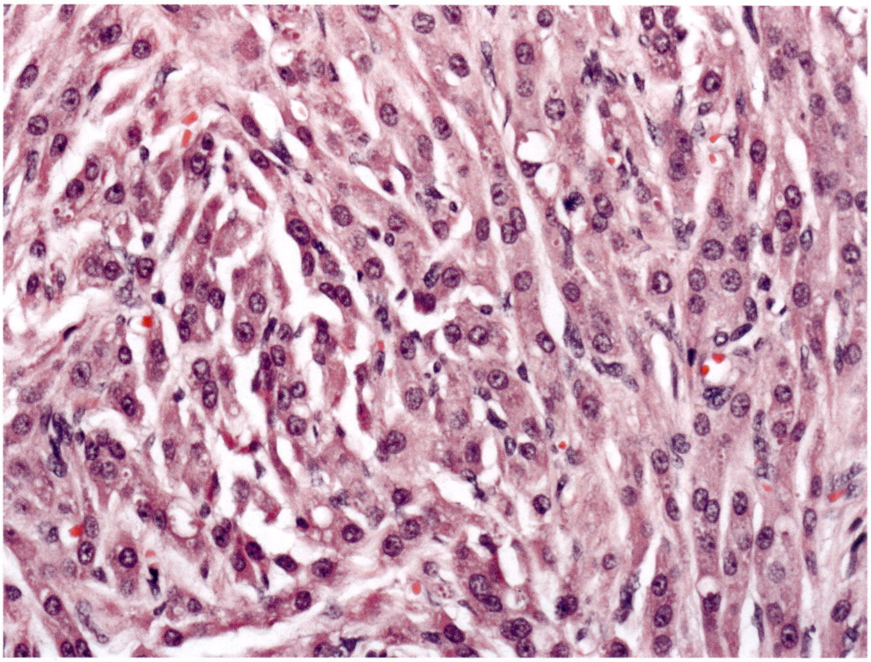

Figure 17-19.
Hyperplastic Leydig cell nodule in AIS.

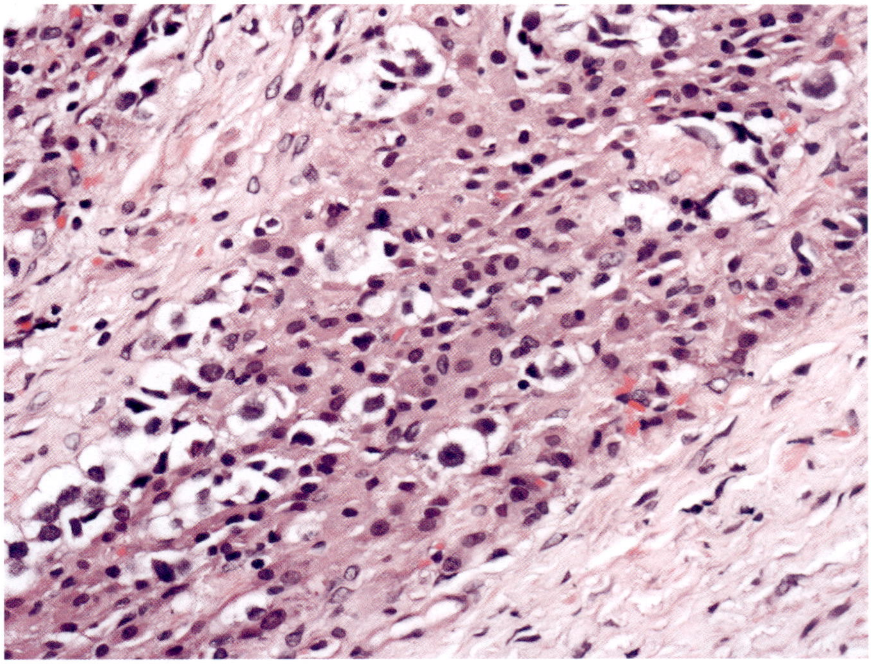

Figure 17-20.
Seminoma developing in a patient with androgen insensitive syndrome is characterized by large atypical cells with a perinuclear halo infiltrating hyperplastic Leydig cells.

TESTIS IN PATIENT WITH CYSTIC FIBROSIS

Definition

- Testis involved by cystic fibrosis (CF), which is an autosomal recessive genetic disorder

Other terms

- Mucoviscidosis

Pathogenesis

- Caused by the mutation of the gene encoding cystic fibrosis transmembrane conductance regulator (*CFTR*), which regulates chloride and sodium ions across the cell membrane
- CF particularly involves the lung, gastrointestinal tract, kidney, pancreas, and other endocrine organs
- Malfunction of *CFTR* leads to the thick mucus and secondary infection, and eventually organ failure

Clinical features

- CF is characteristic of cystic formation and fibrosis in multiple organs
- A small percentage of CF patients are associated with undescended testis, absence of vas deferens, and aspermia
- Malfunction of testicular function in CF patients may be nutritional factors or obstruction related

Histology

- Findings may not be specific
- Sloughing caused by obstruction is the most common finding (Figs. 17-21 and 17-22)
- In late stage, hypospermatogenesis can be seen

Immunohistochemistry

- Not contributory

Molecular analysis

- Mutation analysis for *CFTR* gene is necessary to establish the diagnosis

Clinical relevance (prognosis and treatment options)

- There are many contributing factors for infertility of CF patients
- The majority of mortality conditions are caused by lung failure and pancreatic failure

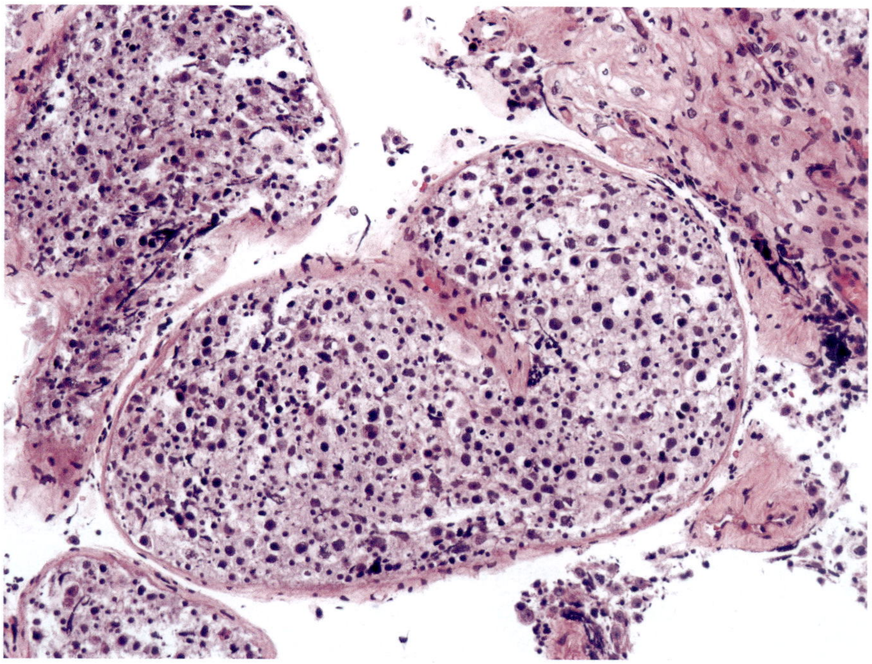

Figure 17-21.
Cystic fibrosis (CF) patient with several seminiferous tubules filled with sloughed germ cells, which are detached and disorganized.

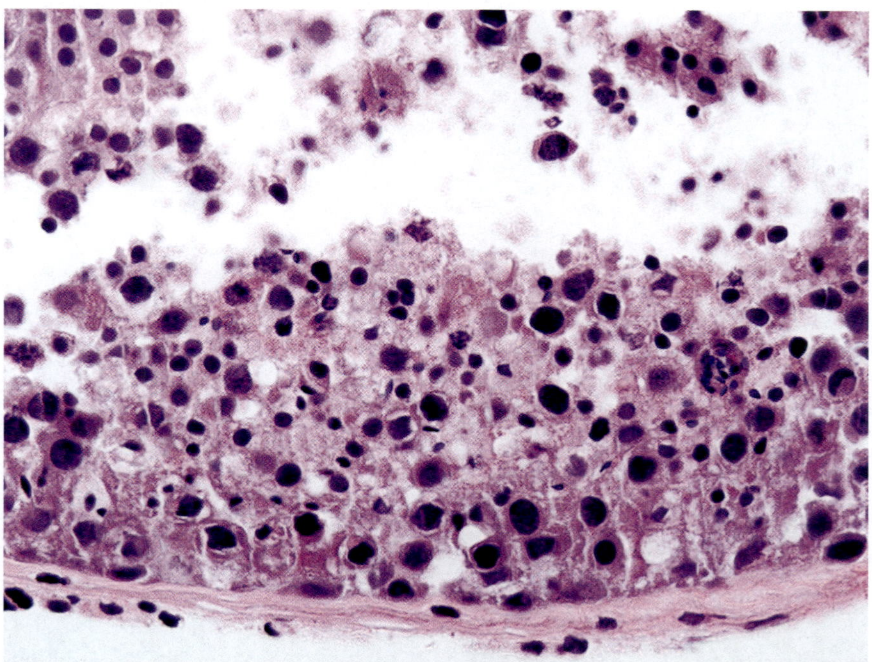

Figure 17-22.
Sloughing in CF. High magnification shows a seminiferous tubule containing spermatozoa (sperm) close to the basal layer instead of their normal central position.

KLINEFELTER SYNDROME

Definition

- Klinefelter syndrome is a genetic disorder of a male caused by an additional X chromosome(s)
- Typical karyotype of 47, XXY
- Variants include XXYY, XXXY, XXXXY, and various mosaic patterns

Clinical features

- The most common sex chromosome disorder in males (1/1000)
- Variable degrees of masculinization, reduced body, and public hair
- Infertility with decreased sperm counts or azoospermia
- Gynecomastia very common
- Increased serum level of gonadotropins (FSH)

Gross pathology

- Small firm testis caused by extensive hyalinization of the tubules with fibrotic cut surface

Histology

- Nonspecific histological changes including variable degree of hypospermatogenesis
- Atrophic testis with fibrosis and hyalinization of the majority of seminiferous tubules (Fig. 17-23)
- Some tubules showing Sertoli-cell-only patterns (Fig. 17-23*b*)
- A small percentage of tubules with decreased spermatogenesis (Fig. 17-24)
- Leydig cells hyperplasia present (Fig. 17-23*b*)

Immunohistochemistry

- Not applicable

Molecular and genetic analysis

- Cytogenetic studies to determine the karyotype are necessary to establish diagnosis

Clinical relevance (prognosis and treatment options)

- Histological changes are not specific; therefore, clinical and molecular genetic correlation is necessary
- Sperm retrieval may apply with success in some cases
- Increased risk for breast cancer

Figure 17-23.
Klinefelter syndrome. A portion of the testis is replaced by hyalinized tubules (*a*) and another part of testis showing Sertoli-cell-only patterns in tubules (*b*) along with Leydig cell hyperplasia.

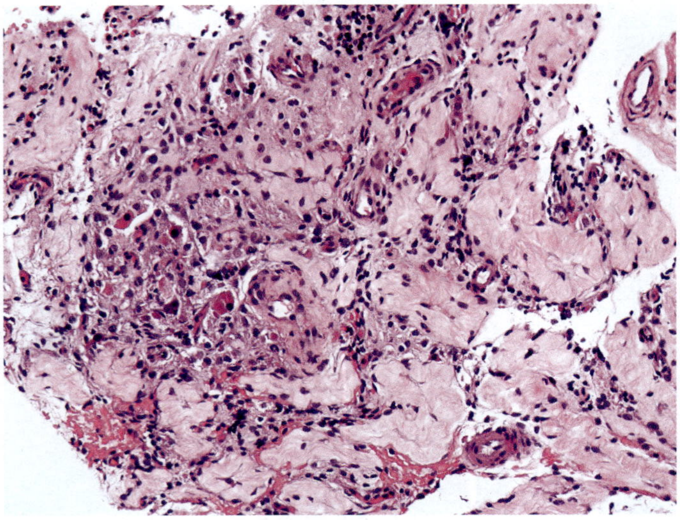

a

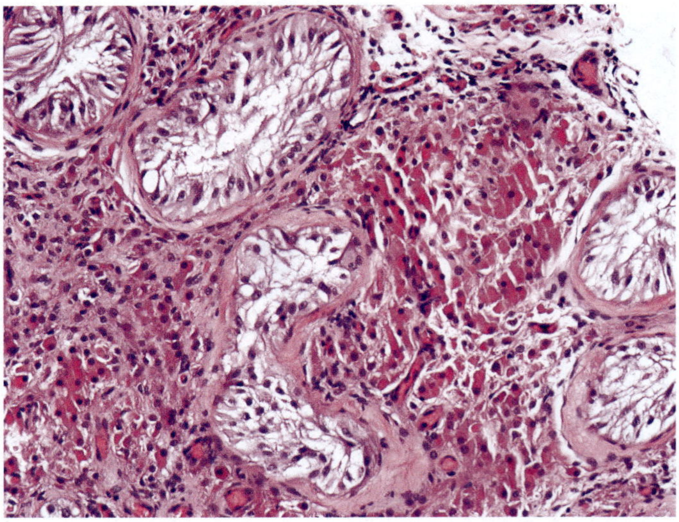

b

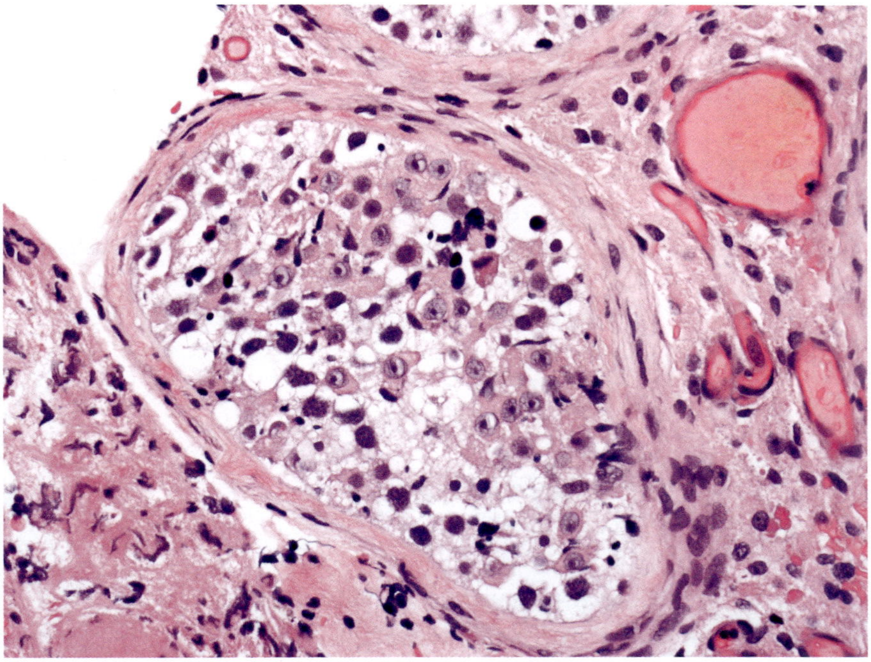

Figure 17-24.
Klinefelter syndrome with only a minority of tubules showing reduced spermatogenesis and sloughing germ cells.

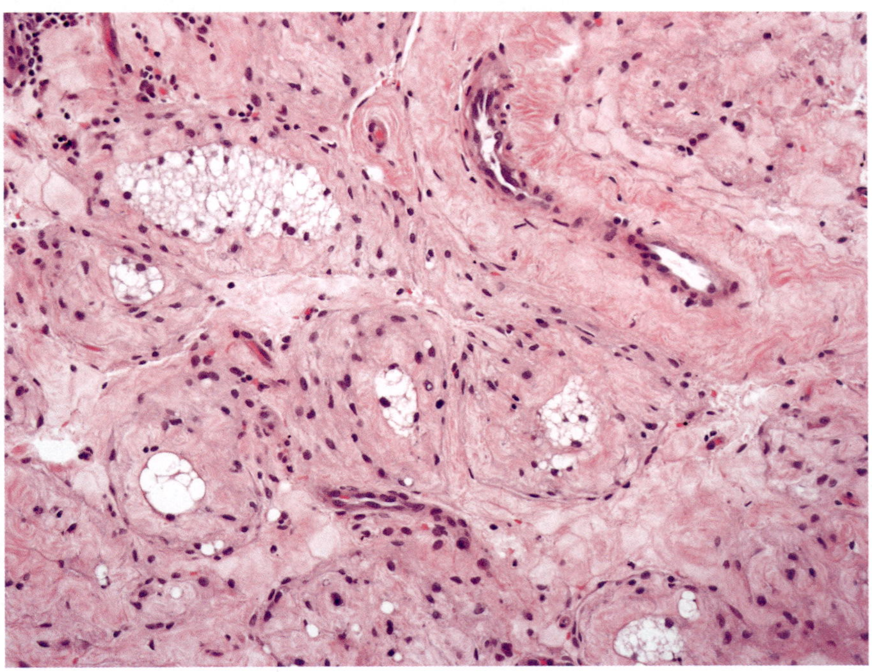

Figure 17-25.
The testis postandrogen ablation contains partially hyalinized tubules with Sertoli cells with foamy cytoplasm without germ cells.

TESTIS AFTER ANDROGEN ABLATION

Definition

- Testis undergoing changes after androgen ablation treatment
- A number of chemical methods have been used to reach androgen ablation (deprivation)

Other terms

- Testis in men with chemical castration, androgen deprivation

Pathogenesis

- Androgen deprivation by antihormonal agents is typically used as a treatment for patients with prostate cancer
- Occasionally chemical castration is used as punishment for sex offender criminals
- Gonadotropin-releasing hormone antagonists such as Lupron lead to atrophic changes in hormonal-producing Leydig cells and depletion of germ cells in the seminiferous tubules

Clinical features

- History of administration of antiandrogen agents
- Small bilateral testes

Gross pathology

- Atrophic testis

Histology

- Most seminiferous tubules are hyalinized without germ cells or Sertoli cells (Fig. 17-25)
- Some tubules contain a small number of Sertoli cells with foamy cytoplasm (Fig. 17-26)
- Leydig cells almost totally disappear (Fig. 17-25)
- Testis may show similar appearance with aging, radiation, or other insults

Immunohistochemistry

- Not indicated

Clinical relevance (prognosis and treatment options)

- Most patients are older with advanced prostate cancer; fertility is not an issue for them
- If reactivation of spermatogenesis in these men is an issue, the severity of atrophy in the testis could have an impact

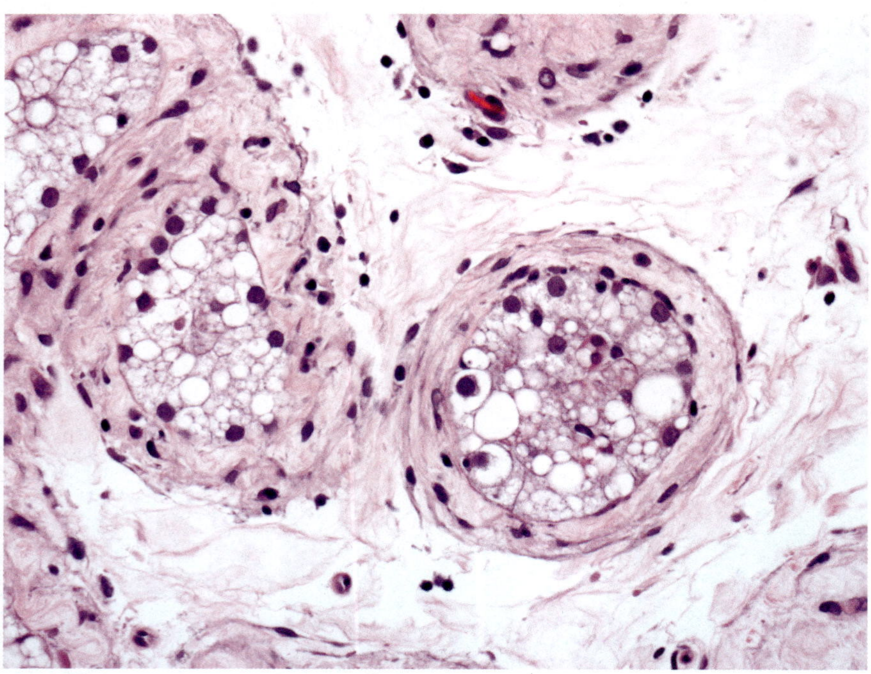

Figure 17-26.
Atrophic tubules postandrogen ablation are filled with Sertoli cells with foamy cytoplasm. Occasional germ cells are seen but reduced in number.

TESTIS UNDER LONG-STANDING EXOGENOUS ESTROGEN ADMINSTRATION

Definition

- The testes on a man with excessive and long-standing exogenous estrogen usage
- A male undergoing sex change surgery to become a female does not fit this entity since the testis is removed during the surgical procedure

Other terms

- Testes from a group of males, so-called "lady boys," that are popular in some cultures

Pathogenesis

- Exogenous estrogen induces the development of breasts and female secondary organs
- By feedback, excess estrogen inhibits the production of FSH
- Suppressed FSH prevents the normal development of germ cells in the testis

Clinical features

- Prominent female appearance with well-developed breasts
- Normal appearance of male external genital organs with small testes present
- Increased risk for germ cell tumors

Gross pathology

- Small testes, with a firm and fibrotic cut surface (Fig. 17-27)
- Should be serially sectioned and carefully examined, because of the possibility of germ cell tumor in the suppressed testes

Histology

- Hypospermatogenesis with reduced numbers of tubules and germ cells (Figs. 17-28 and 17-29)
- Extensive fibrotic tubules
- ITGCNU or germ cell tumor may be present

Immunohistochemistry

- C-kit or OCT-4 may be necessary to rule out ITGCNU

Clinical relevance (prognosis and treatment options)

- Orchiectomy is performed in two situations
  - Requested by the patient
  - Suspicion for development of a germ cell tumor
- Treatment is the same as the patients with conventional germ cell tumor

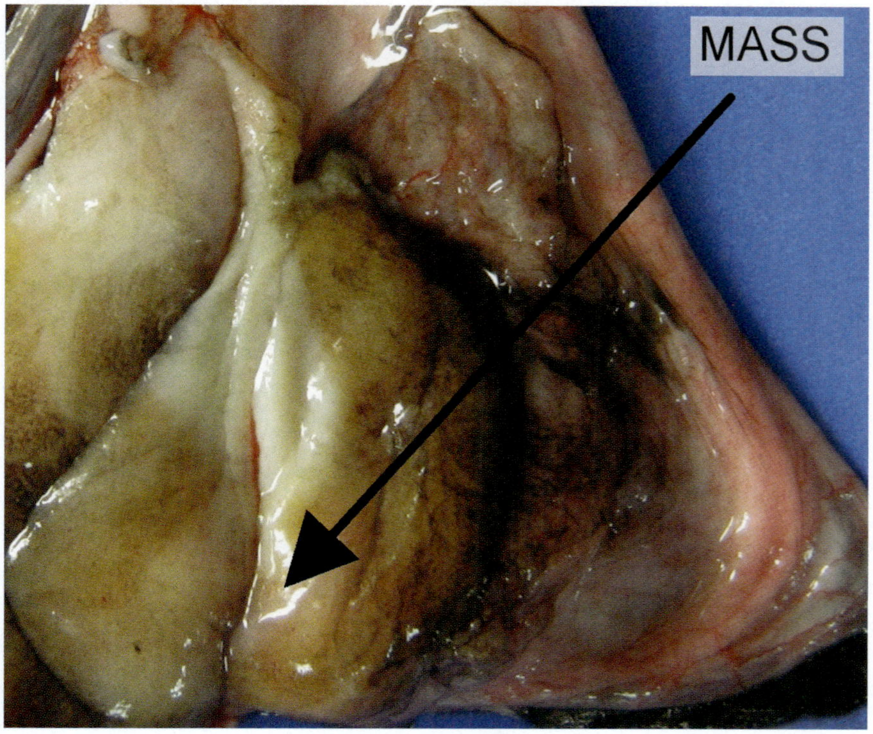

Figure 17-27.
Gross appearance of a testis from a male with long-standing exogenous estrogen influence. The testis was removed with the suspicion of a mass lesion (indicated in the photo), which is actually a fibrotic area.

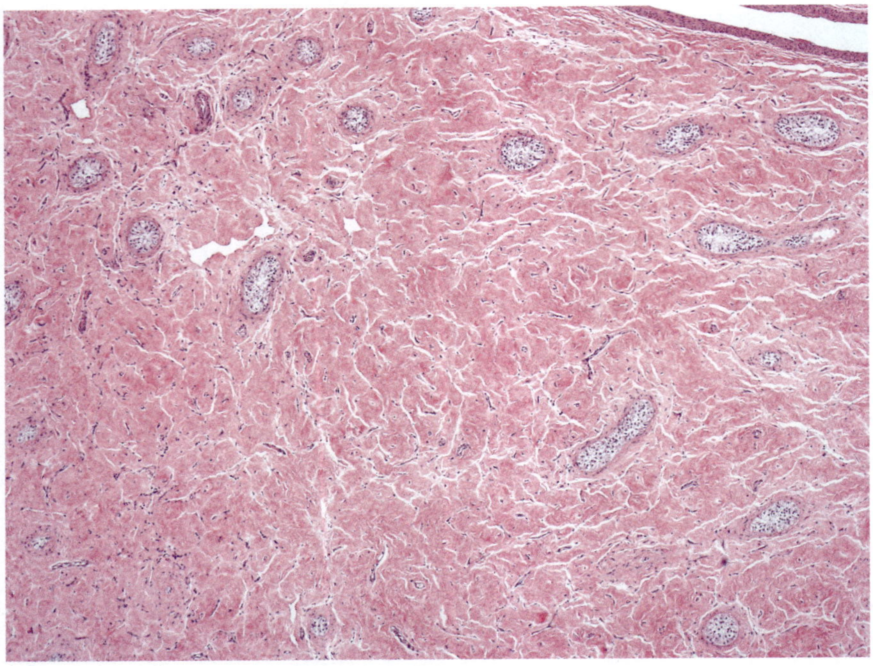

Figure 17-28.
The fibrotic area with only scattered atrophic seminiferous tubules separated by abundant fibrous tissue.

Figure 17-29.
Testis under estrogen influence showing edematous stroma separating tubules (*a*), which are significantly reduced in the number and size. Higher magnification (*b*) shows the atrophic tubule contains mostly Sertoli cells with occasional germ cells.

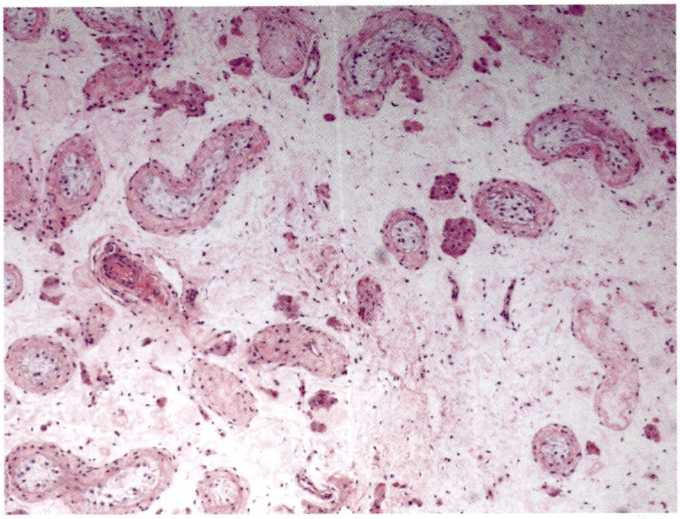

a

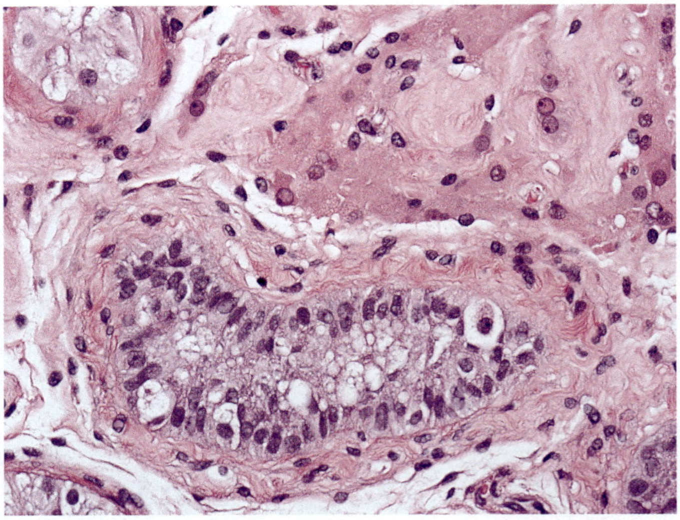

b

TRAUMA

Definition

- Testicular trauma is an injury to one or both testes. The types of injuries include blunt, penetrating, and degloving (scrotum being sheared off from the testis)

Pathogenesis

- Blunt trauma accounts for the majority of the cases of cases, and penetrating trauma accounts for 10% to 20% of cases

Clinical features

- History of trauma
- Extreme scrotal/testicular pain, frequently associated with nausea and vomiting
- Hematocele (blood in the tunica vaginalis) is associated with testicular rupture
- Sometimes, a visible hematoma or scrotal ecchymosis may be seen
- An organized hematoma may be detected as a mass lesion

Gross pathology

- Blunt trauma shows focal hemorrhage in the testis
- Ruptured testis (broken tunica albuginea) or a tear of scrotum may be present, which will cause severe hemorrhage
- Injury could be unilateral or bilateral
- Hematoma can be seen within the testicular parenchyma or paratesticular tissue (Fig. 17-30)
- Late stage trauma is characterized by scar or fibrosis replacing the testicular parenchyma (Fig. 17-31)

Figure 17-30.
Testicular hematoma (*a*) caused by trauma is mimicking a tumor (*a*). High magnification (*b*) shows the organizing granulation tissue (on the left) surrounding the hematoma (on the right).

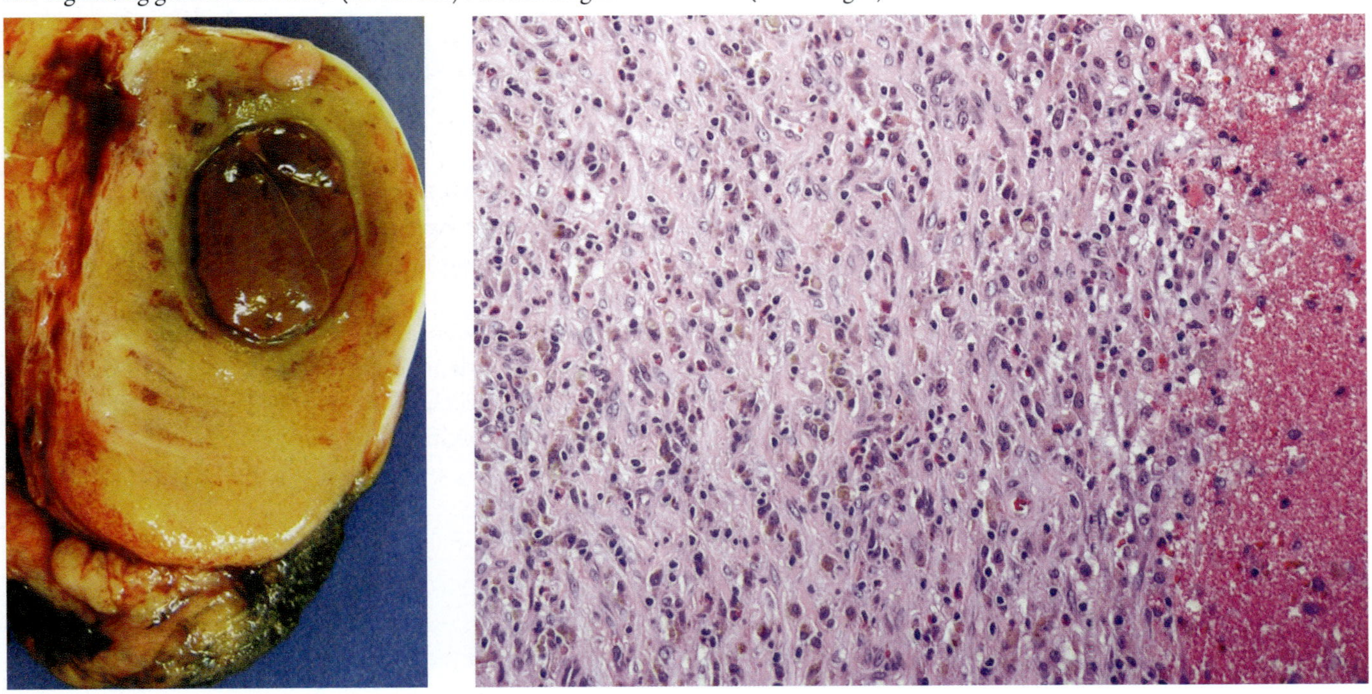

a **b**

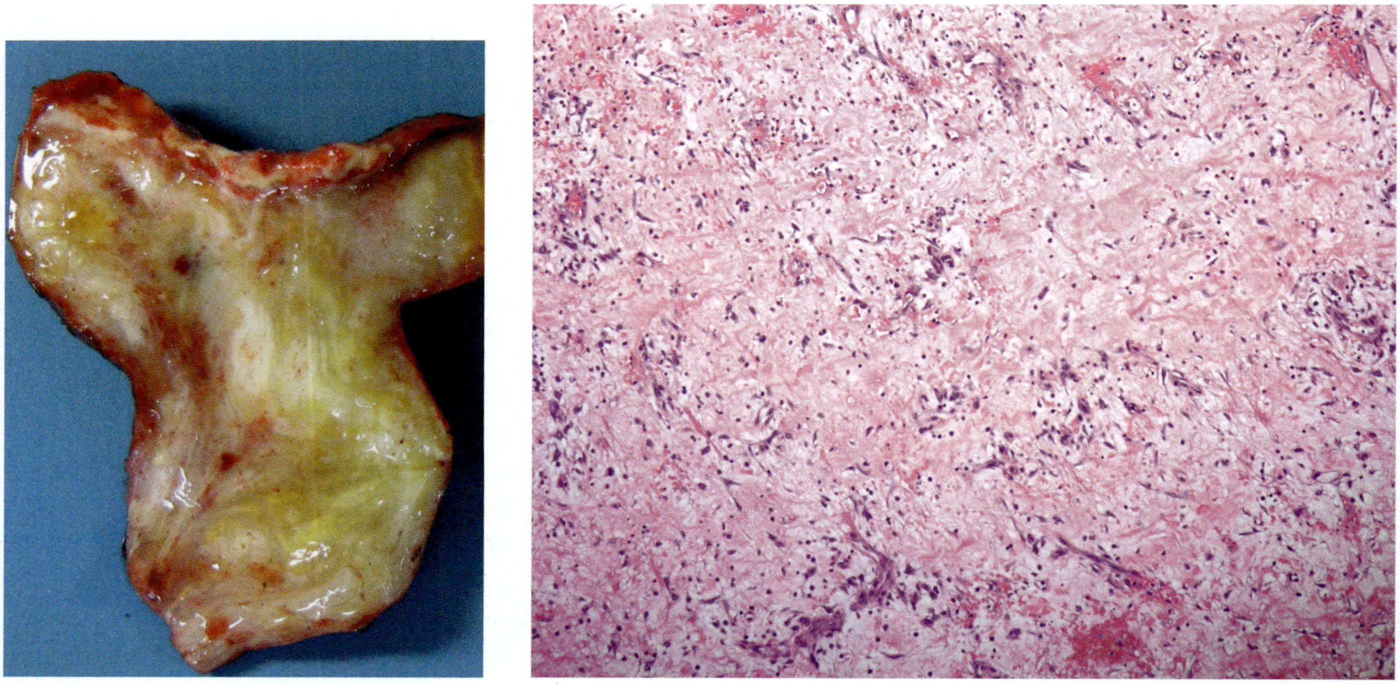

a b

Figure 17-31.
Severe fibrosis of the testis after trauma. Grossly the testis is almost entirely replaced by fibrous tissue with severe distortion (*a*). Microscopy shows the presence of fibrous tissue only (*b*).

Histology

- Hemorrhage, either focal or extensive. A hematoma is localized collection of blood (Fig. 17-30*b*)
- Necrosis is associated with hemorrhage
- Organized hemorrhage is characterized by the presence of macrophages and granulation tissue
- Over time, organization with granulation tissue, inflammatory cells, and fibrosis will replace the damaged tissue and may cause distortion of the testis (Fig. 17-31*b*)

Clinical relevance (prognosis and treatment options)

- Conservative treatment for patients with minor testicular trauma
- Surgical repair would be necessary if the testis is ruptured, testicular debridement and surgical closure of the tunica albuginea are necessary to save the testis
- In severe case, orchiectomy may be necessary

CHAPTER 18

Intratubular Germ Cell Neoplasia, Unclassified

Definition

- Intratubular germ cell neoplasia, unclassified (ITGCNU) is defined as neoplastic germ cells developing within the seminiferous tubules
- It is considered to be the precursor lesion of the majority of malignant germ cell tumors
- ITGCNU is called *unclassified* in order to distinguish from other germ cell neoplasms, which may be present in tubules

Other terms

- Testicular carcinoma in situ (not recommended since it is not an epithelial neoplasm); testicular intraepithelial neoplasia

Pathogenesis and etiology

- Highest incidence seen in Denmark and some European countries
- The latent period to develop into malignant germ cell tumor from ITGCNU is uncertain, but is estimated approximately 10 years
- Presence of germ cell tumor in contralateral testis and cryptorchidism are major risk factor for developing ITGCNU

Clinical features

- Asymptomatic and not forming a mass lesion
- Not known to be associated with elevated serum markers as seen in germ cell tumors
- ITGCNU can only be diagnosed by histological evaluation on tissue, in either testicular biopsy or orchiectomy specimens because it is a microscopic finding

Gross pathology

- Diffuse process, no obvious gross abnormality
- Most commonly seen in the testis harboring a malignant germ cell tumor (80% to 90% of cases)

Histology

- The hallmark of intratubular germ cell neoplasia, unclassified (ITGCNU) is the presence of large atypical neoplastic germ cells within seminiferous tubules (Fig. 18-1)
- The neoplastic cells are similar to seminoma cells with abundant clear cytoplasm and enlarged hyperchromatic nuclei, described as "fried-egg" appearance (Fig. 18-2)
- The tubules with ITGCNU are typically atrophic with decreased spermatogenesis

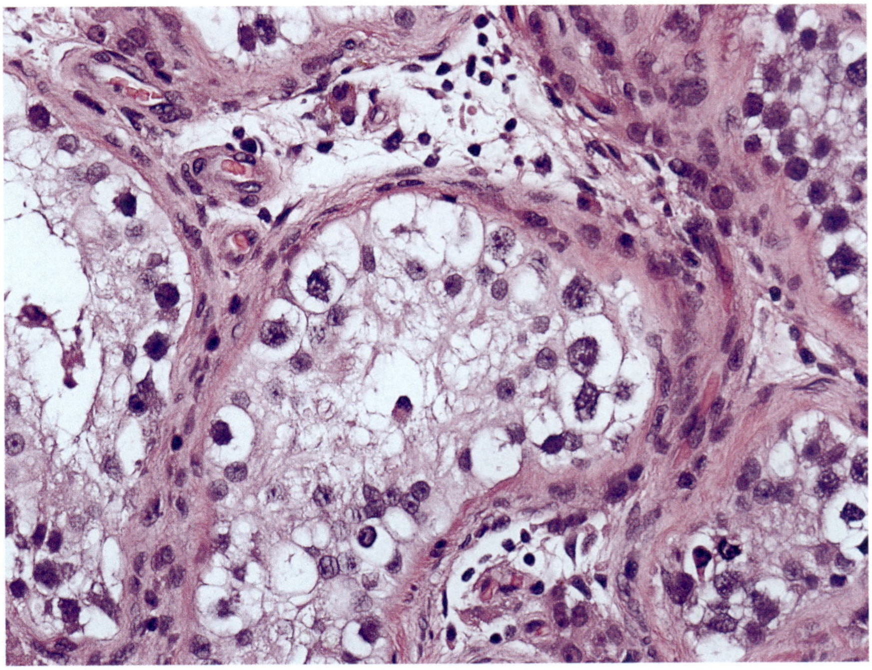

Figure 18-1. Intratubular germ cell neoplasia, unclassified (ITGCNU). A seminiferous tubule with a significantly reduced number of germ cells. Several large atypical germ cells with halo are the neoplastic cells in ITGCNU.

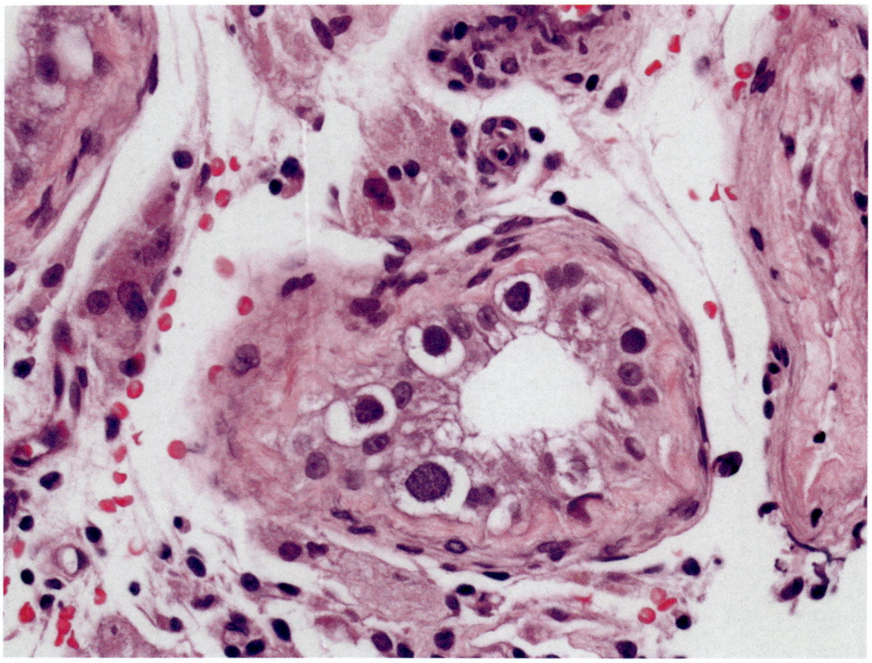

Figure 18-2.
ITGCNU in an atrophic seminiferous tubule with thin germ cell layers. Several large atypical neoplastic germ cells with a halo can be seen.

Immunohistochemistry

- C-kit positive (Fig. 18-3), OCT-4 positive (Fig. 18-4), and SALL4 positive
- Inhibin negative, glypican 3 negative
- Double immunostaining with C-kit and inhibin can highlight the lesional cells better (Fig. 18-5)

Differential diagnosis

- In some benign conditions such as maturation arrest, the abnormal germ cells may have a perinuclear halo mimicking ITGCNU, but they are negative for C-kit, OCT-4, or PLAP

Clinical relevance (prognosis and treatment options)

- Because of uncertain latent period, there are different opinions and approaches regarding the management of patients with unilateral ITGCNU

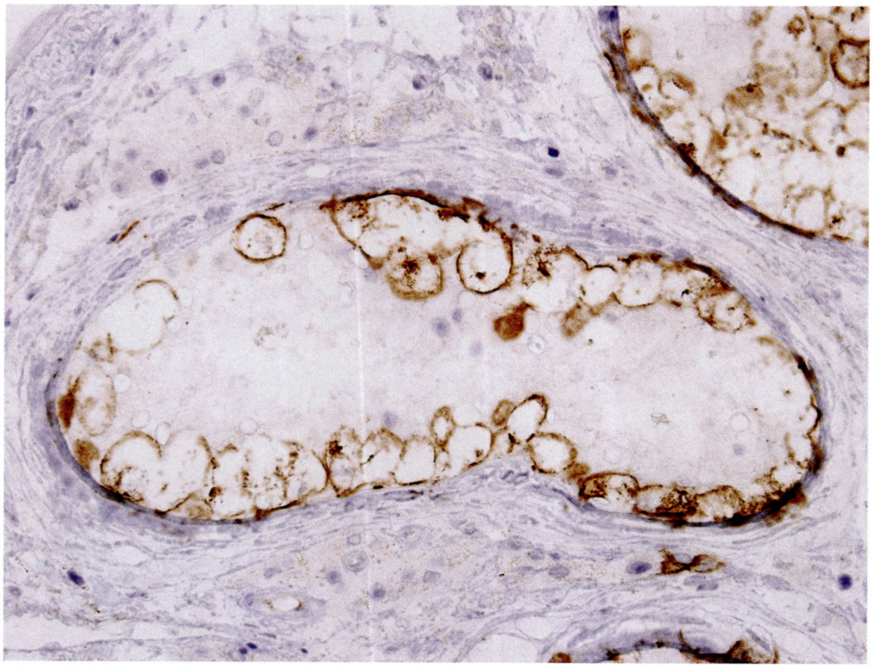

Figure 18-3.
C-kit positive neoplastic germ cells (membrane staining) in ITGCNU.

- In the United States, the presence ITGCNU is not indicative of any radical treatment for malignant germ cell tumors such as surgery or radiation. The patients with isolated ITGCNU (without germ cell tumors) should be clinically followed
- In some European countries, radiation and routine contralateral testicular biopsy will be performed on patients with unilateral ITGCNU. These measures may cause unnecessary damages to the patients

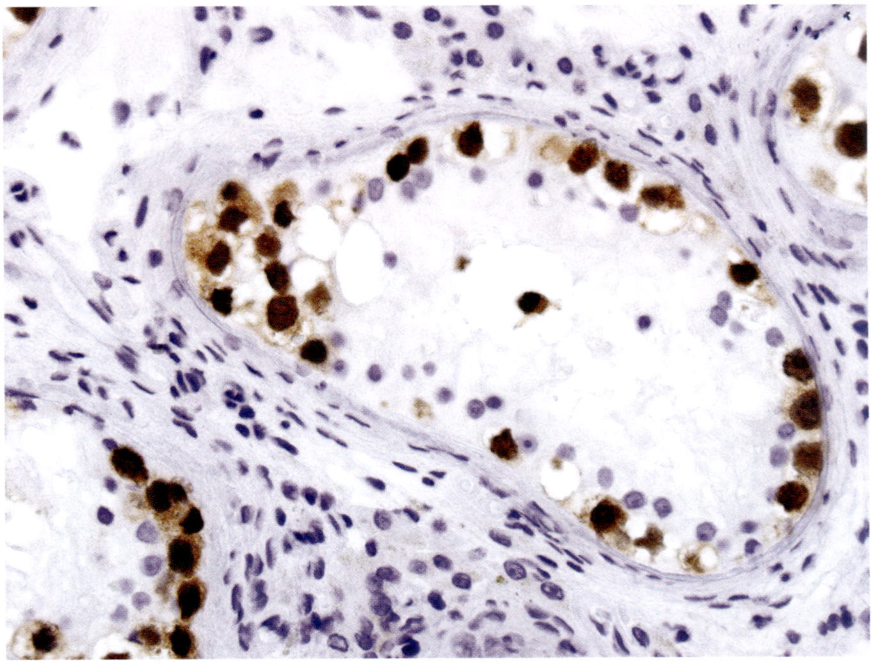

Figure 18-4.
OCT-4 positive neoplastic germ cells (nuclear staining) in ITGCNU.

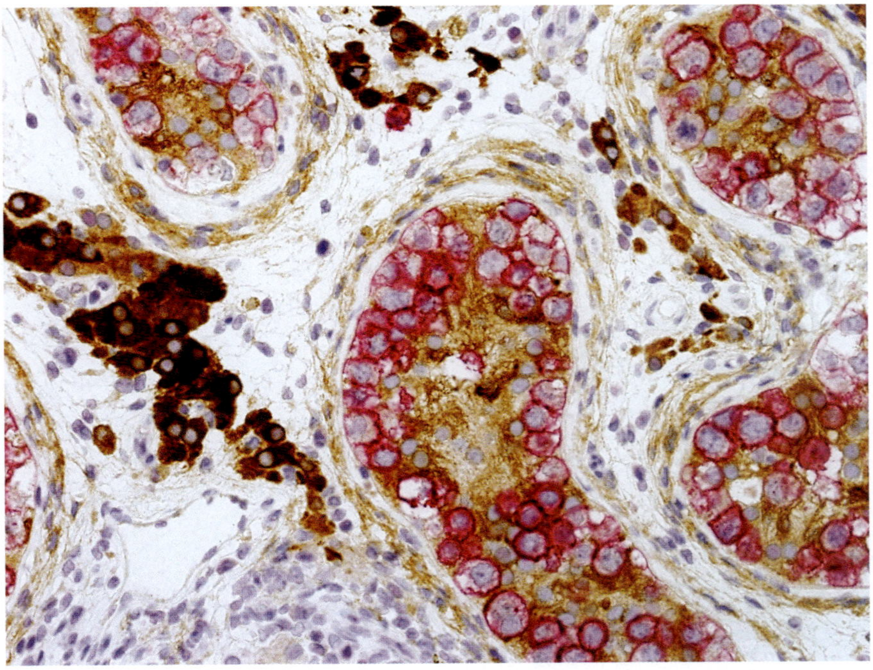

Figure 18-5.
Double immunostaining shows the presence of neoplastic germ cells (red for CD117) and Sertoli cells (light brown for inhibin) in seminiferous tubules and Leydig cells (brown for inhibin) outside the tubules.

CHAPTER 19 Seminoma

SEMINOMA, CLASSIC TYPE

Definition

- Malignant germ cell tumor composed of uniform primitive cells

Other terms

- Generally speaking, seminoma refers to seminoma classic type
- Germinoma: same tumor if it develops in the extragonadal sites; dysgerminoma: same tumor if it develops in females

Pathogenesis

- Progresses from intratubular germ cell neoplasia, unclassified (ITGCNU)
- Malignant germ cell tumors of the testis include several subtypes: seminoma and nonseminomatous germ cell tumors (which are discussed in Chapter 20)
- Seminoma is the most common histological type of malignant germ cell tumor in adults

Clinical features

- Typically a unilateral painless mass
- Mostly seen in patient 30 to 40 years old
- Lactate dehydrogenase (LDH) elevation, which is associated with the tumor load. Occasionally, β-HCG is mildly increased, but no elevation of other serum markers

Gross pathology

- Large, single (Fig. 19-1) lobulated mass, or multiple nodules (Fig. 19-2)
- Mostly well-circumscribed mass without a capsule
- Cut surface is homogeneous, creamy or fleshy color (Fig. 19-1)
- Hemorrhage or necrosis (Fig. 19-2) is less common than nonseminomatous germ cell tumors

Histology

- Common patterns: solid sheets or nests (Figs. 19-3 and 19-4)
- Tumor cells typically push away the residual tubules, but they may surround the tubules (Fig. 19-3)

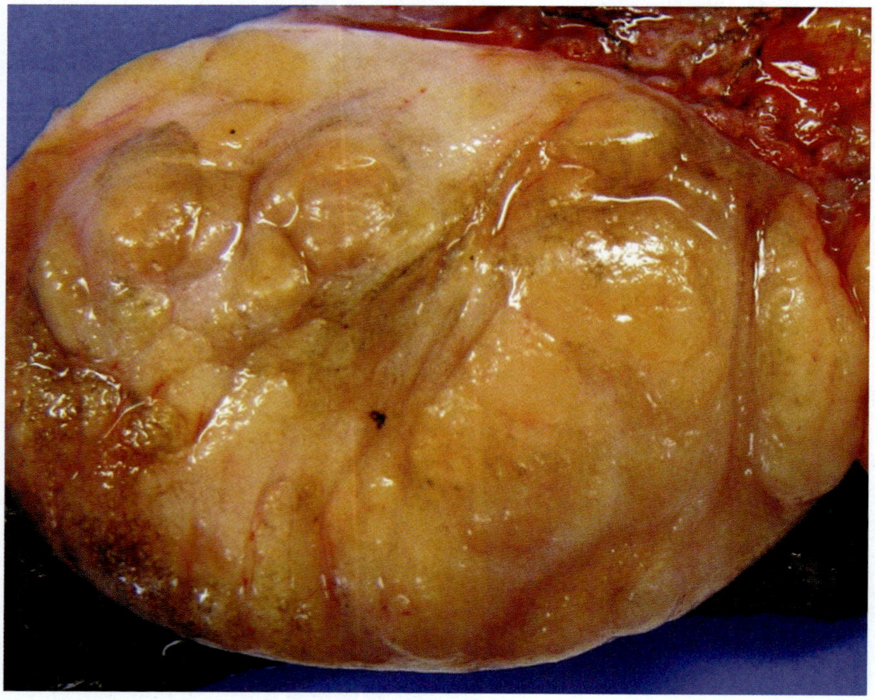

Figure 19-1.
A large seminoma is replacing the entire testis with a smooth and homogeneous cut surface, without hemorrhage and necrosis.

- Rare patterns: trabecular, ribbon like, sclerotic, or pseudoglandular (Figs. 19-5 and 19-6)
- Tumor cells are large polygonal, uniform in size and shape, with clear cytoplasm because of rich glycogen content (Fig. 19-4)
- Large nuclei with prominent nucleoli (Figs. 19-5*a* and 19-6)
- Cell membrane can be seen with a good fixation
- Occasionally, isolated syncytiotrophoblasts are present in seminoma (Fig. 19-5*b*), which should not be confused with choriocarcinoma (containing both cytotrophoblasts and syncytiotrophoblasts)
- Lymphocyte infiltrates are common in the thin septa (Fig. 19-5*c*) and granulomatous reaction can be seen in some cases (Fig. 19-5*d*)
- Morphologically, individual seminoma cells are similar to those in ITGCNU (which is noninvasive)
- Intratubular seminoma refers to cases in which seminoma cells grow within preexisting tubules. However, it is difficult to prove this because of similarity between seminoma cells and neoplastic cells in ITGCNU

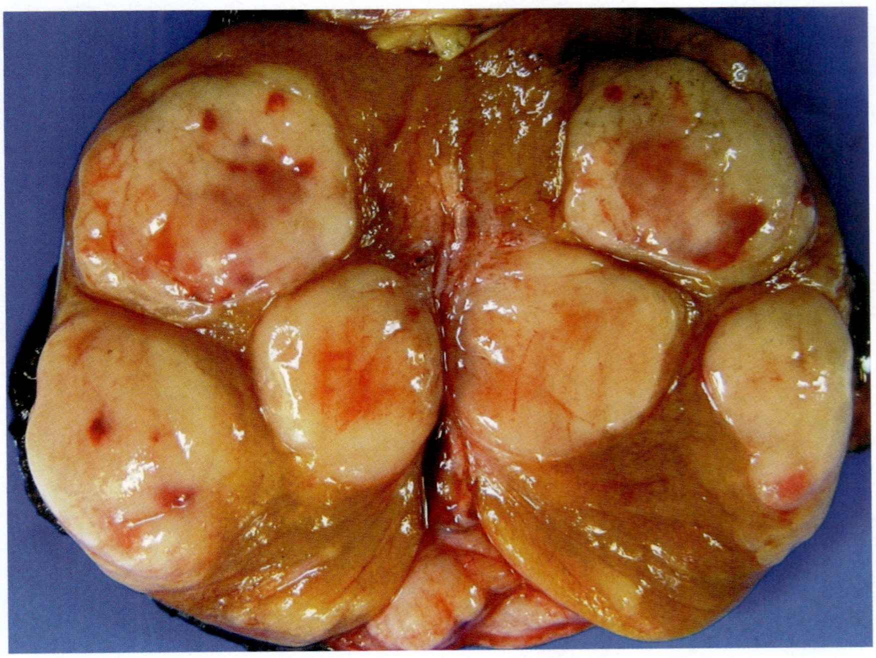

Figure 19-2.
Seminoma with multiple well-circumscribed nodules and a fleshy-colored cut surface. Focal hemorrhage can be seen.

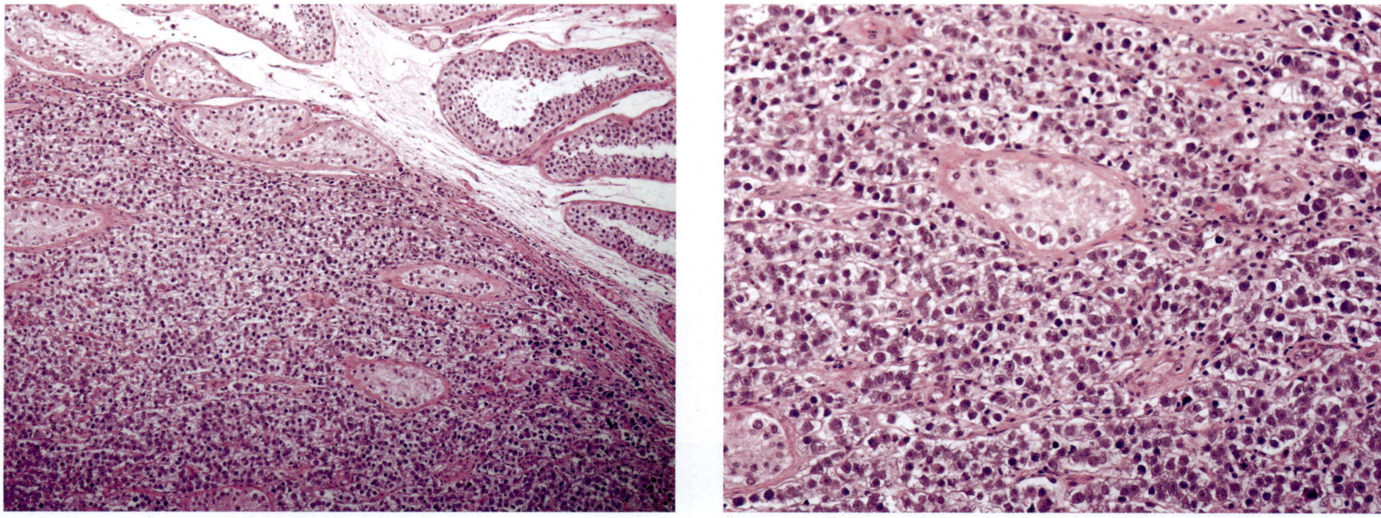

a *b*

Figure 19-3.
Seminoma with the typical well-defined pushing border (*a*); in some area, tumor cells diffusely infiltrate (*b*) around seminiferous tubules.

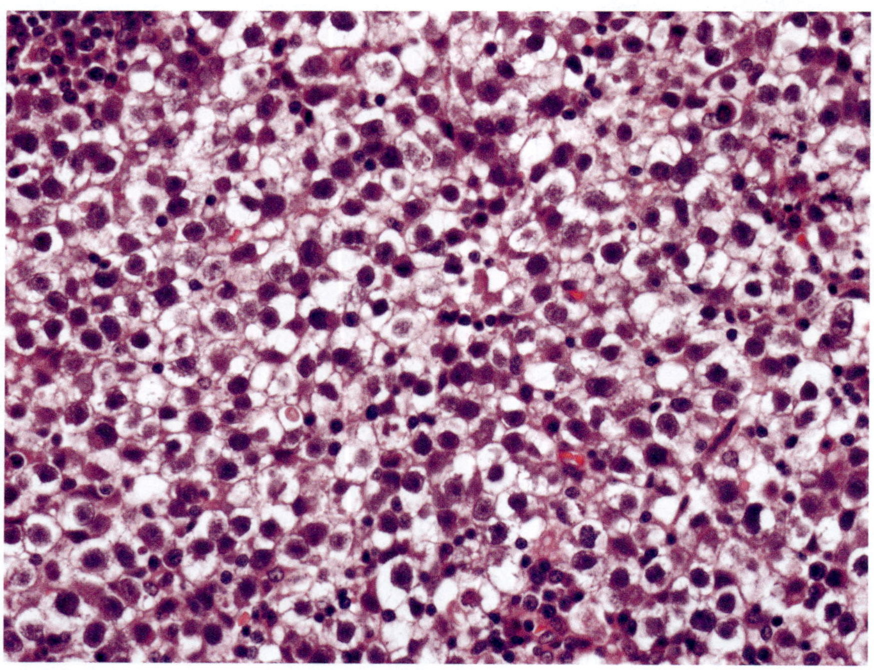

Figure 19-4.
A seminoma is composed of large polygonal tumor cells with clear cytoplasm, large round or slightly irregular nuclei, and prominent nucleoli.

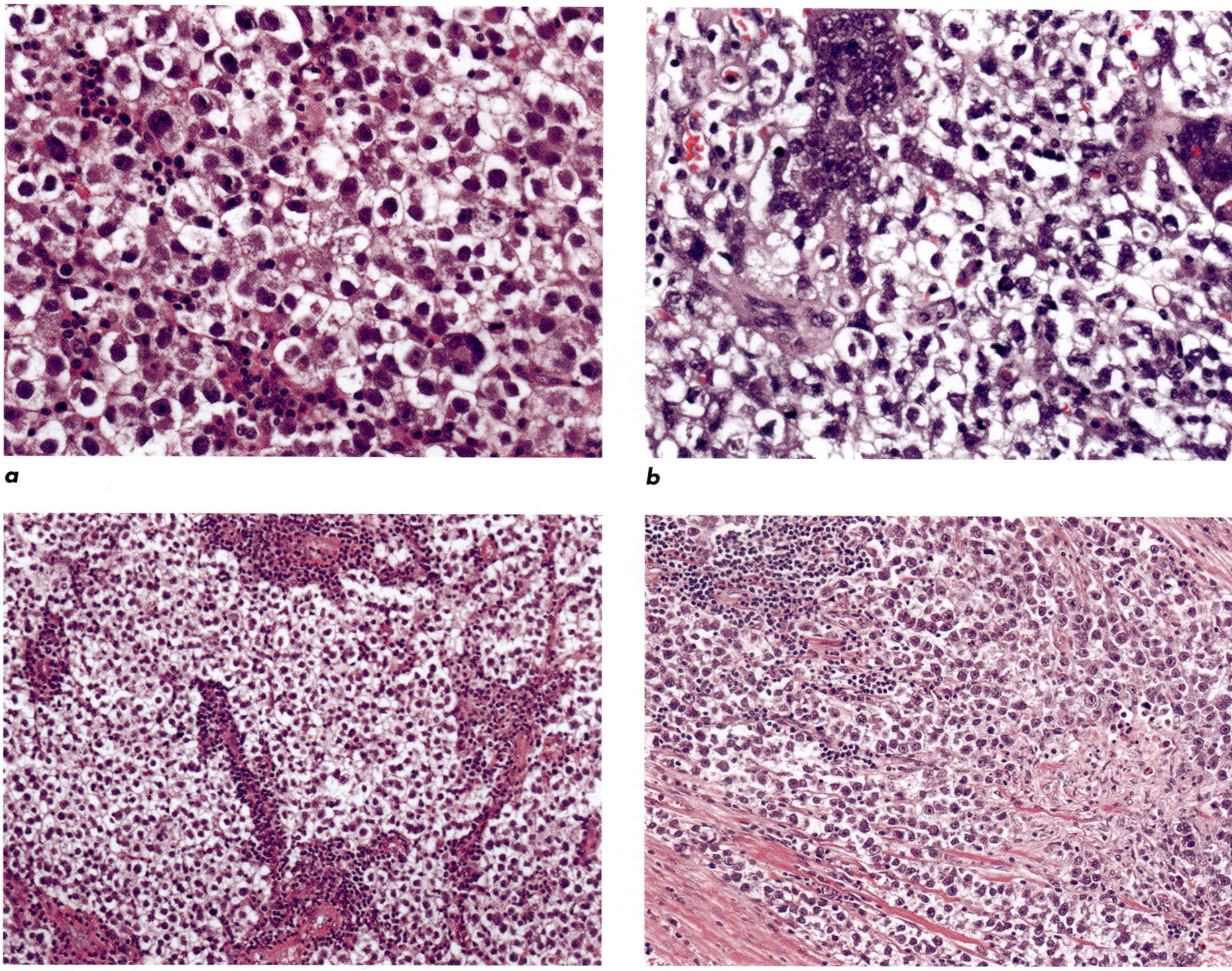

a *b* *c* *d*

Figure 19-5.
Classic seminoma is composed of large tumor cells with clear cytoplasm (*a*). Occasional multinucleated syncytiotrophoblasts can be seen in a seminoma (*b*). Seminoma is associated with prominent lymphocytic infiltrates (*c*) or granulomas (*d*).

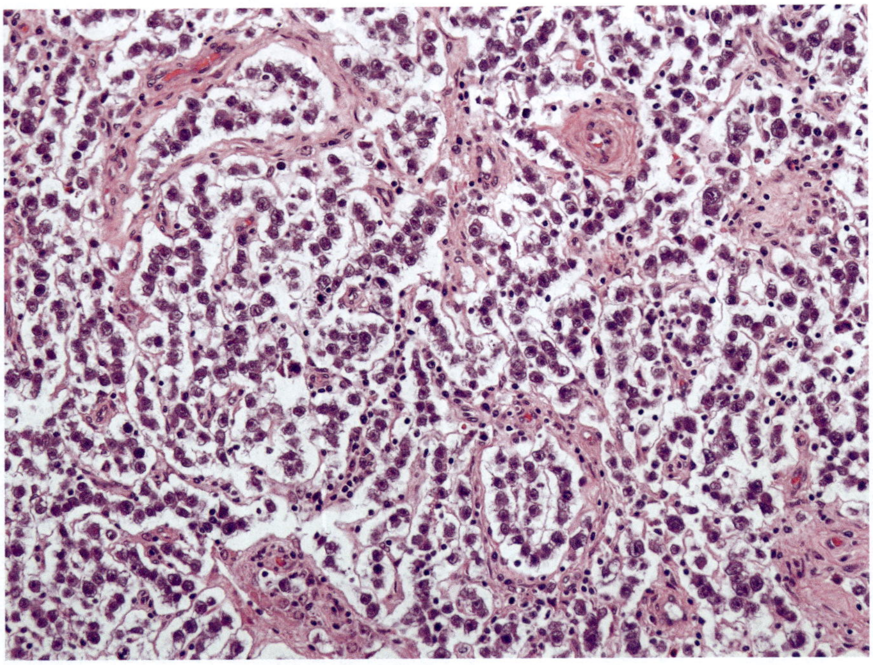

Figure 19-6.
A seminoma with a ribbon-like pseudoglandular pattern.

Immunohistochemistry

- CD117 (C-kit) and OCT-4 positive (Fig. 19-7)
- PAS positive, PLAP positive, SALL4 and D2-40 positive
- Negative for keratin, CD30 negative, HCG rarely positive

Molecular analysis

- Isochromosome 12p can be detected in the majority of cases but rarely necessary because of the typical histologic features

Clinical relevance (prognosis and treatment options)

- Fast growing tumor if untreated
- Radical orchiectomy is the treatment of choice
- Seminoma is sensitive to radiation and chemotherapy, which can be used for a high-stage tumor
- Sometimes, a seminoma may show more prominent cytological atypia. However, the term *atypical* or *anaplastic* seminomas does not have clinical significance in our experience
- Stages of testicular cancer (including seminoma and other germ cell tumors): T1 (tumor confined to the testis, including invasion of the epididymis or tunica albuginea, without lymphovascular invasion); T2 (tumor confined to the testis with lymphovascular invasion); T3 (tumor invades the spermatic cord); and T4 (tumor invades the stroutum)

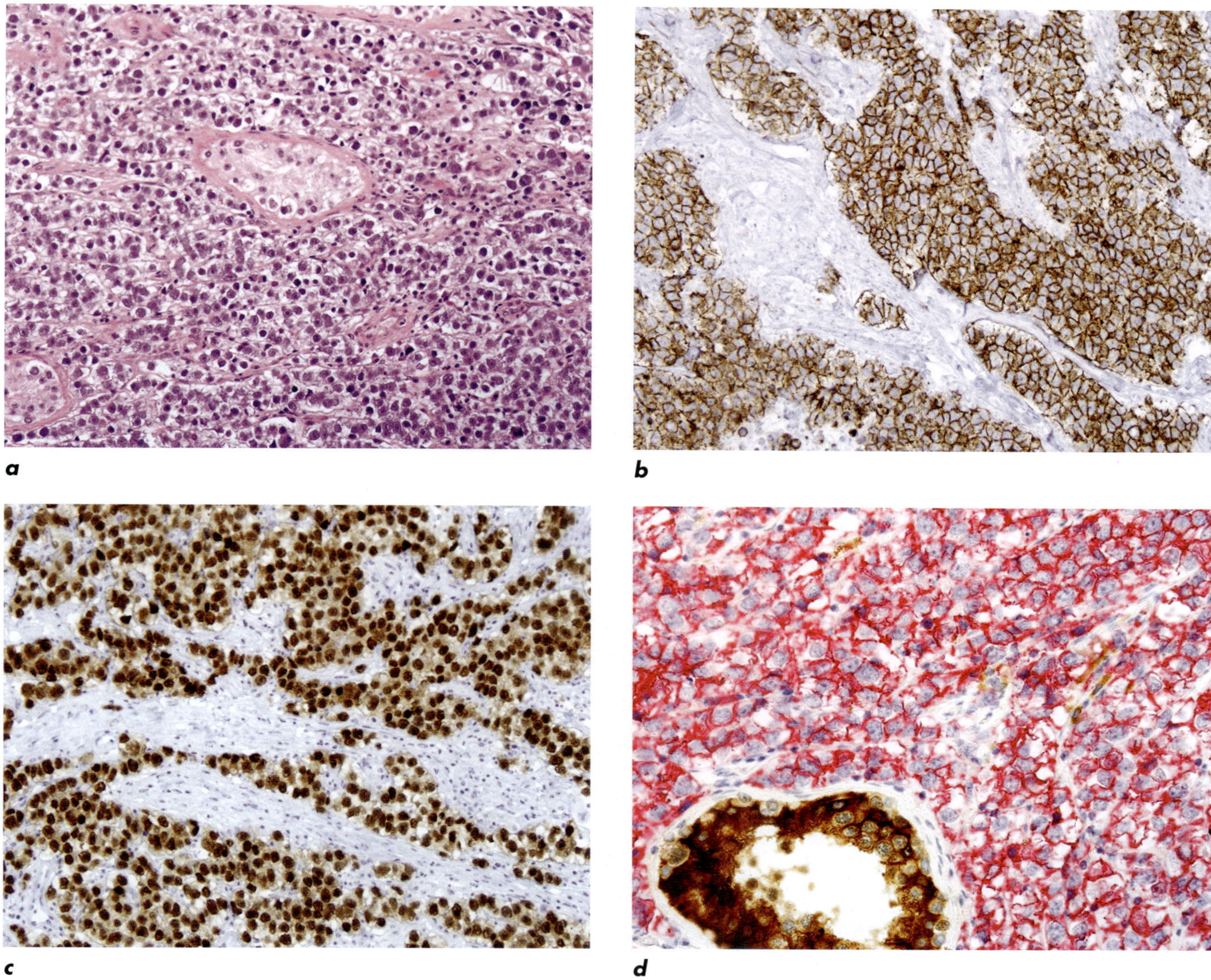

Figure 19-7.
A seminoma (*a*, H&E) shows C-kit positivity (*b*) and OCT-4 positivity (*c*). Double staining (*d*, C-kit = red; inhibin = brown) showing tumor cells positive for C-kit (red) and Sertoli cells positive for inhibin in a benign seminiferous tubule.

SPERMATOCYTIC SEMINOMA

Definition

- A low-grade germ cell tumor composed of three types of primitive germ cells

Pathogenesis

- Etiology is unknown. It is not associated with ITGCNU

Clinical features

- Develops in a wide age range, mostly in a man 50 to 70 years old
- No elevation of specific serum markers
- Testicular swelling

Gross pathology

- Well circumscribed with soft friable cut surface less homogeneous than classic seminoma
- May have gelatinous appearance

Histology

- Diffuse sheet patterns with scant fibrous septa
- Three types of tumor cells (Figs. 19-8 and 19-9)
  - Giant cells (50 to 100 μm) with distinctive filamentous chromatin pattern (Fig. 19-8)
  - Intermediate cells (20 μm) similar to classic seminoma cells (Fig. 19-9)
  - Small cells (size of lymphocytes)
- Typically no lymphocytic infiltrates or granulomatous reaction

Immunohistochemistry

- Occasional positivity for CD117 and SALL14
- Germ cell markers and keratin markers are typically negative

Key differential diagnosis

- Seminoma: seen in younger age, more homogenous cell population, presence of lymphocytes and granulomas, PLAP, CD117, and OCT-4 positive
- Lymphoma: with tubule sparing interstitial growth pattern, and lymphoid markers positive

Clinical relevance (prognosis and treatment options)

- Good prognosis, rarely metastasizes
- Orchiectomy to cure

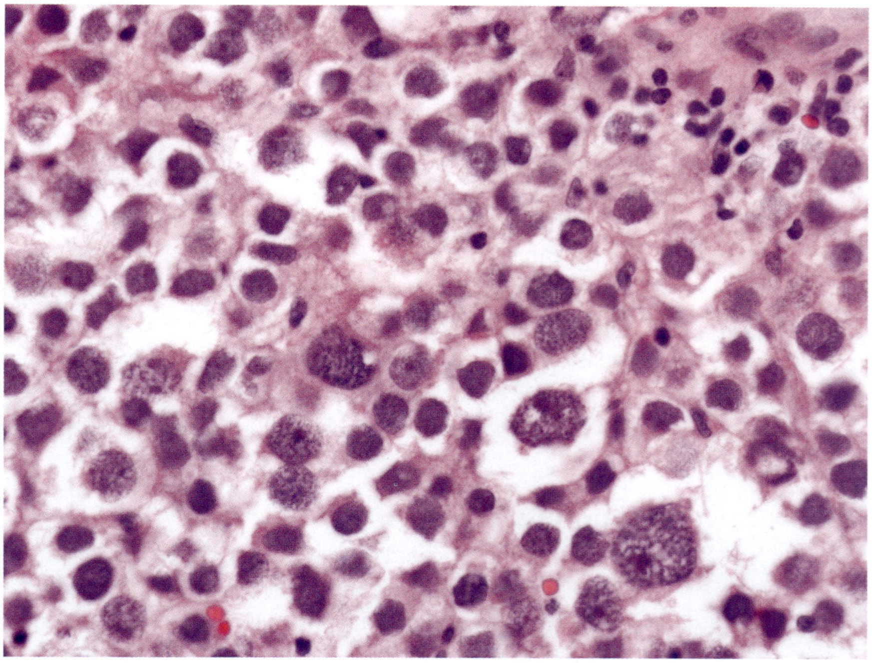

Figure 19-8.
Spermatocytic seminoma consisting small, intermediate, and large tumor cells.

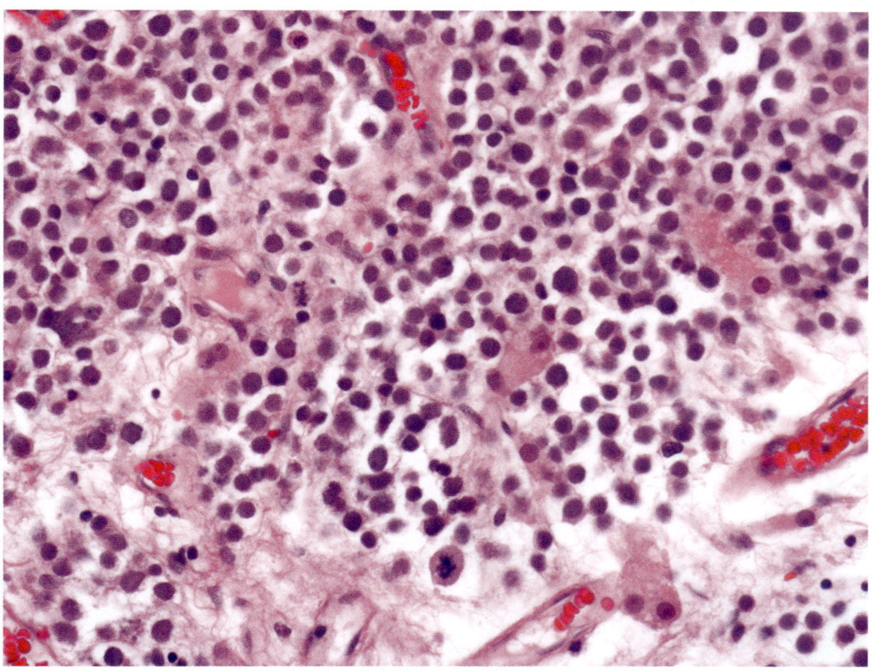

Figure 19-9.
Spermatocytic seminoma with mostly intermediate-sized tumor cells and occasional small-sized tumor cells with mitotic figures similar to classic seminoma.

CHAPTER 20

Nonseminomatous Germ Cell Tumors

Ximing J. Yang, Sean K. Wang

CHORIOCARCINOMA

Definition

- Malignant germ cell tumor (GCT) composed of neoplastic trophoblasts
- Pure choriocarcinoma of the testis is rare. More than 90% of cases present as a component of mixed germ cell tumors

Clinical features

- Small testicular mass in young men (20 to 30 years old)
- Associated with significant increase of serum β-HCG, which could cause gynecomastia

Gross pathology

- Hemorrhagic small nodule in the testicular parenchyma
- Often present within a large mass of mixed germ cell tumor as a minor component

Histology

- Background of prominent hemorrhage and necrosis, caused by the invasiveness of trophoblasts (Fig. 20-1)
- Three cellular components
  - Syncytiotrophoblasts are multinucleated with abundant amphophilic (purple) cytoplasm (Figs. 20-1 and 20-2)
  - Cytotrophoblasts exhibit pale or clear cytoplasm and a large nucleus (Fig. 20-2)
  - Intermediate trophoblasts are slightly larger than cytotrophoblasts, difficult to distinguish from cytotrophoblasts. The identification of intermediate trophoblasts is not required for establishing the diagnosis
- Vascular invasion and hemorrhage are common findings

Immunohistochemistry

- β-HCG and glypican 3 positive in syncytiotrophoblasts
- Keratins may be positive in trophoblasts
- Intermediate trophoblasts positive for human placental lactogen

Clinical relevance (prognosis and treatment options)

- Only 10% of choriocarcinomas are present in a pure form
- Early metastasis may develop. Surgery and possible chemotherapy are required
- Prognosis is worse than choriocarcinoma that develop in the uterus, but similar to other nonseminomatous germ cell tumors of the testis

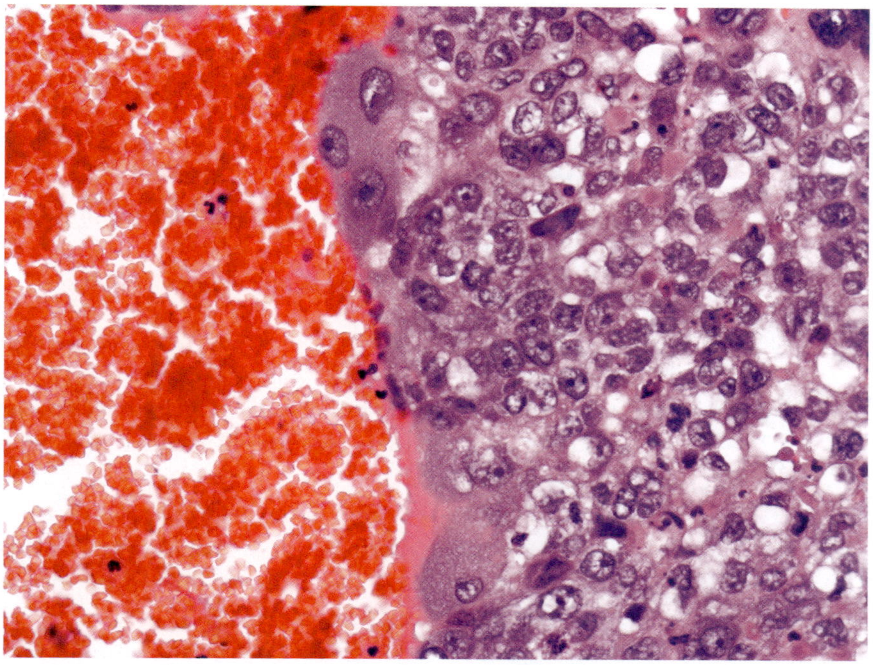

Figure 20-1.
Testicular choriocarcinoma with neoplastic multinuclear syncytiotrophoblasts and cytotrophoblasts (right), associated with an area of hemorrhage.

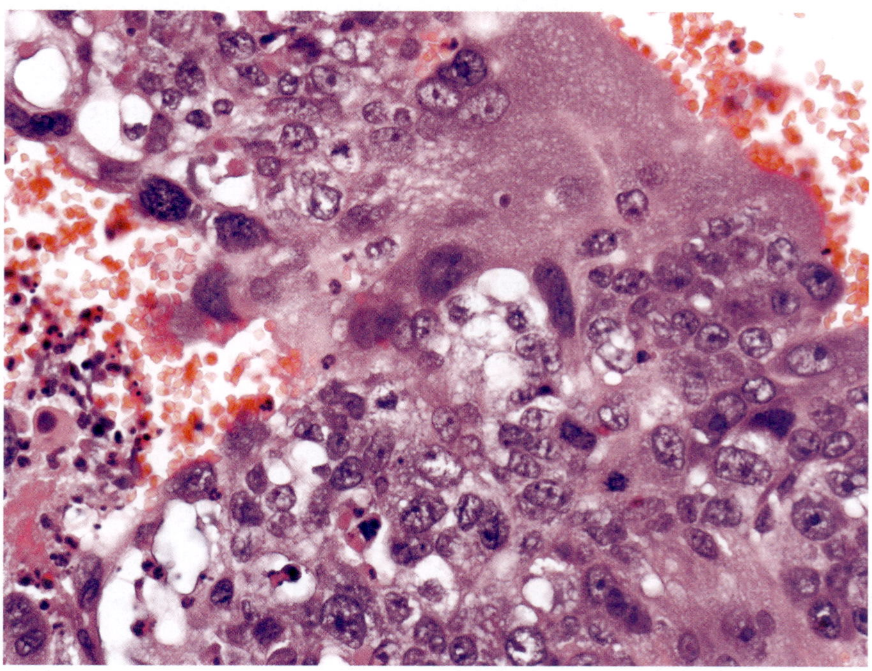

Figure 20-2.
Choriocarcinoma containing large syncytiotrophoblasts with abundant cytoplasm and multiple nuclei (on top) and smaller cytotrophoblasts with vacuolated cytoplasm (on bottom).

YOLK SAC TUMOR

Definition

- A malignant germ cell tumor resembling the yolk sac in embryonic development

Other term

- Endodermal sinus tumor

Pathogenesis

- Yolk sac tumor (YST) of the testis is observed in two forms in two age groups
  - Pure YST is the most common testicular neoplasm in prepubertal children, accounting for 80% to 90% of testicular germ cell tumors in this age group with a median age of 1.5 years
  - In adults, YST presents as a component of mixed germ cell tumor, with an average age of 20 to 30 years. YST components can be seen in 30% to 50% of mixed germ cell tumors in adults

Clinical features

- Children with YST usually present with painless bulky testicular masses. Metastasis is uncommon at presentation, occurring in less than 10% of cases
- In adults, YST tumor is typically mixed with other germ cell components such as embryonal carcinoma, choriocarcinoma, teratoma, and seminoma as a part of a mixed germ cell tumor
- No specific symptoms except testicular mass are present. Almost all the patients with YSTs in either pure form or mixed form have a significantly elevated serum AFP level

Gross pathology

- YST is solid gray-white mass with a gelatinous, myxoid, or mucoid appearance
- Necrosis, cystic changes, and hemorrhage are often seen

Histology

- Composed of primitive tumor cells, which are relatively small (Fig. 20-3) and less pleomorphic compared to embryonal carcinoma cells
- Most common pattern seen in the majority cases of YST is the microcystic pattern, which is characterized by the presence of spider web–like network formed by tumor cells with vacuolated cytoplasm (Fig. 20-3)
- Schiller-Duvall body (Fig. 20-4), an endodermal sinus-like structure pathognomonic of YST, consists of a central fibrovascular core, covered by malignant epithelioid cells, suspended in a cystic space that is lined by flattened tumor cells. However, they are present only in 50% of YST cases
- Other patterns include papillary, solid, glandular, festoon, myxomatous, sarcomatoid, macrocytic, polyvesicular, hepatoid, and parietal patterns (Fig. 20-5). These patterns do not relate to prognosis but can cause difficulty in distinguishing YST from other tumors or other subtypes of germ cell tumors

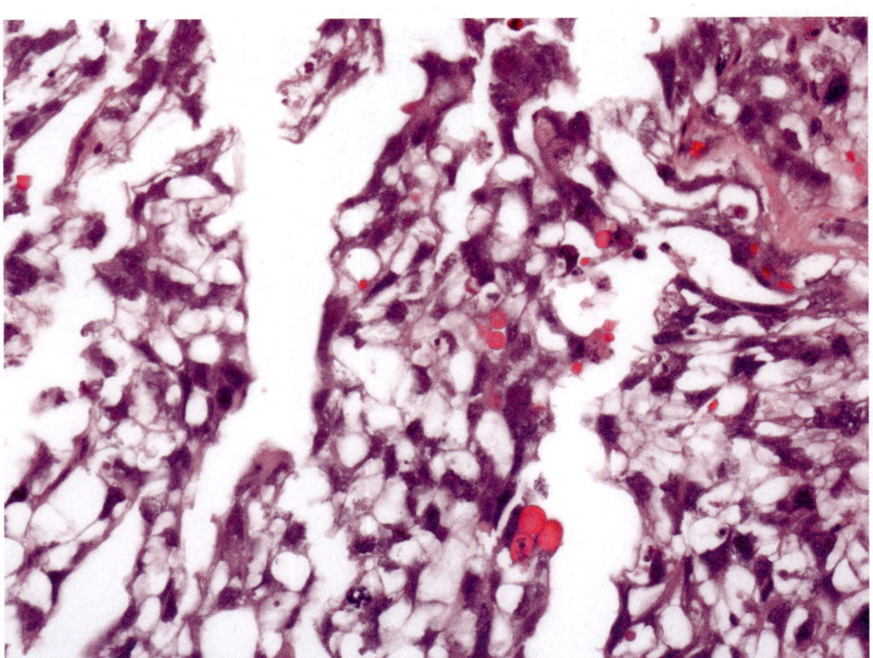

Figure 20-3.
Yolk sac tumor exhibits microcystic pattern, in which tumor cells form network with small cystic space.

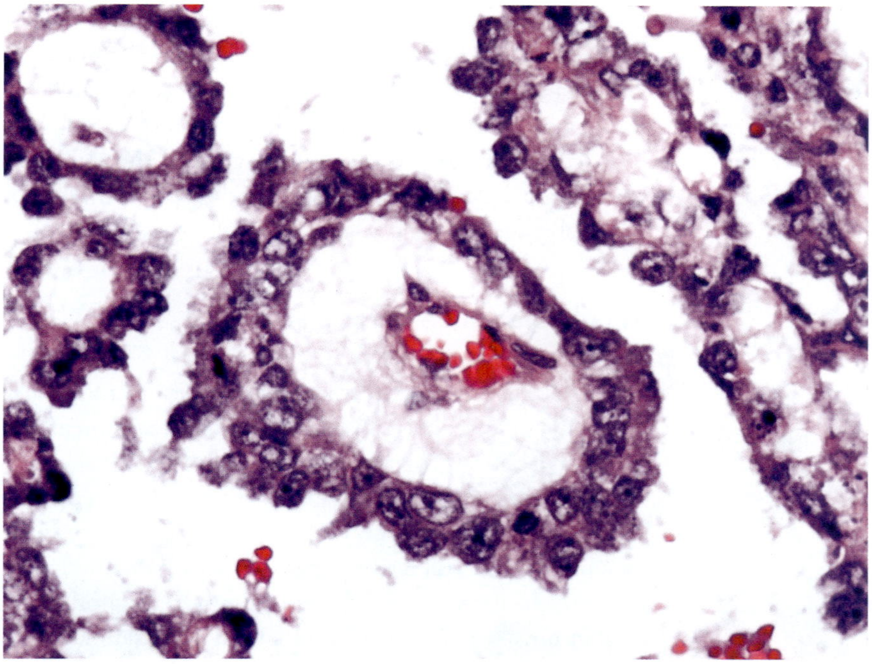

Figure 20-4.
Schiller-Duvall body of YST is composed of central fibrovascular core surrounded by tumor cells, situated in a space.

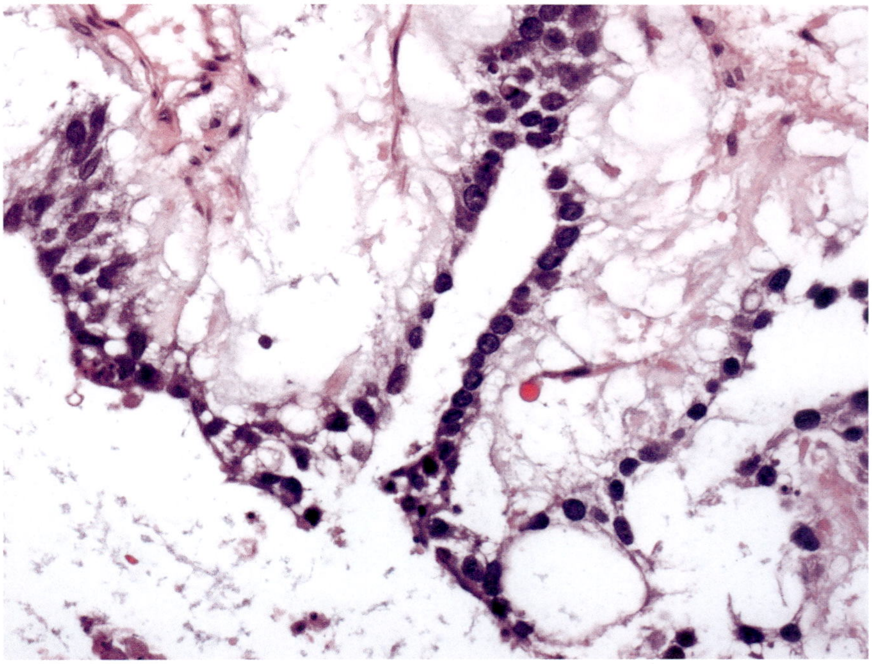

Figure 20-5.
Yolk sac tumor cells forming glandular structures are less pleomorphic than embryonal carcinoma cells. A hyaline globule can be seen.

- Hyaline globules ranging from 1 to 50 μm can be seen in YST (Fig. 20-5), which are PAS positive (diastase-resistant) and occasionally positive for AFP. Eosinophilic bands (extracellular basement membrane material) are also frequent findings in YST. Neither hyaline globules nor eosinophilic bands are specific for YST

Immunohistochemistry

- α-Fetoprotein (AFP) positive in YST cells (Fig. 20-6), which can be detected on tissue sections as well as in the serum of the patient with YST
- Glypican 3 positive in YST cells
- PLAP positive, a marker also present in several different subtypes of germ cell tumors
- Cytokeratin and vimentin can be positive

Differential diagnosis

- Embryonal carcinoma: form nests and islands of tumor cells similar to carcinoma, with larger and more pleomorphic tumor cells
- Seminoma: typically consists of sheets of cells without specific patterns, but often associated with lymphocytic infiltrates

Molecular studies

- Isochromosome 12p, which is characteristic of other malignant testicular germ cell tumors, can be detected
- Loss of short arm of chromosome 1 (1p36) and long arm of chromosome 6 (6q) as well as gain of the long arm of chromosomes 1 and 20 have been reported, but not applicable for clinical practice

Clinical relevance (prognosis and treatment options)

- Stage is also an important prognostic factor. Early detection of lower stage disease and prompt treatment will result in a better prognosis
- Eighty percent to 90% of YST in children are stage I disease. Without treatment, this tumor is highly aggressive in children and will lead to death. With a combination of modern surgical treatment and adjuvant chemotherapy (cisplatin based), the survival rate is greater than 90%
- The prognosis of a malignant germ cell tumor with a YST component in adults is dependent on the tumor stage and its response to therapy

Figure 20-6.
Yolk sac tumor cells (*a*) are surrounded by embryonal carcinoma cells are highlighted by positive α-fetoprotein immunostaining (*b*).

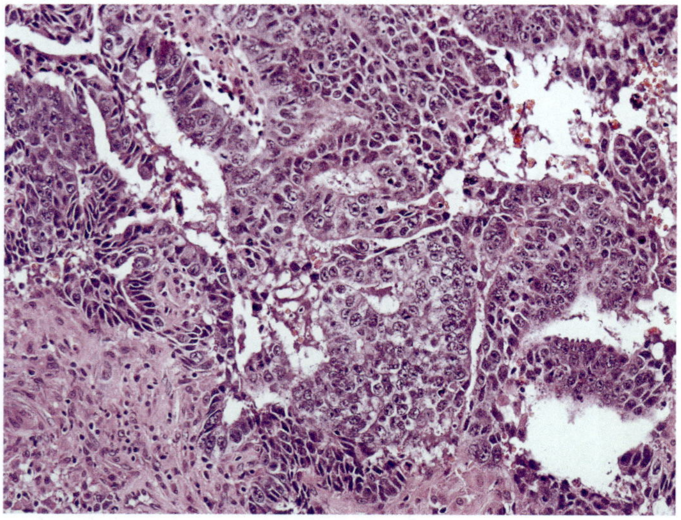

a

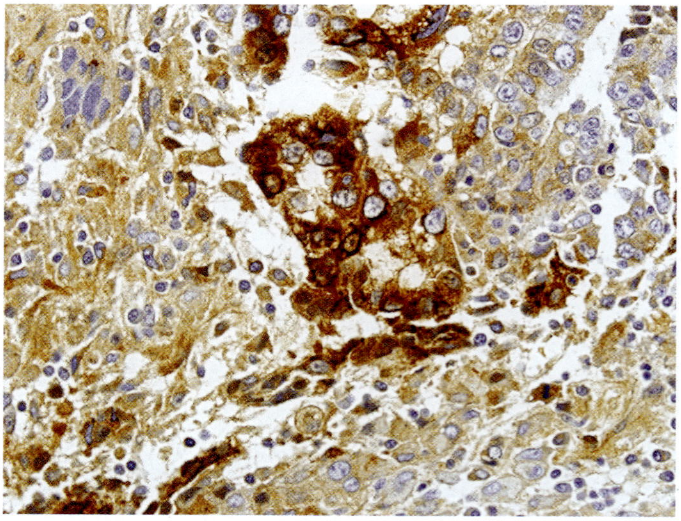

b

EMBRYONAL CARCINOMA

Definition

- Malignant germ cell tumor composed of primitive carcinoma cells

Other terms

- Embryonic carcinoma

Pathogenesis

- Possibly derived from intratubular germ cell neoplasia unclassified (ITGCNU), although intratubular embryonal carcinoma has been reported

Clinical features

- Peaking incidence is 20 to 30 years of age
- Presents with fast-growing, painless testicular swelling
- A well-circumscribed nodule can be palpated in the testicular parenchyma
- Early metastasis can be detected

Gross pathology

- A well-defined or poorly defined solid mass with heterogeneous, yellow, and white cut surface (Fig. 20-7)
- Hemorrhage and necrosis are common

Histology

- Epithelial differentiation is prominent. Embryonal carcinoma (EC) cells form solid sheets, islands, or papillary configuration (Figs. 20-8 and 20-9)
- Tumors cell are highly pleomorphic with abundant granular cytoplasm (Fig. 20-9)
- Vascular invasion is commonly seen (Fig. 20-10)
- In most cases, EC is present as a component of a mixed germ cell tumor

Immunohistochemistry

- CD30 positive (Fig. 20-11). OCT-4 positive and keratins positive
- Glypican 3 negative and CD117 (C-kit) negative

Differential diagnosis

- Yolk sac tumor (see Table 20-1)
- Metastatic adenocarcinoma: OCT-4 and CD30 negative

Molecular analysis

- Isochromosome 12p

Clinical relevance (prognosis and treatment options)

- Aggressive disease if untreated
- Orchiectomy is the treatment of choice
- Pelvic lymph node dissection may be considered for metastatic cases or EC with vascular invasion
- Cisplatin-based modern chemotherapies result in a good survival rate

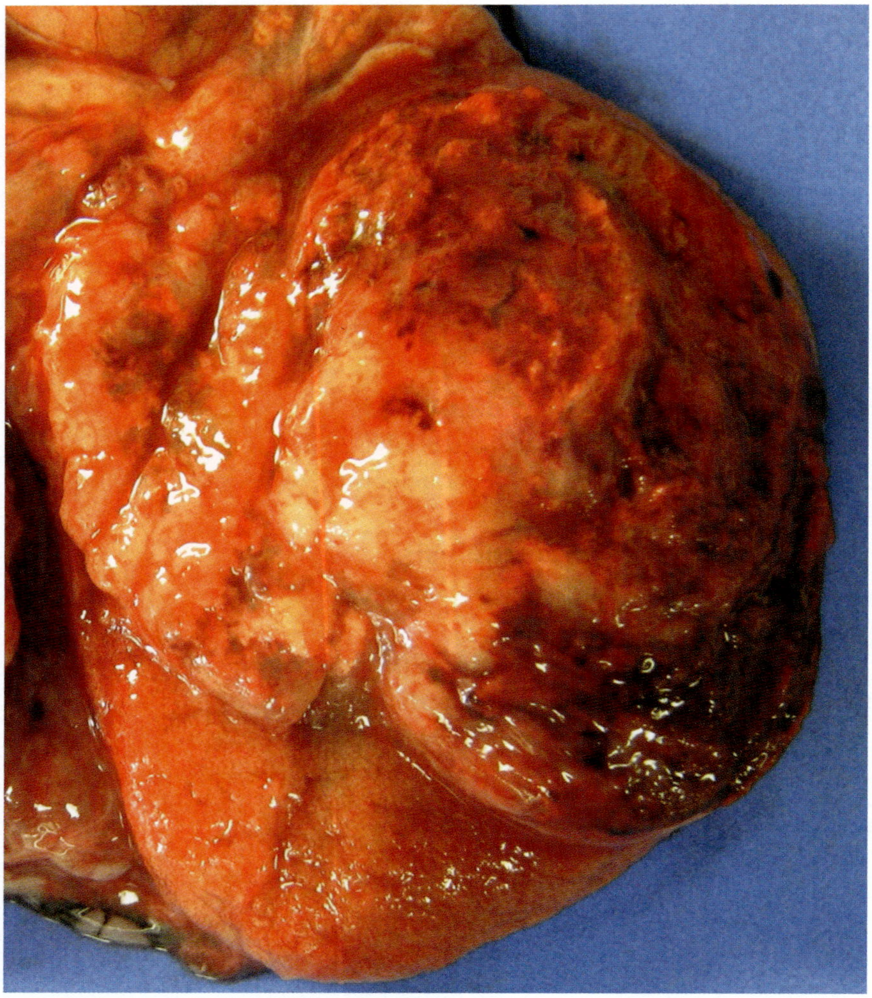

Figure 20-7.
Gross photo of embryonal carcinoma shows a large heterogeneous mass occupying most of the testis. This appearance is not specific for embryonal carcinoma but consists of nonseminomatous germ cell tumor.

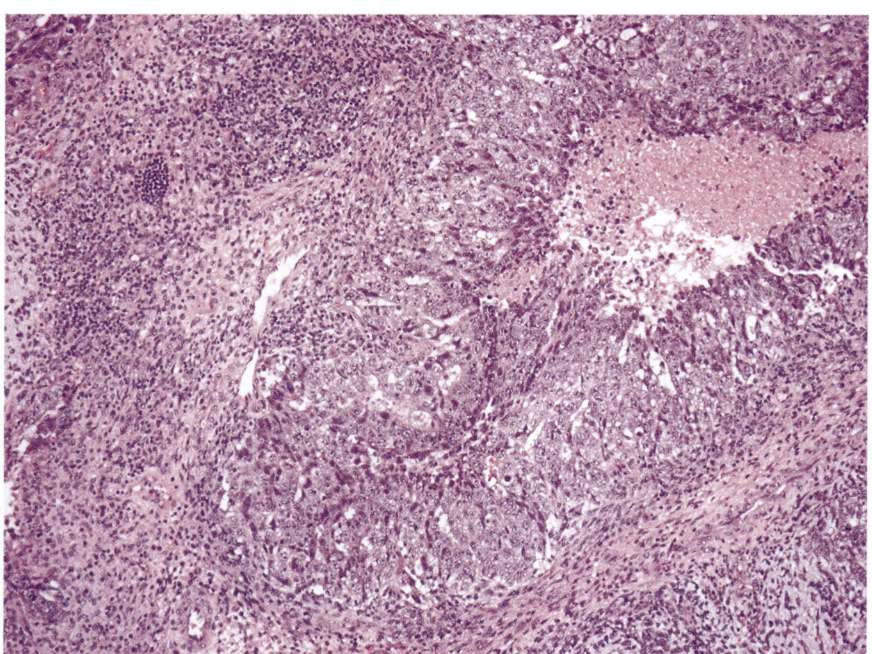

Figure 20-8.
Embryonal carcinoma consist of tumor cells forming islands or large nests with areas of necrosis.

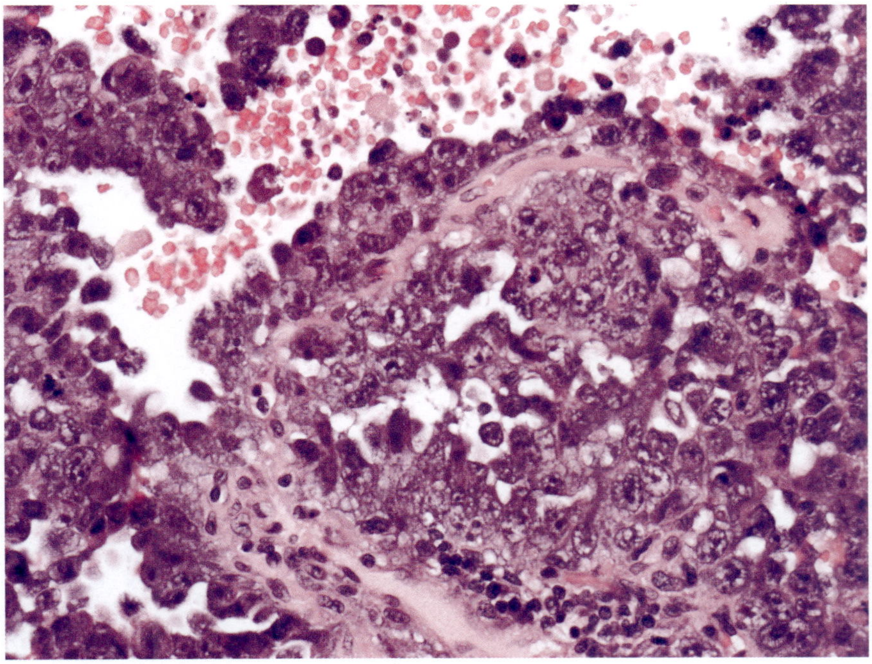

Figure 20-9.
Embryonal carcinoma cells are large and pleomorphic with prominent nucleoli.

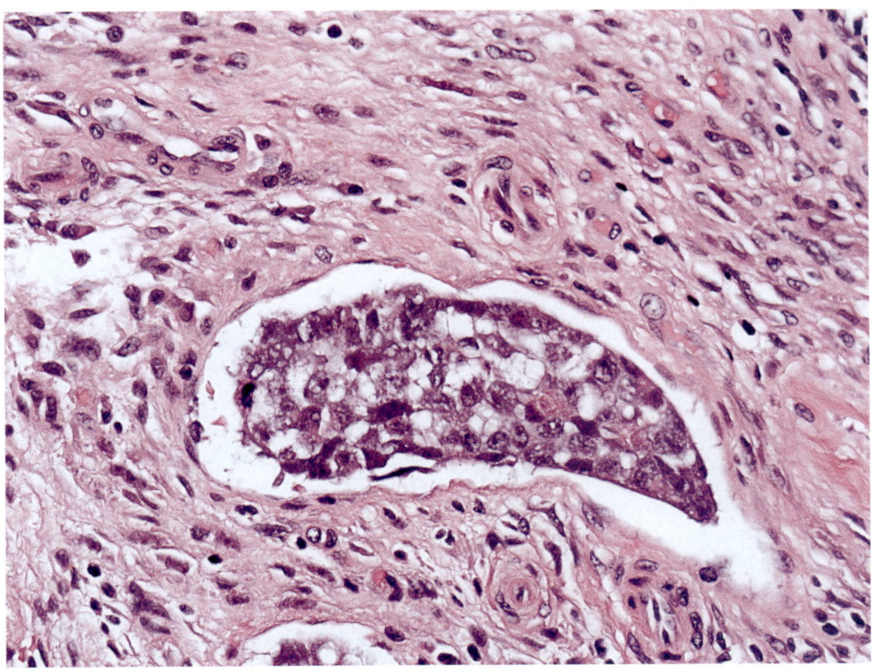

Figure 20-10.
Embryonal carcinoma showing intravascular invasion.

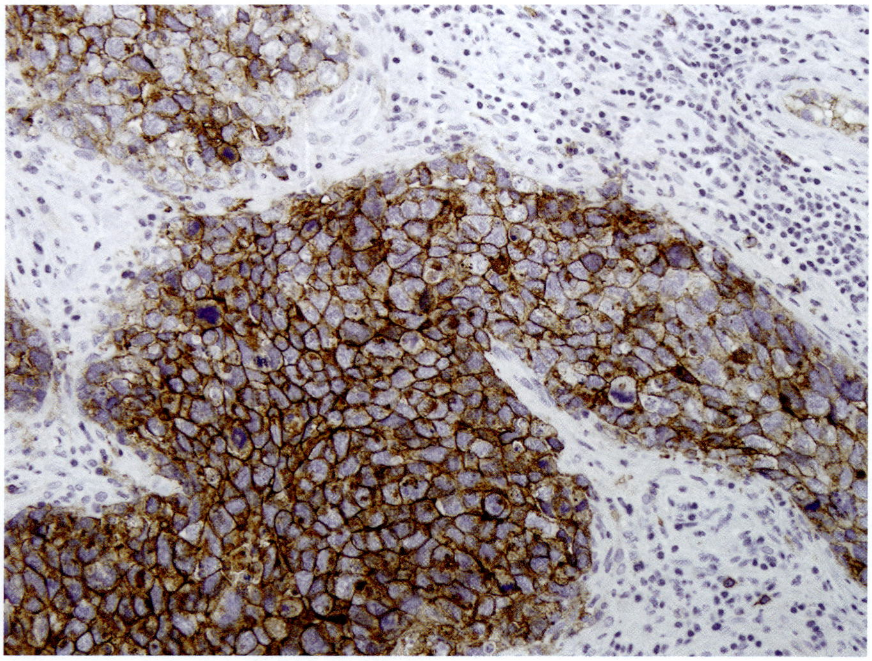

Figure 20-11.
Positive CD30 immunostaining in embryonal carcinoma.

Table 20-1. Comparison of Embryonal Carcinoma and Yolk Sac Tumor

	Embryonal carcinoma	*Yolk sac tumor*
Pure form	Adults	Children
Patterns	Nests, glandular	Microcystic and many other patterns
Cell size	Large	Small
Pleomorphism	More prominent	Less prominent
Schiller-Duvall body	No	Yes
Hyaline globule	No	Yes
Positive markers	CD30, keratins	Glypican 3, AFP

AFP, α-fetoprotein.

IMMATURE TERATOMA

Definition

- Malignant germ cell tumor resembling various immature or fetal somatic tissues of endoderm, mesoderm, or ectoderm

Pathogenesis

- Derived from multipotent stem cells

Clinical features

- Fast growing and painless mass

Gross pathology

- Similar to mixed germ cell tumor, rarely as a pure form
- Large mass of heterogeneous appearance with myxoid, solid, cystic areas (Fig. 20-12)
- Hemorrhage and necrosis are common

Histology

- Various type of immature tissues (Figs. 20-13 to 20-18)
    - Cellular stromal cells (Fig. 20-14)
    - Primitive and cellular epithelial cells without significant cytological atypia (Figs. 20-13 and 20-14)
    - Other immature tissue such as nerve tissue (Fig. 20-15), retina (Fig. 20-16), cartilage (Fig. 20-17), connective tissue, or neuroendocrine cells
- Other types of germ cell tumor or mature teratomatous components may be coexisting
- Immature tumor stromal or epithelial elements should not be considered somatic sarcomas or carcinomas, which will display significant cytological atypia and dominant growth patterns

Immunohistochemistry

- Only useful to confirm the presence of other GCT components

Clinical relevance (prognosis and treatment options)

- Malignant tumor, relatively fast growing
- Almost never present alone, always associated with other malignant germ cell component

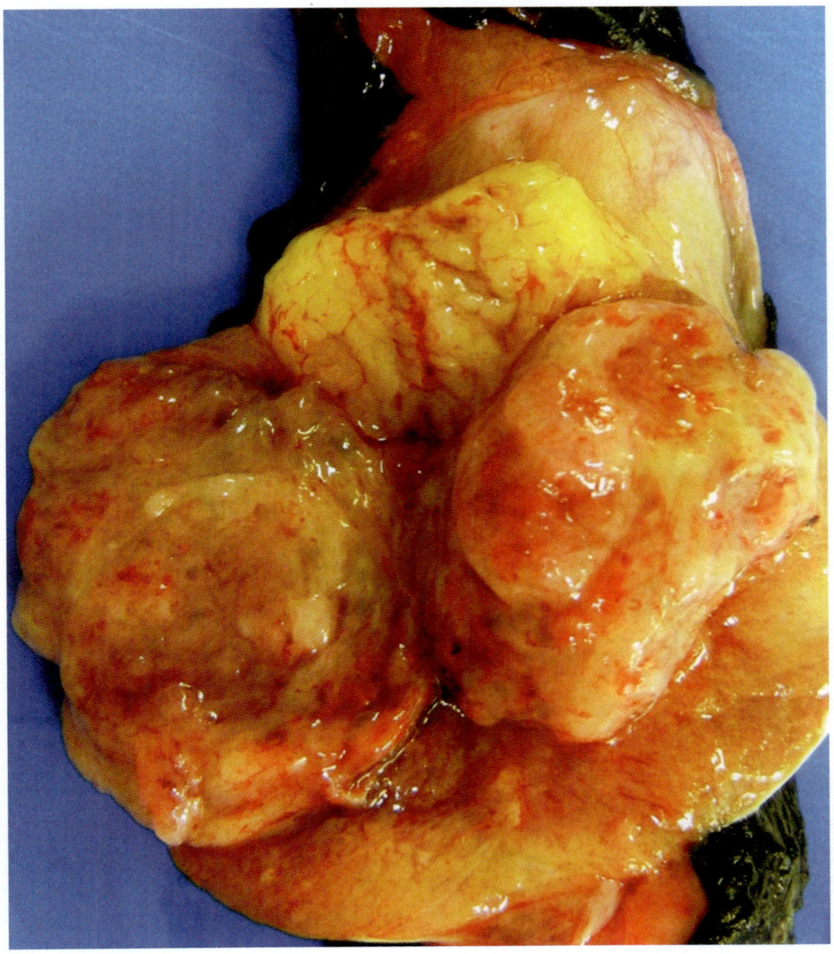

Figure 20-12.
Gross photo of a mixed germ cell tumor, composed primarily of immature teratoma (95%), displays heterogeneous appearance with myxoid areas.

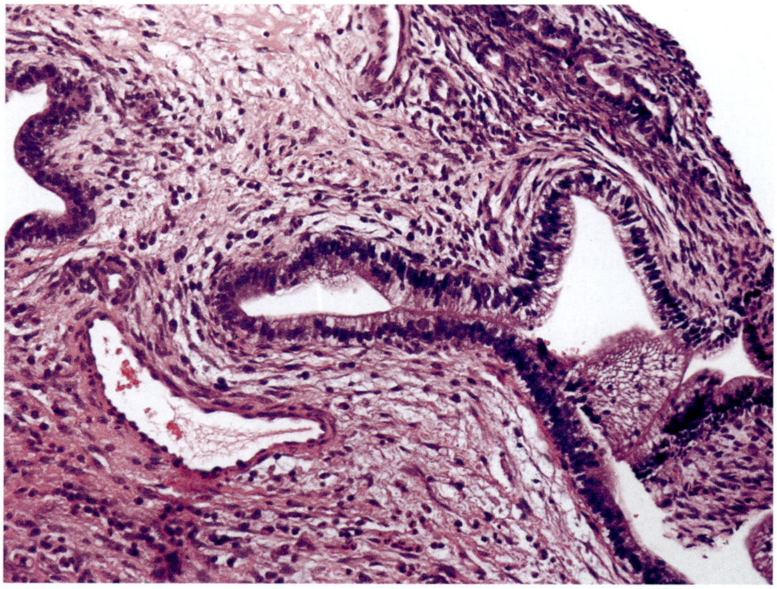

Figure 20-13.
Immature teratoma with immature epithelial cells forming glandular structures.

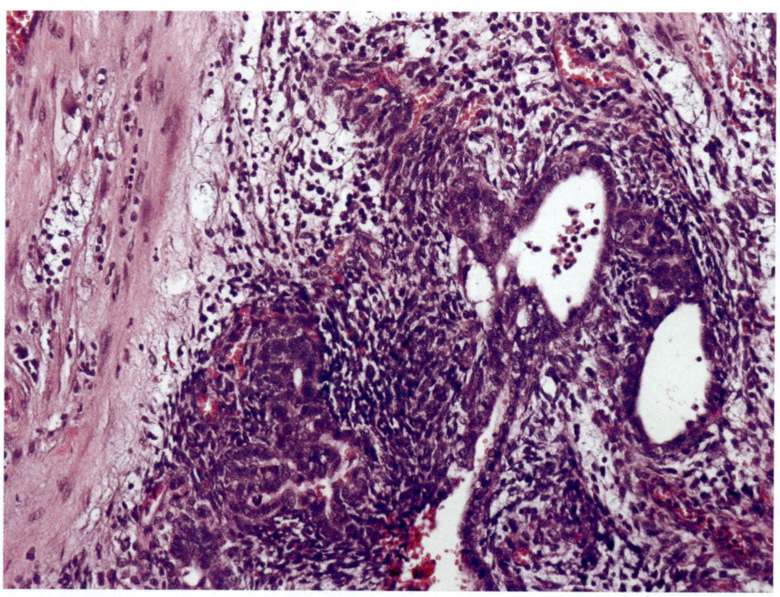

Figure 20-14.
Immature teratomatous component with primitive glandular epithelial cells and stromal cells.

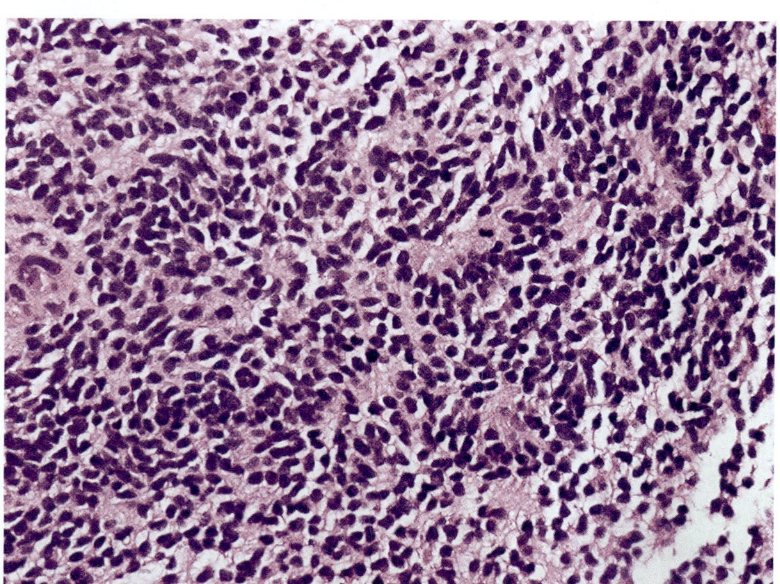

Figure 20-15.
Primitive neuronal cells with rosette formation in an immature teratoma.

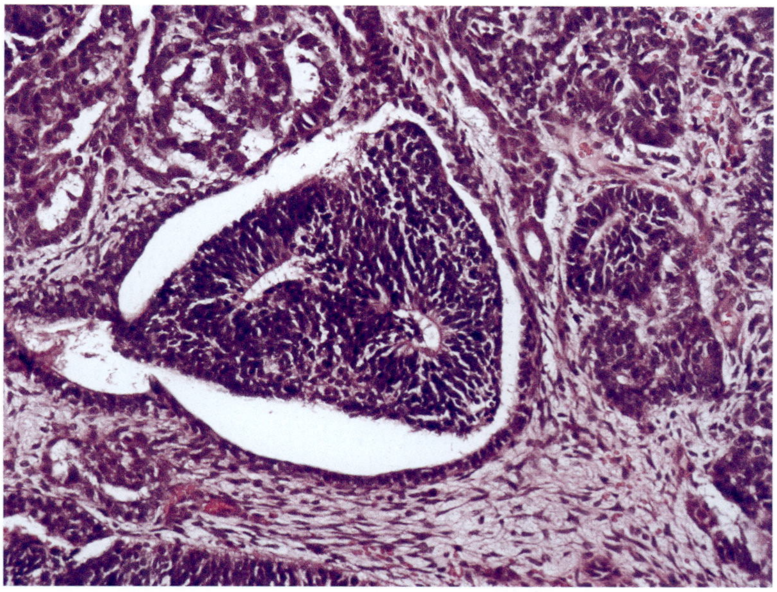

Figure 20-16.
Immature teratomatous component with primitive structures resemble an eyeball with retinal tissue.

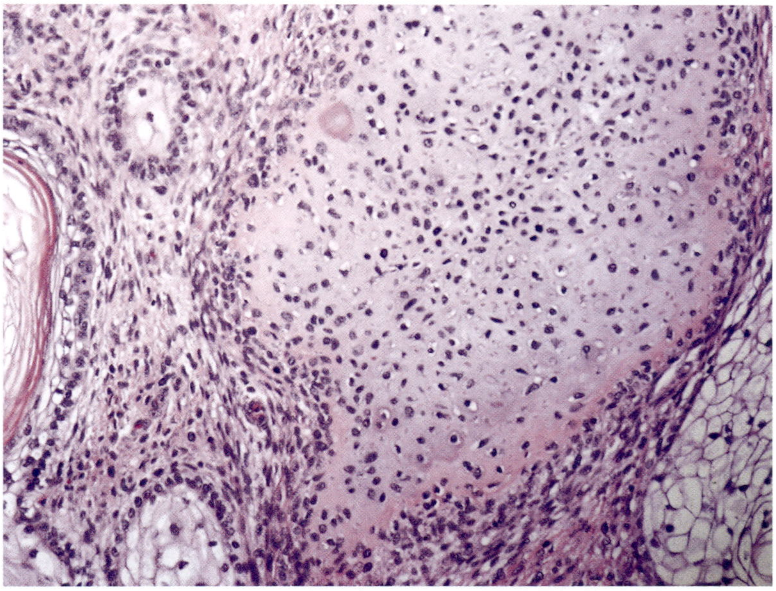

Figure 20-17.
Immature cartilage in an immature teratoma.

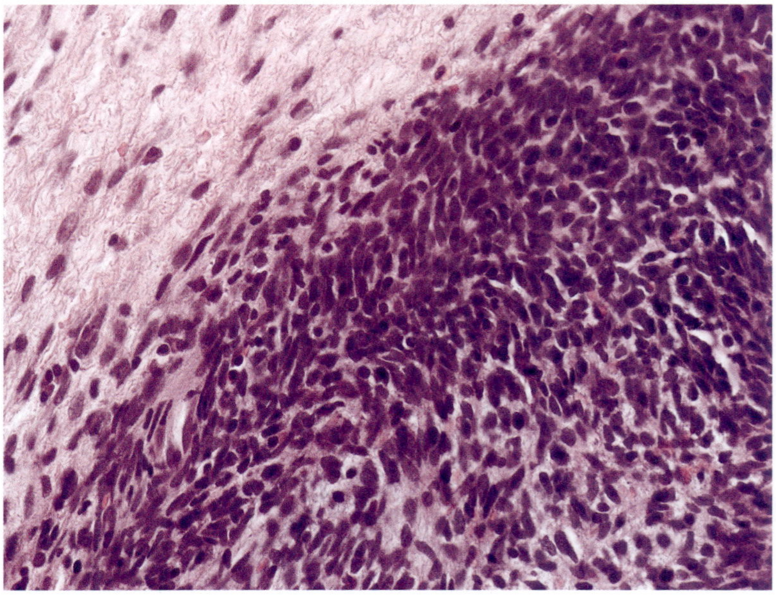

Figure 20-18.
Immature teratoma with primitive stroma with a high cellularity, resembling a sarcoma.

MATURE TERATOMA

Definition

- Germ cell tumor composed of various mature tissues from endoderm, mesoderm, or ectoderm

Other terms

- Many confusing terms that are not correct. We listed some of these in Table 20-2

Pathogenesis

- Different neoplastic tissue components are derived from multipotent stem cells
- Mature teratoma in prepubertal boys are benign
- Mature teratoma in postpubertal males are all malignant
- Dermoid tumor is a mature teratoma
- Some people have used malignant teratoma for nonseminomatous germ cell tumor, which should be avoided
- For the same reason, the Gonzalez-Crussi grading system for extragonadal teratomas (0 for mature or benign; 1 for immature, probably benign; 2 for immature, possibly malignant; and 3 for frankly malignant for a teratoma) is not applicable for testicular teratomas

Clinical features

- Pure mature teratoma is uncommon in adults, most likely because other germ cell tumor components are too small to be sampled
- In the majority cases, mature teratoma is present as a component of mixed malignant germ cell tumors. Therefore, sufficient sampling is necessary
- Painless swollen testis in a young man
- Serum markers negative or only slightly elevated
- Significant elevation of HCG or AFP is indicating a mixed germ cell tumor

Gross pathology

- Well-defined mass with heterogeneous cut surface with cystic and solid areas (Fig. 20-19)
- Hair, cartilage, keratin, or sebaceous material are common finding in the mass lesion (Fig. 20-20)

Histology

- Common components of a mature teratoma are as follows:
  - Skin including hair follicles and sweat glands (Fig. 20-19*b*)
  - Cartilage (Fig. 20-20*b*)
  - Glandular structures of GI or respiratory tracts (Fig. 20-19*c*)
  - Smooth and skeletal muscle (Fig. 20-19*d*)
  - Neural tissue
  - Some mature epithelium cannot be defined to a specific organ
- In a metastatic tumor, mature teratomatous components can be confused with benign tissues (Fig. 20-20)
- Diagnosis of teratoma in the testis does not require the presence of more than two embryonal layers
- A diagnosis of *benign teratoma* should not be made in the postpubertal testis because both mature and immature teratomas in the testis are all malignant in this age group
- To avoid these confusing terminologies such as *teratoma*, *benign teratoma*, and *malignant teratoma*, we use the following terminology in our diagnosis:
  - Malignant germ cell tumor of the testis, composed of immature and mature teratoma
  - Malignant germ cell tumor of the testis, composed of 90% immature teratoma, 5% seminoma, and 5% YST

Immunohistochemistry

- Germ cell markers may be used to confirm the other germ cell tumor components

Molecular analysis

- Isochromosome 12p in postpubertal patient

Table 20-2. Clarification of the Confusing Terminology for Testicular Germ Cell Tumors

	Term	*Preferred term*
US terminology	Teratoma	Mature teratoma
UK terminology	Teratoma	Immature teratoma
US terminology	Immature teratoma	Immature teratoma
UK terminology	Mature teratoma	Mature teratoma
Incorrect terminology	Benign teratoma	Mature teratoma
Incorrect terminology	Malignant teratoma	Mixed nonseminomatous germ cell tumor

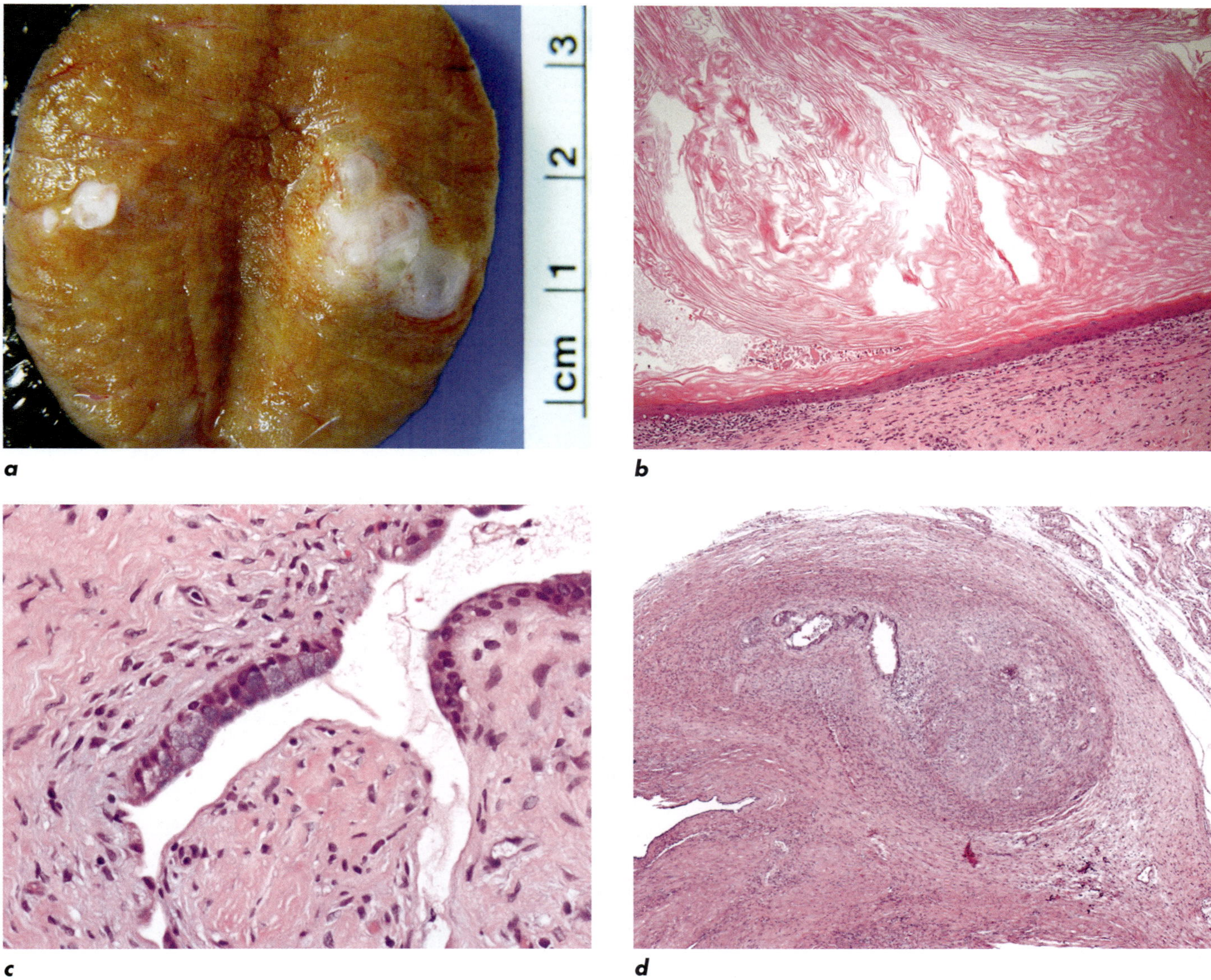

Figure 20-19.

A testicular mature teratoma that has a white cartilaginous and white fibrotic appearance (*a*). Microscopically, the malignant tumor is composed of mature squamous epithelium (*b*), mature glandular epithelium with goblet cells (*c*), and a cluster of mature glands surrounded by disorganized smooth muscle bundles (*d*).

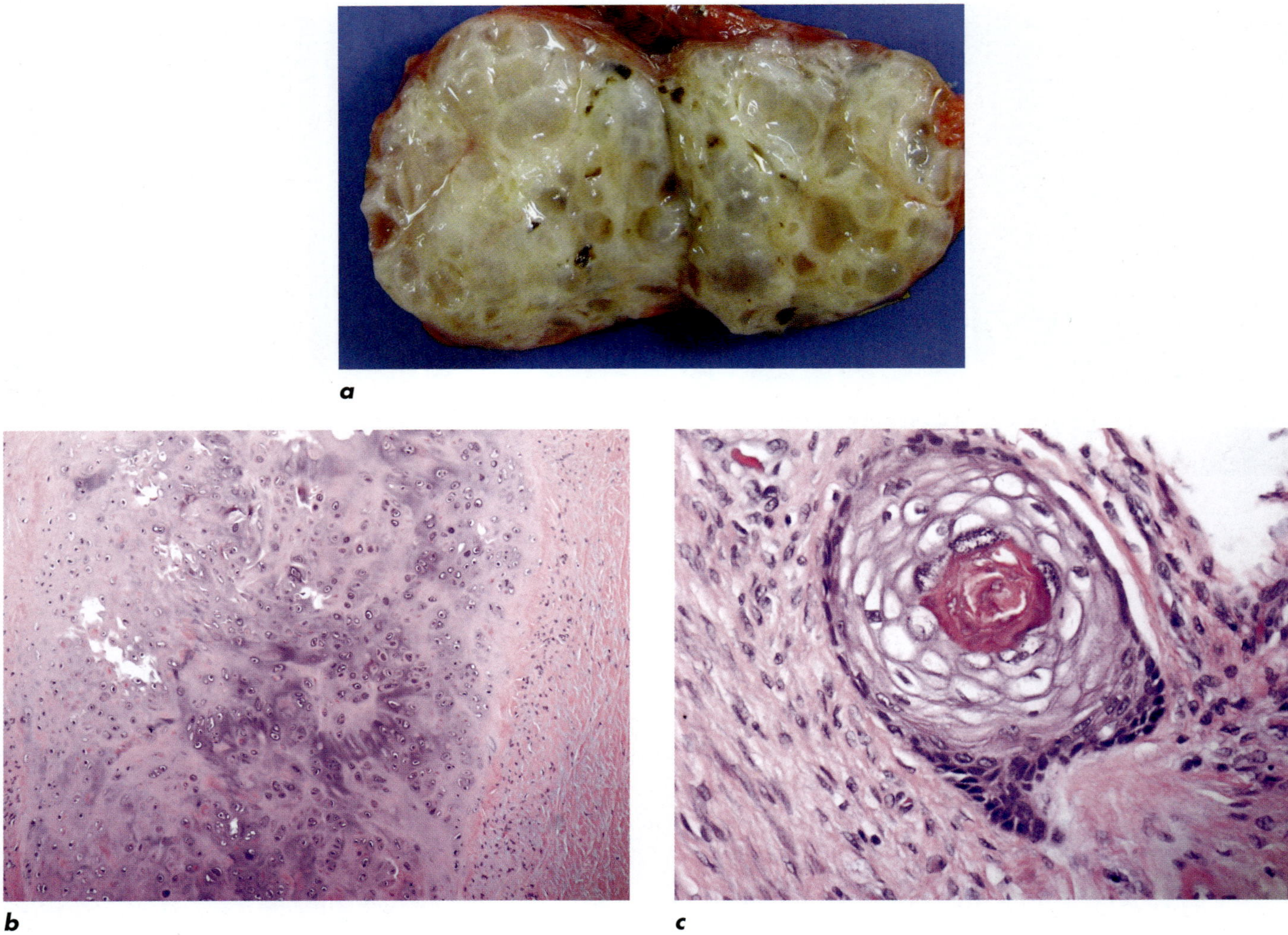

Figure 20-20.
Metastatic testicular malignant germ cell tumor (mature teratoma) in a pelvic lymph node (*a*). Microscopically, the presence of mature cartilage (*b*) and squamous epithelium (*c*) confirms the diagnosis.

Clinical relevance (prognosis and treatment options)

- Very important to know that testicular mature teratoma in a postpubertal boy is a malignant tumor, although the teratomatous tissue components are deceivingly benign-looking morphologically
- When a mature teratomatous component metastasizes to pelvic lymph nodes, these tumor cells are slow growing and resistant to chemotherapy
- Often, dissection of pelvic lymph nodes is necessary if mature teratomatous components are present in the primary tumor or the nodes
- To avoid confusion, we typically report the following:
  - Malignant germ cell tumor with predominant component of mature teratoma
  - The percentage of mature teratomatous component in a mixed GCT

MIXED MALIGNANT GERM CELL TUMOR

Definition

- Malignant germ cell tumor composed of more than two germ cell tumor components

Pathogenesis

- Derived from multipotent stem cells
- In reality, the majority (approximately 80%) of nonseminomatous germ cell tumors are mixed type in adults, which may include components of seminoma, EC, choriocarcinoma, YST, immature or mature teratomas in variable proportions

Clinical features

- Large fasting-growing mass
- Elevated serum markers such as LDH, β-HCG, or AFP

Gross pathology

- Large mass with heterogeneous appearance (Fig. 20-21) with myxoid, solid, cystic cut surface (Fig. 20-22)
- Hemorrhage and necrosis common
- Key to making a correct diagnosis is sufficient sampling
- In many instances, a large germ cell tumor may not be adequately sampled for financial reasons, which leads to the wrong classification of the tumor
- If the tumor is less than 3 cm, we recommend that it is entirely submitted. If it is larger than 3 cm, at least two blocks for each centimeter of the tumor (10 blocks for a 5-cm germ cell tumor), which is two times more than conventional tumor sampling

Histology

- Because of sufficient sampling, each tumor component even a small portion will get evaluated histologically
- Many different combinations of germ cell tumor components are possible such as seminoma + teratoma (Fig. 20-21), yolk sac tumor + embryonal carcinoma (Fig. 20-22), seminoma + yolk sac tumor + immature teratoma + mature teratoma, etc
- Different testicular tumors are compared in Table 20-3

Clinical correlation

- We also recommend to give the percentage for each component (Table 20-4 as examples), since some component may not require special therapies
- Application of immunohistochemical markers is recommended if the classification is inconclusive by morphology alone, particularly EC and YST may have morphological overlapping
- With modern therapies, patients with mixed germ cell tumors have very good prognosis with the vast majority of cases being cured

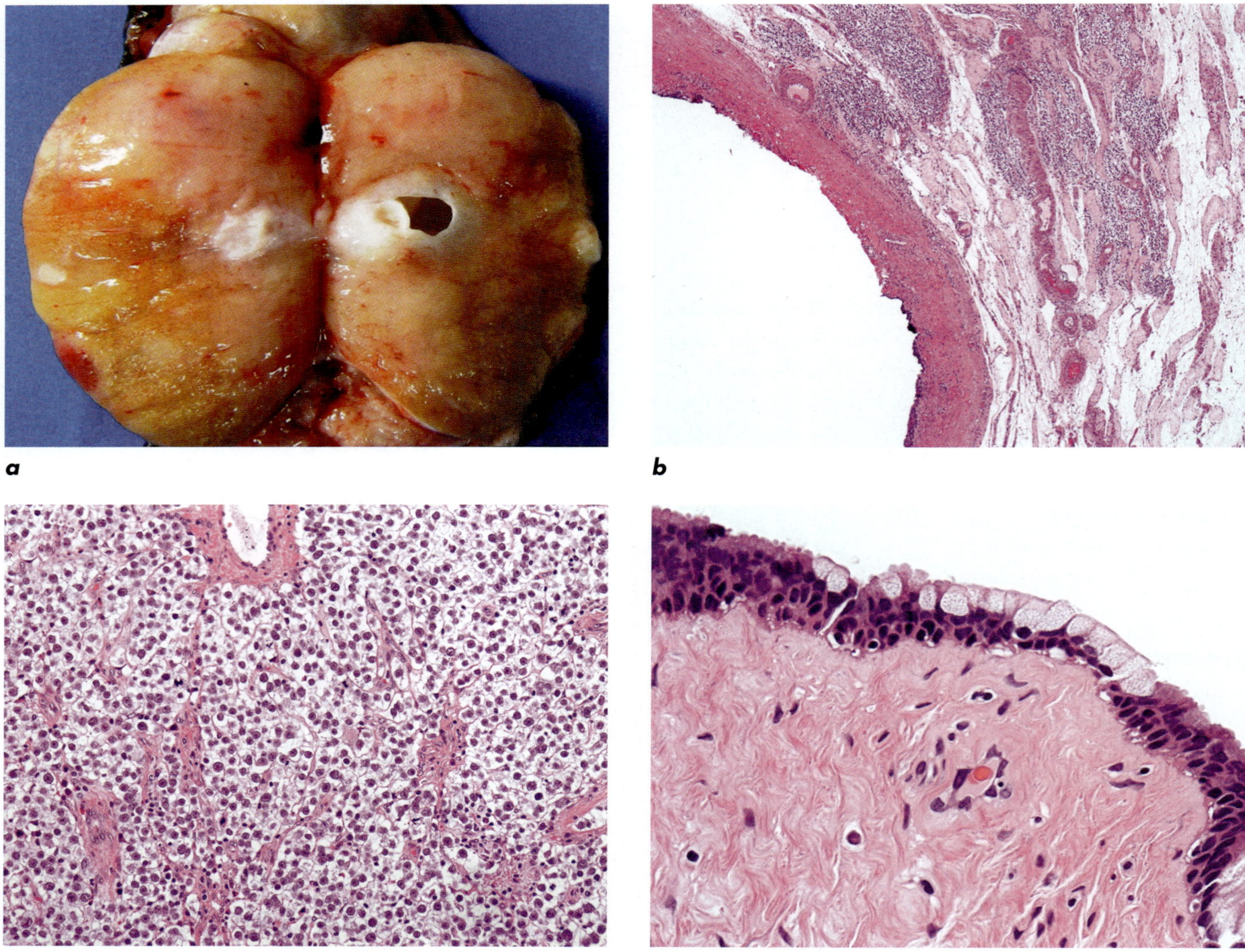

a b c d

Figure 20-21.
A mixed malignant germ cell tumor containing a large solid fleshy-colored mass (seminomatous component) and a cystic structure in the middle (teratomatous component) (*a*). Microscopically, cystic structure is surrounded by seminoma (*b*). High magnification confirms both seminomatous (*c*) and mature teratomatous epithelial components (*d*).

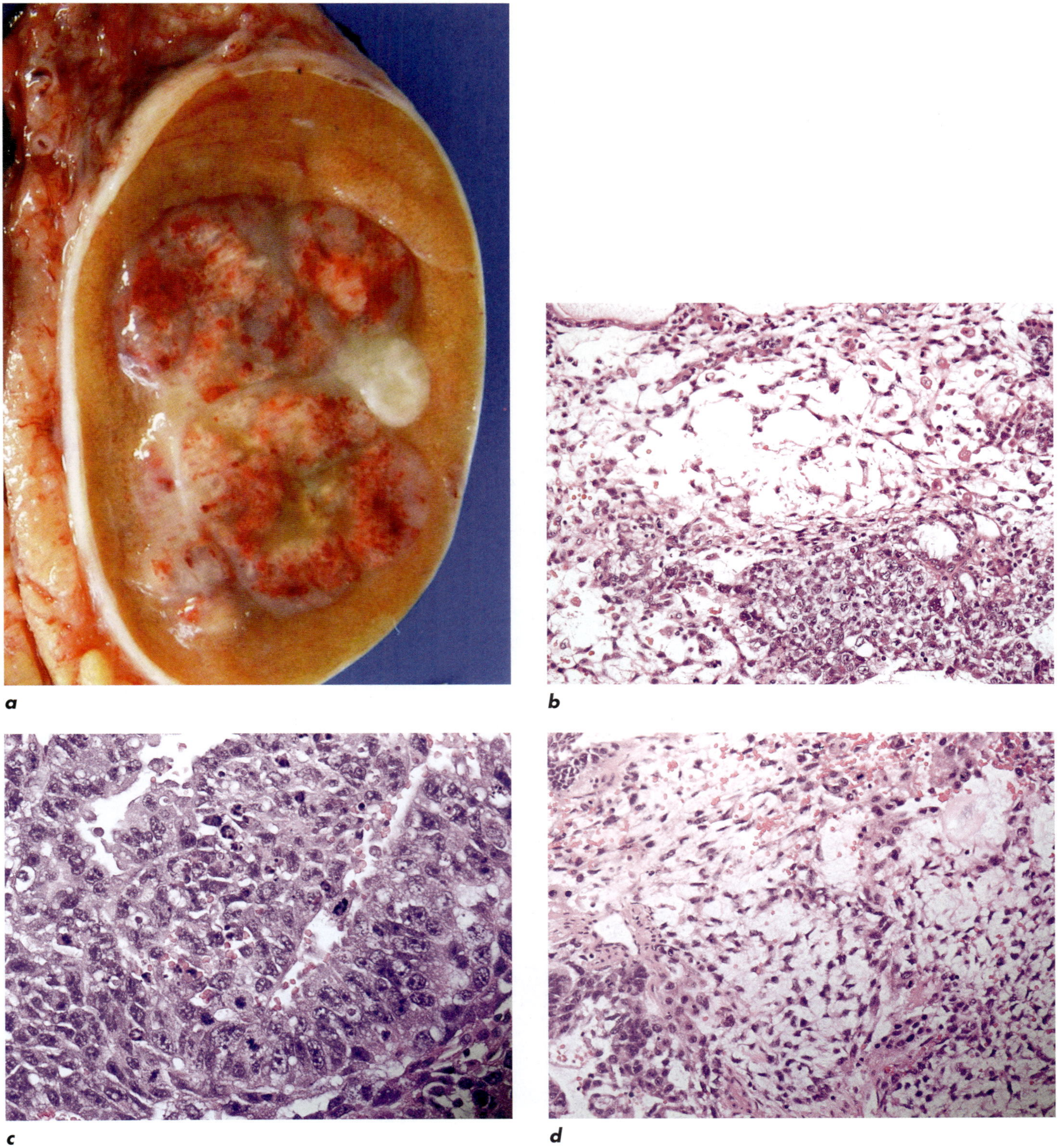

Figure 20-22.
A mixed malignant germ cell tumor with heterogeneous appearance composed of solid, myxoid, and hemorrhagic areas (*a*). Microscopically, the tumor consists of myxoid yolk sac tumor (upper) and embryonal carcinoma components (lower). High magnification shows both embryonal carcinoma (*c*) and yolk sac tumor component (*d*).

Table 20-3. Comparison of Testicular Tumors

Features	*Seminoma*	*Spermatocytic seminoma*	*Lymphoma*	*Carcinoid*	*Merkel cell carcinoma*	*Metastatic prostatic adenocarcinoma*
Age (years)	30 to 40	60 to 70	50 to 70	Any age		60 to 80
Hemorrhage and necrosis	No	No	Possible	No	Yes	Possible
Nesting	No	No	No	Yes	Yes	Yes
Tumor cells	Large polygonal	Three types of cells	Monotonous	Salt-and-pepper chromatin	Small cell neuroendocrine	Prominent nucleoli
Special structures	Diffuse	Diffuse	No	Rosette gland like	Large nests	Cribriform
Small lymphocytes	Many	No	Possible	No	No	No
Granuloma	Yes	No	Possible	No	No	No
Markers	C-kit, OCT-4	Not certain	CD20	NE marker	CK20 NE marker	PSA AMACR
Prognosis & treatment	Good	Excellent	Poor	Poor	Poor	Poor

AMACR, α-methylacyl-CoA racemase; NE, neuroendocrine; OCT-4, octamer-binding transcription factor 4; PSA, prostatic-specific antigen.

Table 20-4. Samples of Pathology Reports of Testicular Germ Cell Tumors

4A

Malignant germ cell tumor, mixed type, composed of

Embryonal carcinoma	30%
Seminoma	20%
Mature teratoma	20%
Immature teratoma	20%
Yolk sac tumor	5%
Choriocarcinoma	5%

4B

Malignant germ cell tumor, mixed type, composed of

Immature teratoma	90%
Embryonal carcinoma	5%
Mature teratoma	5%

EPIDERMOID CYST

Definition

- Benign cyst lined by mature squamous epithelium
- The presence of epidermoid cyst with skin appendages (demoid cyst) is considered to be mature teratoma
- Difference between epidermoid cyst and mature teratoma is listed in Table 20-5

Pathogenesis

- Some cases may arise from the inclusion of overlying skin, and other cases may represent a monophasic teratoma

Clinical features

- Painless slow growing mass

Gross pathology

- Cystic lesion within the testicular parenchyma with a thin wall, without solid areas
- Cystic content is greasy material (keratin debris) (Fig. 20-23)
- Although calcification may be present, no hair, bone, or cartilage should be present
- Entire lesion of epidermoid cyst should be submitted for microscopic evaluation

Histology

- Lesion is composed of mature keratinizing squamous lining of a simple cyst (Figs. 20-24 and 20-25)
- Evidence suggestive of a teratoma (which is malignant in postpubertal males) rather than an benign epidermoid cyst
  - Elevated serum markers
  - Presence of ITGCNU
  - Chromosomal abnormality
  - Presence of any other mature tissues such as smooth muscle, glandular epithelium, or skin appendage, which should not be present within the testis
  - Presence of a small focus of trophoblasts, seminoma, or any other germ cell components

Clinical relevance (prognosis and treatment options)

- In prepubertal males, epidermoid cysts and dermoid cysts are benign
- In our experience, most so-called epidermoid cysts in postpubertal males are malignant germ cell tumors by insufficient sampling
- Close clinical follow-up of a postpubertal patient with the diagnosis of testicular epidermoid cyst is highly recommended

Table 20-5. Comparison of Mature Teratoma and Epidermoid Cyst in the Adult Testis

	Malignant germ cell tumor (mature teratoma)	*Epidermoid cyst*
Serum marker elevation	Yes or no	No
Presence of ITGCNU	Yes	No
Chromosomal abnormality	I(12p)	No
Presence of benign glandular cells	Yes	No
Presence of smooth muscle in the testis	Yes	No
The lesion needs to be entirely submitted	Yes	Yes
Risk for developing metastasis	Yes	Yes
Risk for developing germ cell tumor in contralateral testis	Yes	No

I(12p), Isochromosome 12p.

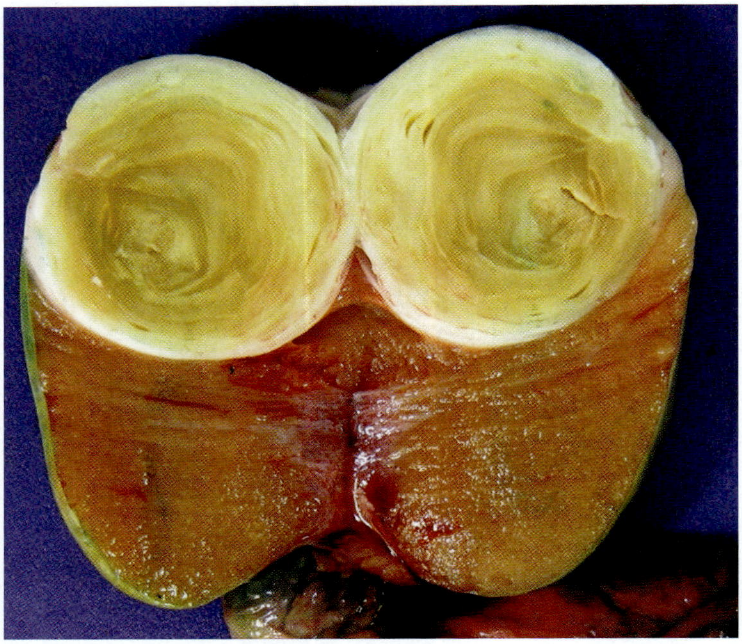

Figure 20-23.
Gross photo of a testicular epidermoid cyst in a young man shows a single cyst filled with keratin material.

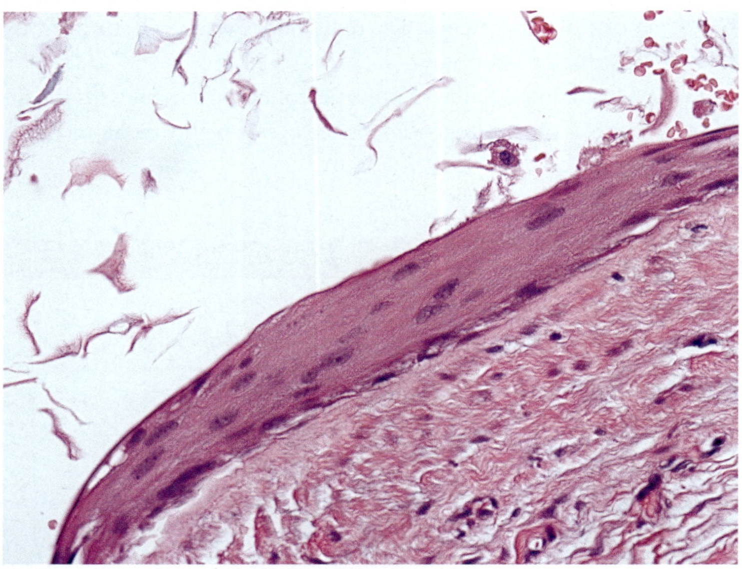

Figure 20-24.
Under microscope, the cyst is lined by mature squamous epithelium without sweat glands, sebaceous glands, or other mature tissues.

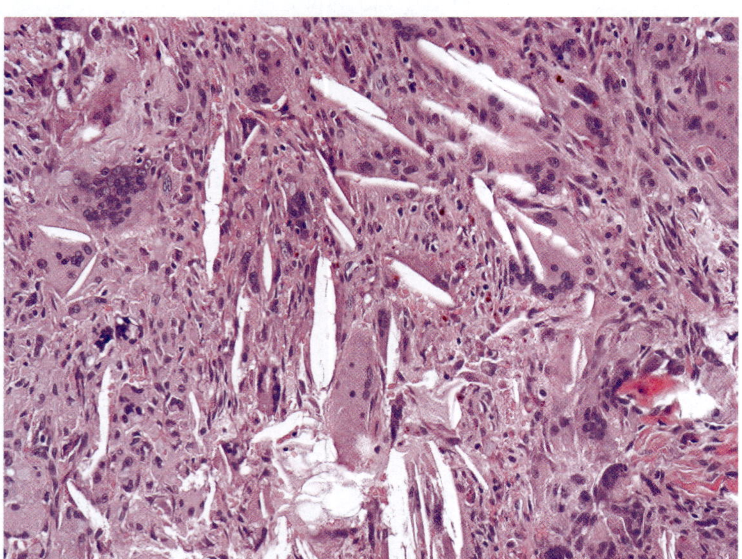

Figure 20-25.
Cholesterol clefts and foreign body giant cell reaction in the ruptured area of an epidermoid cyst.

BURNED-OUT (GERM CELL) TUMOR

Definition

- Well-defined testicular mass composed entirely of fibrous tissue, without any viable germ cell tumor component

Pathogenesis

- Spontaneous regression of testicular germ cell tumors (GCTs) is a well-recognized phenomenon
- A primary germ cell tumor in the testis can under regression result in a scar without any viable tumor cells
- Regression may happen in the primary tumor, while the metastasis is detected

Clinical features

- A testicular painless, palpable mass without change in size

Gross pathology

- Well-defined round fibrotic area, a few centimeters in diameter (Fig. 20-26)
- Lesion should be entirely submitted and evaluated carefully under microscope

Histology

- Area of fibrotic tissue without viable epithelial or germ cells (Fig. 20-26*b*)
- May contain inflammatory cells and hemosiderin-laden macrophages (Fig. 20-26*c*)
- Presence of ITGCNU
- Occasionally, a few neoplastic germ cells (outside seminiferous tubules) can be found within the fibrotic lesion, which can be highlighted by C-kit, OC-4, or other germ cell tumor markers. In that case, the diagnosis is a (regressing) malignant germ cell tumor (Fig. 20-27) rather than burned-out germ cell tumors
- Several findings suggest a burned-out tumor associated with germ cell tumor
  - Presence of ITGCNU in the adjacent tubules
  - Presence of totally necrotic but recognizable tumor cells (ghost cells)
  - Presence of germ cell tumors at multiple extratesticular sites
  - Absence of irregular starlet-shaped scar (which will be favoring trauma)
  - Absence of orchitis

Immunohistochemistry

- Germ cell markers negative
- C-kit and OCT-4 may be positive in seminiferous tubules (ITGCNU)

Clinical relevance (prognosis and treatment options)

- Other factors such as trauma to the testis, radiation, and/or chemotherapy may also result in scar without the presence of a prior germ cell tumor
- A germ cell tumor may develop in extratesticular sites such as mediastinum or retroperitoneum with a viable germ cell tumor in the testis
- In a patient with extratesticular germ cell tumor and the presence of a testicular mass by imaging, orchiectomy should be considered
- In the situation of an extratesticular germ cell tumor, it is important to determine whether the coexisting scar in the orchiectomy is a burned-out germ cell tumor
- The presence of a burned-out (germ cell) tumor in the testis may support the origin of a metastatic germ cell tumor instead of an extratesticular primary
- Clinical follow-up with imaging studies and serum markers is necessary

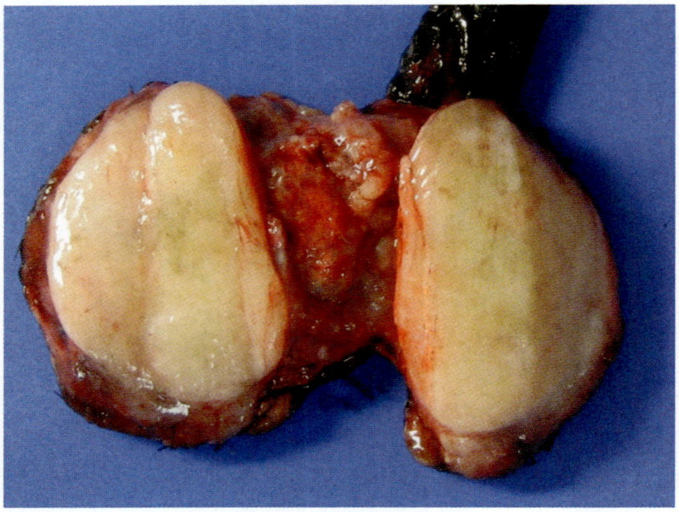

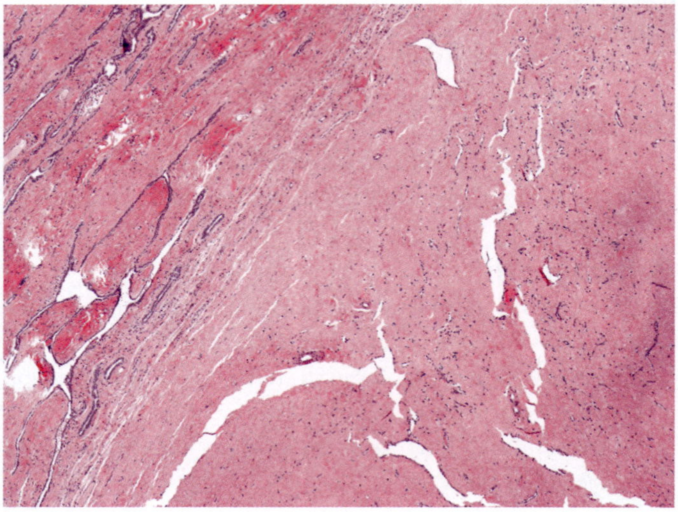

a *b*

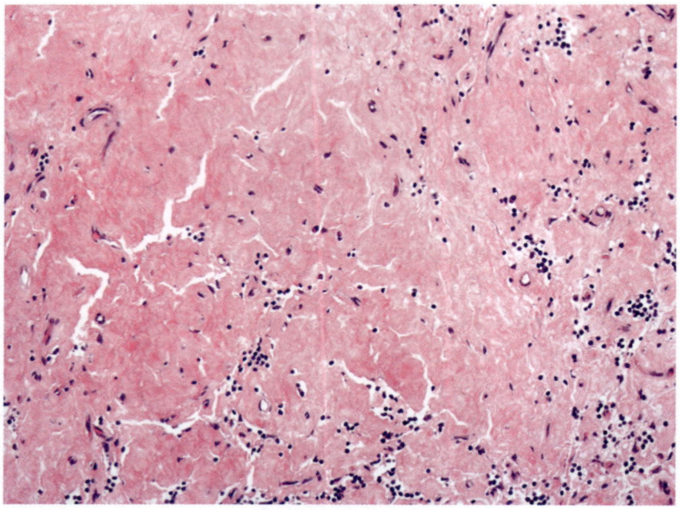

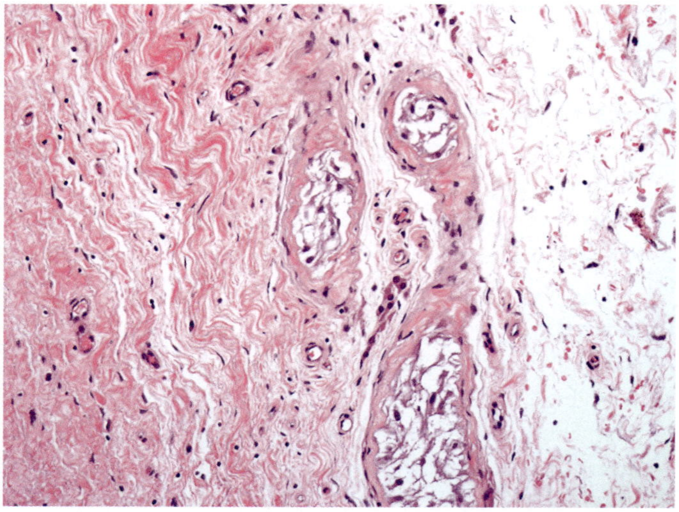

c *d*

Figure 20-26.
Burned-out tumor of the testis. Gross photo of a large mass almost replacing the entire testis (*a*). This lesion is well circumscribed unlike a scar. Under the microscope, the lesion is composed entirely of hyalinized fibrous tissue (*b*) with very low cellularity (*c*). Some areas showing chronic inflammatory infiltrates (*d*).

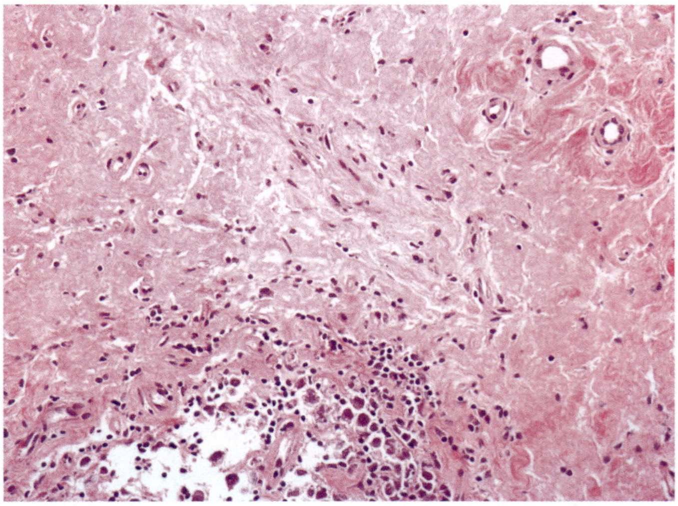

a

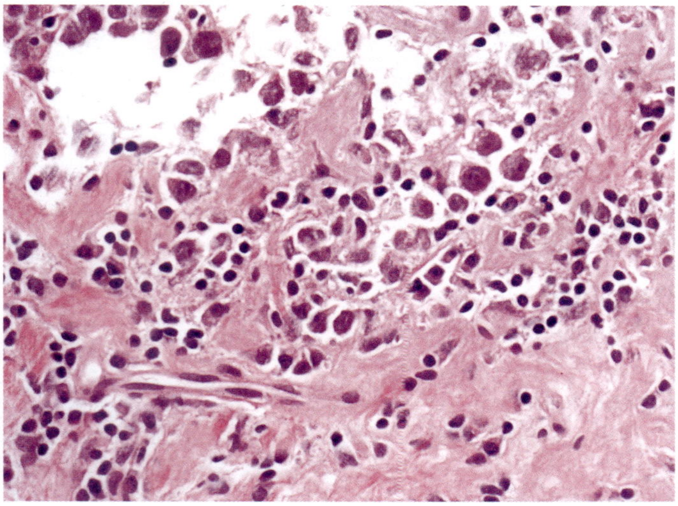

b

Figure 20-27.
Seminoma with extensive fibrosis mimicking a burned-out tumor. The lesion is composed mostly of fibrotic tissue; however there is a small focus of large cells in the low portion of the photo (*a*). High magnification firms the seminoma, rather than a burned-out tumor (*b*).

CHAPTER 21

Sex Cord Stromal Tumors of the Testis

SERTOLI CELL ADENOMA

Definition

- Nodular proliferation of Sertoli cells

Other terms

- Pick adenoma, Sertoli cell nodule, Sertoli cell hyperplasia

Clinical features

- Similar to Sertoli-cell-only syndrome. These lesions are found incidentally in orchiectomy specimens for other diseases

Gross pathology

- Small atrophic testis, typically less than 1 to 2 mm; therefore, they are not visible in gross examination

Histology

- In the background of Sertoli-cell-only patterns
- A well-defined group or small clusters of uniform Sertoli cells proliferation in the tubules (Fig. 21-1)
- Nodule typically consists of 10 to 30 nests with a well-defined border, which may represent a lobule (Fig. 21-1*a*)
- Higher cellularity than the adjacent tubules with Sertoli-cell-only patterns (Figs. 21-1*b* and 21-2*a*)
- No cytological atypia, no necrosis or infiltrating patterns
- Sertoli cell adenoma can be involved by intratubular germ cell neoplasia, unclassified (ITGCNU) with large atypical cells with a perinuclear halo (Fig. 21-2*a*)

Immunohistochemistry

- Inhibin positive (same as Sertoli cell only) (Fig. 21-2*c*)

Clinical relevance (prognosis and treatment options)

- Often as incidental findings in orchiectomy specimens
- It is uncertain whether Sertoli cell adenoma is a neoplasm or reactive change
- Benign, no treatment is necessary

Figure 21-1.
Sertoli cell adenoma is characterized by a group of seminiferous tubules with Sertoli cell proliferation (*a*). Higher magnification shows multiple layers of proliferating Sertoli cells without cytological atypia (*b*).

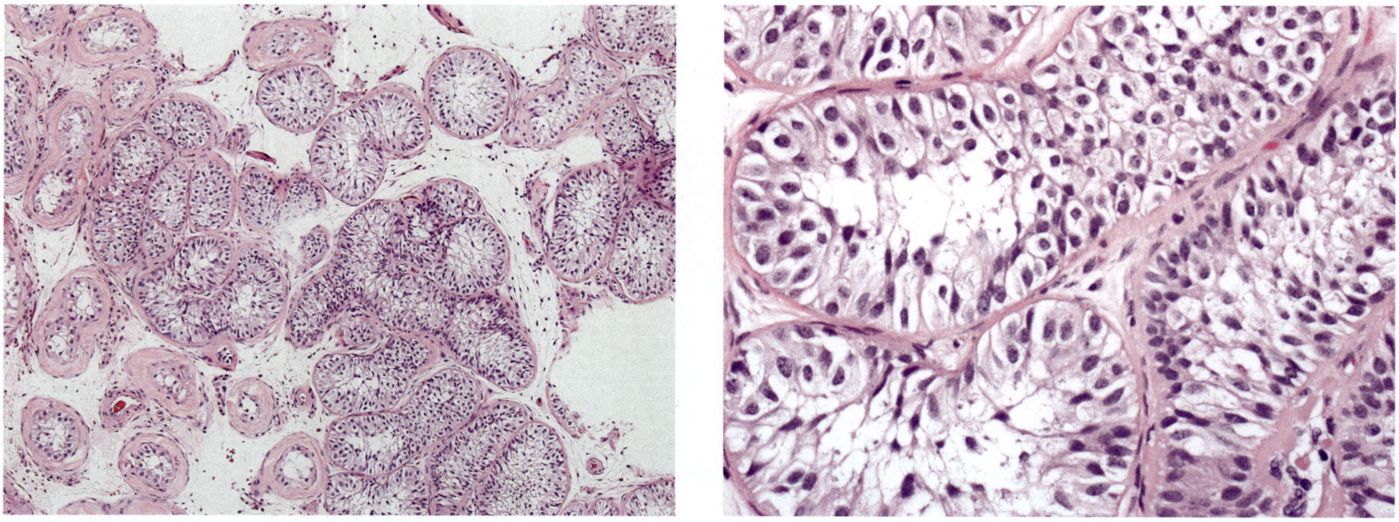

a b

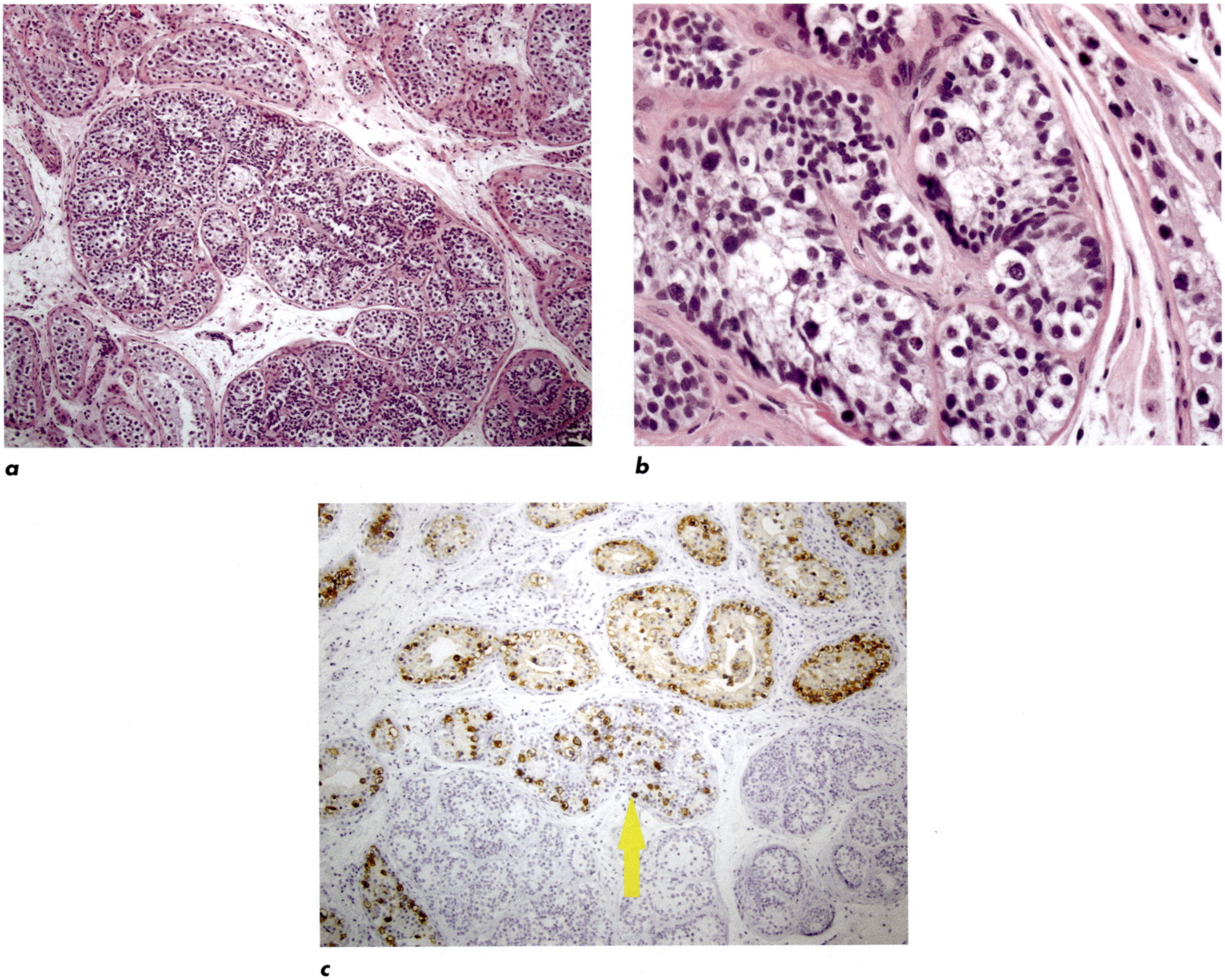

Figure 21-2.
Sertoli cell adenoma involved by ITGCNU (*a*). High magnification shows neoplastic germ cells (*b*) present in the background of proliferating Sertoli cells. C-kit immunostaining highlights neoplastic germ cells (*c*, arrow) in the Sertoli cell adenoma along with other tubules with ITGCNU.

LEYDIG CELL TUMOR

Definition

- Neoplasm of the Leydig cells, which is the most common sex cord stromal neoplasm of the testis

Clinical features

- Majority of Leydig cell tumor (LCT) cases are seen in prepubertal boys and younger men
- Typically slowly growing and painless mass in which many of the cases are incidental findings on imaging
- Precocious puberty is only seen in prepubertal boys with androgen-producing LCT

Gross pathology

- Well-circumscribed mass lesions, typically small, ranging from 2 to 5 cm
- Cut surface showing a brown (Fig. 21-3) or bright yellow mass (Fig. 21-4)
- Rare hemorrhage or necrosis

Histology

- Tumor cells are large polygonal with prominent eosinophilic granules in the cytoplasm (Fig. 21-5)
- Crystals of Reinke and lipofuscin can be seen (Fig. 21-6) in the cytoplasm, which can be also seen in normal or hyperplastic Leydig cells
- Occasionally tumor cells may show lipid vacuoles or xanthomatous changes in the cytoplasm because of their nature as lipid-producing cells (Fig. 21-7)
- Nuclei are round with centrally located nucleoli. Isolated cytological atypia can be seen, which is not an indication of malignancy
- Tumor cells may sometimes form pseudo glandular patterns (Fig. 21-7)
- Seminiferous tubules are atrophic, but negative for intratubular germ cell neoplasia
- Histological criteria for malignancy are not established. However, the presence of large size, necrosis, or extending to paratesticular tissue should suggest a malignant potential

Immunohistochemistry

- Inhibin positive, calretinin positive; vimentin, melan A may be positive
- Keratins and germ cell markers negative

Clinical relevance (prognosis and treatment options)

- Only less than 10% of cases are malignant
- The only evidence of malignancy is the presence of metastasis

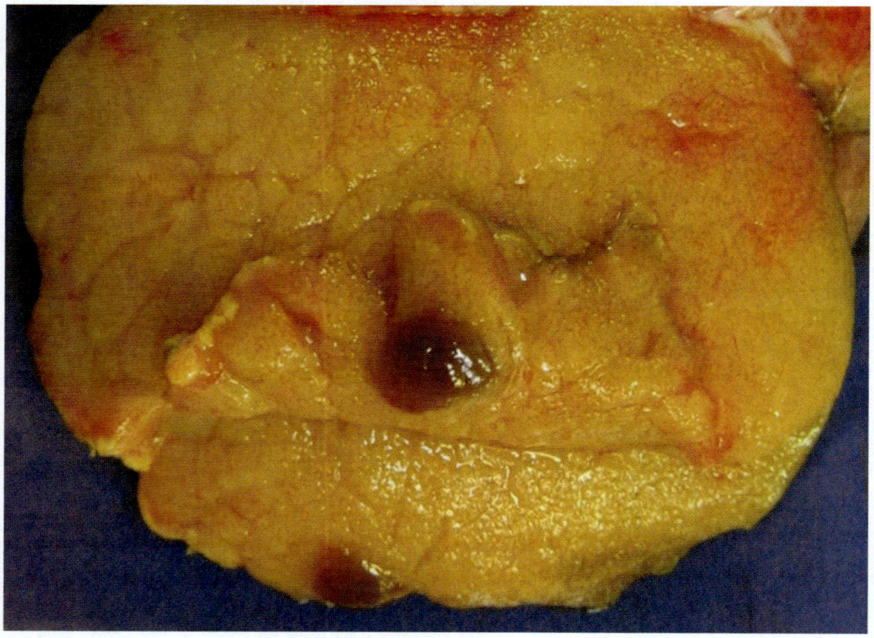

Figure 21-3.
Leydig cell tumor (less than 1 cm) is a well-circumscribed mass with brown cut surface.

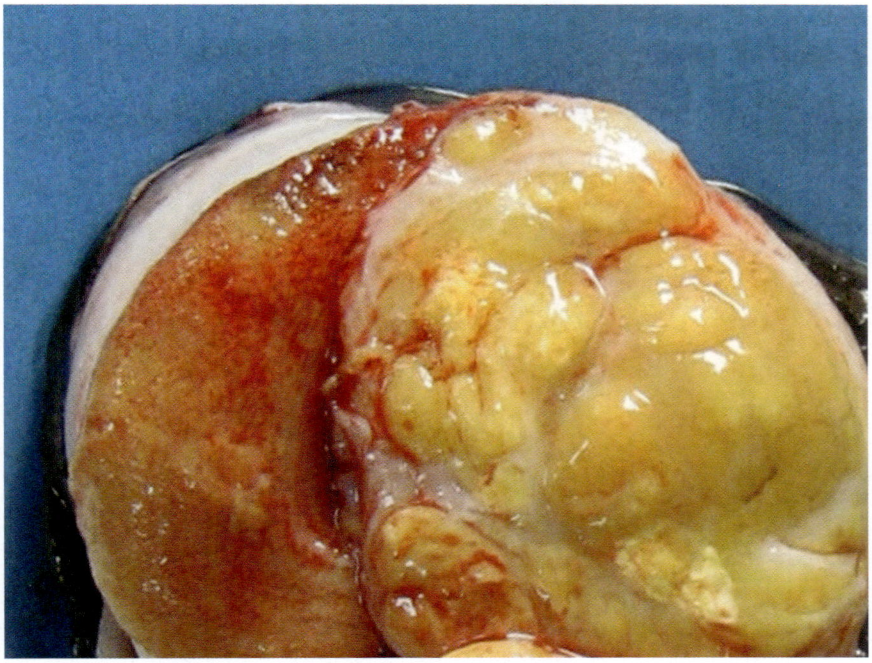

Figure 21-4.
Another Leydig cell tumor with a capsule and yellow cut surface.

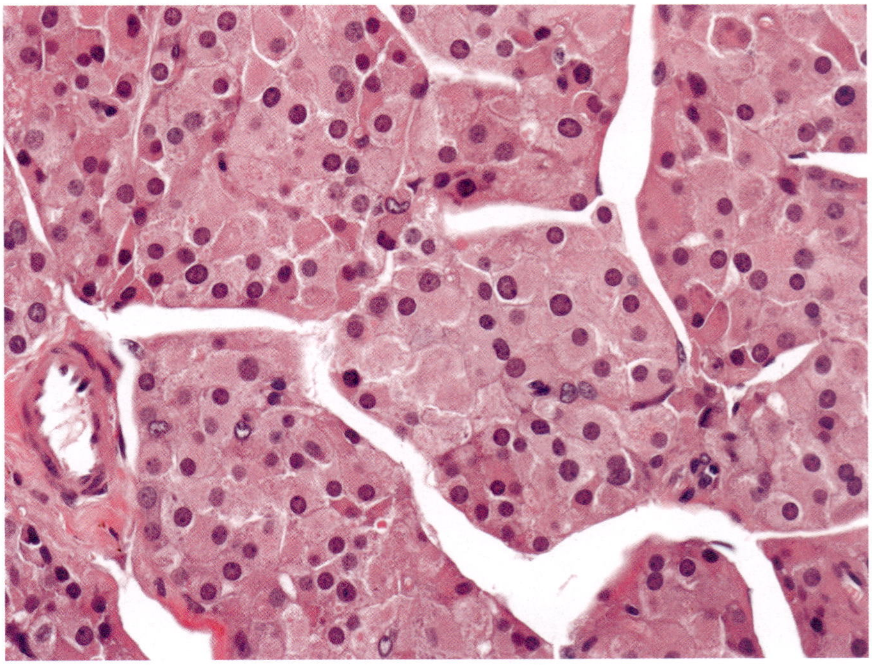

Figure 21-5.
Leydig cell tumor composed of large polygonal cells with eosinophilic cytoplasm. The tumor cells form nests with thin fibrovascular septa.

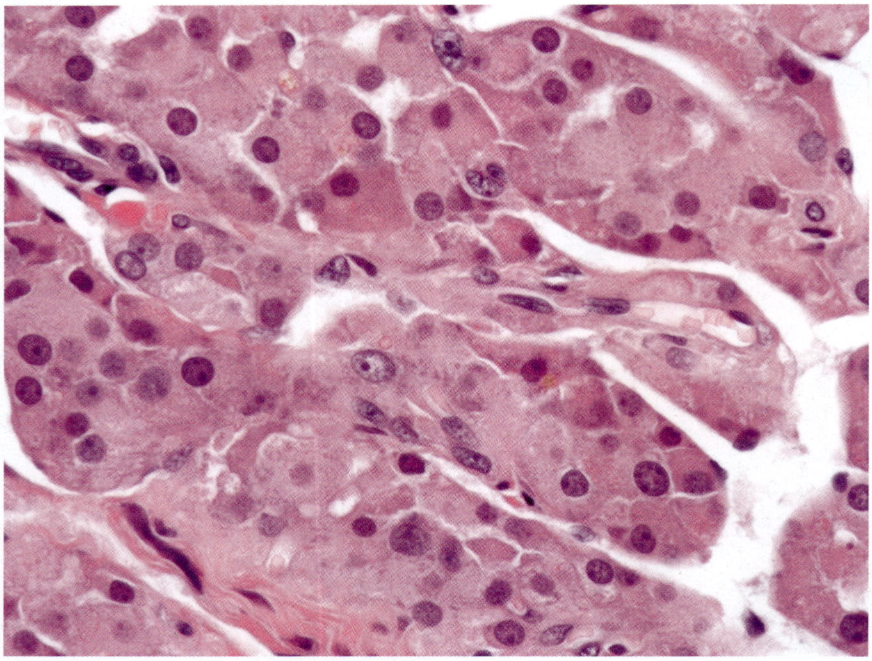

Figure 21-6.
A higher magnification of a Leydig cell tumor showing the tumor cells with abundant eosinophilic cytoplasm, round nuclei with a prominent nucleolus. Some of the tumor cells also contain lipofuscin pigment granules in the cytoplasm.

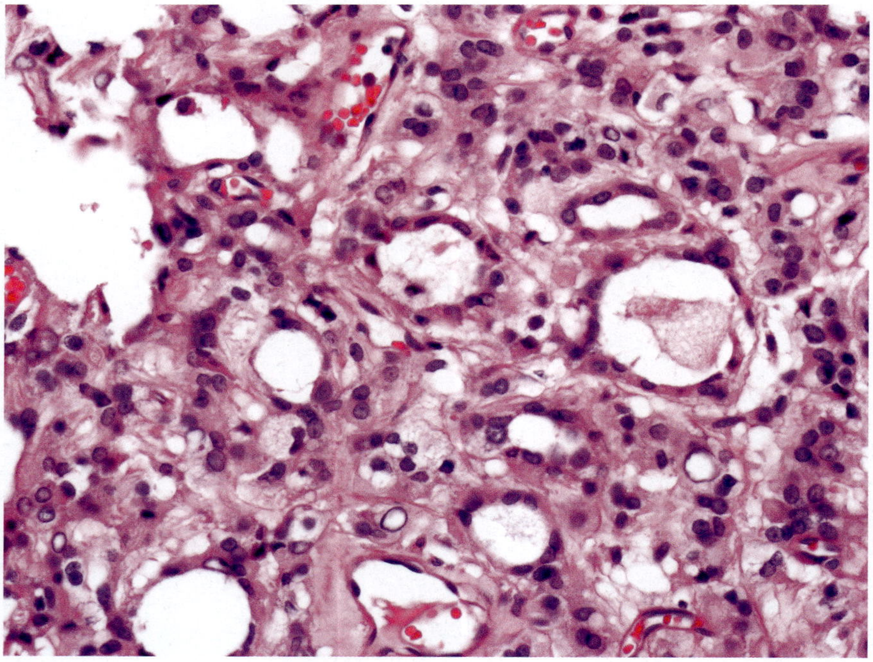

Figure 21-7.
Leydig tumor cells display the pseudogranular formation and the presence of cytoplasmic vacuoles in the tumor cells.

SERTOLI CELL TUMOR

Definition

- Neoplasm of Sertoli cell, or a sex cord stromal tumor composed of tumor cells with the phenotype of Sertoli cells

Other terms

- Androblastoma (not appropriate since Sertoli cells do not produce androgens)

Pathogenesis

- Uncommon tumor, only 1% of testicular neoplasms. Most cases are sporadic
- Tumor may be related to syndromes including Peutz-Jeghers syndrome, androgen insensitivity syndrome, and Carney syndrome

Clinical features

- Most tumors found in adult (mean age = 45 years)
- Slowly growing mass, typically no hormone-related syndromes
- Imaging studies show the tumor to be hypoechoic, sometimes cystic
- Occasionally, the tumor contains calcification (such as large in cell calcifying variant)

Gross pathology

- Well-circumscribed masses, round or lobulated in shape, typically small
- Cut surface is tan-yellow (Fig. 21-8)
- Necrosis or hemorrhage uncommon
- Most sporadic cases are unilateral, some cases associated with genetic syndromes are bilateral

Histology

- Many different patterns of tumor cells forming solid, tubular, or cord-like patterns (Fig. 21-9)
- Tumor cells are small round or spindle shaped; nuclei and prominent, but small nucleoli
- Cytoplasm is scant and may be clear or contain lipid droplets (Fig. 21-10)
- Variable amount of stroma in the tumor. Sometimes, stromal hyalinization is prominent
- Histological diagnosis of a malignant Sertoli cell tumor is difficult
- Large size, cellular atypia, high mitotic counts, and infiltrating pattern of extratesticular extension should be suspicious sign for malignancy (Fig. 21-11)
- Only the presence of a metastasis is definitive evidence of malignancy

Immunohistochemistry

- Positive for inhibin (Fig. 21-11), WT1, calretinin and melan-A

Clinical relevance (prognosis and treatment options)

- More than 90% cases are benign. Surgical excision is treatment of choice

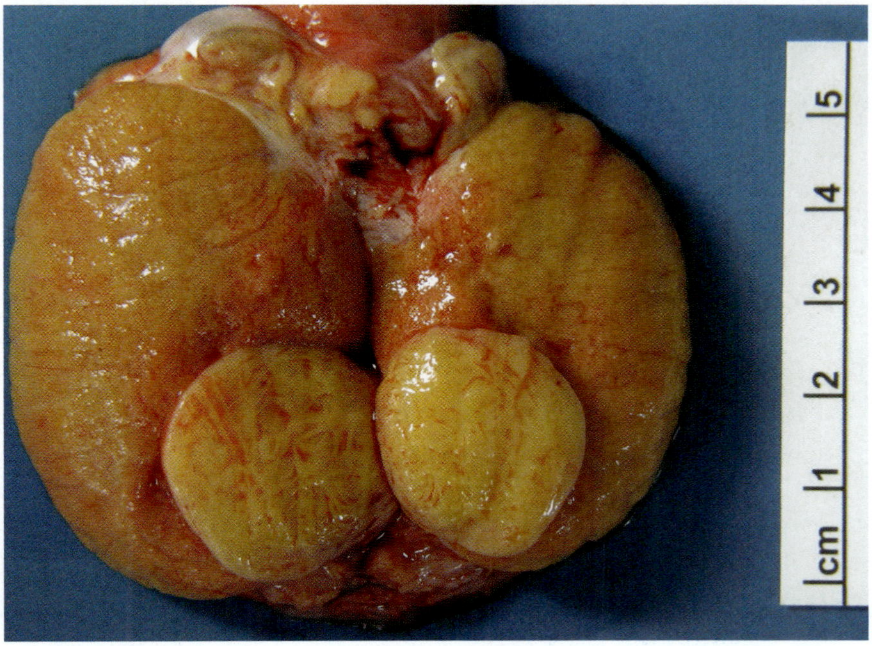

Figure 21-8.
A Sertoli cell tumor as a 2.2-cm well-circumscribed mass with a yellow cut surface, which appears to contain fibrous bands.

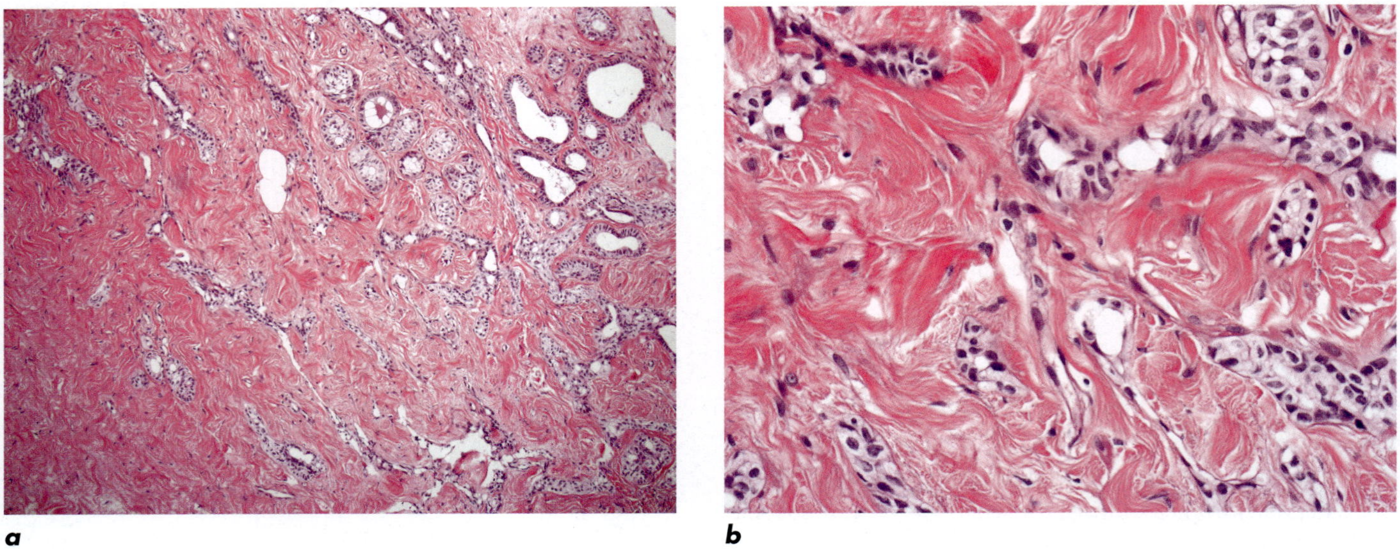

Figure 21-9.
Sertoli cell tumor is composed of tumor cells arranged in cords, or glandular structures (*a*). High magnification shows small ovoid-shaped tumor cells with glandular or cord patterns (*b*).

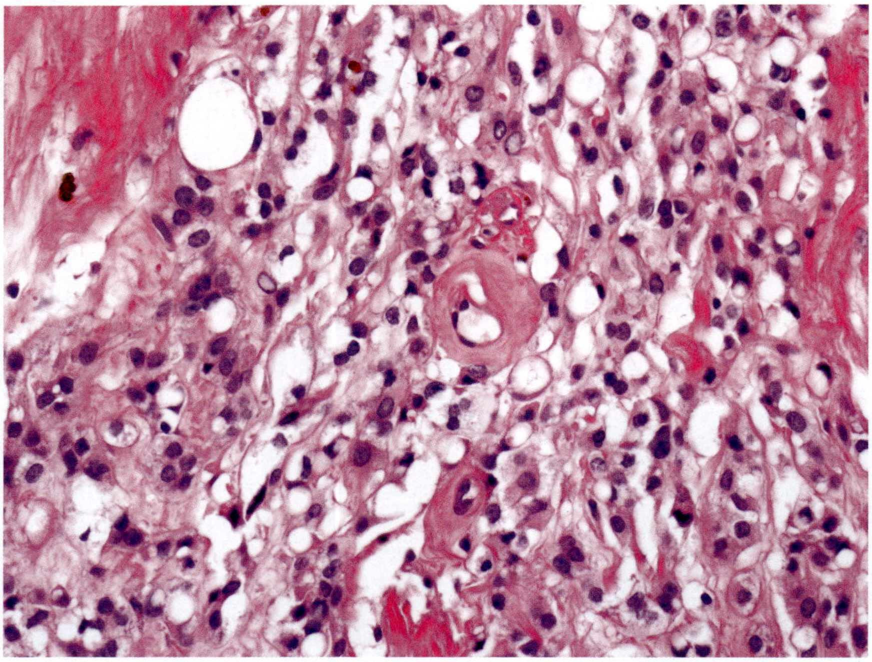

Figure 21-10.
A Sertoli cell tumor consists of tumor cells containing cytoplasmic vacuoles.

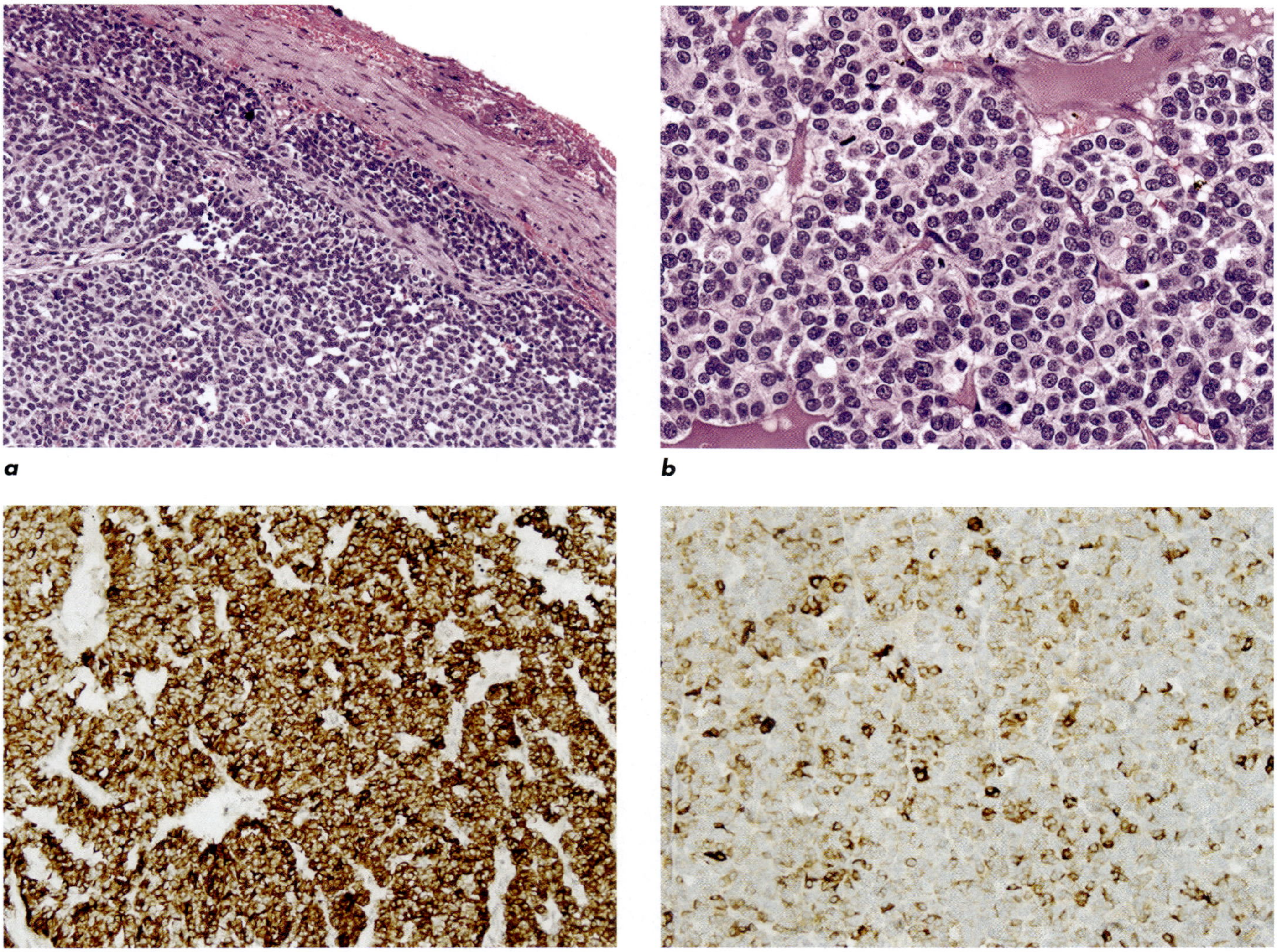

a *b* *c* *d*

Figure 21-11.
Malignant Sertoli cell tumor (with metastatic disease at the time of diagnosis) is hypercellular and composed of tumor cells forming a large nest (*a*). High magnification shows tumor cells with scant cytoplasm with brisk mitoses (*b*). Tumor cells are positive for AE1/AE3 (*c*) and inhibin (*d*).

CHAPTER 22

Other Benign Tumors and Tumor-Like Lesions in the Testis and Paratesticular Tissue

ADENOMATOID TUMOR

Definition

- Benign mesothelial proliferation, mostly seen in the male genital system, particularly epididymis or testis. Rare cases are also seen female genital organs

Other terms

- Adenofibromyoma, Recklinghausen tumor

Clinical features

- Firm nodule in the upper portion of testis or epididymis, typically smaller than 2 to 3 cm

Gross pathology

- Rubbery small fibrotic lesion, often located in the periphery of the testis or epididymis
- White to yellow cut surface, which may have mucinous appearance (Fig. 22-1)

Histology

- Tumor is composed of fibrous tissue, smooth muscle, and cords of epithelioid cells (Figs. 22-2 and 22-3)
- The epithelioid tumor cells have vacuolated cytoplasm and small nucleolus without significant cytological atypia (Fig. 22-2*b*)
- The tumor cells are arranged in nests, glandular or cribriform patterns, and appear infiltrating the wall of epididymis or smooth muscle (Fig. 22-4)

Immunohistochemistry

- Mesothelial markers such as calretinin and WT1 are positive
- CK5 and CK6 positive
- CD31 negative

Clinical relevance (prognosis and treatment options)

- Benign lesion, no treatment necessary if asymptomatic. Treatment of choice is surgical removal

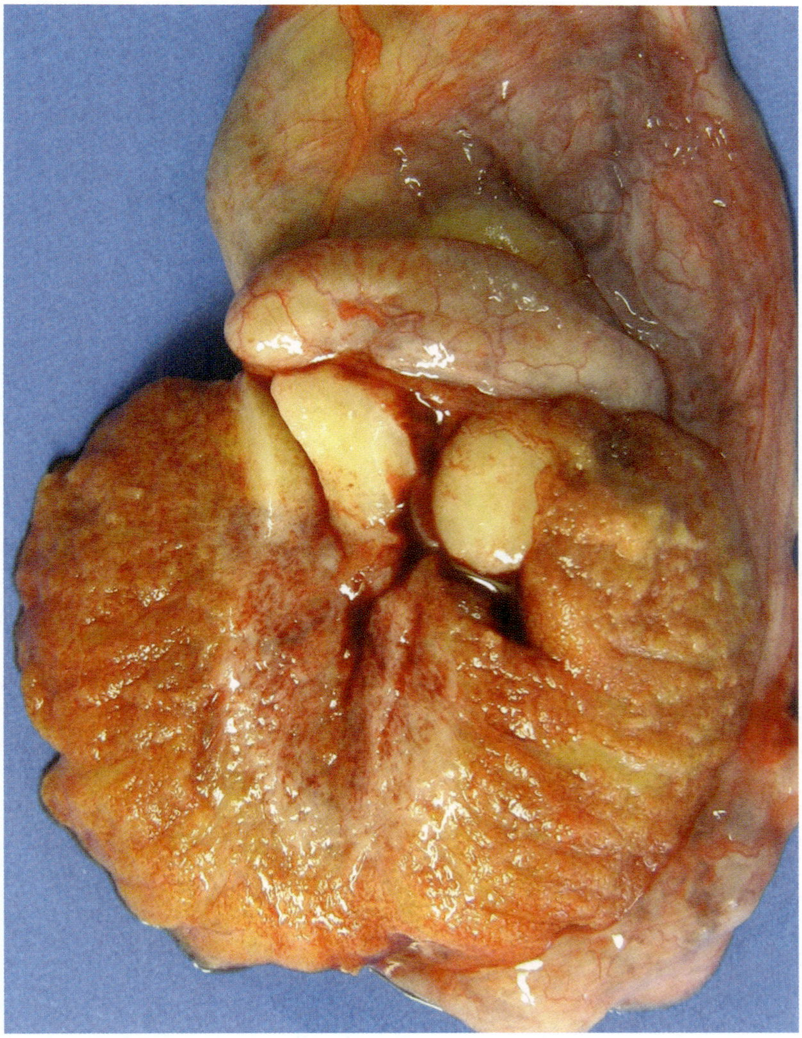

Figure 22-1.
Adenomatoid tumor in the testis is a well-circumscribed small yellow nodule located in the testis hilar region close to the epididymis.

Figure 22-2.
Adenomatoid tumor composed of small irregular nests of epithelioid cells (*a*). High magnification shows the tumor cells are cuboidal with bland nuclei and small nucleoli (*b*).

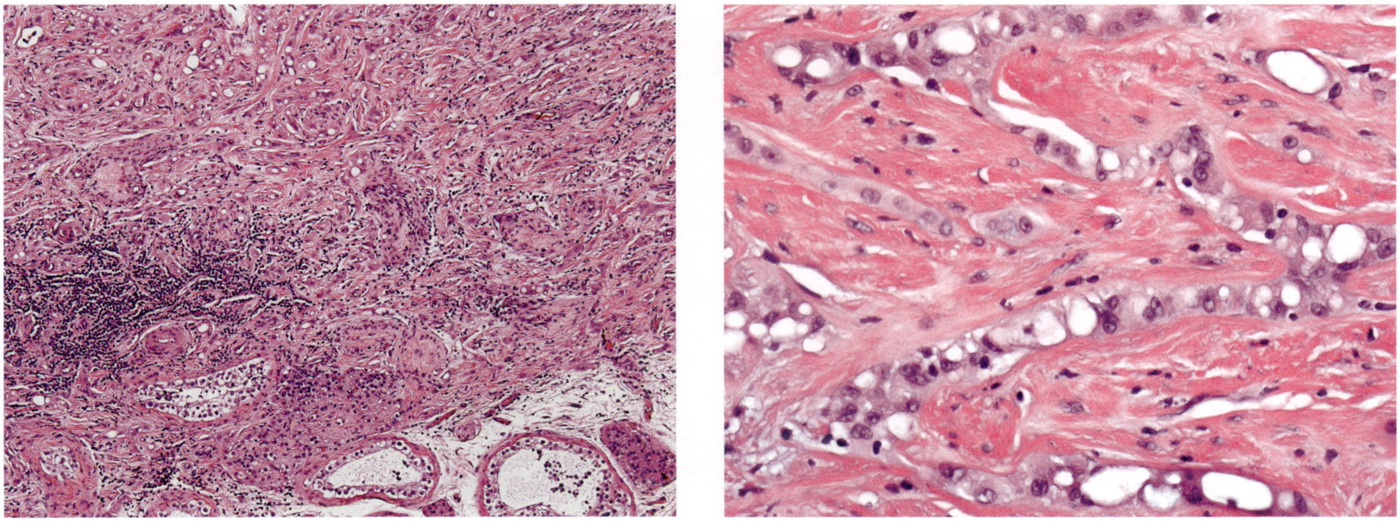

a *b*

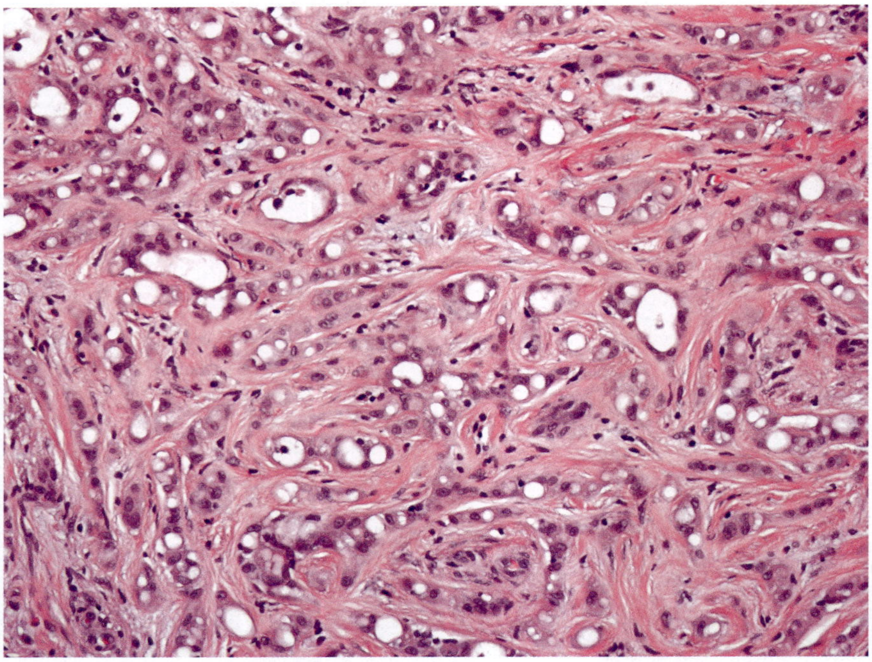

Figure 22-3.
Adenomatoid tumor cells with cytoplasmic vacuoles, forming tubular structures and haphazardly infiltrative patterns, mimicking adenocarcinoma.

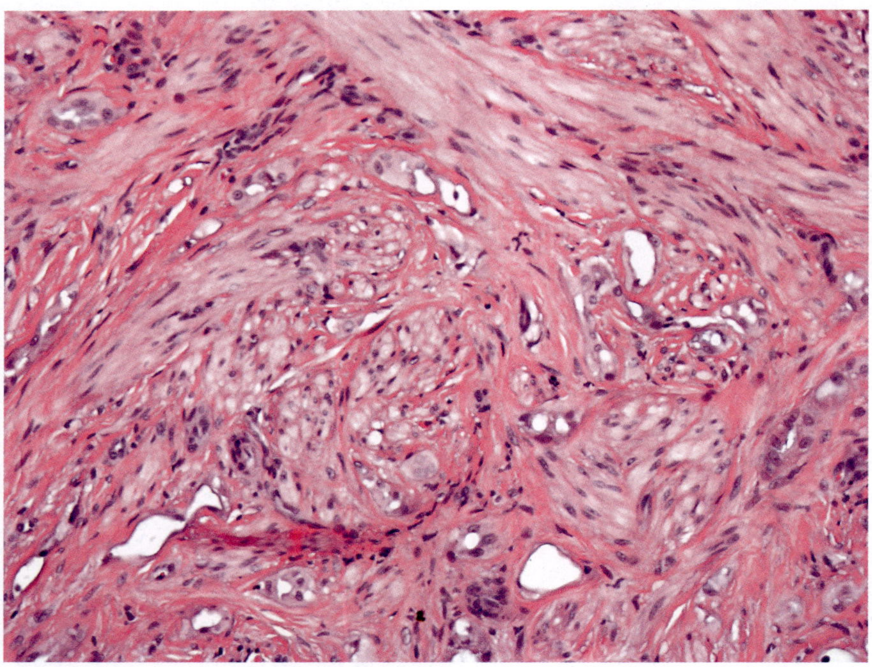

Figure 22-4.
Adenomatoid tumor cells infiltrating epididymal smooth muscle.

TESTICULAR FIBROMA

Definition

- Benign testicular fibrous stromal tumor resembling the ovarian counterpart

Other terms

- Fibrothecoma (this term is not correct because these testicular tumor cells are not related to estrogen production)

Pathogenesis

- Although the tumor histologically resembles fibroma or the ovary, there is no evidence that this tumor produces estrogen or other hormones

Clinical features

- Slowly growing, painless firm mass, no evidence of hormonal abnormality

Gross pathology

- Well-circumscribed nodule with white or yellow fibroid cut surface (Fig. 22-5)

Histology

- Tumor is composed of bland spindle cells without cytological atypia or mitosis (Fig. 22-6), which may have vacuolated cytoplasm, similar to ovarian stromal cells (Fig. 22-7)

Immunohistochemistry

- Vimentin positive and smooth muscle actin positive

Clinical relevance (prognosis and treatment options)

- Benign. Surgical removal for cure in the cases with symptoms or suspicion for malignancy

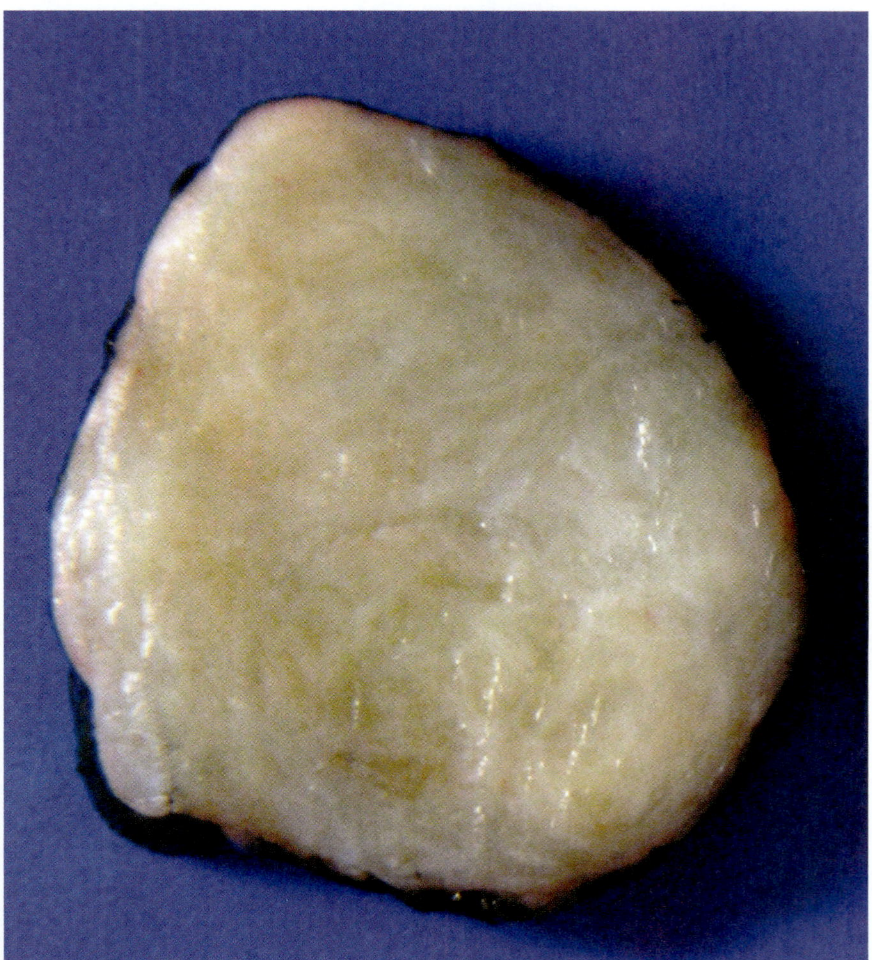

Figure 22-5.
Testicular fibroma showing white cut surface with fibrous bands in the tumor.

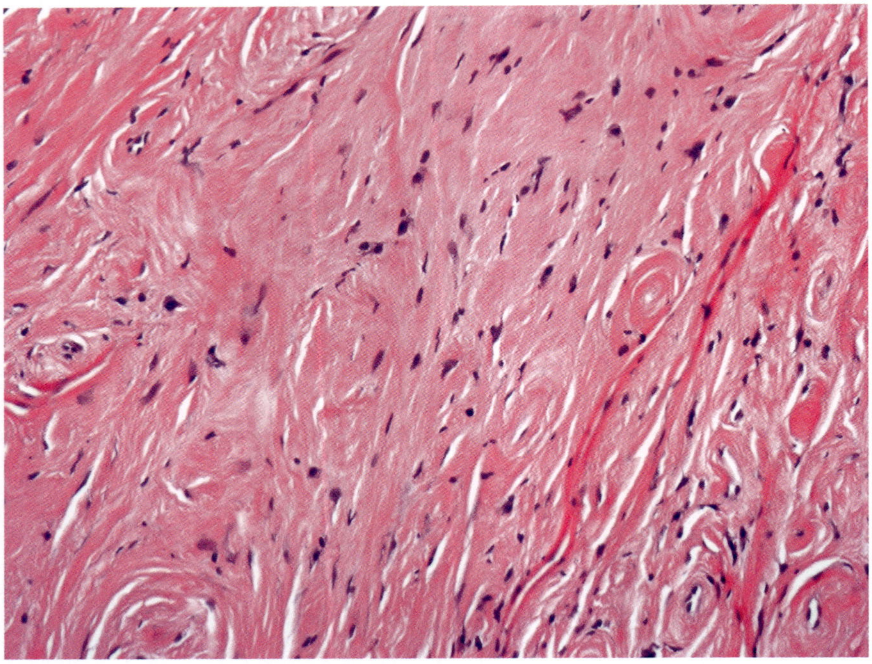

Figure 22-6.
Testicular fibroma is composed of spindle cells at a low cellularity and bland cytology.

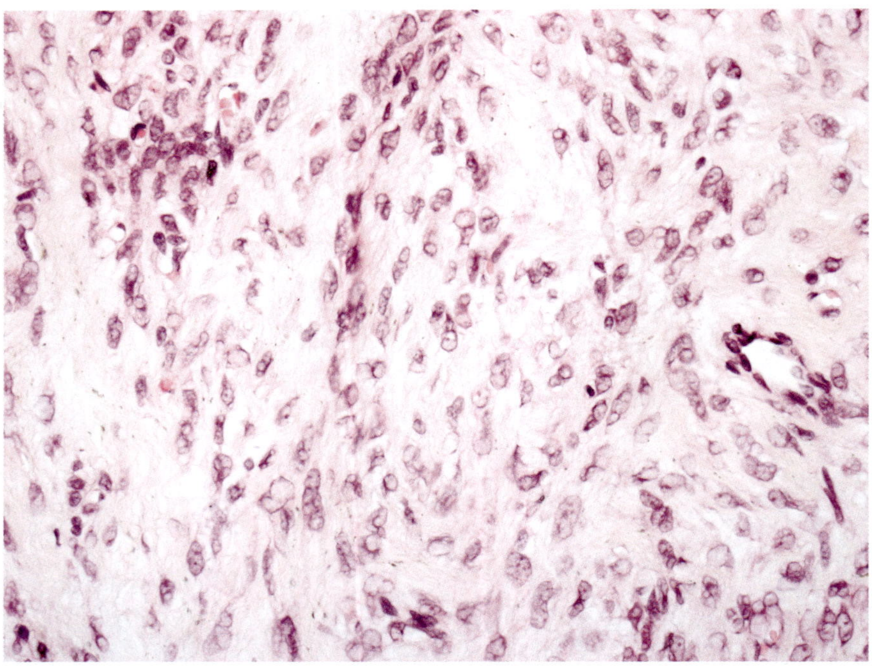

Figure 22-7.
Testicular fibroma cells with vacuolated cytoplasm, resembling ovarian stroma.

LIPOMA OF SPERMATIC CORD

Definition

- Benign stromal tumor composed of mature adipose tissue
- True lipoma is rare in the spermatic cord. The majority of cases of *lipoma of the spermatic cord* are herniated fibroadipose tissue in an inguinal hernia sac

Clinical features

- Painless mass in spermatic cord or scrotum, which may be palpable
- High lipid content by imaging studies

Gross pathology

- Lobular mass with capsule with bright yellow cut surface

Histology

- True lipoma has a thin capsule. In most cases, there is mature lobulated adipose tissue similar to normal fat without a capsule (Fig. 22-8)

Differential diagnosis

- Atypical lipoma contains lipoblasts in the septa and chicken wire vasculature

Clinical relevance (prognosis and treatment options)

- Benign. Surgical repair and resection of the lesion

Figure 22-8.
A spermatic cord lipoma is composed of mature adipose tissue (*a*). High magnification shows mature adipocytes with no atypia (*b*).

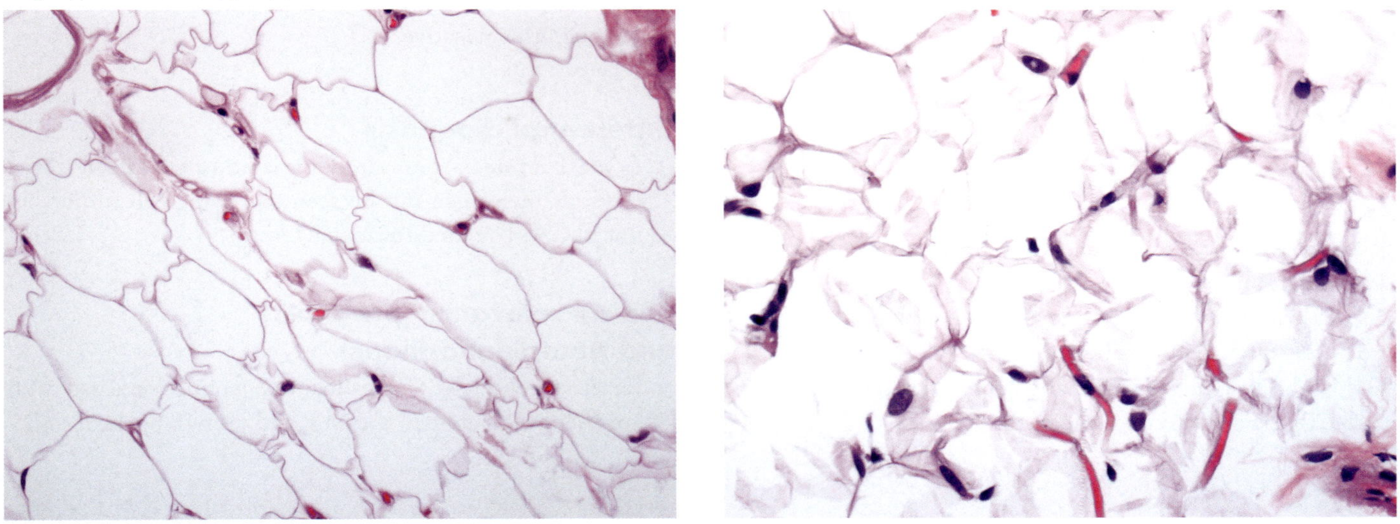

a b

TESTICULAR TUMOR OF CONGENITAL ADRENAL HYPERPLASIA

Definition

- Benign bilateral testicular masses in patients with congenital adrenal hyperplasia (CAH)
- Lesional cells are similar to adrenal or Leydig cells in morphology
- Most likely a hyperplastic condition rather than a neoplasm

Other terms

- Testicular tumor of adrenogenital syndrome

Pathogenesis

- CAH is a group of autosomal recessive diseases caused by the mutation of the enzymes essential for steroid hormone synthesis, which results in adrenal hyperplastic changes and changes in other organs
- Cellular origin of this tumor is unclear; possible candidates include stem cells, adrenal rest cells, or Leydig cells of the testis

Clinical features

- The deficiency of the enzyme hinders the normal production of adrenal hormones and accumulation of precursor adrenocortical hormones
- Precursors act as excess androgen, which leads to resultant virilization
- Salt losing symptom in two of three patients because of loss of mineral steroid hormone
- Bilateral testicular masses and orchialgia (testicular pain) due to the expansion of the testes

Gross pathology

- Well-circumscribed mass with no capsule, ranging from 0.5 to 10 cm in size (Fig. 22-9*a*)
- Often bilateral and multiple

Histology

- Mass is composed of cells with eosinophilic cytoplasm forming sheets, nest, cored separated by septa (Fig. 22-9*b*), trapped adipose tissue may be seen
- Sometimes, there are numerous nodules, which is suggestive of hyperplasia
- Abundant eosinophilic cytoplasm with lipofuscin (Fig. 22-9*c*)
- No crystal of Reinke in the cytoplasm (Fig. 22-10)

Immunohistochemistry

- Inhibin positive
- Melan-A positive, synaptophysin positive, and vimentin positive
- Cytokeratins negative

Differential diagnosis

- *Leydig cell tumor,* sporadic, not related to CAH syndrome. Crystals of Reinke can be seen in Leydig cell tumor but not in CAH-related testicular tumors

Clinical relevance (prognosis and treatment options)

- Reactive condition. High-dose exogenous corticosteroids are effective to control the pain and growth of the lesion

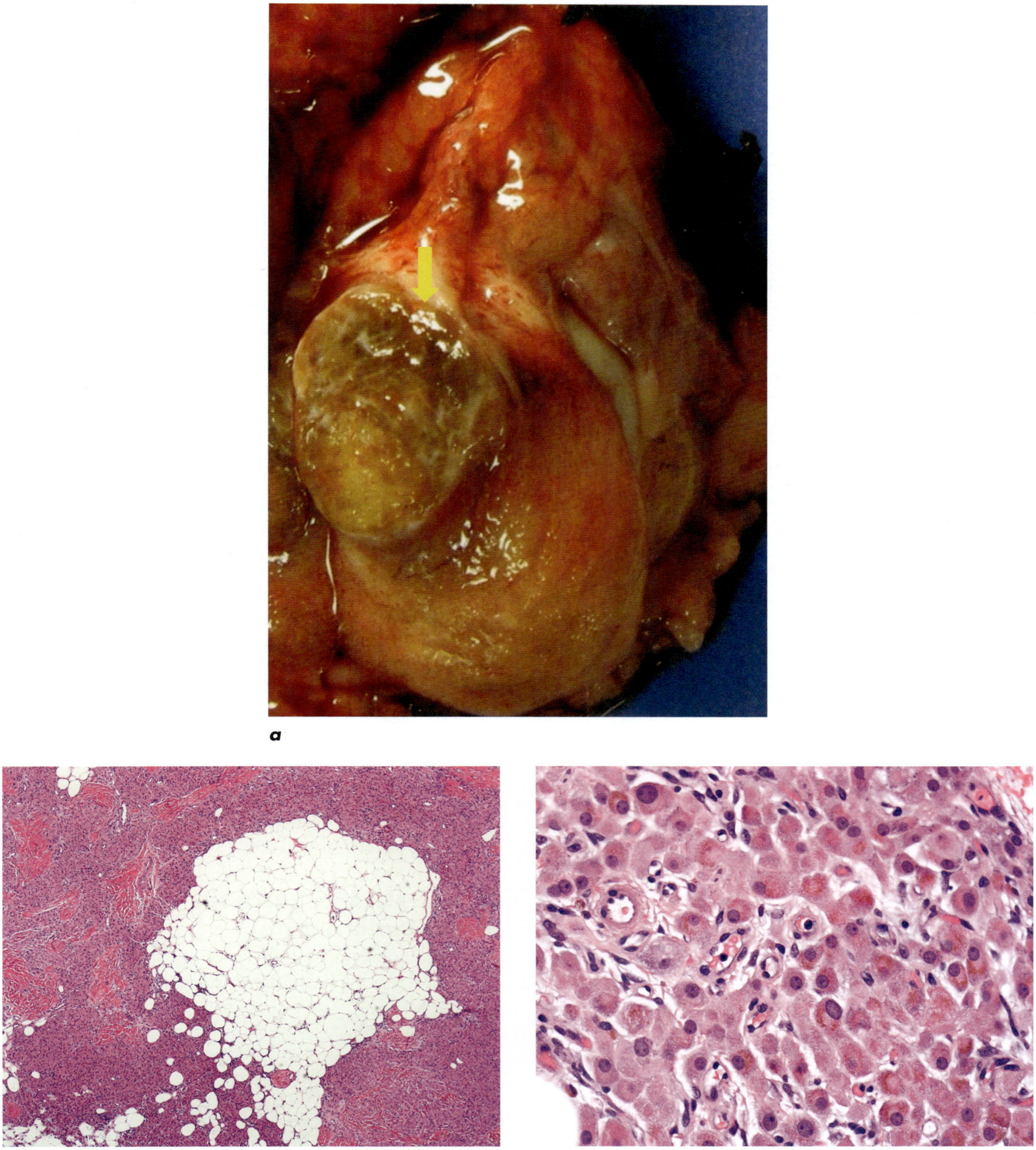

a

b

c

Figure 22-9.
Testicular tumor associated congenital adrenal hyperplasia (CAH) contains multiple nodules. One of the tumor nodules is well circumscribed with light brown cut surface (*a*, arrow). The tumor contains entrapped adipose tissue (*b*). The tumor cells have abundant eosinophilic cytoplasm containing lipofuscin (*c*).

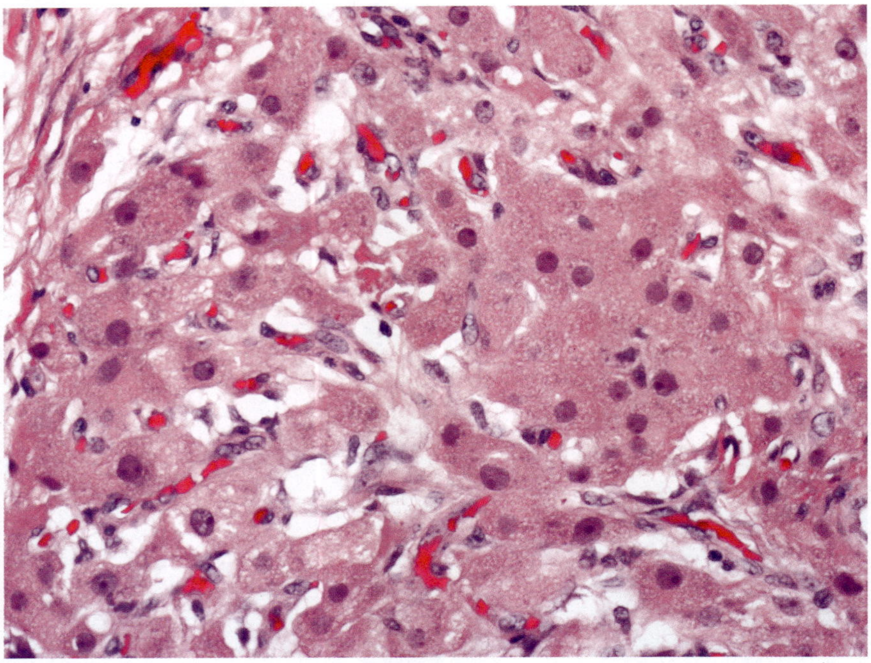

Figure 22-10.
Testicular tumor in CAH composed of large polygonal cells with abundant granular cytoplasm, similar to Leydig cells but no crystal of Reinke.

HEMANGIOMA

Definition

- Benign mesenchymal tumor composed of disorganized mature blood vessels

Clinical features

- Mass lesion in the testicular parenchyma
- Imaging studies may provide suggestion of hemangioma because of the blood component
- No other specific clinical symptoms except testicular enlargement and compression

Gross pathology

- Irregular infiltrating border with red spongy cut surface containing blood

Histology

- Cavernous type: the lesion is composed of dilated thin wall vessels (Fig. 22-11)
- Capillary type: the lesion is composed of small capillaries
- Thrombosis can be seen in cavernous hemangioma
- Old lesion may have organized thrombosis (Fig. 22-11*a*), rechannelization (Fig. 22-12), fibrosis, and calcification

Immunohistochemistry

- CD31 and CD34 positive for endothelium

Differential diagnosis

- Angiosarcoma: with anastomosing channels and cytological atypia in endothelial cells

Clinical relevance (prognosis and treatment options)

- Benign, no treatment necessary if asymptomatic
- Surgical removal if clinically suspicious

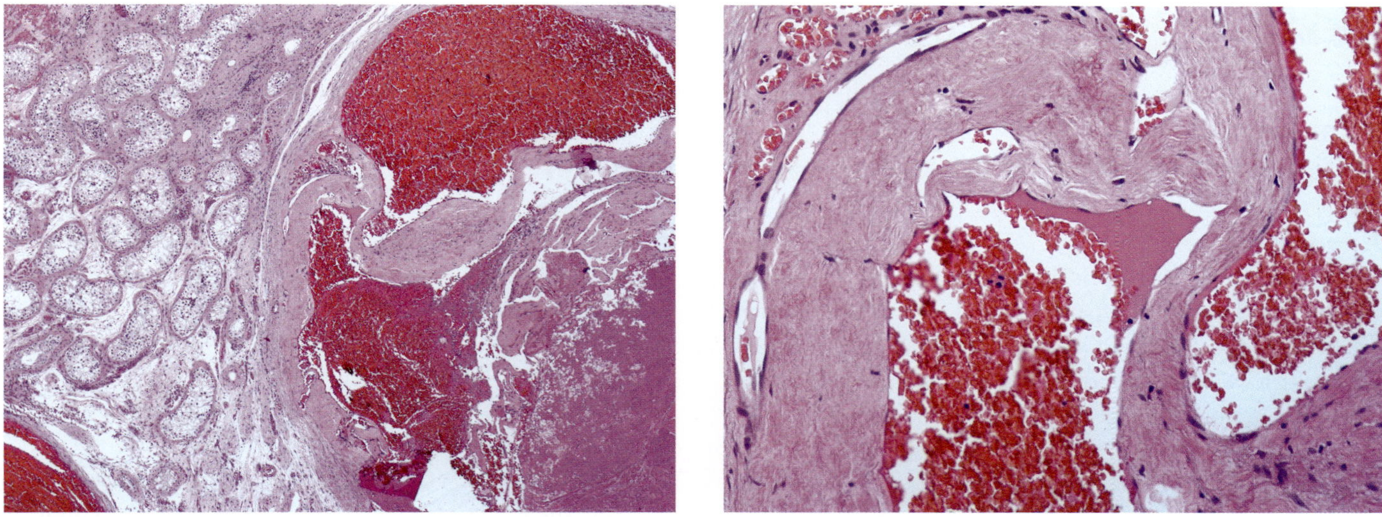

a ***b***

Figure 22-11.
Testicular hemangioma, cavernous type, is composed of large dilated vessels with thrombosis (*a*). The vessels are lined by benign endothelium (*b*).

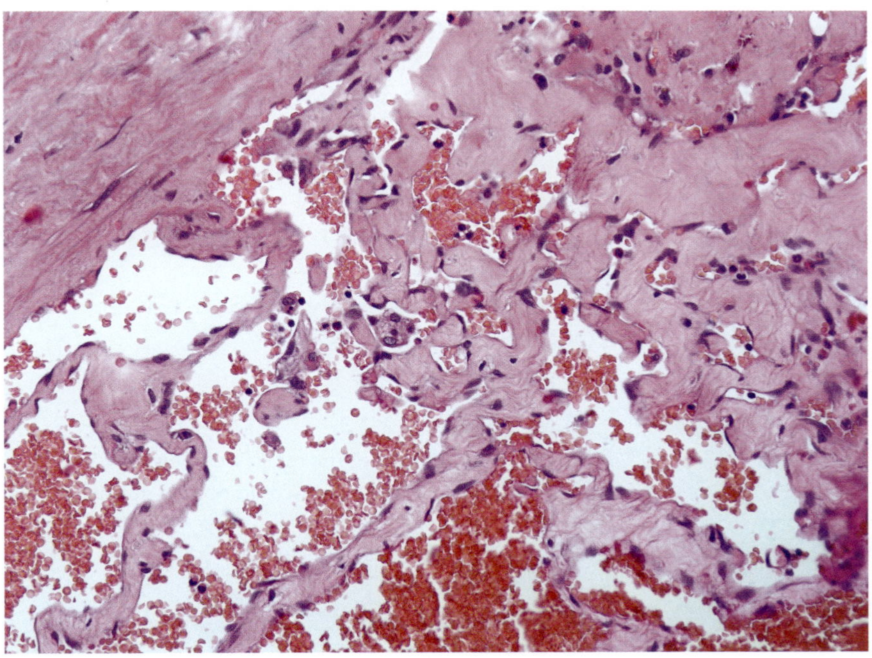

Figure 22-12.
In a cavernous hemangioma, organization of thrombosis, rechannelization, and endothelial papillary hyperplasia can be seen.

ADENOMATOUS HYPERPLASIA OF THE RETE TESTIS

Definition

- Benign nodular proliferation of epithelium of the rete testis

Other terms

- Adenoma of the rete testis, hyperplasia of the rete testis
- Distinction between hyperplasia and adenoma of the rete testis is not well defined. If lesion is a small focus without forming a well-circumscribed mass, we would use the term of adenomatous hyperplasia

Pathogenesis

- The etiology of adenomatous hyperplasia of the rete testis (AHRT) in adults is unknown
- AHRT can be also seen as congenital cases
- Majority of the cases are associated with some testicular abnormalities, suggesting a reactive process
- An uncommon condition, with only a few dozens of cases reported in the literature, although it may be underreported

Clinical features

- Most cases are associated with cryptorchidism
- Other associated conditions include benign cysts, hernia, germ cell tumors, and prostate cancer
- Mostly as incidental findings during procedures for other conditions

Gross pathology

- This lesion is located in the hilar region of the testis. Because of its small size, it may not be seen grossly

Histology

- Most cases are multifocal without formation of a defined mass
- Proliferating cells form complex channels, papillary or solid patterns (Fig. 22-13)
- Epithelial nests, ranging from a few cells to 2 mm in size, adjacent or connected to rete testis epithelial channels (Figs. 22-14 and 22-15)
- Proliferating cells are bland, with scant cytoplasm and occasional nuclear grooving (Fig. 22-14*b*)
- The lesional cells of the adenomatoid hyperplasia are disorganized, but similar to those covering the cuboidal epithelium of the rete testis
- Some of the adjacent rete testis channels show partial or focal proliferation
- Other associated lesions such as cryptorchidism can be seen

Immunohistochemistry

- PAX8 positive. PAX8 normally present in the epithelial cells of Wolffian duct derivatives in male such as the rete testis, efferent ducts, epididymis, vas deferens, seminal vesicles, and ejaculatory ducts, but not in germ cells or sex stromal cells (Fig. 22-15*b*)
- Keratin markers such as AE1/AE3 positive
- Inhibin negative
- Germ cell tumor markers negative such as C-kit, PLAP, and OCT-4

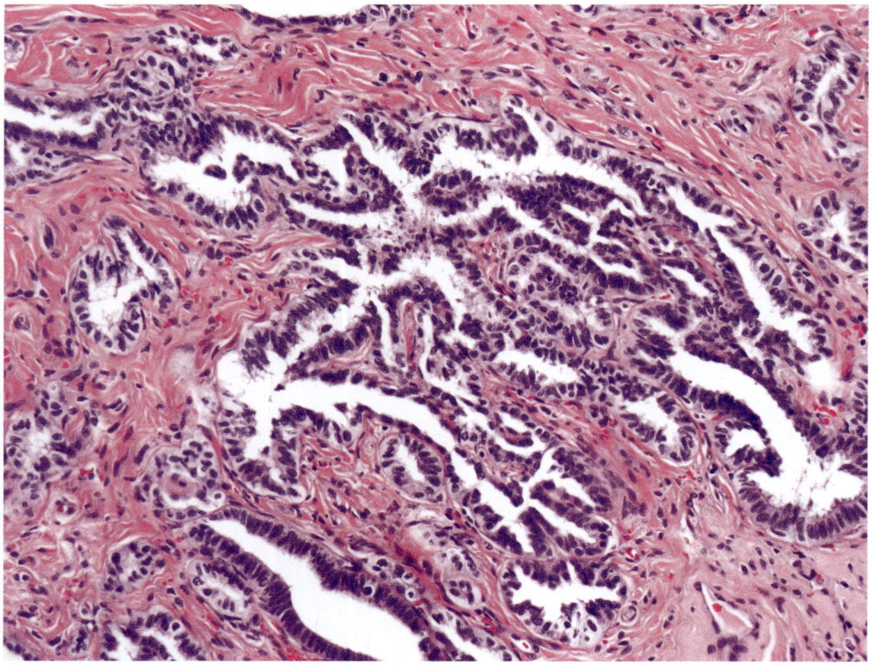

Figure 22-13.
Hyperplasia of the rete testis showing complex channels and increased number of epithelial cells.

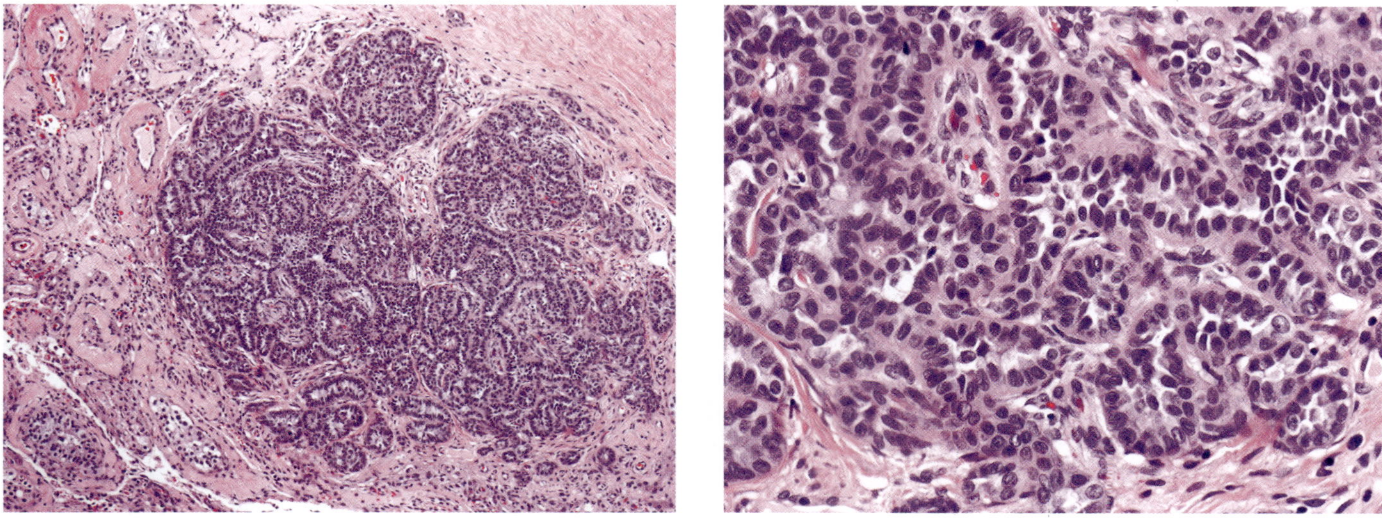

a **b**

Figure 22-14.
Adenomatous hyperplasia of rete testis is well-circumscribed nodule composed of bland columnar cells with scant cytoplasm (*a*). High magnification shows lesional cells with minimal cytological atypia and occasional nuclear grooves (*b*).

Figure 22-15.
Adenomatous hyperplasia of rete testis with papillary configuration (*a*). The lesional cells and the residual rete testis are positive for PAX8 (*b*).

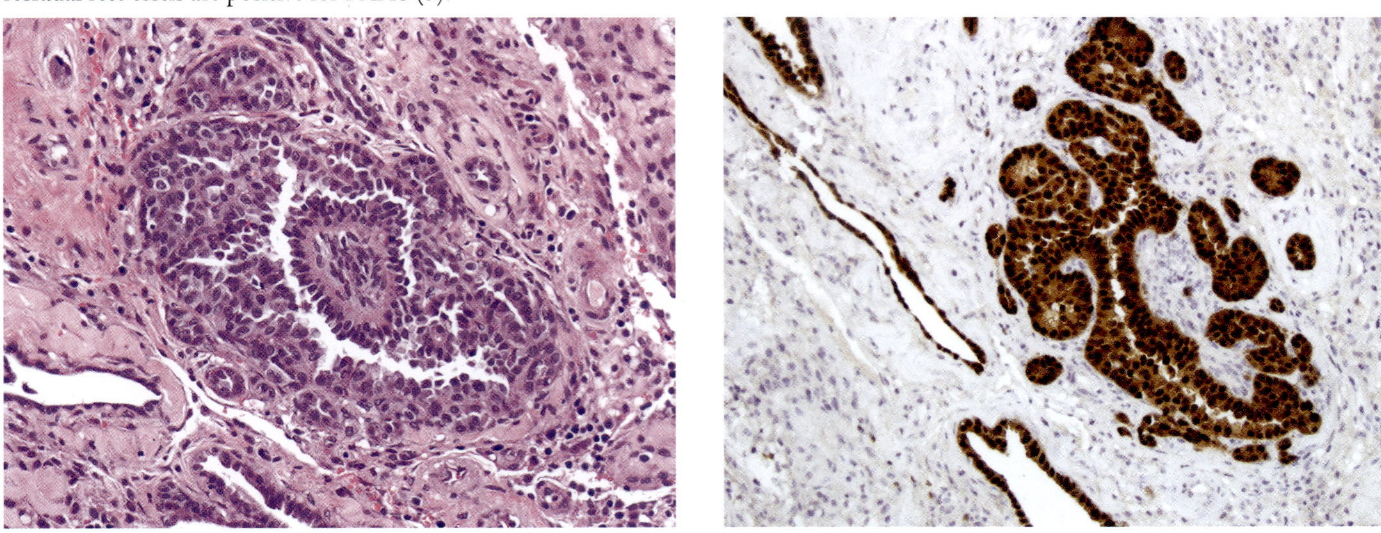

a **b**

Differential diagnosis

- Primary adenocarcinoma of the rete testis: larger mass lesion with invasion. Significant cytological atypia and frequent mitoses are present
- Metastatic adenocarcinoma to the rete testis: history of a primary adenocarcinoma in another organ. A metastatic adenocarcinoma is very rare in the rete testis, almost never to be the first site of metastasis. Morphologically, AHRT resembles type 1 papillary RCC; however, that tumor is usually low grade and rarely contributes to metastasis. Other features suggesting metastatic adenocarcinoma include mucin production, cribriform patterns, or significant cytological atypia. Immunostains may be helpful

Clinical relevance (prognosis and treatment options)

- Incidental findings. Orchiectomy is usually performed for other testicular conditions

CHAPTER 23

Other Malignant Neoplastic Lesions in the Testis and Paratesticular Tissues

Ximing J. Yang, Shan Zheng, Ning Lu

CARCINOID TUMOR

Definition

- Neuroendocrine (carcinoid) tumor develops in the testis, either primary or secondary

Other terms

- Neuroendocrine tumor

Pathogenesis

- Carcinoid tumor cells have the features of neuroendocrine cells producing serotonin, which can lead to carcinoid syndrome

Clinical features

- Painless testicular mass
- If the tumor is functional, the carcinoid syndrome will be present, such as flushing, diarrhea, bronchoconstriction, and heart failure
- If it is metastatic, a history of a primary tumor in another organ should be present

Gross pathology

- Yellow white well-circumscribed nodule with a homogeneous cut surface, occasionally with spotty hemorrhage

Histology

- Tumor cells are uniform in size and shape, form regular ribbons or islands (Fig. 23-1)
- Fine chromatin with "salt-and-pepper" appearance in tumor cells (Fig. 23-2)
- Rosettes or glandular-like structures can be seen
- No evidence of intratubular germ cell neoplasia
- Absence of lymphocytes or granulomas that are often associated with seminoma
- A metastatic carcinoid (Fig. 23-3) is difficult to be distinguished from a primary testicular carcinoid by morphology or immunohistochemistry

Immunohistochemistry

- Neuroendocrine markers (chromogranin, NSE, or synaptophysin) positive
- Keratins positive
- Germ cell and lymphoma markers negative

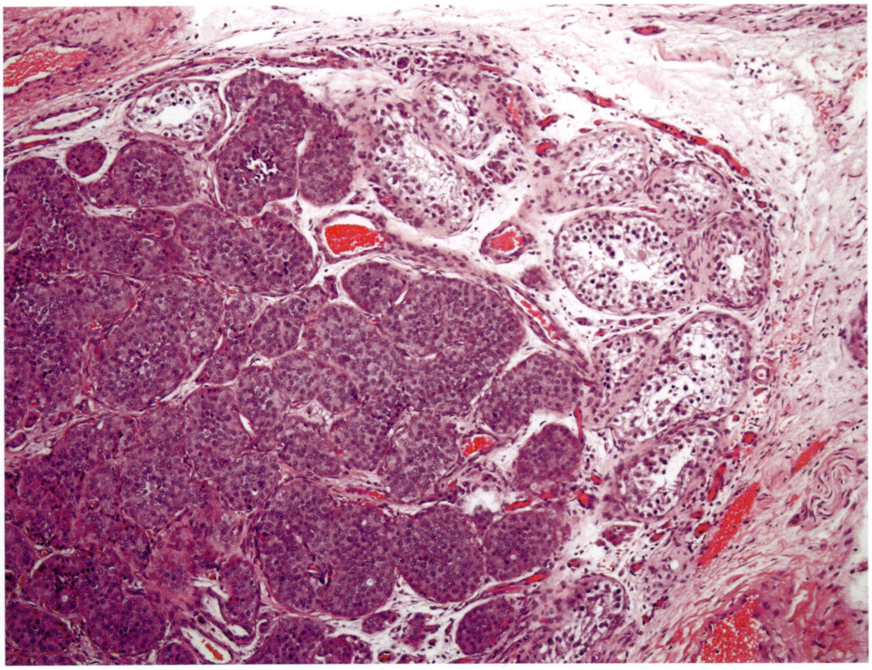

Figure 23-1.
Primary carcinoid tumor consists of tumor cells in lobular patterns forming a defined border from seminiferous tubules.

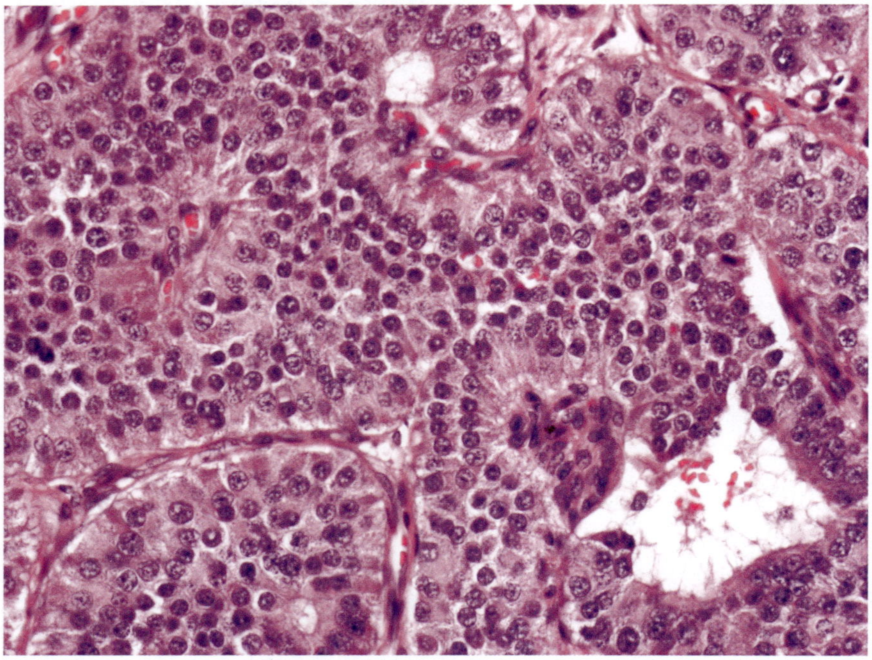

Figure 23-2.
Primary carcinoid tumor cells with salt-pepper chromatin, forming rosette-like and pseudoglandular structures.

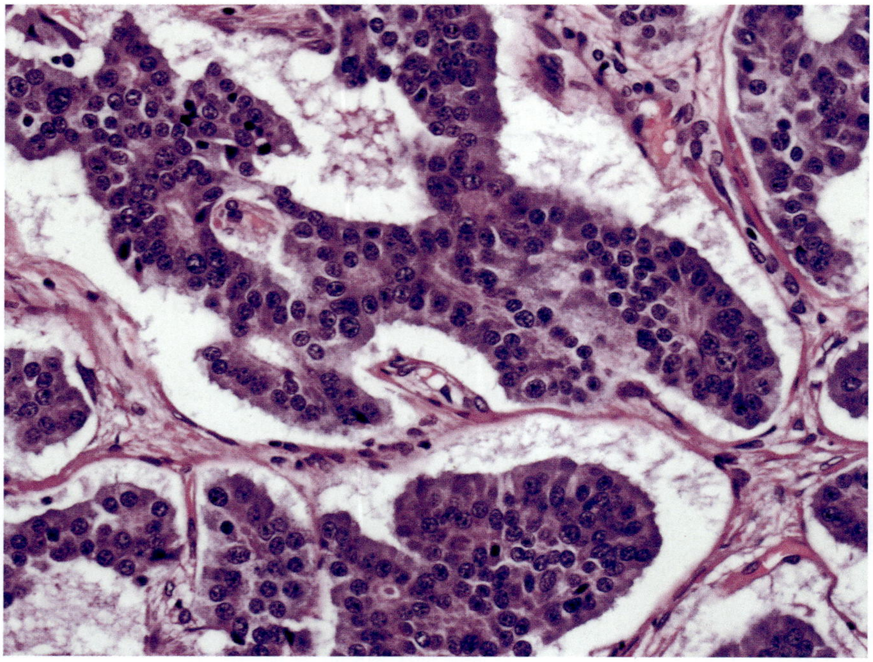

Figure 23-3.
A metastatic carcinoma from the small bowel displays typical neuroendocrine features arranged in ribbons and islands.

Differential diagnosis

- Seminoma: tumor cells are larger, more atypical, with diffuse patterns not forming ribbons or islands, salt-and-pepper chromatin pattern is absent
- Carcinoma, more pleomorphic and infiltrative. No salt-and-pepper chromatins

Clinical relevance (prognosis and treatment options)

- Primary carcinoid is a low-grade malignancy, and orchiectomy is an option for treatment
- Secondary carcinoid is a part of systemic disease, and systemic treatment is necessary to control metastatic carcinoid

TESTICULAR LYMPHOMA

Definition

- Malignant neoplasm of lymphocytes involving the testis

Pathogenesis and epidemiology

- Testicular lymphoma usually represents a secondary involvement of the testis by a lymphoma originated from the lymph node
- Rarely, primary lymphoma may develop in the testis before or without nodal involvement
- Testicular lymphomas account for only 5% of testicular tumors
- However, in men over 60 years old, 50% of the testicular malignancies are lymphoma

Clinical features

- Testicular lymphomas can be seen in any age of men ranging from 16 to 90 years old, but mostly in older patients with a mean age of 60 years
- In contrast, patients develop testicular germ cell tumors such as seminoma (mean age = 40 years) and nonseminomatous germ cell tumors (mean age = 20 to 30 years) at younger ages
- Majority cases presented with a painless testicular mass
- Some patients may have systemic symptoms such as fever, sweats, and weight loss
- Most patients with testicular lymphomas will be found to have nodal or other organ involvement during a complete clinical work-up

Gross pathology

- In some cases, testicular lymphoma (Fig. 23-4) may form a single or multiple mass lesions, similar to the appearance of a seminoma
- More often, however, testicular lymphoma is diffuse and replacing the entire testis without a discrete mass (Fig. 23-5)
- Cut surface is homogenous, solid fine granular, tan to pink in color (Fig. 23-6)

Histology

- Most common type of lymphomas of the testis in adults is diffuse large B-cell lymphoma, which accounts for up to 50% to 75% of all testicular lymphomas
- Other types such as small lymphocytic lymphoma, T-cell lymphoma and NK-cell lymphoma can be seen in younger patients
- Tumor cells usually exhibit interstitial growth patterns, encasing but not replacing the seminiferous tubules giving the appearance of "tubules sparing" (Fig. 23-7)
- Large B-cell lymphoma is typically composed of large tumor cells with diffuse growth patterns. The tumor cells have vesicular nuclei and prominent nucleoli. Mitotic activities are brisk (Figs. 23-8 and 23-9)
- Presence of granulomas (common in seminoma) is not commonly seen

Immunohistochemistry and special study

- Variable depending on the type of lymphoma
- Large diffuse B-cell lymphoma, CD45 positive, CD20 positive (Fig. 23-9*b*), CD3 negative
- Lymphomas are negative for germ cell markers such as AFP, HCG, C-kit, or OCT-4
- Lymphomas are also negative for epithelial markers such as AE1/AE3, Cam5.2

Main differential diagnoses

- Seminoma: typically seen in younger patients with a well-circumscribed mass. Histologically, seminoma will be replacing not sparing tubules. Seminoma markers such as C-kit, OCT-4 are confirmative
- Reactive lesions: lymphoid hyperplasia and chronic orchitis will display germinal centers, often with mixed inflammatory cell infiltrates

Clinical relevance (prognosis and treatment options)

- The stage of the testicular lymphoma is the most important factor for the prognosis
- Patients with early stage lymphoma will have better prognosis. The five-year tumor-free survival is 60% for early stage patients, and less than 20% for patients in the advanced stage
- The prognosis of testicular lymphoma is typically worse than nodal lymphoma with high recurrence rate, up to 80%, which depends on the type; T-cell lymphoma is worse than B-cell lymphoma
- With contemporary chemotherapy, survival rate for testicular lymphoma is improving
- Orchiectomy is not a treatment of choice for testicular lymphomas. However, the majority of the testicular lymphomas encountered in surgical pathology are found in orchiectomy specimens

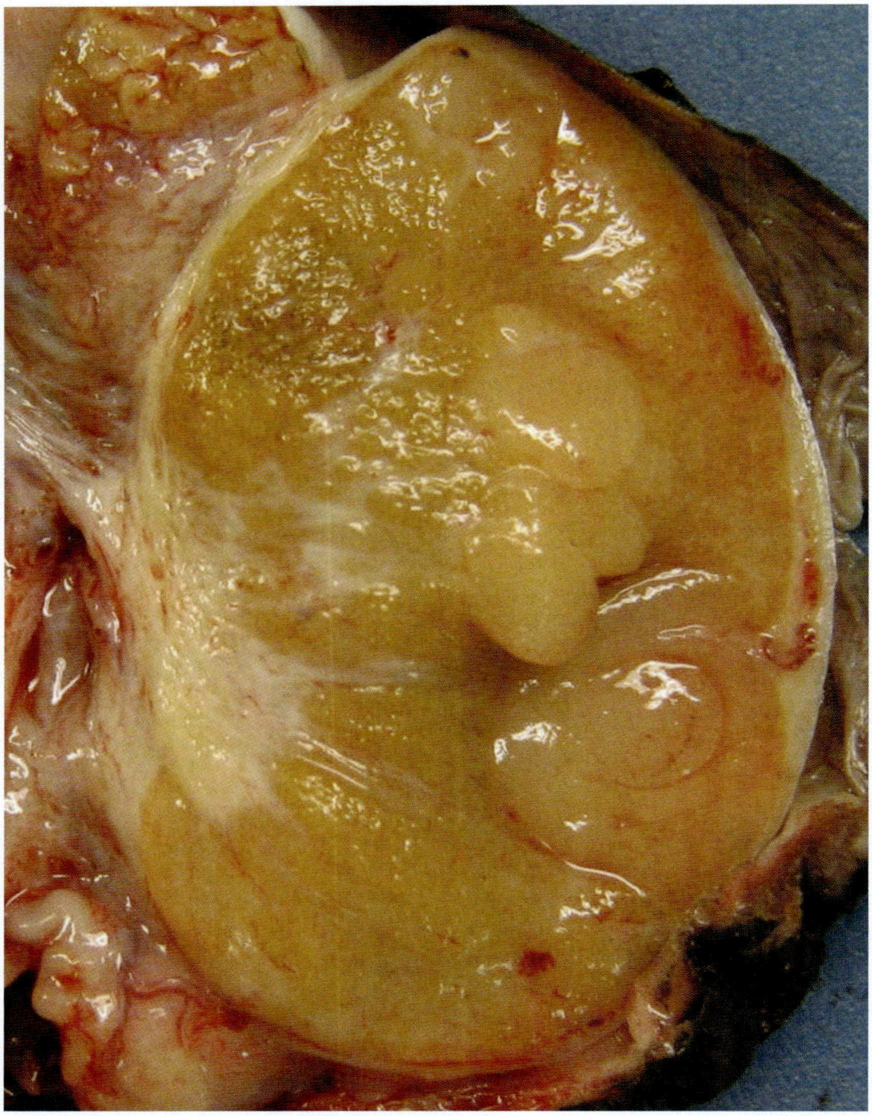

Figure 23-4.
A testicular lymphoma contains multiple tumor nodules with fleshy homogenous cut surfaces.

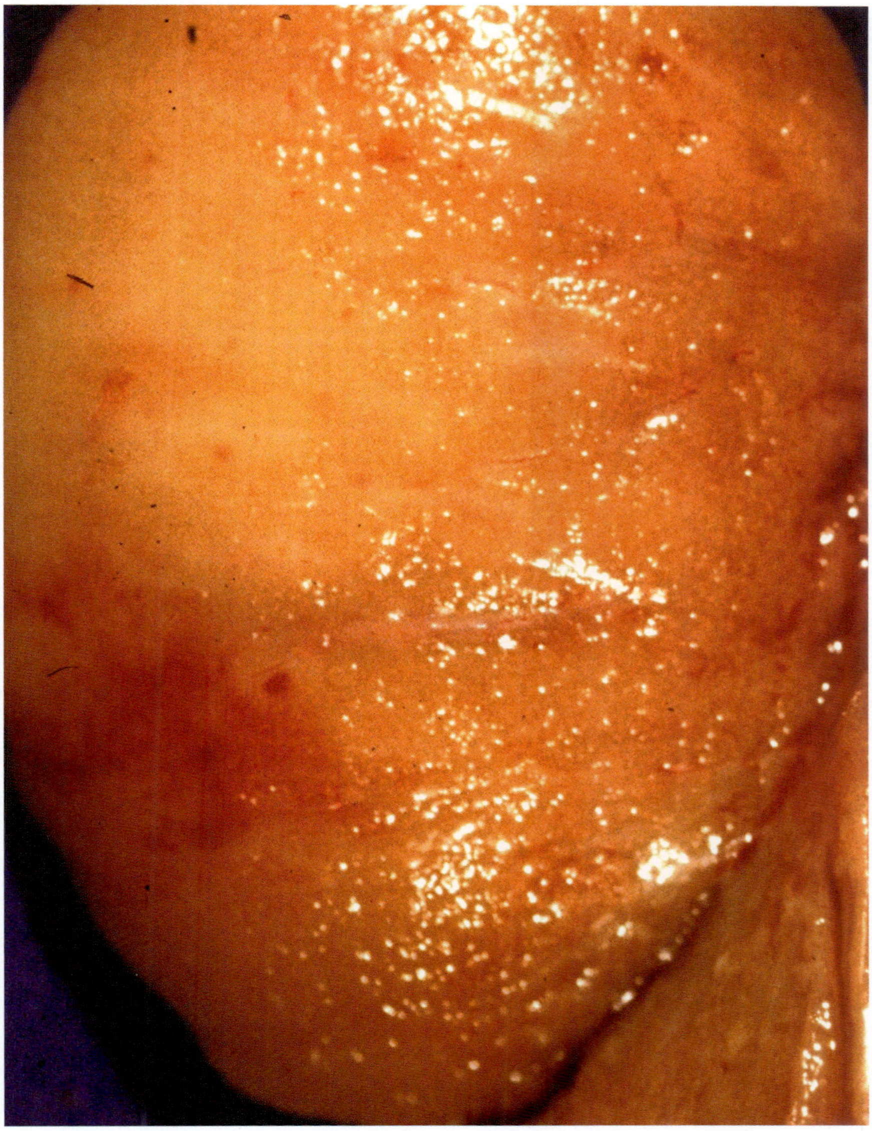

Figure 23-5.
Large B-cell lymphoma diffusely infiltrating the testis parenchyma.

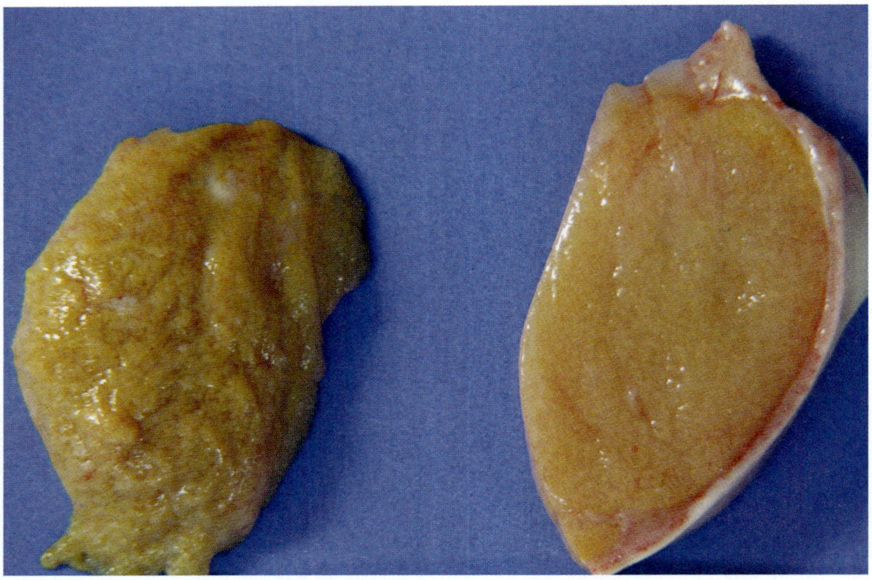

Figure 23-6.
Testicular lymphoma (right), in comparison to normal testicular parenchyma (left), is more solid and fleshy, with finer granular appearance.

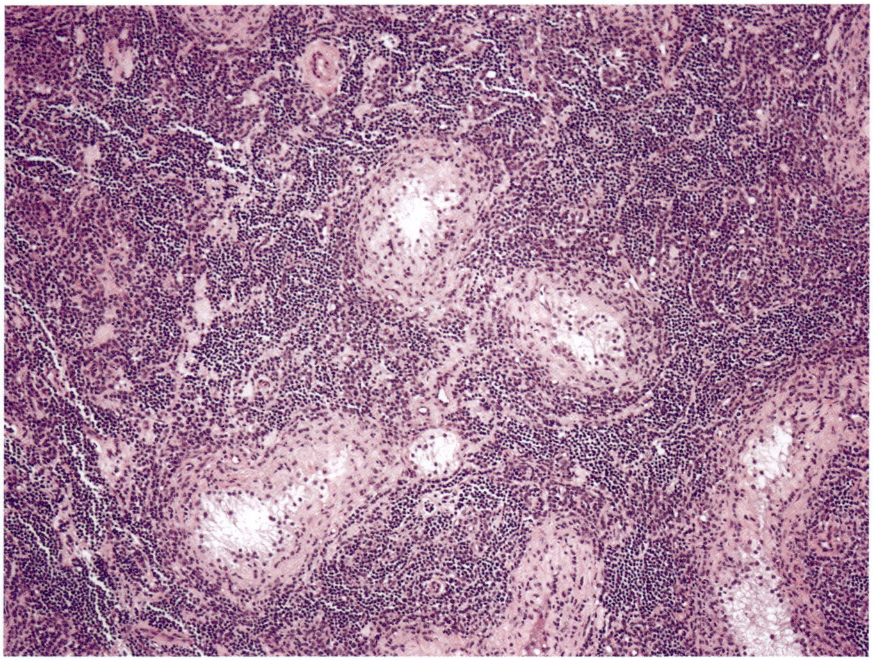

Figure 23-7.
Typically lymphoma cells demonstrate interstitial growth patterns, sparing of seminiferous tubules that contain only Sertoli cells. ITGCNU is absent.

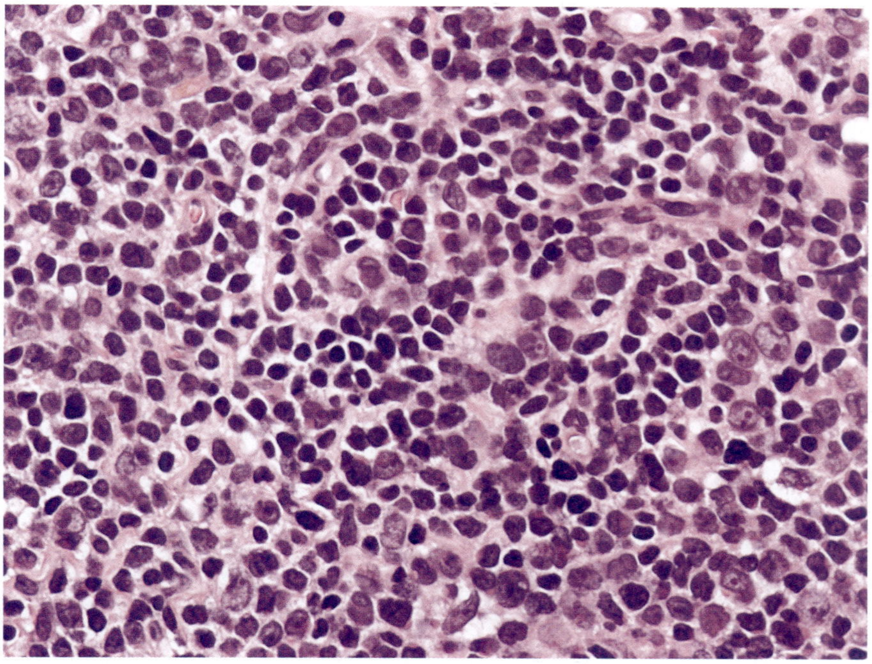

Figure 23-8.
Testicular large B-cell lymphoma with large atypical lymphoma cells in the background of small reactive lymphocytes.

Figure 23-9.
High magnification shows large malignant cells with cytological atypia (*a*), and CD20 positivity (*b*) confirmed the diagnosis of large B-cell lymphoma.

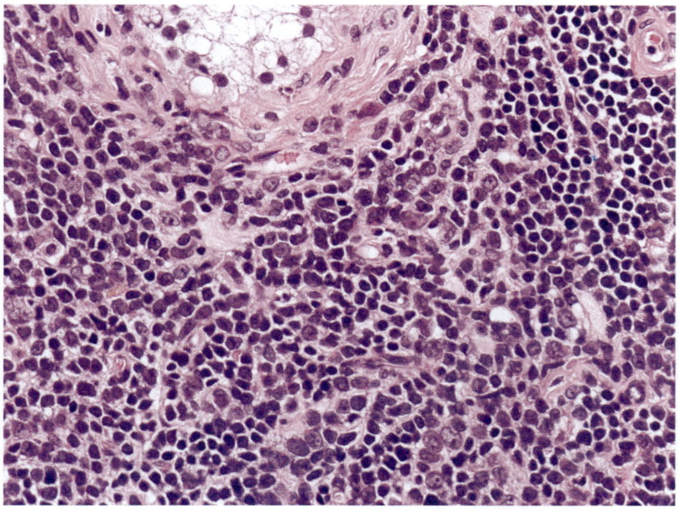

a

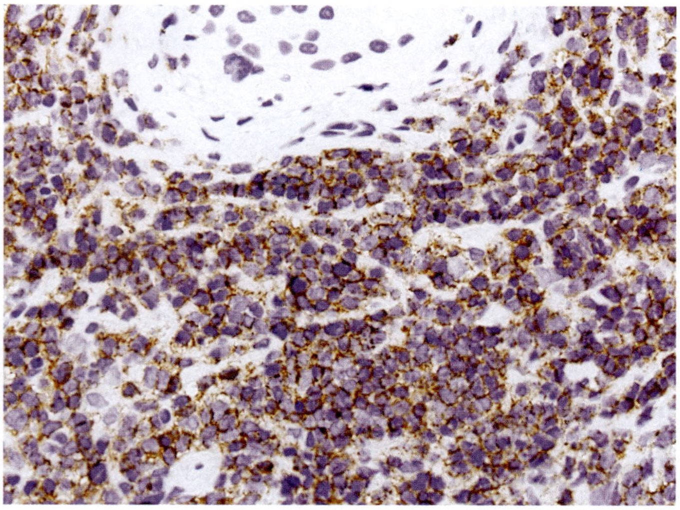

b

LIPOSARCOMA

Definition

- Malignant adipose neoplasm that develops in the paratesticular tissue

Other terms

- Atypical lipoma (low-grade superficial)

Pathogenesis

- The most common location of low-grade liposarcoma in the genitourinary (GU) system is paratesticular tissue
- High-grade sarcoma is rare in paratesticular tissue. They are mostly derived from dedifferentiation of a low-grade liposarcoma
- Liposarcoma can be found in the perirenal tissue and any other parts of the body

Clinical features

- Typically a large mass lesion located in paratesticular tissue particularly spermatic cord

Gross pathology

- Lobulated large mass, well-defined or infiltrating borders, with yellow to tan cut surface (Fig. 23-10*a*)
- Fleshy appearance or the presence of hemorrhage and necrosis suggests the presence of a high-grade tumor (Fig. 23-11)

Histology

- Well-differentiated (low-grade) liposarcoma
  - Mostly mature adipocytes; occasional atypical lipoblasts (Fig. 23-10*b*)
  - Complex "chicken-wire" vascular patterns seen in some cases
- High-grade sarcoma
  - Coexistence of both high-grade sarcoma and low-grade liposarcoma is the evidence of dedifferentiation (Fig. 23-11)
  - High-grade sarcoma shows high cellularity, increased mitoses, and cytological atypia, resembling malignant fibrous histiocytoma, fibrosarcoma, or pleomorphic sarcoma (Fig. 23-11*d*)

Figure 23-10.
Gross photo of a liposarcoma located above the testis with white-yellow cut surface (*a*). Microscopically, this well-differentiated liposarcoma showing chicken-wire patterns and the presence of lipoblasts in the middle (*b*).

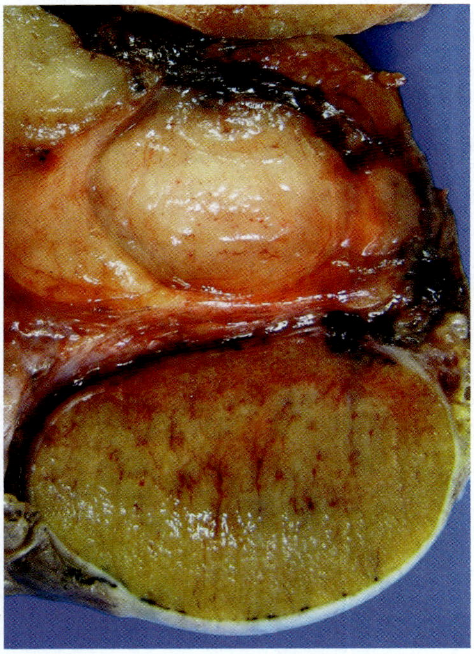

a

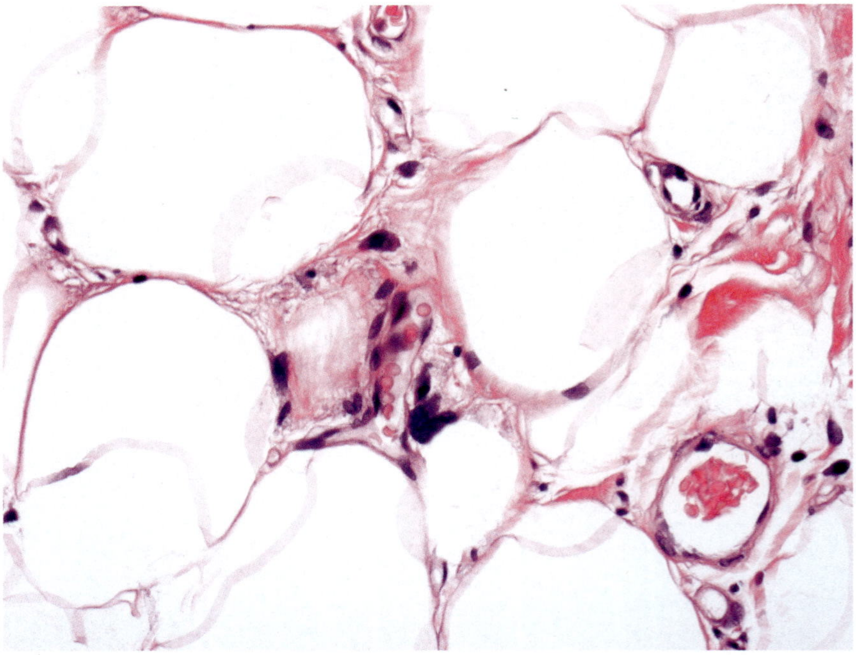

b

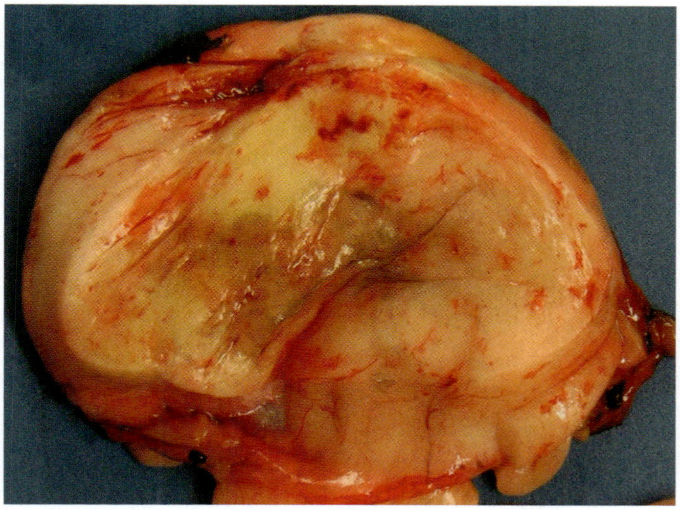

a

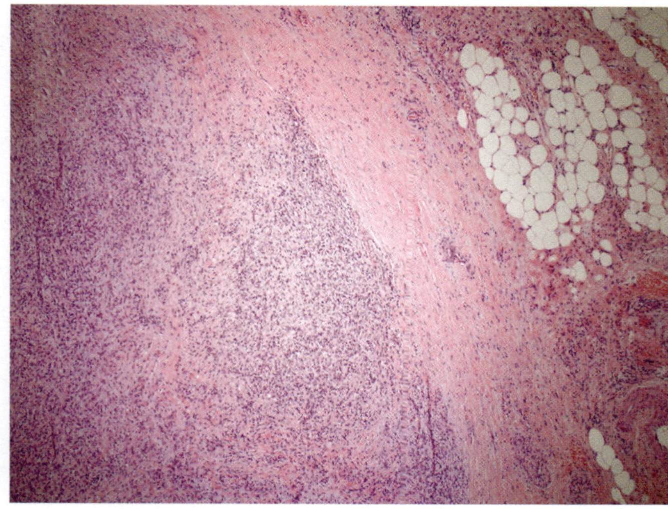

b

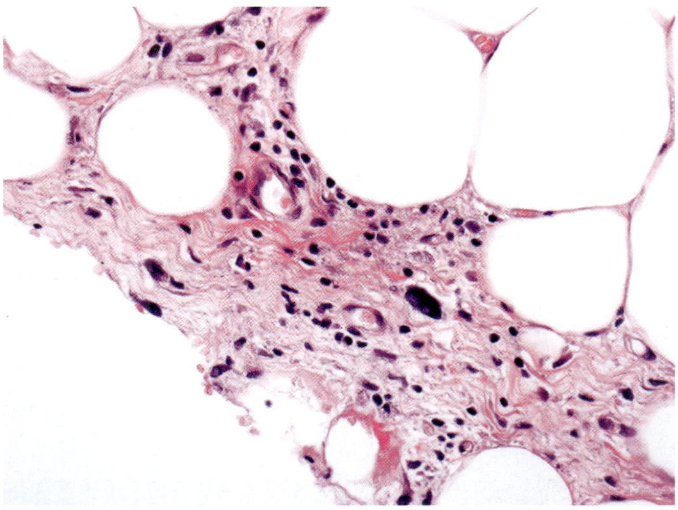

c

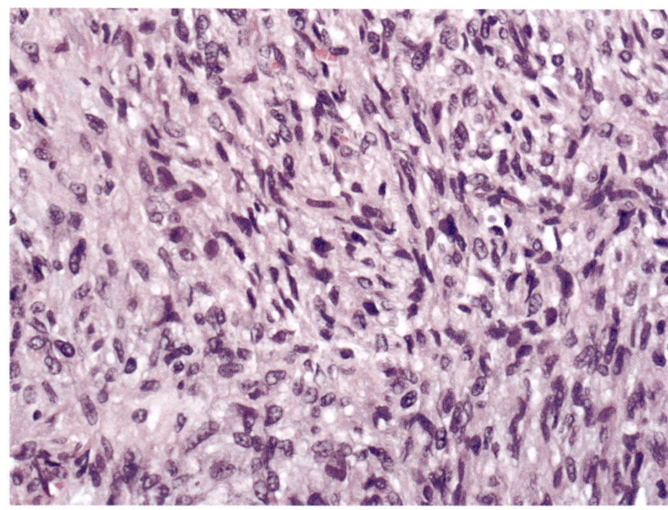

d

Figure 23-11.

Dedifferentiated liposarcoma. Paratesticular tumor showing yellow and fleshy areas with spotty hemorrhage in cut surface (*a*). Low magnification (*b*) shows two components: low-grade liposarcoma (right) and high-grade sarcoma (left). High magnification confirms the presence of low-grade liposarcomatous (*c*) and cellular high-grade sarcomatous (*d*) components.

Immunohistochemistry

- Vimentin, S100 positive
- CD 36, MDM2 and CDK 4 positive

Differential diagnosis

- Spermatic cord lipoma: lipoma is much more common. Bright yellow gross appearance. No cytological atypia, particularly in the septa

Molecular analysis

- 12q12-q15 amplification

Clinical relevance (prognosis and treatment options)

- Surgical resection is the treatment of choice, good prognosis if complete resection
- Recurrent rate is relatively high
- High-grade sarcoma carries much worse prognosis

METASTATIC PROSTATIC ADENOCARCINOMA IN TESTIS

Definition

- Prostatic adenocarcinoma metastasizes to the testis

Clinical features

- A history of prostate cancer, typically high-grade adenocarcinoma (Gleason score 8-10)
- Elevated serum PSA, older age (not typical age for germ cell tumor)

Gross pathology

- The testis is usually small and atrophic particularly with posthormonal treatment
- Well-circumscribed mass or diffusely replacing entire testis with white or tan cut surface
- Hemorrhage and necrosis commonly present

Histology

- Very important to obtain clinical history of the prostate cancer for a more accurate diagnosis including (1) the age of the patient; (2) the time of diagnosis; (3) the Gleason grade of the original prostate cancer; (4) the treatment history
- Clues suggesting metastatic carcinoma rather than germ cell tumors include: history of another primary cancer, age, bilateral involvement, lack of ITGCNU, and lack of other components of germ cell tumor such as seminoma or teratoma
- Some metastatic prostatic adenocarcinomas may display typical features such as cribriform patterns, fused glands, less pleomorphic appearance, and prominent cherry red nucleoli (Fig. 23-12)
- Metastatic prostatic adenocarcinomas, particularly those hormonal resistant and/or postradiation, may exhibit greater cytological pleomorphism (Fig. 23-12*b*), which can mimic embryonal carcinoma or choriocarcinoma

Immunohistochemistry

- PSA positive but often focal in high-grade prostatic adenocarcinoma (Fig. 23-12*c*)
- AMACR positive in both low-grade and high-grade prostatic adenocarcinoma (Fig. 23-12*d*), but it can be also positive in other cancers such as colonic adenocarcinoma
- AE1/AE3, CAM5.2 positive and germ cell markers (PLAP, C-kit, OCT-4, CD30) negative

Molecular analysis

- Not indicated for diagnosis

Clinical relevance (prognosis and treatment options)

- Metastatic carcinoma can be easily misdiagnosed as germ cell tumor, embryonal type, which is primitive carcinoma with marked pleomorphism
- Clinical information is important. One should be extremely cautious to make a diagnosis of seminoma/germ cell tumor in a man older than 60 years
- Metastatic carcinoma in the testis has poor prognosis. However, it may respond better to different therapies than a germ cell tumor

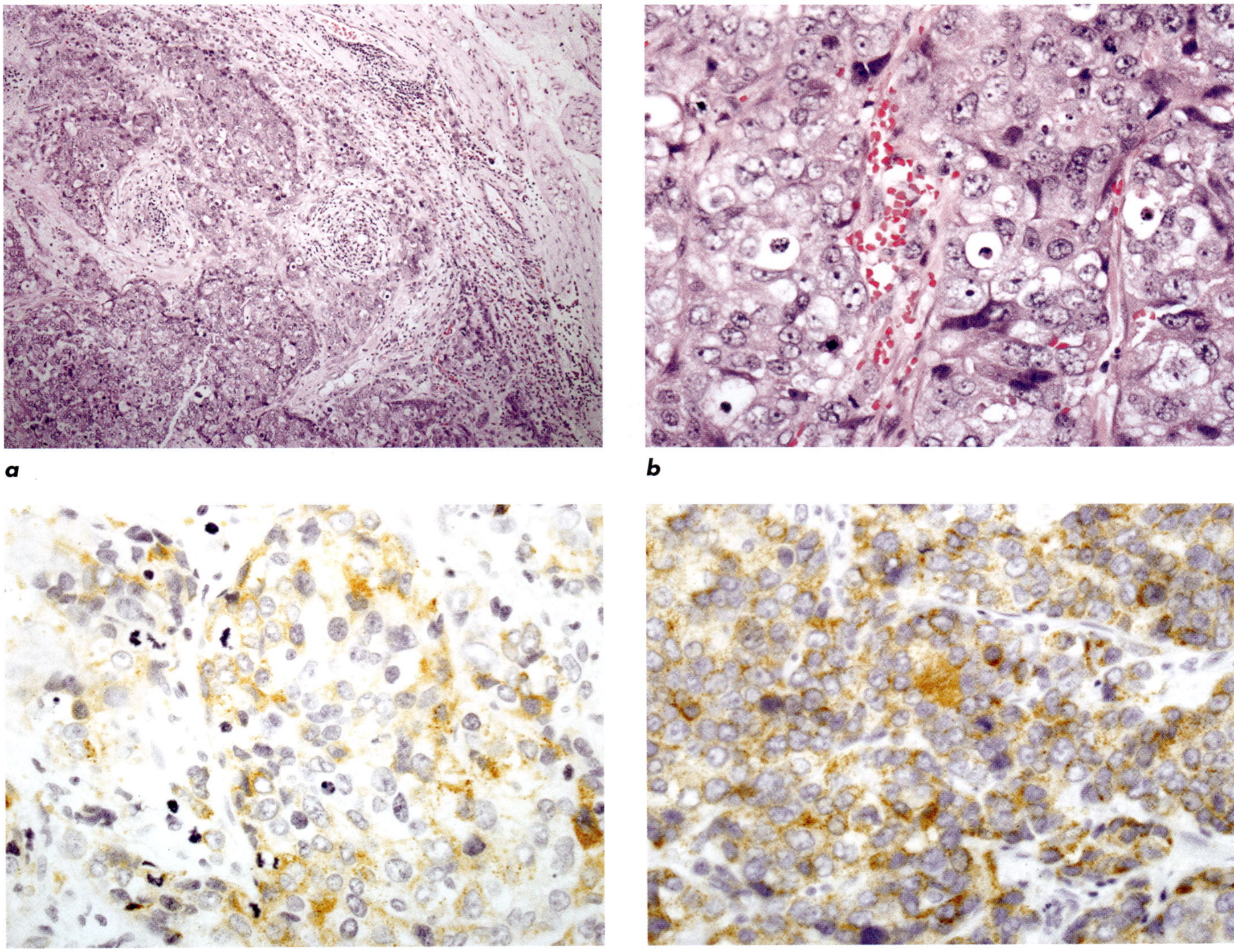

a b c d

Figure 23-12.

Metastatic prostatic adenocarcinoma in the testis. The tumor cells form island and sheets, without glandular formation (*a*). The tumor cells are large and pleomorphic with prominent nucleoli, which can be easily confused with embryonal carcinoma (*b*). They are positive for PSA (*c*) and AMACR (*d*), which confirms the diagnosis of high-grade (Gleason 5 + 5) metastatic prostatic adenocarcinoma.

MERKEL CELL CARCINOMA INVOLVING THE TESTIS

Definition

- Neuroendocrine carcinoma, primarily developing in the skin, involves the testis

Other terms

- Cutaneous APUDoma, small cell carcinoma of the skin, neuroendocrine carcinoma of the skin, trabecular carcinoma of the skin

Pathogenesis

- The development of Merkel cell carcinoma is probably related to a virus named Merkel cell polyoma virus
- Testicular Merkel cell carcinoma can be metastatic from a distant skin site or direct extension from penis/scrotum skin

Clinical features

- This tumor typically develops in the sun-exposed areas, but it can be seen in the penis or scrotal skin as a primary tumor
- Presents as a firm painless nodule growing rapidly

Gross pathology

- Nodules or mass with red-blue or flesh color with or without ulceration

Histology

- Primary tumor is located in the deep scrotal skin, centered around the dermis and subcutaneous, which may be on the surface of tunica vaginalis (Fig. 23-13*a*)
- The epidermis is spared
- Tumor cells are monotonous, round small tumor cells with scant cytoplasm, and vesicular nuclei with fine granular chromatin and multiple nucleoli (Fig. 23-13*b*)
- Brisk mitotic activities and apoptosis similar to small cell carcinoma of the lung

Immunohistochemistry

- CK20 shows a unique perinuclear dot-like staining pattern
- Neuroendocrine markers, keratins markers, and EMA are positive

Clinical relevance (prognosis and treatment options)

- Tumor is aggressive
- Treatments include wide surgical excision, lymph node dissection and radiation
- Small and early tumor without metastasis has better prognosis (5-year survival more than 80%)
- With effective treatment, the survival rate has been improving

Figure 23-13.
Merkel cell carcinoma secondarily involving the testis, composed of small blue cells (*a*). Tumor cells are small cells with vesicular nuclei, "salt-and-pepper" chromatin and scant cytoplasm (*b*).

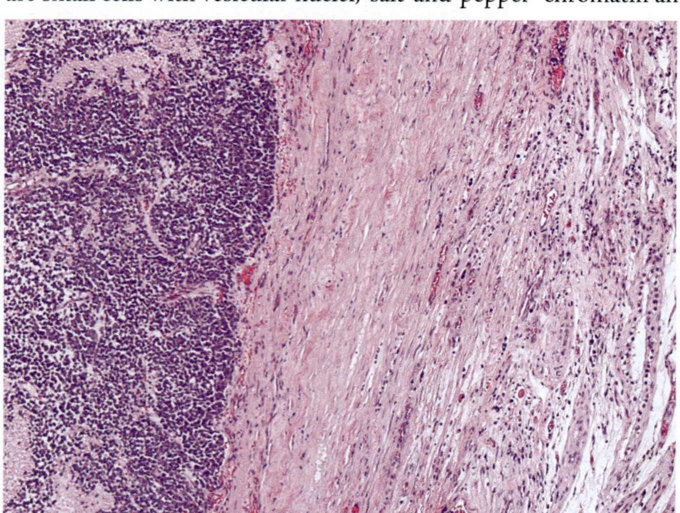

a

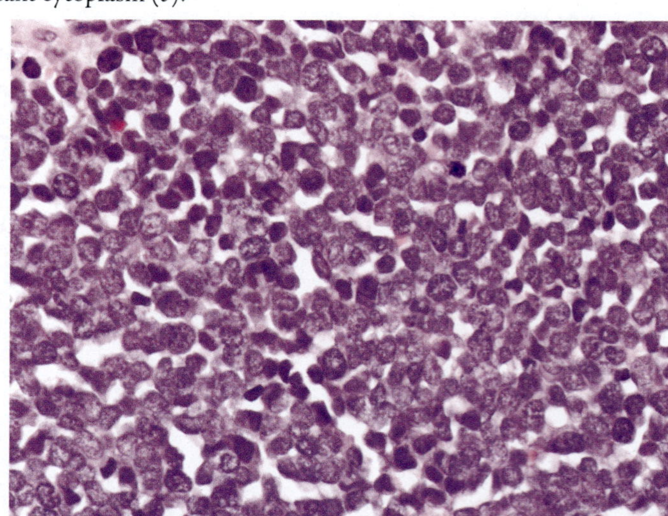

b

PARATESTICULAR MALIGNANT MESOTHELIOMA

Definition

- Malignant neoplasm arising from the mesothelial lining in the paratesticular region including, tunica vaginalis, spermatic cord, or epididymis
- This tumor may also develop in the other GU organs

Pathogenesis

- May be associated with exposure to asbestos, although this association is weaker than that of pleural mesothelioma

Clinical features

- Rare but highly aggressive tumor, mostly affecting older men (mean age = 65 years)
- Presenting as intrascrotal mass, and it may be associated with secondary hydrocele

Gross pathology

- Multiple masses involving the surface of tunica vaginalis
- The tunica vaginalis is significantly thickened
- The lesion may invade testis or adjacent tissues

Histology

- Tumor involving the surface of tunica vaginalis rather than testicular parenchyma (Fig. 23-14*a*)
- Tumor cells exhibit nuclear atypia with vesicular nuclei and variable amount of eosinophilic cytoplasm, forming tubular and papillary patterns (Fig. 23-14*b*) infiltrating surrounding tissues

Immunohistochemistry

- Positive for cytokeratins, EMA, calretinin, WT1, CK5/6
- Negative for CEA, CK20

Clinical relevance (prognosis and treatment options)

- Aggressive with a capacity of widespread with a high mortality rate and high recurrence rate
- Radical orchiectomy required, with possible chemotherapy

Figure 23-14.
Malignant mesothelioma involving the testis. The tumor is composed of mostly epithelioid cells and some spindle cells (*a*). Higher magnification shows the epithelioid tumor cells form slit-like structures (*b*). The tumor cells are positive for calretinin (not shown).

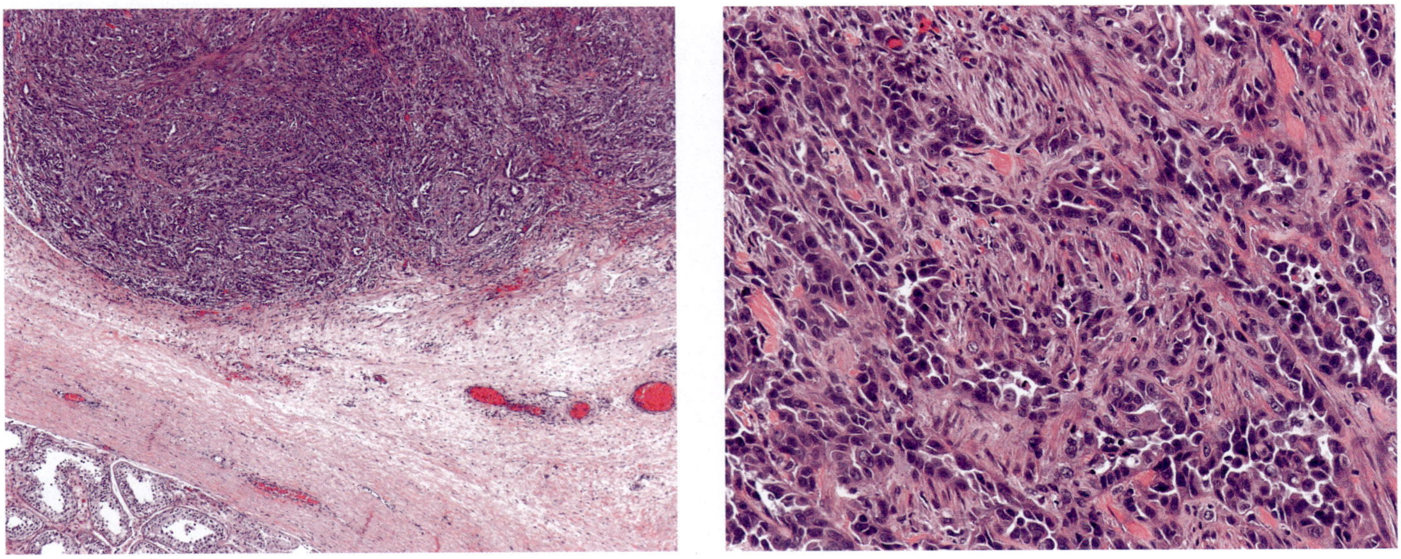

a *b*

PARATESTICULAR RHABDOMYOSARCOMA

Definition

- A malignant neoplasm with skeletal muscle differentiation develops in the paratesticular region
- May develop in other GU organs or regions such as spermatic cord, bladder, and prostate

Pathogenesis

- PAX3/FKHR fusion may be related to the tumor development

Clinical features

- Typically young patients (mean age = 9)
- Mass located in spermatic cord or tissue adjacent to the testis
- Fast-growing tumor with metastasis in lung and other organs

Gross pathology

- Lobulated large mass with white, gray, or tan cut surface with gelatinous appearance
- Focal hemorrhage and cystic changes

Histology

- Embryonal type: small round cells with myoblasts and myxoid background (Fig. 23-15)
- Other types include spindle cell type, alveolar type, and pleomorphic type
- Strap-shape myoblasts can be seen in some cases
- Some tumor cells will show cross-striations

Immunohistochemistry

- Muscle markers MyoD1 and myogenin are positive
- Desmin is positive although not specific for skeletal muscle

Molecular analysis

- PAX3/FKHR fusion

Clinical relevance (prognosis and treatment options)

- Poor prognosis for alveolar and pleomorphic types
- Better prognosis for spindle cell type and embryonal types
- Surgery with radiation and chemotherapy

Figure 23-15.
Testicular rhabdomyosarcoma composed of small primitive cells and large tadpole-shaped myoblasts with abundant eosinophilic cytoplasm (*a*). The positive desmin immunostaining in the tumor cells confirms diagnosis of rhabdomyosarcoma (*b*).

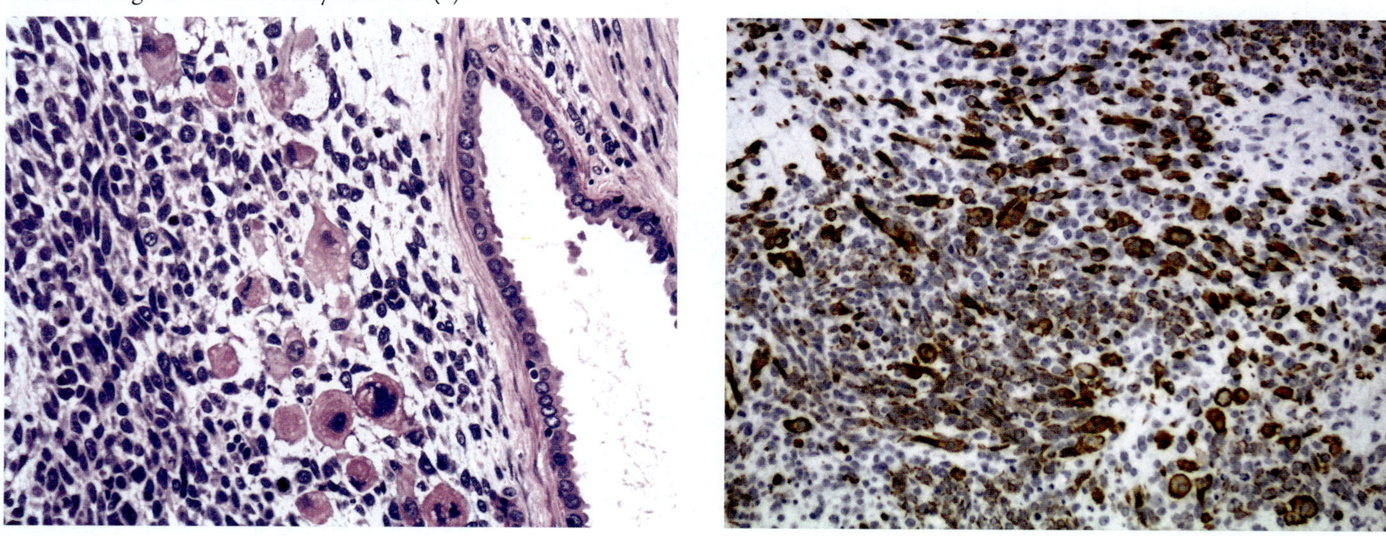

a **b**

SECTION 3
The Penis and Scrotum

CHAPTER 24 Normal Histology of the Penis and Scrotum

PENIS

Anatomy

- The penis contains three cylindrical-shaped erectile structures
  - Two corpora cavernosa in the dorsal aspect of the penis
  - One corpus spongiosum (also known as corpus carvernosum urethrae) in the midline of the ventral aspect of the penis with the penile urethra passing through
- The outside layers of the penis are skin and subcutaneous tissue
- The enlarged portion of penis is the glans penis, which is covered by the foreskin
- The meatus is the urethral opening at the tip of the glans penis

Histology

- Foreskin is covered by nonpigmented mucosa (inside) and heavily pigmented skin (outside), associated with hair, sweat glands, and small smooth muscle bundles (Fig. 24-1)
- The corpora cavernosa are surrounded by the dense connective tissue sheet: tunica albuginea that is approximately 2 mm in thickness
- Erectile tissue of the penis, in both corpora cavernosa and corpus spongiosum, consists of large cavernous vascular channels (cavernosal spaces) lined by endothelium, separated by fibromuscular septa (Fig. 24-2)
- The amount of blood in the erectile tissue channels essentially determine the size of an erected penis
- There are numerous thick-walled arteries called helicine arteries (Fig. 24-3), in the erectile tissue, which supply the blood to the channels of the erectile tissue
- Penile urethra is lined by urothelium with the presence of outpouching periurethral glands
- The penile skin also contains skin adnexa including hair follicles, sebaceous glands, sweat glands, and smooth muscle bundles of erector pilli
- Therefore, the penis is subjected to conventional skin lesions, sexually transmitted lesions such as condylomas, and urothelial lesions

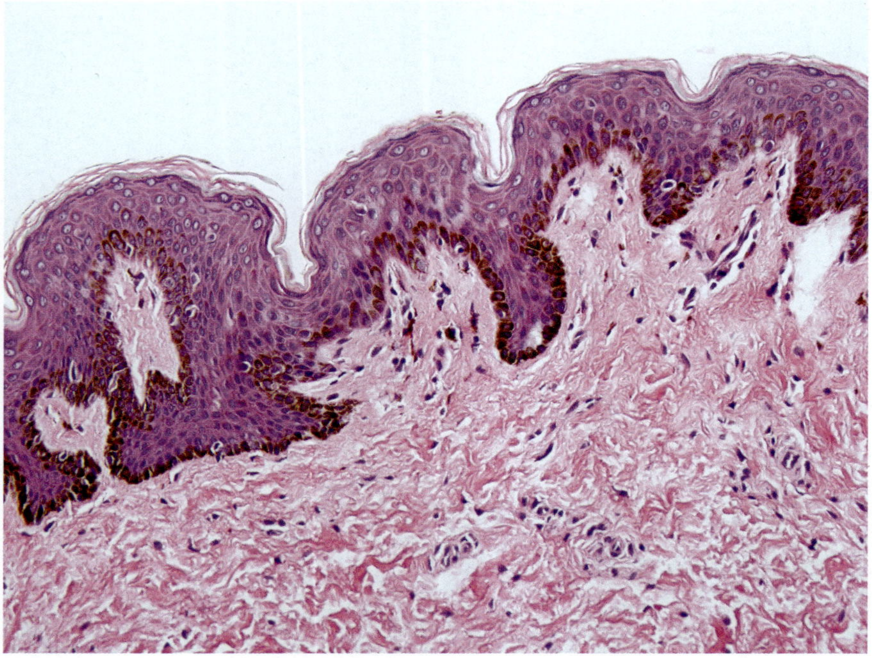

Figure 24-1.
Adult foreskin. The outside portion of the foreskin is heavily pigmented skin with keratinization.

Figure 24-2.
The corpus cavernosum consists of erectile tissue (*a*, right) surrounded by thick tunica albuginea (*a*, left). High magnification shows the erectile tissue of the penis is composed of vascular spaces separated by smooth muscle septa (*b*).

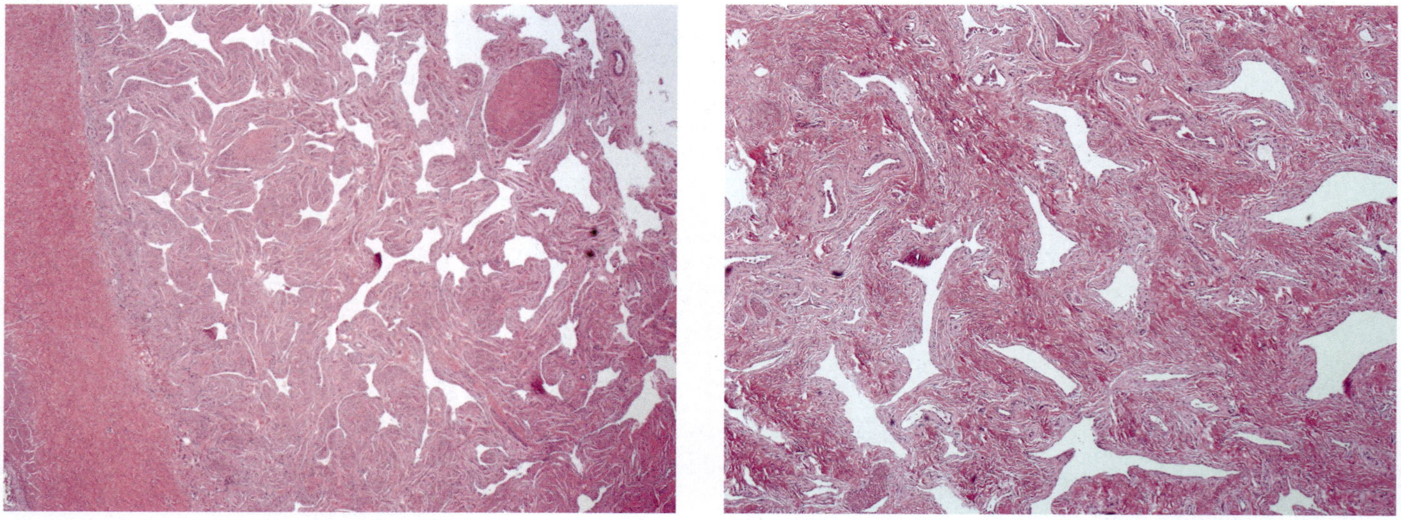

a **b**

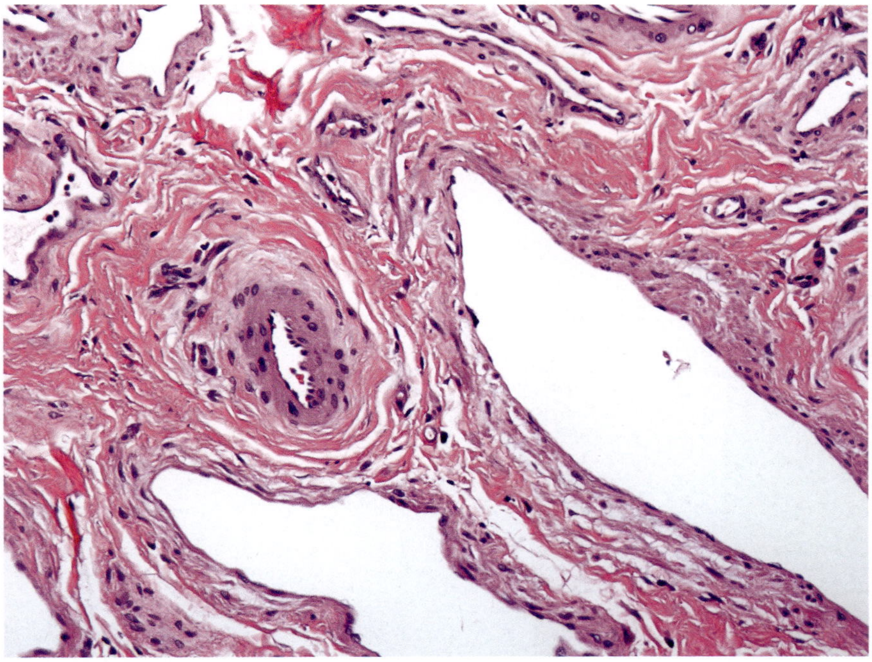

Figure 24-3.
A thick-walled artery (helicine artery) present in the corpus erectile tissue.

SCROTUM

- The scrotum is a specialized skin, with hair, sweat glands, sebaceous glands, and apocrine glands as well as subcutaneous tissue for protection of the testes (Fig. 24-4).
- The function of the scrotum is to keep the temperature of the testes slightly lower than that of the rest of the body at 35°C to 36°C.
- The scrotum skin is specialized with abundant smooth muscle bundles called the *elevator muscle* (Fig. 24-5)
- When the outside temperature gets cold, these smooth muscle bundles contract and elevate the scrotum and testes, resulting in the wrinkled appearance of the scrotum
- Scrotum skin is subjected to other skin lesions

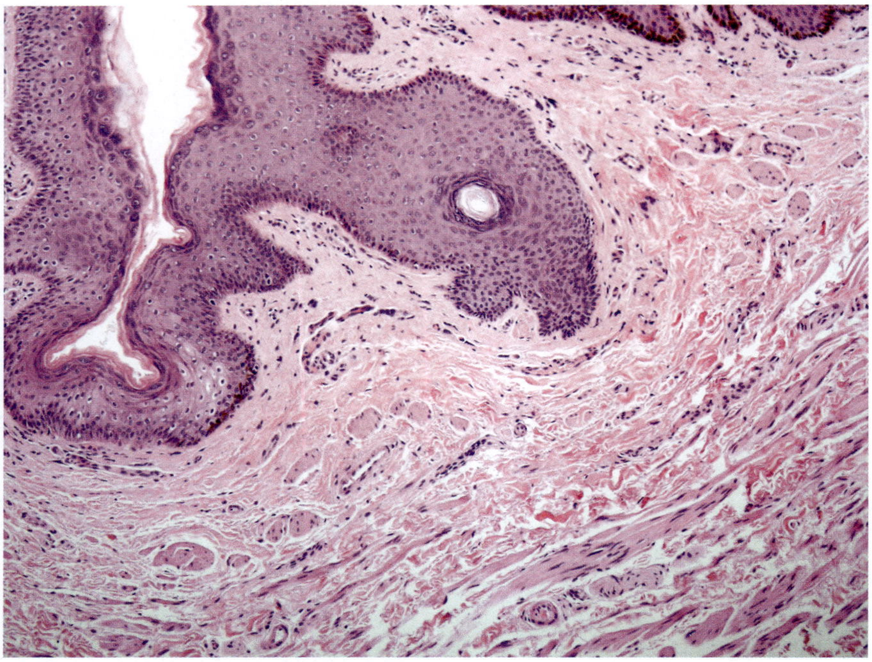

Figure 24-4.
Scrotal skin is slightly thicker than the penile skin and with many epidermal folds. In the dermis there are numerous smooth muscle bundles (elevator muscle) seen in the lower portion of the photo.

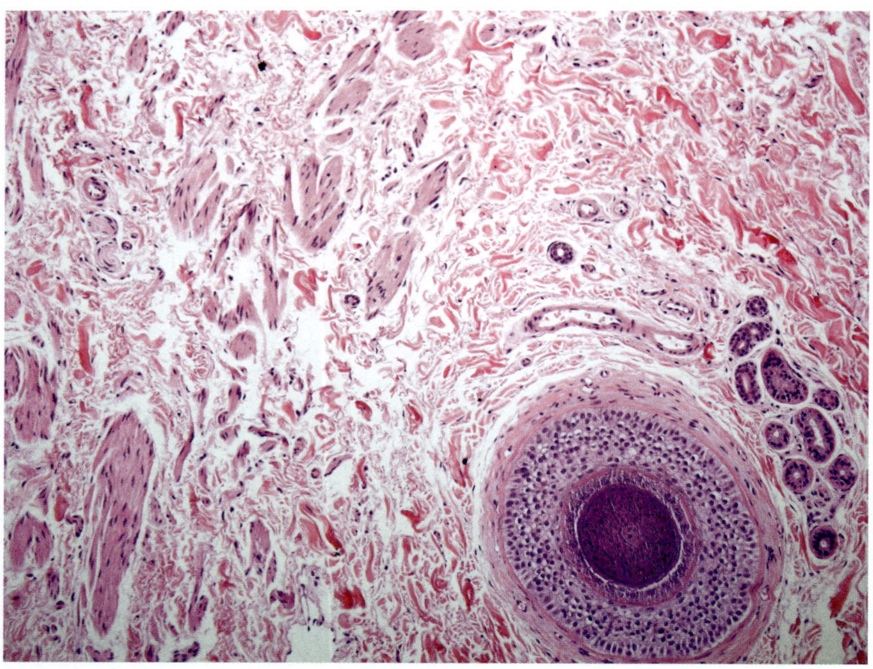

Figure 24-5.
In addition to elevator muscles, there are skin adnexa in the scrotal skin such as hair follicle, sweat glands, and sebaceous glands (not shown here).

CHAPTER 25

Benign Reactive Lesions of the Penis and Scrotum

FIBROEPITHELIAL POLYP

Definition

- A benign polypoid lesion composed of fibrovascular core covered by benign squamous epithelium
- Chronic stimulation or prior low-risk HPV infection may contribute to its development

Other terms

- Skin tag, acrochordon, cutaneous tag

Clinical features

- A polypoid (tag-like) painless skin lesion, typically no change of color or shape over time
- Mostly seen in the areas with skin creases, such as scrotum, vulva, and other groin areas, armpit, head and neck region

Gross pathology

- Small skin-colored lesions less than 1 to 2 cm in size, with smooth surface, may have a stalk

Histology

- Polypoid lesion with two components including (Fig. 25-1)
  - Fibrovascular core with prominent small dilated vessels
  - Squamous epithelium with variable thickness without koilocytic changes

Immunohistochemistry and molecular analysis

- Typically not necessary, negative for p16 and HPV tests

Differential diagnosis

- Condyloma: koilocytic changes present
- Squamous dysplasia: squamous epithelium with cytological atypia
- Seborrheic keratosis: with thickened epidermis and horn cysts

Clinical relevance (prognosis and treatment options)

- Benign lesion, treatment not necessary unless symptomatic or suspicious for other lesions
- Surgical resection may be necessary if it is frequently broken, hemorrhage, or associated with infection
- Methods of removal include surgical excision, cryosurgery, or cauterization by lesser or other physical measures

Figure 25-1.
Fibroepithelial polyp is a polypoid lesion with fibrovascular core with prominent small dilated vessels covered by squamous epithelium (*a*). The squamous epithelium of a fibroepithelial polyp is variable in thickness without HPV changes or dysplasia (*b*).

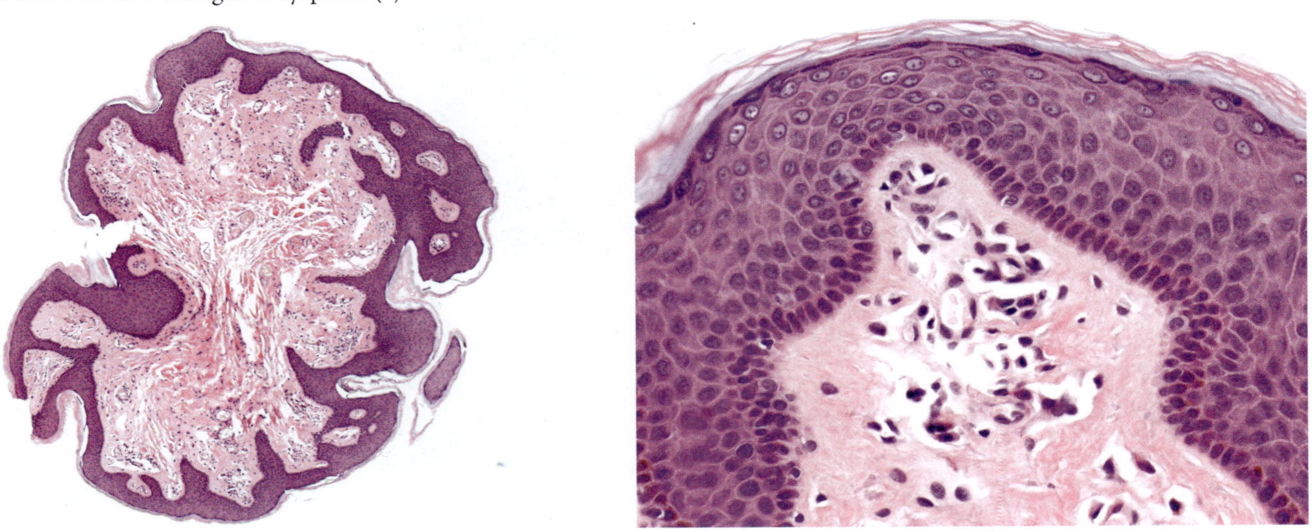

a *b*

SEBORRHEIC KERATOSIS

Definition

- Benign squamous proliferative lesion of the skin

Clinical features

- One of the most common lesions of the skin. Mostly located on face, but also on the extremities, not in the palms and soles
- Uncommonly seen in external genital areas.
- Typically a small slow growing lesion, a few millimeters in diameter
- It develops in the middle age, single or multiple painless, slightly itching
- Some lesions may be inflamed as irritated seborrheic keratosis

Gross pathology

- Dark-brown, waxy surface, slightly raised lesion with "stuck-on-surface" appearance

Histology

- Several patterns have been described with some common features
- Hyperkeratosis and acanthosis (thickening) (Fig. 25-2) present, may also display papillomatous changes
- Composed of predominantly benign basaloid cells and some squamous cells
- *Horn cysts* are keratin tunnels, which contain whorls of keratin in the middle (Fig. 25-2)
- Irritated seborrheic keratosis shows irregularity and disorganization of the squamous epithelial cells

Differential diagnosis

- Basal cell carcinoma: neoplastic basal cells forming nests with a palisading periphery, with invasive growth patterns
- Squamous cell carcinoma: significant cytological atypia and loss of polarity, with keratin pearls, and invading dermis and other tissue

Clinical relevance (prognosis and treatment options)

- Benign condition

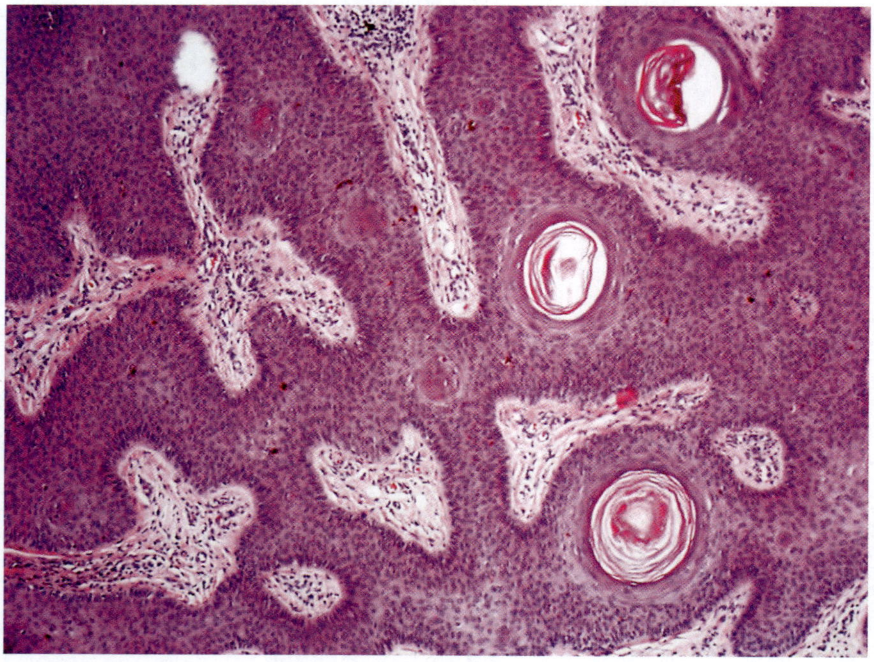

Figure 25-2.
Seborrheic keratosis. Islands of squamous cells form anastomosing nests, without cytological atypia, and the presence of multiple horn cysts containing whorls of keratin is characteristic.

LICHEN SCLEROSUS

Definition

- Lichen sclerosus (LS) is a chronic inflammatory condition of the skin, which leads to development of white plaques with epidermal atrophy and eventually sclerosis of the dermis

Other terms

- Lichen sclerosus et atrophicus, balanitis xerotica obliterans (when the lesion is confined to the glans penis)

Pathogenesis

- LS occurs in men of a wide range of age groups, essentially the same type of lesion affecting women genital areas
- LS mostly involves genital areas, particularly foreskin, glans penis, meatus, and distal urethra. The extragenital presentations may occasionally occur
- The etiology is not defined. HPV infection or autoimmune have been speculated but not confirmed

Clinical features

- One of the most common causes of urethral stricture. It may lead to phimosis in adults

Gross pathology

- White plaques involving penile skin, most commonly in the foreskin, but can be seen in glans penis, penile urethra, and bulbar urethra

Histology

- Two types of lesions can be seen in various proportions, which may represent early and late stage of the disease
- Inflammatory (early) phase
  - Chronic inflammation: lichenoid band-like inflammatory cells in the upper dermis (Fig. 25-3)
  - Epidermal changes: variable thickness of epidermis, atrophy of epidermis coexisting with hyperkeratosis, and variable degree of basal cell loss (Fig. 25-3*b*)
- Sclerosing (late) phase
  - Prominent atrophic epidermis and loss of basal cells (Fig. 25-4)
  - Hyalinized stroma (sclerosing) in the upper dermis (Fig. 25-5)
  - Calcification and ossification may be also present in the advanced LS (Fig 25-6)
  - Early phase and late phase changes may be seen in one case
  - Presence of dysplasia or squamous cell carcinoma should be carefully evaluated in both early and late phases

Immunohistochemistry

- P16 is often positive in early phase, but negative in the late phase

Clinical relevance (prognosis and treatment options)

- Topical medication may relieve symptoms for the early phase
- The sclerosing stage of the lesions would be difficult to reverse. Surgical excision if involving foreskin or urethral stricture present. Buccal mucosa transplant has shown some success
- There is an increased risk for developing squamous cell carcinoma; therefore, follow-up and rebiopsy may be necessary

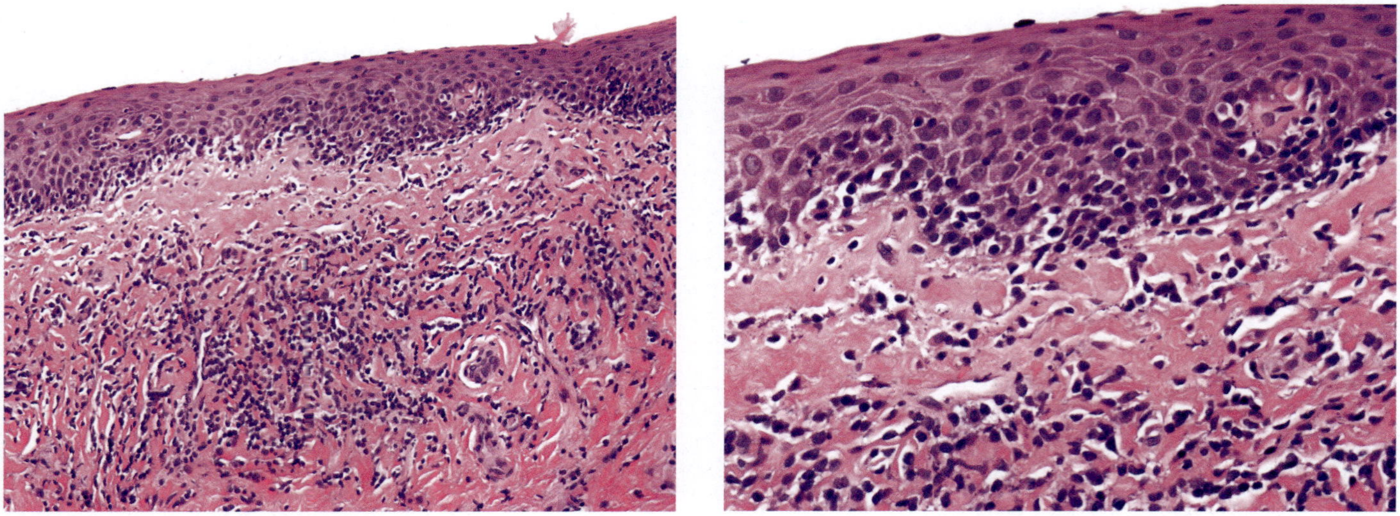

a *b*

Figure 25-3.
Early phase lichen sclerosus, with band-like chronic inflammation in the dermis and the epidermis with uneven thickness (*a*). High magnification shows intraepithelial lymphocytes, loss of basal cells, and early fibrosis of the upper dermis (*b*).

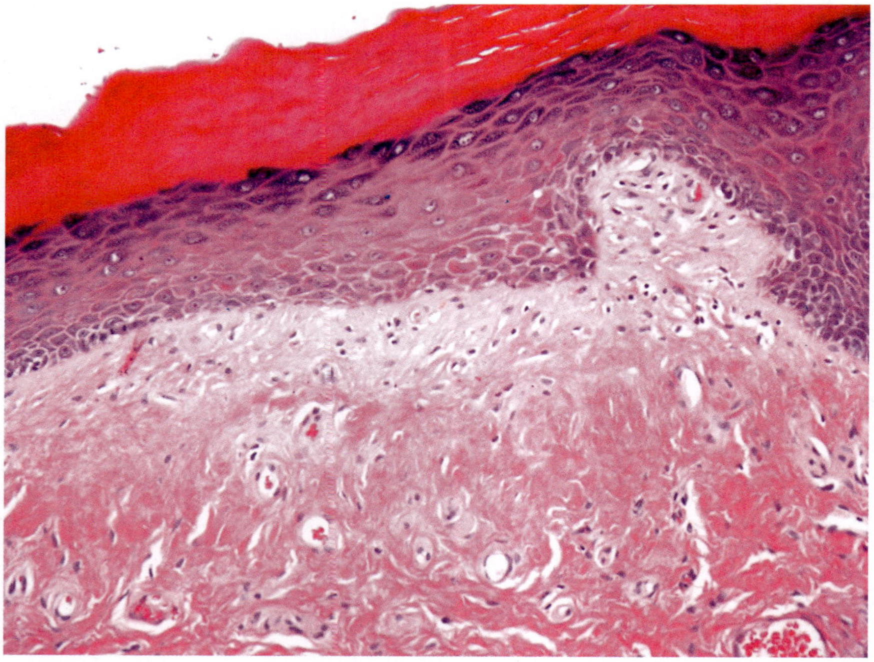

Figure 25-4.
Late phase lichen sclerosus, showing atrophy and hyperkeratosis of the epidermis. The loss of basal cell and dermal fibrosis are evident.

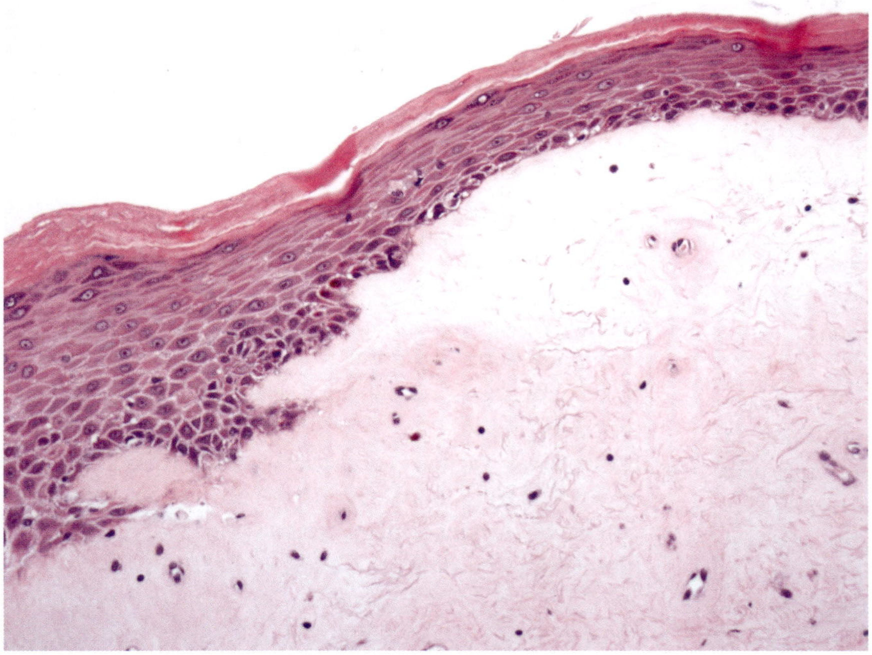

Figure 25-5.
Late phase lichen sclerosus shows prominent hyalinized dermis and complete loss of basal cells.

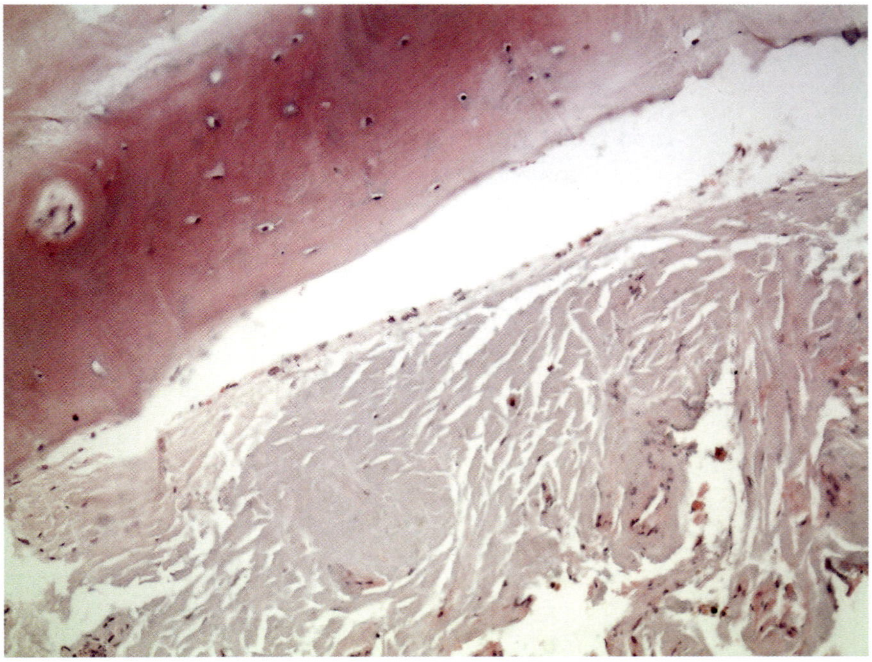

Figure 25-6.
Ossification in a hyalinized fibrotic area in late lichen sclerosus.

LIPOGRANULOMA OF THE PENIS

Definition

- Granulomatous reaction to the presence of foreign lipid material

Other terms

- Sclerosing lipogranuloma when fibrosis present; primary lipogranuloma if injection history cannot be found

Pathogenesis

- Lipogranuloma is mostly caused by reaction to an injection of exogenous lipid-rich material in the penis, which may also occur in the scrotum, testis, or other male genital organs
- Typically this is a self-administered process in order to enhance the appearance or performance of male genitalia. The injected material may contain paraffin, silicon, or other oily material
- Occasionally, trauma or surgical procedures to the penis or genital areas induce fat necrosis, which leads to lipogranulomatous reaction

Clinical features

- A history of injection or trauma should be present; however, it may not be provided initially
- A painless mass lesion in the penis, often common in young or middle-age males, typically
- When associated with secondary trauma, hemorrhage, or infection, the lesion will be painful, red, or swollen

Gross pathology

- Mass lesion with yellow cut surface

Histology

- Granulomatous inflammation composed mainly of histiocytes, foreign body giant cells, and other inflammatory cells (Fig. 25-7)
- Presence of vacuoles of variable sizes (dissolved lipid material during histology tissue processing) inside or outside histiocytes is characteristic (Fig. 25-7)
- Fibrosis may become prominent in the later phase

Immunohistochemistry

- CD68 positive for histiocytes

Clinical relevance (prognosis and treatment options)

- Symptomatic cases may need surgical removal. Some cases may be inactive or spontaneously resolved

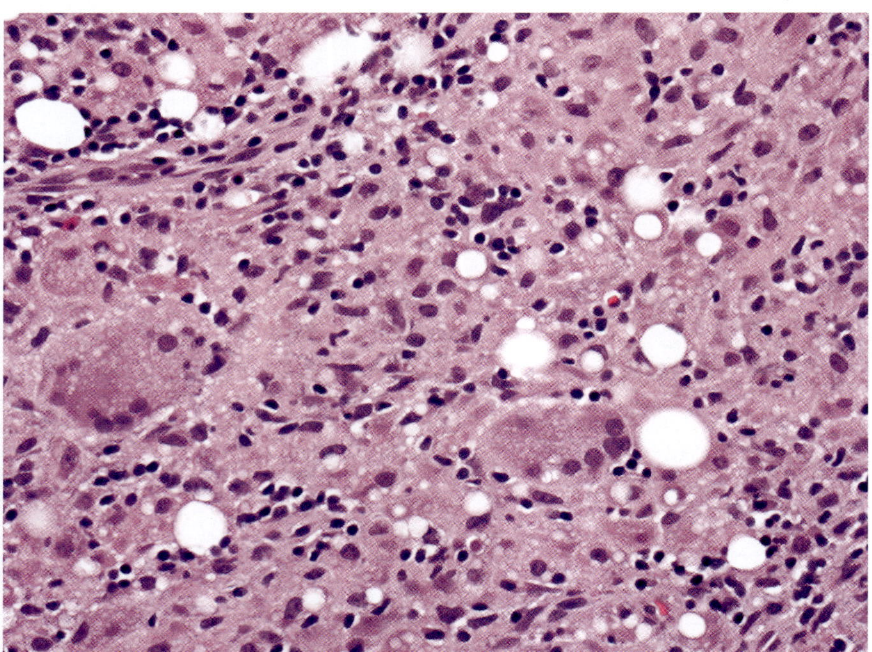

Figure 25-7.
Lipogranuloma composed of histiocytes containing lipid droplets in the cytoplasm, several multinucleated giant cells, and lymphocytes.

LYMPHEDEMA OF THE PENIS OR SCROTUM

Definition

- Edema caused by lymphatic blockage

Pathogenesis

- Lymphatic obstruction is the direct cause of lymphedema. The blockage of the lymphatics will lead lymph fluid accumulated in tissue, which is lymphedema
- Penile lymphedema is either primary or secondary
  - Secondary lymphedema includes parasite infection (filariasis), radiation, bacterial infections; lymph node removal for treatment of cancer or trauma
  - Primary lymphedema: unknown cause
  - Congenital lymphedema is present at birth

Clinical features

- Persistence of penile or scrotal swelling. Leg swelling may be also present in extensive cases

Gross pathology

- Penile or scrotal swelling

Histology

- Dilated lymphatic channels, with or without proteinaceous (lymphatic) fluid (Fig. 25-8)
- Tissue edema caused by the accumulation of lymphatic fluid
- Lymphangitis signified by lymphocytic infiltrates (Fig. 25-9), which is the cause of lymphedema in this case

Clinical relevance (prognosis and treatment options)

- The major complication is widespread cellulitis and secondary infection
- Other complications include loss of sexual function and difficulties in urination
- Conservative treatment including compression with bandages or manual lymph drainage may not be applicable in penile lymphedema
- Less invasive surgery such as fasciectomy may preserve the sexual function

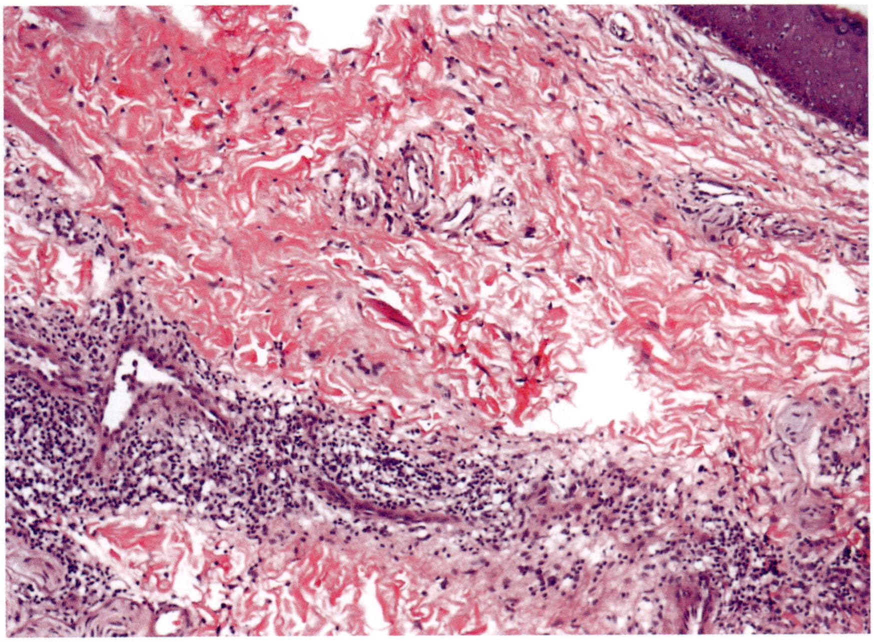

Figure 25-8.
Lymphedema with a portion of penile skin and subcutaneous tissue showing chronic inflammation around lymphatics (lymphangitis).

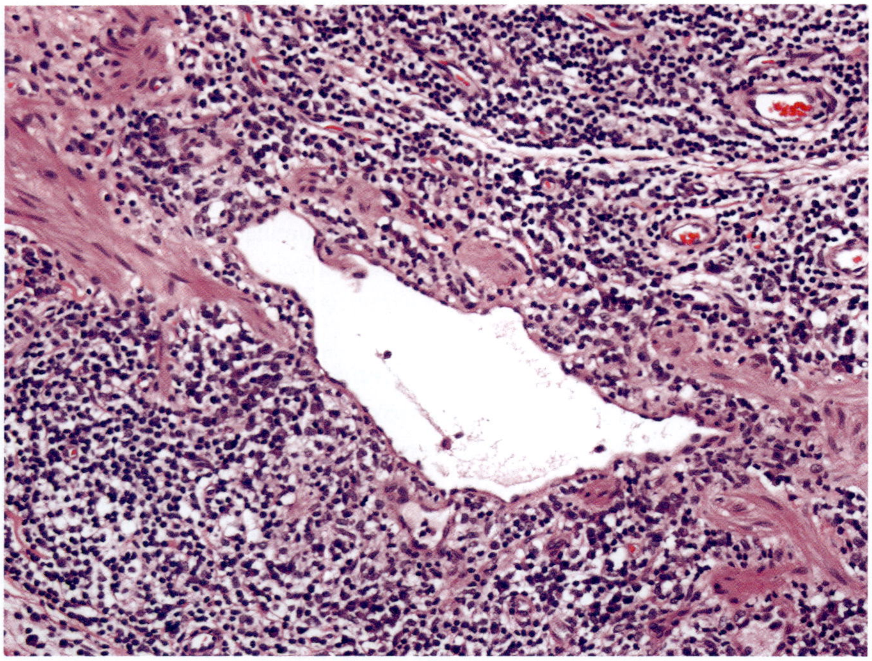

Figure 25-9.
A lymphatic channel with marked chronic inflammation and dilation.

PENILE ULCERATION

Definition

- An ulcer develops in the penis skin with a wide range of causes

Pathogenesis

- The majority of chronic penile ulcers are caused by sexually transmitted diseases such as syphilis, chancroid, or *Chlamydia trachomatis*
- Other infectious etiology may occur caused by bacteria, TB, or fungi
- Noninfectious etiology may include injury, autoimmune connective tissue disease such as lupus, rheumatoid arthritis, or Behcet disease
- In most cases, it is not possible to identify the pathogen in the biopsy specimens by histological examination alone, microbiology studies are often essential to determine the etiology

Clinical features

- Painful or painless penile ulcers, mostly located in the glans penis or shaft

Gross pathology

- Ulceration or defect of skin

Histology

- Defect and necrosis of the penile skin with granulation tissue, associated with acute or chronic inflammation and fibrosis (Fig. 25-10)
- The presence of special etiology such as bacteria, or virus effect may be identified histologically (see Chapter 27)

Immunohistochemistry

- May be useful to identify specific infectious etiologies

Clinical relevance (prognosis and treatment options)

- Pathological features often are not specific
- Identification of etiology by microbiology and serology will lead to the best treatment

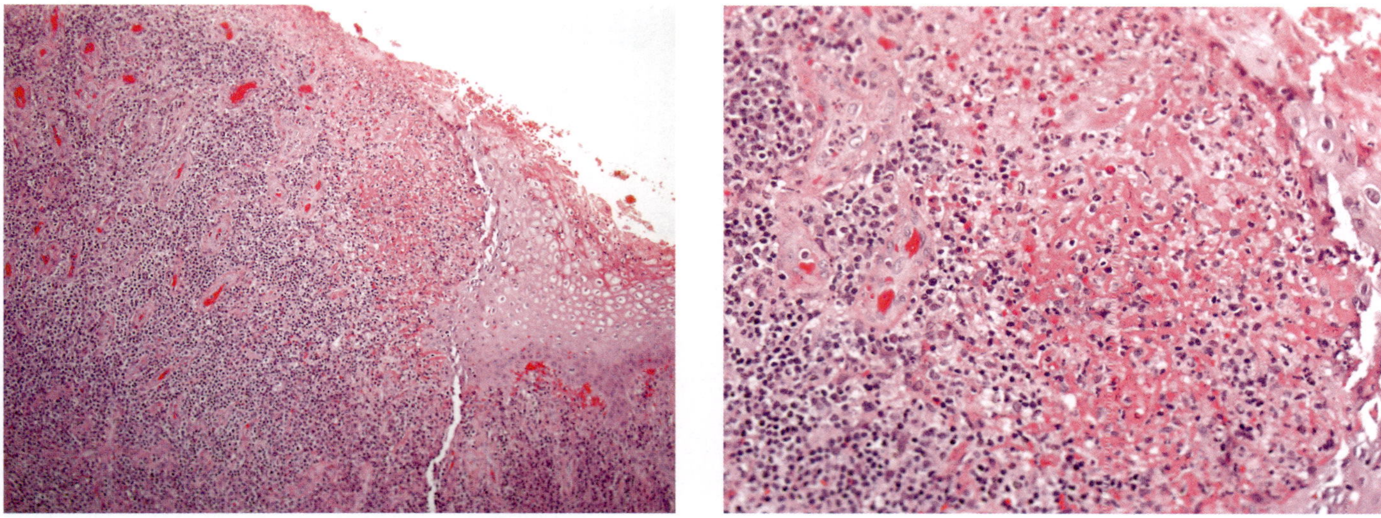

a **b**

Figure 25-10.
Penile ulcer. A portion of skin is replaced by necrotic tissue and fibrinoid exudate, granulation tissue, and chronic inflammation (*a*). High magnification shows the presence of necrotic tissue and chronic inflammatory infiltrates in the base of the ulcer (*b*).

CHAPTER 26

Benign Neoplasms and Tumor-Like Lesions of the Penis and Scrotum

LYMPHANGIOMA CIRCUMSCRIPTUM OF THE PENIS

Definition

- Congenital malformation of lymphatics in the superficial areas such as the penis, and other external genital areas or head and neck areas
- Similarly, hemangioma circumscriptum is congenital malformation of blood vessels (angiokeratoma circumscriptum)

Other terms

- Lymphangioma, superficial lymphatic malformation

Clinical features

- Papules on the skin occur at birth or develop early in childhood

Prognosis and treatment

- Surgical resection may be necessary for cosmetic reason or relief of symptoms associated with compression

Gross pathology

- Vesicle-like skin lesions, resembling frog spawn

Histology

- The lesion is composed of cystically dilated lymphatics, lined by endothelium (Fig. 26-1*a*)
- Typically involving stratum papillae (papillary dermis) of the skin
- The contents of the cysts are lymphocytes and pink proteinaceous lymph fluid (Fig. 26-1*b*)

Immunohistochemistry

- Positive endothelial cell markers such as CD31 or lymphatic marker D2-40

Clinical relevance

- Benign, no treatment unless symptomatic or for cosmetic reasons

Figure 26-1.
Lymphangioma circumscriptum of the penis, as a polypoid lesion of the upper dermis pushing the epidermis, consists of a dilated lymphatic channel (*a*). High magnification shows the dilated lymphatics containing lymph fluid and lymphocytes (*b*).

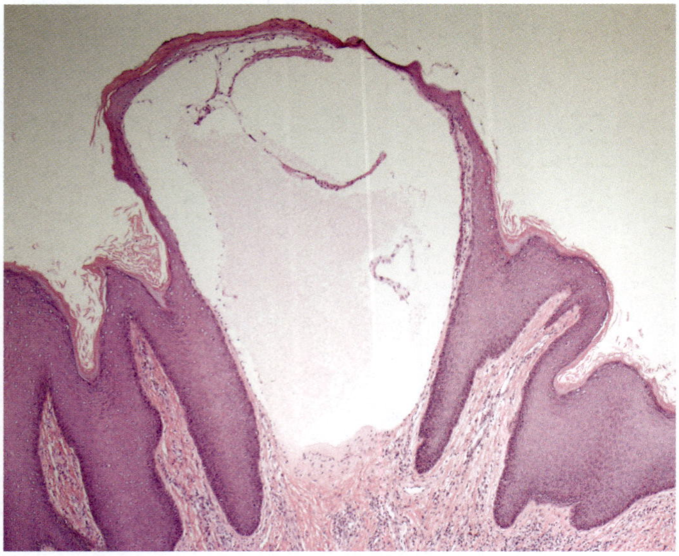

a

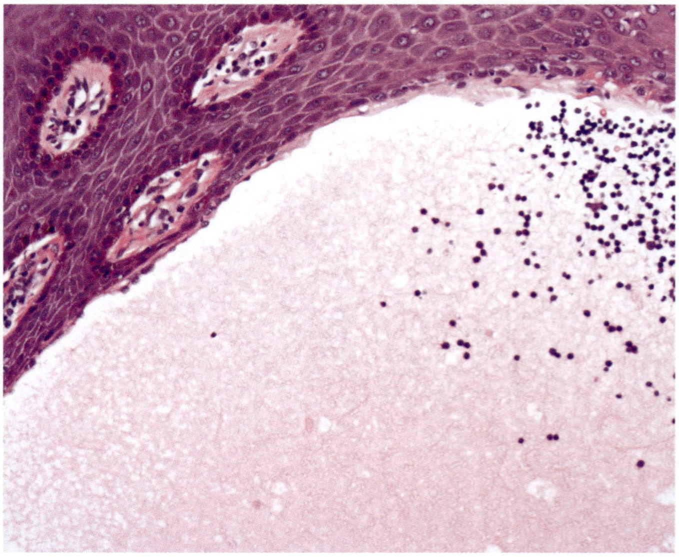

b

HEMANGIOMA OF THE PENIS

Definition

- Benign vascular tumor arising in the penis, which can be seen in other GU organs

Clinical features

- Most commonly affects young or middle-age men
- Asymptomatic and solitary lesion, occasionally can be associated with symptoms such as bleeding or infection

Gross pathology

- Red and purple papule or slightly elevated skin lesion or it may present as a mass lesion deep in the penis

Histology

- The tumor is composed of disorganized blood vessels in several forms (Fig. 26-2)
  - Capillary type: composed of small capillaries (Fig. 26-2*b*)
  - Cavernous type: composed of dilated mature vessels (Fig. 26-2*d*)
- Mixed of different types of blood vessels

Immunohistochemistry

- CD31 positive for endothelial cells (Fig. 26-2*c*)

Clinical relevance (prognosis and treatment options)

- Surgical removal rarely necessary unless symptomatic

Figure 26-2.
Penile hemangioma as a dome-shaped capillary hemangioma consists of many small dilated capillaries (*a*), which are lined by benign endothelium (*b*), positive for CD31 (*c*). Cavernous hemangioma deeply located in penile erectile tissue is composed of larger disorganized blood vessels containing blood (*d*).

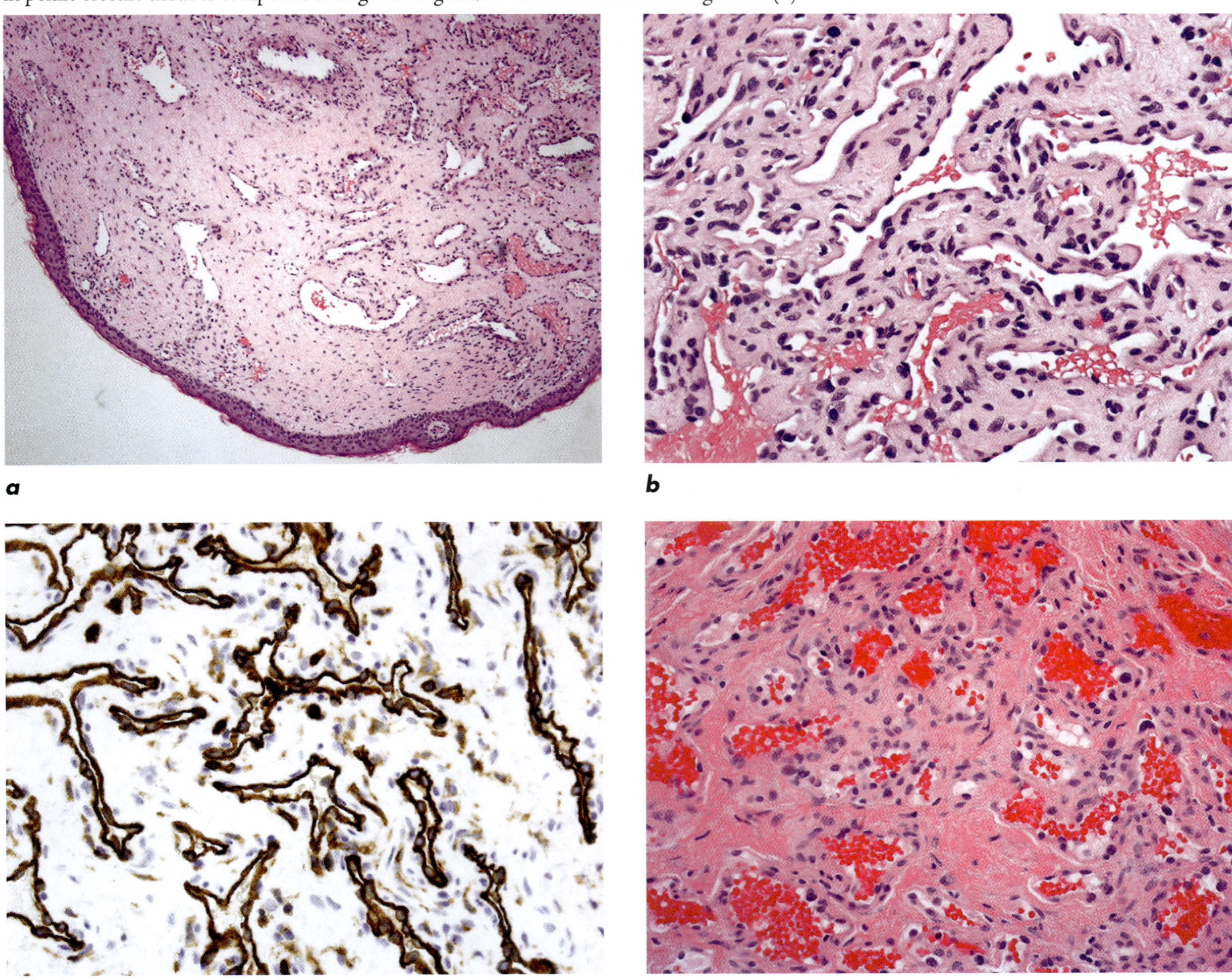

a b c d

ANGIOKERATOMA OF THE SCROTUM

Definition

- Benign skin lesion with vascular component and hyperkeratosis

Other terms

- Angiokeratoma of Fordyce

Clinical features

- Asymptomatic 2 to 5 mm blue or red with scaly papules on the scrotum, penis, or inner thigh

Gross pathology

- Red-blue papules on the skin surface

Histology

- Dilated thin wall vessels in superficial dermis with overlying hyperplastic epidermis (Fig. 26-3)

Differential diagnosis

- Fordyce disease: 1 to 3 mm while bumps in scrotum, representing ectopic sebaceous glands without follicles
- Angiokeratoma may include a spectrum of diseases
- Localized forms: (1) solitary papular angiokeratosis (leg); (2) localized angiokeratoma of the scrotum (Fordyce type); (3) congenital form (angiokeratoma circumscriptum); and (4) bilateral finger angiokeratomas
- Systemic form: angiokeratoma corposis diffusum is associated with a metabolic disorder such as fucosidosis

Clinical relevance (prognosis and treatment options)

- Benign lesion, a destructive therapy (such as laser, excision, or cryotherapy) is only needed when symptomatic

Figure 26-3.
Localized angiokeratoma of the scrotum is composed of dilated blood vessels in the upper dermis and hyperkeratosis of the epidermis (*a*). High magnification shows the papillary hyperplasia of the endothelium (*b*).

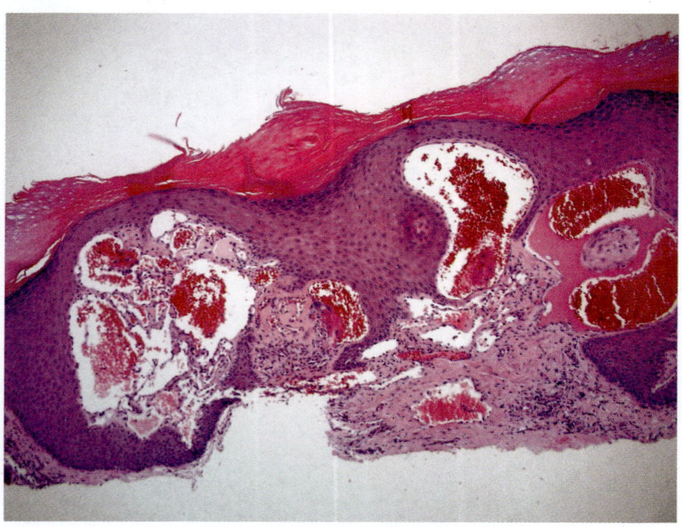

a

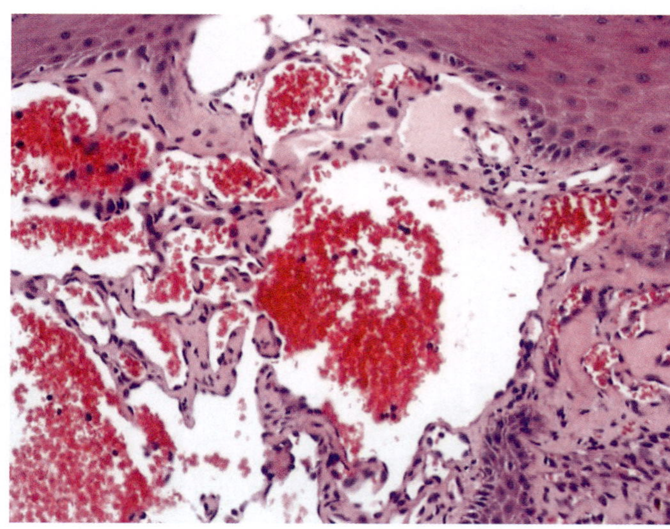

b

LEIOMYOMA OF THE PENIS

Definition

- Benign smooth muscle neoplasm develops in the penis
- It can been also seen in other GU organs such as the bladder, scrotum, kidney, or prostate

Clinical features

- Small slow-growing lesion, which can be polypoid if occurs in the mucosal side

Gross pathology

- Small firm or rubbery well-circumscribed mass, with white and fibrotic cut surface

Histology

- Well-defined mass composed of interlacing bundles of spindle cells (Fig. 26-4*a*). Benign smooth muscle cells with a low cellularity and with no evidence of cytological atypia, necrosis or increased mitosis (Fig. 26-4*b*)

Immunohistochemistry

- Positive for desmin and smooth muscle actin, negative for S100 or keratins

Clinical relevance (prognosis and treatment options)

- Benign, no surgery necessary unless symptomatic

Figure 26-4.
Penile leiomyoma is a solid mass composed of bland spindle cells (*a*). High magnification shows benign spindle cells with smooth muscle features without atypia (*b*).

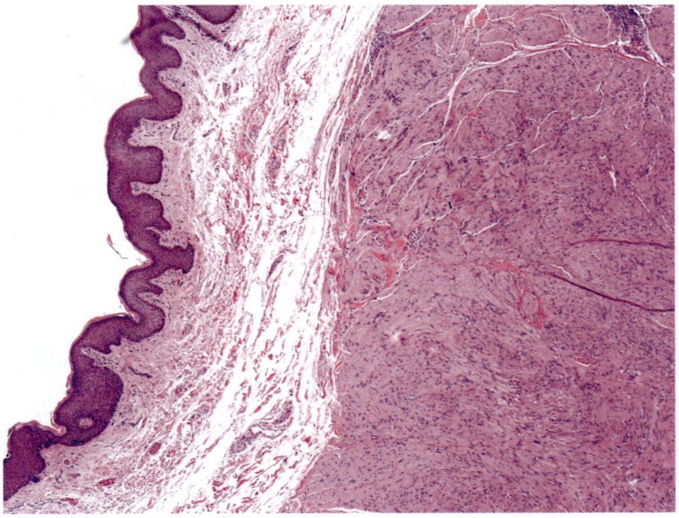

a

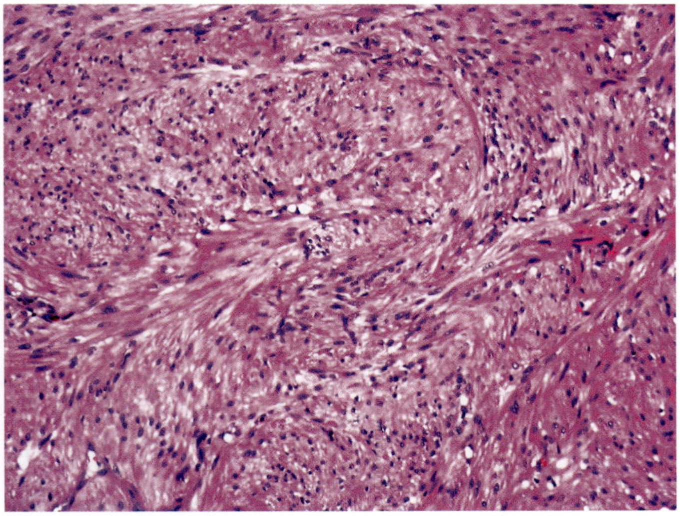

b

GRANULAR CELL TUMOR OF THE PENIS

Definition

- Benign neoplasm composed of cells containing abundant eosinophilic granules in the cytoplasm, which is believed to be derived from the nerve

Clinical features

- Painless, ill-defined nodules and slow growing, typically smaller than 3 to 4 cm
- The common locations in the GU system are penis, scrotum, and bladder
- Overlying skin is thickened and may have a cobblestone appearance due to the epidermal proliferation

Gross pathology

- Poorly circumscribed firm lesion with an infiltrative border
- White or tan solid cut surface, necrosis, or hemorrhage is uncommon

Histology

- This tumor is not encapsulated, infiltrating mass, which may infiltrate the penile erectile tissue (Fig. 26-5)
- The tumor cells arranged in sheets, nests, or solid patterns surrounded by variable stroma septa (Figs. 26-5 and 26-6)
- Tumor cells are polyhedral in shape, uniform in size, and containing abundant cytoplasm full of eosinophilic granules (lysosomes) in the cytoplasm (Fig. 26-6). Epidermal squamous proliferation can be prominent, showing pseudoepitheliomatous appearance (Fig. 26-7*a*)
- Rare cases associated with squamous cell carcinoma

Immunohistochemistry and cytohistochemistry

- S100 positive (Fig. 26-7*b*)
- Neuron-specific enolase positive, PAS positive and resistant to diastase

Clinical relevance (prognosis and treatment options)

- The vast majority of cases are benign, but recurrence may occur if the tumor is not completely excised
- The malignant granular cell tumor is rare. The presence of a large size, frequent mitoses, nuclear atypia, and aggressive growth, leading to necrosis, hemorrhage may indicate malignancy

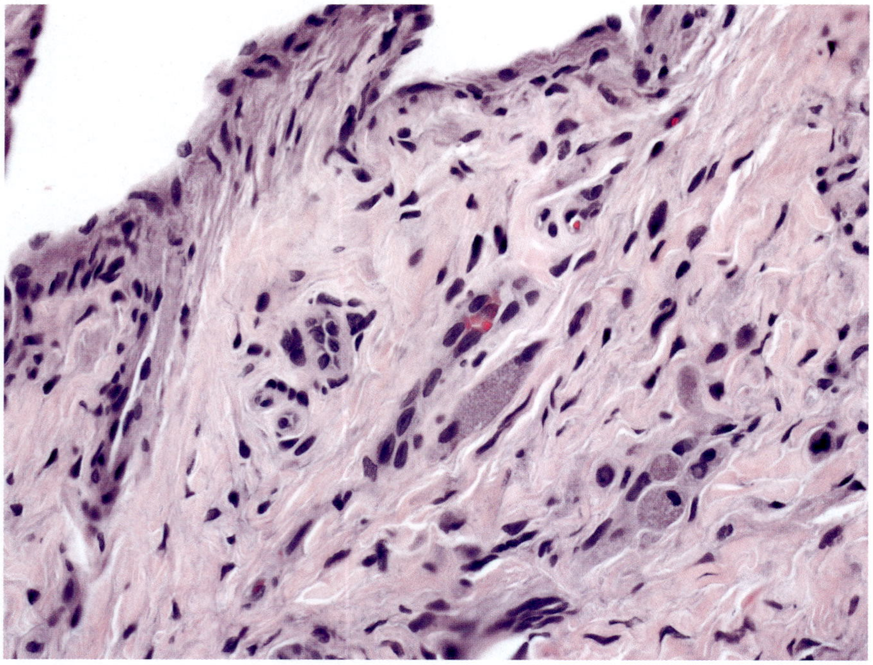

Figure 26-5. Penile granular cell tumor infiltrating penile erectile tissue.

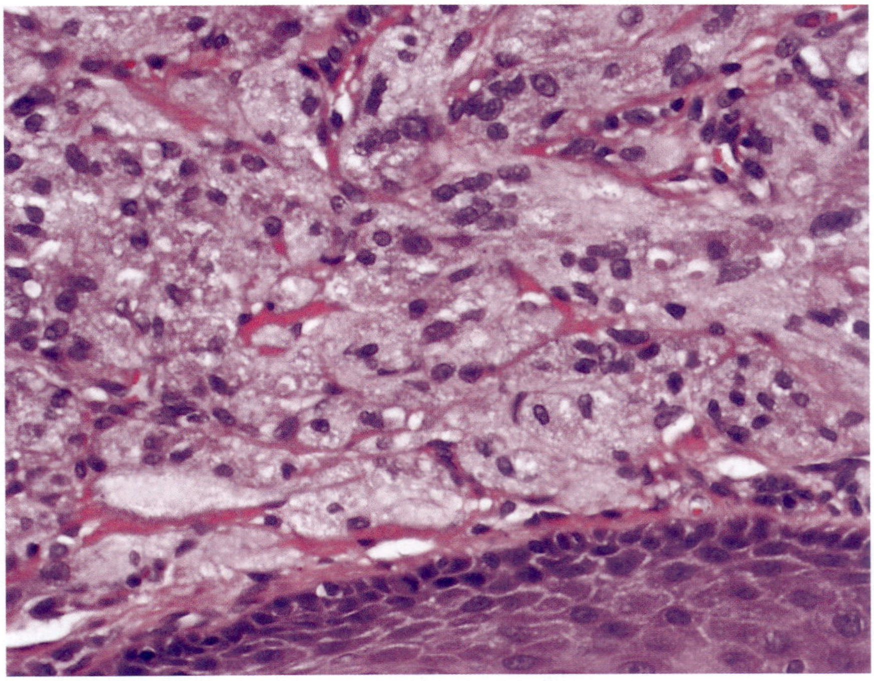

Figure 26-6.
Penile granular cell tumor cells contain abundant cytoplasmic granules.

Figure 26-7.
Penile granular cell tumor composed of cells with abundant eosinophilic cytoplasm and small nuclei (*a*). The tumor cells are positive for S100 immunostaining (*b*).

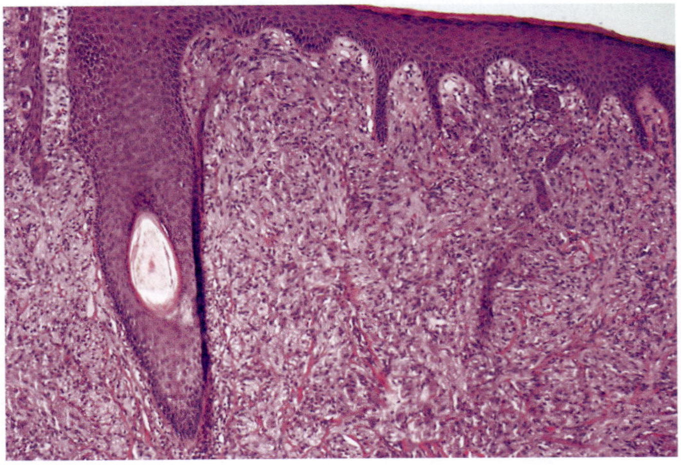

a

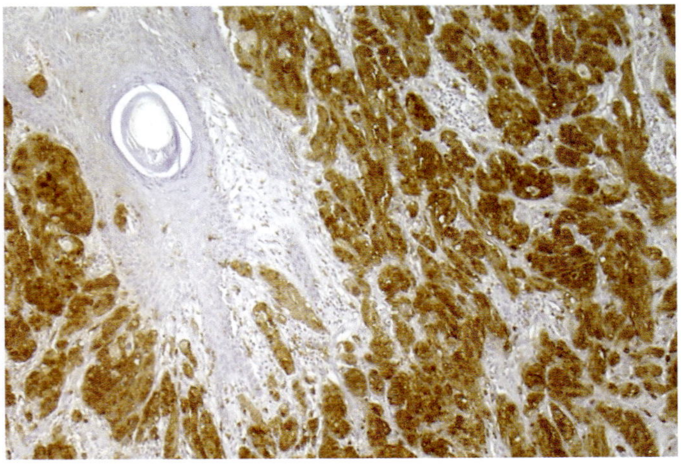

b

PENILE FIBROMATOSIS

Definition

- Superficial fibroblastic lesion characterized by nodular or diffuse proliferation of fibroblasts and myofibroblasts
- Fibromatosis is a group of benign fibroblastic proliferative lesions including palmar, plantar, and penile fibrosis

Other terms

- Superficial fibromatosis, Peyronie disease, or Peyronie fibromatosis

Pathogenesis

- Unknown, traumatic cause has been speculated but not confirmed

Clinical features

- Palpable firm nodule, or cord-like soft tissue lesion, usually in the dorsolateral aspect of the penis
- A painful lesion can be associated with difficulty in sexual function such as painful intercourse, or erectile dysfunction
- Abnormal curvature of the penile shaft, or urethral stricture may occur in the advanced cases

Gross pathology

- Poorly defined lesions without capsule, located in the dorsolateral aspect, white-tan firm cut surface

Histology

- Fascicles of benign-looking spindle cells (Fig. 26-8) intermingled with adjacent fibrous tissue, which makes it difficult to define the border of the tumor
- No cytological atypia, mitosis can be seen occasionally

Immunohistochemistry

- β-Catenin diffusely positive (Fig. 26-8*d*), while scar tissue can be weakly positive for β-catenin

Clinical relevance (prognosis and treatment options)

- Penile fibromatosis is a bothersome, however, not a life-threatening condition
- It is a slowly progressive disease, regression may occur in a small number of cases
- Over the time, it may cause sexual dysfunction and anatomic distortion of the penis, such as abnormal curvature of the penile shaft, or urethral stricture
- Treatment options include medical therapy, physical therapy, or surgery, but none of them are totally satisfactory

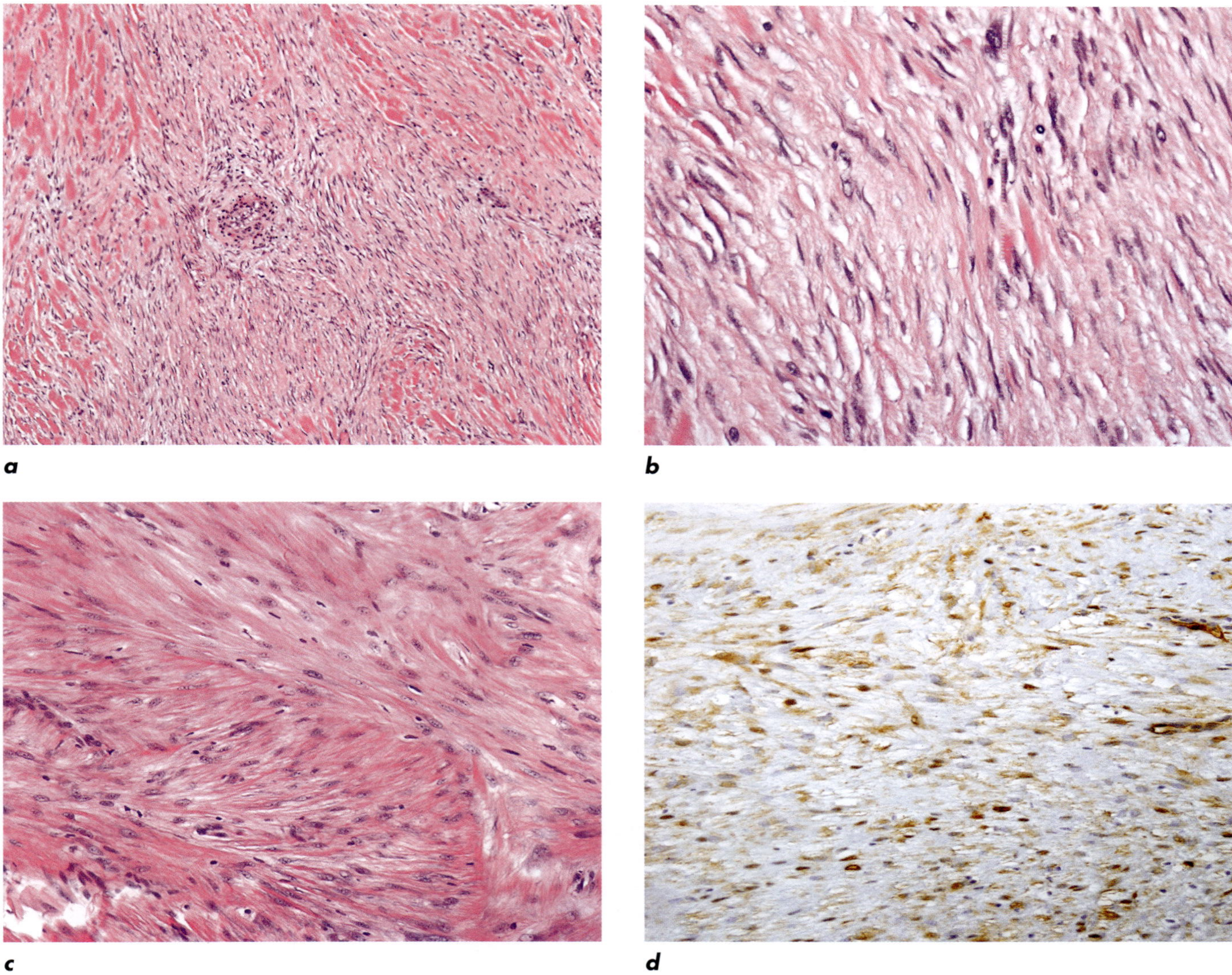

Figure 26-8.
Penile fibromatosis consists of fascicles of bland spindle cells (*a*). The spindle cells show no cytological atypia; mitotic figures can be seen occasionally (*b*). Another case of penile fibromatosis composed of fascicles of benign-appearing spindle cells with infiltrating patterns (*c*), which are positive for β-catenin (*d*).

SYRINGOMA

Definition

- Syringoma is a benign skin adnexal neoplasm forming well-differentiated tubular structures (*syrinx*: Greek word meaning tube)
- It is believed to be derived from eccrine (sweat) or apocrine gland ducts

Clinical features

- Multiple small yellow papules, mostly seen in the face and trunk, but also in other areas of skin, rarely seen in the penis

Gross pathology

- Small well-circumscribed lesions

Histology

- Nonencapsulated lesions located in the upper dermis, but with noninfiltrating borders
- Tumor is composed of small island of epithelium-lined ducts without atypia or mitosis (Fig. 26-9)
- Two layers of thick epithelial cells lining the ductal structures (Fig. 26-10)
- Several forms of syringoma have been recognized clinically: localized form, associated with Down syndrome, generalized form that encompasses multiple and eruptive syringomas, and familial form

Differential diagnosis

- Malignant syringoma: significant cytological atypia and infiltrating patterns with desmoplastic reaction
- Squamous cell carcinoma: cytological atypia, invasive nature, and keratin pearl formation

Clinical relevance (prognosis and treatment options)

- Benign condition, treatment includes laser, dermabrasion, and curettage

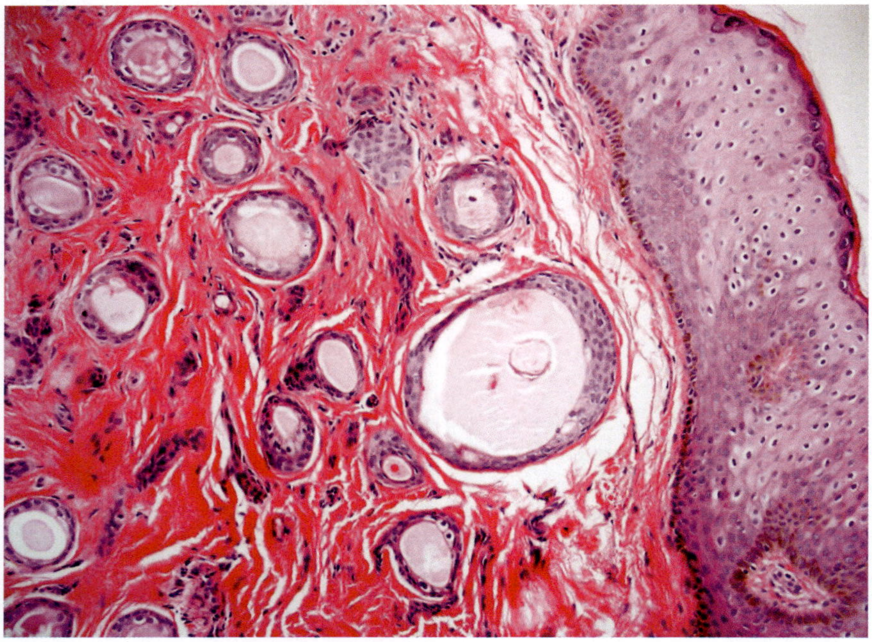

Figure 26-9.
Syringoma is composed of tumor cells forming small islands or epithelium-lined ducts.

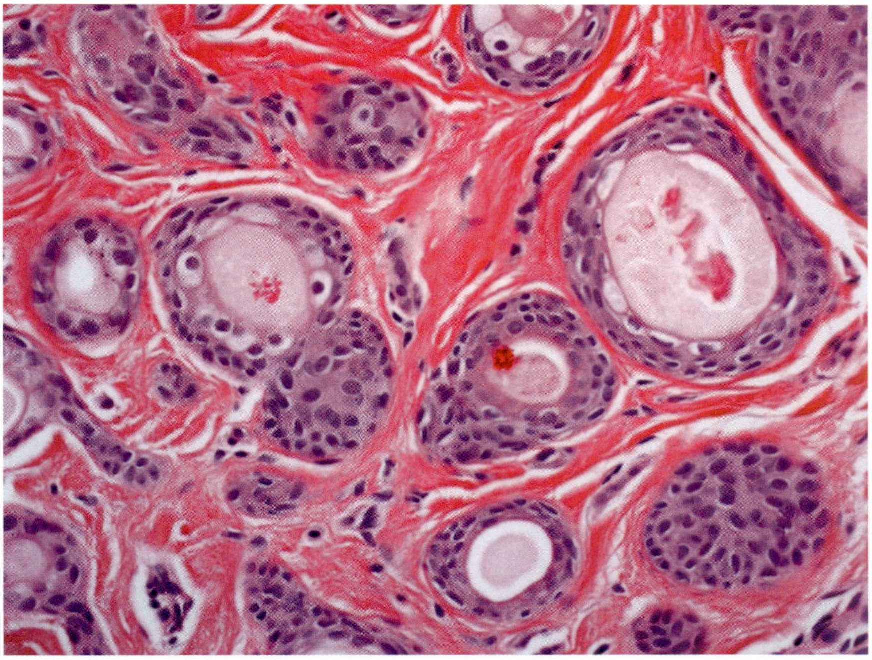

Figure 26-10.
High magnification shows that the tumor cells form two to three layers covering ducts.

NEVI AND OTHER BENIGN MELANOCYTIC LESIONS

Definition

- Nevus is a congenital or acquired benign melanocytic proliferation
- A number of benign melanocytic lesions can occur (listed in Table 26-1) in the skin of penis and scrotum as well as mucosa (bladder and urethra)

Other terms

- Nevus = birthmark in Latin

Pathogenesis and epidemiology

- Nevi are more common in Caucasians, but they can occur in anyone
- Some nevi are congenital and others developing late in life are probably neoplastic, because they are clonal

Clinical features

- Usually clinically evident between ages 2 and 6 years
- More common on head, neck, and trunk in Caucasians
- More common on acral sites in Asians and Afro-Caribbeans
- More common in the skin, but they can occasionally develop in the mucosa

Gross pathology

- Small in size, well-circumscribed and symmetrical lesions. Occasional congenital nevi can be very large
- Black color if located in the upper dermis, blue or gray if located in the deep dermis
- Hemorrhage and color changes are not common. If they occur, they would be the suspicious signs for malignance

Histology

- There are more than 20 different types of nevi, only the most common types of benign and atypical melanocytic lesions will be discussed here (see Table 26-1)
- Several benign hyperpigmented lesions can be seen in the external genital areas

Genital melanosis

- Large, single pigmented flat skin lesion as a macule or patch
- Basal cell hyperpigmentation without melanocytic hyperplasia (Fig. 26-11)

Genital lentiginosis

- Scattered irregular variegated pigmented lesions
- Basal cell hyperpigmentation in the rete ridges and the presence of melanocytic hyperplasia (Fig. 26-12)

Table 26-1. Summary of Benign and Atypical Melanocytic Lesions

Lesion	*Histology*	*Behavior*	*Management option*
Melanosis	Basal cell hyperpigmentation No melanocytic hyperplasia	Benign	Biopsy if suspicious No additional treatment
Lentiginosis	Basal cell hyperpigmentation No melanocytic hyperplasia	Benign	Biopsy if suspicious No additional treatment
Intradermal nevus	Nevus cells confined within dermis	Benign	Biopsy if suspicious No additional treatment
Junctional nevus	Nevus cells present at the epidermal-dermal junction	Benign	Biopsy if suspicious No additional treatment
Compound nevus	Both intradermal and junctional nevus components present	Benign	Biopsy if suspicious No additional treatment
Nevus with mild atypia	Hyperchromatic nuclei, small nucleoli, no mitosis	Benign	Treated as benign
Nevus with moderate or severe atypia	Nuclear enlargement, pagetoid atypical melanocytes, increased mitosis	High risk for melanoma	Wider excision
Atypical melanocytic hyperplasia	Individual atypical melanocytes, peripheral of melanoma	Possible melanoma recurrence	Observation or wider excision

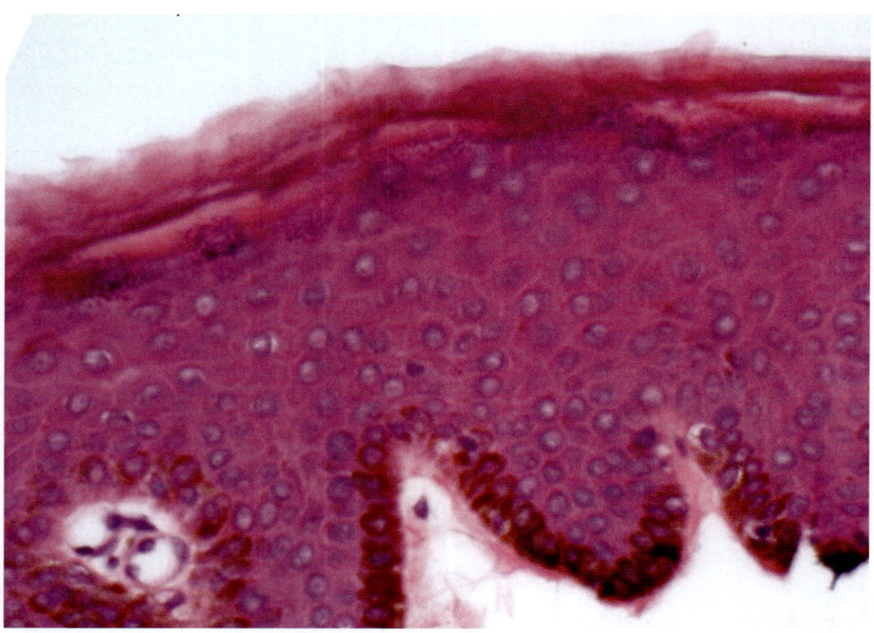

Figure 26-11.
Genital melanosis is characterized by the hyperpigmentation of basal cells without melanocytic hyperplasia.

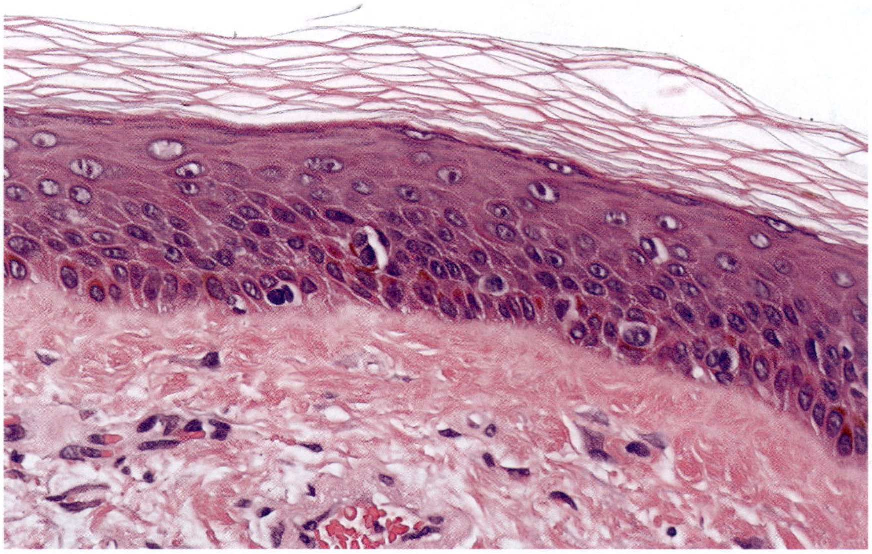

Figure 26-12.
Genital lentiginosis is characterized by the presence of basal cell hyperpigmentation and melanocytic hyperplasia.

Intradermal nevus

- Nevus cells confined in the dermis (Fig. 26-13*a* and *b*)

Junctional nevus

- Nevus cells present in the epidermis and dermis junction

Compound nevus

- Presence of both junctional and intradermal components (Fig. 26-13*c* and *d*)

Atypical nevus (dysplastic nevus)

- Any nevus with cytological or architectural atypia
- Atypical nevi in the genital areas as well as on the scalp of adolescents have apparent benign behavior
- Solitary dysplastic nevus is a controversial entity. Some believe a solitary nevus with dysplastic features should be treated as clinically benign. Others believe that a dysplastic nevus may represent a transition between benign nevus and melanoma
- Mild atypia
  - At high power, hyperchromatic nuclei of melanocytes with small nucleoli; perinuclear halo common with minimal pagetoid melanocytes, no mitotic figures in dermal component
- Moderate atypia
  - At high power, nevus nuclei are variable in size (Fig. 26-14), although some have *mild atypia* plus small nucleoli
  - Enlarged cytoplasm compared to melanocyte with a few mitotic figures (Fig. 26-15)
- Severe atypia
  - Usually asymmetrical nests of nevus cells, not individual cells, but still well circumscribed in epidermis
  - Some central upward migration of individual nevus cells
  - Crowded nests in dermis
  - Enlarged nuclei, often bizarre hyperchromatic nuclei mixed with small nuclei, prominent nucleoli
  - No confluent atypia as seen with melanoma
  - Frequent mitoses in junctional component but not in deep dermal component

Atypical melanocytic hyperplasia

- Atypical individual melanocytes limited to epidermis (Fig. 26-16), which can be seen at periphery of classic melanoma
- Different form melanoma in situ, only focal confluence at the dermoepidermal junction, limited pagetoid spread
- Involvement of only the upper part of the hair follicles

Immunohistochemistry

- Melan-A positive, HMB45 generally negative, low Ki67 proliferative activity (Fig. 26-15*b*)

Clinical relevance (prognosis and treatment options)

- Biopsy will be performed for any lesions suspicious for melanomas
- Pathologically confirmed benign nevi and mildly atypical nevi do not require additional treatment
- Nevi with moderate and severe atypia usually are excised with negative margins

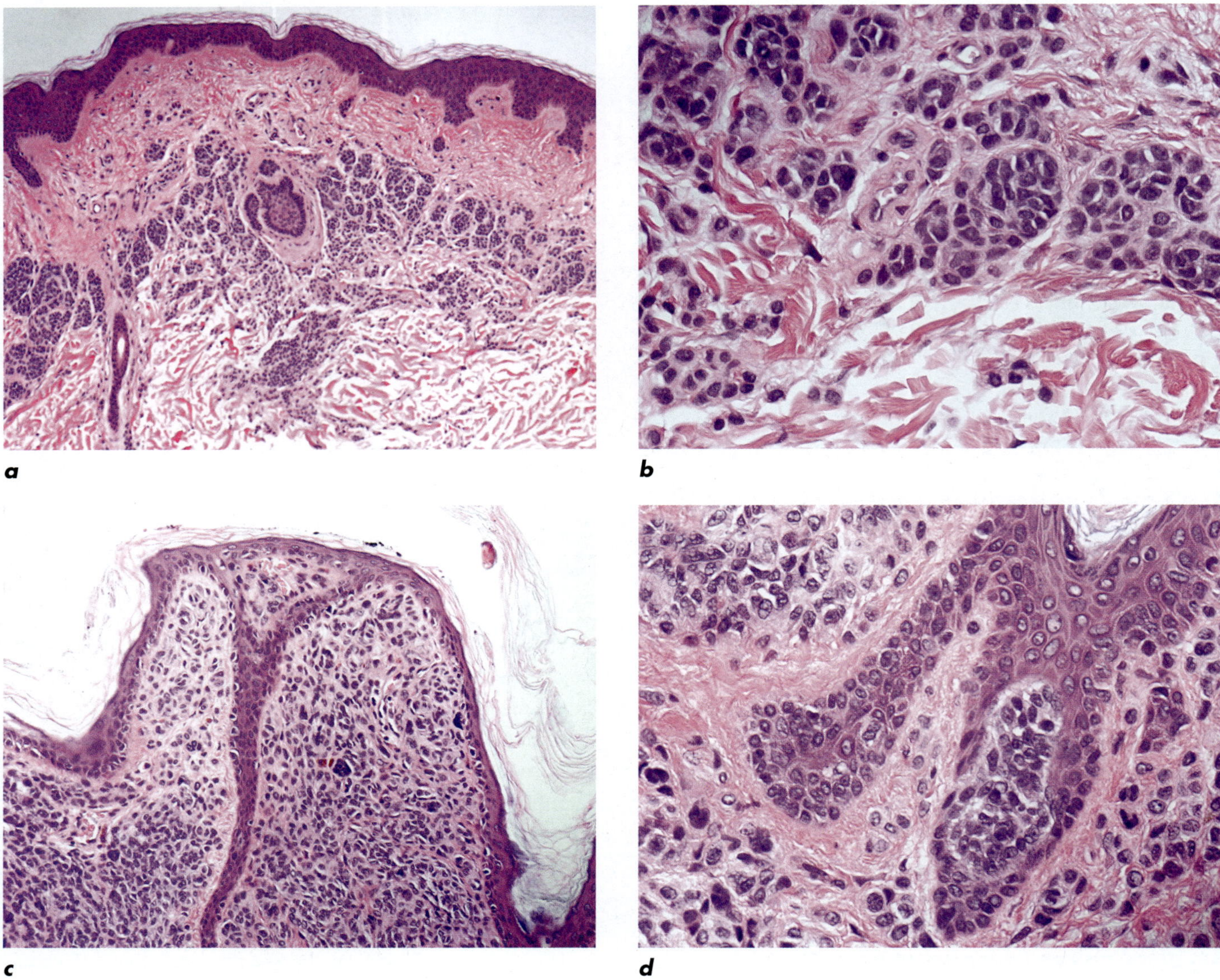

Figure 26-13.
Intradermal nevus (*a* and *b*). The nevus cells are confined in the dermis (*a*). High magnification shows the regular shape of the nevus nests, and nevus cells have no cytological atypia (*b*). Compound nevus (*c* and *d*) contains both intradermal component and junction component that are between the epidermis and upper dermis (*c*). High magnification shows a nest of nevus cells in the in junction area between the dermis and epidermis (*d*).

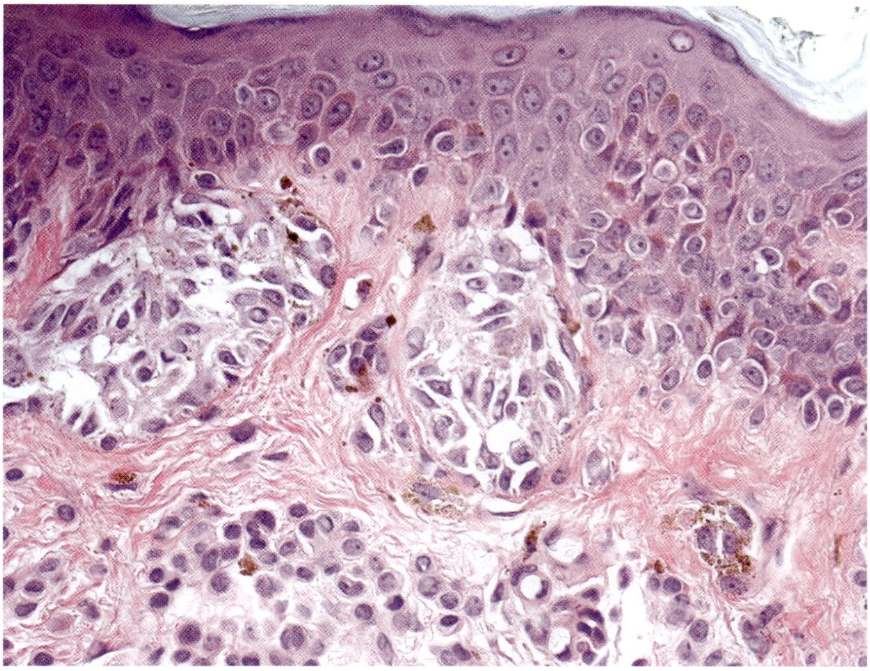

Figure 26-14.
Atypical compound nevus. The junctional component of nevus cells showing moderate cytological atypia.

Figure 26-15.
Atypical compound nevus. The junctional nevus component contains individual atypical melanocytes (*a*). The Ki67 immunostaining shows that the proliferative activity of the atypical nevus cells is relatively low (*b*).

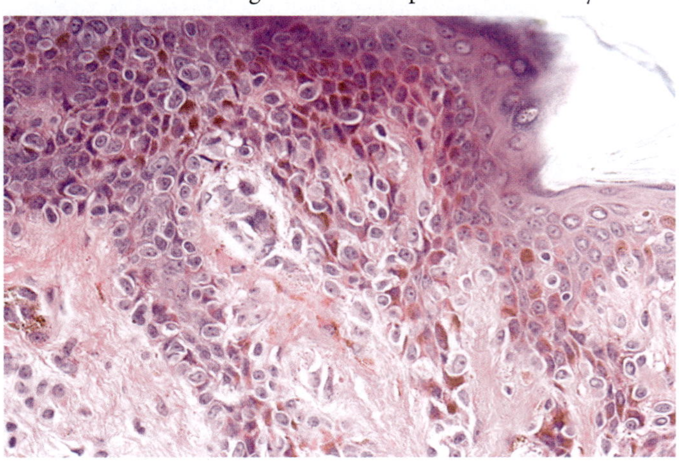

a

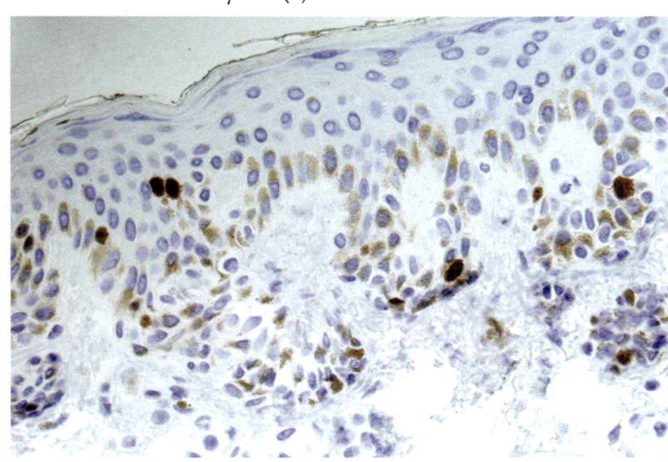

b

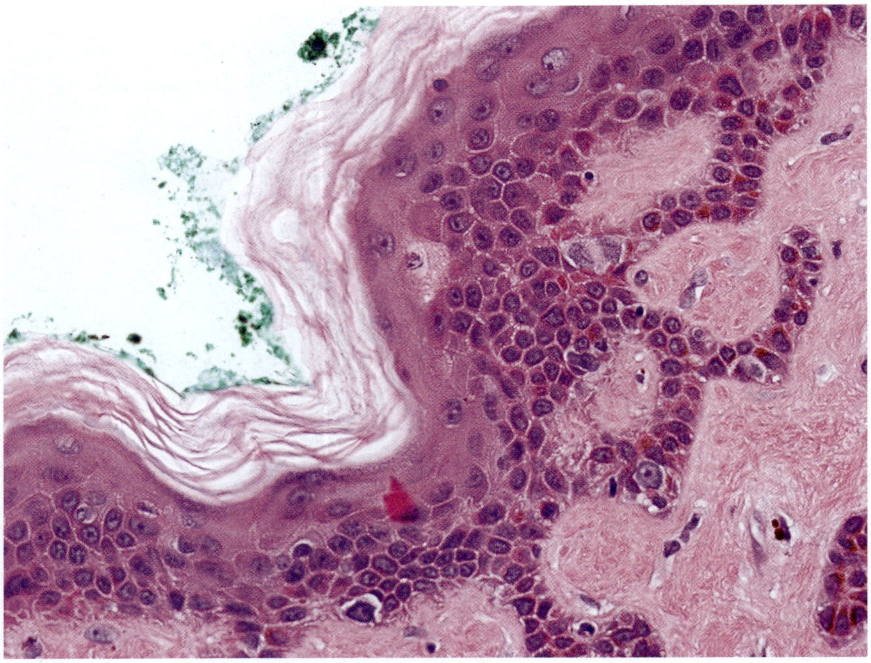

Figure 26-16.
Atypical melanocytic hyperplasia presents in the area adjacent to a melanoma and contains scattered atypical melanocytes in the dermis.

NEUROFIBROMA

Definition

- Benign mesenchymal tumor with nerve sheet differentiation

Clinical features

- Usually develops during childhood but may not be noticed until adulthood
- A small percentage may undergo malignant transformation
- Either sporadic or as a part of type 1 neurofibromatosis syndrome

Gross pathology

- Often present as single or multiple plaque-like or pedunculated lesions in skin, deep lesions are typically associated with the nerve

Histology

- Neurofibroma does not have a capsule, which appears infiltrative in the dermis (Fig. 26-17*a*)
- The tumor is composed of spindle nerve sheet cells with loose background
- Dermal neurofibromas may lead to entrapment of skin adnexa such as follicles or sweat glands (Fig. 26-17*b*)
- The lesion may be localized or diffuse

Immunohistochemistry

- S100 positive
- Epithelial (AE1/AE3, EMA) and smooth muscle markers (desmin, SMA) negative

Clinical relevance (prognosis and treatment options)

- Benign, no treatment unless symptomatic or for cosmetic reasons
- Surgical resection may be necessary if suspicious for other neoplasms or malignant transformation

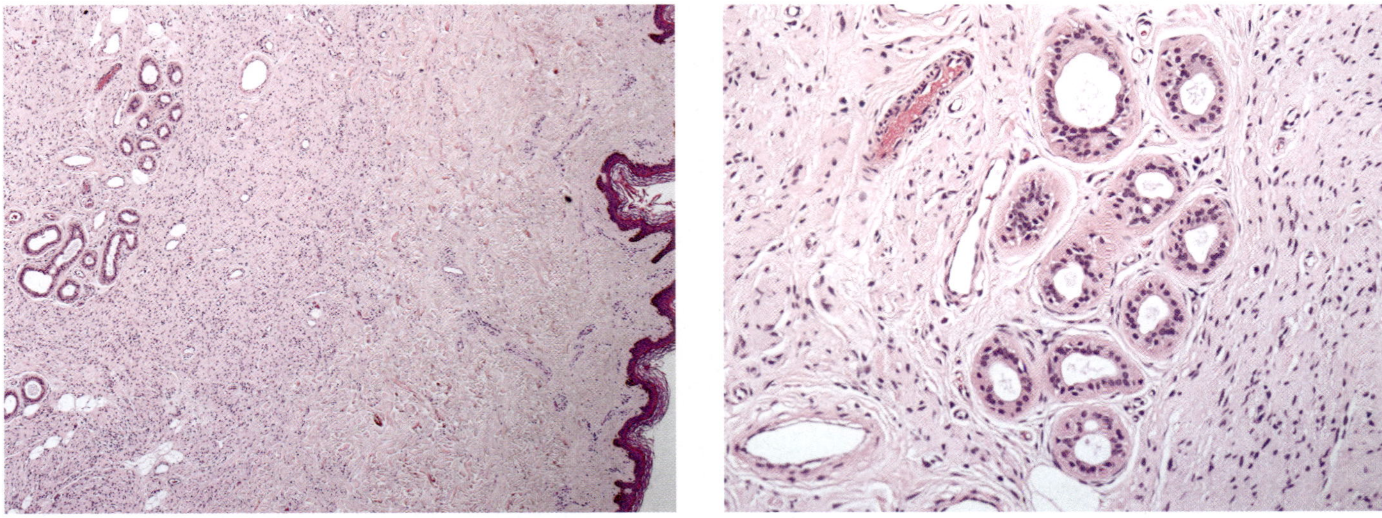

a b

Figure 26-17.
Neurofibroma of the scrotum. Spindle cell proliferation without a capsule in the dermis entrapping sweat glands (*a*). High magnification shows the presence of spindle neurofibromatous cells without cytological atypia, surrounding the sweat glands (*b*).

CHAPTER 27 Condyloma and Other Viral Infectious Lesions of the Penis and Scrotum

CONDYLOMA ACUMINATUM

Definition

- Skin lesions caused by human papilloma virus (HPV)

Other terms

- Condyloma acuminata (plural), genital wart, venereal wart, HPV, or koilocytic changes

Clinical features

- Condyloma acuminatum is the most common penile lesion encountered in our surgical pathology practice in the United States
- This is a highly contagious sexually transmitted disease, transmitted through direct skin-skin contact during oral, genital, or anal sex with an infected person
- Early lesions are present in the tip of the penis where the sex contact happened
- They may also be found on the shaft of the penis, the scrotum, or other genital and anal areas

Gross pathology

- Fleshy, polypoid, and cauliflower-like skin lesions, either single or multiple lesions in a cluster

Histology

- Papillomatosis: squamous epithelium covers fibrovascular cores, most condylomas are papillary (Figs. 27-1 and 27-2)
- Koilocytosis: HPV-specific cellular changes characterized by the presence of nuclear enlargement, raisinoid nuclei, and presence of perinuclear halos (Fig. 27-1*b*)
- Parakeratosis: thickened squamous epithelium, condyloma can be flat (Fig. 27-3)

Immunohistochemistry and molecular analysis

- Immunostain for HPV can be used for detection, although the sensitivity is not very high
- Polymerase chain reaction (PCR)–based tests are available for HPV types 6 and 11, which are responsible for 90% of condylomas
- Whereas HPV types 16 and 18 are strongly associated with cervical cancer development

Figure 27-1.
Penile condyloma acuminatum with a cauliflower appearance (*a*) and typical koilocytosis characterized by raisinoid nuclei and perinuclear halos (*b*).

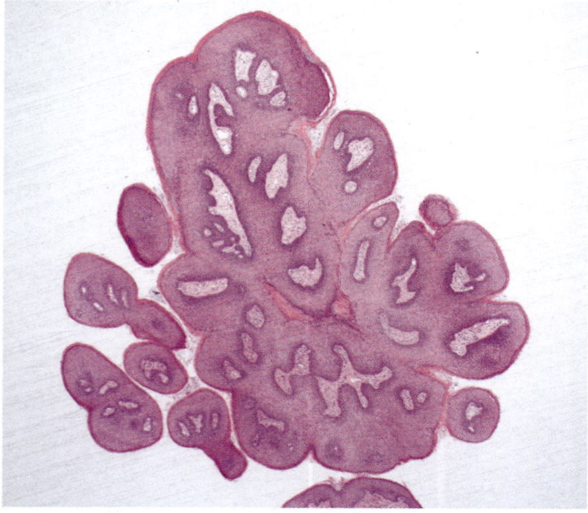

a

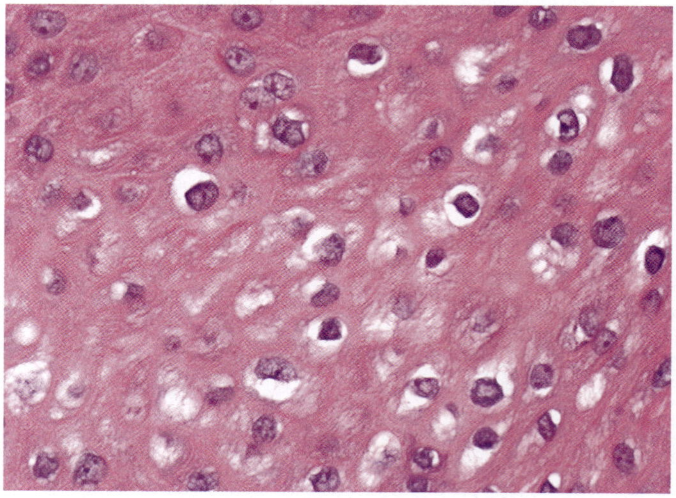

b

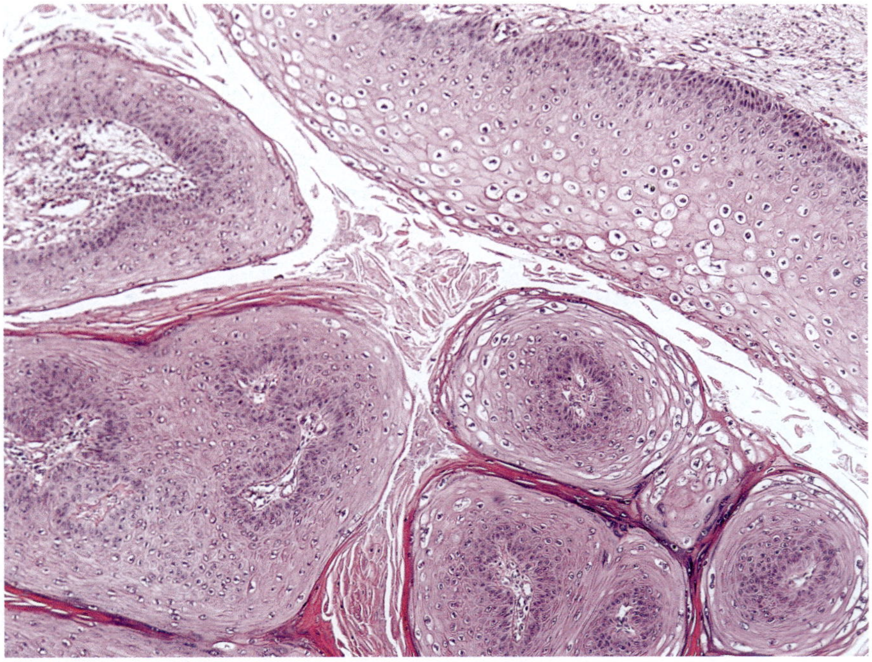

Figure 27-2.
Penile condyloma with papillomatosis.

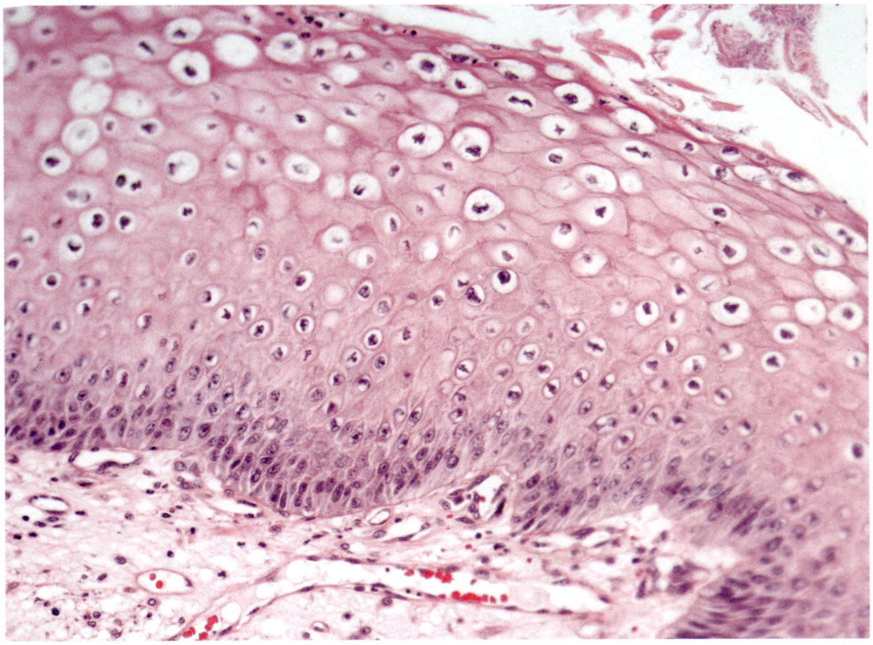

Figure 27-3.
Penile flat condyloma shows acanthosis, thickening of squamous epithelium containing koilocytes.

Clinical relevance (prognosis and treatment options)

- Condyloma acuminatum is a precursor lesion of squamous dysplasia and subsequent squamous cell carcinoma
- For prevention, HPV vaccines are available. Gardasil, an HPV vaccine (by Merck) protects against HPV types 6, 11, 16, and 18
- A wide range of methods can be used to remove condylomas, such as surgery, laser electrocauterization, cryosurgery, or topical medication. However, the presence of latent HPV in the affected cells may not be eradicated
- So that the recurrence rate of condylomas is high in proximately 50% of cases

SQUAMOUS DYSPLASIA IN CONDYLOMA

Definition

- Squamous dysplasia or/and carcinoma in situ (severe dysplasia) developing in the background of condyloma

Clinical features

- Similar lesions to condyloma grossly but this condition represents an early phase of carcinoma development

Gross pathology

- Cauliflower-like skin lesions, same as condyloma

Histology

- Presence of dysplasia in the background of condyloma (Fig. 27-4)
- Mild (basal one-third involvement), moderate (basal two-third involvement), and severe (full thickness involvement)
- The presence of atypical mitoses and severe pleomorphism are helpful in establishing the diagnosis of dysplasia
- A condyloma associated with dysplasia can be flat or papillary (Fig. 27-5*a* and *b*)
- Carcinoma in situ is full thickness involvement by dysplastic cells, often used interchangeably with severe dysplasia (Fig. 27-5*c* and *d*)

Immunohistochemistry

- P16 positive and P53 may be positive (more so in moderate or severe dysplasia), Ki67 proliferative index may be increased

Clinical relevance (prognosis and treatment options)

- Mild and moderate dysplasia is the precursor of carcinoma
- Squamous severe dysplasia = carcinoma in situ
- Mild dysplasia will be treated as condyloma
- Moderate and severe dysplasia require treatment such as resection

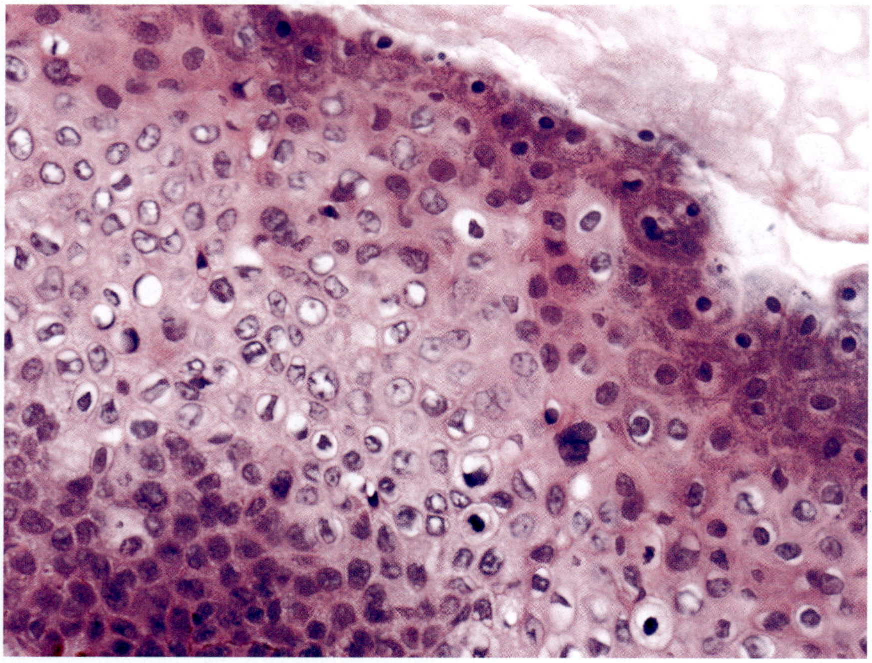

Figure 27-4.
Presence of mild dysplasia in a condyloma is characterized by the nuclear enlargement, hyperchromasia, and mitoses present in the lower portion of the squamous epithelium.

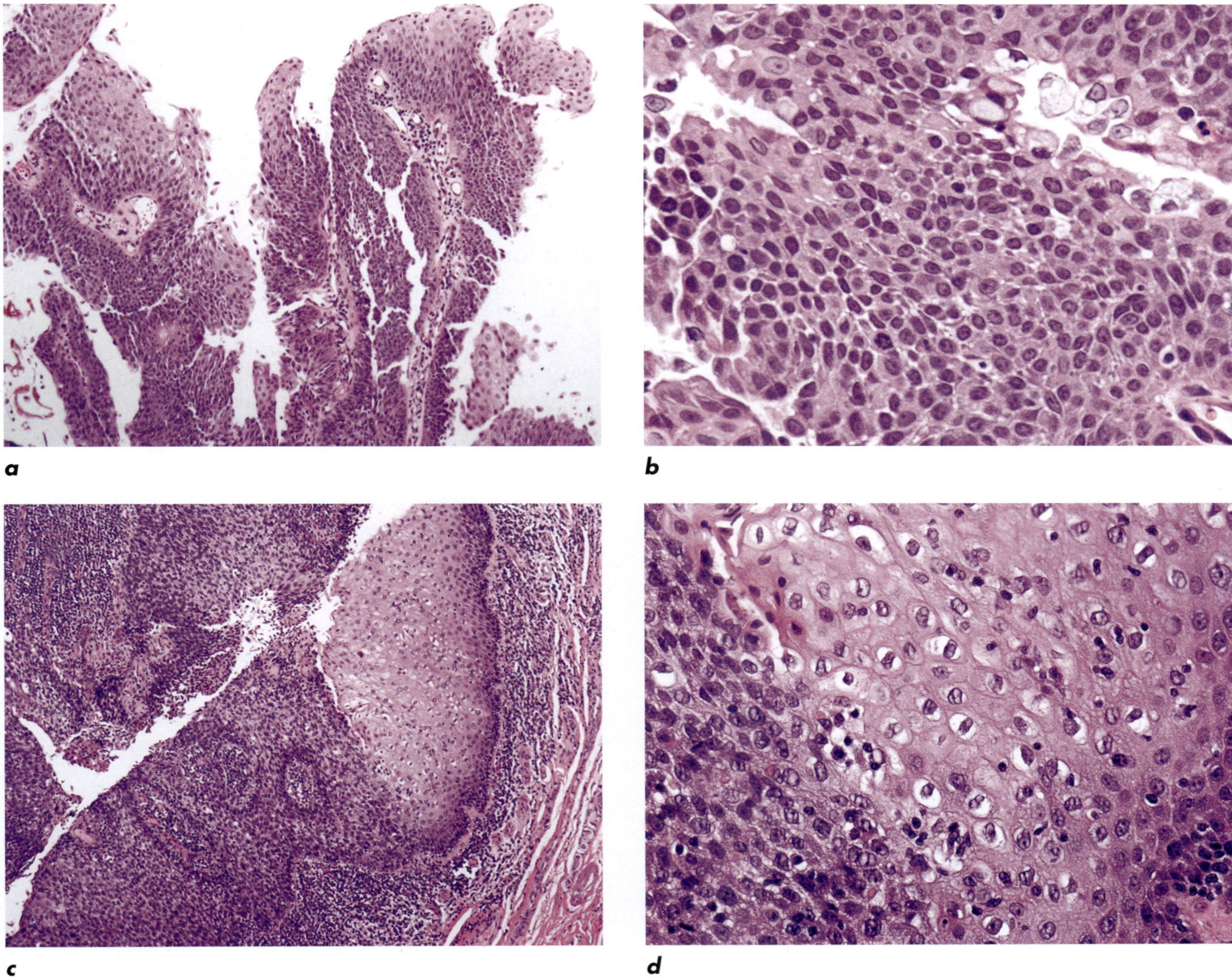

Figure 27-5.
Penile condyloma acuminata with dysplasia. A condyloma with papillary configurations (*a*) and moderate squamous dysplasia (*b*). Another penile condyloma associated with severe squamous dysplasia (*c*). High magnification shows the presence of koilocytic changes (*d*, right) and the full thickness involvement by dysplastic cells (*d*, left).

MOLLUSCUM CONTAGIOSUM

Definition

- Molluscum contagiosum is the skin lesion caused by poxvirus infection

Other term

- Mouse nipple

Pathogenesis

- The virus responsible for this lesion is molluscum contagiosum virus (MCV), which belongs to the poxvirus family
- Molluscum contagiosum is infectious and typically transmitted by skin-skin contact
- It commonly affects children, sexually active adults, and immunocompromised patients
- The incubation time from infection to the appearance of lesions ranges from 2 weeks to a few months
- MCV is a double-stranded DNA virus with four subtypes of MCVs 1-4. MCV-2 usually seen in sexually transmitted, which is responsible for the majority cases of penile molluscum contagiosum
- Unlike HPV, MCV will be cleared if skin lesion is removed, so it is not going to recur unless the person is reinfected again

Clinical features

- Molluscum contagiosum is usually small lesion ranging 1 to 5 mm in diameter
- It may be itchy but not painful. Secondary bacterial infection may develop
- Autoinoculation, a process in which virus spreads to adjacent areas, is often seen in children

Gross pathology

- Typically a skin-colored, round elevated pearly lesion, solitary of multiple
- The central waxy core contains the virus

Histology

- Typically a dome-shaped lesion composed of islands of affected squamous cells (Fig. 27-6*a*)
- An island is called molluscum body that contains large infected squamous cells with eosinophilic inclusions in the cytoplasm (Fig. 27-6*b*)

Immunohistochemistry and molecular analysis

- The gross and histologic features of molluscum contagiosum are so characteristic that additional tests are usually not necessary

Clinical relevance (prognosis and treatment options)

- Most lesions will disappear without treatment within a year or two. So that treatment may not be necessary if it is single without complications
- Occasionally they spread to other skin areas (autoinoculation)
- Treatment options include surgery, laser, or other medical and physical modalities
- The confirmation of diagnosis can be made by excisional biopsy

Figure 27-6.
Molluscum contagiosum is a dome-shaped lesion, composed of several squamous cell islands in the dermis (*a*). A high magnification reveals a molluscum body containing numerous infected squamous cells with large eosinophilic inclusions in the cytoplasm (*b*).

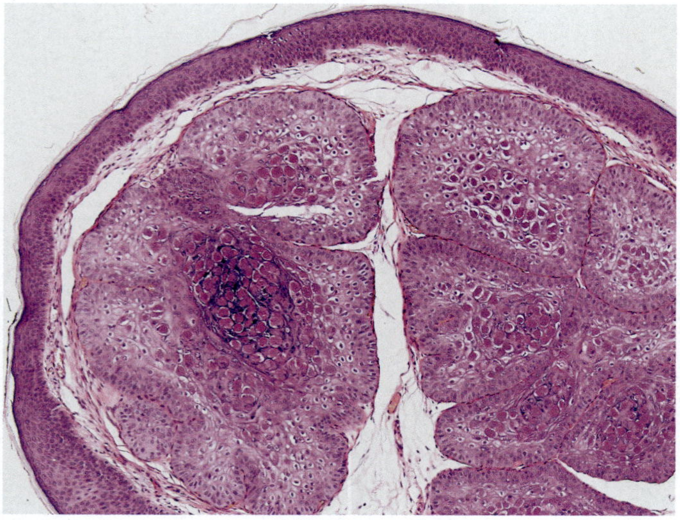

a

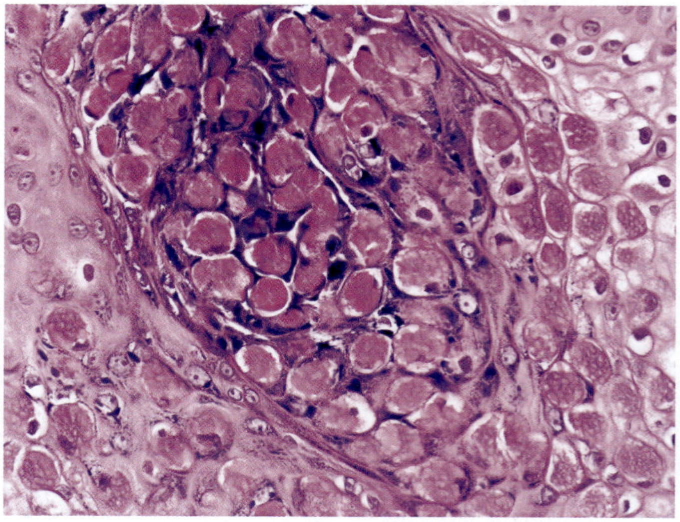

b

HERPES SIMPLEX INFECTION

Definition

- Skin inflammatory lesion caused by herpes simplex virus (HSV)

Pathogenesis

- HSV is a DNA virus that belongs to the herpes virus family, which may cause other infections (summarized in Table 27-1)
- Penile HSV infection, primarily caused by HSV2, is sexually transmitted and spreads by direct contact with lesions
- Latent virus present in the cells can be responsible for recurrence

Clinical features

- Primary infection may have flu-like symptoms or asymptomatic
- Initially, groups of blisters appear in the genital areas
- The blisters contain large number of viral particles and are highly contagious, and the rupture of blisters will cause painful ulcers, usually at tip of penis or on shaft
- The ulcers are large and persistent in immunocompromised patients. Occasionally, a destructive mass lesion can be present, mimicking penile cancer

Gross pathology

- Multiple blisters or ulcers on the skin surface. The lesion can destroy penile tissue, mimicking a malignant tumor (Fig. 27-7*a*)

Histology

- Blister with prominent tissue necrosis and ulceration if a blister is ruptured
- Inflammatory cell infiltrates, predominantly neutrophils associated with blisters or ulceration (Fig. 27-7*b*)
- Presence of multinuclear giant cells with nuclear molding (Fig. 27-7*c* and *d*)

Immunohistochemistry and molecular analysis

- HSV immunostaining or PCR for viral DNA can be confirmative

Clinical relevance (prognosis and treatment options)

- Recurrent infection may occur years after primary outbreak, usually milder than the initial outbreak
- Treatment as antiviral medicines such as valacyclovir or acyclovir. Surgery is an option for larger and resistant lesions

Table 27-1. Herpes Viruses and Their Related Lesions

Herpes family	*Conditions related*
HSV1	Oral blister lesions
HSV2	Penile blister lesions or genital ulcer
EBV	EBV inflammation, NPC, Burkitt lymphoma
CMV	Inflammatory lesion with CMV inclusions
VZV	Zoster
Human herpes virus 6	Exanthem subitum or roseola infantum
Human herpes virus 7	
Human herpes virus 8	Kaposi sarcoma

CMV, cytomegalovirus; EBV, Epstein-Barr virus; HSV, herpes simplex virus; NPC, nasopharyngeal carcinoma; VZV, varicella-zoster virus.

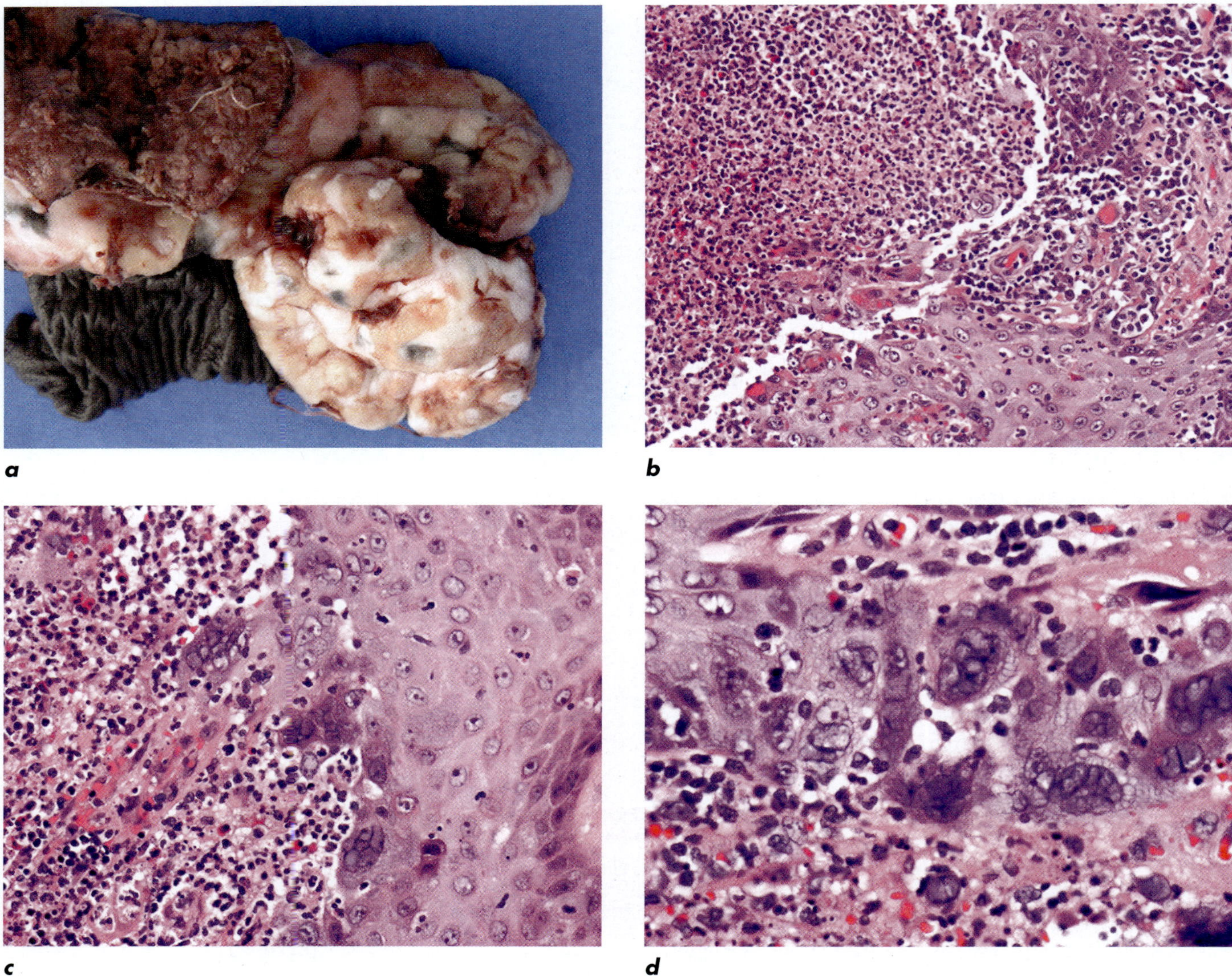

Figure 27-7.
Herpes simplex viral (HSV) infection. Multiple HSV lesions destroy the glans penis (*a*), mimicking a malignant tumor. The biopsy shows extensive necrosis and ulceration in the skin (*b*). Infected squamous epithelial cells are transformed to multinuclear cells with molding characteristic of HSV infection (*c* and *d*).

CHAPTER 28

Noninvasive Carcinomas of the Penile and Scrotal Skin

SQUAMOUS CELL CARCINOMA IN SITU

Definition

- Noninvasive squamous cell carcinoma is an early form of squamous cell carcinoma that develops within penile and scrotal epidermis, without penetrating through the basement membrane

Other terms

- In situ = in place, in Latin
- Severe squamous dysplasia, condyloma with severe dysplasia: carcinoma in situ may develop within a condyloma
- Bowen disease: single well-demarcated plaque-like lesion
- Bowenoid papulosis: multiple or solitary, macular, or papular lesion
- Erythroplasia of Queyrat, named after Louis Queyrat, is a squamous cell carcinoma in situ of the glans penis

Pathogenesis

- Squamous cell carcinoma in situ (CIS) is associated with HPV16 and the precursor for invasive carcinoma

Clinical features

- Solitary or multiple lesion, plaque-like lesions or papules

Gross pathology

- Flat or slightly elevated lesion that does not form a mass
- Polypoid if associated with a condyloma
- When it is located in the glans, it has erythematous appearance known as *erythroplasia of Queyrat* (Fig. 28-1)

Histology

- Full thickness involvement of squamous epithelium (Fig. 28-2) by malignant or dysplastic squamous cells, which are characterized by the nuclear enlargement, nuclear membrane irregularity, hyperchromasia, and atypical mitosis (Figs. 28-3 and 28-4)
- With (Fig. 28-4) or without keratinization (Fig. 28-2)
- CIS may be associated with condyloma, as in Bowenoid papulosis (Fig. 28-5)
- The major forms of squamous CIS are compared in Table 28-1. However, histologically they are almost identical
- CIS may be associated with invasive components. If that is the case, it confirms the primary site or origin of the invasive carcinoma

Immunohistochemistry

- P53 positive
- Higher Ki67 proliferative activity, and p16 positive if associated with HPV

Clinical relevance (prognosis and treatment options)

- Because of the risk to develop into an invasive disease, CIS should be treated
- Treatment options include surgical excision and removal by other methods

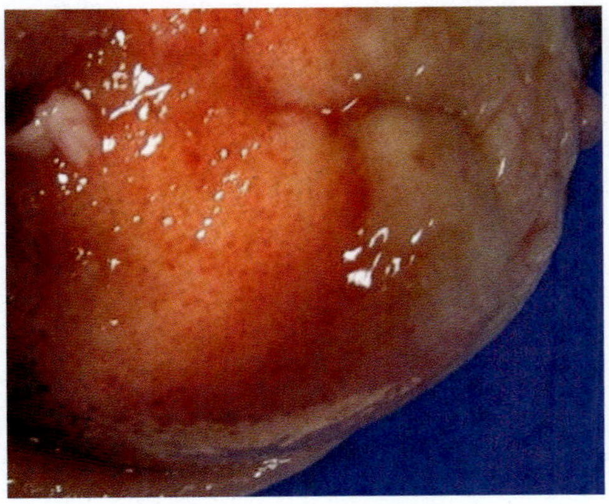

Figure 28-1.
Gross photo of squamous cell carcinoma in situ (CIS) in the glans penis (erythroplasia of Queyrat) showing red granular area of the glans penis.

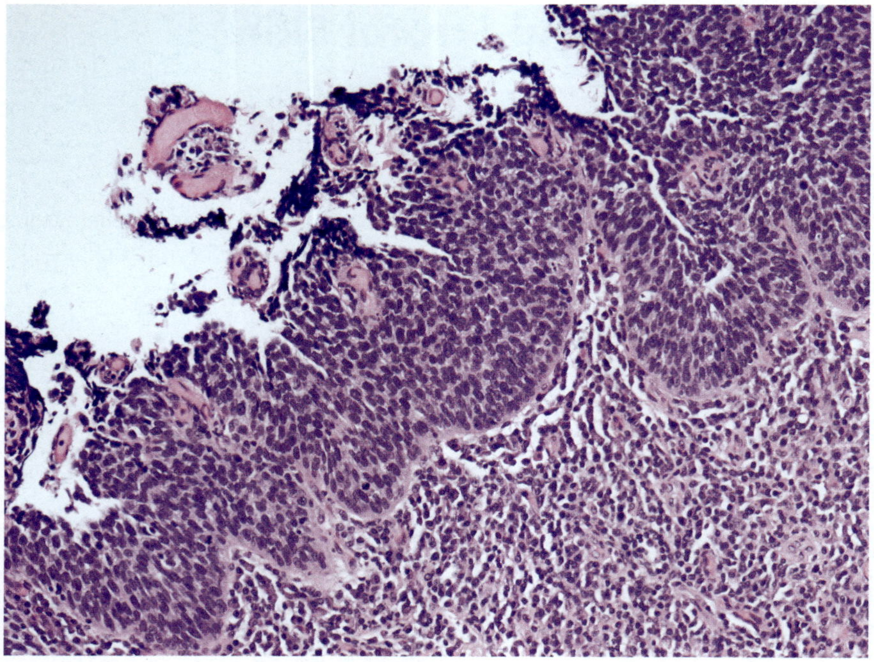

Figure 28-2.
Squamous cell CIS shows nonkeratinized malignant squamous cells involving full thickness of the epithelium, but confined within basement membrane. It is associated with marked chronic inflammation.

Figure 28-3.
Squamous cell CIS (Bowenoid papule) with acanthosis and "epitheliomatous" growth patterns without invasion (*a*). High magnification shows dysplastic squamous cells involving the full thickness of the epidermis (*b*).

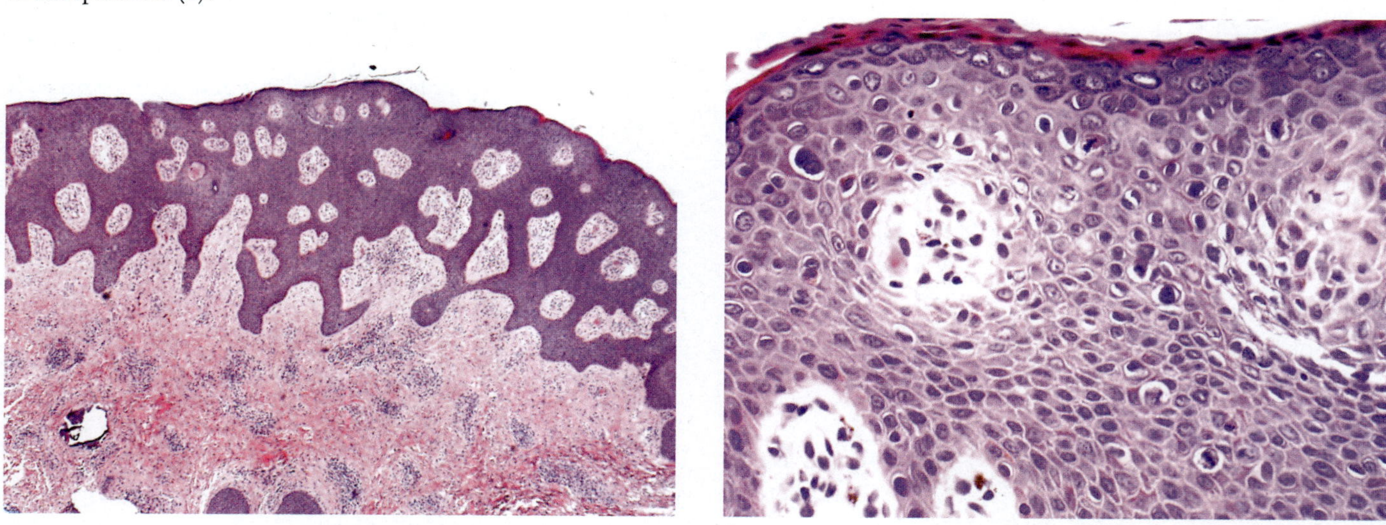

a b

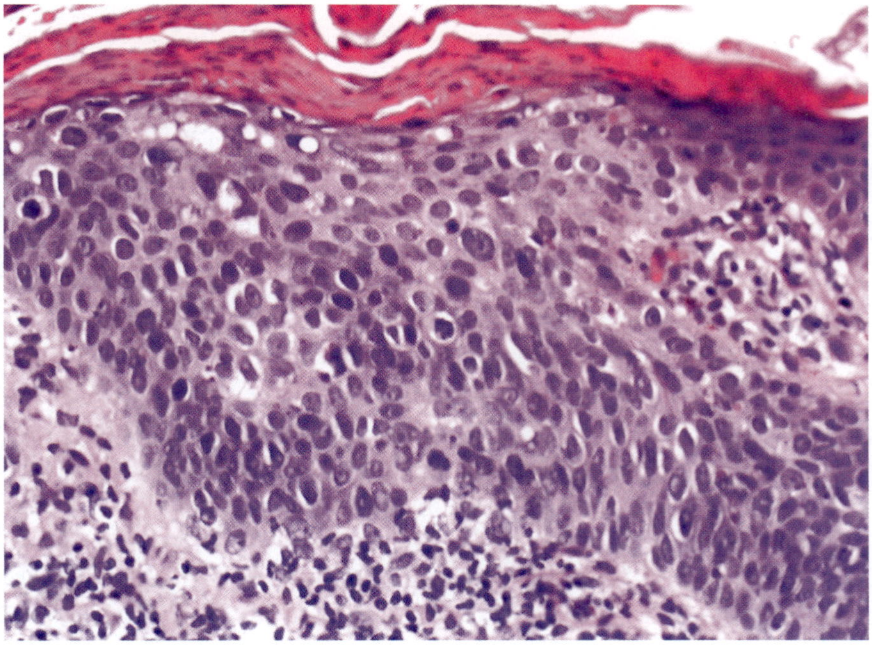

Figure 28-4.
Squamous cell CIS with keratinization.

Figure 28-5.
Squamous cell CIS associated with a condyloma. The full thickness involvement of the epidermis by dysplastic squamous cells (*a*). High magnification shows both koilocytes (*b*, right side) and high-grade dysplastic cells (*b*, left side).

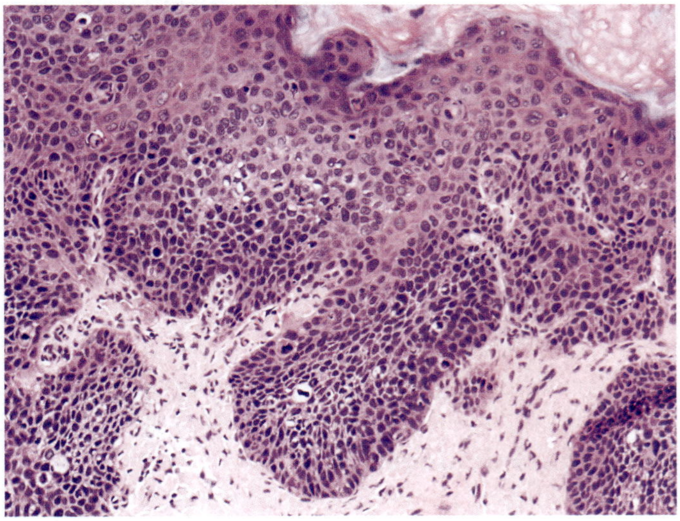

a

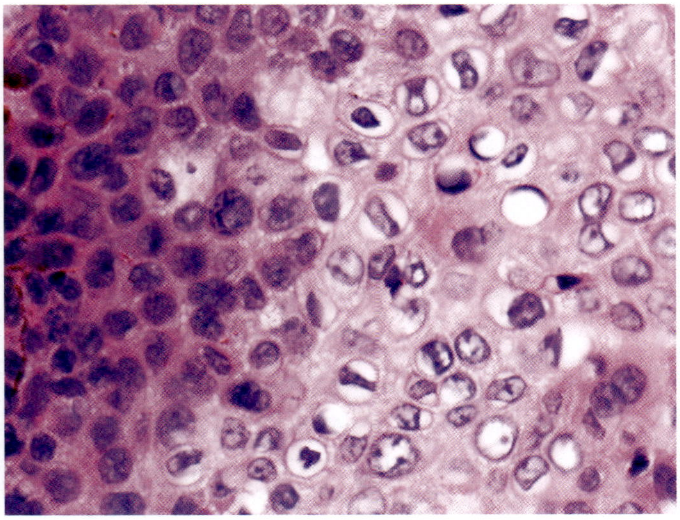

b

Table 28-1. Comparison of Different Forms of Squamous Cell Carcinoma In Situ (CIS)

Features	*Bowen disease*	*Bowenoid papulosis*	*Erythroplasia of Queyrat*
Histology	Squamous cell CIS	Squamous cell CIS	Squamous cell CIS
Location	Anywhere on skin	External genital areas	Glans penis
Gross	Solitary lesion up to several centimeters	Multiple lesions	Reddish lesion of glans penis
Associated with HPV	Mostly not	Yes	Mostly not
Progression to invasive carcinoma	Likely	Possible, maybe small percentage	Likely
Histology	Full thickness involvement by dysplastic cells	Full thickness involvement by dysplastic cells	Full thickness involvement by dysplastic cells
Treatment	Necessary	Necessary	Necessary
Other features		Koilocytes seen	

CIS, carcinoma in situ; HPV, human papilloma virus.

PAGET'S DISEASE

Definition

- Intraepidermal carcinoma, usually adenocarcinoma, present in the skin of penis or scrotum

Other terms

- Extramammary Paget disease (EMPD)

Pathogenesis

- Primary: unlike in mammary Paget disease where an underlying breast cancer is always present, in the majority of cases of extramammary Paget disease, the underlying carcinoma cannot be identified
- Secondary: a small percentage of cases (20% to 25%), an underlying carcinoma of the skin adnexa, colonic adenocarcinoma, or bladder urothelial carcinoma can be seen associated with Paget disease

Clinical features and gross pathology

- The lesion may involve the penile shaft, scrotum, inguinal and perineal regions
- Red or pale plaque-like lesion with scaling or oozing

Histology

- Scattered individual or clusters of malignant epithelial cells within the epidermis, distinct from the background benign squamous cells (Fig. 28-6)
- The Paget cells have pale cytoplasm, large nuclei, which may be arranged in apparent or subtle glandular patterns (Figs. 28-6 and 28-7)
- In the case of bladder cancer as underlying carcinoma, it can be either adenocarcinoma or pagetoid urothelial carcinoma
- When Paget cells invade the dermis, it will become invasive adenocarcinoma, which may lead to metastasis to other distal organs (Fig. 28-8)

Immunohistochemistry

- Depending on the nature of primary carcinoma. CEA and low molecular weight keratin (Fig. 28-7*b*) can be positive
- EMA or Mucicarmine stain can be positive (Fig. 28-7*c*)
- High molecular weight cytokeratin may be negative (Fig. 28-7*d*)

Differential diagnosis

- Bowen disease (squamous cell CIS): are malignant squamous cells without glandular formation. CEA, MUC will be negative
- Melanoma in situ: melanoma cells may have intracytoplasmic pigment, S100 and melanin A are positive, but keratins are negative

Clinical relevance (prognosis and treatment options)

- If an underlying adenocarcinoma can be identified by a clinical work-up, the treatment should be focused on the control of the primary tumor
- Primary Paget disease (if no primary adenocarcinoma can be identified) is usually treated by surgical resection

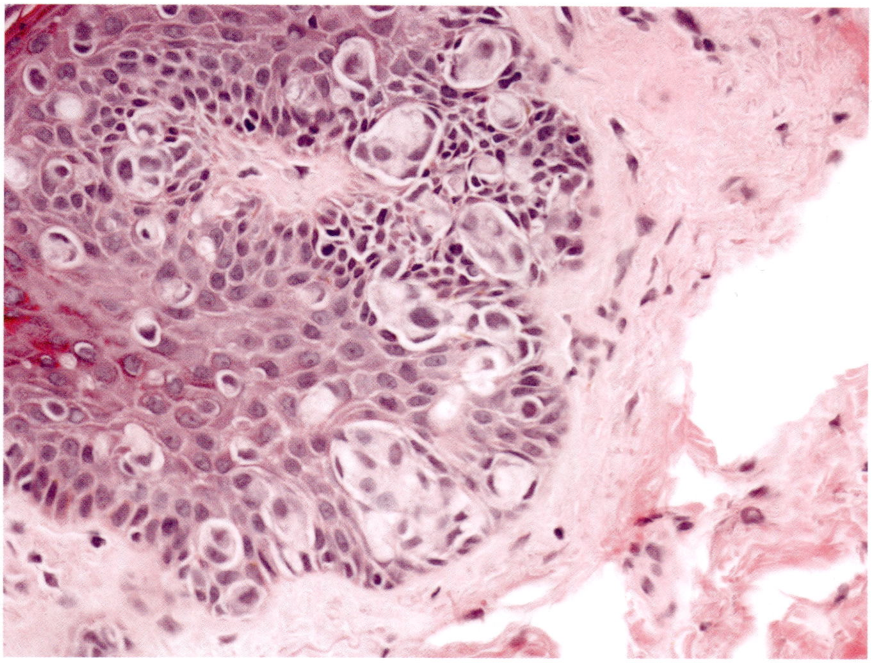

Figure 28-6.
Primary Paget disease of the scrotum exhibits individual or clustered carcinoma cells in the epidermis, with subtle glandular formation.

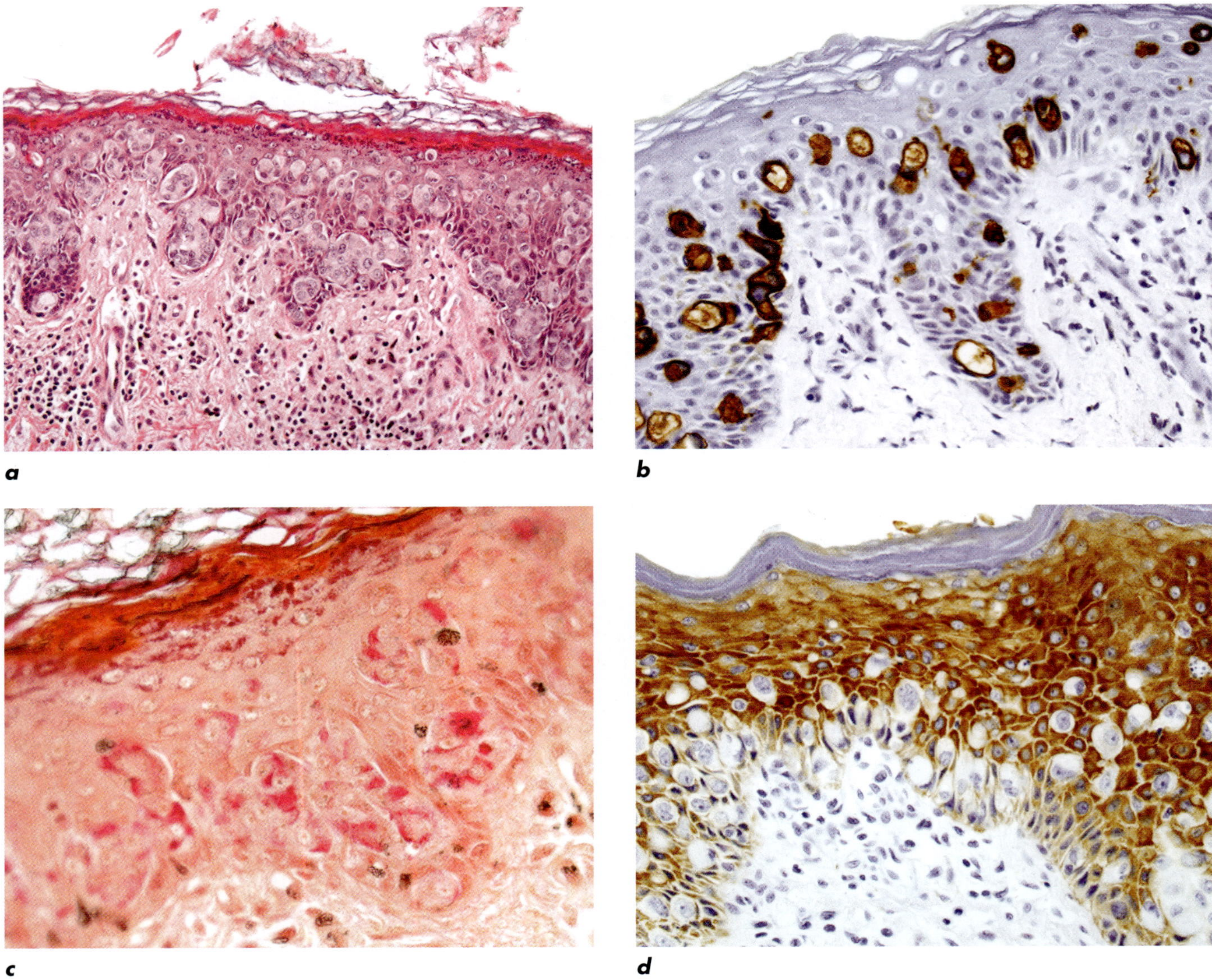

Figure 28-7.
Paget disease of the scrotum (*a*). The tumor cells are positive for AE1/AE3 (*b*) and mucicarmine staining (*c*), negative for high molecular keratins (*d*).

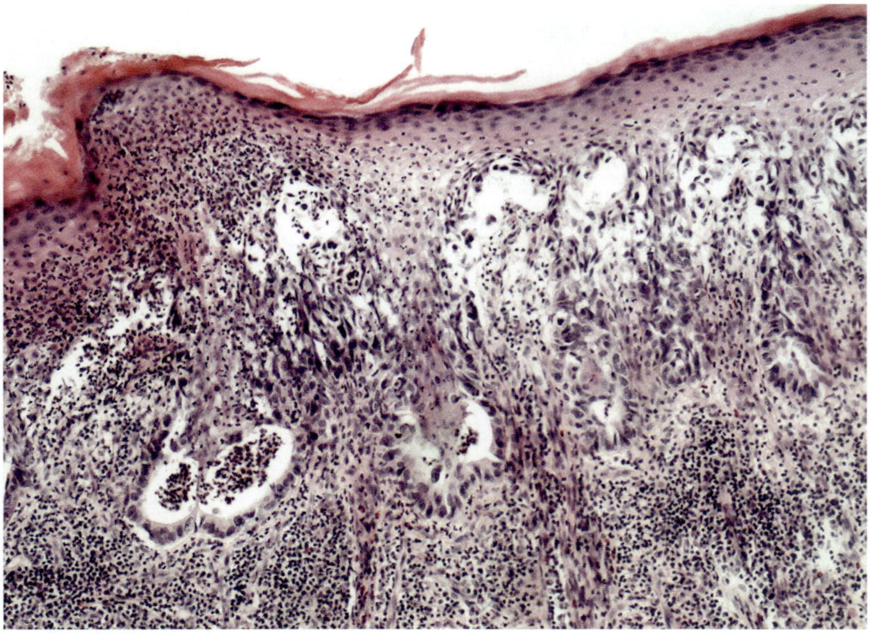

Figure 28-8.
Primary Paget disease of the penis with an invasive component. Tumor cells demonstrating glandular formation, involving the rete ridges of the epidermis and extending to the upper dermis (left).

CHAPTER 29

Invasive Carcinoma of the Penis and Scrotum

VERRUCOUS CARCINOMA

Definition

- An uncommon malignant squamous neoplasm, locally invasive but nonmetastasizing
- Anogenital-type verrucous carcinoma is defined as Type II verrucous carcinoma
- Verrucous carcinoma (Type I) may occur in other locations, such as head and neck regions

Other terms

- Carcinoma cuniculatum, epithelioma cuniculatum, Ackerman tumor

Pathogenesis

- Verrucous carcinoma is an essentially unusual variant of low-grade invasive squamous cell carcinoma

Clinical features

- It is a slow-growing lesion with large exophytic appearance, usually occurs in men older than 60 years
- It may be painful if deeply invasive

Gross pathology

- An exophytic and papillary mass on the skin, which may discharge malodorous debris through several sinus tracts

Histology

- Diffuse and broad-based papillary lesions composed of elongated fronds (Figs. 29-1 and 29-2)
- Well-differentiated squamous epithelium on the surface of the tumor (Figs. 29-3 and 29-4), which is difficult to make the diagnosis when specimen is limited
- Presence of deeply invading fronds is required to establish diagnosis (Figs. 29-2 and 29-5)

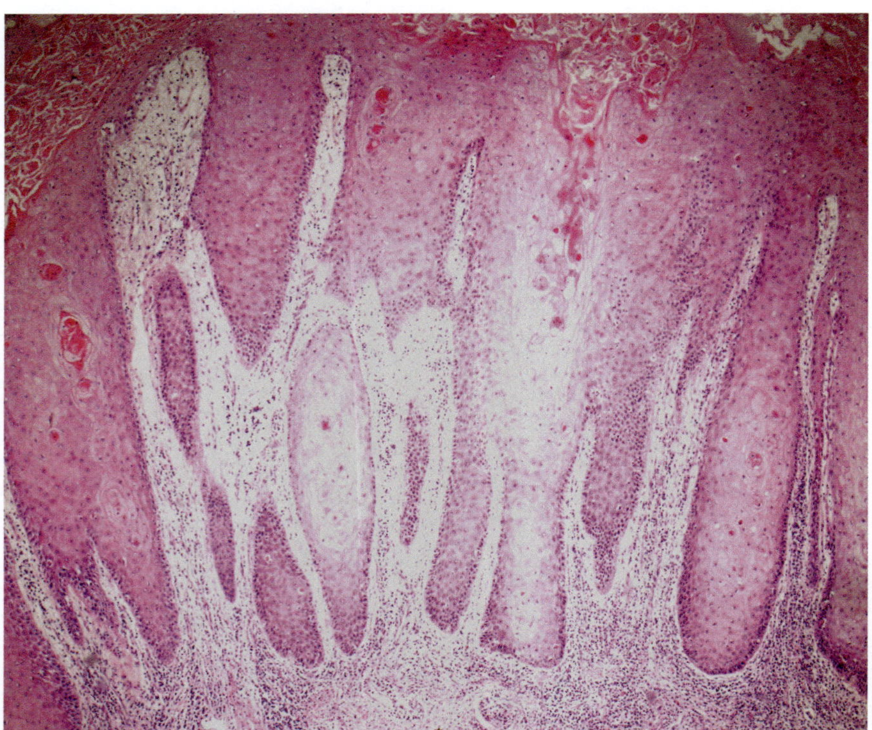

Figure 29-1.
Verrucous carcinoma of the penis is composed of the well-formed elongated and paralleled papillary fronds.

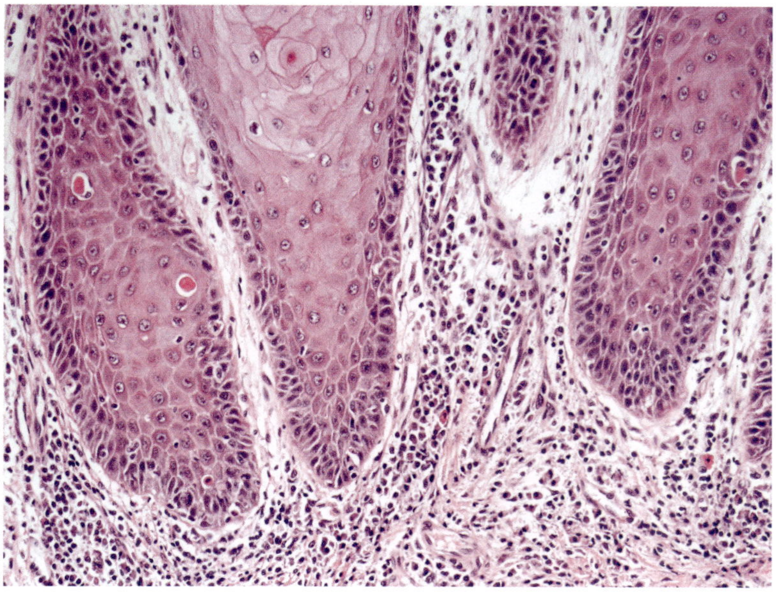

Figure 29-2.
Verrucous carcinoma shows the well-differentiated squamous islands along with the invasive fronds.

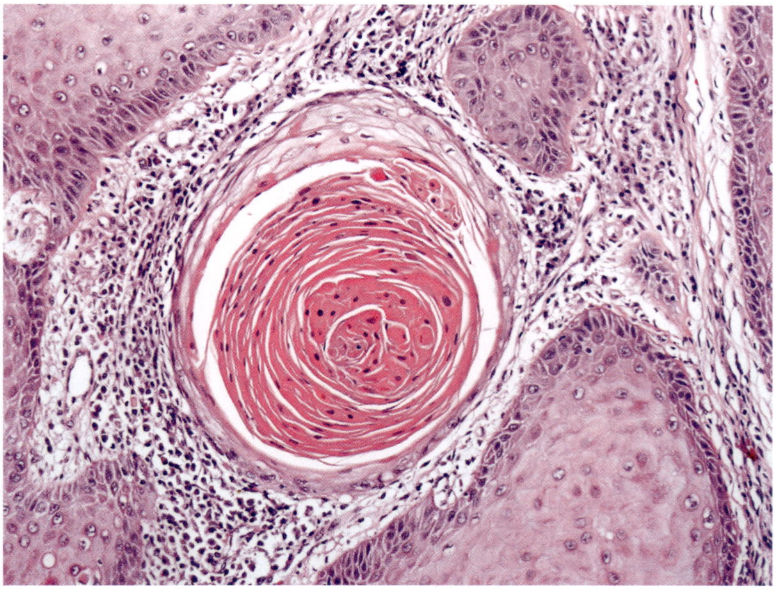

Figure 29-3.
Verrucous carcinoma with a keratin pearl and well-differentiated squamous islands.

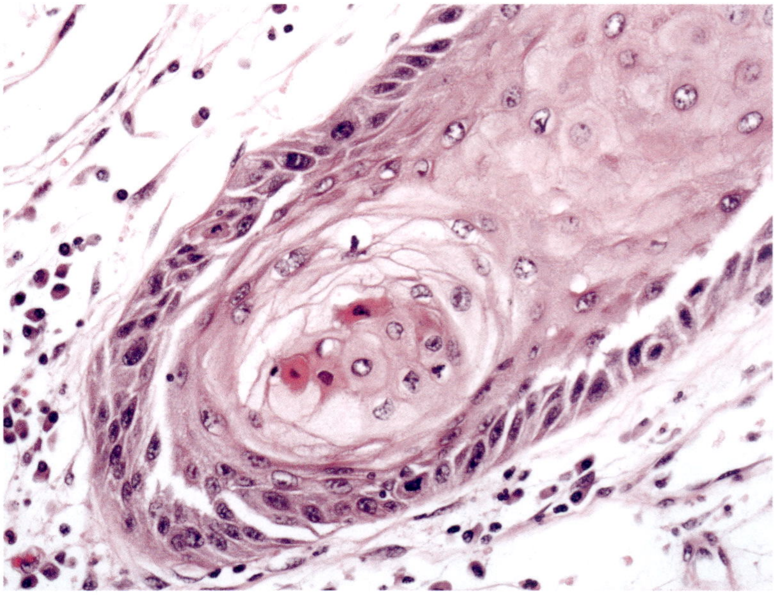

Figure 29-4.
The invasive fronds of a verrucous carcinoma displays minimal cytological atypia.

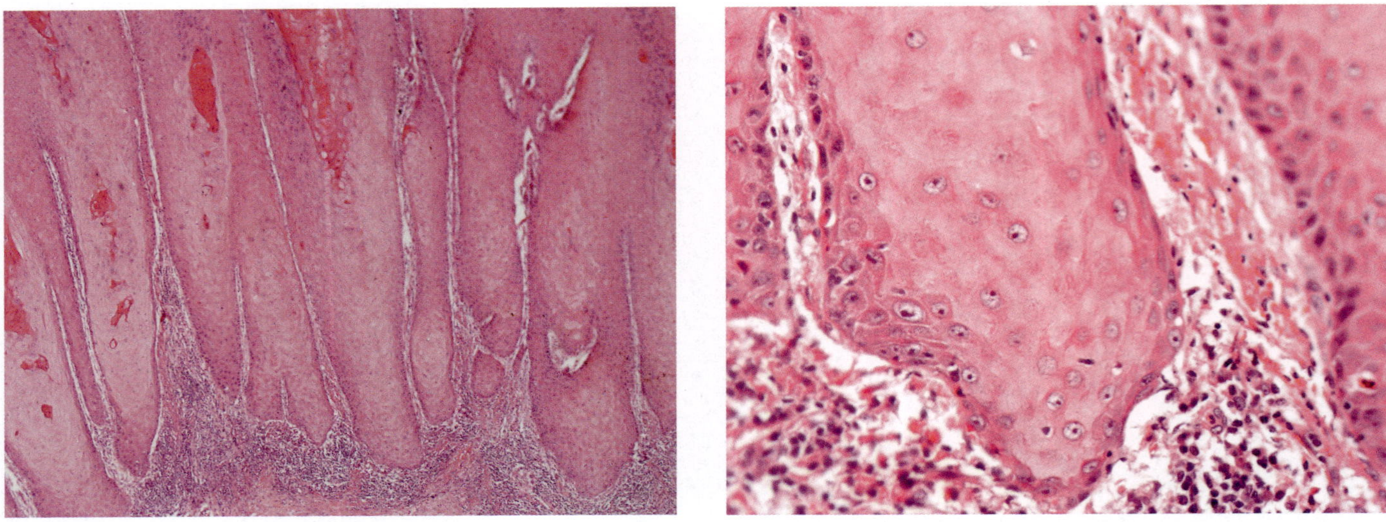

a b

Figure 29-5.
Penile verrucous carcinoma characterized by the paralleled long papillary fronds (*a*). High magnification shows the invasive cells with no cytological atypia (*b*).

- No significant cytological atypia is present (Figs. 29-2 to 29-5)
- If there is mild cytological atypia in a verrucoid lesion, we sometimes use the diagnosis of *verruciform squamous cell carcinoma, well-differentiated,* which basically covers both verrucous carcinoma and well-differentiated invasive squamous cell carcinoma

Clinical relevance (prognosis and treatment)

- Surgical excision or laser therapy are the treatments of choice
- Penile cancer stage: Ta
- Most patients with a good prognosis. Local recurrence is common but metastasis is rare

SQUAMOUS CELL CARCINOMA, INVASIVE

Definition

- A malignant epithelial neoplasm derived from squamous epithelium
- Typically, this is an invasive tumor (CIS described previously)

Pathogenesis

- Risk factors include phimosis, chronic inflammation, lichen sclerosus, and condyloma

Clinical features

- The mean presentation age is 60 years
- Either exophytic or ulcerated mass. In the advanced stage, the tumor may have necrosis
- First metastatic site is superficial inguinal lymph node

Gross pathology

- Typical large mass greater than 3 cm (Fig. 29-6). A firm base indicates desmoplastic reaction and invasion. Necrosis and ulceration are commonly seen

Histology

- Squamous cell carcinoma, from well to poorly differentiated, nonkeratinized (Fig. 29-7) or keratinized tumor cells (Fig. 29-8)
- Tumor cells are present at the base or edges of an ulcerated mass
- Tumor invasion and desmoplastic reaction by the stroma (Fig. 29-9) or perineural invasion can be seen (Fig. 29-10)
- Two distinct features of squamous cell carcinoma are keratin pearls (Fig. 29-8*b*) and intercellular bridges (tight junctions, Fig. 29-10), although these features sometimes are not obvious (Fig. 29-11)
- Tumor cells may invade erectile tissue of the corpus (Fig. 29-12)

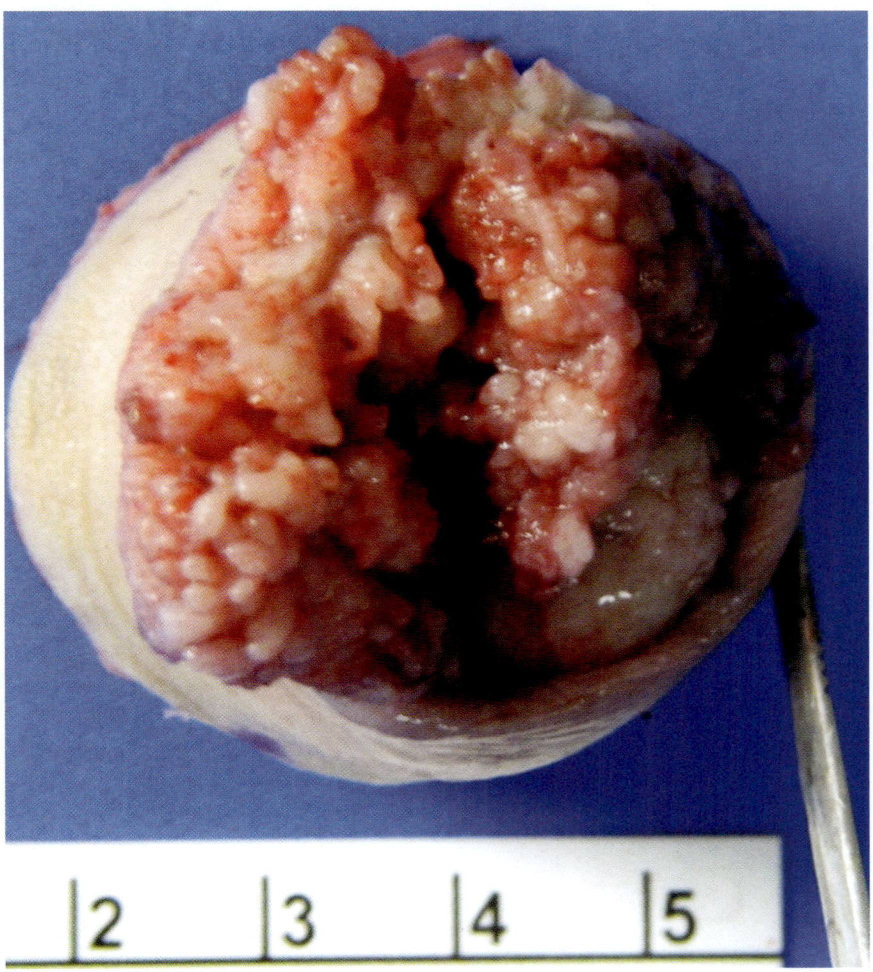

Figure 29-6.
Gross photo of a penile invasive squamous cell carcinoma shows a large mass replacing a portion of the glans penis.

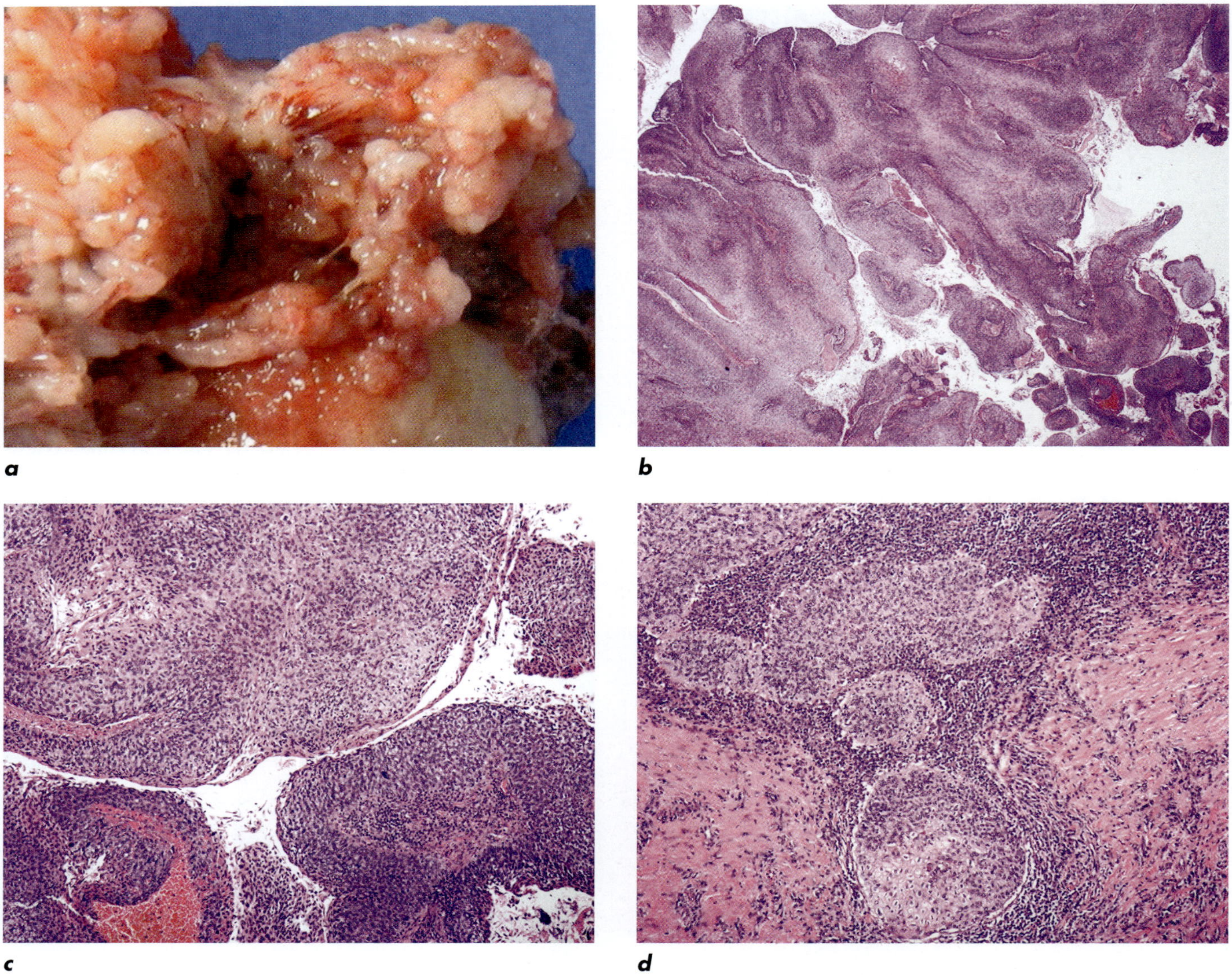

Figure 29-7.
Invasive squamous cell carcinoma with a papillary appearance (*a*). Microscopically, the tumor shows extensive papillary projections (*b*). High magnification shows the malignant squamous cells covering the papillary structures (*c*) and invasive component of the tumor (*d*).

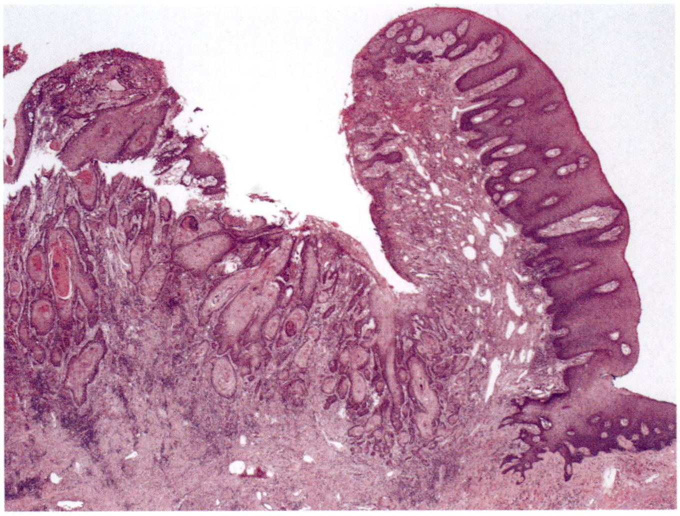

a

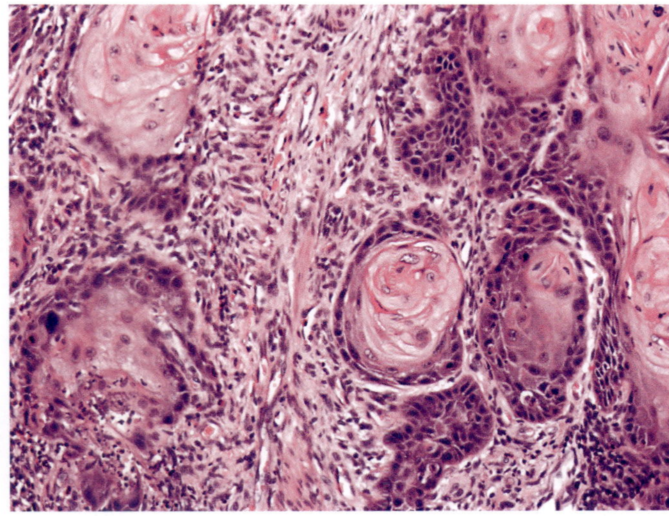

b

Figure 29-8.
Invasive squamous cell carcinoma of the penis is a large fungating mass with a crater-like center (*a*). High magnification shows invasive tumor cells forming keratin pearls, and associated desmoplastic reaction and chronic inflammation (*b*).

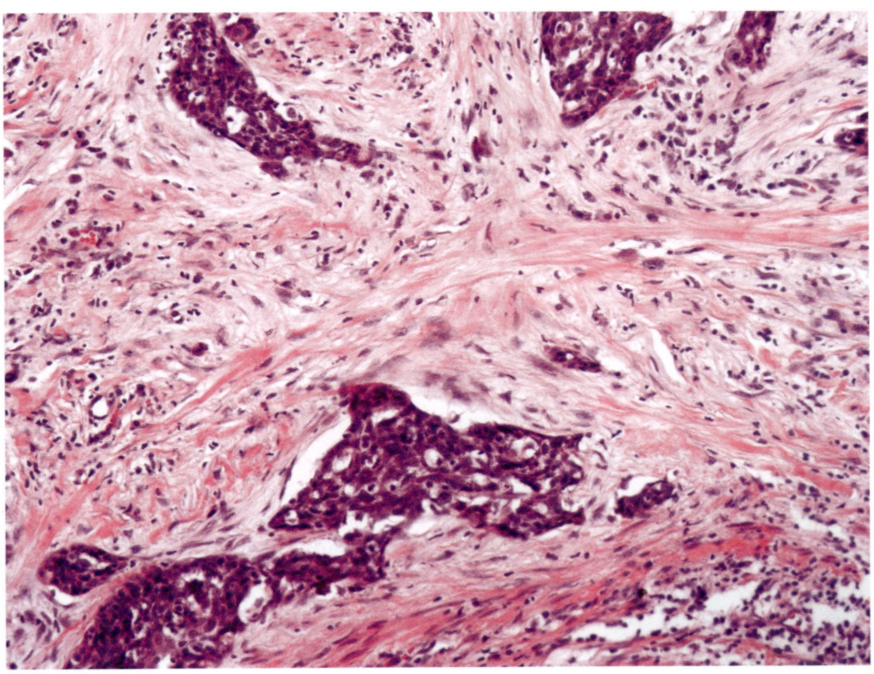

Figure 29-9.
Invasive squamous cell carcinoma with basaloid features showing strong desmoplastic reaction.

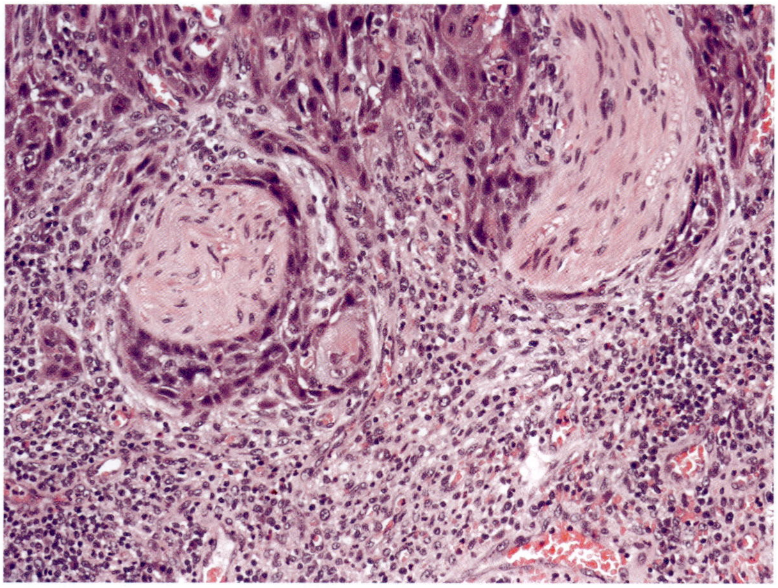

Figure 29-10.
Squamous cell carcinoma with perineural invasion.

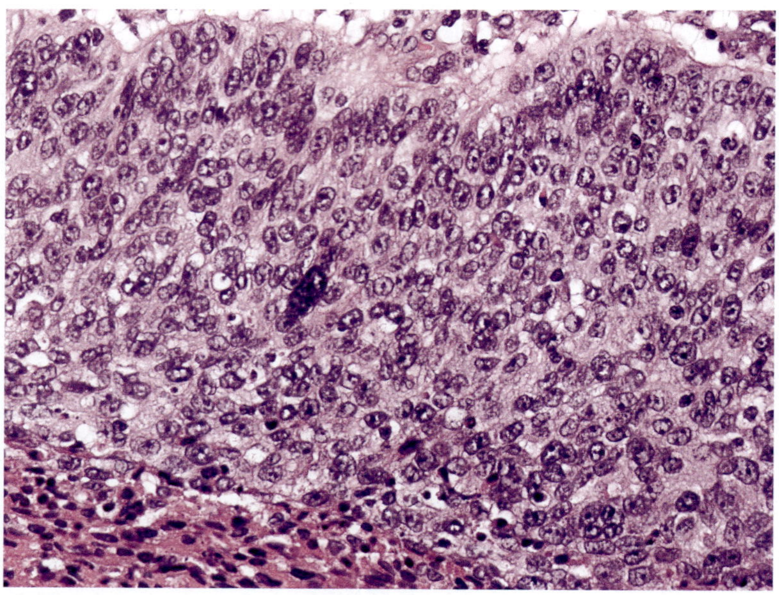

Figure 29-11.
Nuclear atypia of squamous cell carcinoma, keratinization, and intercellular bridges are difficult to see in this case.

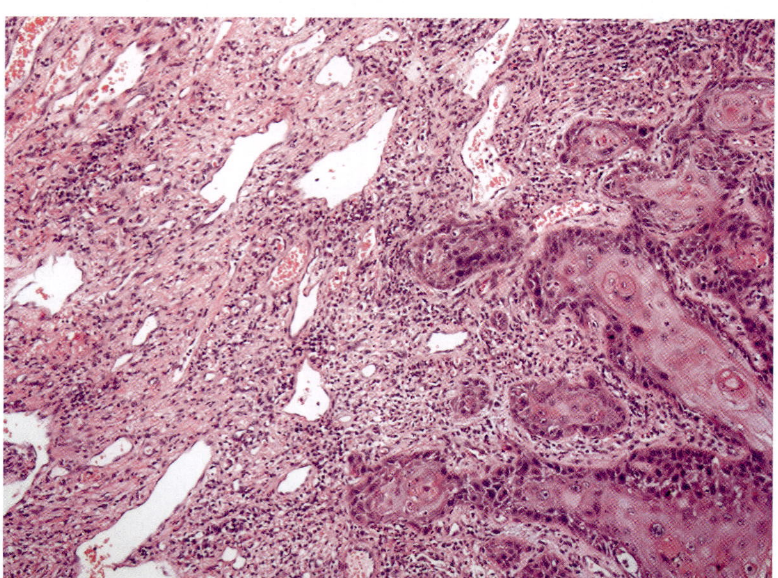

Figure 29-12.
Squamous cell carcinoma of the penis invading the corpus erectile tissue.

- Histological variations
  - Basaloid carcinoma (different from basal cell carcinoma)
  - Warty (condylomatous) carcinoma
  - Papillary carcinoma, not otherwise specified
  - Sarcomatoid carcinoma
  - Adenosquamous carcinoma

Immunohistochemistry

- P16 positive and p53 positive

Clinical relevance (prognosis and treatment options)

- Prognosis is related to the tumor site, size, growth pattern, histological type and grade, as well the depth of invasion. The prognostic factors of penile squamous cell carcinoma are summarized in Table 29-1
- Treatment of choice is surgical resection, local excision, or penectomy (Table 29-1)
- Penile cancer staging
  - **Tx**: primary tumor cannot be assessed; **T0**: no evidence of primary tumor; **Tis**: carcinoma in situ; **Ta**: noninvasive verrucous carcinoma (broad pushing invasion permitted); **T1**: tumor invades subepithelial connective tissue; **T1a**: without lymph vascular invasion, not poorly differentiated; **T1b**: with lymphovascular invasion, or poorly differentiated; **T2**: tumor invades corpus spongiosum or carvernosum; **T3**: tumor invades urethra; **T4**: tumor invades other adjacent organs

Table 29-1. Prognostic Factor for Penile Squamous Cell Carcinoma

Factors	*Better*	*Worse*
Site	Foreskin	Other penile locations
Growth patterns	Superficial spread	Vertical
Tumor size	Small	Large
Grade	Well differentiated	Poorly differentiated
Depth of invasion	Superficial	Deep
Histological type	Verrucous Verruciform	Sarcomatoid (Carcinosarcoma)

BASAL CELL CARCINOMA

Definition

- Malignant cutaneous tumor characterized by the presence of lobule or cord of neoplastic basaloid cells

Other terms

- Basal cell epithelioma, trichoblastic carcinoma

Clinical features

- Basal cell carcinoma is the most common skin carcinoma, which typically develops on the sun-exposed areas
- Basal cell carcinoma in the skin of penis or scrotum is rare

Gross pathology

- Slow-growing lesions
- Mostly seen in the shaft of the penis
- Elevated pearly nodules
- May be associated with ulceration

Histology

- More than 10 histological subtypes, such as superficial, invasive types, have been described for BCC, most of these types do not correlate with tumor behaviors
- Tumor lobules can be attached to the epidermis (Fig. 29-13) or infiltrative in the dermis (Fig. 29-14)
- Evident palisading cells located in the periphery of the tumor lobule (Fig. 29-14*b*)
- Desmoplastic or myxoid stromal changes are frequently seen (Fig. 29-15)

Clinical relevance (prognosis and treatment options)

- Locally invasive disease, its metastatic potential extremely low
- If there is an evidence of metastasis, the diagnosis of basaloid squamous cell carcinoma or other types of carcinoma rather than basal cell carcinoma should be considered
- Local excision is the treatment of choice

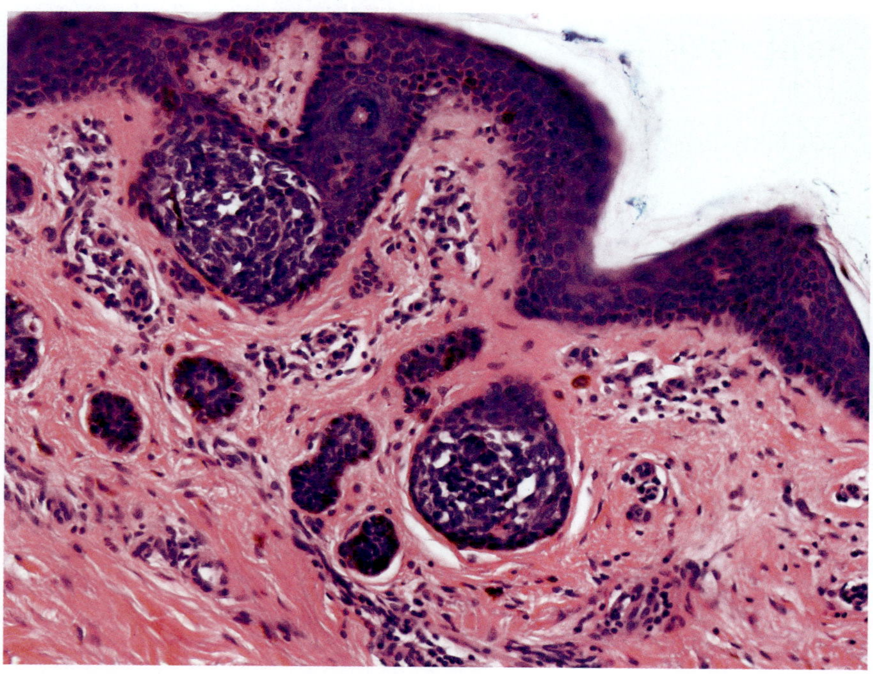

Figure 29-13.
Basal cell carcinoma, superficial type, composed of small nests of tumor cells in the junction of epidermis and dermis.

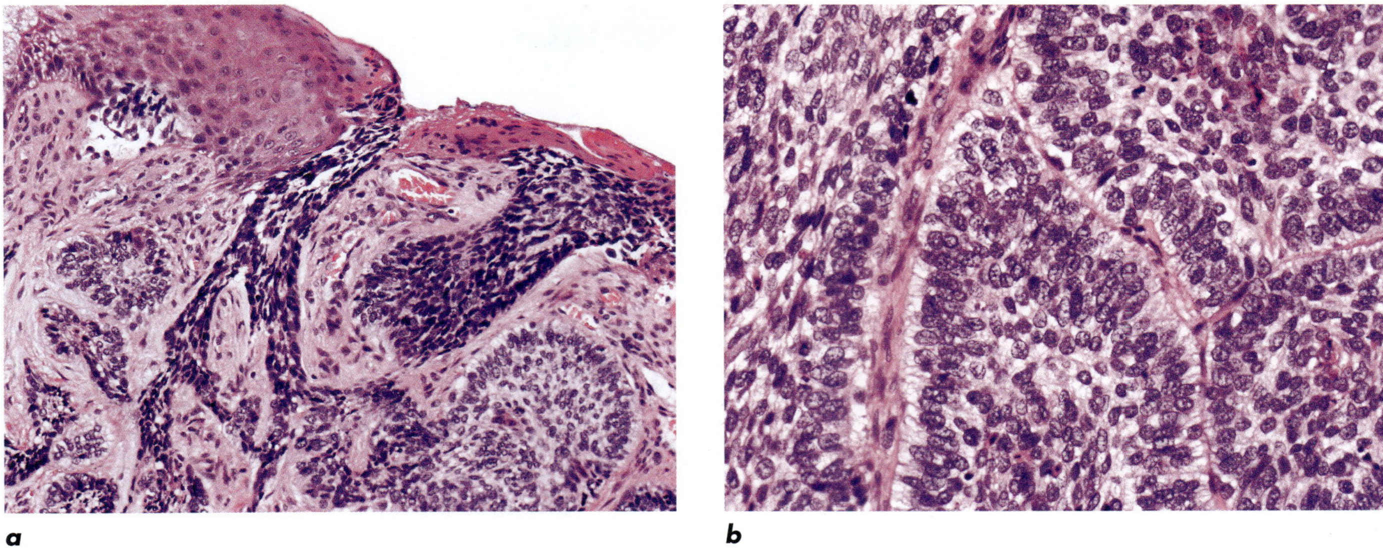

Figure 29-14.
Basal cell carcinoma, invasive type, with multiple tumor lobules present in the basal layers and island of basaloid tumor cells invading the dermis (*a*). High magnification shows palisading periphery and scant cytoplasm of basaloid tumor cells (*b*).

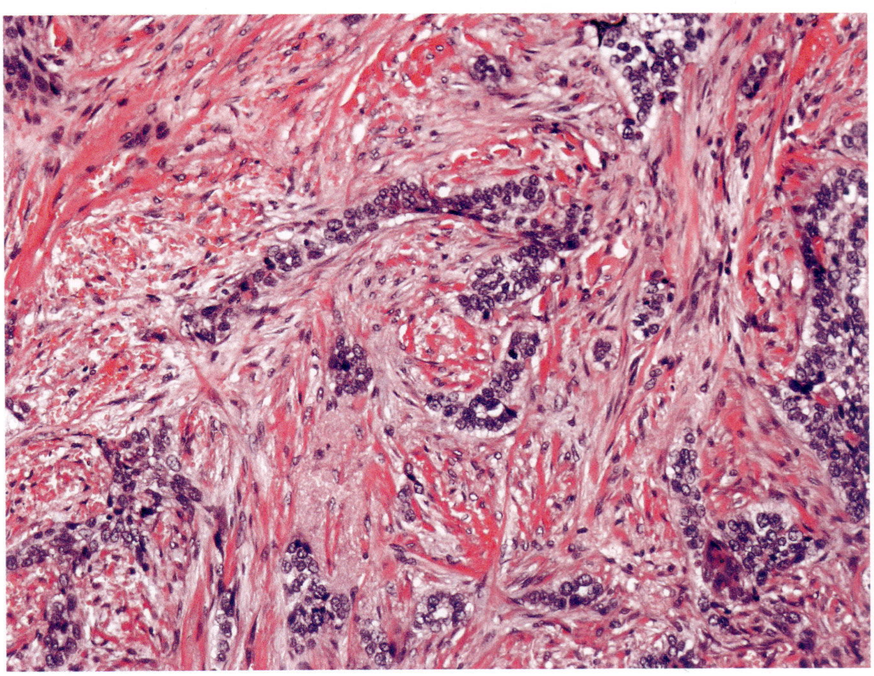

Figure 29-15.
Basal cell carcinoma with cords of invasive tumor cells with scant cytoplasm and associated with marked desmoplastic reaction.

CHAPTER 30

Other Malignant Tumors of the Penis and Scrotum

METASTATIC CARCINOMAS

Definition

- Carcinoma originated from other organs metastatic to the penis or scrotum
- A rare condition, and difficult to diagnose without clinical history of the primary carcinoma

Clinical features

- Because of its location, the GU primary such as bladder or prostate primary should be considered first
- Typically, only high-grade and high-stage carcinoma will cause metastasis, therefore, the symptoms related to the primary tumor may be detected
- One exception is low-grade clear cell RCC, which may develop early metastasis although the penile/scrotal location is uncommon

Histology

- If carcinoma in the penis or scrotum is not a squamous cell carcinoma, but a poorly differentiated carcinoma (Fig. 30-1) or an adenocarcinoma, a secondary carcinoma should be excluded particularly if the patient has a history of another malignancy
- If a tumor resembles melanoma, work-up is necessary to exclude a melanoma

Immunohistochemistry

- Necessary for confirmation of diagnosis
- Urothelial carcinoma positive for CK20 and p63 (Fig. 30-1)
- Colonic adenocarcinoma positive for CK20 and CDX2

Clinical relevance (prognosis and treatment options)

- Biopsy is necessary to establish a definitive diagnosis
- Radical surgery such as penectomy is unlikely beneficial for a patient with metastatic tumor. Systemic treatment is necessary

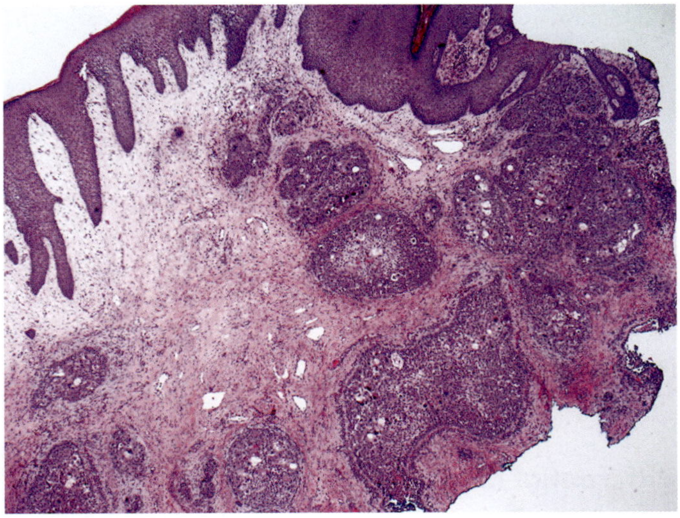

a

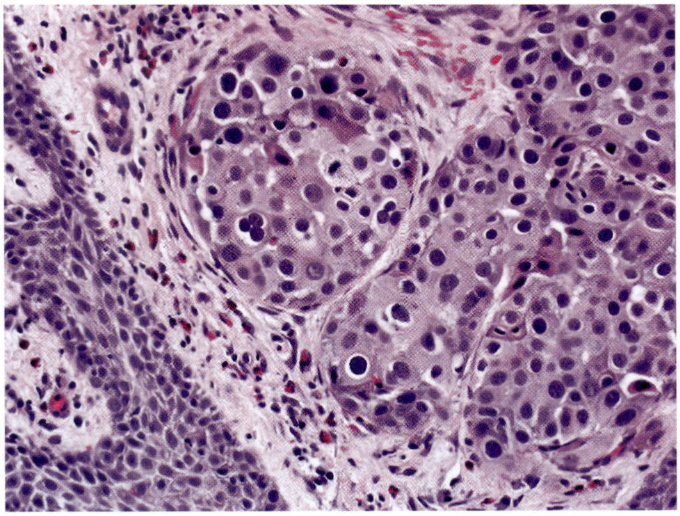

b

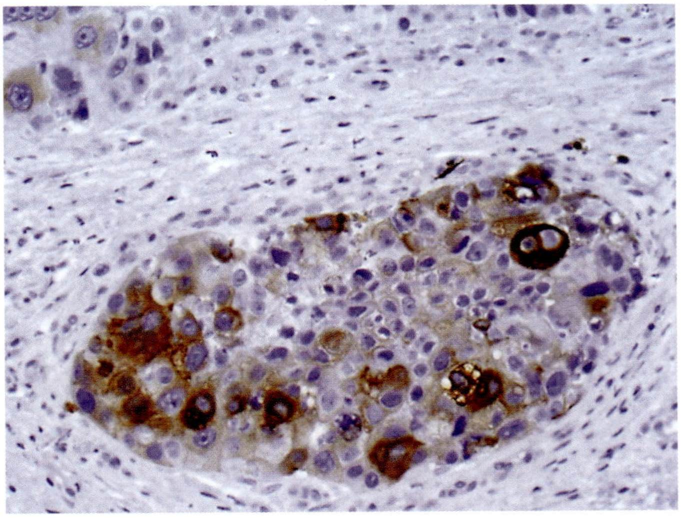

c

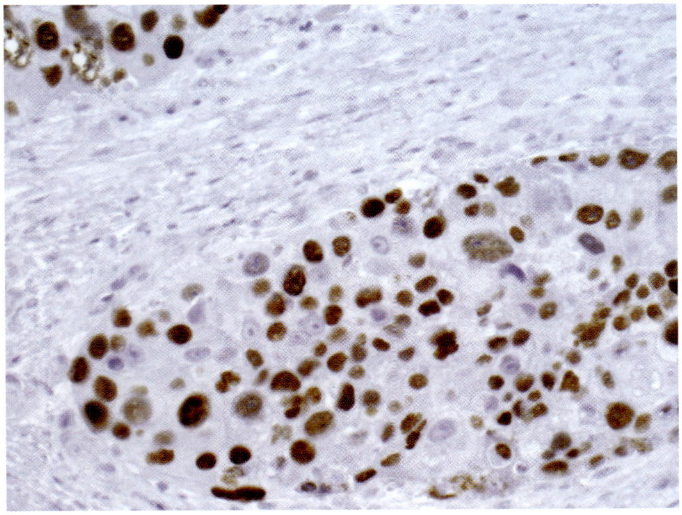

d

Figure 30-1.

Metastatic urothelial carcinoma in the penis with multiple nests of invasive tumor cells in dermis (*a*). High magnification shows the difference between the normal squamous epithelium and urothelial carcinoma cells (*b*, right). The tumor cells do not form glands or exhibit squamous features. The diagnosis is confirmed by immunoreactivity of CK20 (*c*) and p63 (*d*) in the tumor cells.

MELANOMA OF THE PENIS

Definition

- Malignant melanocytic neoplasm develops in the penis or scrotum
- Can be primary or secondary (metastasis or direct extension). Primary melanoma may develop in the penile/scrotal skin or the penile urethral mucosa
- Melanoma can be also seen in other GU organs such as urethra and bladder

Clinical features

- Fast-growing mass with or without pigment, may be associated with spontaneous hemorrhage or change of color
- Mean age 65 years

Gross pathology

- Typically a large lesion, necrosis or hemorrhage may be present

Histology

- Melanoma cells are large polygonal, with abundant cytoplasm, which often form large nests, but they can form many other patterns, mimicking other malignant neoplasms
- Pagtoid melanoma in situ may be present (Figs. 30-2 and 30-3)
- Tumor cells may contain cytoplasmic pigment granules or dusty appearance (Figs. 30-3 and 30-4)
- Prominent nucleoli with other marked cytological atypia (Fig. 30-5) and brisk mitoses
- Clark level (Table 30-1) refers to the extent of an invasive melanoma
- Melanoma in situ refers to malignant melanocytes confined within the epidermis (Clark level 1)
- The Breslow thickness (Table 30-2) is defined as the total vertical thickness of a melanoma, measuring from the epidermal granular layer to the deepest invasive area in the dermis

Immunohistochemistry

- S100, HMB45 positive and keratin negative

Differential diagnosis

- *Bowen disease* (squamous carcinoma in situ), p16, and p63 positive
- *Paget disease* (adenocarcinoma), CEA, CDX2, or PAS positive
- IHC may be necessary in the difficult cases
- Melanoma in situ, Bowen disease, and Paget disease are compared in Table 30-3

Clinical relevance (prognosis and treatment options)

- Generally poor prognosis, also depending on the stage, Breslow depth (thickness, in mm), and Clark level
- It is not clear whether the Breslow system does apply to the mucosa melanoma and its correlation with prognosis
- Wide excision with lymph node dissection as a treatment option

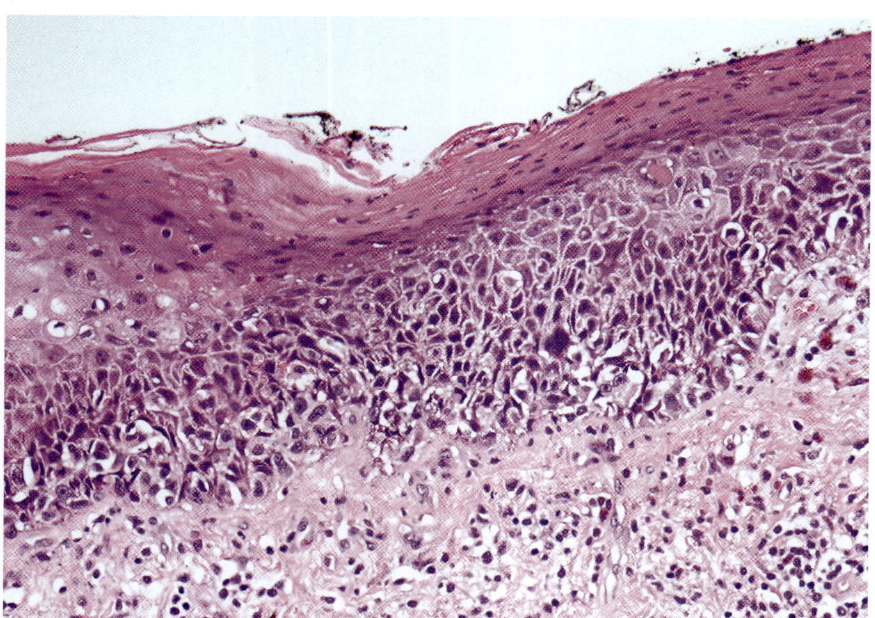

Figure 30-2.
Melanoma in situ of the penile skin involving the basal layer of the epidermis.

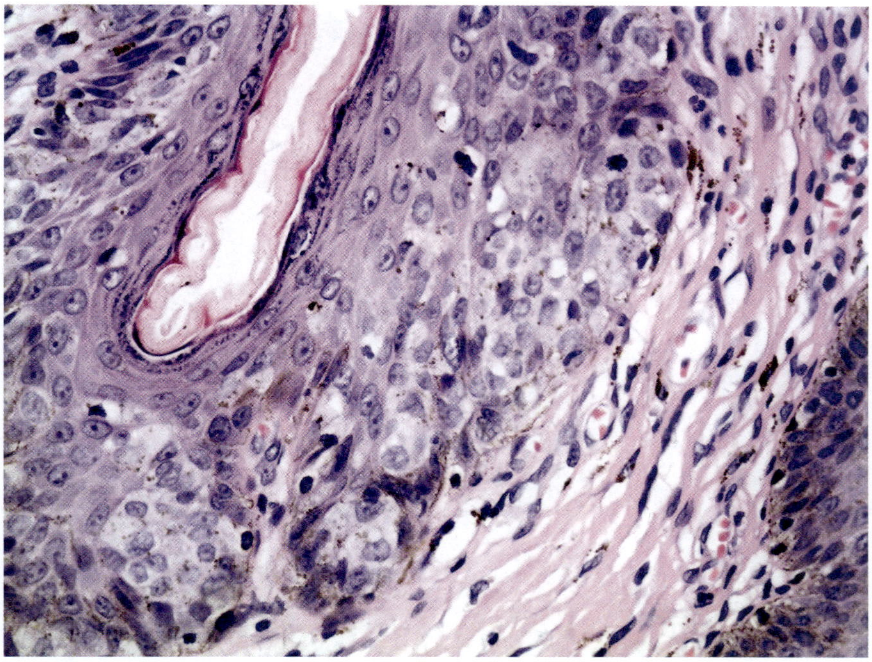

Figure 30-3.
Melanoma in situ consists of nests of cells involving a follicle, but still no invasion of the dermis.

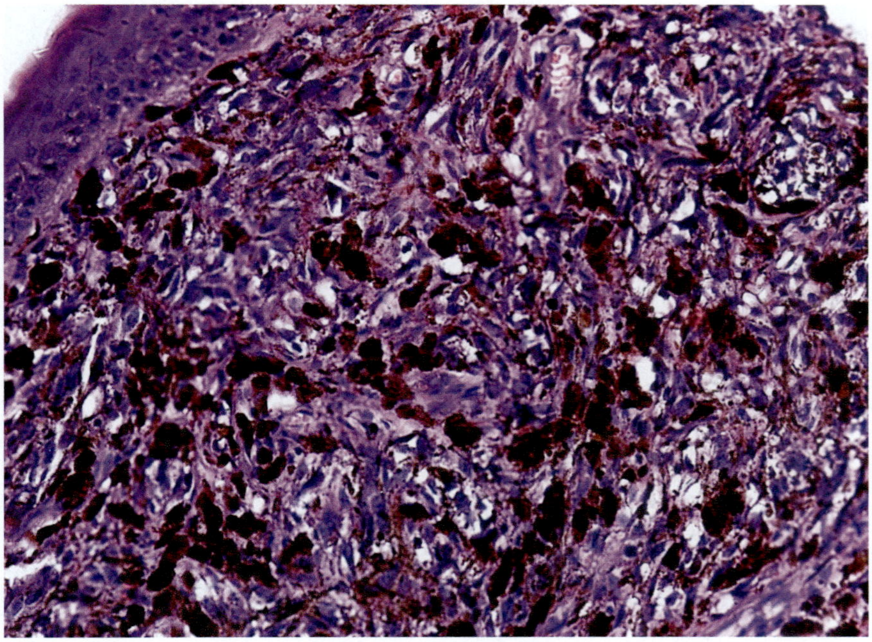

Figure 30-4.
A heavily pigmented melanoma of the penis showing the presence of spindle-shaped tumor cells with pigment.

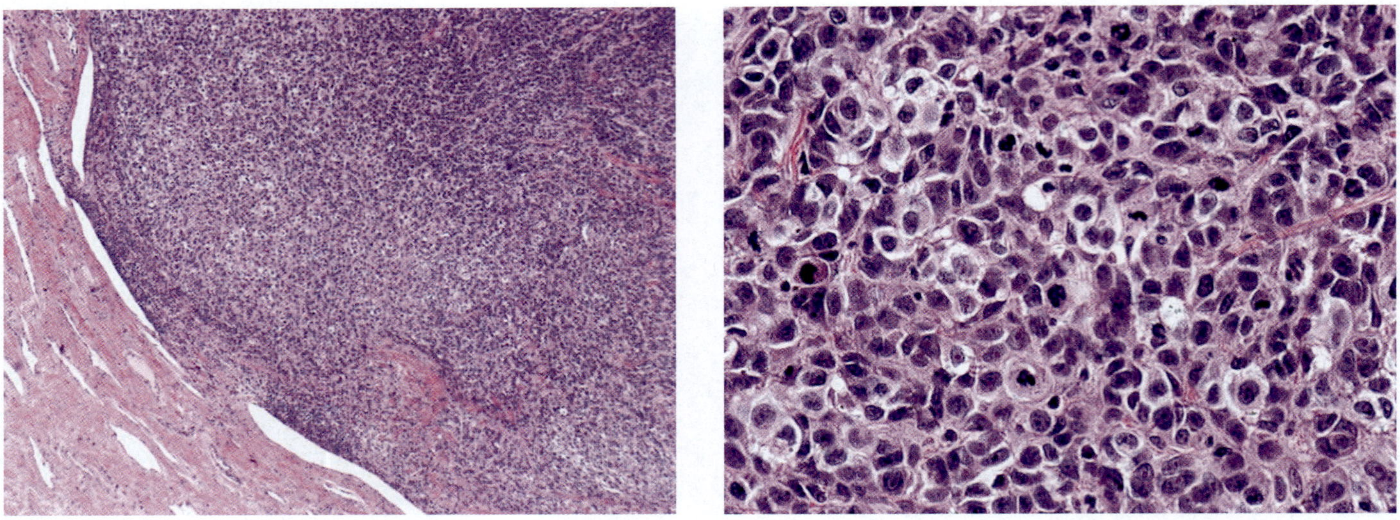

a b

Figure 30-5.
Invasive melanoma of the penile urethra invading to erectile tissue (*a*). High magnification shows the epithelioid tumor cells with significant cytological atypia and fine pigment particles (*b*).

Table 30-1. The Clark Level of Melanoma

The Clark level	*Invasion level*
I	Epidermis (in situ)
II	Papillary (upper) dermis
III	Filling of the papillary dermis
IV	Reticular (lower) dermis
V	Subcutaneous tissue

Table 30-2. The Breslow Thickness and Its Associated Prognosis

Breslow thickness	*5-year survival*
<1 mm	95% to 100%
1 to 2 mm	80% to 95%
2.1 to 4 mm	60% to 80%
>4 mm	<50%

Table 30-3. Comparison of Melanoma In Situ, Squamous Cell Carcinoma In Situ, and Paget Disease in the Skin

	Melanoma in situ	*Squamous cell carcinoma in situ*	*Paget disease*
In epidermis	Malignant melanoma cells	Squamous carcinoma cells	Adenocarcinoma cells or urothelial carcinoma cells
Dermal invasion	No	No	No
Possible associated conditions	Nevus	HPV-associated changes	Internal organ invasive carcinoma
Cell features	Nests of individual melanocytes with or without pigment	Full thickness of dysplastic squamous cells mixed with background nonneoplastic squamous cells	Glandular structures or individual carcinoma cells
Markers	S100, Melanin A	P63, p53	CEA, CDX2 for gastrointestinal primary
	HMB45		HWMCK and p63 for urothelial carcinoma

CEA, carcinoembryonic antigen; HPV, human papilloma virus; HWMCK, high molecular cytokeratins.

KAPOSI SARCOMA

Definition

- Malignant vascular neoplasm caused by human herpesvirus 8 (HHV8)

Pathogenesis

- Kaposi sarcoma (KS) is arising from the endothelium
- The infectious agent HHV8 is sexually transmitted in AIDS patients or other immunocompromised patients

Clinical features

- Several different forms
  - Classic KS, indolent disease in elderly men from Mediterranean region
  - Endemic KS: affecting lower limbs of young Africans
  - Transplant related KS: may be enhanced by the immunosuppression (T-cell inhibitor) drugs such as cyclosporine
  - Epidemic KS: 300 times more common in AIDS patients than in transplant patients
- KS is a defining symptom of AIDS

Gross pathology

- Can affect genital areas as well as lower limbs, face, and back
- Skin: red, purple, black papular, or plaque-like lesions
- GI or respiratory tract can be affected
- May be associated with inflammation or erosions

Histology

- KS is composed of atypical spindle cells with high cellularity and frequent mitoses (Fig. 30-6*a*)
- High vascularity, dense, and irregular vessels mixed with atypical endothelial cells (Fig. 30-6*b*)
- Extravasated red blood cells (RBCs) are characteristic of KS (Figs. 30-6*b* and 30-7*a*), which gives the red color of the tumor. Sometimes, hyaline globules can be seen (Fig. 30-7*a*)
- In some rare cases, KS is composed entirely of anastomosing channels, which is mimicking lymphangioma or low-grade angiosarcoma, the lining cells of the channels show mild to moderate atypia (Fig. 30-7*c*)

Immunohistochemistry

- HHV8 protein LANA immunostaining positive (Fig. 30-7*b* and 30-7*d*)

Molecular analysis

- Not necessary

Clinical relevance (prognosis and treatment options)

- Localized KS can be removed by surgery, cryotherapy, radiotherapy, etc
- KS may be difficult to cure, but it can be effectively palliated over long time
- Extensive skin lesions and internal KS need chemotherapy
- Highly active antiretroviral therapy is effective in preventing and inducing regression of KS

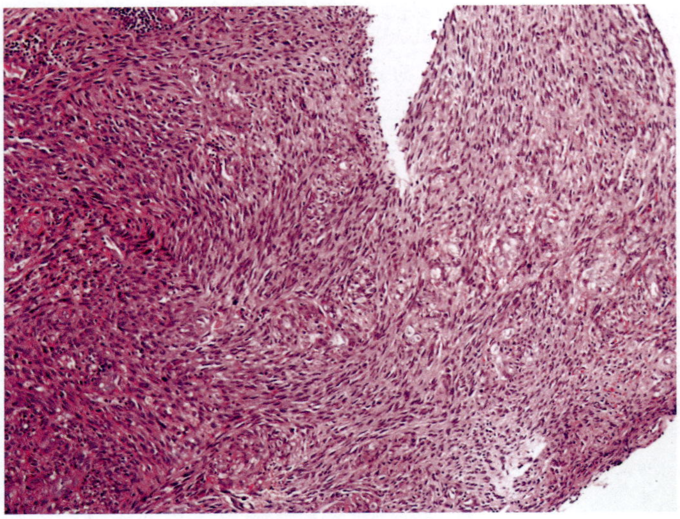

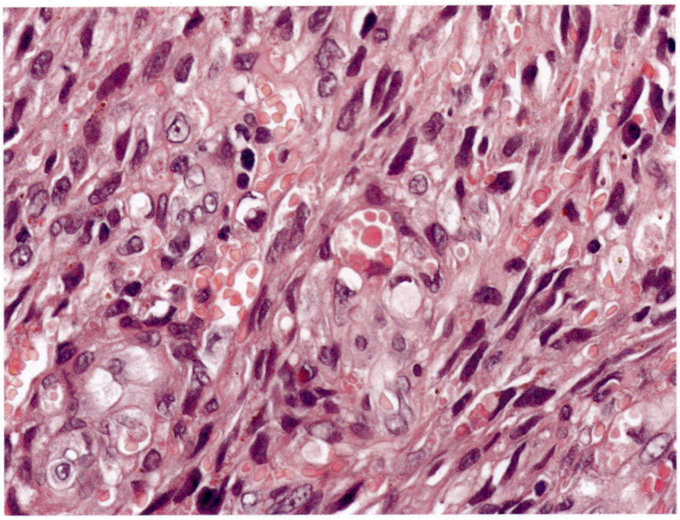

a b

Figure 30-6.
Kaposi sarcoma of the penis from an HIV patient. The tumor is composed of cellular spindle cells (*a*). High magnification shows atypical spindle cells associated with hyaline globules and extravasated red blood cells (*b*).

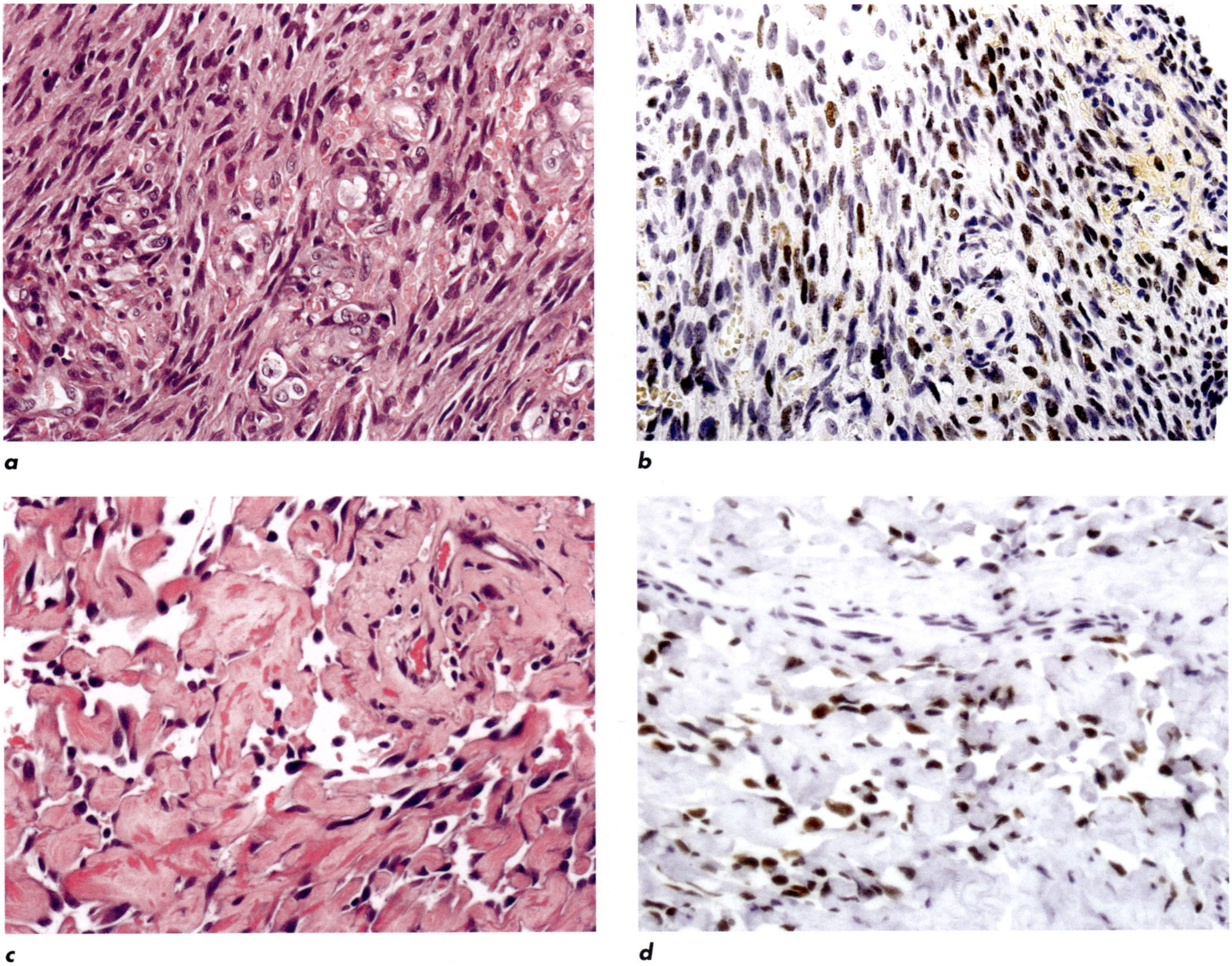

Figure 30-7.

Kaposi sarcoma with abnormal spindle-shaped endothelial cells and extravasated RBCs (*a*). Immunostaining for HHV8 protein LANA1 demonstrates the nuclear positivity in Kaposi sarcoma cells (*b*). Lymphoangiomatoid Kaposi sarcoma of the penis exhibits anastomosing channels lined by slightly atypical endothelial cells (*c*). LANA1 immunostaining is positive in tumor cells, negative in benign endothelium (*d*).

PART II
Urinary Tract Surgical Pathology

INTRODUCTION

The urinary system can be divided into several functional units including

Kidney (pair)

- Function: nonstop filtration of the blood, production of urine and secretion of important hormones such as renin, erythropoietin

Ductal structures

Ureter (pair)

- Function: transport urine to the storage space—bladder

Urethra

- Function: transport urine from the bladder to outside the body. The urethra also functions as a duct to transport semen in men

Bladder (urinary bladder)

- Function: store urine temporarily and release when it is full or there is a chance of urination

Exocrine glands

- Periurethral glands

SECTION 4
The Kidney

CHAPTER 31 Normal Histology of the Upper Urinary Tract

KIDNEY

Location

- Retroperitoneum surrounded by fibroadipose tissue

Histology (from outer to inner layers)

- Renal fascia also known as Gerota fascia
  - A thin layer of dense connective tissue encasing the kidney and adrenal
  - This layer is often used in the nephrectomy process to determine the extent of renal tumor
  - But it can be hardly recognized in the nephrectomy specimen
- Perinephric adipose tissue
- Renal capsule: thick fibrous capsule covering the renal parenchyma and embedded in perinephric fat
- Parenchyma
  - Renal parenchyma is composed of the outer layer (cortex) and the inner portion (medulla) (Fig. 31-1)
  - Major components of the cortex (Fig. 31-2)
    - Glomeruli (Fig. 31-3)
    - Proximal and distal convoluted tubules (Fig. 31-4)
  - Major components of the medulla (Fig. 31-5)
    - Collecting ducts, lined by cuboidal epithelium
    - Duct of Bellini, the large diameter collecting ducts, lined by cuboidal epithelium
    - In practice, we use collecting ducts and collecting ducts of Bellini interchangeably since these two structures cannot be distinguished by routine light microscopy
    - Loops of Henle, smaller tubules lined by cuboidal or flattened epithelium. Different portions of loops of Henle include descending and ascending loops, which are similar in histology
- Glomerulus
  - A small knot of capillaries and related structures suspended within Bowman capsule (Fig. 31-3)
  - *Cell populations* present within a glomerulus
    - Endothelial cells line the fenestrated glomerular capillaries
    - Podocytes attaching to the outer side of the glomerular capillaries
    - Mesangial cells are concentrated between capillaries at the vascular pole

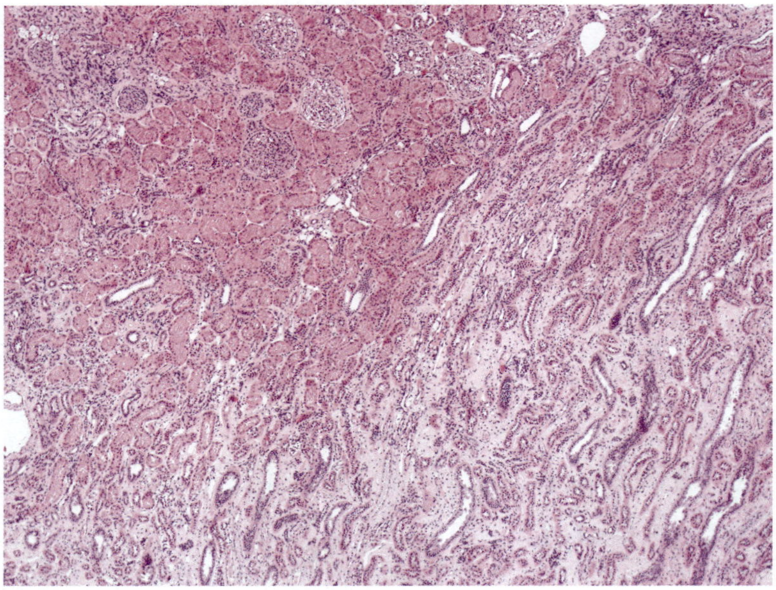

Figure 31-1.
Low magnification of the kidney showing the cortex (left) and medulla (right).

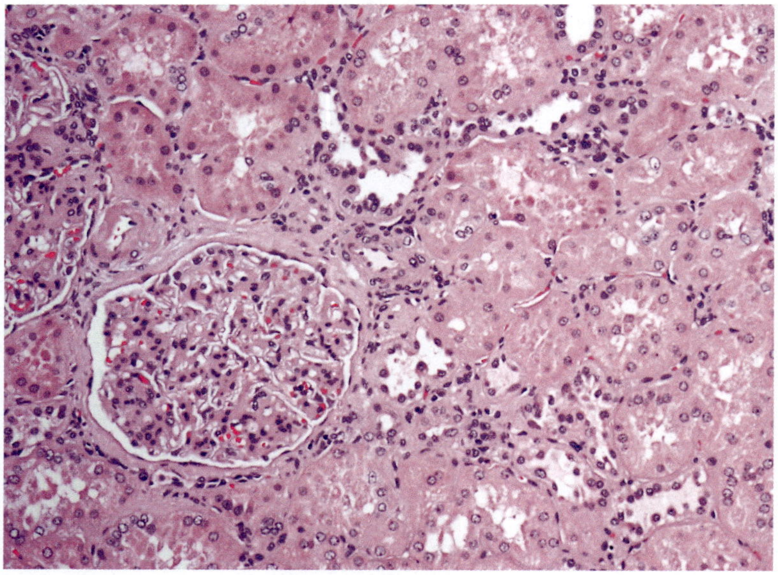

Figure 31-2.
Renal cortex containing glomeruli, proximal and distal convoluted tubules.

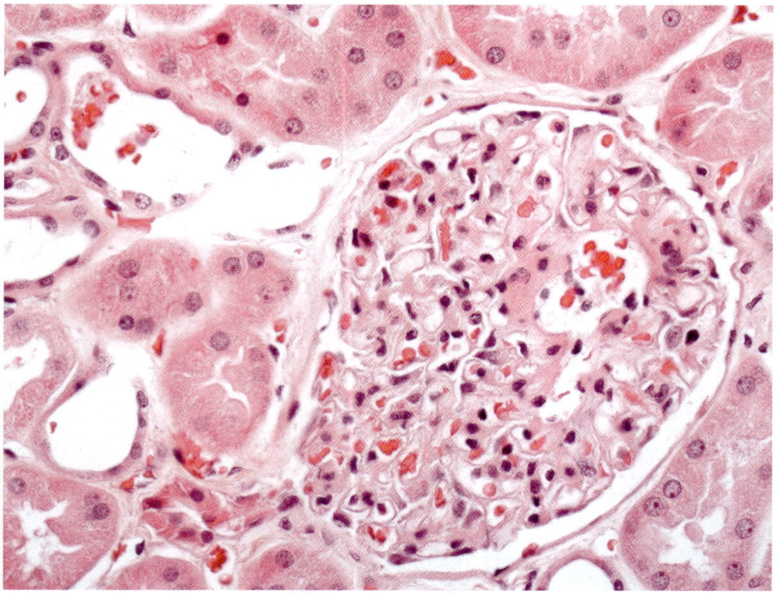

Figure 31-3.
High magnification of a glomerulus shows the glomerular capillaries in the middle surrounded by Bowman space and Bowman capsule.

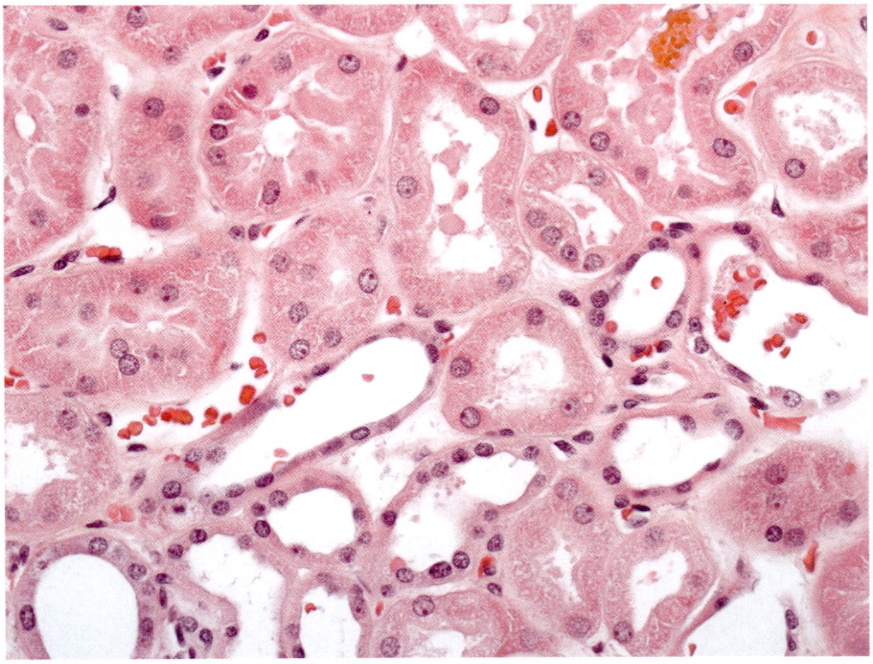

Figure 31-4.
The proximal convoluted tubules lined by larger cuboidal epithelial cells with abundant eosinophilic granular cytoplasm; while the distal tubules lined by low cuboidal epithelial cells.

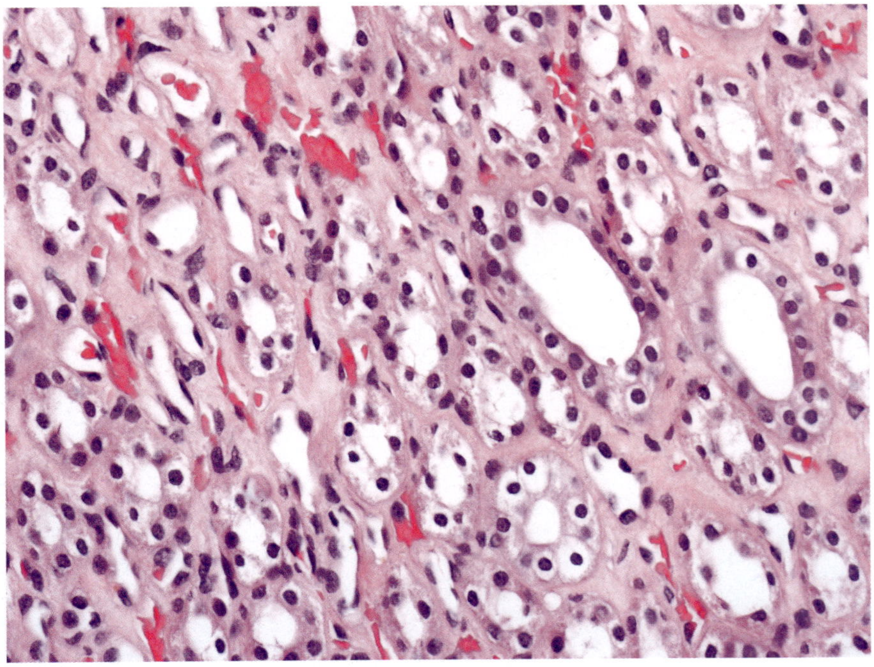

Figure 31-5.
Renal medulla composed of collecting ducts (with a larger diameter) and descending and ascending loops of Henle (smaller tubules).

- Extracellular material
  - The base membrane is composed of endothelial and podocyte basement membranes
  - Mesangial matrix is a special form of connective tissue
- Juxtaglomerular apparatus (Fig. 31-6)
  - Macula densa of the distal convoluted tubule
  - Smooth muscle cells of the afferent arteriole
  - Juxtaglomerular cells
  - Function: producing renin that plays a key role in regulating renal blood flow and glomerular filtration rate
- Renal hilar region and pelvis
  - Renal pelvis (Fig. 31-7) is a funnel-shaped structure that occupies the major portion of the hilar region of the kidney
  - Renal pelvis branches to renal calyces and collects urine from the collecting duct system (Fig. 31-8)
- Other structures in the hilar region (medial portion)
  - Renal vein
    - The renal vein drains to inferior vena cava
    - The presence of tumor thrombus in the renal vein is a major risk factor for distal metastasis
  - Renal sinus
    - The renal sinus can be a confusing term and a poorly defined structure
    - It generally refers to a space within the renal hilar region including the renal pelvis, renal calyces, renal veins and arteries, nerves, and fat
    - However, when the term *renal sinus involvement* is used in kidney cancer staging, it specifically refers to the perinephric fat and connective tissue in the hilar region
    - If the adipose tissue in the renal sinus is invaded by a renal cell tumor, it would be stage T3 disease (outside the kidney)

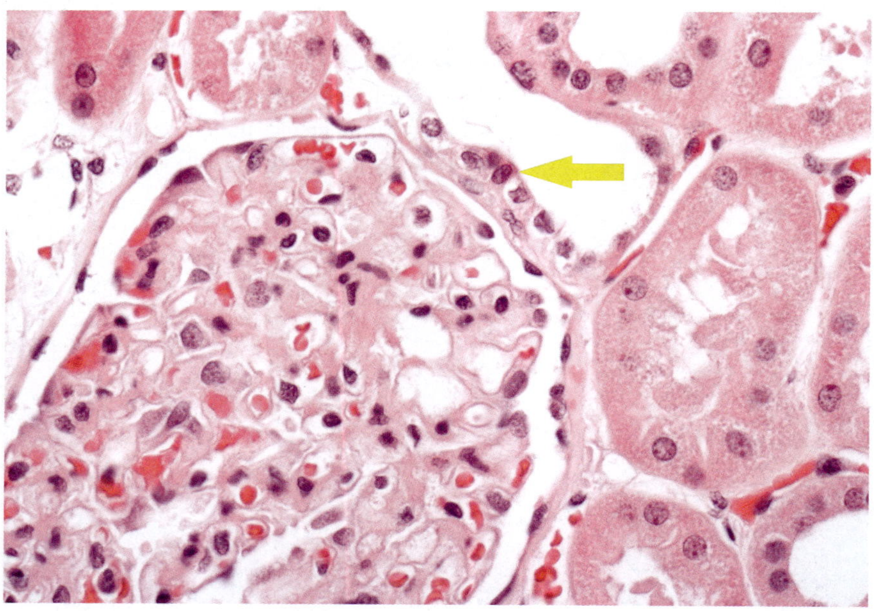

Figure 31-6.
Portion of the juxtaglomerular apparatus: specialized cells in the distal convoluted tubule (macula densa). These cells (arrow) are capable of producing renin.

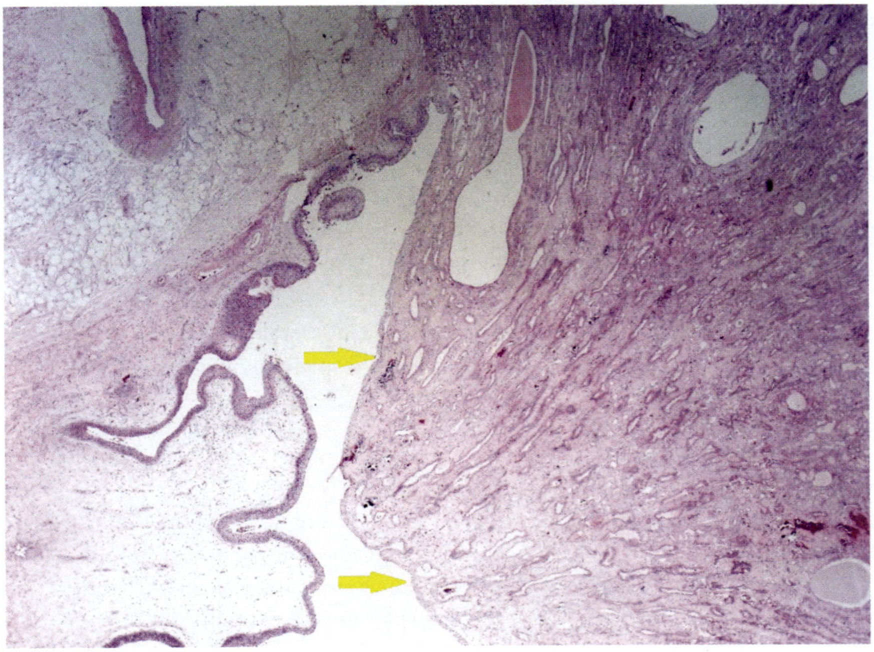

Figure 31-7.
The relationship between the funnel-shaped renal pelvis (left) and renal papilla (right, arrows).

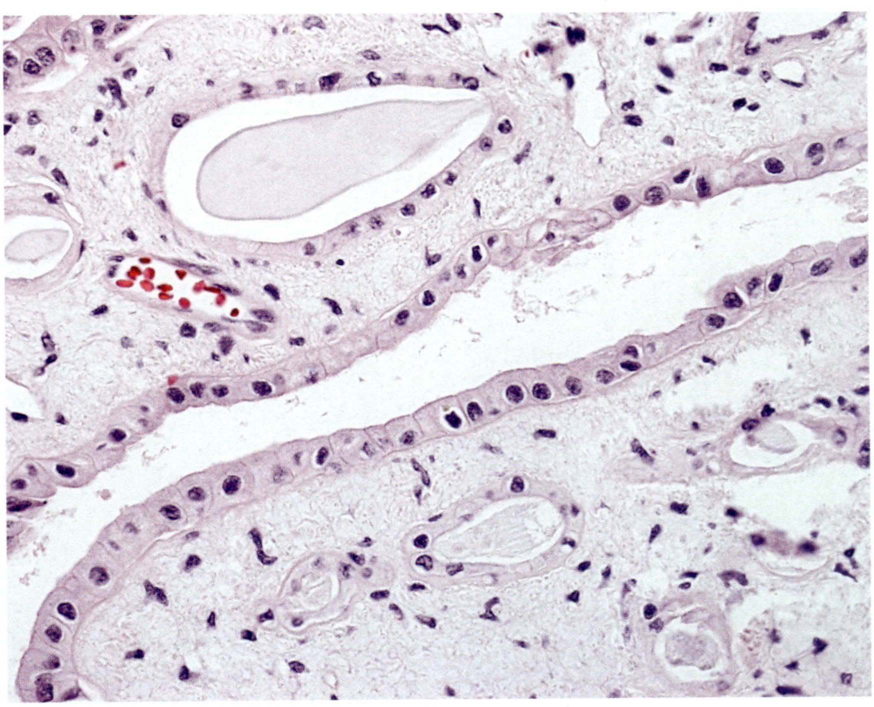

Figure 31-8.
Collecting duct is lined by cuboidal epithelial cells.

RENAL PELVIS

- A funnel-like structure lined by urothelium (Figs. 31-7 and 31-9)
- Surrounded by thin layer of loose connective tissue
- Muscularis propria is thin and often discontinuous (Fig. 31-9)
- Therefore, renal pelvis does not provide thick protective muscular wall as the bladder does
- Renal calyces
  - Branches of renal pelvis, also lined by urothelium (Fig. 31-10)
  - Microscopically, they can't be distinguished from renal pelvis
- The urothelium of the renal pelvis is essentially the same as the urothelium covering the ureter and bladder, composed of the umbrella cells and basal cells (Figs. 31-11 and 31-12). The urothelium covering the renal papilla is very close to the renal tubules (Fig. 31-11)
- Because of the presence of urothelium, the renal pelvis and calyces are often involved by diseases different from the ones involving renal parenchyma, but similar to those involving the bladder
- The common conditions of renal pelvis and calyces are urothelial carcinoma, stone, pyelonephritis

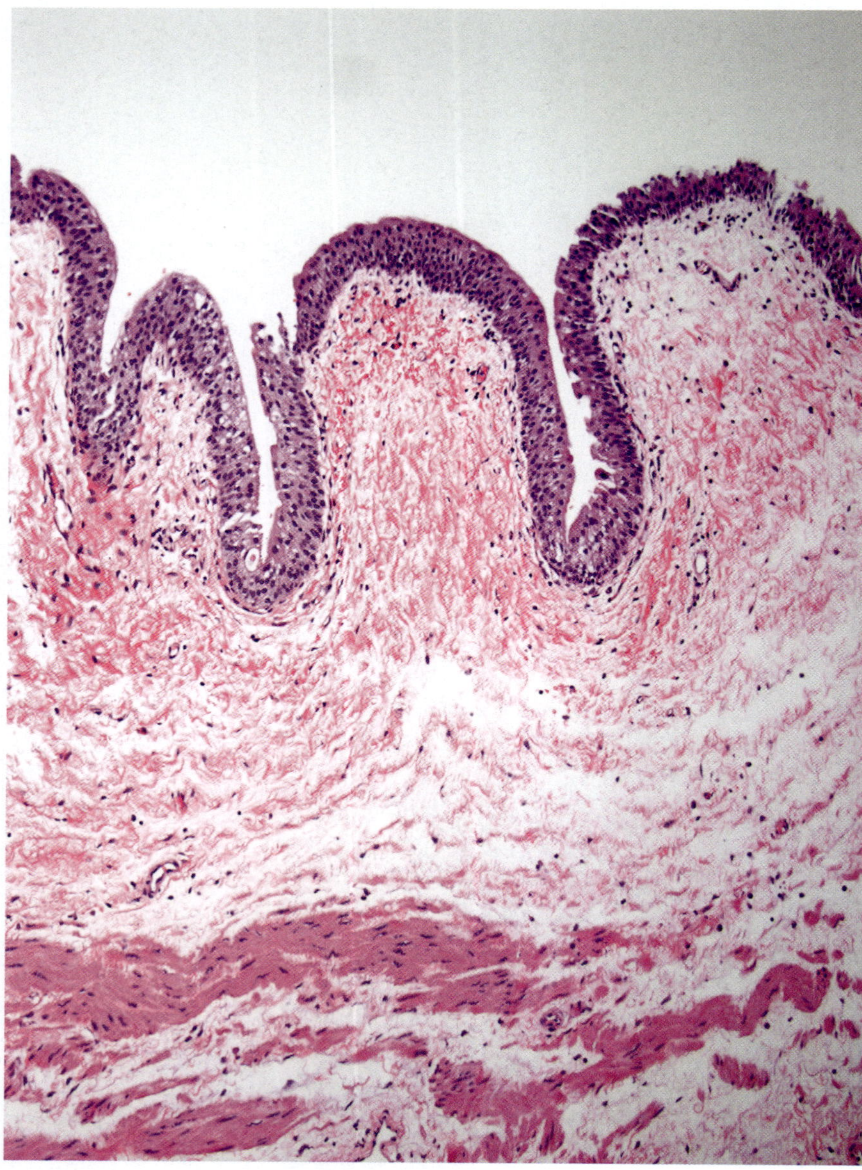

Figure 31-9.
The renal pelvis composed of urothelium on the surface, lamina propria connective tissue, and discontinuous small smooth muscle bundles without thick muscularis propria.

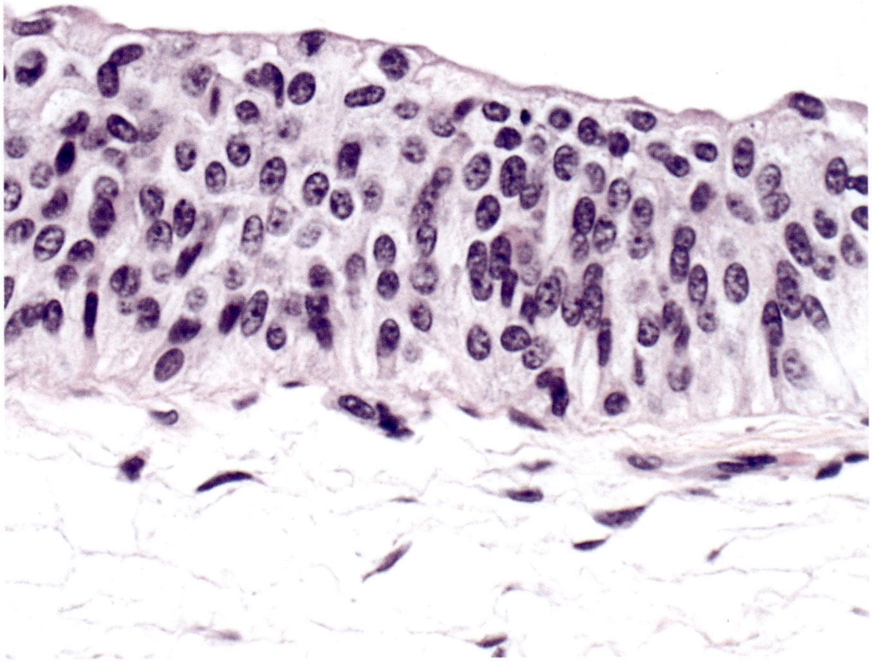

Figure 31-10.
Urothelium of the renal pelvis and lamina propria.

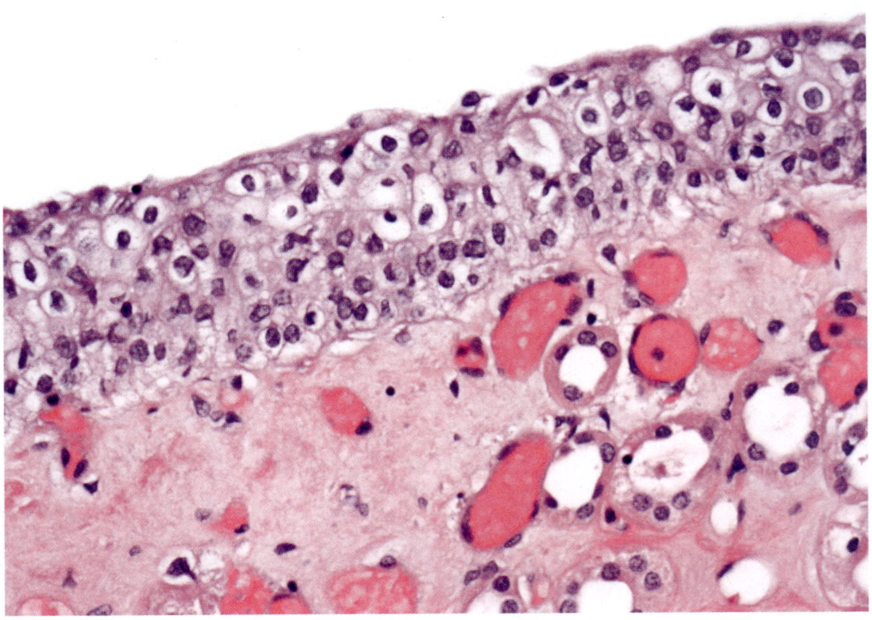

Figure 31-11.
The renal pelvic urothelium covering the renal papilla (visceral pelvis) is very close to the renal tubules.

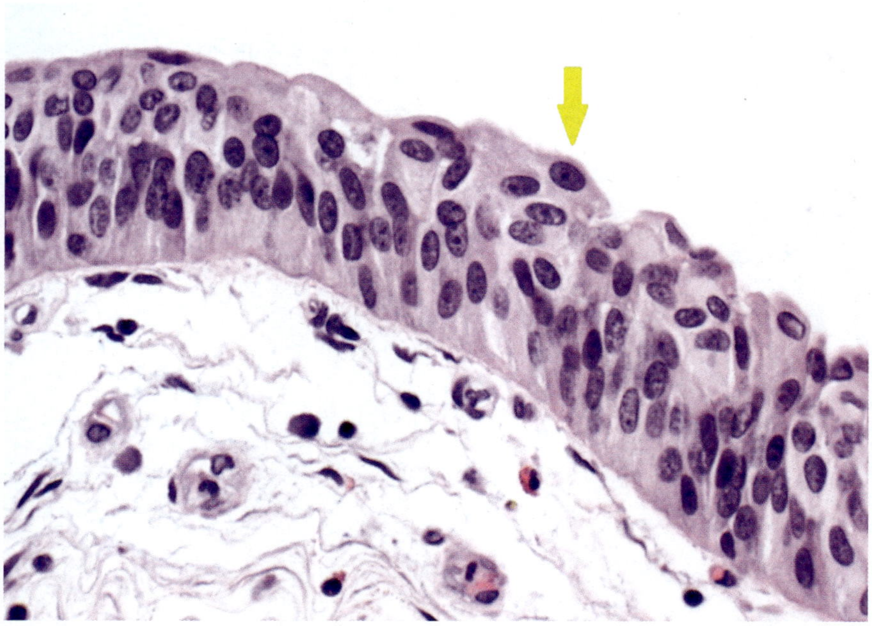

Figure 31-12.
Urothelium of the renal pelvis is composed of umbrella cells on the surface (arrow) and basal cells.

URETER

- A pair of tubular structures connecting the kidney (renal pelvis) to the bladder
- The two ureteral openings in the bladder are called ureteral orifices
- Histology
  - The urothelial lining of the ureter is in continuation with the urothelia of the renal pelvis proximally and the bladder distally (Figs. 31-13 and 31-14)
  - The lamina propria present
  - The muscularis propria consists of circular inner and longitudinal outer layers (Fig. 31-13), much thinner than the counterparts of the bladder
  - The adventitia is the outermost layer of connective tissue surrounding the ureter
- Ureter specimens are often received for evaluation of the surgical margin status in urothelial carcinoma

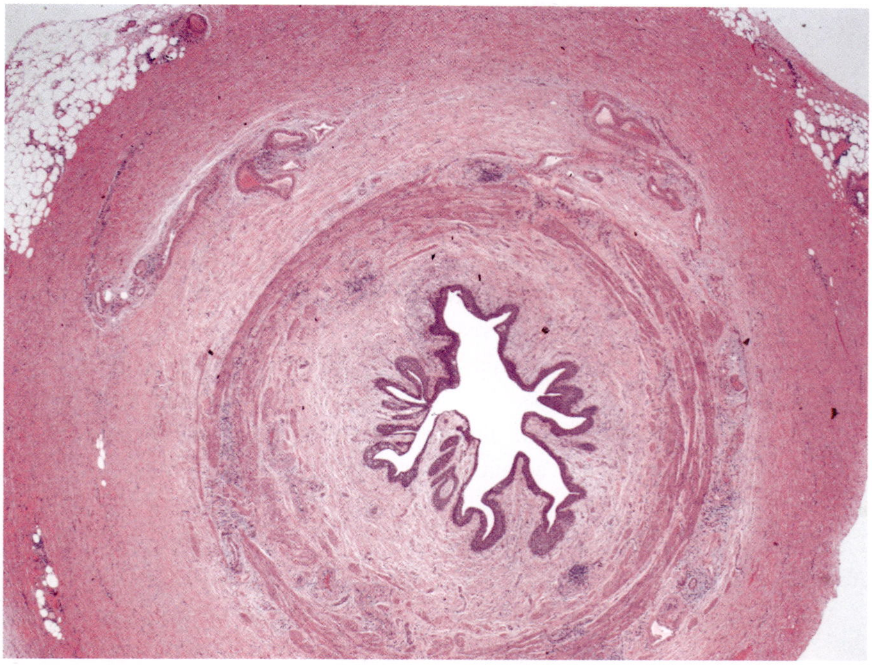

Figure 31-13.
Cross-section of ureter showing (from inside to outside) urothelial lining, lamina propria, muscularis propria, and adventitia (fibroadipose tissue).

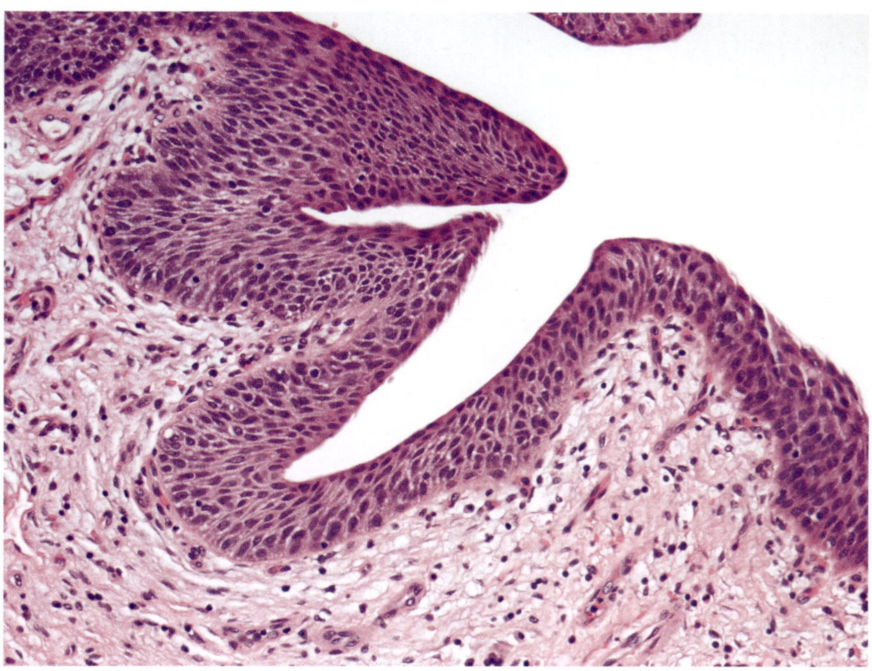

Figure 31-14.
Urothelial lining of the ureter is similar to the bladder urothelium.

CHAPTER 32

Medical Renal Diseases

Ximing J. Yang, Kirtee Raparia, Nedjema Sustento-Reodica, Yashpal Kanwar

DIABETIC NEPHROPATHY

Definition

- Diabetic nephropathy (DN) is a long-term insidious complication of diabetes mellitus
- It is the most common cause of chronic renal failure in the United States and accounts for more than one-third of patients enrolled in long-term dialysis
- The specific glomerular lesions associated with diabetes mellitus were first recognized by Kimmelstiel and Wilson in 1936, and since then they have been referred to as Kimmelstiel-Wilson (KW) nodules

Pathogenesis

- The kidney is the major target organ affected by complications of both type 1 and 2 diabetes mellitus. In both instances the lesions are similar and are characterized by amassing of extracellular matrix in the glomerular and tubulointerstitial compartments and by the thickening and hyalinization of intrarenal vasculature, albeit the basic pathogenetic mechanisms for evolution of renal lesions differ to a certain degree
- Various cellular events occur in the kidney secondary to hyperglycemia, including excessive channeling of glucose intermediaries into various metabolic pathways with generation of advanced glycation products, activation of protein kinase C, increased expression of transforming growth factor-β and GTP-binding proteins, and generation of reactive oxygen species
- Hyperglycemia also impairs autoregulation within the glomerulus by activating the local intrarenal renin-angiotensin aldosterone system, thus compounding the hyperglycemia-induced injury

Clinical features

- It is characterized clinically by the onset of microalbuminuria progressing to overt nephrotic range proteinuria, a steady decline in the glomerular filtration rate and elevation of systemic blood pressure

Histology

- Morphological changes in DN affect all the four renal compartments: glomeruli, tubules, interstitium, and vessels (Fig. 32-1*a* to *d*). The glomeruli shows a constellation of findings including a diffuse form with mesangial sclerosis and uniform thickening of capillary loops, nodular lesions recognized as KW lesions, exudative or segmental hyalinosis lesions, and the subcapsular capsular drops
- The tubules show changes that are usually accompanied with glomerular alterations, and they include tubular

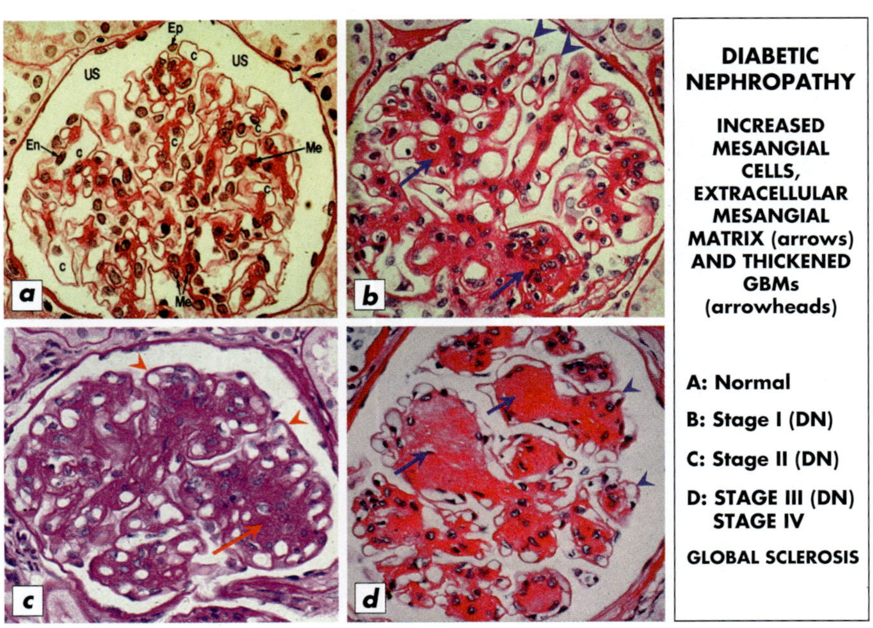

Figure 32-1. Light photomicrographs highlighting the progression of pathologic lesions in a patient with diabetic nephropathy (*a*–*d*).

atrophy, apoptosis, and thickened tubular basement membrane with occasional splitting and lamination

- The arteries show varying degrees of intimal thickening along with reduplication of the elastic lamina. Hyaline arteriolosclerosis is more pronounced in patients with diabetes than in any other disease, except those associated with chronic transplant glomerulopathy
- Interstitial fibrosis along with increased chronic inflammatory infiltrates composed of T lymphocytes and macrophages are commonly seen in a diabetic kidney

Immunofluorescence

- Typical immunofluorescence findings include linear staining of glomerular and tubular basement membranes (GBMs and TBMs) with reactivity toward immunoglobulin G (IgG) although staining with IgM, complement C1q, fibrinogen, and albumin has also been reported. Hyalinotic lesions in the glomeruli and arterioles also stain with IgM and C1q

Electron microscopy

- Electron microscopy (EM) shows thickened GBMs, variable degree of effacement of the foot processes of the visceral epithelial cells (podocytes), and increase in the mesangial matrix (Fig. 32-2). The lesions of hyalinosis appear as homogenous electron-dense material between the endothelial cells and GBM, and the capsular drop is similar between Bowman capsular basement membrane and the parietal epithelium

Differential diagnosis

- Lesions similar to DN can be seen in other glomerulonephritides, such as light chain deposition disease, amyloidosis, immunotactoid nephropathy, membranoproliferative form of diffuse glomerulonephritis, and idiopathic nodular glomerulosclerosis. These lesions should be excluded by pathologists by performing special stains on histologic sections, immunofluorescence, and electron microscopic studies

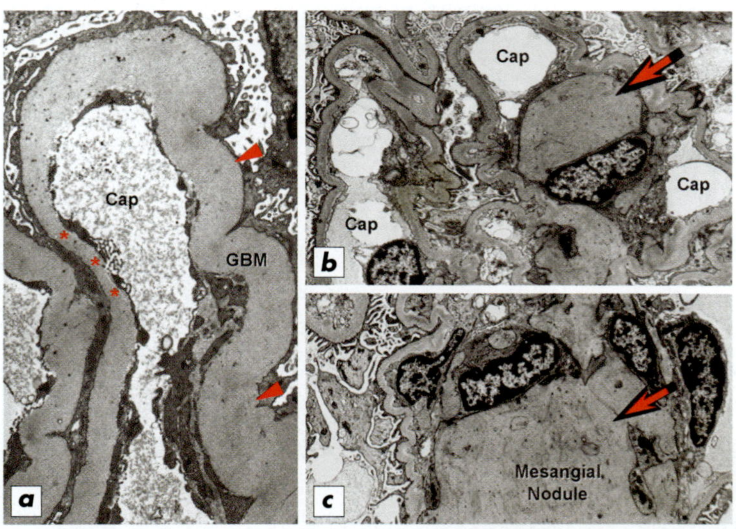

DN: A. THICKENED GBM (▲), COMPARED TO THE NORMAL SIZE (*) ON THE LEFT SIDE OF THE CAPILLARY. B. BEGINNING OF THE FORMATION OF A NODULE IN THE MESANGIUM (↙). C. WELL ESTABLISHED MESANGIAL NODULE (↙)

Figure 32-2.
Electron photomicrographs highlighting the thickened glomerular basement membrane (GBM) (*a*) and expanded mesangium (*b*) and formation of mesangial nodule (panel *c*) in a patient with diabetic nephropathy.

FOCAL SEGMENTAL GLOMERULOSCLEROSIS AND HYALINOSIS

Definition

- Focal segmental glomerulosclerosis (FSGS) is a pattern of glomerular disease that occurs in primary form of unknown cause and secondary to many known conditions
- Diagnosis of FSGS implies that some of the glomeruli are normal (focal) and the affected glomeruli are involved partially (segmental)
- Secondary causes of FSGS include drugs, viruses, immunologic diseases, physical agents, and hereditary diseases

Pathogenesis

- The pathogenetic process in FSGS still remains unknown; however, hypothesis includes several mechanisms including genetic disease of the podocyte, humoral factors, hemodynamic injury, glomerular hypertrophy, podocyte injury, and hyperlipidemia

Clinical features

- The frequency of FSGS is highly variable in the world, ranging from 2% to 41% of primary glomerulopathies
- There is increase in prevalence of FSGS in the United States, perhaps due to the broadened definition of FSGS and new environmental causes and transplantation
- Patients with FSGS tend to be older with increased incidence of hematuria, hypertension, renal insufficiency, and less selective proteinuria that is steroid unresponsive

Histology

- The glomerular lesions are focal (some but not all glomeruli) and segmental (partial glomerular involvement) and are characterized by variable scarring, cellularity, and hyaline deposits. Glomerular enlargement is characteristic of FSGS in both children and adults. The segmental lesion tends to involve the hilum or the origin of proximal convoluted tubule where it leaves Bowman space in the glomeruli. The segmental lesions are often hypercellular caused by proliferation of intrinsic glomerular cells or infiltration of leucocytes (Fig. 32-3). The visceral epithelial cells overlying the sclerotic lesions can show hypertrophy
- Focal tubular atrophy is often seen in these patients proportional to the glomerular injury
- Interstitial fibrosis accompanies tubular loss and atrophy
- Arterial and arteriolar thickening and hyaline deposition can be seen, which may be related to hypertension frequently present at presentation

Immunofluorescence

- The deposits usually IgM and C3 are localized in the sclerotic segment without any obvious granular or linear pattern. Other proteins such as C1q, C4, IgG, and IgA can also be seen in FSGS, but are variable and stain less intensely than IgM and C3

Electron microscopy

- Podocyte foot process effacement is often seen in FSGS
- The sclerotic segment may contain foamy macrophages, cellular debris, lipid droplets, granular matrix, fibrils, and electron-dense deposits (Fig. 32-4)

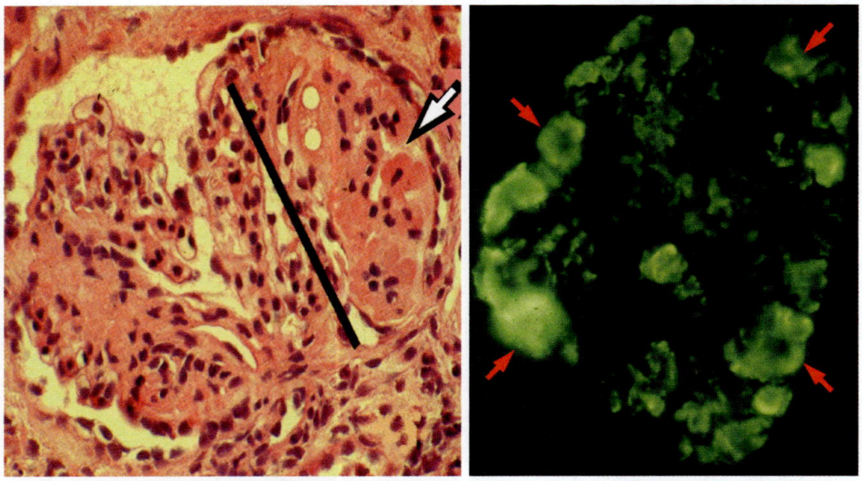

FSGS: SEGMENTAL HYALINOSIS OF THE GLOMERULUS (ARROW)

FSGS: LARGE SEGMENTAL IgM OR C1q DEPOSITS IN THE GLOMERULUS (ARROWS)

Figure 32-3.
Light photomicrograph highlighting segmental lesions in focal segmental glomerulosclerosis and hyalinosis (FSGS, left panel). Immunofluorescence photomicrograph depicting large segmental IgM and C1q deposits in a patient with FSGS (right panel).

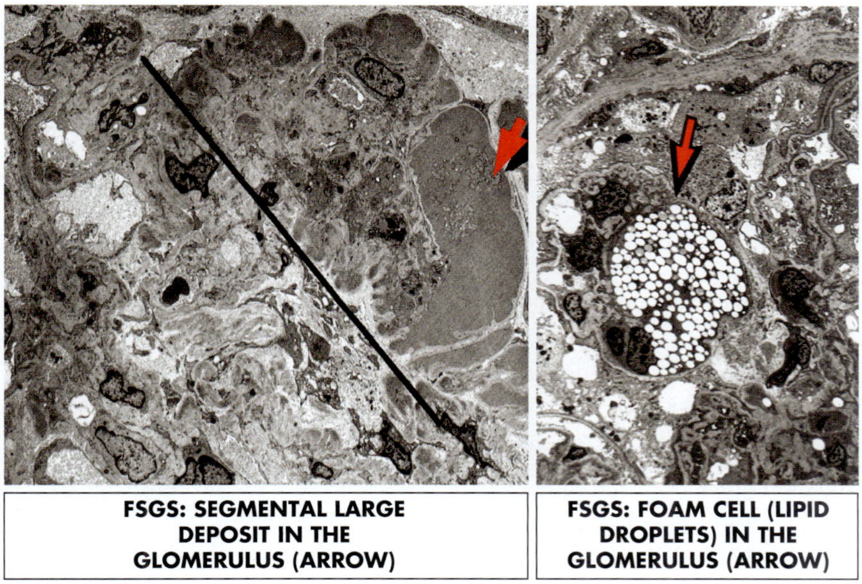

Figure 32-4.
Electron photomicrograph highlighting segmental lesions as dark dense deposits in focal segmental glomerulosclerosis and hyalinosis (FSGS, left panel) and a mesangial cell loaded with lipid droplets (foam cell, right panel).

Differential diagnosis

- Lesions similar to FSGS can be seen in heroin nephropathy and chronic transplantation rejection. Lesions in these entities at times are accompanied with global sclerosis. To distinguish them from primary FSGS, one needs to carefully examine the juxtamedullary regions of the kidney biopsy since in primary FSGS the lesions initially develop in this location

MINIMAL CHANGE DISEASE

Definition

- A disease process with usually abrupt onset of nephrotic range proteinuria
- The proteinuria may be accompanied with lipiduria
- Patients usually are children presenting with marked swelling of feet, face, and ascites
- Glomeruli by light microscopy appear normal, thus the name coined as minimal change disease (MCD)

Pathogenesis

- The pathogenesis of MCD remains unknown. However, one of the theories is the combination of abnormal immune response leading to the production of a circulating factor, which results in increased glomerular permeability

Clinical features

- MCD can be seen in both children and adults with nephrotic syndrome being the presenting feature in these patients

Histology

- Light microscopy of this disease shows no or minimal glomerular abnormality with few glomeruli showing increase in mesangial cellularity or matrix (Fig. 32-5)
- Tubular and interstitial pathologic lesions are not classic features of MCD, but clear vacuoles or hyaline PAS-positive droplets can be seen in the tubular epithelial cells

Immunofluorescence

- Most studies have reported absence of immune deposits in the glomeruli of patients with MCD. Immunoglobulins and complement (C3) when present are of low intensity and localized to mesangium without any associated electron deposits

Electron microscopy

- Effacement of the foot processes of the epithelial cells is the key finding seen by EM (Fig. 32-6)

Differential diagnosis

- FSGS: segmental lesions can be seen in patients with long-standing MCD, usually 5 to 10 years, but they are usually not associated with interstitial fibrosis or significant tubular atrophy
- IgM nephropathy, C1q nephropathy, and congenital nephrotic syndrome. The first two can be distinguished from the MCD by the positive immunofluorescence findings. The congenital syndrome may be associated with biochemical abnormalities in the GBM

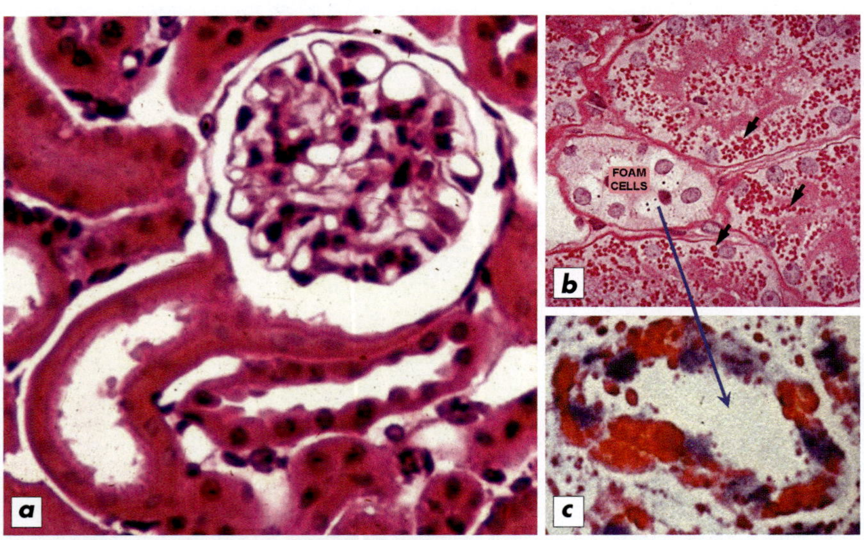

MCD: A. NORMAL GLOMERULAR MORPHOLOGY, B. TUBULAR PROTEIN ABSORPTION DROPLETS, C. TUBULAR LIPID DROPLETS (OIL RED O STAIN)

Figure 32-5.
Light photomicrograph highlighting normal morphology of the glomerulus in a patient with minimal change disease (*a*), PAS-positive absorption droplets in tubules (*b*), and oil red–stained droplets in tubular epithelia (*c*).

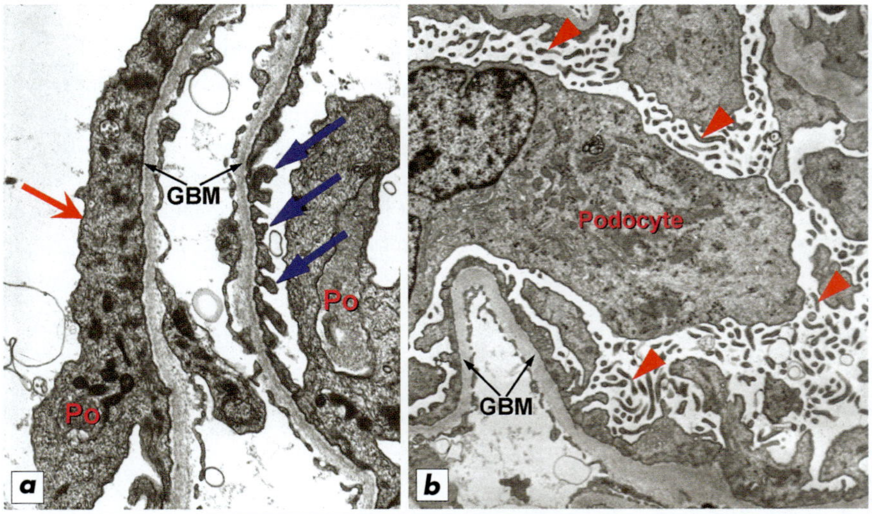

Figure 32-6.
Electron photomicrograph highlighting fusion of foot processes of the podocytes (Po) (*a*, red arrow) compared to normal interdigitating pattern (blue arrows), and reactive villous transformation of the podocytes (*b*, arrow heads).

IDIOPATHIC MEMBRANOUS GLOMERULONEPHRITIS

Definition

- Membranous glomerulonephritis (MGN) is a pathologic diagnosis characterized by a spectrum of changes in the GBM; defining feature being the subepithelial immune deposits
- MGN is most common in primary or idiopathic form, but may occur secondary to many diseases, such as infections, drug toxicity, neoplasms, and autoimmune disorders

Pathogenesis

- The subepithelial immunoglobulin deposits in MGN supports a chronic immune complex pathogenesis, but the mechanism of immune complex formation and nature of the antigen are still unknown. The possibility of megalin or phospholipase A2 receptor acting as nephritogenic antigens has been reported in the literature

Clinical features

- MGN is seen throughout the adult life with a peak incidence in the fourth and fifth decades
- It is the most common cause of the nephrotic syndrome in Caucasian adults

Histology

- The glomerular architecture is preserved in early cases; however, as the disease progresses, the glomerular capillary walls appear thicker. Eventually, the thickened GBM, increased mesangial matrix, and accumulation of immune deposits give the glomeruli a solid appearance. Eventually, segmental scarring and global sclerosis develop (Fig. 32-7, left panel)
- Special stains such as periodic acid-Schiff (PAS), Jones, or trichrome stains can highlight the abnormal GBM. Jones stain yields spiky tooth-comb appearance of the GBM, while immune-complex stains red with trichrome in blue background of the GBM
- Tubules may show hyaline droplet changes and mild atrophy associated with interstitial fibrosis as the glomerular lesion progresses

Immunofluorescence

- Diffuse global granular (discrete and uniform) deposit of IgG following the contour of GBM is the typical finding in MGN (Fig. 32-7, right panel)
- The other immunoglobulin and complement components may also show a weaker staining reaction

Electron microscopy

- EM demonstrates subepithelial and intramembranous electron-dense deposits in the GBM (Fig. 32-8)

Differential diagnosis

- Patients with chronic glomerulonephritis, arterial and arteriolar nephrosclerosis, and chronic allograft glomerulopathy can show thickened GBM. While considering patients with nephrotic syndrome differential diagnosis includes MCD, FSGS, MPGN, diabetes, and amyloidosis. The main diagnostic issue is distinguishing primary (idiopathic) MGN from secondary forms

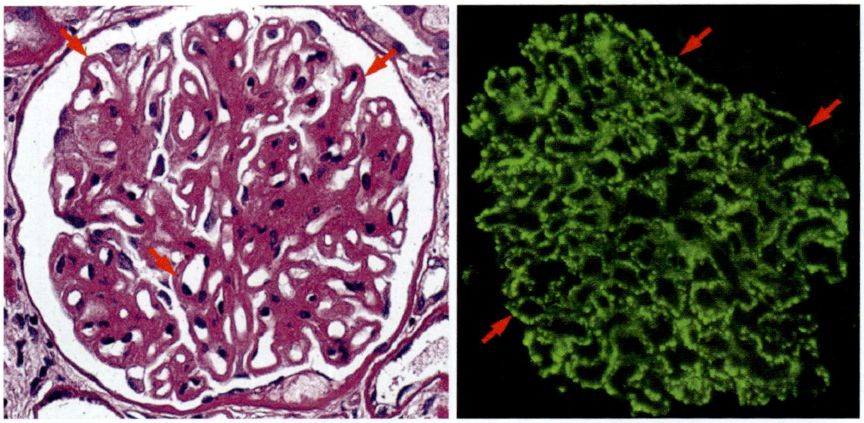

IMN: THICK CAPILLARY BASEMENT MEMBRANES (ARROWS) WITHOUT PROLIFERATION OF CELLS

IMN: CAPILLARY DEPOSITS WITH GRANULAR APPEARANCE OF IgG DEPOSITS (ARROWS)

Figure 32-7.
Light photomicrograph highlighting normal morphology of the glomerulus with thick basement membranes in a patient with membranous nephropathy (left panel, arrows). While the immunofluorescence photomicrograph shows the presence of IgG with beaded granular appearance of the glomerular capillaries (right panel).

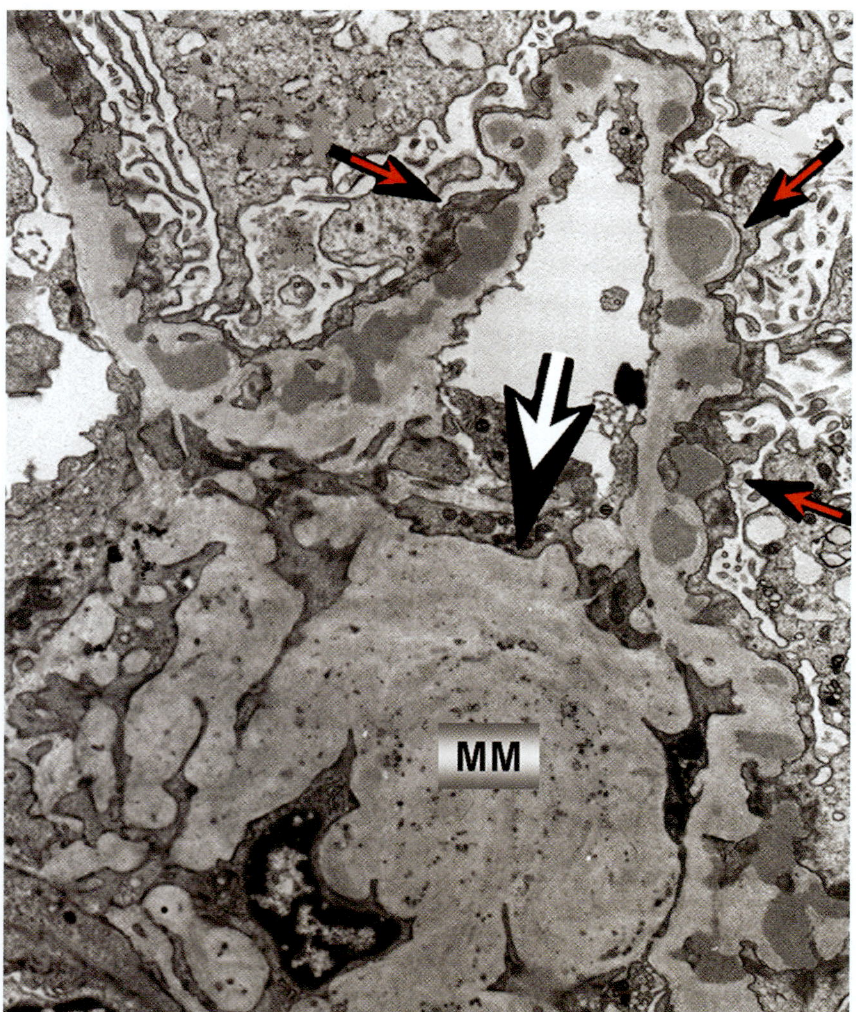

IMN: SUBEPITHELIAL DEPOSITS (➘). NOTE THAT THERE ARE NO DEPOSITS IN MESANGIAL MATRIX (MM) (⇙)

Figure 32-8.
Electron photomicrograph highlighting the presence of subepithelial electron-dense deposits (red arrows) in the glomerular basement membrane, while no electron dense deposit is seen in the mesangial matrix (MM) of the glomerulus.

LUPUS NEPHROPATHY

Definition

- The renal manifestations of systemic lupus nephritis (SLE) called lupus nephritis (LN) show a variable clinical and morphologic expression

Pathogenesis

- The pathogenesis of SLE is quite complex involving susceptible genetic background combined with particular environmental factors, abnormalities of B- and T-cell functions, and dysregulation of the immune response

Clinical features

- SLE is a chronic inflammatory autoimmune disease affecting multiple organ systems, including skin, joints, heart, lungs, kidneys, central nervous system, and serous membranes. Renal complications in SLE pose the greatest risk of morbidity and mortality
- Patients may present with microhematuria and mild proteinuria or full blown nephrotic syndrome or rapidly progressive renal failure

Histology

- The pathologic manifestations of LN are quite diverse and may affect any or all the renal compartments, including glomeruli, tubules, interstitium, and blood vessels (Figs. 32-9 to 32-12). The mesangial hypercellularity and extent of glomerular involvement are interpreted in the context of the immune deposits as detected by light microscopy, immunofluorescence, and electron microscopy. The most recent classification (2004) proposed by International Society of Nephrology (ISN) and Renal Pathology Society (RPS) includes the following categories:
    - Class I: minimal mesangial LN
    - Class II: mesangial proliferative LN
    - Class III: focal LN
    - Class IV: diffuse LN (Fig. 32-11)
    - Class V: membranous LN (Fig. 32-9)
    - Class VI: advanced sclerosing LN
- Tubulointerstitial lesions may be encountered in all classes of LN
- Vascular lesions are also commonly seen in LN including arteriosclerosis, arteriolosclerosis, noninflammatory necrotizing vasculopathy, thrombotic microangiopathy, and necrotizing vasculitis. At times accompanied with anti-phospholipid syndrome

Immunofluorescence

- Immune deposits can be detected in all the renal compartments including the glomeruli, tubules, interstitium, and blood vessels. IgG is found universally in all cases with codeposits of IgM and IgA. C3 is the most frequent complement component followed by C1q and sometimes C4. Fibrin-related antigens can be seen in areas corresponding to necrotizing lesions and in active crescents. Tissue antinuclear antibody (ANA) can be frequently identified in these patients, as manifested by nuclear staining of immunoglobulins (Figs. 32-10 and 32-11)

Electron microscopy

- Electron microscopic findings of LN patients are diverse. Glomerular deposits may range from sparse and small to

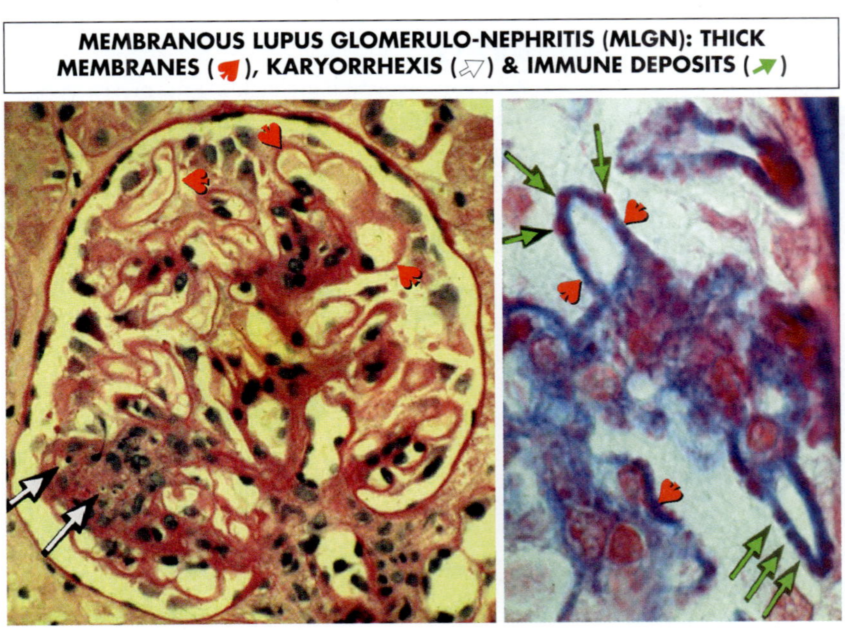

Figure 32-9.
Light photomicrograph highlighting thickened GBM (arrowheads) karyorrhexis (arrows) in a patient with lupus membranous nephropathy (left panel). Trichrome stain highlights the presence of reddish deposits (arrows) with blue background of the GBM (right panel).

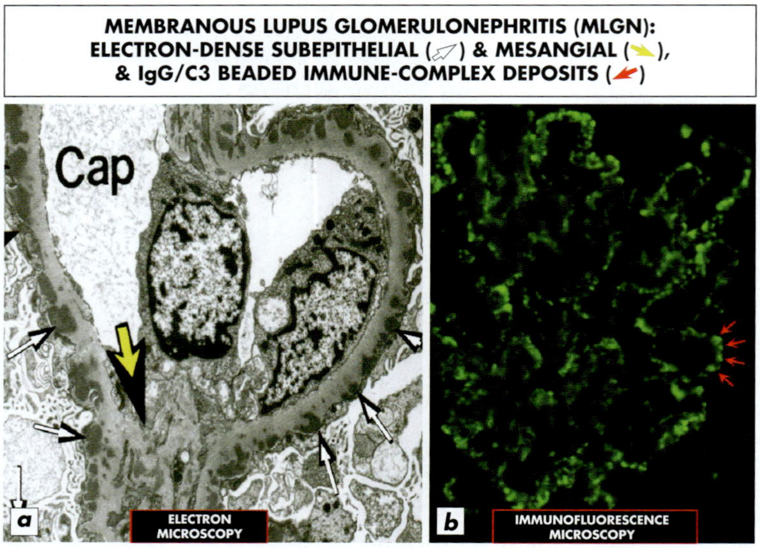

Figure 32-10.
Electron photomicrograph highlighting the presence of subepithelial (small arrows) and mesangial (big arrow) electron-dense deposits in a patient with lupus membranous nephropathy (*a*). The nature of deposits (IgG/C3) are confirmed by immunofluorescence microscopy (red arrows, *b*).

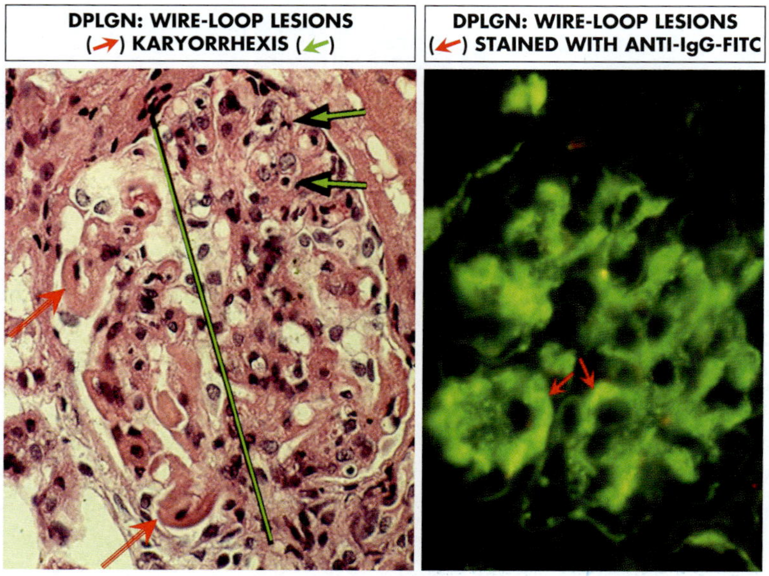

Figure 32-11.
Light photomicrograph highlighting segmental proliferative lesions with karyorrhexis (green arrows) and wire-loop appearance of the glomerular capillaries (red arrows) in a patient with diffuse proliferative glomerulonephritis (DPGN, left panel). Immunofluorescence microscopy delineates the nature of immune deposits (IgG/C3) in the thick wire loops (red arrows, right panel).

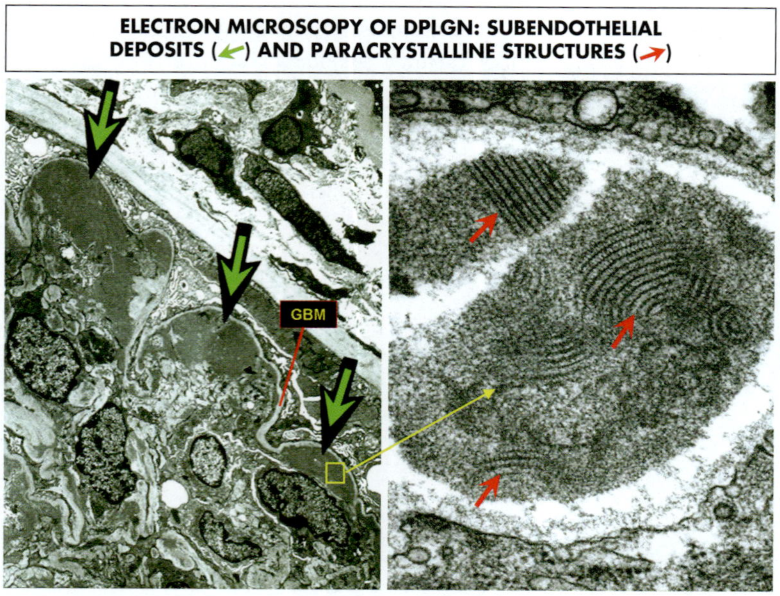

Figure 32-12.
Electron photomicrograph highlighting the presence of subendothelial (green arrows) and electron-dense deposits in a patient with DPGN (left panel). Higher magnification shows the presence of paracrystalline structures (red arrows) in the subendothelial electron-dense deposits (right panel).

abundant and large. In LN class I and II, the electron dense deposits are small and discrete, located in the mesangia. In severe cases, copious electron dense deposits are seen in the mesangia and also involve subendothelial, intramembranous, and subepithelial locations, at times obliterating the glomerular capillary lumen (Figs. 32-10 and 32-12)

Differential diagnosis

- Patients with IgA nephropathy and Schonlein-Henoch purpura need to be carefully evaluated for lupus. In the presence of other immunoglobulins such as IgG or IgM and especially C1q along with IgA, it is likely the patient has lupus disease
- Similarly, membranous lupus nephropathy needs to be distinguished from idiopathic membranous nephropathy. In the latter, the mesangial or subendothelial deposits are absent

MEMBRANOPROLIFERATIVE GLOMERULONEPHRITIS

Definition

- Membranoproliferative glomerulonephritis (MPGN) includes several different pathologically distinct forms of glomerulonephritis in which there is thickening of the GBM (membrano-) and increase in the number of cells in the glomerular tuft (-proliferative)
- MPGN is characterized by profound hypocomplementemia, mesangial cell proliferation, mesangial interposition, and deposition of immunoglobulins and complement in the peripheral portion of the nodules (fringe) formed by merging of glomerular capillaries
- This entity includes three subtypes: MPGN type 1(with subendothelial deposits, classic type, mesangiocapillary glomerulonephritis), MPGN type II (dense deposits in the GBMs), and MPGN type III (mixed membranous and proliferative glomerulonephritis)

Pathogenesis

- In the pathogenesis of MPGN both classical and alternate pathways of the complement may be involved. Besides complement, the immune complex deposits made up of IgG or IgM may be seen
- In the alternate pathway, properdin system and C3 nephritic factor (C3NeF) may be involved, and such an involvement leads to profound hypocomplementemia
- Association of chronic hepatitis associated with persistent hepatitis B antigenemia with MPGN has been also described

Clinical features

- MPGN type 1 is commonly seen in children with clinical presentation being of a nephritic or nephrotic syndrome or both
- MPGN type II is also seen commonly in children and young adults, with clinical picture quite similar to that of MPGN type I

Histology

- Light microscopy findings in type I MPGN include enlarged glomeruli with a diffuse increase in glomerular tuft cellularity, creating an accentuation of the lobular pattern
- There is marked diffuse thickening of the glomerular capillary walls with reduplication of the basal lamina (mesangial interposition), which can lead to narrowing of the capillary lumens (Fig. 32-13)
- The histologic findings in MPGN type II can have a variety of light microscopic findings with some similarities to MPGN type I including lobular glomerulonephritis (Fig. 32-14) or glomerular sclerosis, pure mesangial cellularity (focal and segmental or diffuse), MGN-like pattern, crescentic glomerulonephritis, minimal changes, focal and segmental necrotizing glomerulonephritis, and diffuse proliferative glomerulonephritis
- Morphologic changes in the tubules, interstitium, and vessels can be seen, but are secondary to the changes in the glomeruli

Immunofluorescence

- Immunofluorescence findings in type I MPGN is typical of a fine to coarse granular pattern along the glomerular capillaries with C3 while of lesser intensity with immunoglobulins (Fig. 32-15). Intense linear, granular, or nodular staining for C3 is seen along the glomerular capillary walls and in the mesangial regions in type II MPGN (Fig. 32-14)

Electron microscopy

- EM demonstrates the presence of subendothelial or mesangial immune deposits in type I MPGN (Fig. 32-16) and dense black intramembranous ribbon-like deposits in the GBMs, and Bowman capsule, and TBMs in type II form of MPGN (Fig. 32-17)

Differential diagnosis

- Poststreptococcal glomerulonephritis (PSGN) needs to be distinguished from MPGN since one would encounter proliferative component along with certain degree of lobular accentuation. The distinguishing feature would be high antistreptolysin O (ASO) titer in PSGN
- DN needs to be distinguished as well since in DN there is proliferation and lobular accentuation of the capillary tuft. The absence of hypocomplementemia and high blood sugar levels would distinguish DN from MPGN

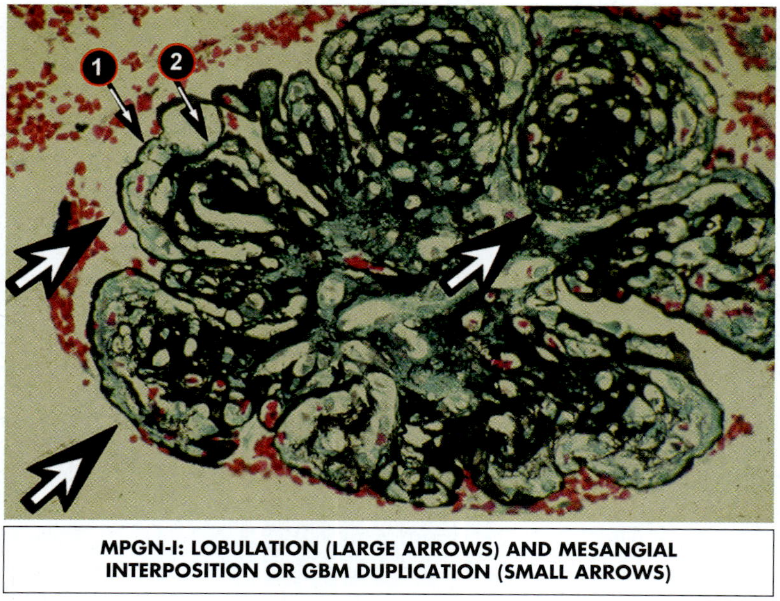

Figure 32-13.
Light photomicrograph highlighting lobular accentuation of the glomerulus (big arrows) and double contour of the basement membrane (small arrows) in a patient with membranoproliferative form of glomerulonephritis (MPGN-I).

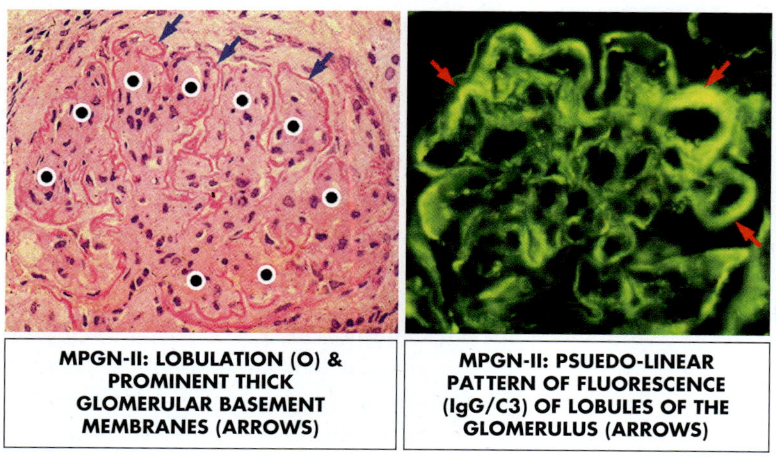

Figure 32-14.
Light photomicrograph showing accentuated lobules (circles) of the glomerulus with prominent basement membranes (arrows) in a patient with MPGN-II (left panel). Immunofluorescence photomicrograph highlighting the reactivity of IgG/C3 with GBM of the lobules (arrows, right panel).

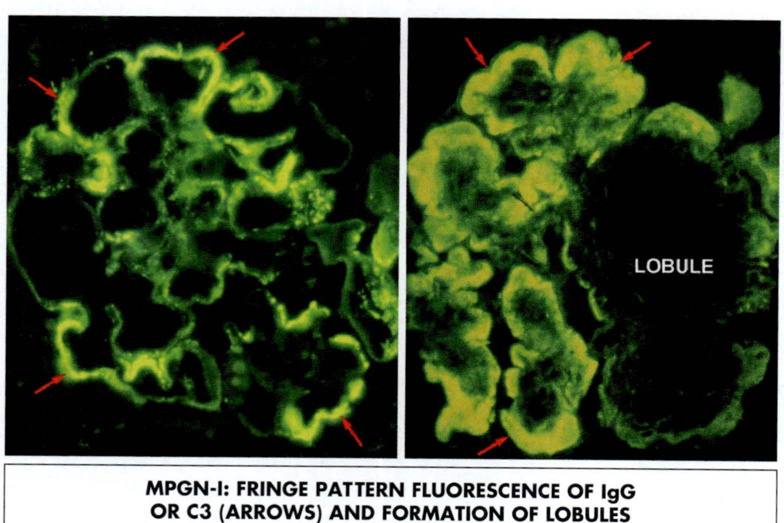

Figure 32-15.
Light immunofluorescence photomicrograph highlighting the reactivity of IgG/C3 with periphery of the lobules (fringe pattern, arrows) of the glomerulus in a patient with MPGN-I.

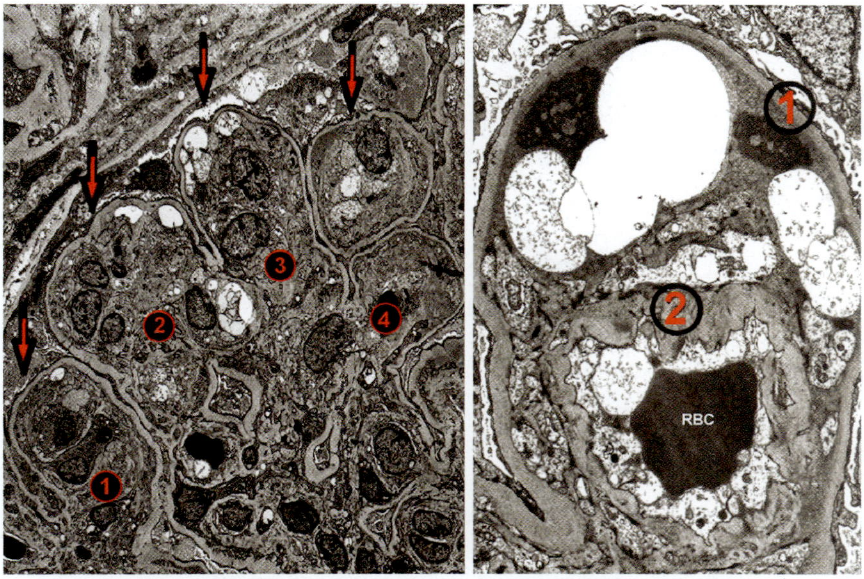

MPGN-I: PROLIFERATION OF MESANGIAL & ENDOTHELIAL CELLS AND LOBULATION (1–4 LOBULES) OF THE GLOMERULUS (↗)

MPGN-I: MESANGIAL INTERPOSITION OR GBM DUPLICATION (1 & 2)

Figure 32-16.
Electron photomicrograph highlighting the presence of lobular accentuation of the glomerulus (arrows, left panel) and double contour of the basement membrane (mesangial interposition, right panel) in a patient with MPGN-I.

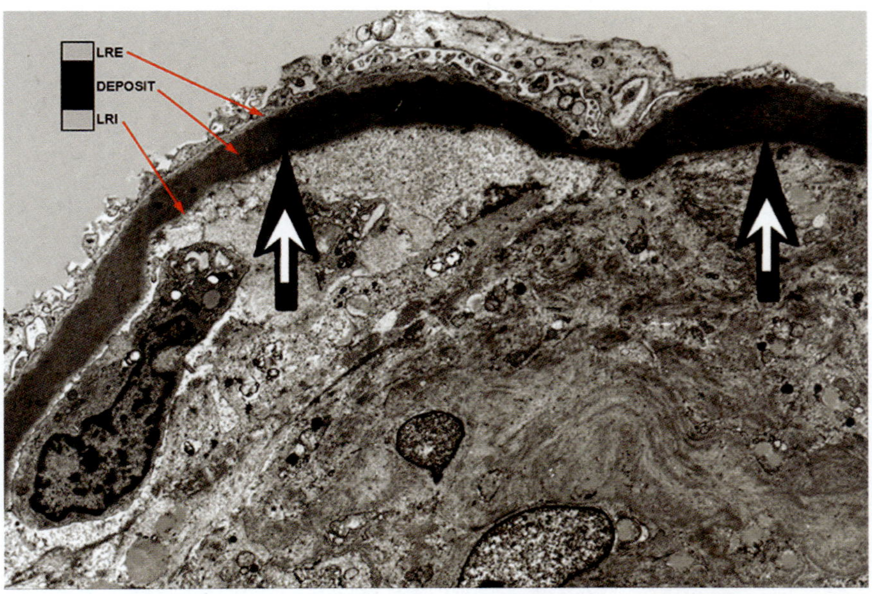

MPGN-II: THICK BLACK ELECTRON DENSE LINEAR DEPOSITS IN GLOMERULAR BASEMENT MEMBRANE (WHITE ARROWS)

Figure 32-17.
Electron photomicrograph highlighting the presence of linear electron-dense black deposit in the lamina densa of the GBM (arrows) in a patient with MPGN-II.

ACUTE POSTINFECTIOUS GLOMERULONEPHRITIS

Definition

- Acute postinfectious glomerulonephritis is a type of glomerulonephritis that follows infection, PSGN being the most common and best understood

Pathogenesis

- Acute postinfectious glomerulonephritis stems from an immunologic phenomenon. The immune reactions could occur in several ways: circulating or local immune complexes or both consisting of streptococcal antigen-antibody complex or autologous antigen-antibody complexes

Clinical features

- Acute postinfectious glomerulonephritis most commonly affects children and young adults. A preceding infectious episode is the sine qua non for the clinical diagnosis. The onset of clinical symptoms is abrupt with presentation being of nephritic syndrome and time microscopic hematuria

Histology

- There is a diffuse involvement of all the glomeruli showing endocapillary hypercellularity with numerous neutrophils and narrowing of lumina of all the glomerular capillaries. The individual lobules of the glomeruli are wider than normal assuming a clubbed appearance (Fig. 32-18)
- Changes in tubules and blood vessels are not as pronounced as in glomeruli. Variable interstitial involvement can be seen

Immunofluorescence

- Large coarse, granular deposits are seen along the glomerular capillary walls with anti-IgG and C3. At times, no immune complex deposits are seen (Fig. 32-19, right panel)

Electron microscopy

- The most consistent finding of EM is the presence of glomerular subepithelial electron-dense deposits, referred to as "humps." Discrete electron dense deposits are also seen in mesangial regions (Fig. 32-19, left panel)

Differential diagnosis

- Acute postinfectious glomerulonephritis of nonstreptococcal origin
- Membranoproliferative glomerulonephritis
- Cryoglobulinemic glomerulonephritis
- Membranous glomerulonephritis
- Diffuse proliferative (Class IV) lupus nephritis

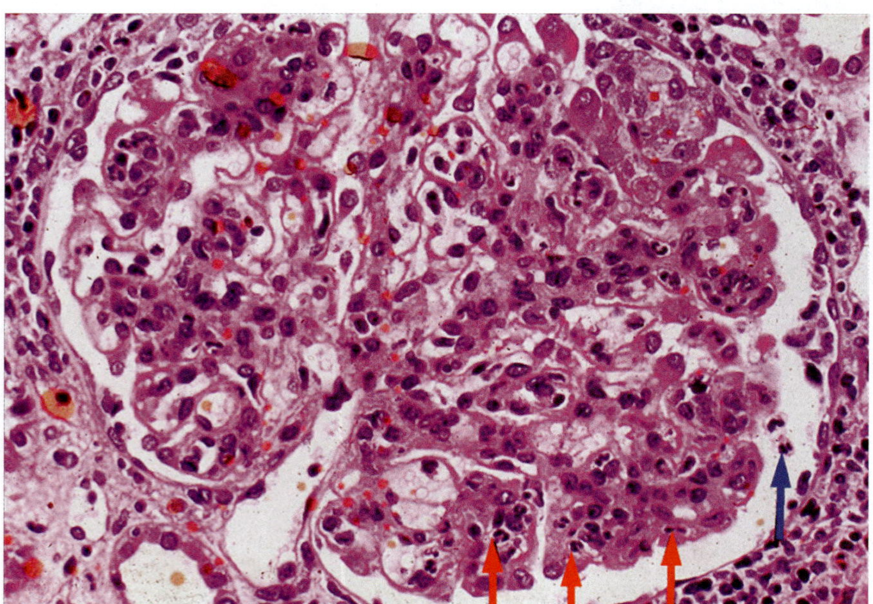

POST-STREP. GN: HYPERCELLULAR GLOMERULUS WITH PMNS IN THE CAPILLARY (↑) & URINARY SPACE (↑).

Figure 32-18.
Light photomicrograph showing hypercellular glomerulus with influx of polymorphonuclear neutrophil (PMN) in the capillaries (red arrows) in a patient with poststreptococcal nephritis. Some PMNs are present in the urinary space.

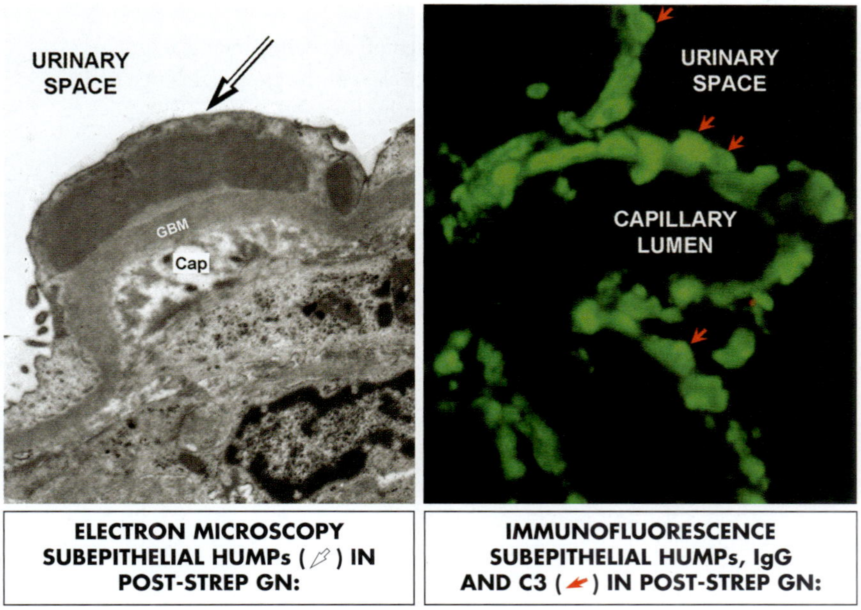

Figure 32-19.
Electron photomicrograph highlighting the presence of electron-dense subepithelial humps (arrow) in a patient with PSGN (left panel). By immunofluorescence microscopy subepithelial humps are confirmed to be made up of IgG/C3 (red arrows, right panel).

IGA NEPHROPATHY

Definition

- IgA nephropathy is one the most common forms of primary glomerulonephritis characterized by hematuria with preceding history of respiratory or gastrointestinal problems

Pathogenesis

- IgA nephropathy is commonly described as an immune-complex-mediated glomerular disease, the immune complexes being either circulating or forming locally with antigens planted in the mesangia. The IgA deposition leads to activation and proliferation of mesangial cells in response to IgA binding to receptors on these cells and subsequent cross-linking of receptors and activation of complement

Clinical features

- IgA nephropathy can occur in individuals of all ages, although most commonly between ages of 10 and 40 years with male predominance. The major clinical presentations include asymptomatic urinary abnormalities and macroscopic hematuria

Histology

- The histologic presentation of IgA nephropathy is highly diverse, ranging from no detectable histologic lesions, minimal histologic lesions (minimal increase in mesangial cellularity) to FSGS like, focal proliferative glomerulonephritis and diffuse proliferative and crescentic glomerulonephritis, similar to LN (Fig. 32-20)

Immunofluorescence

- Deposits of IgA in the mesangia with or without staining of capillary loops are diagnostic for IgA nephropathy. C3 is also detected in majority of cases of IgA nephropathy (Fig. 32-21, lower panel)

Electron microscopy

- Uniform electron dense deposits are seen in the mesangial or paramesagial regions in IgA nephropathy (Fig. 32-21, upper panel)

Differential diagnosis

- Schonlein-Henoch purpura nephritis can be distinguished from IgA nephropathy only on clinical grounds
- Lupus nephropathy
  - C1q nephropathy
  - HIV-associated lupus-like glomerulonephritis
- IgA dominant postinfectious glomerulonephritis
- Incidental (latent) mesangial IgA deposits

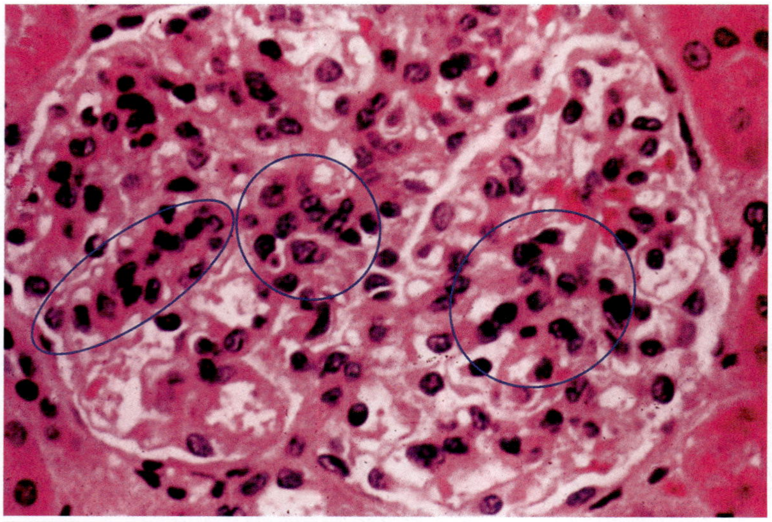

IgA NEPHROPATHY: MESANGIAL CELL PROLIFERATION (CIRCLES)

Figure 32-20.
Light photomicrograph showing mesangial hypercellularity (circles) of the glomerulus in a patient with IgA nephropathy.

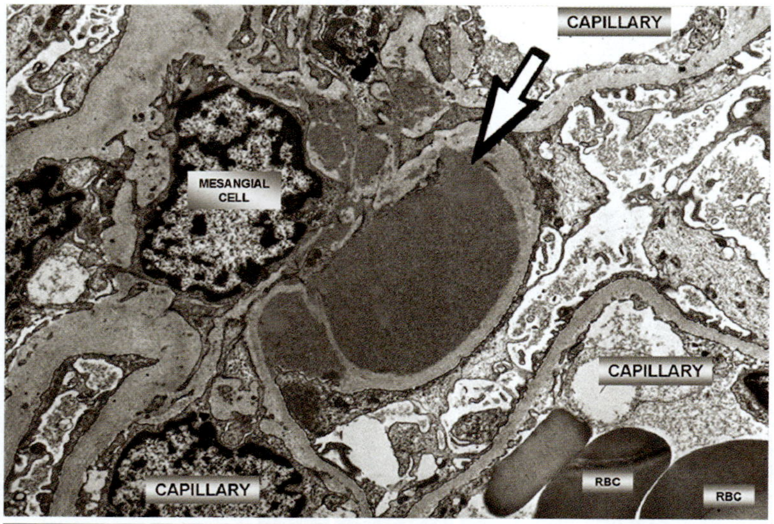

IgA NEPHROPATHY: PARAMESANGIAL DEPOSIT (ARROW)

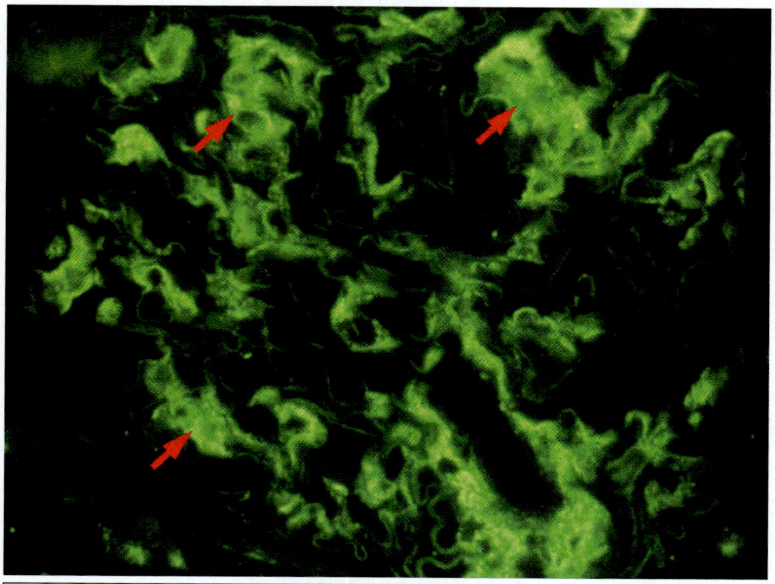

IgA NEPHROPATHY: MESANGIAL FLUORESCENCE (ARROWS)

Figure 32-21.
Electron photomicrograph depicting the presence of paramesangial electron-dense deposit (arrow) in a patient with IgA nephropathy (upper panel). By immunofluorescence microscopy, the IgA deposits are seen confined to paramesangial and mesangial regions of the glomerulus (arrows, lower panel).

ANCA-ASSOCIATED GLOMERULONEPHRITIS

Definition

- Pauci-immune crescentic glomerulonephritis (ie, ANCA crescentic glomerulonephritis) is associated with anti-neutrophilic cytoplasmic autoantibodies (ANCA) and includes patients with and without systemic vasculitis

Pathogenesis

- ANCA IgG plays a role in the induction of pauci-immune glomerulonephritis and small vessel vasculitis. The reason why patients develop an autoimmune response against neutrophils proteins is unknown
- The antibodies/autoantibodies may be directed against myeloperoxidase (MPO) or proteinase 3 (PR3)
- Occasionally, antibodies against matrix metalloproteinase (MMP) may be present

Clinical features

- Patients with ANCA-associated glomerulonephritis usually presents with rapidly progressive glomerulonephritis, hematuria, proteinuria, and elevated serum creatinine

Histology

- The hallmark histologic lesions of acute pauci-immune ANCA glomerulonephritis are crescents and fibrinoid necrosis of the glomeruli. The severity of the lesions can range from focal to severe diffuse necrotizing and crescentic glomerulonephritis with global necrosis of virtually all the glomeruli (Fig. 32-22)
- Necrotizing small vessel vasculitis causing renal arteritis, arteriolitis, and medullary angiitis can be seen in these patients
- Interstitial edema and interstitial leukocytic infiltration (tubulointerstitial and periglomerular) are commonly seen

Immunofluorescence

- Pauci-immune crescentic glomerulonephritis does not have immunofluorescence findings diagnostic of anti-GBM disease or immune complex disease; however, many patients have a low level of staining for immunoglobulins

Electron microscopy

- These patients have no or scanty glomerular or vascular immune-complex-type electron deposits
- At times disruption in the GBMs may be seen

Differential diagnosis

- Pauci-immune crescentic glomerulonephritis must be distinguished from immune-complex-mediated glomerulonephritis and small-vessel vasculitis and anti-GBM disease. Immunofluorescence and serology are helpful in making a definitive diagnosis

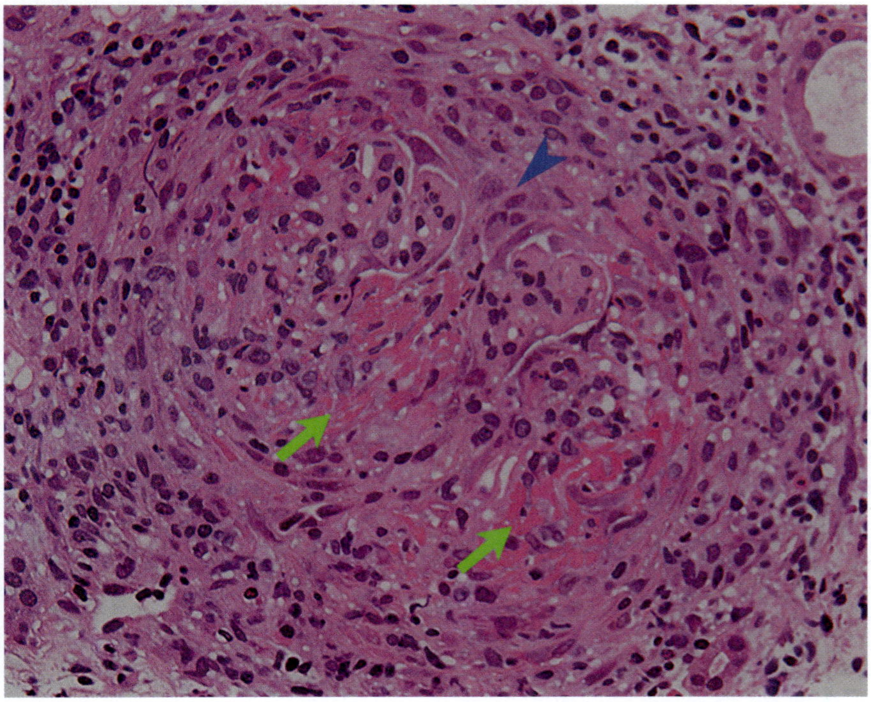

Figure 32-22.
Light photomicrograph showing necrotizing lesions (green arrows) and small crescent (blue arrowhead) with marked influx of inflammatory cells in and around the glomerulus in a patient with pauci-immune crescentic glomerulonephritis.

TUBULOINTERSTITIAL NEPHRITIS

Definition

- Primary tubulointerstitial nephritis refers to cases where the inflammation is limited to tubules and interstitium; glomeruli and vessels are uninvolved or show minor changes. Secondary tubulointerstitial nephritis is associated with primary glomerular, vascular, or systemic disease; the most frequent cause being drug related followed by infections and or may be idiopathic

Pathogenesis

- Pathogenesis of tubulointerstitial nephritis appears to result from systemic release of lymphokines promoting chemoattraction and activation of mononuclear cells in the kidneys. In underlying infections, microbial release of degradative enzymes and toxic molecules, direct penetration of host cells by microbes and inflammatory response mediated by antibodies, T cells, or both can cause tubulointerstitial nephritis. Drug-induced tubulointerstitial nephritis is most likely immunologically mediated, with drugs acting as haptens

Clinical features

- Tubulointerstitial nephritis has two common clinical presentations: sudden onset and rapid decline in renal function (acute tubulointerstitial nephritis) and protracted onset and slow decline in renal function (chronic tubulointerstitial nephritis)

Histology

- The interstitium contains cellular infiltration with neutrophils and mononuclear cells, predominately T cells in acute tubulointerstitial nephritis. Eosinophils are common in drug-induced cases, which is reflective of hypersensitivity reaction. Tubular injury including tubulitis, breaks of TBM, necrosis of tubular cells, and atrophy and loss of tubules can be seen (Fig. 32-23)
- In chronic tubulointerstitial nephritis, atrophic tubules are seen, secondary to which tubules frequently undergo compensatory hypertrophy and interstitial fibrosis

Immunofluorescence

- Immunofluorescence is rarely helpful in determining the underlying cause. Granular or linear TBM staining for C3 is a frequent nonspecific finding, especially in the basement membrane of atrophic tubules

Electron microscopy

- EM is of limited value and occasionally may show electron-dense immune deposits along the TBM or in the interstitial compartment

Differential diagnosis

- The major entity that needs to be distinguished from acute or chronic interstitial nephritis is the cellular infiltrates related to lymphoma, leukemia, or plasma cell disorders. In these cases use of various molecular diagnostic markers are usually very helpful
- Along these lines the entities related to posttransplant lymphoproliferative disorders (PTLD) and polyoma virus infection in immunosuppressed patients should be ruled out. Various molecular diagnostic markers and immunohistochemical stains are helpful in distinguishing them from traditional acute or chronic interstitial nephritis

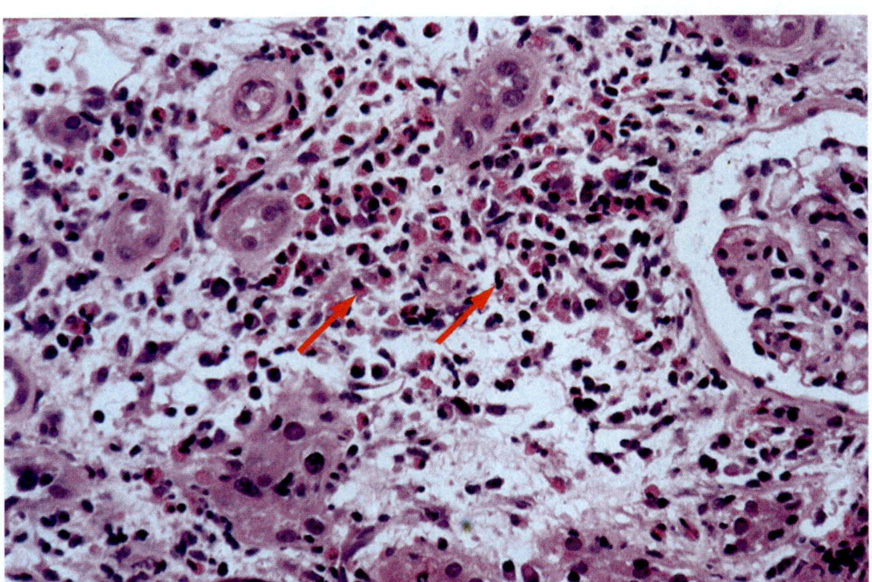

DITIN: INTERSTITIAL EDEMA AND INFLUX OF EOSINOPHILS (ARROWS)

Figure 32-23. Light photomicrograph showing interstitial edema, influx of eosinophils (red arrows), and destruction of tubules in a patient with drug-induced tubulointerstitial nephritis.

KIDNEY TRANSPLANTATION

Definition

- The most common indications for renal transplantation are end-stage renal disease due to diabetes, nephrosclerosis associated with hypertension, polycystic kidney disease, and various glomerulopathies most common being IgA nephropathy. Therapy for graft dysfunction is primarily based on renal biopsy findings, which remain the gold standard to determine the cause of dysfunction

Pathogenesis

- The principal alloreactive initiators of graft rejection are T cells and antibodies (cellular or humoral rejection), which trigger various secondary mediators (activation of macrophages and complement)

Clinical features

- Monitoring of graft dysfunction is usually performed by measuring the serum creatinine value
- At times, the patients may develop hemolytic uremic syndrome, in which case haptoglobin levels and examination of peripheral smear would be helpful

Histology

- The usual major findings in acute cellular rejection are infiltration of activated T-lymphocytes and monocytes in the edematous interstitium and tubules and in more severe cases, similar infiltrate is seen in the arterial intima and glomeruli. Hemorrhage and necrosis are seen in more severe cases (Figs. 32-24 to 32-27)
- Neutrophils in peritubular capillaries are often seen in acute antibody-mediated rejection (Fig. 32-24)
- Tubulitis is considered a hallmark of acute cellular rejection (Fig. 32-26)

Immunofluorescence

- There is minimal immunoglobulin deposition in acute cellular rejection. Peritubular capillaries lack C4d deposition in "pure" cellular rejection cases; however, it is the diagnostic

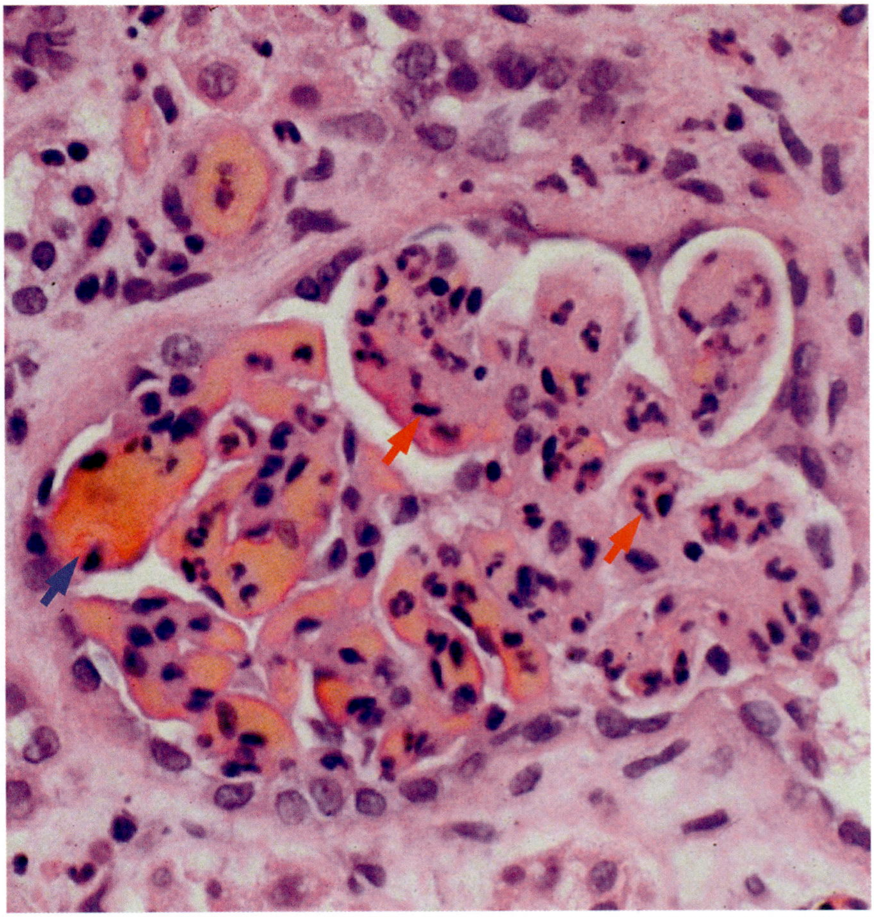

HY-AR: INFLUX OF PMNS (↗) & SLUDGING OF RBCs (↗) IN THE GLOMERULUS

Figure 32-24. Light photomicrograph showing marked influx of PMNs (red arrows) and sludging of RBCs in glomerular capillaries in a patient with hyperacute antibody-mediated rejection.

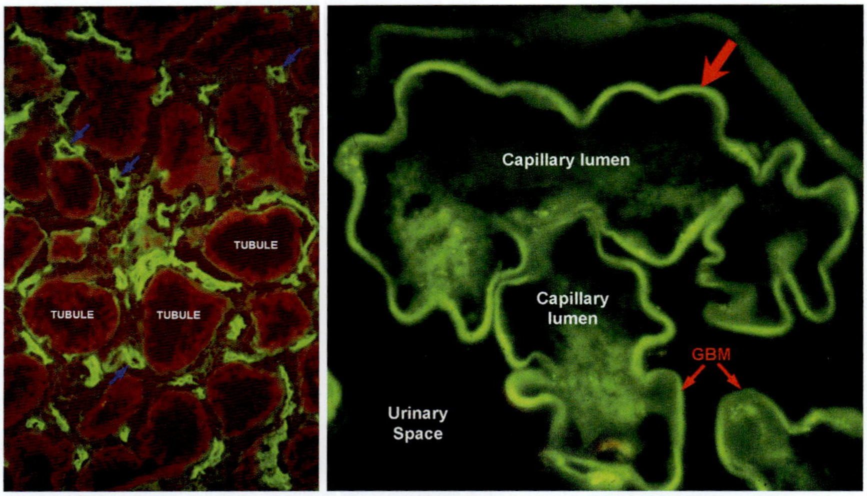

C4d TEST (COMPLEMENT FRAGMENT): PERITUBULAR CAPILLARY REACTIVITY (↗) TO PREFORMED DONOR SPECIFIC ANTIBODIES

HY-AR: LINEAR IMMUNFLUORESCENCE (ARROW) DUE TO THE BINDING OF PREFORMED ANTIBODIES (IgG) TO GLOMERULAR BASEMENT MEMBRANE (GBM, ARROWS)

Figure 32-25.
Light immunofluorescence photomicrograph highlighting the reactivity of C4d with interstitial capillaries (blue arrows, left panel) and linear GBM staining (red arrows, right panel) in a patient with antibody-mediated rejection.

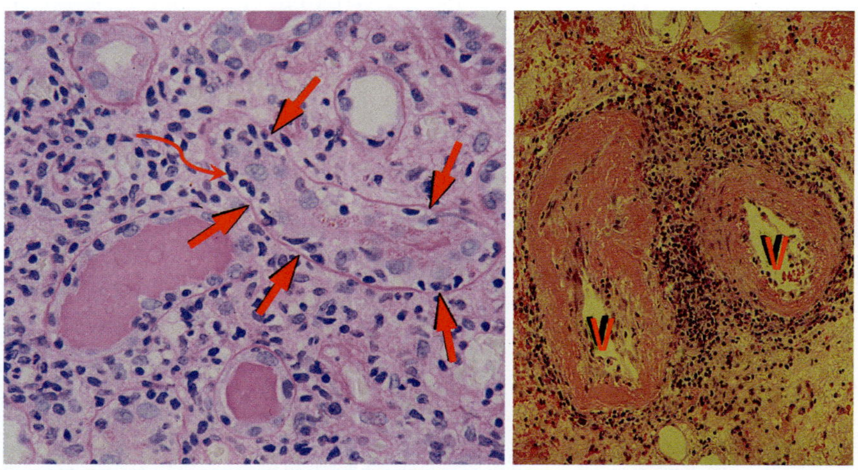

AR: TUBULITIS, INFLUX OF CELLS INTO THE TUBULES AFTER CROSSING THE BASEMENT MEMBRANE (ARROWS)

ACUTE REJECTION (AR): INTENSE PERIVASCULAR (V) CELLULAR INFILTRATES

Figure 32-26.
Light photomicrograph showing tubulitis (red arrows, left panel) and vascular cuffings and intimal arteritis of blood vessels (V) in a patient with kidney acute cellular rejection.

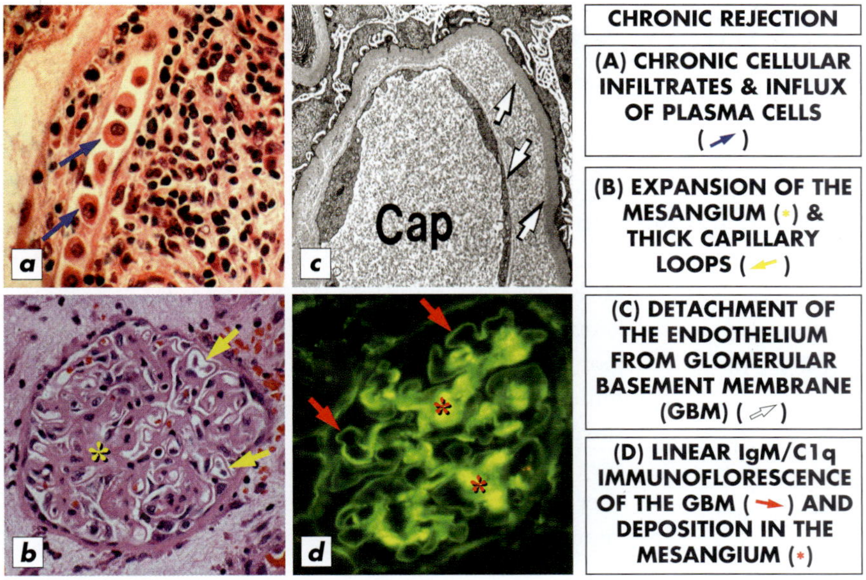

Figure 32-27.
Morphologic features of chronic renal transplant rejection. (*a*) Light photomicrograph showing influx of plasma cells and lymphocytes into the interstitium and capillaries (blue arrows). (*b*) Light photomicrograph showing thickened glomerular capillaries (yellow arrows) and expanded mesangia (asterisk). (*c*) Electron photomicrograph showing detachment of the endothelia from the underlying glomerular basement membrane (white arrows). (*d*) By immunofluorescence microscopy IgM/C1q deposits are seen confined to the mesangial regions of the glomerulus (asterisks) and GBM (red arrows).

feature in acute antibody-mediated rejection (Fig. 32-25). Abundant C3 deposition can be seen along the TBM in segmental linear pattern

Electron microscopy

- EM is generally not performed for diagnostic purposes in acute rejection. However, it may be indicated if glomeruli are notably involved or there is a recurrence of the original disease process

Differential diagnosis

- Tubulointerstitial inflammation
- Infection (polyoma, CMV, and adenovirus)
- Posttransplant lymphoproliferative diseases
- Drug allergy
- Calcineurin inhibitor toxicity and ischemic injury

CHAPTER 33

Other Inflammatory and Reactive Conditions of the Kidney

ACUTE PYELONEPHRITIS

Definition

- Acute suppurative inflammation of the renal pelvis and interstitial parenchyma, characterized by the presence of heavy neutrophilic infiltrate

Pathogenesis and epidemiology

- Infectious etiology, mostly by *E coli* and many gram-negative bacteria
- It can be divided into ascending type and hematogenous type
  - Ascending type: most cases are ascending infections from the lower urinary tract
  - Hematogenous type: sometimes it is caused by systemic infection such as sepsis
- Four to five times more common in women than men
- More frequently seen in younger women of 20 to 50 years old
- Predisposing factors include urinary obstruction, reflux, diabetes, and immunosuppression

Clinical features

- Acute onset of fever and flank pain
- Increased WBCs in urine and positive urine culture
- Renal failure in severe cases

Gross pathology

- Large abscesses or microabscesses in the renal pelvis and renal parenchyma (Fig. 33-1*a*)

Histology

- Diffuse infiltrate of neutrophils with tissue destruction and abscess formation (Figs. 33-1 and 33-2)
- Lesions are involving, but not limited in, the renal pelvic region (Fig. 33-3)
- Glomeruli and tubules in the renal parenchyma are uninvolved initially, but can be involved in the advanced stage (Fig. 33-4)
- Other inflammatory cells can be present as minor components

Differential diagnosis

Acute interstitial nephritis

- May have history of drug reaction
- Presence of numerous eosinophils
- Less severe, abscess uncommon
- Negative urine culture

Clinical relevance (prognosis and treatment options)

- Most cases are caused by bacterial infection, therefore, antibiotics as treatment of choice
- The majority of cases can be controlled by antibiotic administration and will have a benign course. Some cases may progress to chronic pyelonephritis
- Nephrectomy may be considered if medical treatment has failed or the presence of large or extensive abscesses

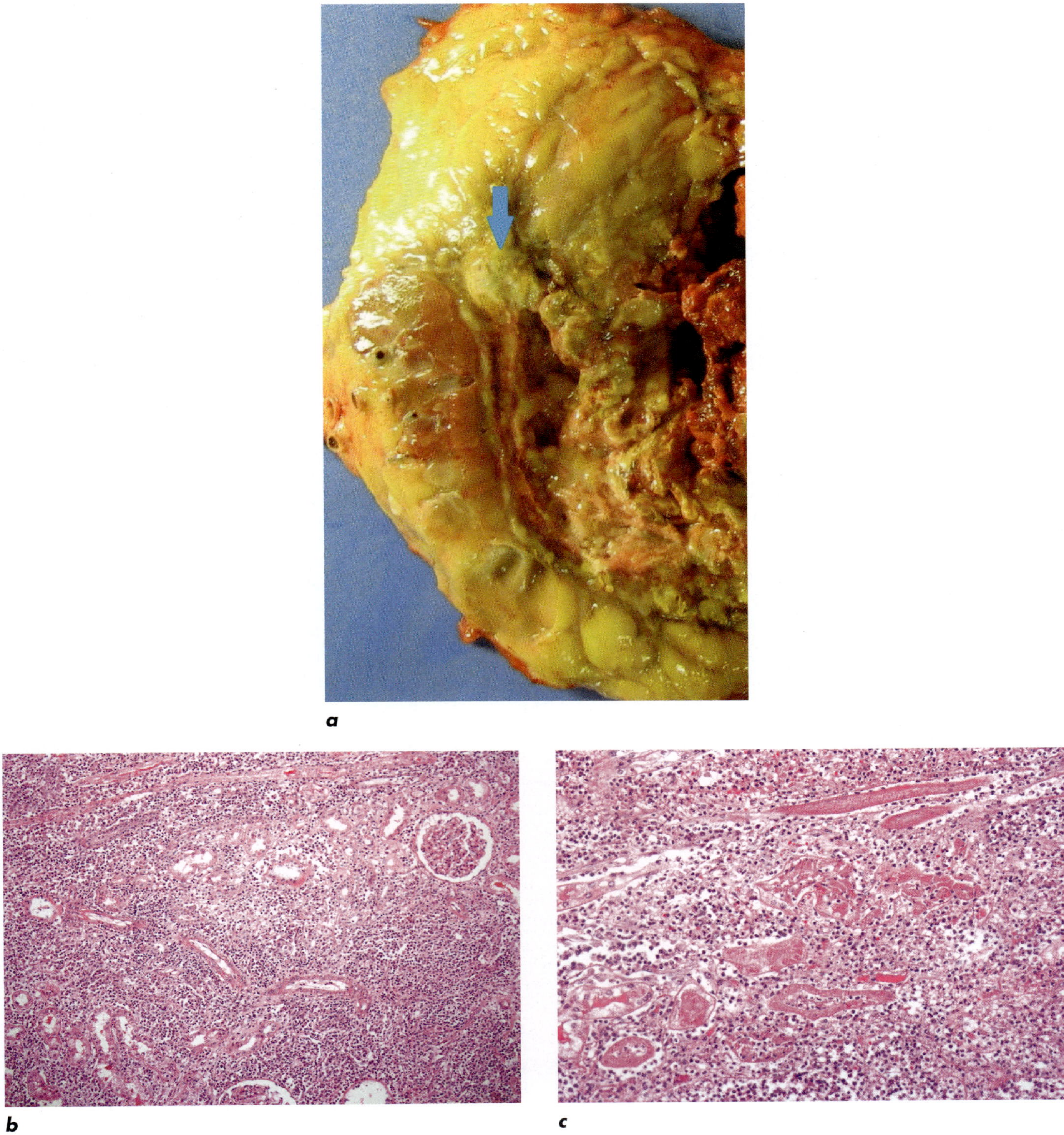

Figure 33-1.
Acute pyelonephritis. Gross photo showing a kidney partially destroyed and replaced by large abscesses. Adjacent to an abscess (arrow), there is residual renal tissue (*a*). Microscopically, the renal tissue is diffusely infiltrated with neutrophils and other inflammatory cells (*b*); some portion has been replaced by an abscess composed of necrotic tissue and degenerative neutrophils (*c*).

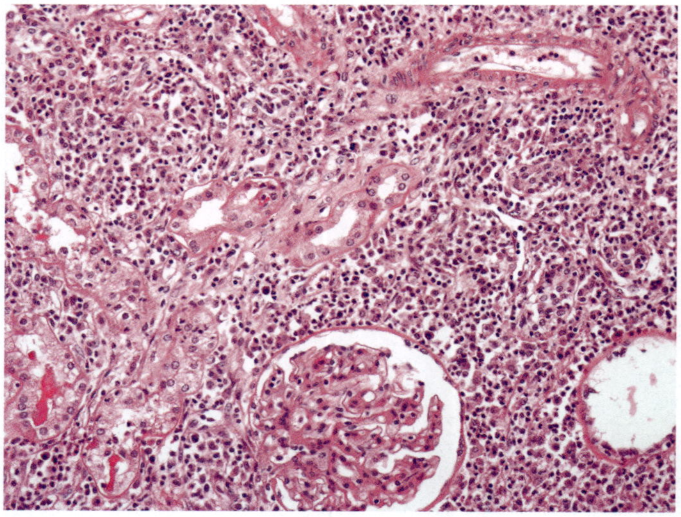

a

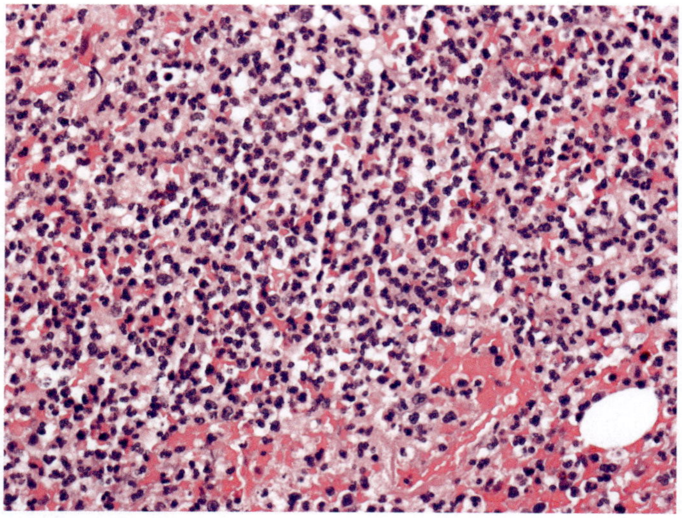

b

Figure 33-2.

Acute pyelonephritis with abscess formation. The inflammatory cells are predominantly neutrophils with some lymphocytes in renal interstitium, surrounding but sparing of glomerulus and renal tubules (*a*). An abscess with tissue destruction is seen (*b*).

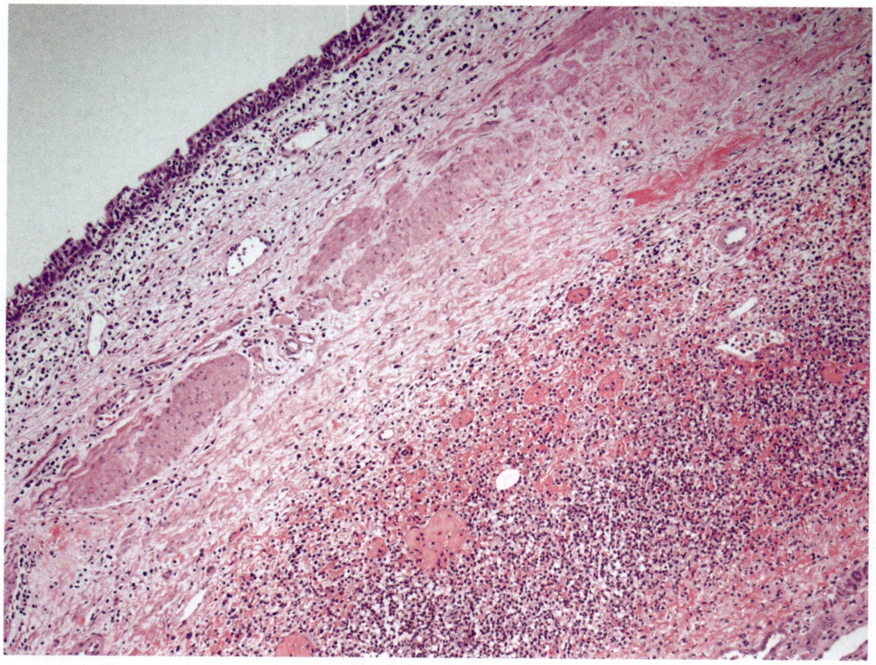

Figure 33-3.

Acute and chronic pyelonephritis. In addition to chronic inflammation on the surface of the renal pelvis, microabscess are seen in the wall of the renal pelvis.

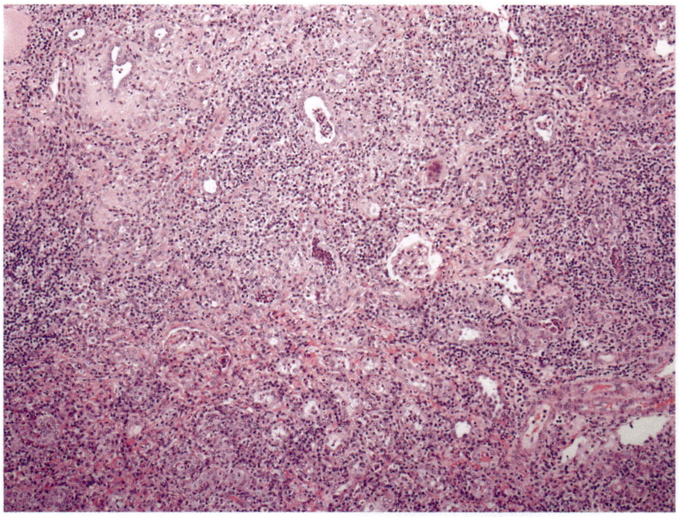

a

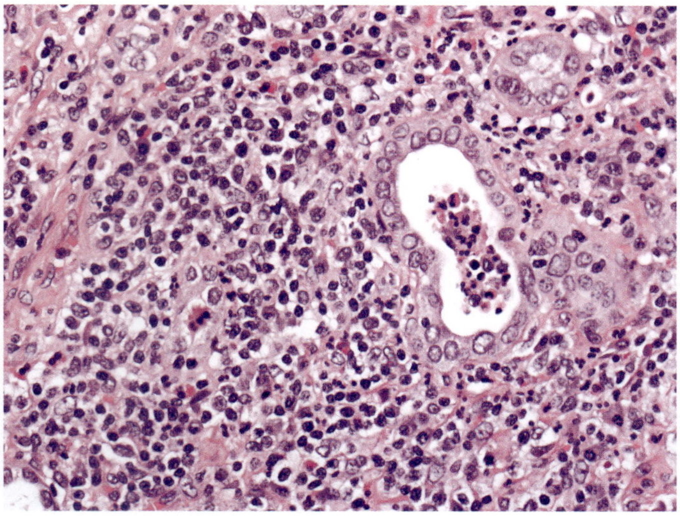

b

Figure 33-4.
Acute and chronic pyelonephritis with extensive inflammatory infiltrates in the renal parenchyma (*a*). High magnification shows the mixed inflammatory cells involving renal interstitial tissue and a renal tubule containing a neutrophil cast (*b*).

CHRONIC PYELONEPHRITIS

Definition

- Chronic inflammation of renal pelvis and interstitial parenchyma of the kidney

Pathogenesis

- Can be divided into obstructive and nonobstructive types
- Most cases are associated with urinary obstruction by stone, or tumors
- Others are hematogenous type, converted from acute pyelonephritis
- Reflux may also be responsible for a subset of the diseases

Clinical features

- Highly variable. Early phase with signs of infection such as fever
- Obstructive symptoms may occur
- Late stage pyelonephritis often associated with hydronephrosis and renal failure

Gross pathology

- Dilated renal pelvis with thickening of mucosa (Fig. 33-5)
- Associated lesions such as stones or tumors may be present
- Renal atrophy with cortical thinning and scaring

Histology

- Chronic lymphocytic infiltrates in the renal pelvis, extending to the interstitium (Figs. 33-5 and 33-6)
- Urothelium may show reactive atypia (Fig. 33-7) or fibrosis (Fig. 33-5*b*)
- Secondary changes include global glomerulosclerosis (Fig. 33-5*c*)
- Diffuse renal parenchymal atrophy including thyroidization of the renal tubules
- Obstructive etiology shows more dilatation of tubules than reflux type
- Acute and chronic inflammatory cells are often coexisting

Immunohistochemistry and molecular analysis

- Not specific

Clinical relevance (prognosis and treatment options)

- Chronic pyelonephritis is commonly seen in surgical specimens, which is often secondary to nephrolithiasis, tumors, or BPH
- Removal of the primary lesion will eliminate the etiology for chronic pyelonephritis
- Severe cases associated with hydronephrosis and end-stage renal disease may require nephrectomy. The prognosis is depending on the causes

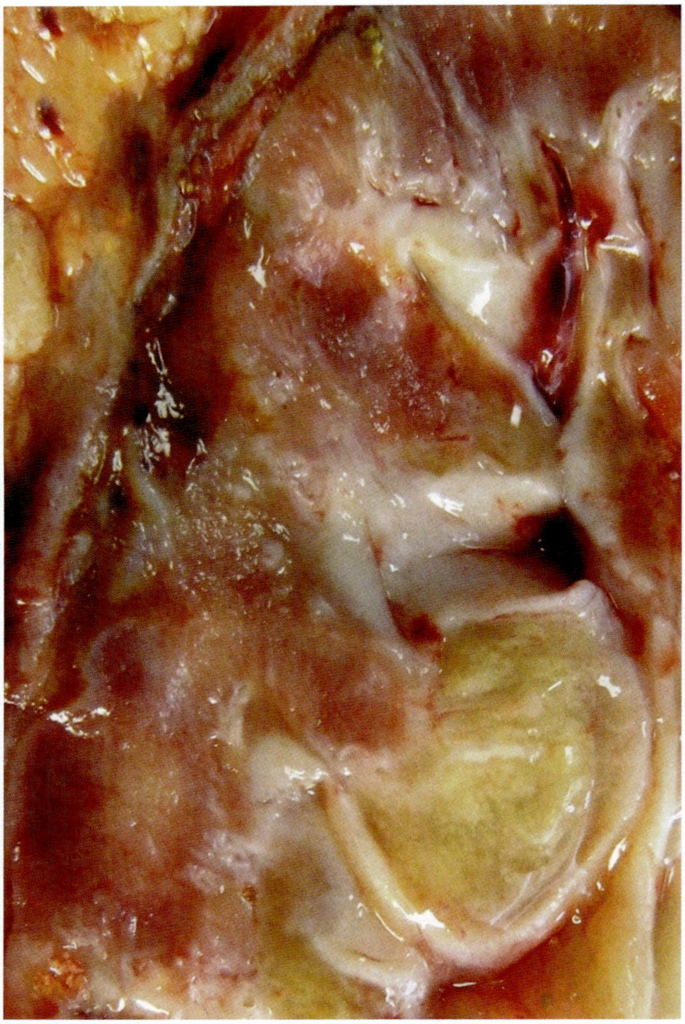

a

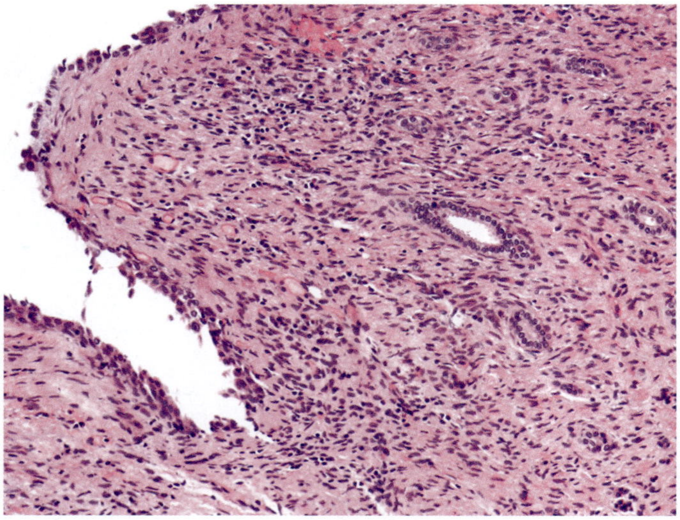

b

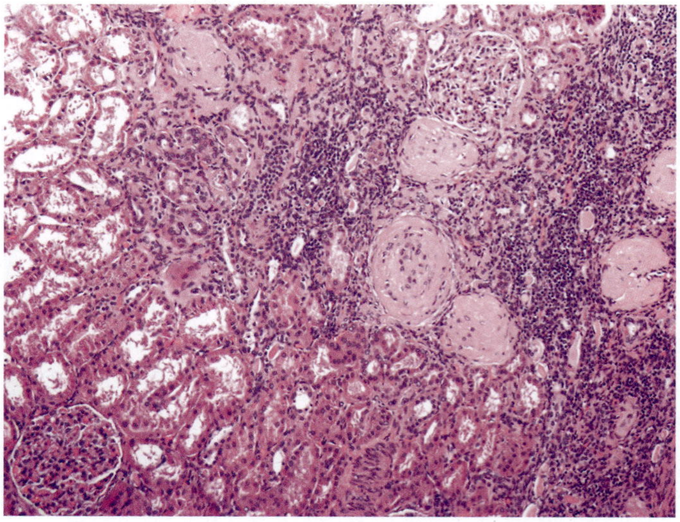

c

Figure 33-5.

Chronic pyelonephritis. Gross photo of chronic pyelonephritis is characterized by the thickening pelvic mucosa, mild hydronephrosis, and atrophic renal parenchyma (*a*). Microscopically, chronic pyelonephritis characterized by the heavy lymphocytic infiltrate and fibrosis in the renal pelvis (*b*) and focal glomerulosclerosis (*c*).

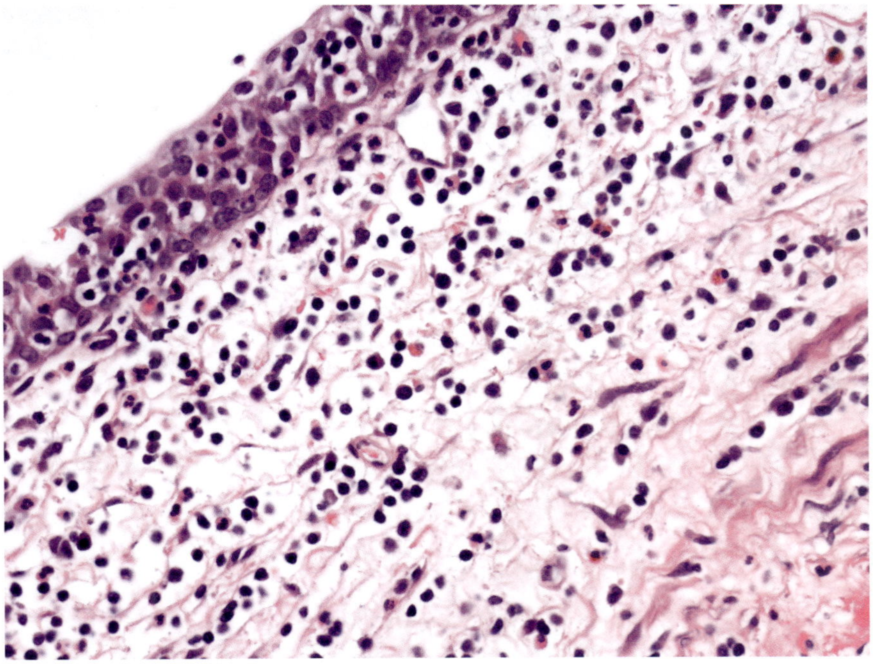

Figure 33-6.
Chronic pyelonephritis showing chronic lymphocytic infiltrate and edema in the renal pelvis.

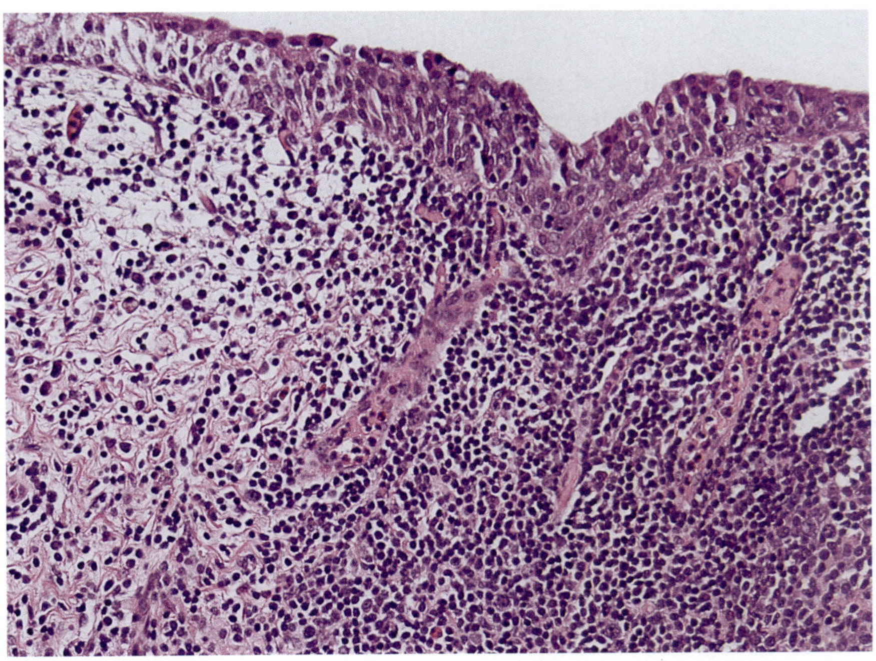

Figure 33-7.
Chronic pyelonephritis exhibiting marked chronic inflammation and reactive atypia of the pelvis urothelium.

HISTOPLASMOSIS OF THE KIDNEY

Definition

- The renal infection caused by a fungal organism—histoplasma

Other term

- Histoplasma infection of the kidney

Pathogenesis

- Histoplasmosis is the infection caused by histoplasma capsulatum
- Initially, it is acquired by inhalation of dust particles contaminated with spores from bird droppings
- Histoplasma capsulatum presents in the human as an intracellular fungal organism within macrophages

Clinical features

- Initial clinical symptoms related to the lung involvement
  - Self-limiting respiratory infection
  - Localized lung lesions
  - Symptoms of lung involvement include cough, fever, and night sweats
- The renal involvement present as
  - Localized renal lesion, as chronic pyelonephritis
  - Widely disseminated disease, as the kidney involvement in a immunocompromised patient
  - Or widely disseminated disease including kidney involvement in an immunocompromised patient

Gross pathology

- Diffuse or localized mass lesions in renal parenchyma with or without associated necrosis (Fig. 33-8) and thickening of renal pelvis if it is involved

Histology

- Chronic interstitial inflammation (Fig. 33-9*a*) and granulomatous inflammation with areas of necrosis (Fig. 33-9*b*)
- Small thin-walled yeasts (2 to 5 μm) may be identified on the H&E sections at high magnification

Histochemistry

- PAS or GMS demonstrates the small yeast organism (Fig. 33-9*c* and *d*)

Differential diagnosis

Bacterial pyelonephritis

- GMS, other fungal staining or microbiology studies are necessary to confirm the diagnosis

Clinical relevance (prognosis and treatment options)

- Acute phase, histoplasmosis can be treated with antifungal drugs
- In chronic renal involvement, surgical resection may be necessary
- In transplant patients and AIDS patients, histoplasmosis is a major opportunistic infection

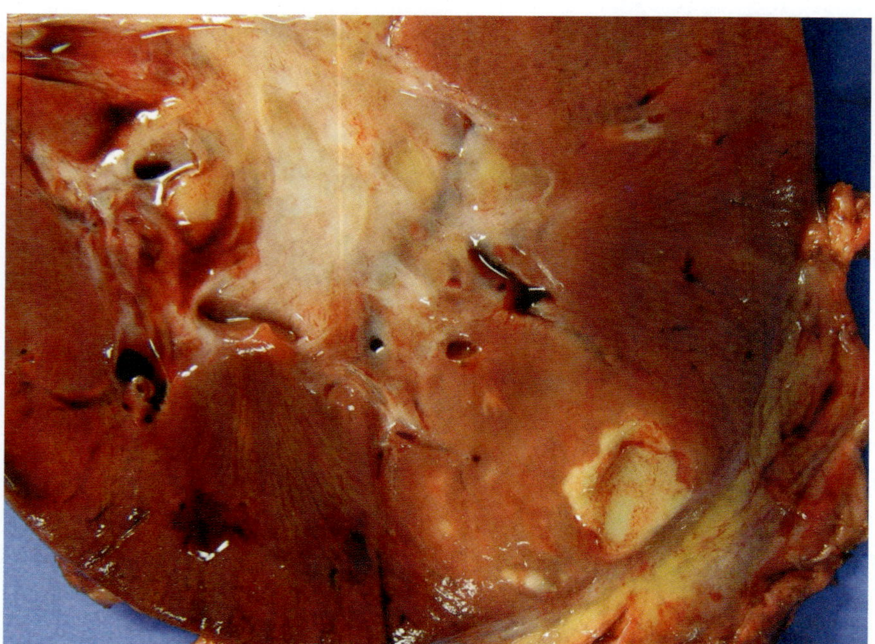

Figure 33-8.
A small nodule can be seen in the renal cortex with a bright yellow cut surface and irregular borders, mimicking renal cell carcinoma.

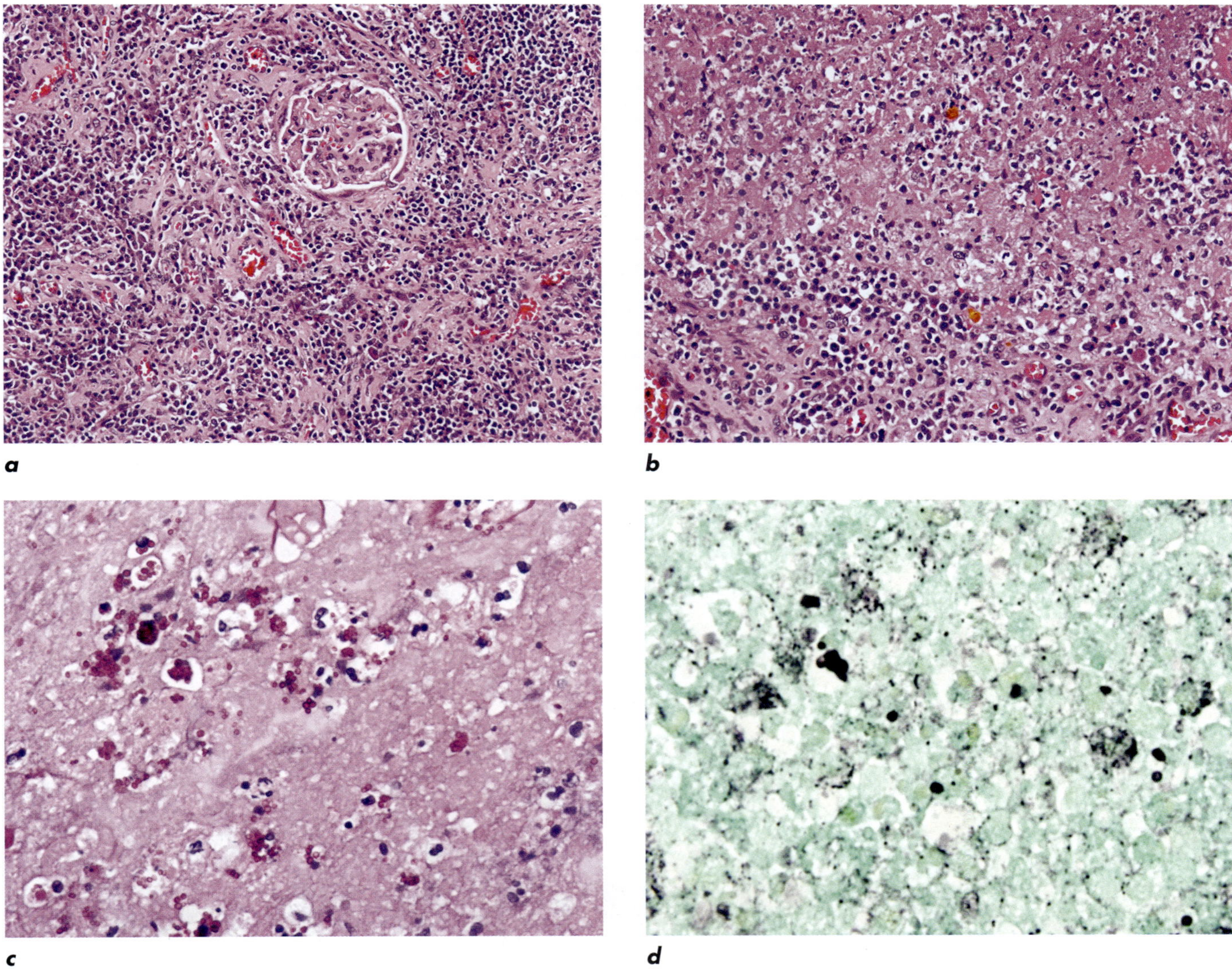

Figure 33-9.
Renal histoplasmosis with chronic interstitial inflammation in the renal parenchyma (*a*). Area of necrosis and granulomatous reaction around necrosis can be seen (*b*). Small thin-wall histoplasma yeasts in necrotic tissue can be seen by using PAS (*c*) and GMS stains (*d*).

XANTHOGRANULOMATOUS PYELONEPHRITIS

Definition

- Xanthogranulomatous pyelonephritis (XGPN) is a granulomatous inflammation of the kidney, characterized by the presence of numerous foamy macrophages in the background of chronic pyelonephritis

Pathogenesis

- The most likely pathogenesis is urinary obstruction induced by acute pyelonephritis
- The inflammatory process leads to tissue necrosis and subsequent foamy macrophage granulomatous reaction to clean up the necrotic material

Clinical features

- The patients often present with obstructive symptoms
- Renal mass or masses resembling neoplasms are detected by imaging studies
- Stones or hydronephrosis may be present in addition to the renal parenchyma mass lesions

Gross pathology

- XGPN is present as single or multiple lesions in the kidney (Fig. 33-10)
- The lesions are poorly circumscribed with golden yellow cut surface (Fig. 33-11)
- Hemorrhage and necrosis are frequent findings
- Calculi, dilated renal pelvis, or hydronephrosis may be seen (Fig. 33-11)
- The lesion(s) can be easily confused with clear cell RCC because of the appearance of a yellow color mass

Histology

- XGPN can be divided into three phases
  - Phase I, renal parenchyma
  - Phase II, renal capsule
  - Phase III, beyond Gerota fascia
- The hallmark of the XGPN is the presence of granulomatous inflammation with a large number of foamy macrophages (Fig. 33-11)
- Giant cells are occasionally seen (Fig. 33-12)
- Numerous macrophages with foamy abundant cytoplasm associated other chronic inflammatory cells are present (Fig. 33-13)
- Reactive residual renal tubules can be observed, but there is no proliferative epithelial lesion present

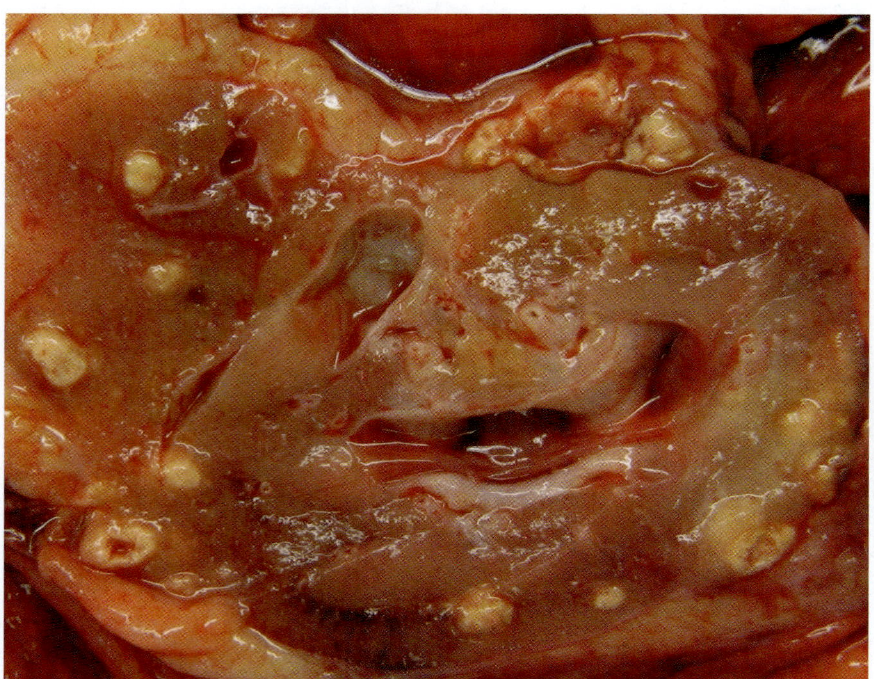

Figure 33-10.
Xanthogranulomatous pyelonephritis (XGPN) with multiple small yellow nodules scattered in the kidney parenchyma.

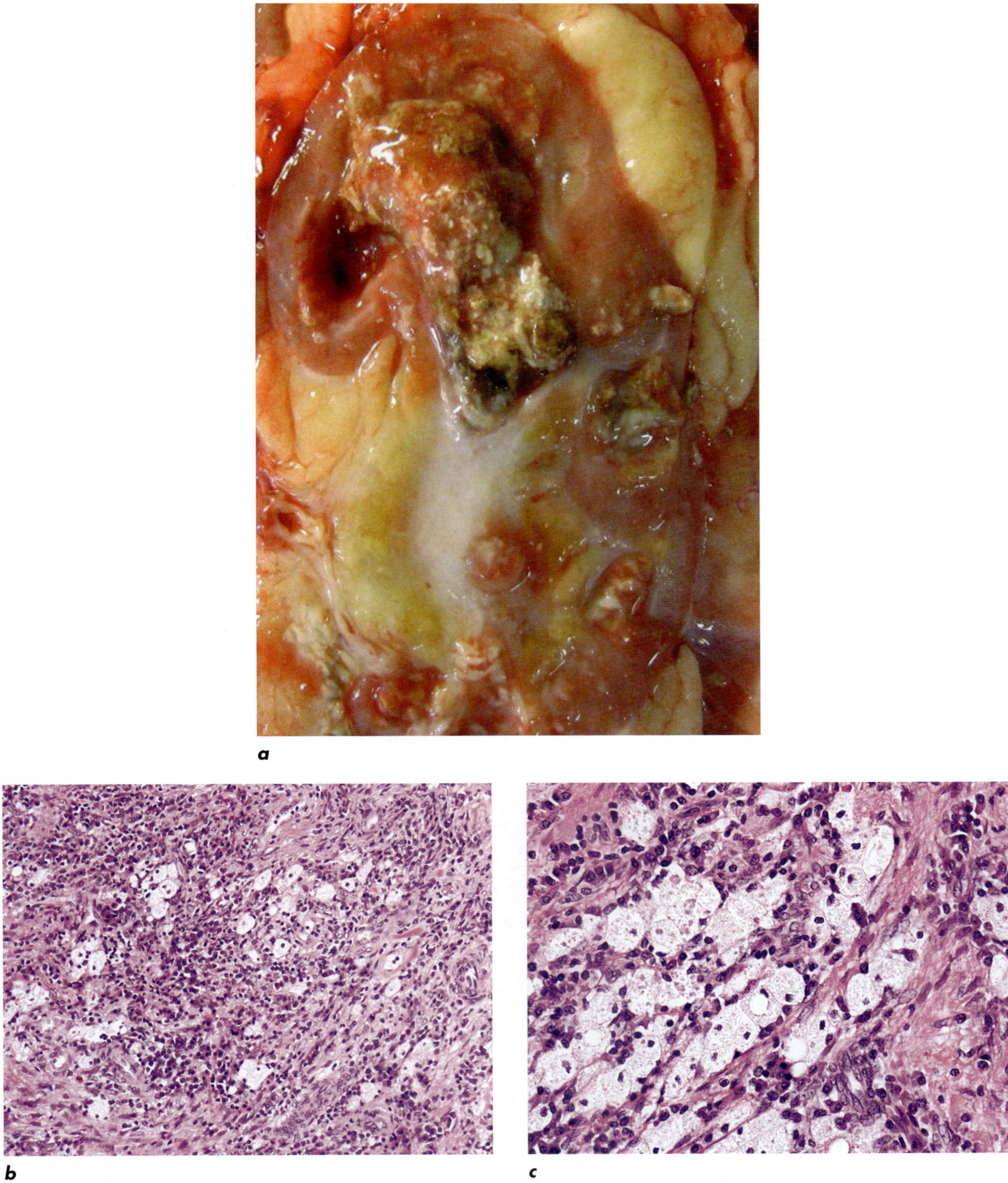

Figure 33-11.
XGPN appears to be a mass lesion with spotty necrotic material in the upper pole of the kidney, mimicking RCC (*a*). Microscopically, it is characterized by the presence of mixed inflammatory cells and numerous foamy macrophages (*b*). High magnification confirms the presence of lipid-laden macrophages (*c*).

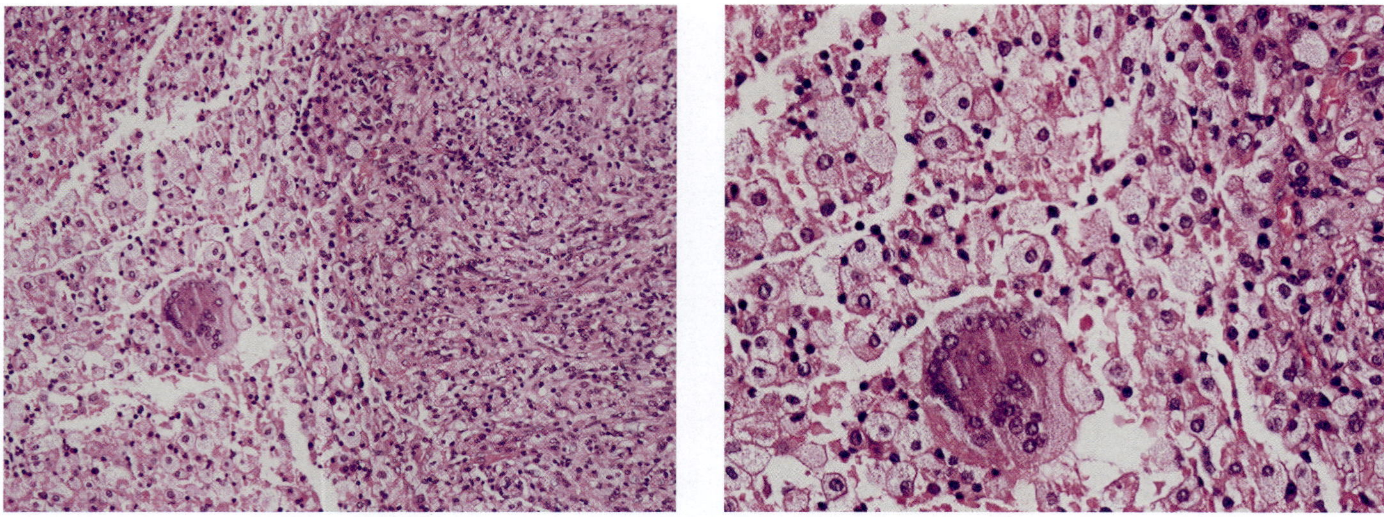

a ***b***

Figure 33-12.
XGPN containing a noncaseating granuloma (*a*) with many foamy macrophages and a multinucleated giant cell (*b*).

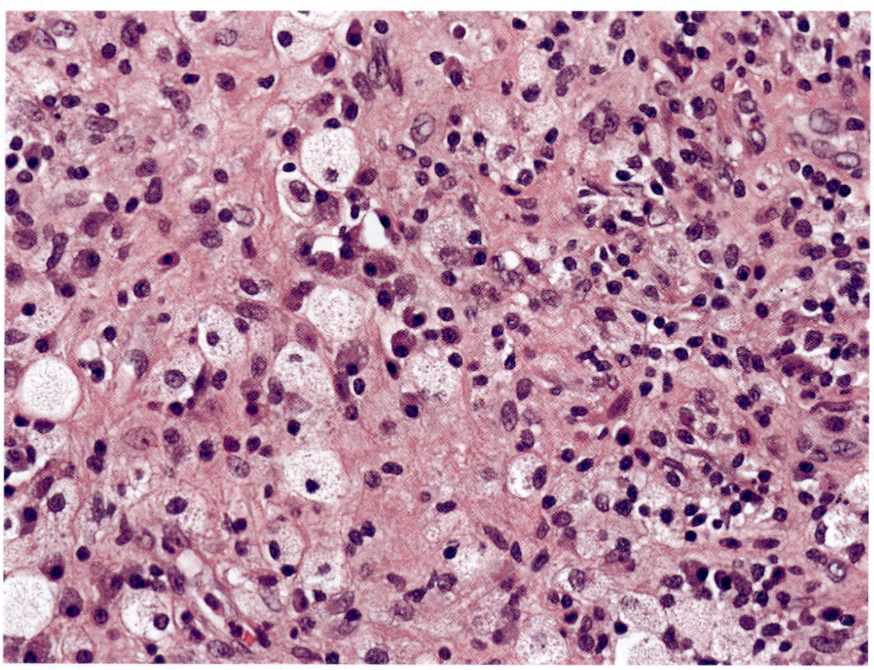

Figure 33-13.
XGPN is signified by the presence of numerous foamy macrophages along with other inflammatory cells.

Immunohistochemistry

- Macrophages are CD68 positive
- They are negative for epithelial markers and keratins
- Other renal cell carcinoma markers are negative

Differential diagnosis

- The renal inflammatory lesions other than inflammation of the glomeruli are listed in Table 33-1

Clinical relevance (prognosis and treatment options)

- If the lesions are persistent and medical treatment has failed to relieve the obstruction symptoms, nephrectomy is necessary
- When clinical suspicion for malignancy is high, nephrectomy can be considered

Table 33-1. Inflammatory Lesions of the Kidney

Lesions	*Causes*	*Inflammatory cells type and location*	*Associated conditions*
Acute interstitial nephritis	Mostly induced by drugs	Predominantly neutrophils Renal interstitial location	Many eosinophils
Chronic interstitial nephritis	Many causes	Predominantly lymphocytes mixed with plasma cells and other inflammatory cells Renal interstitial location	
Ascending acute pyelonephritis	Infection from low track	Suppurative inflammation Centered around renal pelvis and papilla	Abscesses
Hematogenous acute pyelonephritis	Infection from sepsis	Suppurative inflammation Centered around interstitial parenchyma	Abscesses
Chronic obstructive pyelonephritis	Obstruction by stones or tumor	Mixed chronic inflammatory cells Renal pelvis and interstitium	Calculi and hydronephrosis
Chronic nonobstructive pyelonephritis	Mostly related to reflux	Mixed chronic inflammation cells Renal pelvis and interstitium	Scar and distortion of renal pelvis and calyces
Xanthogranulomatous Pyelonephritis	Any causes to tissue necrosis	Granulomatous inflammation with foamy macrophages	Calculi or hydronephrosis may be present

END-STAGE RENAL DISEASE

Definition

- Complete failure of kidney function resulting from progressive chronic kidney diseases of any etiology

Other term

- End-stage kidney disease

Pathogenesis

- Any renal disease that leads to a significant loss of functional nephrons
- The most common causes of end-stage renal disease (ESRD) in the United States are diabetes and hypertension (see Chapter 32)
- Many other chronic renal diseases that may lead to ESRD include glomerular diseases, pyelonephritis, papillary necrosis, polycystic kidney disease, amyloidosis, and transplant chronic rejection

Clinical features

- General ill feeling, fatigue, and headaches
- Weight loss, loss of appetite, and nausea
- Pruritus and edema, most prominent in the extremities
- Low urine production

Gross pathology

- The kidney is small and atrophic (Figs. 33-14 and 33-15*a*)
- Except in adult polycystic kidney disease in which the kidney is massively enlarged
- Acquired cystic disease is a common finding in ESRD and characterized by the presence of multiple cysts

Histology

- Common features present in all ESRD cases (Figs. 33-15 to 33-18)
  - Glomerulosclerosis
  - Thyroidization of renal tubules
  - Chronic interstitial inflammation
  - Calcium oxalate crystals may be seen (Fig. 33-19)
- Specific pathological changes related to a different etiology may be recognized, but in many cases, they are not identifiable
- Diabetic nephropathy: Wilson bodies in glomeruli
- Hypertensive nephropathy: hyalinization of small arteries
- Chronic pyelonephritis: chronic inflammatory cell infiltrates in the renal pelvis

Immunohistochemistry

- Variable

Clinical relevance (prognosis and treatment options)

- ESRD with renal failure may lead to death without proper treatment
- ESRD requires dialysis or renal transplant
- Long-term dialysis may be associated with complications such as renal cell carcinoma
- Renal transplants may be associated with complications such as renal rejections, infection, malignancy, or graft-versus-host disease

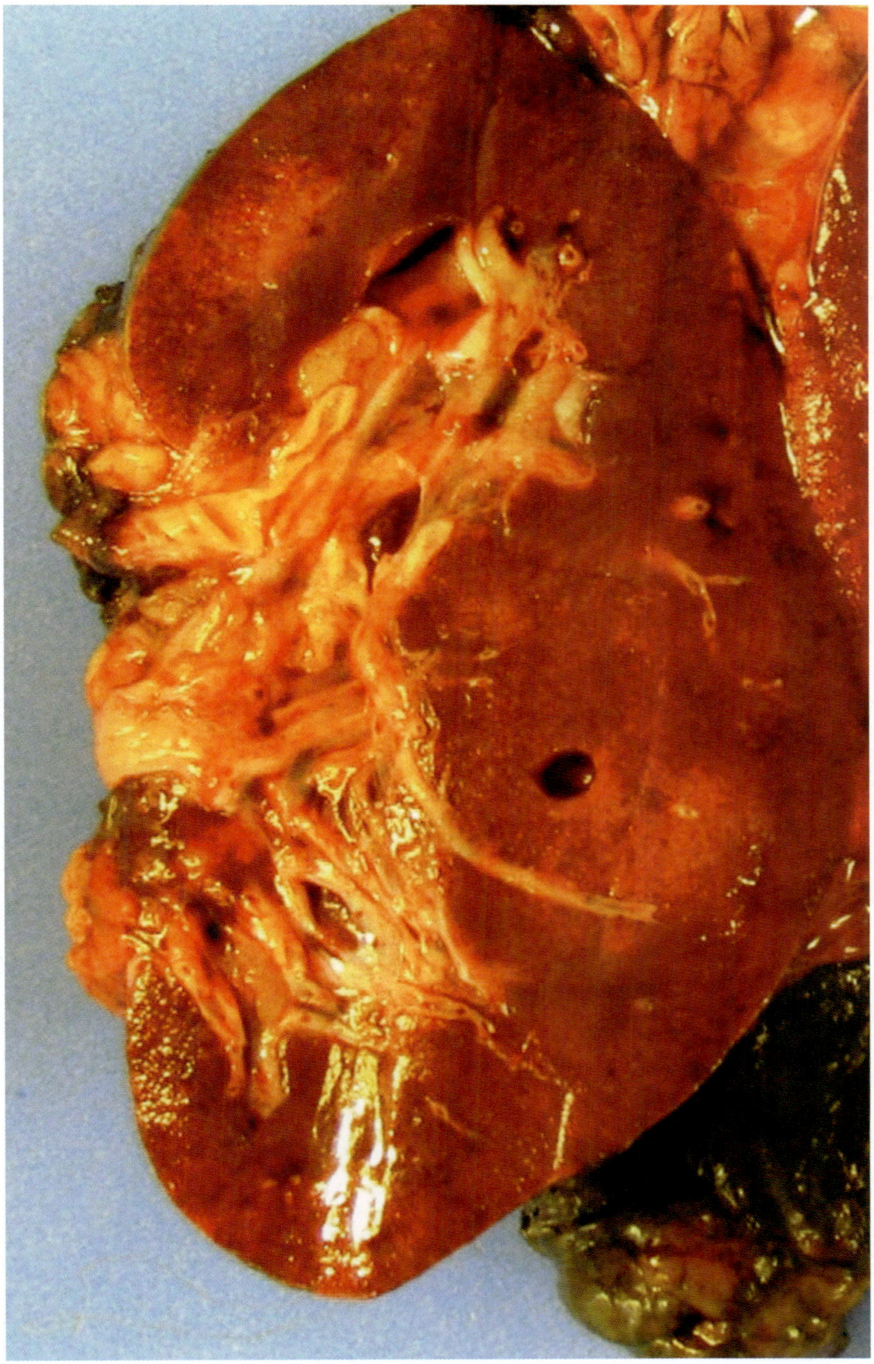

Figure 33-14.
Gross photo of end-stage renal disease (ESRD) displays relatively increased renal hilar tissue due to the reduced renal parenchyma.

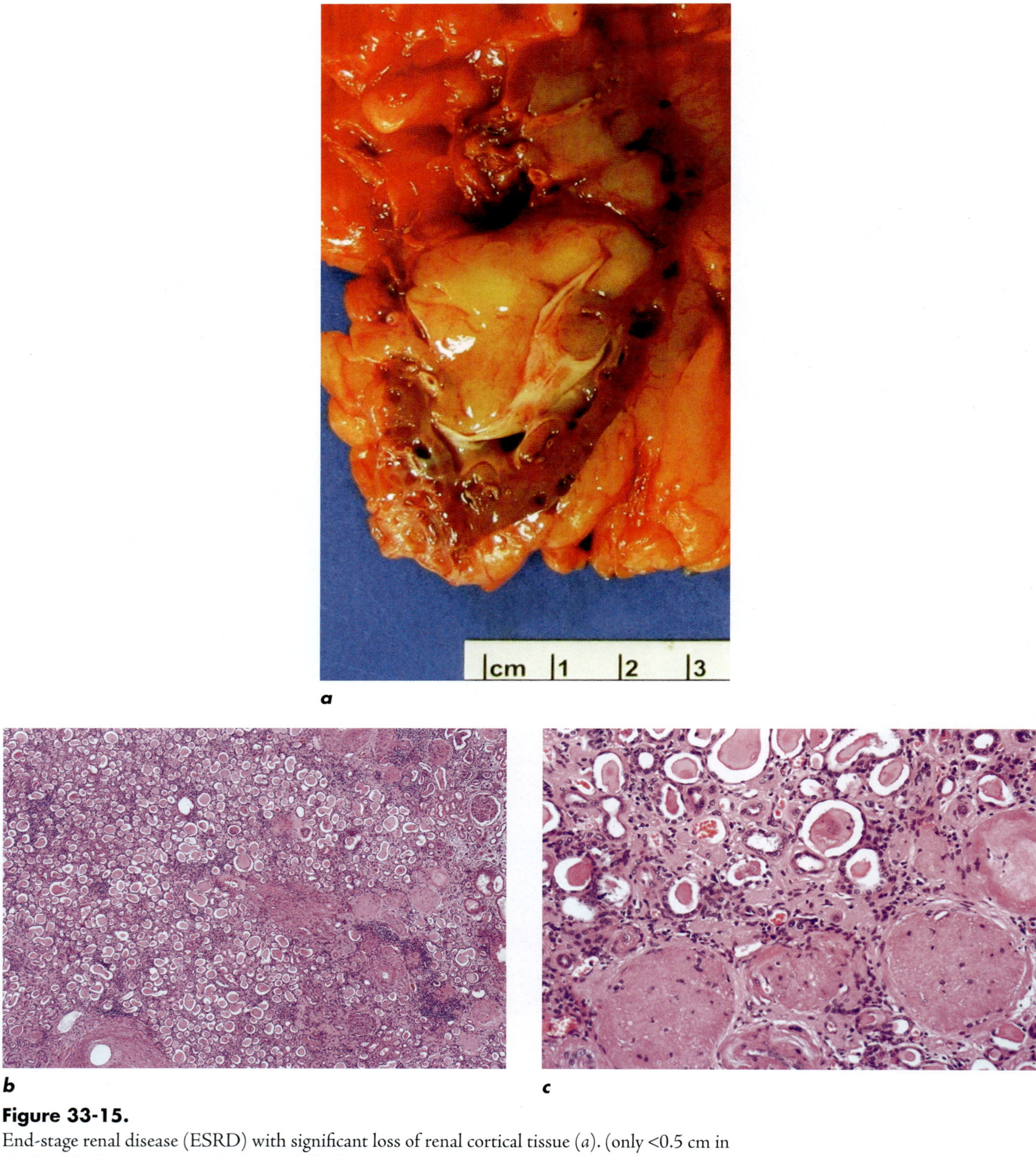

Figure 33-15.
End-stage renal disease (ESRD) with significant loss of renal cortical tissue (*a*). (only <0.5 cm in thickness). The microscopic findings of ESRD include tubular thyroidization, chronic interstitial inflammation (*b*), and glomerulosclerosis (*c*).

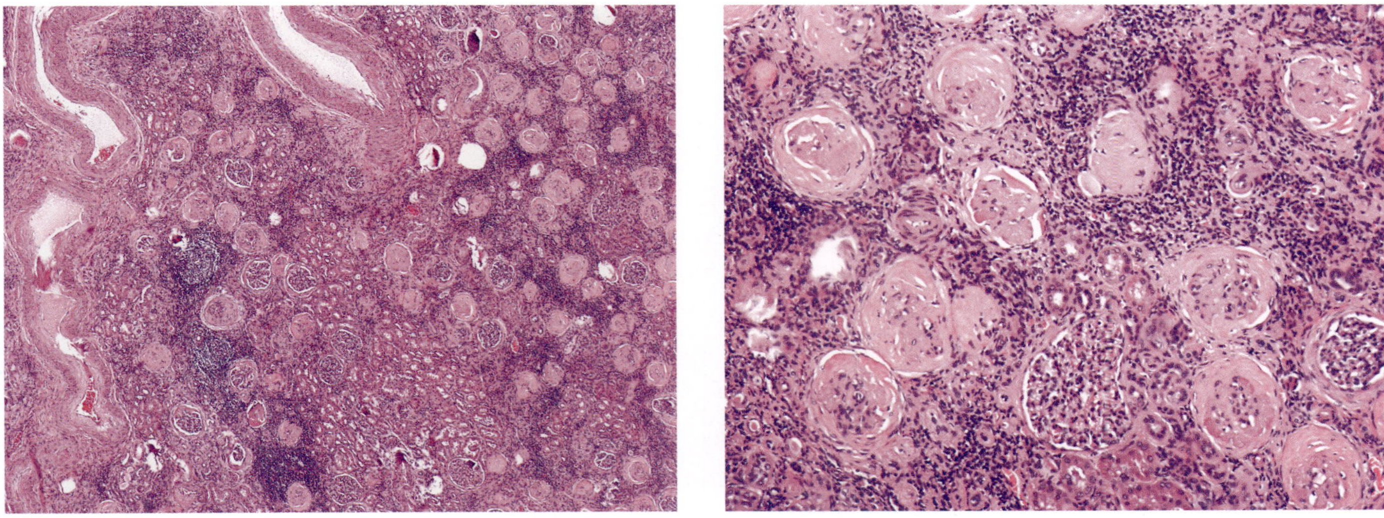

a b

Figure 33-16.
ESRD with extensive glomerulosclerosis (*a*). High magnification shows the presence of hyalinized glomeruli and interstitial lymphocytic infiltrate (*b*).

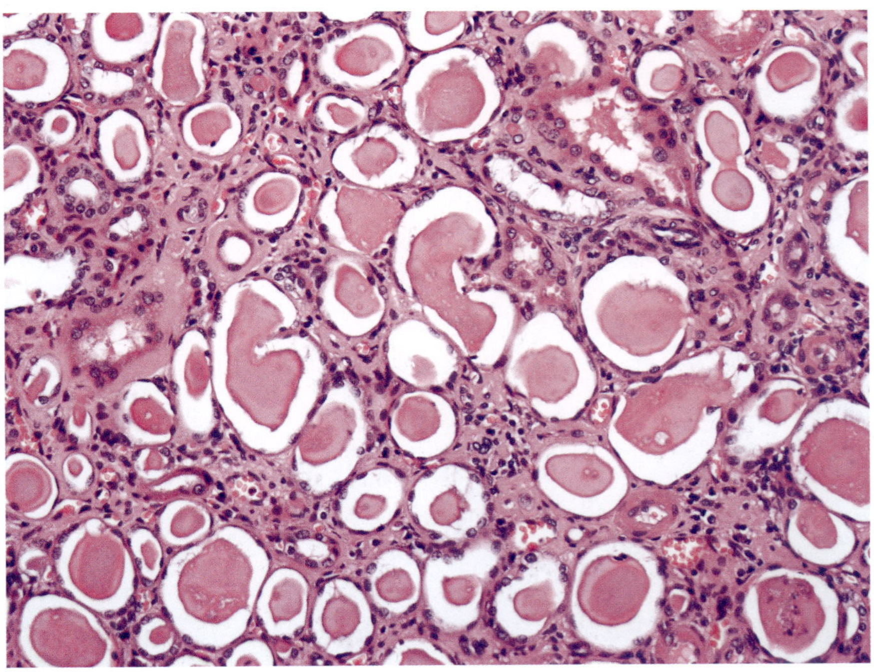

Figure 33-17.
Extensive thyroidization in ESRD is characterized by dilated tubules filled with pink secretion.

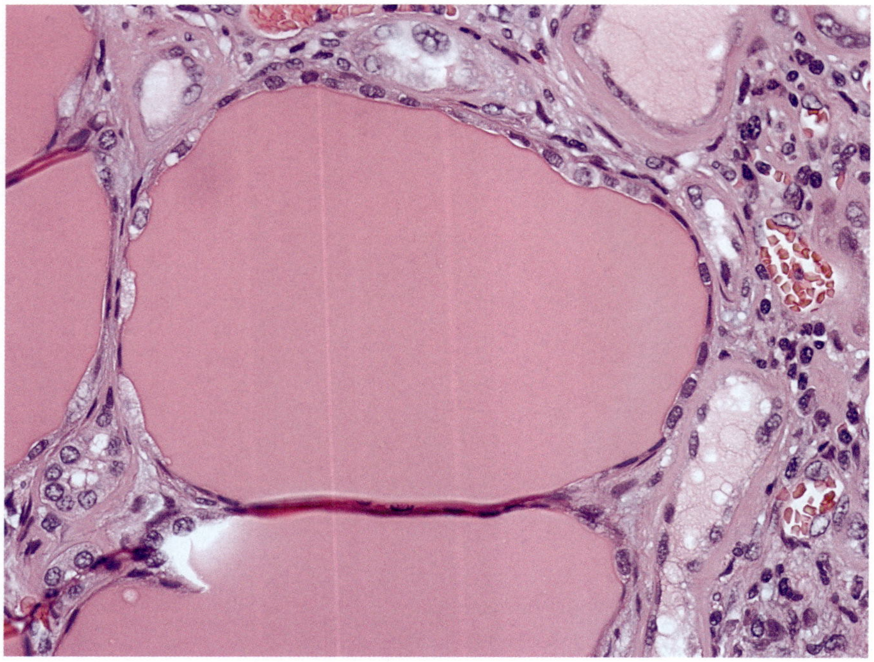

Figure 33-18.
EDRD with high magnification showing eosinophilic material in the tubules lined by flat epithelium, resembling thyroid follicles.

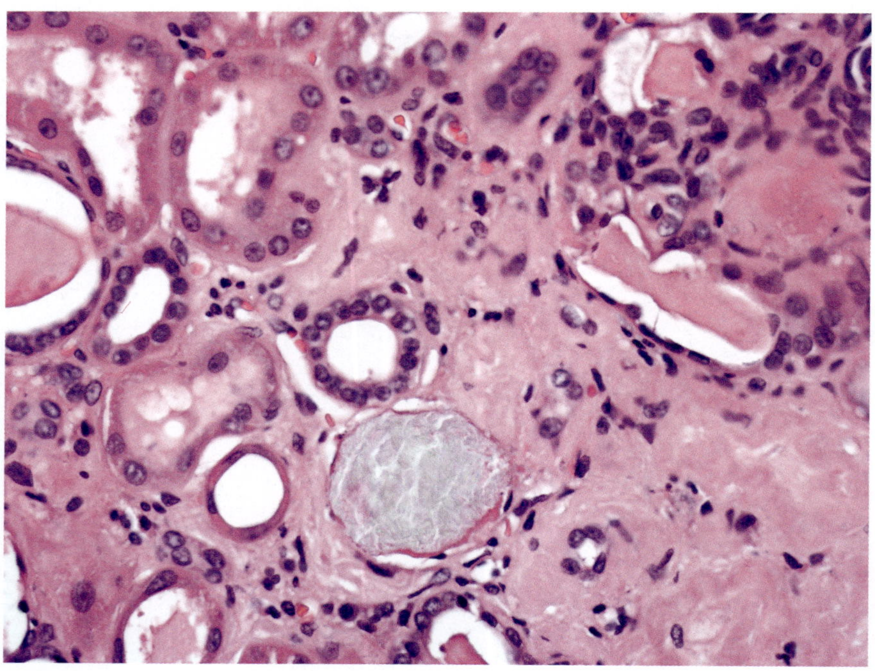

Figure 33-19.
The presence of calcium oxalate crystals in the renal parenchyma in ESRD.

ADRENAL REST IN THE KIDNEY

Definition

- An island of adrenal tissue (typically only cortical tissue) found in the kidney
- Adrenal rest can also be found in retroperitoneal tissues and genital organs such as testis, spermatic cord

Other terms

- Accessory adrenal, ectopic adrenal
- Adrenal heterotopia

Pathogenesis

- Adrenal tissue remnant left in the kidney during early development. It may regress or persist in adults

Clinical features

- Incidental finding, not associated with specific symptoms or signs
- Rare condition, more commonly seen in pediatric population

Gross pathology

- Small yellow nodules in millimeters in diameter in the kidney parenchyma or perirenal tissue

Histology

- A well-circumscribed cluster (without capsule) of adrenal cortical cells in the renal parenchyma (Fig. 33-20)
- The adrenal cortical cells have round nuclei and foamy or vesicular cytoplasm (Fig. 33-20*b*)
- Adrenal medullary tissue is rarely present

Figure 33-20.
Adrenal rest in the kidney is characterized by clusters of cortical cells with foamy cytoplasm in the renal parenchyma (*a*). High magnification shows the foamy cytoplasm of the cortical cells (*b*).

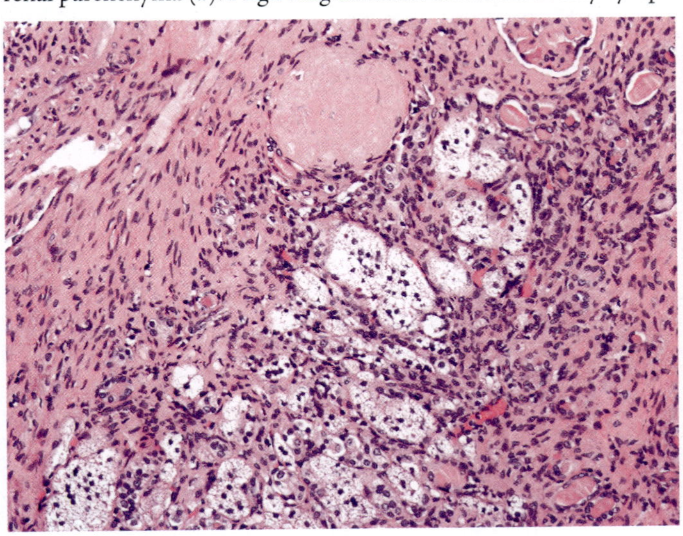

a

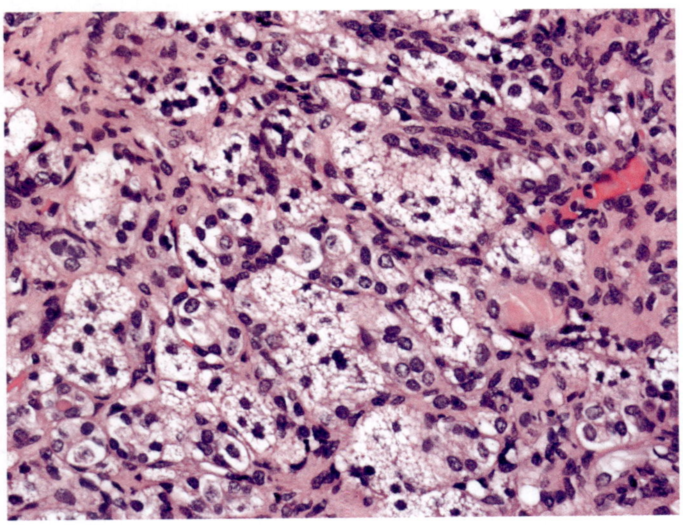

b

Immunohistochemistry

- Inhibin positive (Fig. 33-21), chromogranin may be positive
- Keratin negative and renal markers (such as Pax8) negative

Differential diagnosis

- *Macrophages accumulation* such as in XGPN, macrophages positive for CD68 or CD138, negative for inhibin
- *Clear cell RCC* is a mass lesion composed of malignant epithelial cells with clear cytoplasm that are positive for RCC markers, negative for inhibin

Clinical relevance (prognosis and treatment options)

- The adrenal rest is typically small and an incidental finding, with no clinical significance
- No specific treatment is necessary
- Extremely rare cases of adrenal cortical hyperplasia, cortical adenoma, or even cortical carcinoma may arise in the adrenal rest of the kidney
- It should not be misdiagnosed as clear cell RCC or macrophages especially when present in biopsy specimens

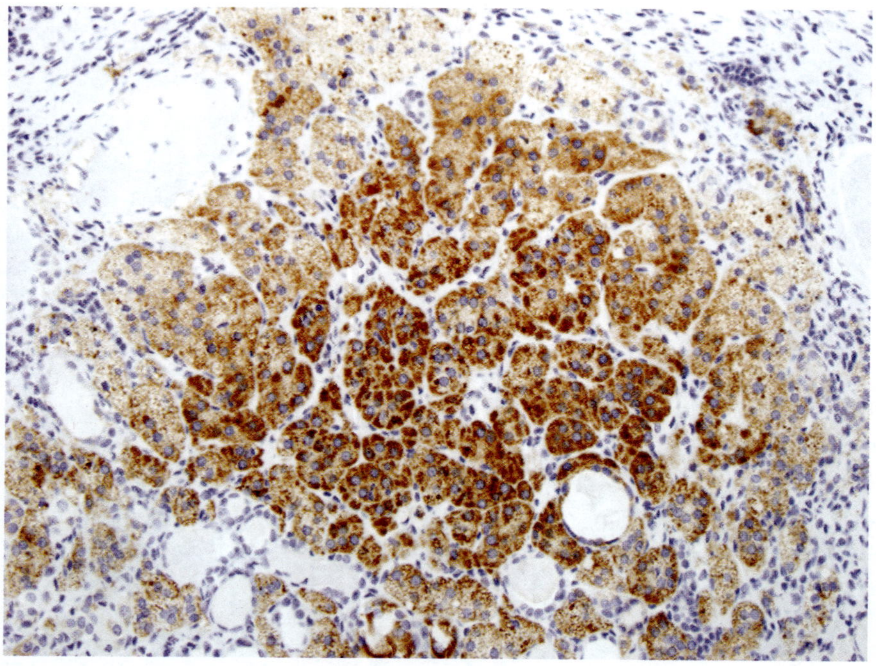

Figure 33-21.
Adrenal rest cells are positive for inhibin.

CLEAR CELL CHANGES IN THE KIDNEY

Definition

- Small clusters of abnormal epithelial cells present in the renal parenchyma with morphological features similar to low-grade clear cell RCC

Pathogenesis

- Unknown
- Because of their similarity to clear cell RCC in morphology and immunohistochemistry, clear cell changes may be one of the precursor lesions of clear cell RCC

Clinical features

- Incidental findings in partial or radical nephrectomy specimens
- Occasionally seen in renal core biopsies for medical renal disease or mass lesions

Gross pathology

- Typically less than 1 mm in size, not visible grossly
- If grossly identifiable, it would be considered clear cell RCC

Histology

- Small clusters, single or multiple, of abnormal epithelial cells forming nests or irregular tubular structures present in the cortex (Figs. 33-22 and 33-23)
- The lesional cells intermingled with renal tubules
- The cytoplasm is clear and abundant similar to that of clear cell RCC (Fig. 33-23)
- There is no nuclear atypia and nucleoli are difficult to identify (Fig. 33-24)

Immunohistochemistry

- Keratin markers such as AE1/AE3 or CK7 may be positive
- CA9 positive or negative

Differential diagnosis

- It should be distinguished from adrenal rests (cortical cells positive for inhibin)

Clinical relevance (prognosis and treatment options)

- Uncertain
- However, the clear cell changes of the kidney as a microscopic finding does not justify any radical treatment
- If the lesion is greater than 0.2 to 0.3 mm in diameter, it should be considered small clear cell RCC although the cutoff value has not been established
- The patients, with clear cell changes found in biopsy with a mass lesion, need to be followed and monitored for the potential risk of development of clear cell RCC

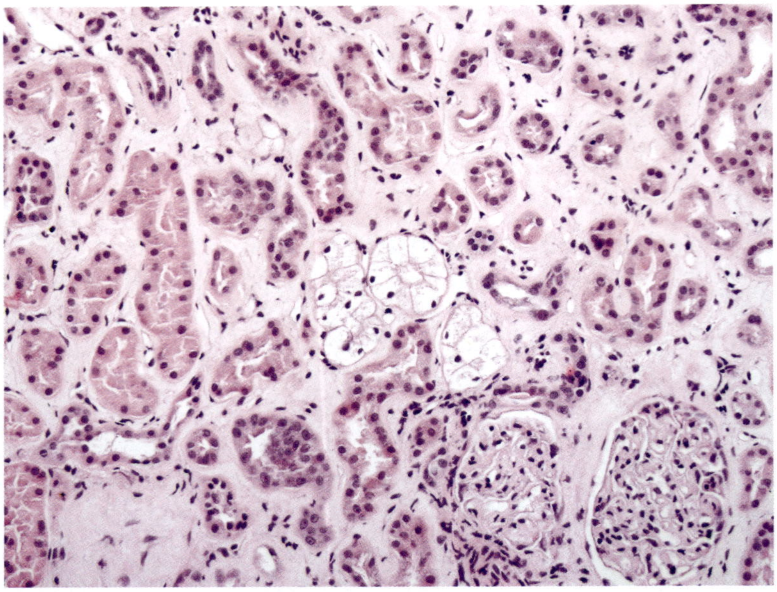

Figure 33-22.
Several small clusters of epithelial cells with clear cytoplasm, distinct from either proximal or distal convoluted tubules.

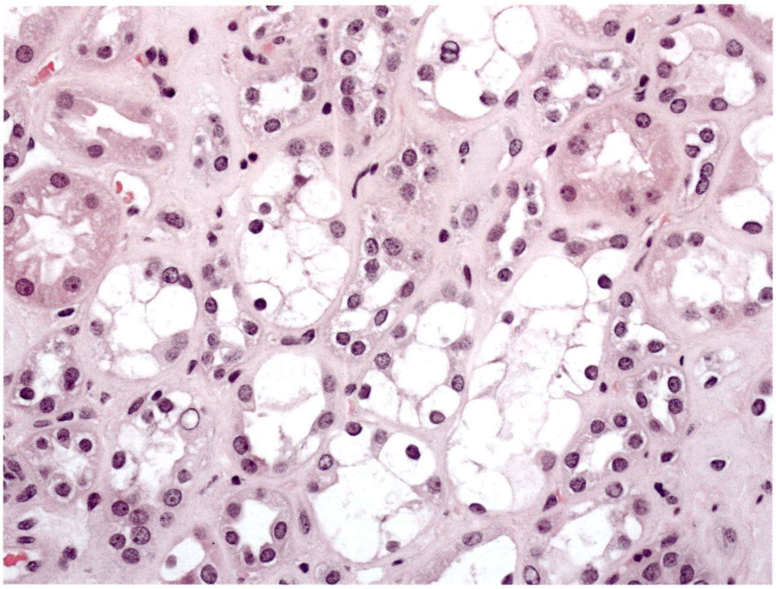

Figure 33-23.
A large focus of epithelial cells with clear cytoplasm. Some of the clear cells are forming glandular or acinar patterns.

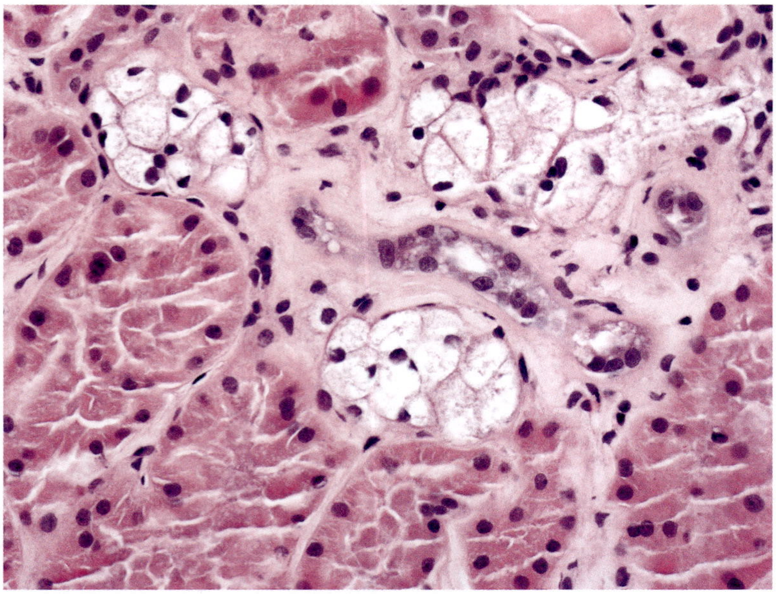

Figure 33-24.
Several small clusters of solid clear cells with subtle glandular formation.

KIDNEY TRAUMA

Definition

- Severe renal injury caused by physical forces
- The common causes include automobile accident, blunt objects such as sport injuries, or penetration wound by sharp objects or bullets (gunshot wound)

Clinical features

- The patient with a history of injury
- Flank pain with or without hematuria

Gross pathology

- The renal capsule can be ruptured (Fig. 33-25)
- Laceration or defects of kidney parenchyma to a different degree
- The lacerated renal tissue with reactive (red) edges (Fig. 33-25)
- Hemorrhage and possible tissue necrosis
- Gross examination and diagnosis is very important, because microscopic examination cannot determine the extent of the damage

Histology

- Rupture of renal capsule (Fig. 33-26)
- Areas of tissue defect, necrosis and hemorrhage (Fig. 33-27)
- Acute inflammatory cell reaction can be seen in an early phase
- Repair changes and fibrosis in the late phase

Clinical relevance (prognosis and treatment options)

- A minor injury to the kidney can stop spontaneously by blood coagulation
- A major injury to the kidney will result in severe bleeding and hemoperitoneum
- In addition, acute peritonitis can be present because of leaking urine to the peritoneal cavity
- The severe trauma to the kidney is a medical emergency and requires prompt surgical repair or nephrectomy

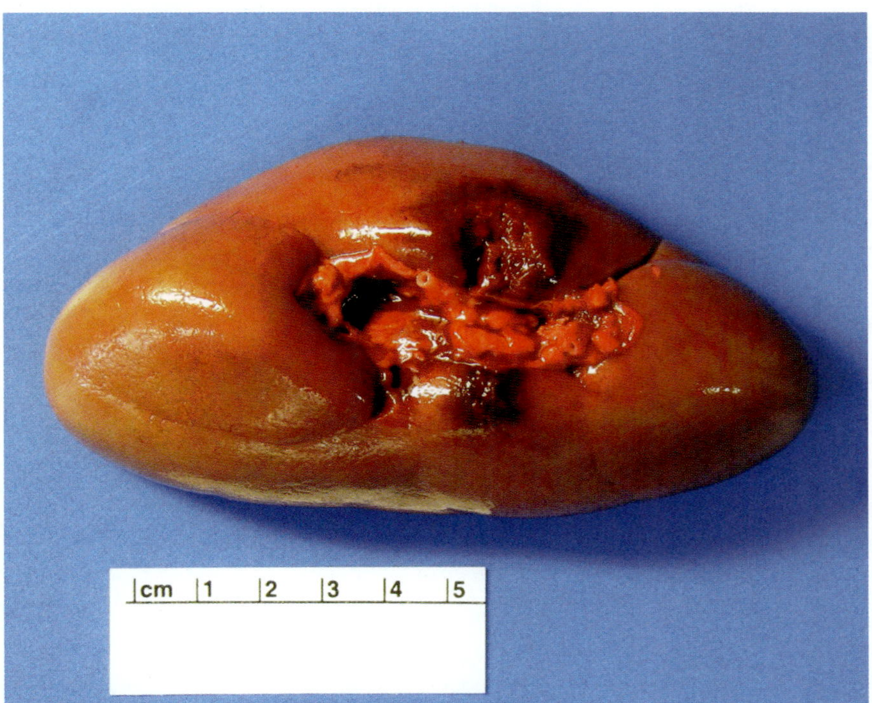

Figure 33-25.
Gross photo of lacerated kidney (gunshot wound) with hemorrhage around the defected areas.

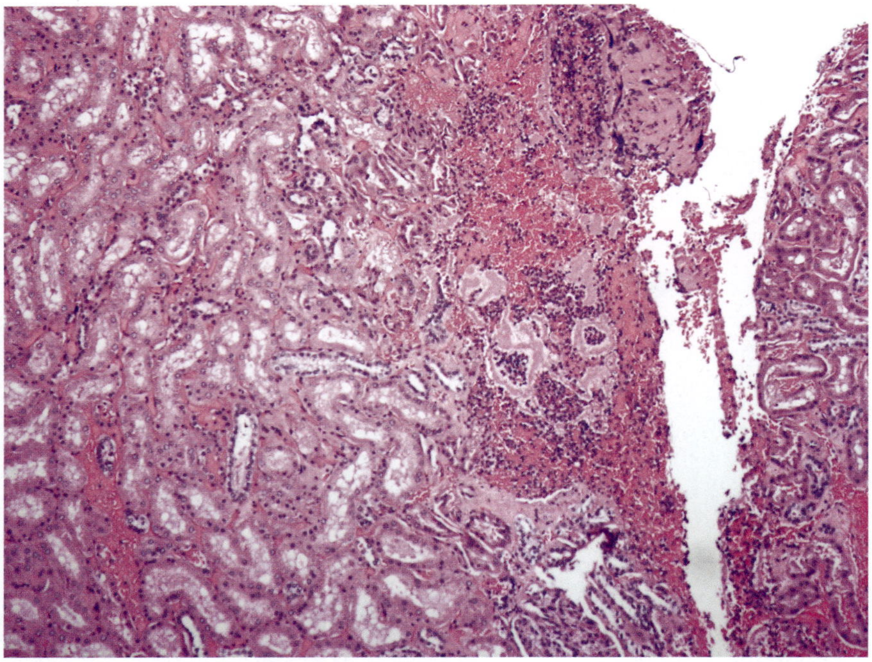

Figure 33-26.
Microscopically, the defect caused by a penetrating bullet is surrounded by necrotic tissue and hemorrhage.

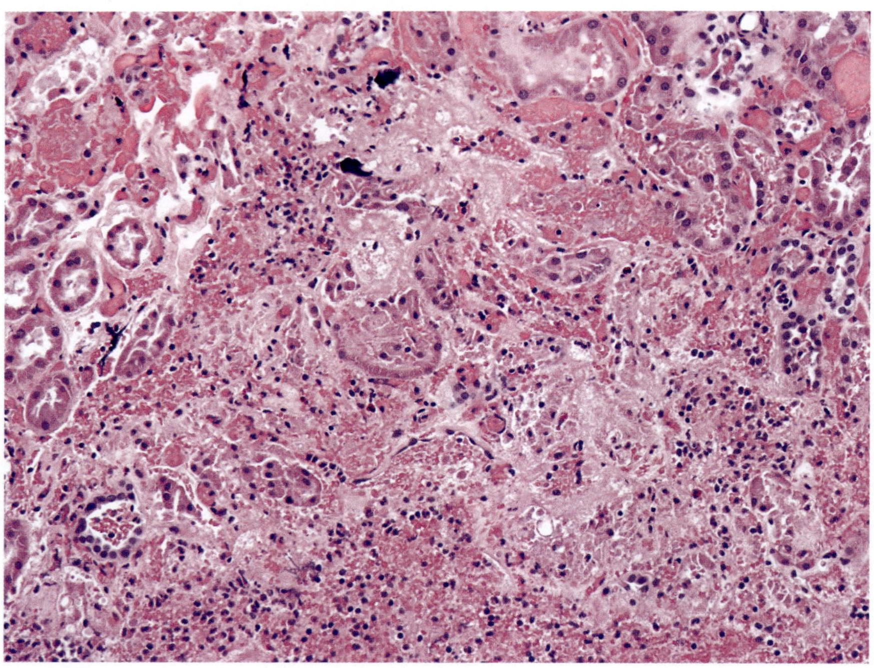

Figure 33-27.
The renal tissue adjacent to the defect displays the tubular necrosis, hemorrhage, and acute inflammatory cell reaction.

CHAPTER 34 Benign Cystic Lesions of the Kidney

Bing Zhu, Ximing J. Yang, Pauline M. Chou

SIMPLE CORTICAL CYST

Definition

- An acquired singular cystic lesion in the kidney lined by a single layer of epithelium similar to the lining of a renal tubule

Pathogenesis and epidemiology

- Probably originated from dilation or diverticulum of the renal tubule
- Very common conditions, present in 30% to 40% of individuals older than 50 years

Clinical features

- Asymptomatic
- Found incidentally by image studies or in nephrectomy specimens for other lesions
- In radiology, the Bosniak classification is based on the complexity of the cyst to predicate the malignant potentials

Gross pathology

- Typically unilocular (Fig. 34-1) or multiple nonfused cysts in the cortex
- Filled with clear fluid, smooth inner surface

Histology

- Cyst is lined by flat or low cuboidal epithelium with no cytological atypia (Fig. 34-2)
- Occasionally, inflammation, hemorrhage, fibrosis, and calcification may be seen

Differential diagnosis

- There are many benign and malignant cystic conditions in the kidney. Their main features are listed in Table 34-1 for differential diagnosis

Clinical relevance (prognosis and treatment options)

- Benign, no treatment necessary
- However, whether some of these simple cysts may develop into multilocular cystic renal cell carcinoma (RCC) or low-grade clear cell RCC is of question. Clinical and imaging follow-up may be necessary

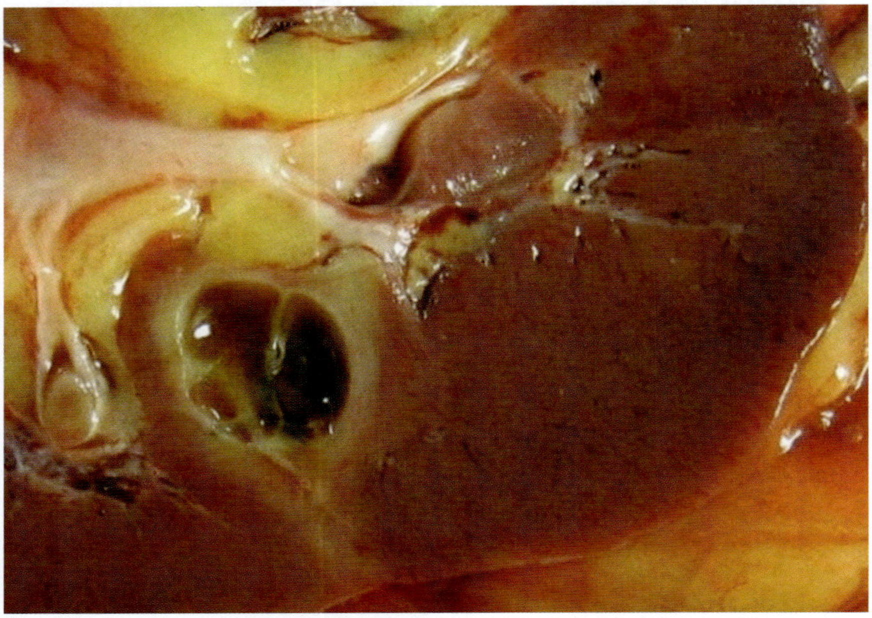

Figure 34-1.
Gross photo of a simple cortical cyst of the kidney.

Figure 34-2.
Microscopic appearance of a cortical cyst surrounded by normal appearing renal cortical tissue (*a*). High magnification shows the cyst lined by flat epithelium with scant cytoplasm (*b*).

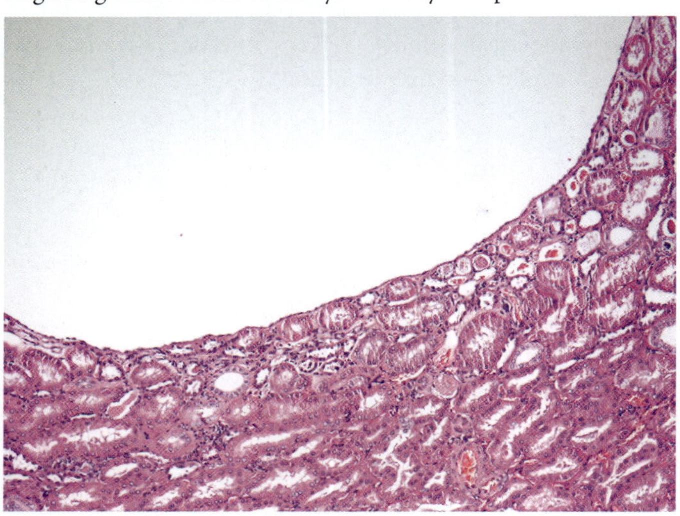

a

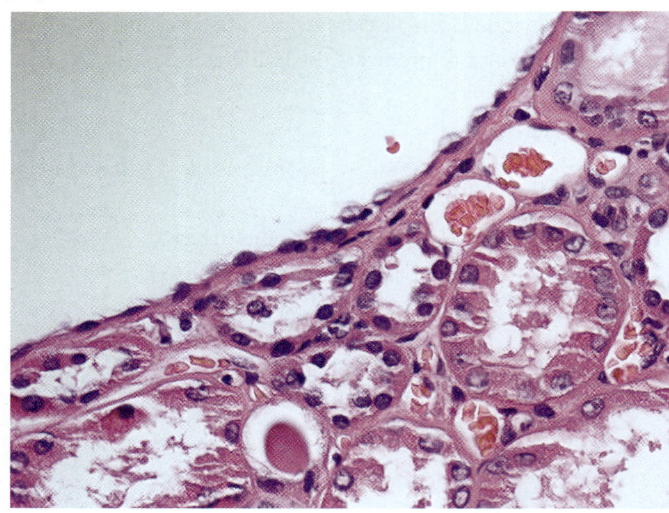

b

Table 34-1. Cystic Lesions of the Kidney

	Cyst distribution	*Nature of the cyst*	*Kidney size*	*Other features*
Benign				
Simple cortical cysts	Localized individual cyst	Reactive	Normal	
Autosomal dominant PKD	Diffusely involving kidney	Genetic disorder	Very large	Leading to renal failure
Autosomal recessive PKD	Diffuse	Genetic disorder	Normal or large	Many are lethal in infants
Medullary spongy kidney	Diffuse, medulla	Reactive or genetic disorder	Normal	Dilated collecting ducts
Acquired cystic kidney disease	Diffuse involving kidney	Reactive, high risk for carcinoma	Small, atrophic	Associated with high risk for RCC
Mixed epithelial and stromal tumor	Localized mass	Benign tumor	Normal	Ovarian stroma
Malignant				
Multilocular cystic RCC	Localized mass	Early malignant neoplasm	Small to medium	Very low-grade RCC
Tubulocystic carcinoma	Localized mass	Special type of malignant neoplasm	Small to medium	Low-grade RCC
RCC with cystic changes	Single or multiple masses	Degenerative changes in RCC	Small or large	Low- or high-grade clear cell RCC

PKD, polycystic kidney disease; RCC, renal cell carcinoma.

AUTOSOMAL DOMINANT POLYCYSTIC KIDNEY DISEASE

Definition

- An autosomal dominant renal disease characterized by numerous cysts diffusely involve the entire kidney
- It is a progressive disease with late onset

Other term

- Adult polycystic kidney disease

Pathogenesis

- Autosomal dominant polycystic kidney disease (PKD) associated with *PKD1* gene mutations (16q13.3) in the majority of cases, and *PKD2* gene (4q21-23) mutations in the minority of cases
- Incidence 1/4000 to 1/10,000 live births

Clinical features

- Most of the patients with a family history of PKD, presented in the fourth or fifth decade
- Hematuria or proteinuria
- Bilateral flank masses (massively enlarged kidneys) and flank pain
- Eventually develop renal failure
- Extrarenal manifestations include intracranial berry aneurysm, hypertension, heart valve abnormality, and colonic diverticulum
- Cysts in other organs such as liver or pancreas may occur

Gross pathology

- Bilateral diffuse renal enlargement, typically each kidney can weigh greater than 1 kg, which is 5 to 10 times bigger than a normal kidney (Fig. 34-3)
- Irregular external surface (Fig. 34-3) and cut surface showing numerous cysts ranging from a few millimeters to a few centimeters, intermingled with residual solid renal parenchyma (Fig. 34-4*a*)
- Cyst filled with clear or occasionally hemorrhagic fluid
- Presence of mass lesions is uncommon

Histology

- Numerous cysts separated by intervening renal parenchyma (Fig. 34-4*b*)
- Intervening renal tissue shows chronic interstitial inflammation, atrophic tubules, and glomerulosclerosis mixed with normal appearing glomeruli (Fig. 34-4*c*)
- Cysts lined by single-layer cuboidal or flat epithelium (Figs. 34-5 and 34-6)
- Focal papillary hyperplasia may be seen, typically less than 1 to 2 mm in diameter (Fig. 34-7*a*). The lining cells of papillary hyperplasia are bland, with scant eosinophilic cytoplasm. The nuclei are located close to the luminal surface (Fig. 34-7*b*)

Molecular analysis

- Mutations of *PKD1* (encoding polycystin 1) or *PKD2* (encoding polycystin 2)

Clinical relevance (prognosis and treatment options)

- Renal failure is irreversible for this condition, which will eventually lead to dialysis
- By 60 years, more than 50% will have renal failure (end-stage renal disease)
- Renal transplant is curative for autosomal dominant PKD

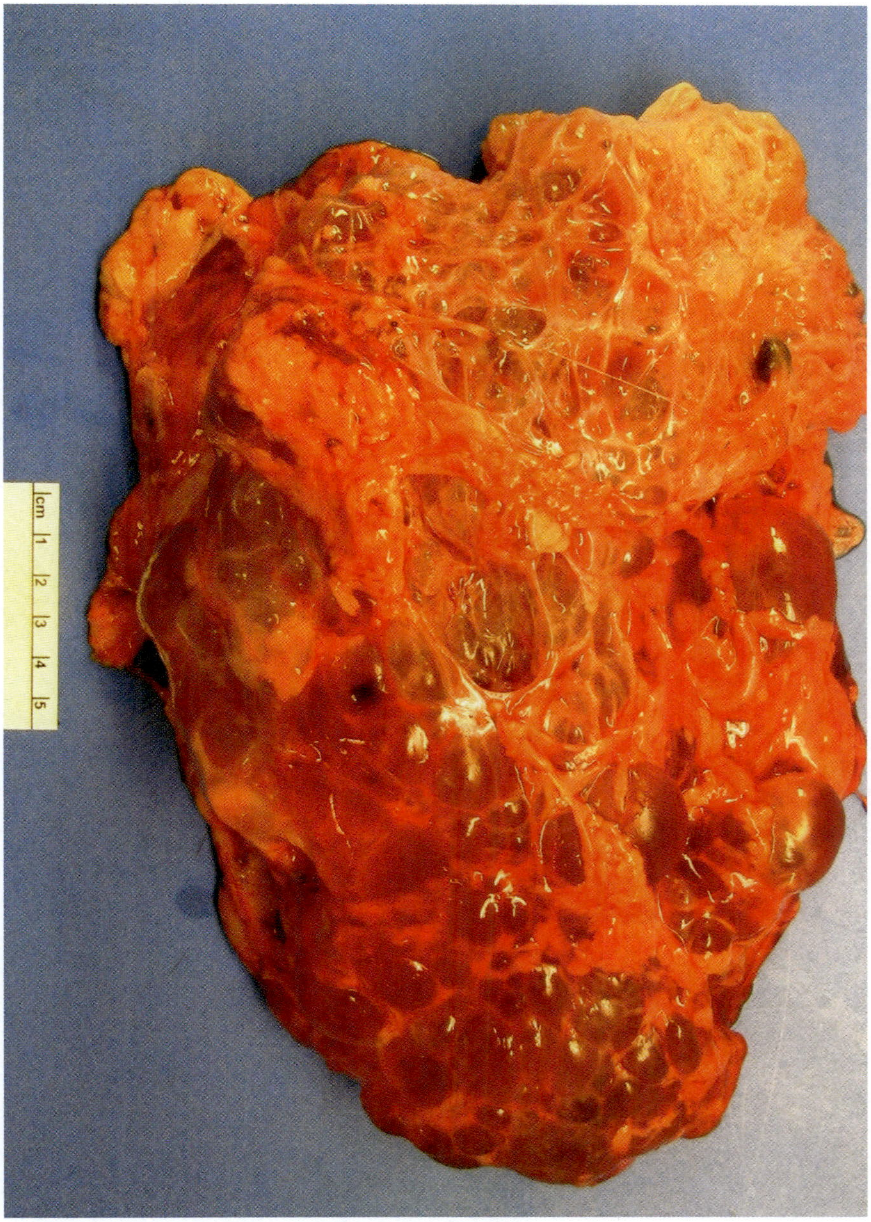

Figure 34-3.
Autosomal dominant polycystic kidney disease (PKD). The kidney, measuring 24 cm in the greatest dimension, is significantly increased in size. Multiple cysts can be seen bulging to the capsular surface of kidney.

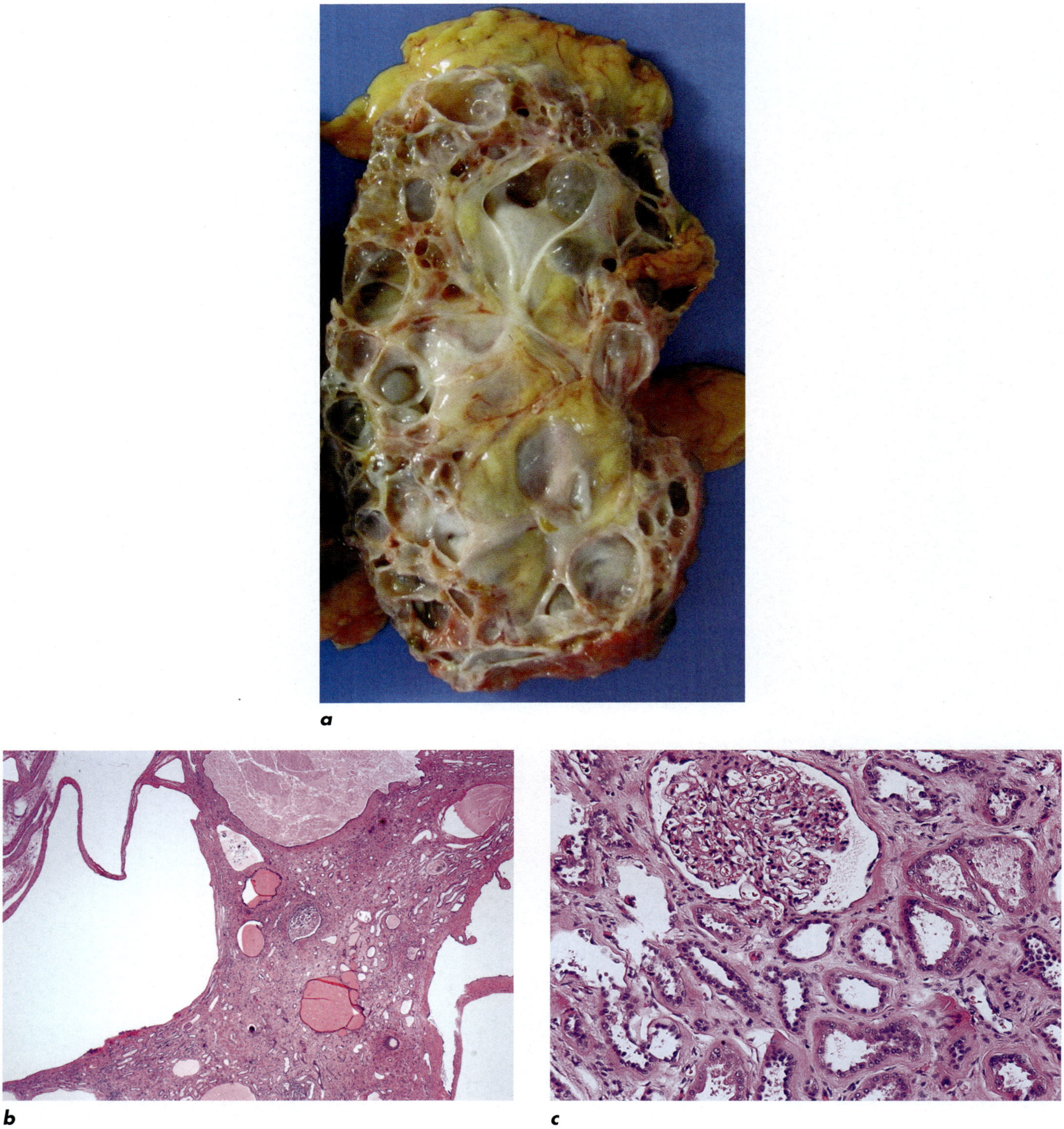

Figure 34-4.
Autosomal dominant PKD. Cut surface of a kidney shows multiple cysts throughout the enlarged kidney (*a*). Microscopically, it is characterized by dilated cysts with cystic septa containing residual renal parenchyma (*b*). The residual renal cortical tissue in the cystic septa appears to be normal (*c*).

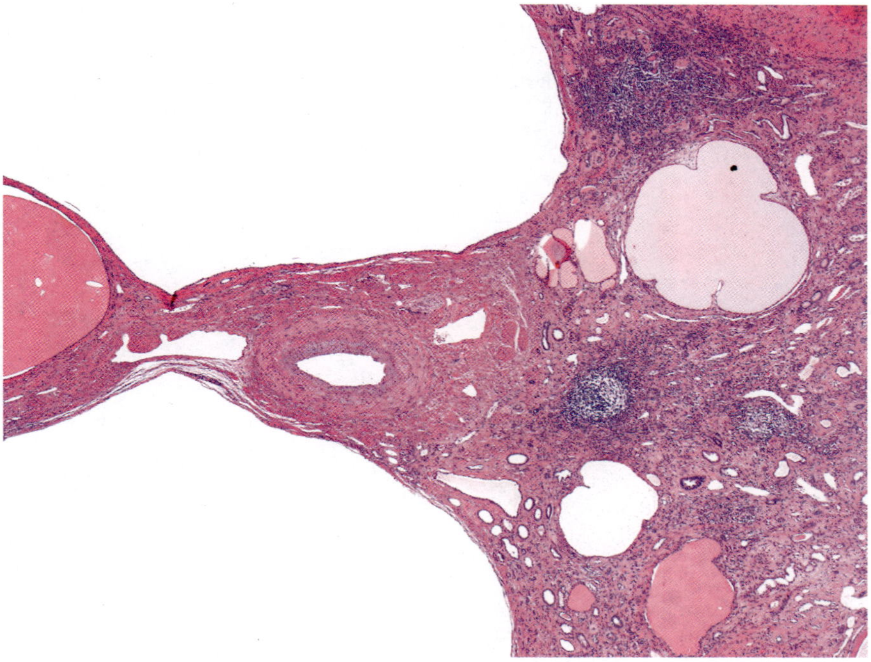

Figure 34-5.
Multiple cysts and septa containing atrophic renal tubules in autosomal dominant PKD.

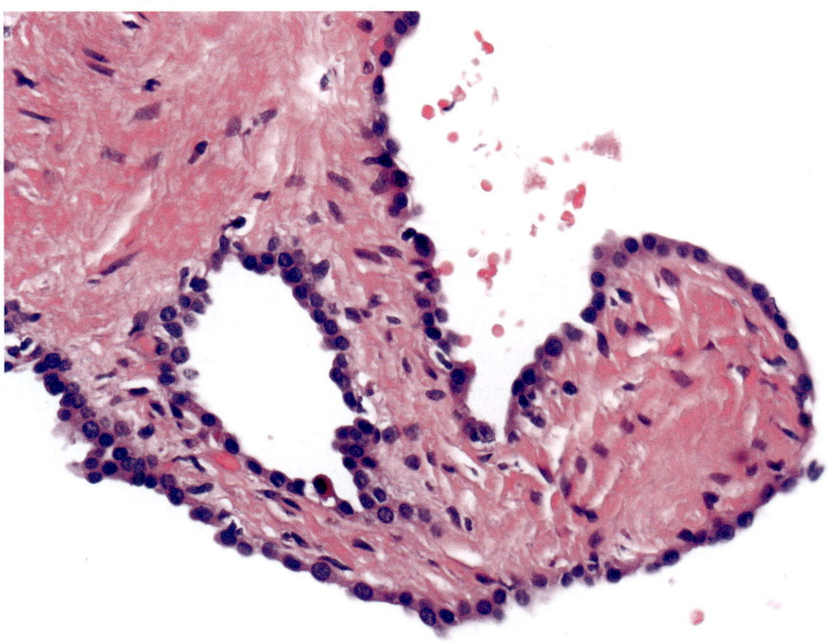

Figure 34-6.
The cystic lining epithelium of the autosomal dominant PKD is cuboidal.

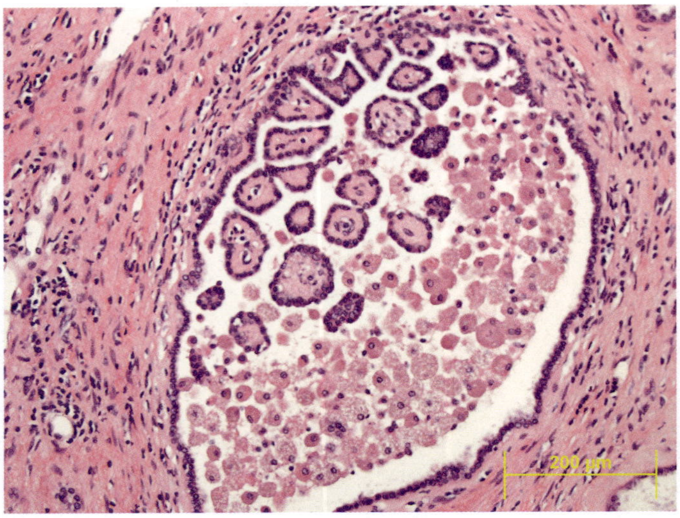

a

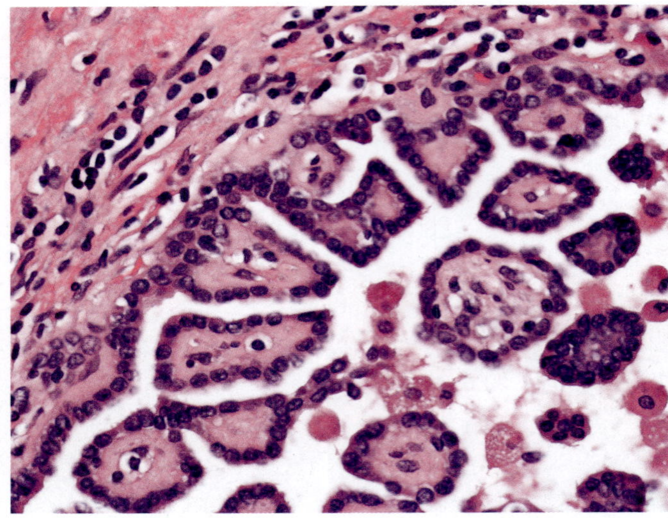

b

Figure 34-7.
Papillary hyperplasia in autosomal dominant PKD, measuring 1 to 2 mm each, is a common finding (*a*). High magnification shows the papillary hyperplasia composed of bland cuboidal cells with scant eosinophilic cytoplasm without cytological atypia (*b*).

AUTOSOMAL RECESSIVE POLYCYSTIC KIDNEY DISEASE

Definition

- A genetic kidney disorder characterized by early onset of polycystic changes
- Inherited in autosomal recessive fashion

Other terms

- Child polycystic kidney disease, infantile polycystic kidney disease

Pathogenesis

- The mutation of PKHD1 gene located on chromosome 6p21-23 is responsible for the disease

Clinical features

- Incidence 1/10,000 to 1/15,000
- Enlargement of bilateral kidneys
- Can be found in the third trimester or in the neonatal period

Gross pathology

- Massively enlargement of bilateral kidneys with a smooth external surface
- Cut surfaces show cystic change with "rays" appearance, in which cystic lines are perpendicular to the external surface (Fig. 34-8)
- Cysts involve both cortex and medulla and are relatively uniform in size

Histology

- Numerous cysts replacing the renal parenchyma (Figs. 34-9 and 34-10*a*)
- Cysts involving the cortex and medullar are radially arranged and oriented perpendicular to the renal capsule (Fig. 34-9)
- The cysts lined by single layer of uniform cuboidal cells of the collecting ducts (Fig. 34-10*b*) may contain proteinaceous secretions

Immunohistochemistry

- No specific findings reported

Molecular analysis

- The PKHD1 gene mutation can be detected in the majority of suspected cases prenatally

Clinical relevance (prognosis and treatment options)

- Fatal in the majority of cases (70% to 80%), either a stillborn or early neonatal death
- The cases that survive to the early childhood may develop renal failure
- Some cases are associated with hepatic fibrosis

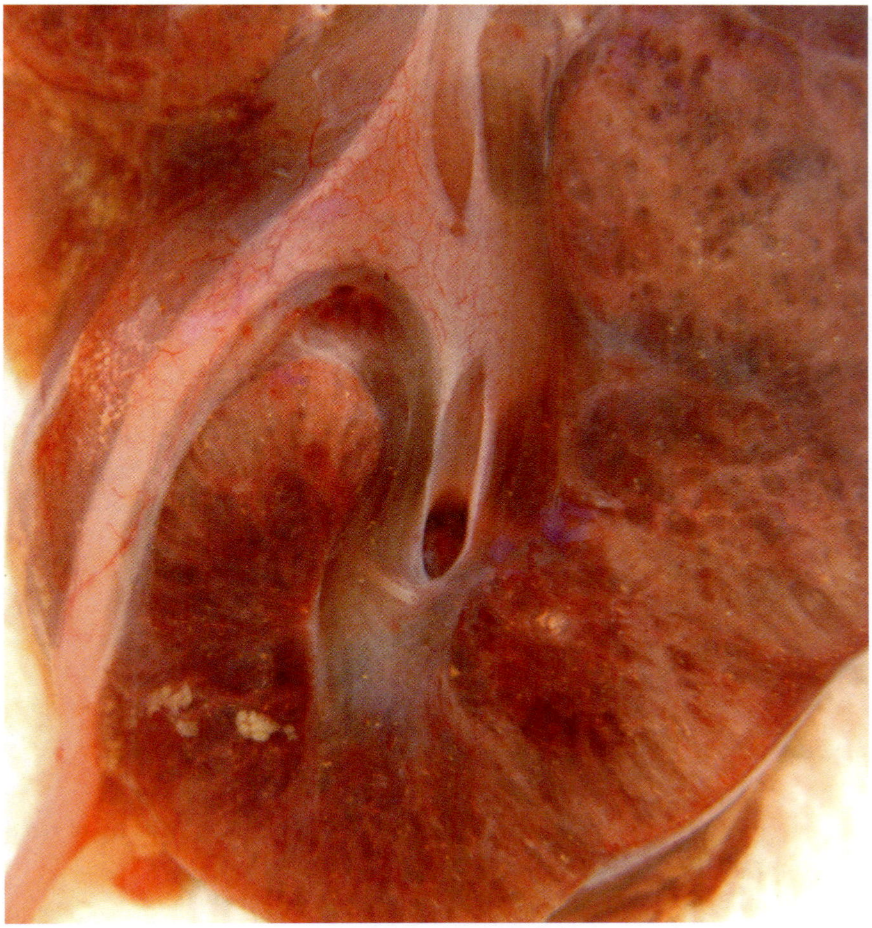

Figure 34-8.
Autosomal recessive polycystic kidney disease (PKD). There are rays in the cortex perpendicular to the renal capsule.

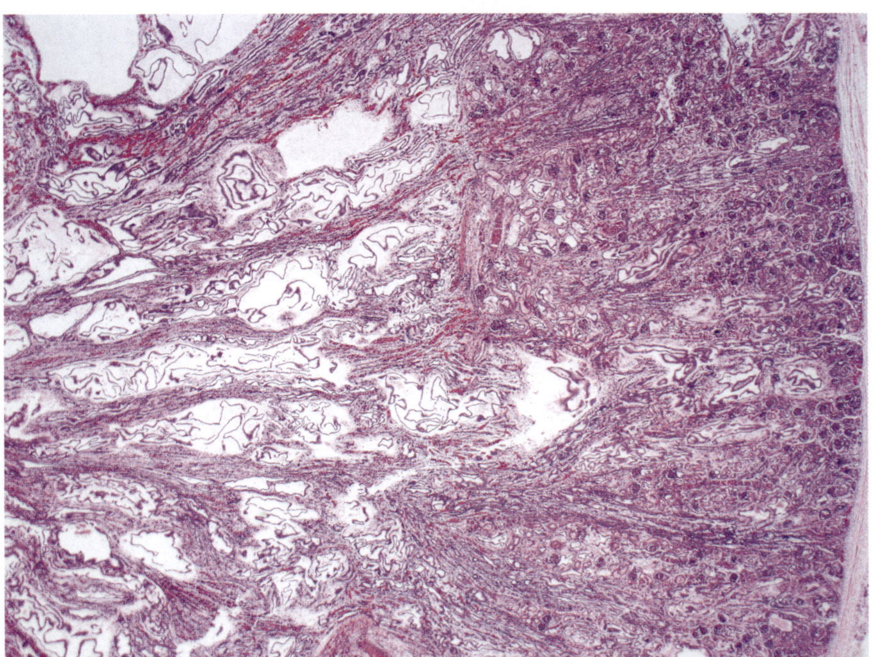

Figure 34-9.
The elongated cysts perpendicular to the renal capsule are responsible for the rays in autosomal recessive PKD.

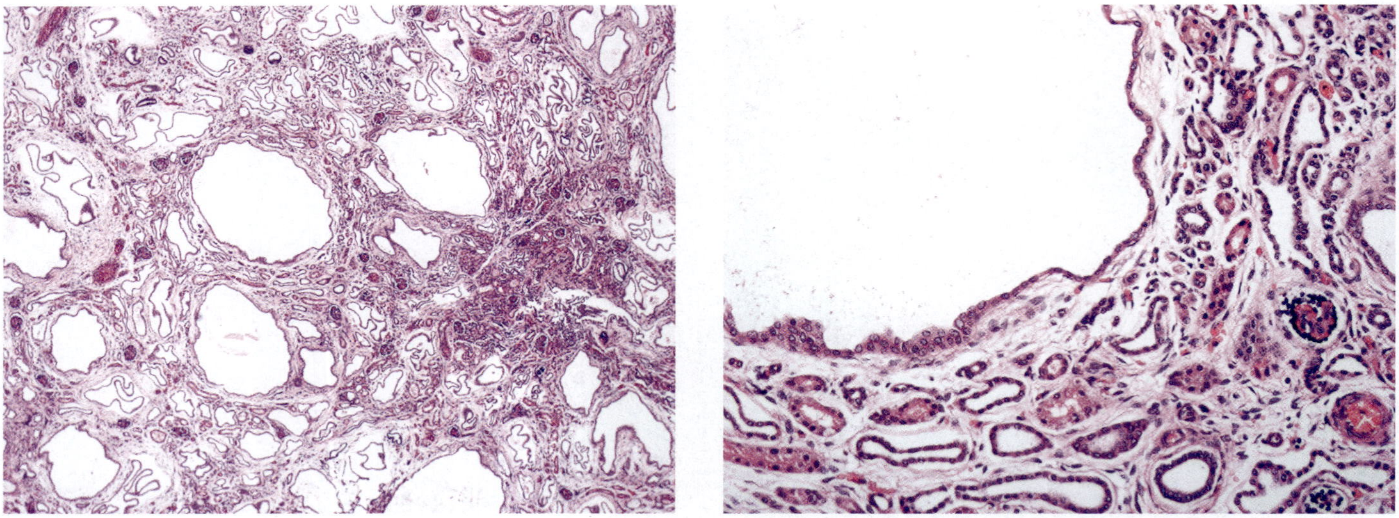

a *b*

Figure 34-10.
Autosomal recessive PKD contains dilated cysts (*a*), which are lined by flat or cuboidal epithelial cells similar to those of renal distal tubules. Several immature glomeruli are also seen (*b*).

MEDULLARY SPONGE KIDNEY

Definition

- Cystic disease characterized by bilateral cystic dilations of medullary collecting ducts, which give the renal medulla a sponge-like appearance; normal cortex

Pathogenesis

- With no evidence of genetic transmission

Clinical features

- One per 5000 births; no gender preference; not familial
- Symptom start between fourth and fifth decades
- Associated with hemihypertrophy of body (25% of cases), Marfan, Caroli, or Ehlers-Danlos syndrome
- Bilateral in 80% cases
- The condition is complicated by nephrolithiasis, infection, hematuria, and hypercalcemia

Gross pathology

- Involved kidney usually normal in size
- Multiple small cysts (1 to 5 mm) involving the tip of renal papillae
- Microcalculi in the dilated collecting ducts

Histology

- Dilated collecting ducts lined with cuboidal or flattened epithelium
- The cysts usually communicate with collecting tubules

Clinical relevance (prognosis and treatment options)

- Treatment focuses on complications

ACQUIRED CYSTIC KIDNEY DISEASE

Definition

- Bilateral and multiple cysts developing in the kidney with chronic renal failure
- This condition is not directly related to polycystic kidney disease or the genetic disorders of the kidney

Pathogenesis

- Acquired cystic kidney disease (ACKD) develops in patients with renal failure or on dialysis at a very high frequency
- Various nongenetic renal diseases can lead to renal failure and ACKD

Clinical features

- Most ACKD patients received dialysis for end-stage renal disease
- Early lesions are asymptomatic, detected by imaging studies
- Symptoms in the late phase ACKD may be related to secondary hemorrhage and infection
- Signs of renal failure such as increase of B-type natriuretic peptide and creatinine
- Risk of developing RCC (renal masses) increases

Gross pathology

- Bilateral renal involvement with a moderate increase or decrease in the kidney size. Renal distortion can be seen because of the presence of cysts (Fig. 34-11)
- Cut surface showing multiple cysts of variable sizes, involving cortex and/or medulla (Fig. 34-12*a*)
- Solid areas and occasionally a mass lesion may be seen

Histology

- Cysts are single or multilocular (Fig. 34-12*b*). Cysts are lined by cuboidal or flat epithelium with eosinophilic or clear cytoplasm (Figs. 34-12*c* and 34-13)
- Calcium oxalate crystals can be seen as a sign of renal failure
- Features of severe end-stage kidney such as thyroidization of tubules, severe glomerular sclerosis can also be seen in the background (Fig. 34-12*c*)
- Most of the cystic lining cells are flat or low cuboidal without cytological atypia
- Some of the cysts are lined by cells with eosinophilic or clear cytoplasm with minimal cytological atypia (Figs. 34-13). These cells in the cysts may give rise to RCC

Clinical relevance (prognosis and treatment options)

- Long-term dialysis is associated with significant risk in development of ACKD
- ACKD is associated with a high risk for RCC in 10% to 20% cases

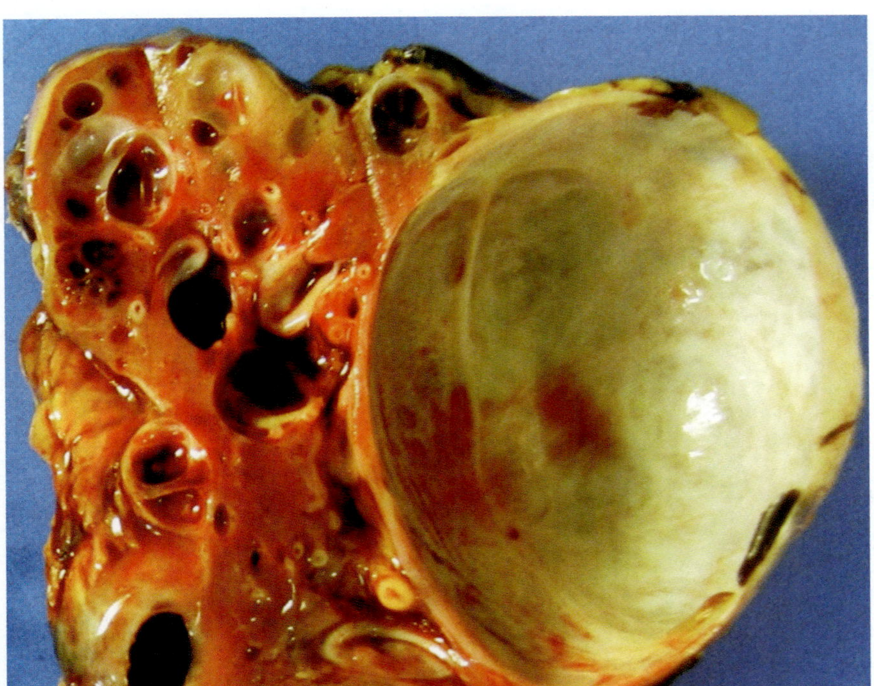

Figure 34-11. Acquired cystic kidney disease shows an atrophic kidney distorted by many cystic lesions of variable sizes.

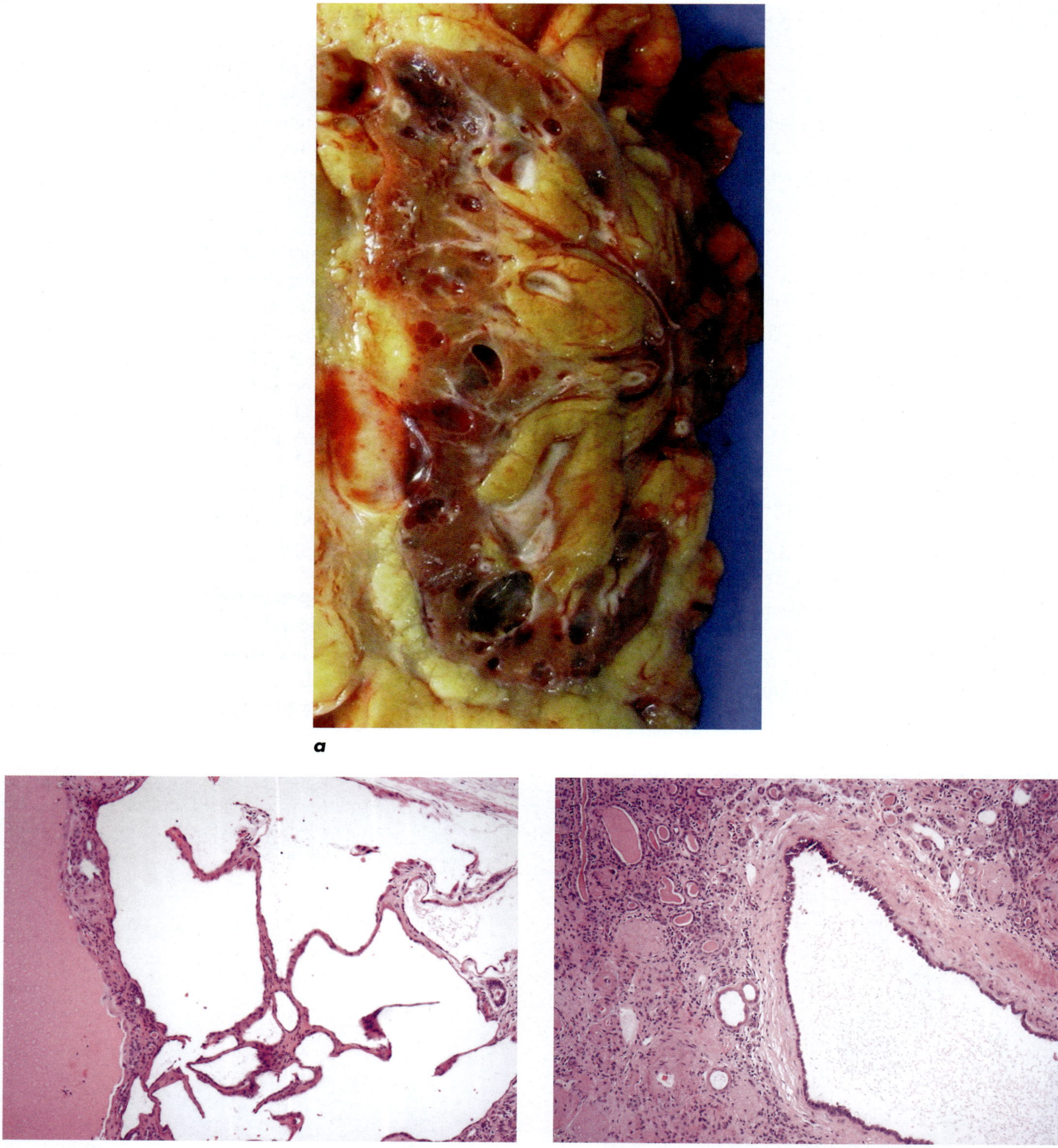

a

b

c

Figure 34-12.

Acquired cystic kidney disease. Gross photo shows multiple cysts dispersed throughout the atrophic kidney (*a*). The cysts are separated by thin septa (*b*) and lined by cuboidal epithelial cells with eosinophilic cytoplasm (*c*) in the background of glomerulosclerosis and thyroidization of the renal tubules.

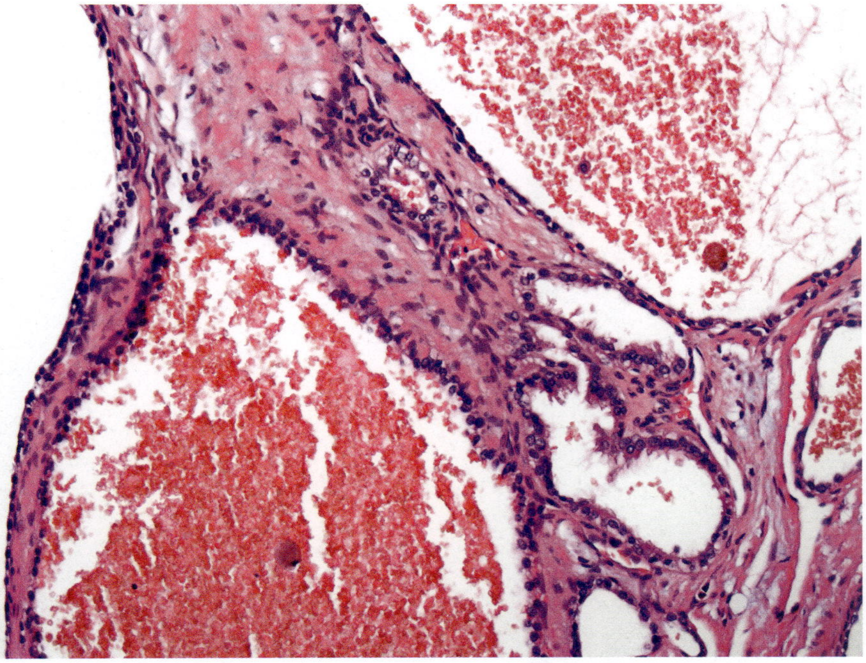

Figure 34-13.
ACKD is composed of cyst lined by epithelial cells with scant clear cytoplasm and no cytological atypia.

MIXED EPITHELIAL AND STROMAL TUMOR (CYSTIC NEPHROMA)

Definition

- Benign neoplasm composed of both epithelial and stromal components

Other terms

- Mixed mesenchymal and epithelial tumors
- Mixed epithelial and stromal tumor (MEST) and cystic nephroma are considered to be within the spectrum of the same disease, so that both terms have been used interchangeably
- Cystic nephroma refers to entirely cystic lesions. MEST may have both cystic and solid areas

Clinical features

- Adult, female to male ratio is 7 to 1, typically in perimenopausal females, rarely in male patients receiving estrogen therapy
- Symptoms associated with renal mass. Image studies will report a renal mass highly suspicious for RCC because of solid areas

Gross pathology

- Cystic nephroma
  - Encapsulated, entirely cystic mass with minimal solid areas or necrosis (Fig. 34-14)
- Mixed epithelial and stromal tumor
  - Partially solid and cystic mass (Fig. 34-15)
- In reality, there are always some stromal components for both lesions. Therefore, we believe that they are within the spectrum of the same disease
- Sometimes, the mass can be very large (Fig. 34-16)

Histology

- The tumor is composed of both epithelial and stromal components (Figs. 34-15*b* and 34-17)
- Hypercellular stroma is a common finding, which is similar to ovarian or endometrial stroma (Figs. 34-17 and 34-18)
- Epithelial cells range among flat (Fig. 34-17*b*), cuboidal, hobnail, columnar (Fig. 34-15*c*), or urothelium like (Fig. 34-18)

Immunohistochemistry

- Epithelial cell components are positive for keratin
- Spindle stromal cells are positive for smooth muscle actin, ER, and PR
- Positive for inhibin in some cases or CD10 in other cases (Fig. 34-19)

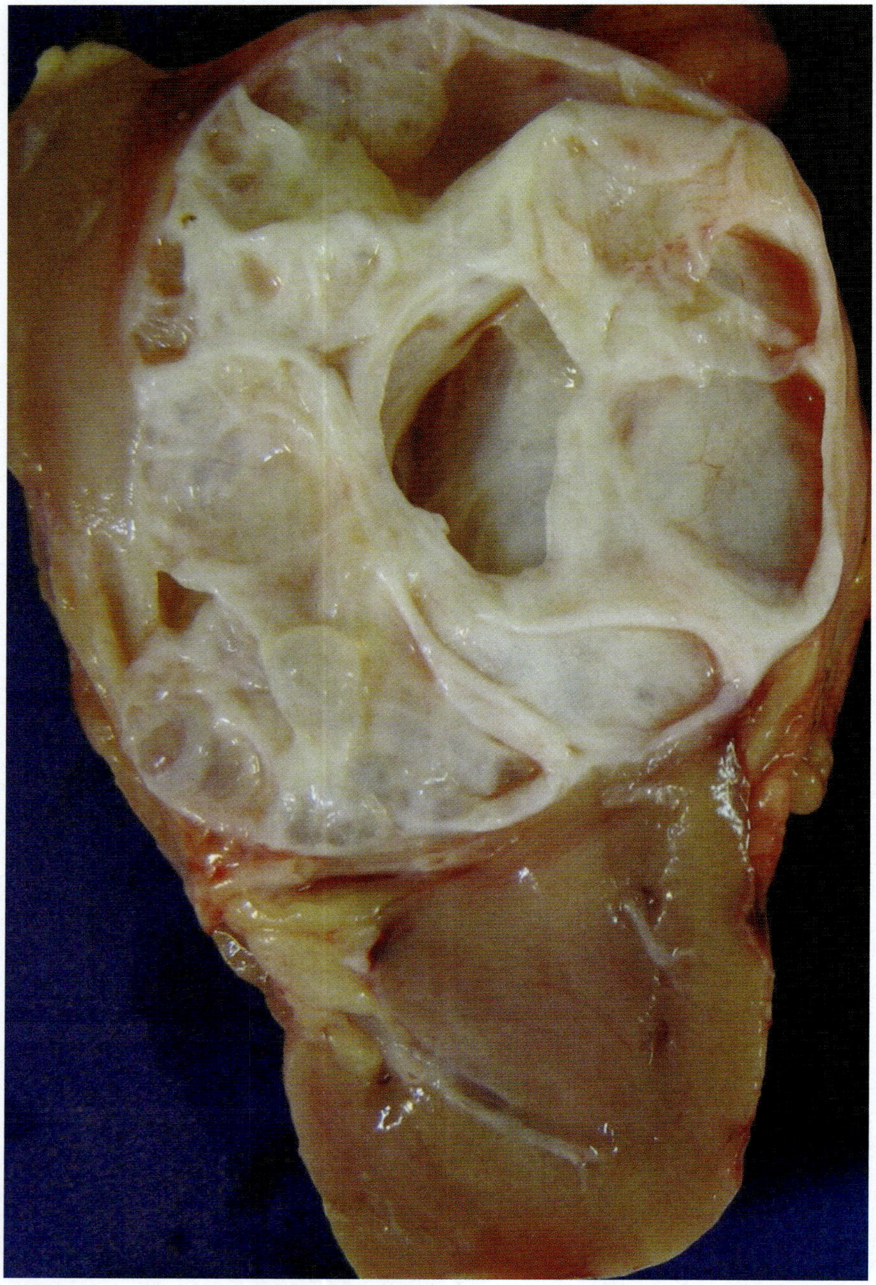

Figure 34-14.
Gross photo of mixed epithelial and stromal tumor (MEST)/cystic nephroma characterized by a multilocular cystic mass with minimal solid areas.

Differential diagnosis

- Should include benign cystic lesions such as PCK or malignant cystic lesions such as multilocular cystic RCC, tubular cystic RCC (see Table 34-1)

Clinical relevance (prognosis and treatment options)

- Prognosis: benign
- Rare cases of sarcoma arising in MEST/cystic nephroma have been reported
- Treatment: partial or radical nephrectomy

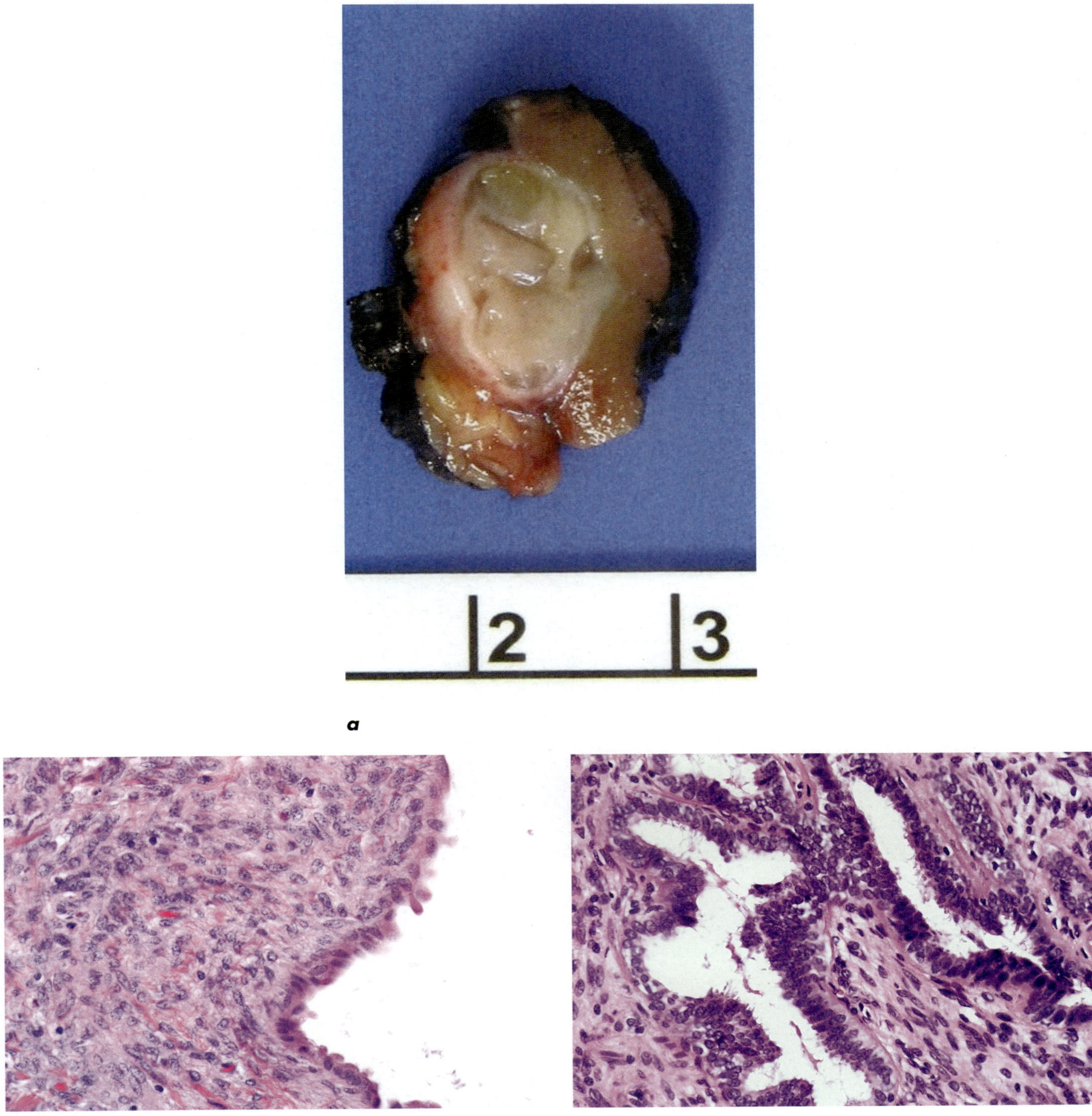

Figure 34-15.
MEST is characterized by the presence of a well-defined mass exhibiting solid and cystic areas (*a*). Microscopically, the tumor is composed of epithelium-lined cysts and ovarian type of stroma (*b*). The micropapillary appearance of columnar epithelial lining with cilia, but no cytological atypia is present (*c*).

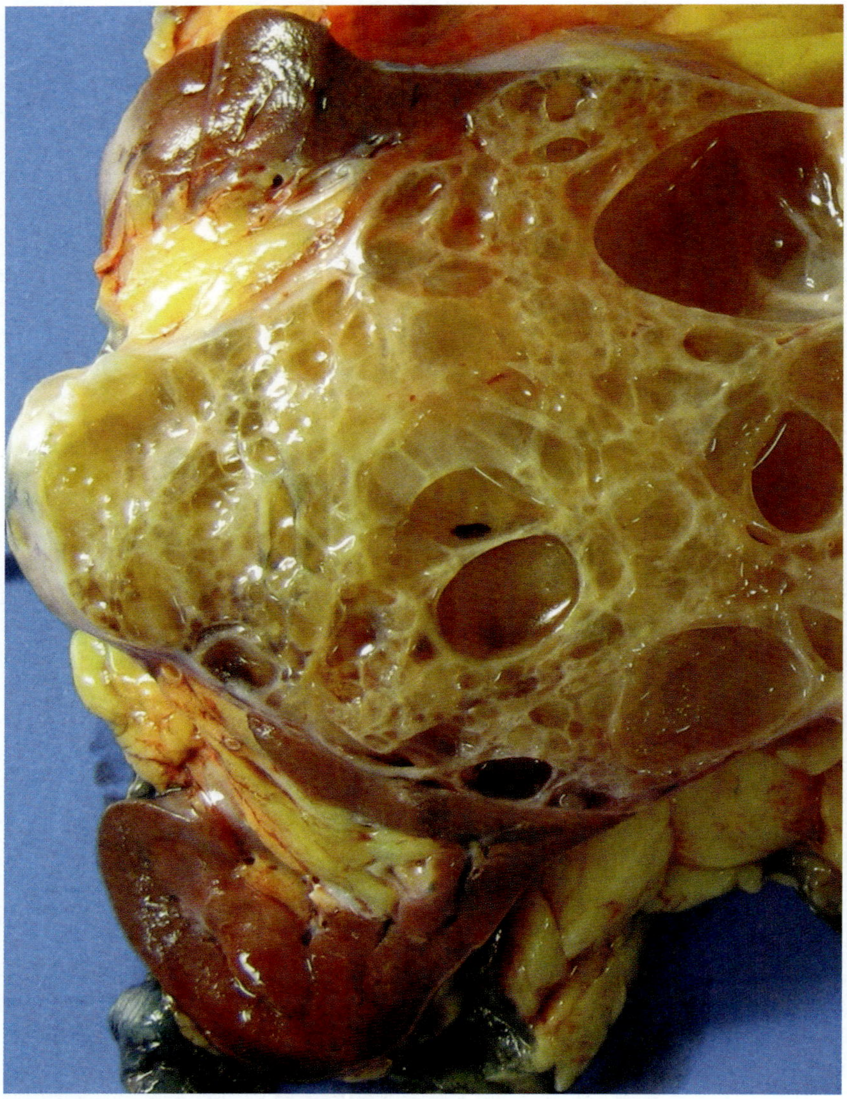

Figure 34-16.
A large MEST composed of multilocular cysts with prominent solid areas of cellular stroma.

Figure 34-17.
MEST with multilocular cyst (*a*) and prominent ovarian type of stroma (*b*).

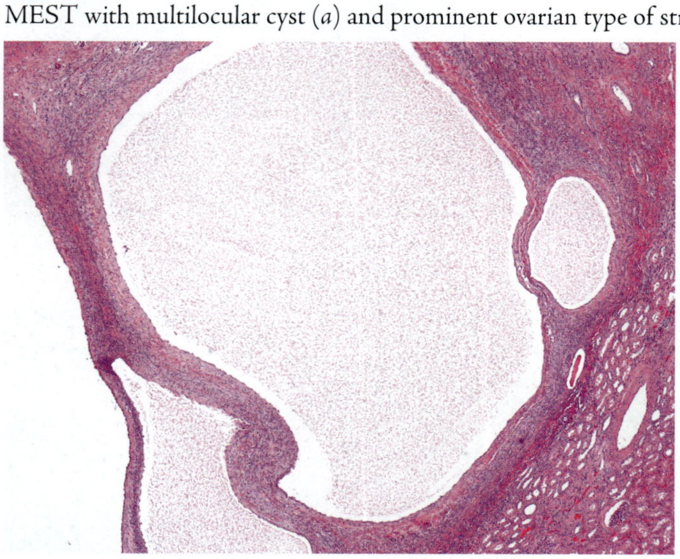

a

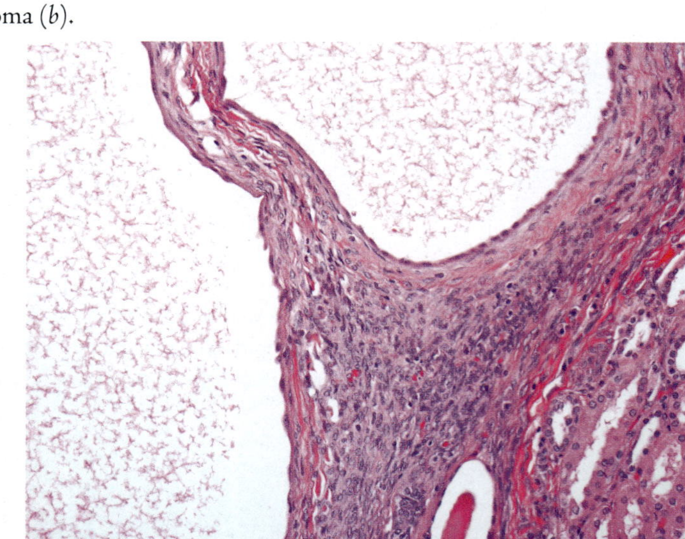

b

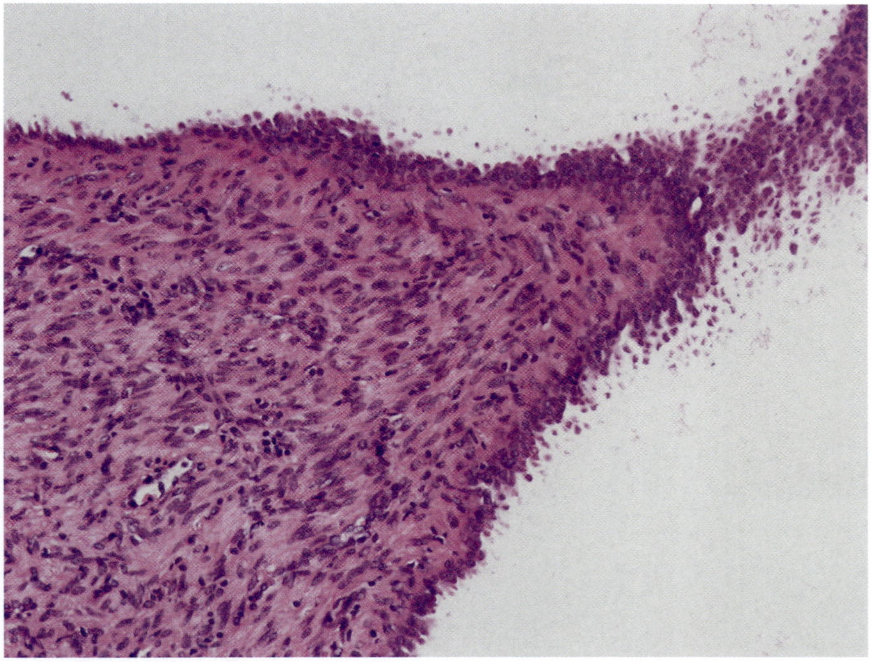

Figure 34-18.
MEST with cellular stroma and stratified epithelial lining resembling urothelium.

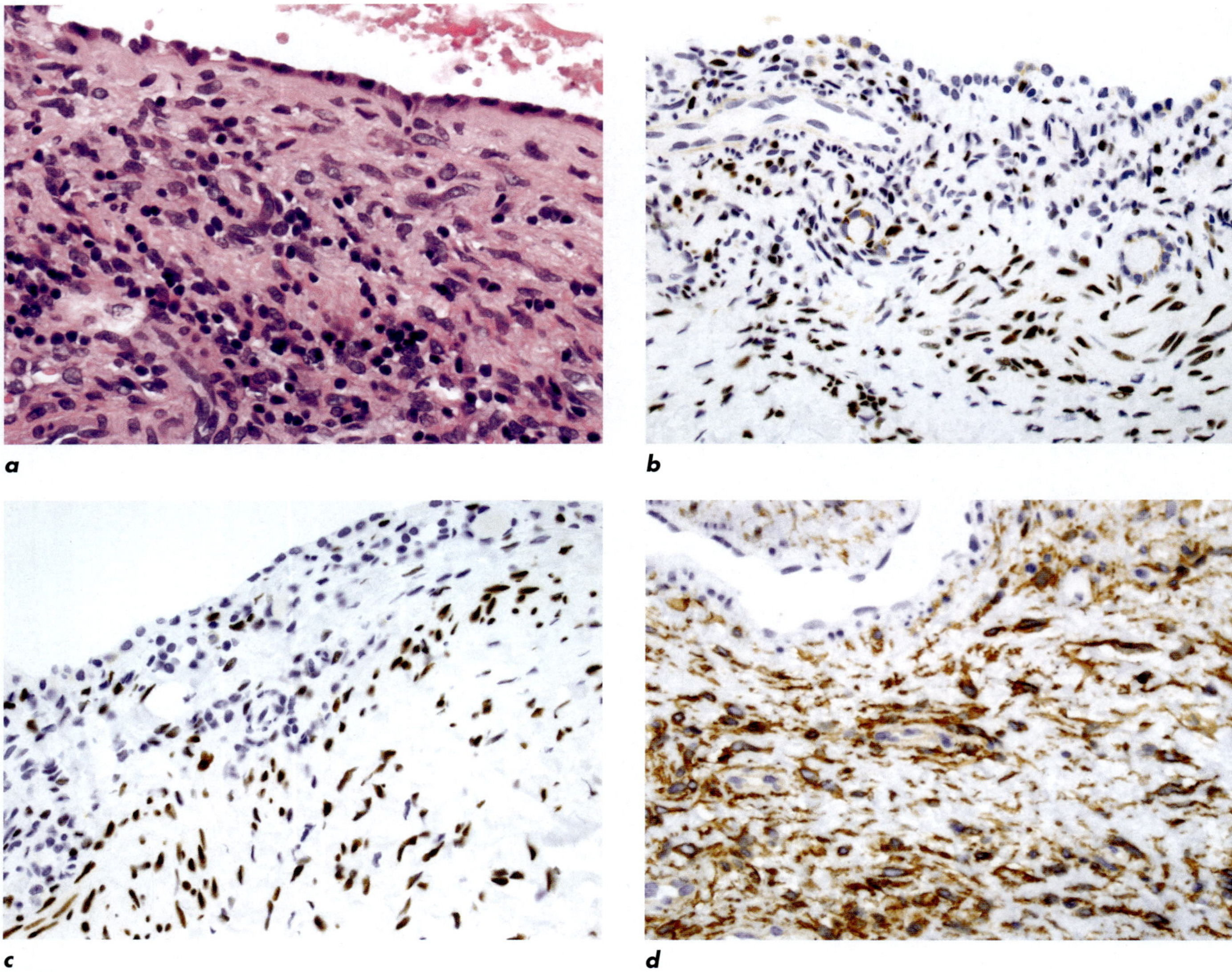

Figure 34-19.
MEST with typical epithelial cell lining and cellular stroma components (*a*), which are positive for ER (*b*), PR (*c*), and CD10 (*d*).

CHAPTER 35

Benign Neoplastic Lesions of the Kidney

Ondrej Hes, Ximing J. Yang, Huiying He

PAPILLARY HYPERPLASIA

Definition

- Small microscopic foci (usually less than 1 mm in diameter) of epithelial lesions in the kidney with papillary configurations and low nuclear grade

Other terms

- Papillary adenomatous changes
- Adenoma is considered if the size of the lesion is between 1 and 5 mm. Papillary hyperplasia is probably more appropriate when the lesion is too small to be called a tumor

Pathogenesis

- Proliferative lesions of the renal tubules, a possible precursor of papillary adenoma and papillary renal cell carcinoma (RCC)
- We have shown that there is a possible progression from papillary hyperplasia → papillary adenoma → papillary RCC

Clinical features

- Incidental findings, commonly seen in nephrectomy specimens harboring papillary RCC or papillary adenoma

Gross pathology

- The lesions are too small to be identified grossly
- Other commonly associated changes are small atrophic kidneys with or without multiple cysts
- Papillary RCC or papillary adenomas may be present as well

Histology

- Small microscopic foci of epithelial proliferation typically less than 1 mm in diameter (Figs. 35-1 and 35-2)
- The lesional cells form tubular, solid, or papillary patterns (Fig. 35-1*b*) similar to those of papillary adenoma or papillary RCC
- Psammoma bodies can be seen in the lesion
- Low nuclear grade equivalent to Fuhrman grade 1 (Fig. 35-2)
- Papillary hyperplasia is commonly seen in adult polycystic kidney disease, which developed from the cystic lining cells (Fig. 35-3)

Immunohistochemistry

- CK7 positive, AMACR positive, and PAX2/PAX8 positive
- CA9 negative

Figure 35-1.
Papillary hyperplasia of the kidney measured less than 1 mm as indicated by the ruler (*a*). High magnification shows the papillary structures covered by cuboidal epithelial cells of low nuclear grade (*b*), similar to low-grade papillary RCC except the size of the lesion.

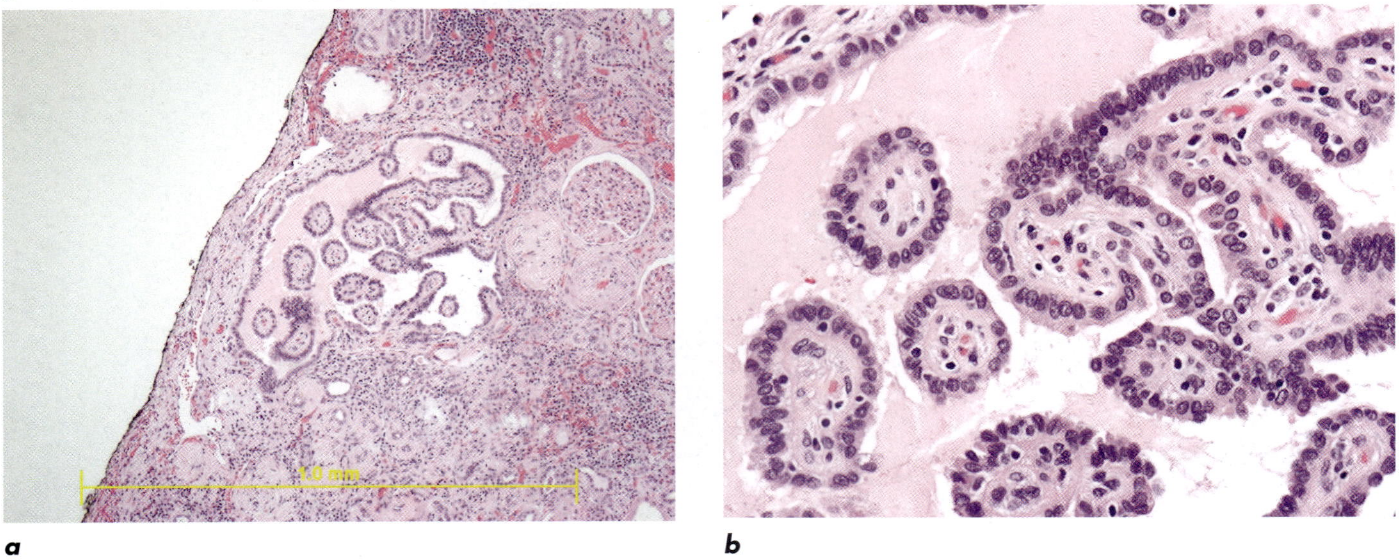

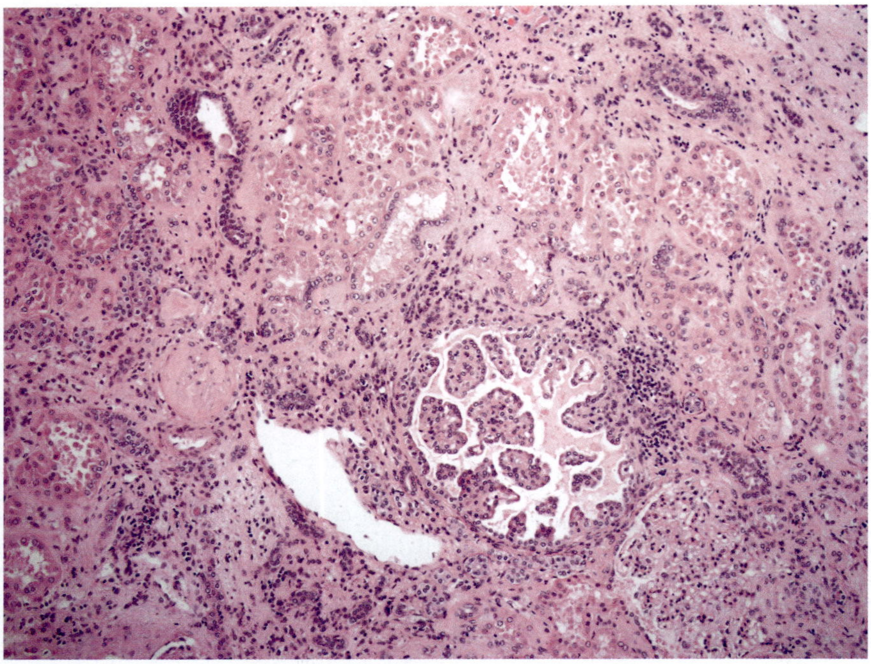

Figure 35-2.
Papillary hyperplasia is composed of a glandular structure with multiple small papillary projections.

Clinical relevance (prognosis and treatment options)

- This is a microscopic finding, not detectable by imaging studies
- Except for its smaller size, the lesion is histologically similar to papillary adenoma, which is the precursor lesion of papillary RCC
- The patient does not need treatment
- However, papillary hyperplasia may be mistaken for papillary RCC in needle core biopsy or on a surgical margin of a partial nephrectomy specimen

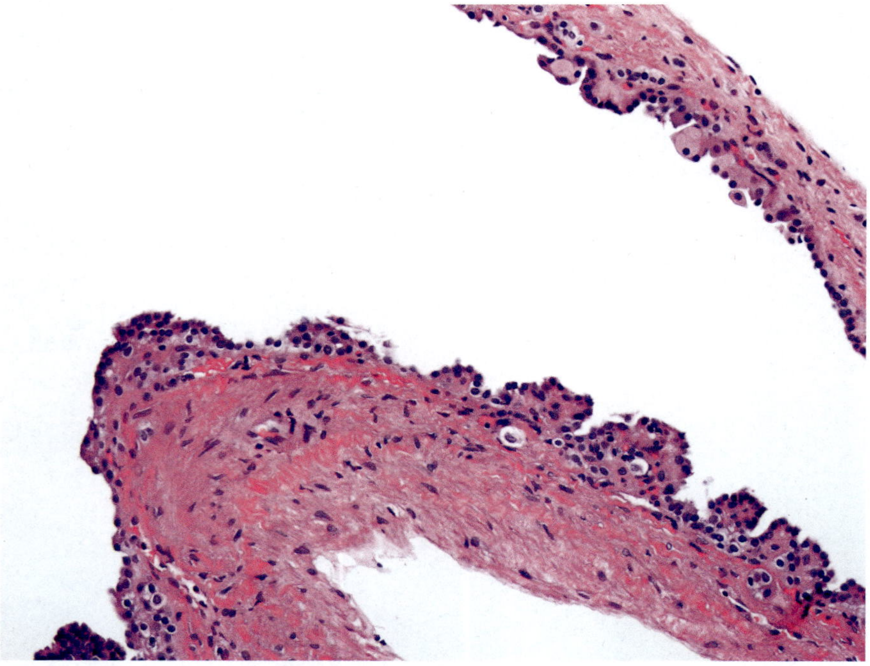

Figure 35-3.
Papillary hyperplasia seen in a case of adult polycystic kidney disease, which appears to be stuck on the surface of the cyst lining.

PAPILLARY ADENOMA

Definition

- Benign epithelial neoplasm composed of papillary and tubular architecture of low nuclear grade tumor cells
- Equal or less than 5 mm in diameter, usually visible grossly (greater than 1 mm)

Pathogenesis

- Because its morphological and immunohistochemical features, papillary adenoma is considered to be the precursor lesion of low-grade papillary RCC

Clinical features

- Incidental findings, more often seen in the areas adjacent to papillary RCC

Gross pathology

- Small, well-circumscribed nodule, visible but not more than 5 mm (Fig. 35-4)
- While, yellow, or tan solid cut surface (Fig. 35-4)
- Hemorrhage and necrosis rare

Histology

- The tumor is equal or less than 5 mm in size (Fig. 35-5*a*)
- Papillary or tubular configuration with fibrovascular cores (Figs. 35-5*b* and Fig. 35-6)
- Scant cytoplasm makes a basophilic appearance (Fig. 35-7)
- Low nuclear grade, small round to oval nuclei with inconspicuous nucleoli (Figs. 35-5*b* and Fig. 35-7)
- Psammoma (sand in Greek) bodies, concentric collection of calcium, commonly seen (Figs. 35-6 and 35-7)
- Psammoma bodies can also been seen in papillary RCC, as well as papillary carcinoma of the thyroid, ovary, or other organs
- Microscopic foci (<1 mm, not visible grossly) lesions with similar low-grade histology can be considered papillary hyperplasia

Immunohistochemistry

- CK7 positive, AMACR positive
- CA9 negative and vimentin positive

Differential diagnosis

- *Clear cell RCC* can be smaller than 5 mm, but it is composed of clear cells
- *High-grade papillary RCC,* mostly type 2, can be smaller than 5 mm, but it has a high nuclear grade

Molecular analysis

- Trisomy chromosome 7 and 17 can be detected

Clinical relevance (prognosis and treatment options)

- Determining the benign or malignant nature of a tumor based on its size is not scientific, but it is clinically relevant and practical if one understands the adenoma to carcinoma progression scenario
- Adenoma is benign without potential for metastasis

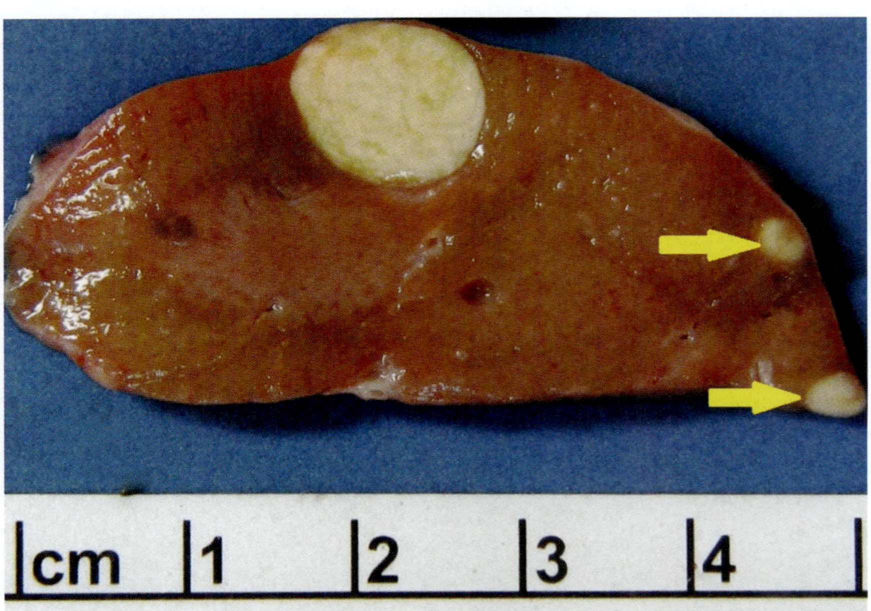

Figure 35-4.
Gross photo of a partial nephrectomy specimen containing a papillary RCC greater than 1 cm and two smaller papillary adenomas (indicated by arrows), each is less than 0.5 cm in diameter; microscopically all three tumors have identical histological features.

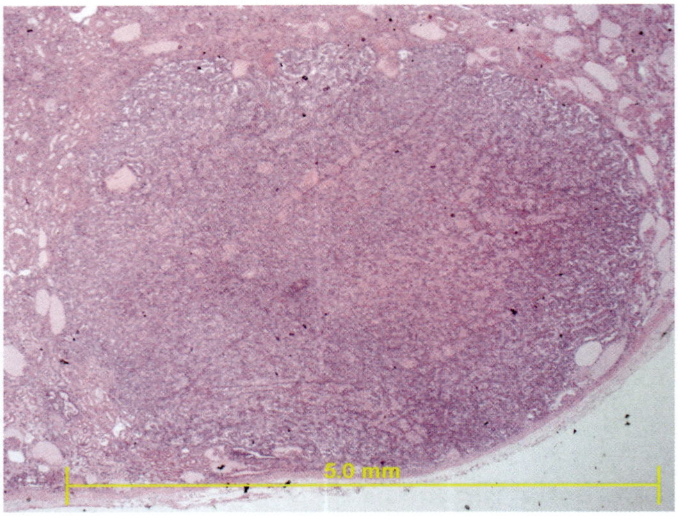

a

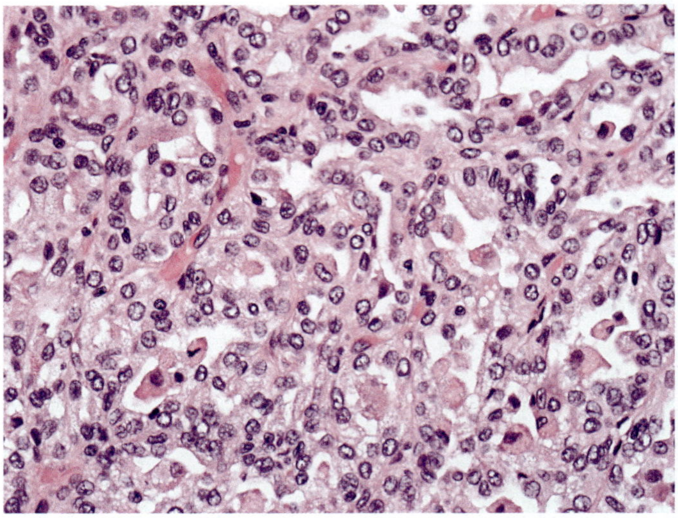

b

Figure 35-5.
Papillary adenoma less than 5 mm is composed of tubular and papillary structures (*a*). High magnification shows the tumor cells with low nuclear grade forming tubular structures (*b*).

- However, it may keep growing and reach 5 mm or larger to become papillary RCC with increasing risk of developing metastasis
- Therefore, a patient with a diagnosis of papillary adenomas of the kidney (either diagnosed in partial nephrectomy specimens or detected by a combination of imaging studies and needle core biopsy) needs to be followed
- Issues with surgical margins. Because of its morphological similarities to low-grade papillary RCC, papillary adenoma can compromise surgical margin evaluation of a nephrectomy specimen. We have seen cases where margins were called positive because of the presence of papillary adenoma

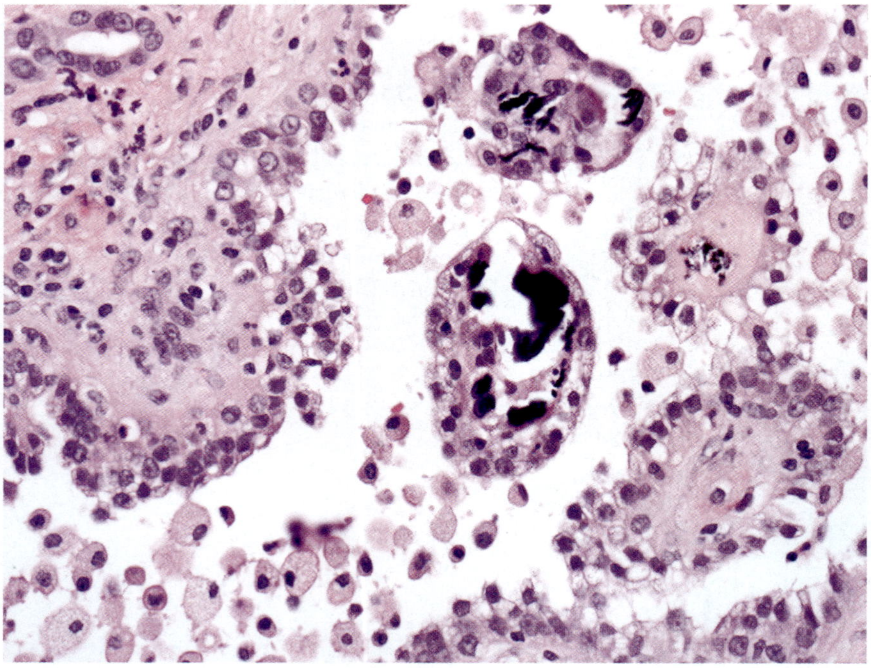

Figure 35-6.
Papillary adenoma with psammoma bodies and clear cell changes.

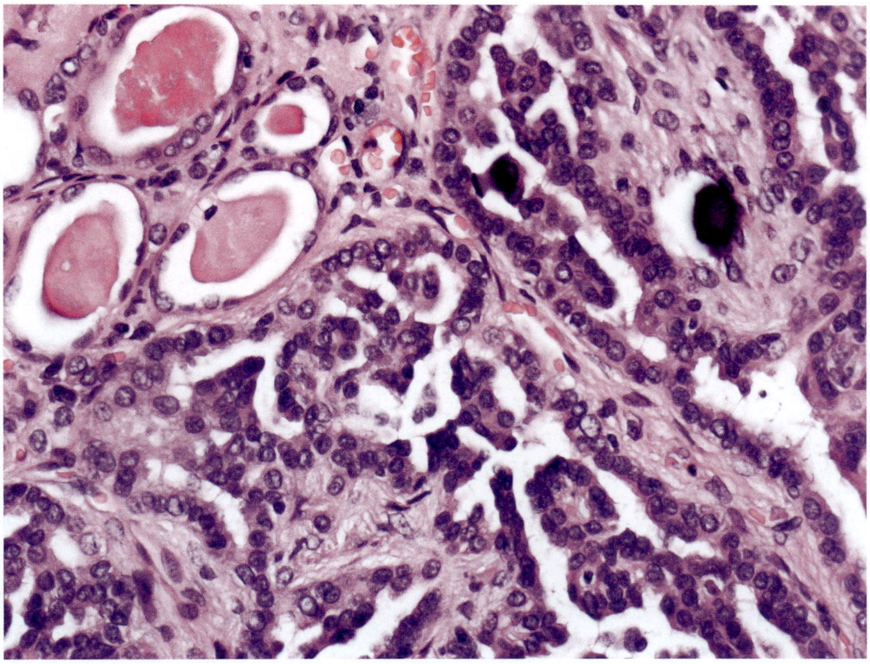

Figure 35-7.
Papillary adenoma with tubular/papillary structures and psammoma bodies, which are identical to those seen in papillary RCC.

- First, the resected renal tumor should be evaluated first if it is papillary RCC, the possibility to have coexisting papillary adenomas increases
- Second, in the frozen section diagnosis of a renal surgical margin specimen, one could specify "the presence of a papillary renal cell neoplasm, which could be either papillary adenoma or low-grade papillary RCC" if the size cannot be evaluated
- On needle core biopsy specimen or fine needle aspirate specimens, papillary adenoma is indistinguishable from low-grade papillary RCC—based morphology or IHC staining. So that it may be over-interpreted as RCC and subjected to unnecessary surgical procedures. Clinical correlation with imaging studies is essential.

METANEPHRIC ADENOMA

Definition

- Benign highly cellular epithelial neoplasm composed of small uniform tumor cells with scant cytoplasm
- It probably belongs to a group of tumors including metanephric adenoma, metanephric adenofibroma (containing cellular stromal cells in addition to epithelial component), metanephric stromal tumor (see Chapter 37)

Clinical features

- Usually asymptomatic, mostly as incidental findings
- Some patients may present with polycythemia
- Female predominance (ratio M:F = 1:2), broad age range 1 to 83 years

Gross pathology

- Well-circumscribed or partly encapsulated solid or partially cystic mass, size ranging from 0.3 to 20 cm
- Variable color, from gray to yellow/tan on cut surface
- Hemorrhage and necrosis are very uncommon

Histology

- Tumor composed of small basophilic cells with scant cytoplasm, forming acini and narrow elongated, branching tubules (Figs. 35-8 and 35-9)
- Hypocellular stroma is generally present, could be edematous with hyalinization (Fig. 35-10)
- Tubular (Fig. 35-11*a*), solid (Fig. 35-11*b*) glomeruloid structures (Fig. 35-11*c*) or papillary structures with tall columnar cells (Fig. 35-11*d*) are invariably present
- Tubules are lined by cuboidal primitive-looking basophilic cells with round uniform nuclei and inconspicuous nucleoli (Figs. 35-12 and 35-13)
- Calcifications and even ossification can be seen. Psammoma bodies are frequently encountered
- Prominent papillary configurations can be occasionally seen (Figs. 35-11*b* and 35-13)
- Some of the tumor cells, so-called high grade, may have nuclear enlargement mimicking RCC (Fig. 35-14)
- Overlapping areas with papillary RCC and Wilms tumor morphology could be focally present

Immunohistochemistry

- PAX-2, PAX8, and CD57 usually positive
- However, WT1 is positive in majority of the cases, but it can be completely negative in large areas of the tumor
- CK7, EMA, and AMACR are generally negative; however, focally in papillary areas could be present
- Vimentin and keratins stains are highly variable and inconsistent

Molecular diagnostics

- Cytogenetic analyses showed normal karyotypes
- Abnormalities in chromosome 2 have been reported
- Deletion of chromosome 11p13 is absent (characteristic feature for Wilms tumor)

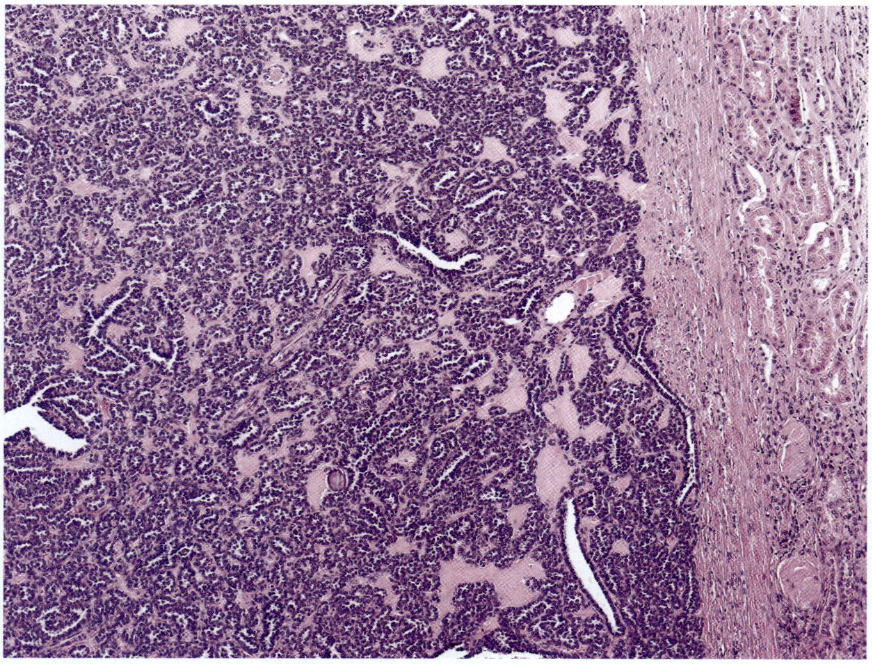

Figure 35-8.
Metanephric adenoma with noninvasive well-defined border. The tumor is composed of small cuboidal epithelial cells forming tubules or acini.

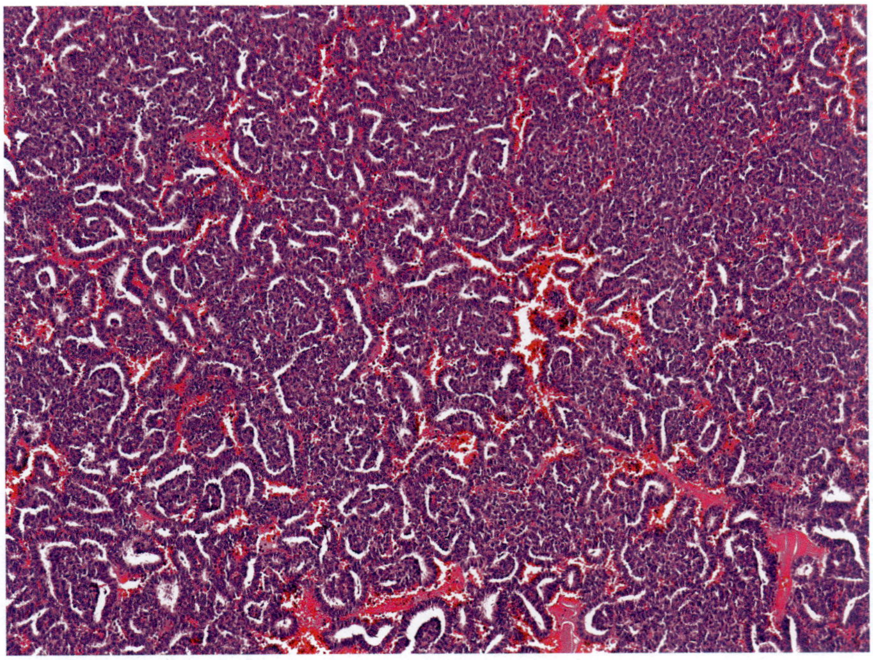

Figure 35-9.
Metanephric adenoma is characterized by the primitive epithelial tumor cells with scant cytoplasm forming small tubular structures.

Figure 35-10.
Metanephric adenoma with small tubules and eosinophilic stroma (*a*). High magnification shows the presence of tubular structures with prominent eosinophilic stroma (*b*).

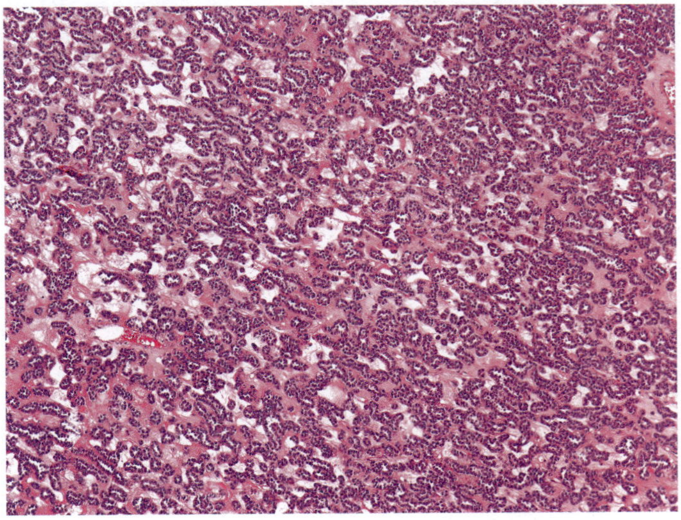

a

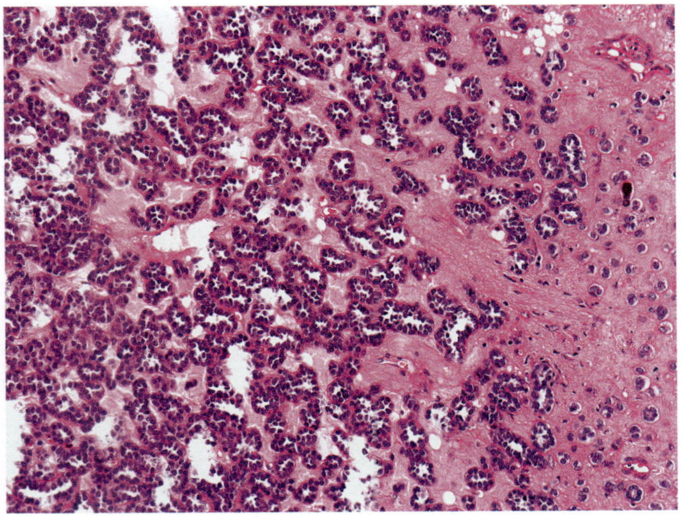

b

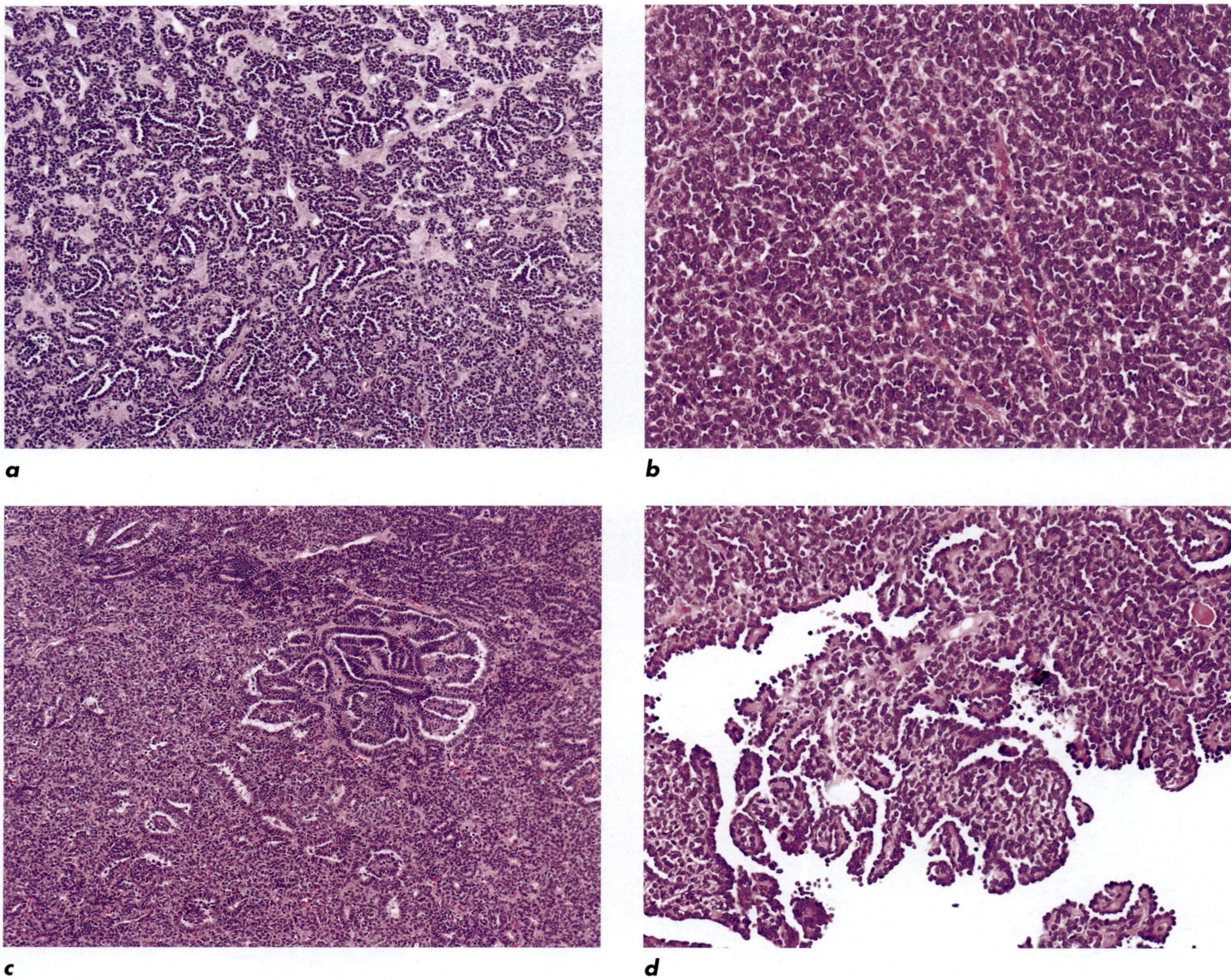

Figure 35-11.
Metanephric adenoma. Tumor cells forming elongated and anastomosing tubular structures (*a*), "solid" pattern (*b*), glomeruloid structures (*c*), or papillary configurations (*d*).

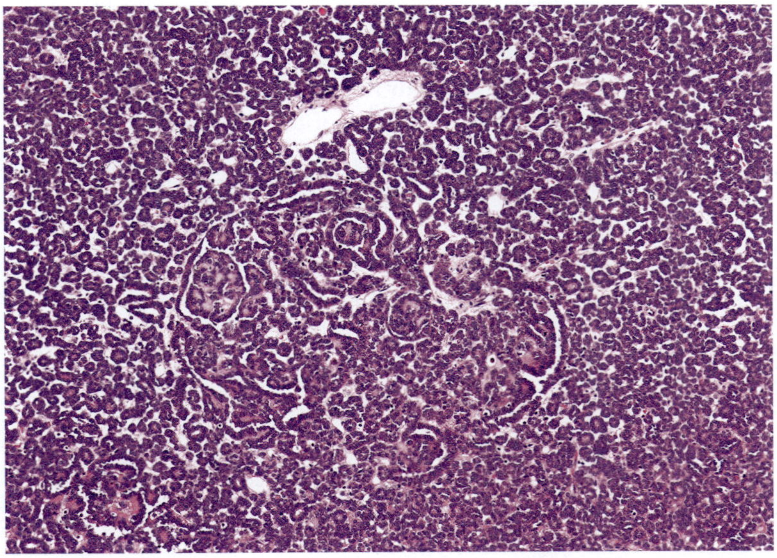

Figure 35-12.
Metanephric adenoma with structures mimicking primitive glomeruli.

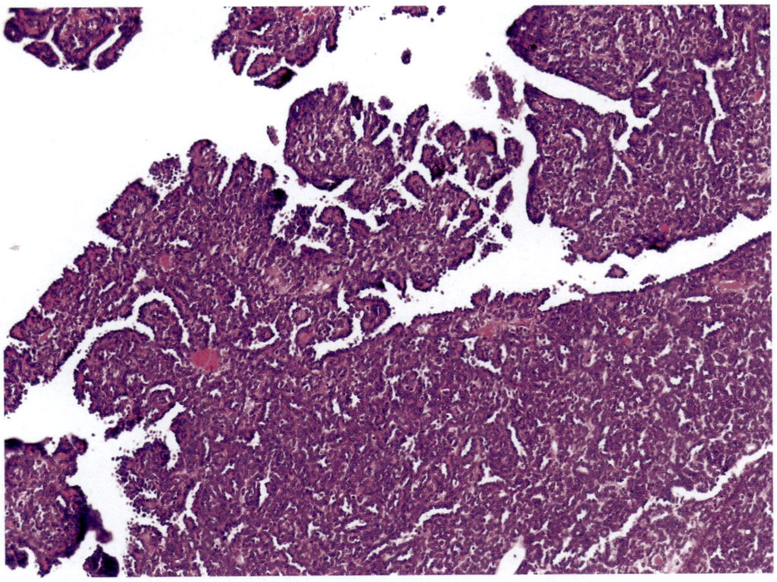

Figure 35-13.
Metanephric adenoma with prominent papillary configurations mimicking papillary RCC.

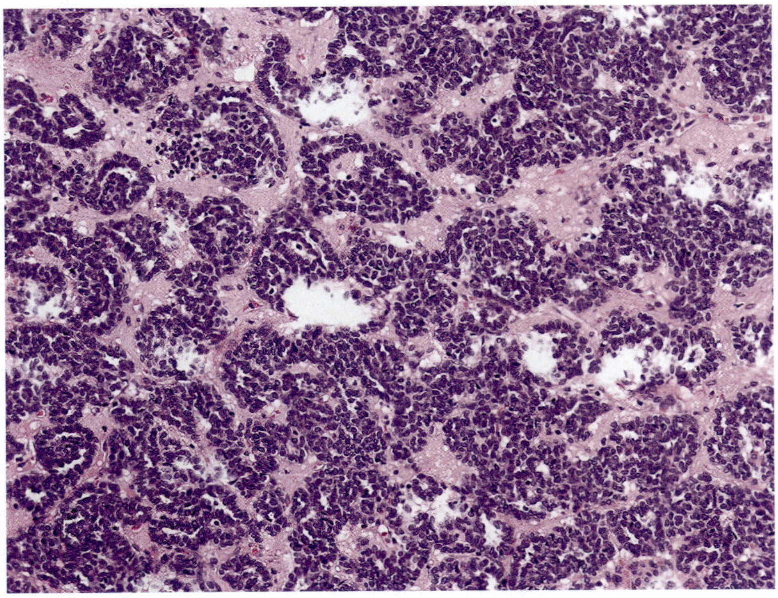

Figure 35-14.
So-called "high-grade" metanephric adenoma composed of primitive cuboidal tumor cells with solid or tubular structures.

Main differential diagnosis

Wilms tumor

- Epithelial predominant Wilms tumor could be morphologically similar to metanephric adenoma
- Wilms tumor cells are generally more primitive, higher degree of polymorphism and higher mitotic activity than metanephric adenoma
- Findings of stromal, blastemal components, or cellular anaplasia favor the diagnosis of Wilms tumor
- However, in rare cases it is extremely difficult to draw a line between "high-grade" metanephric adenoma and very well-differentiated epithelioid Wilms tumor

Papillary RCC

- Short papillae are occasionally seen in metanephric adenoma, long prominent papillary structures are not consistent with picture of metanephric adenoma
- Papillary RCC is rarely composed of small primitive cuboidal cells like metanephric adenoma
- Presence of prominent necrosis, hemorrhage, foamy cells, siderophages, and cholesterol clefts is highly unusual for metanephric adenoma
- Immunohistochemical positivity for AMACR, vimentin, cytokeratins, EMA favors the diagnosis of papillary RCC
- The presence of polysomy/trisomy of chromosomes 7 and 17 is a feature typical for papillary RCC not for metanephric adenoma

Clinical relevance (prognosis and treatment options)

- Treated with nephron sparing or radical nephrectomy

RENAL ONCOCYTOMA

Definition

- Benign renal epithelial neoplasm composed of round-to-polygonal cells with abundant mitochondria-rich eosinophilic cytoplasm

Pathogenesis and epidemiology

- It is believed to arise from the intercalated cells. However, it is most likely derived from the stem cells in the kidney
- Accounting for 4% to 8% of adult renal epithelial neoplasms in most surgical pathology practices
- Wide range of age distribution with a peak incidence in the seventh decade of life. More prevalent in males than females with a ratio of 2:1
- Rare cases of oncocytoma are associated with Birt-Hogg-Dube syndrome (see Chapter 40)

Clinical features

- Asymptomatic presentation and incidental findings on imaging studies in most patients
- Classical triad (hematuria, flank pain, and/or flank mass), similar to those of RCC, seen in a very small subset of patients
- The tumor appears to be a solid homogenous mass on imaging studies and a central irregular scar can be seen

Gross pathology

- Well-circumscribed but nonencapsulated solid mass (Fig. 35-15)
- Color of the tumor ranging from dark yellow, brown to typical "mahogany" (Figs. 35-16 and 35-17)

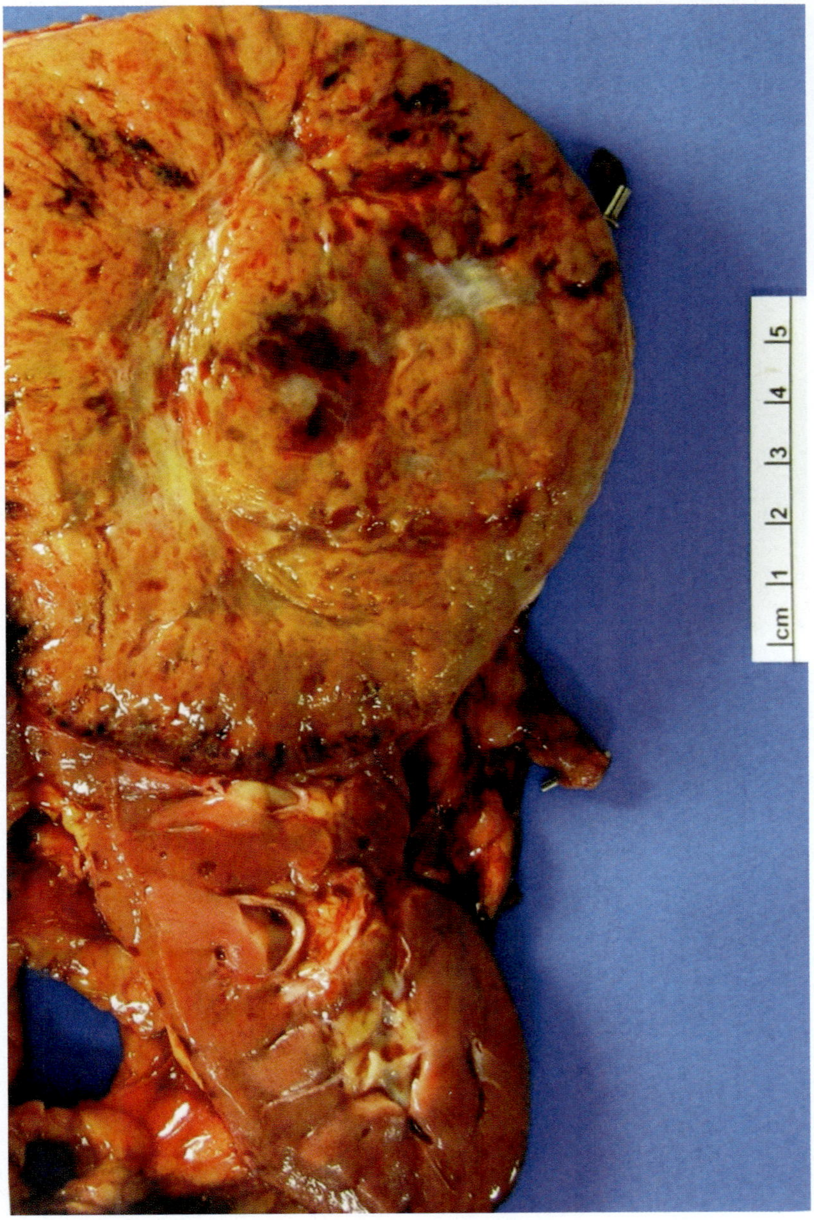

Figure 35-15.
A large oncocytoma with a tan-yellow cut surface displaying an irregular central scar. This case is difficult to be distinguished from RCC grossly.

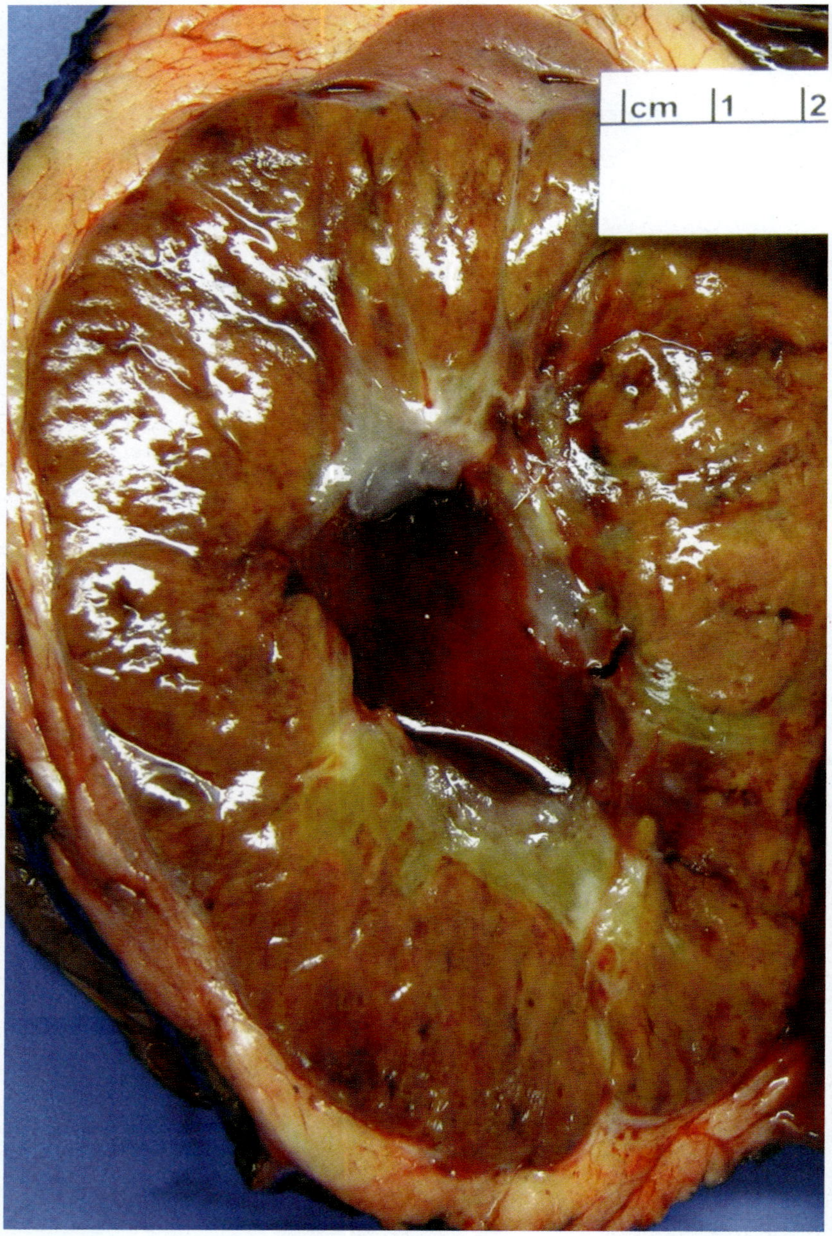

Figure 35-16.
Gross photo of a renal oncocytoma, which shows a large well-circumscribed renal mass with distinct mahogany color and a central scar.

- A central stellate scar may be present only in small percentage of cases (Fig. 35-16)
- Hemorrhage and cystic changes are not very common, necrosis is rare
- Multiple oncocytomas in a kidney can be seen, which is considered to be *oncocytosis*

Histology

- Composed predominantly of large round-to-polygonal cells with abundant eosinophilic cytoplasm (Fig. 35-18) containing cytoplasmic mitochondria, which can be confirmed by electron microscopy
- Areas of edematous stroma with hypocellularity, particularly in the central scar, are frequently seen (Fig. 35-19)

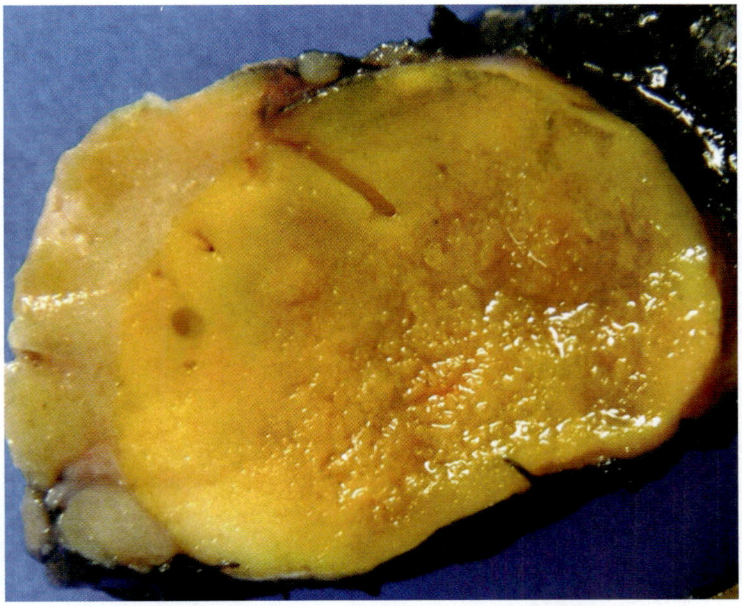

Figure 35-17.
Gross photo of another oncocytoma with unusual yellow cut surface.

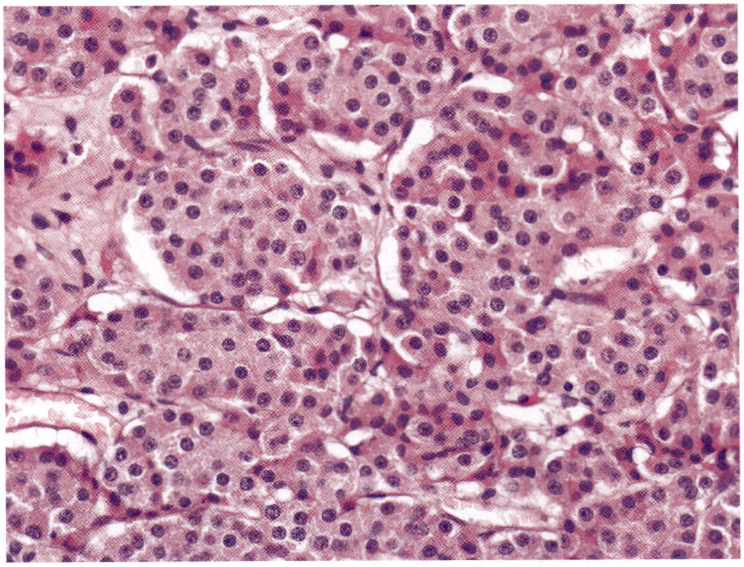

Figure 35-18.
Typical histological appearance of oncocytoma is characterized by nests of large tumor with abundant eosinophilic cytoplasm and round nuclei.

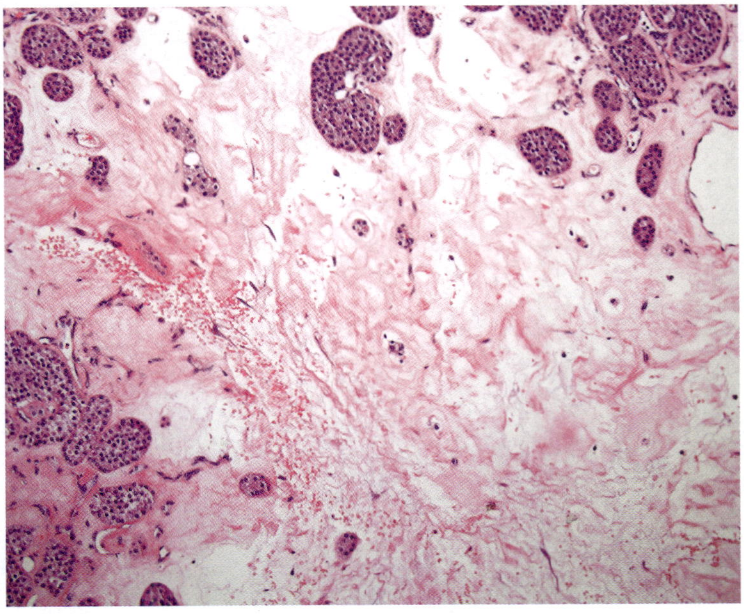

Figure 35-19.
Central scar in oncocytoma showing prominent edematous stroma and scattered nests to tumor cells.

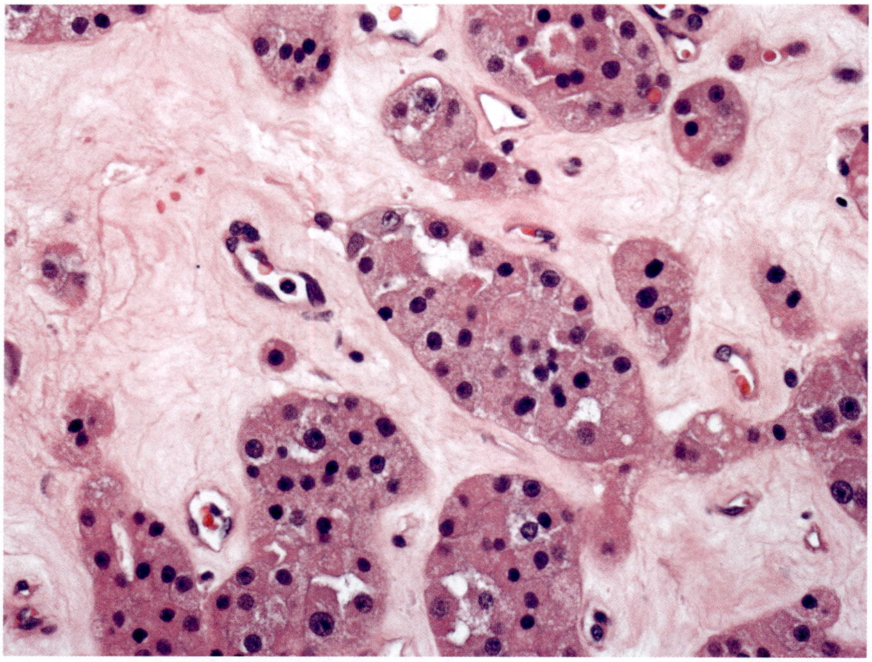

Figure 35-20.
Oncocytoma cells with abundant eosinophilic granular cytoplasm, round nuclei, and occasionally nucleoli. Tumor cells may show focal nuclear atypia.

- Tumor cells frequently form large solid nests, acini, tubules, or microcysts (Figs. 35-20 to 35-22)
- Uniformly round nuclei with inconspicuous nucleoli; scattered but not diffuse degenerative nuclear atypia can be seen (Fig. 35-20)
- Membrane-bound microvesicles (typical of chromophobe RCC) not present in oncocytoma under electron microscope
- Oncoblasts are small tumor cells with minimal cytoplasm, and dense hyperchromatic nuclei can be frequently seen
- Although small papillae may occasionally be seen, the presence of extensive papillary architecture is not a typical of oncocytoma and should raise a suspicion for an oncocytic papillary RCC
- Extension to perinephric fat without stromal response is not uncommon (may be seen in 10% to 20% of cases) (Fig. 35-21)

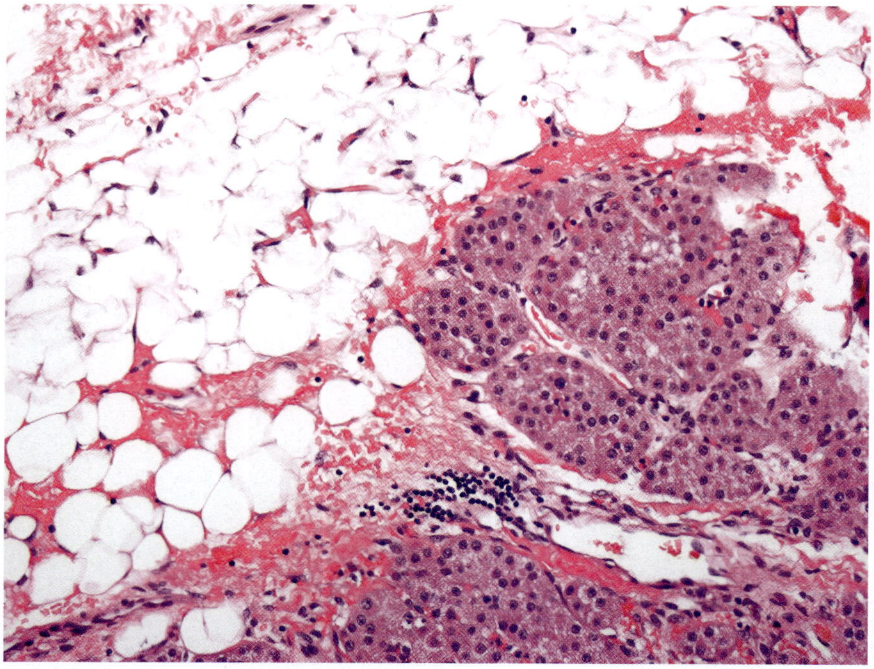

Figure 35-21.
Oncocytoma extending to perinephric adipose tissue but with no desmoplastic reaction.

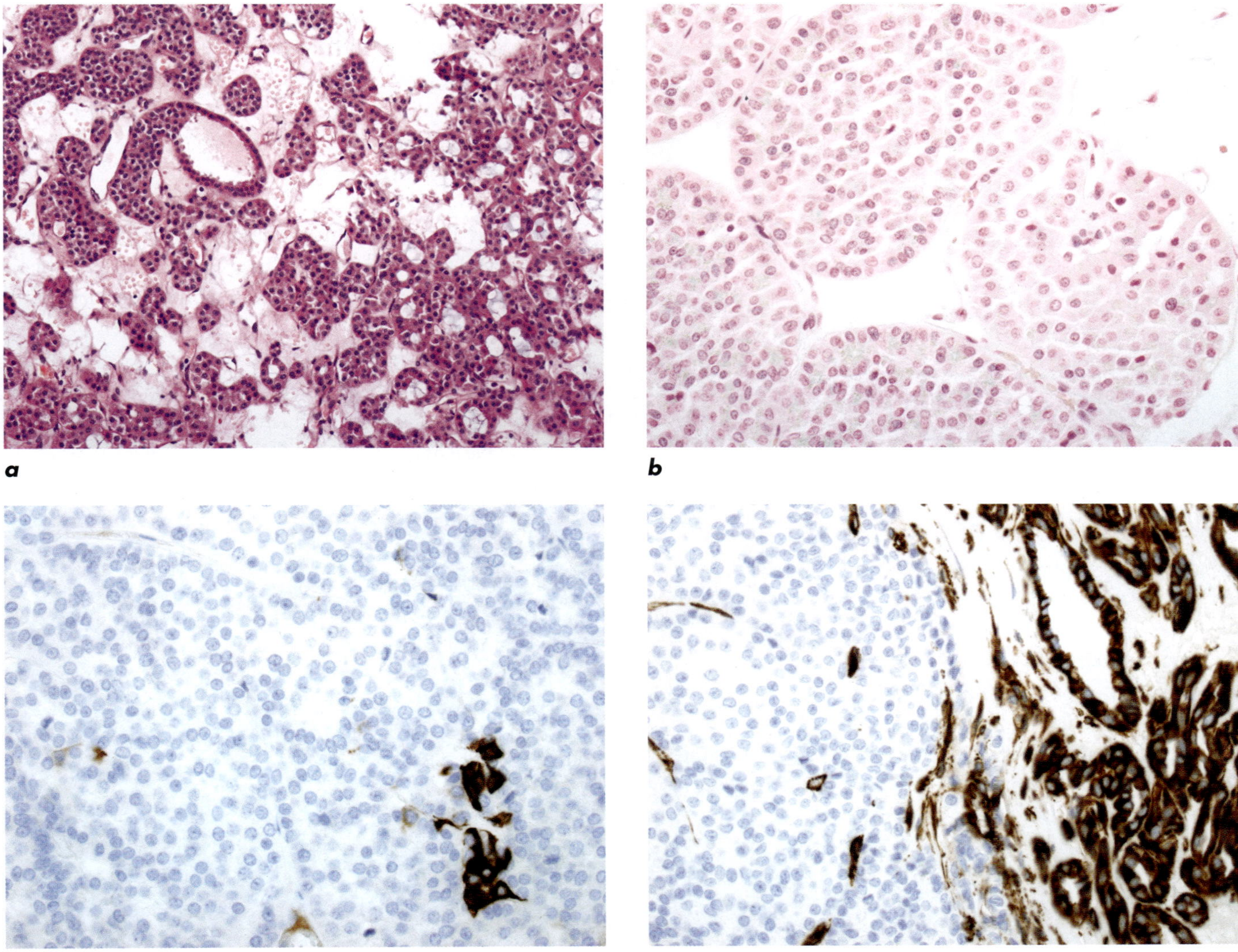

Figure 35-22.
Oncocytoma with tubular, glandular, and solid patterns (*a*), negative Hale colloidal iron staining (*b*), negative CK7 immunostaining, while a few trapped tubules are positive for CK7 (*c*). Vimentin staining is negative (*d*) in the majority of the tumor cells, although it is occasionally positive in oncocytoma cells.

- Extension into renal veins reported in up to 5% of cases. RCC should always be ruled out first in this situation
- Oncocytosis refers to numerous oncocytomas involving the kidney

Immunohistochemistry

- CD117 (C-kit) diffusely positive
- Hale colloidal iron shows luminal staining (Fig. 35-22*b*)
- CK7 negative in oncocytoma, but positive in entrapped tubules (Fig. 35-22*c*)
- Vimentin negative in the majority of tumor cells, although focal positivity can be seen in tumor cells within septa (Fig. 35-22*d*)

Molecular diagnostics

- Unique molecular signature defined by gene expression microarrays and micro-RNA studies
- Minimal chromosomal alterations on cytogenetic studies, in contrast to multiple chromosomal losses seen in chromophobe RCC

Differential diagnosis

Other subtypes of RCC with oncocytic cytoplasm

- The following features should raise a suspicion for an RCC: necrosis (more than focal); papillary architecture (more than focal); frequent mitosis (>1 per 20× filed); atypical mitosis; clear cells or spindle cells; diffusely positivity for CK7, AMACR, or vimentin

Clear cell RCC with eosinophilic cytoplasm

- Grossly clear cell RCC is bright or golden yellow rather than dark brown color of oncocytoma
- Clear cell RCC has a distinctive "chicken-wire" vascular patterns
- It generally has higher Fuhrman grade (grade 3 or 4)

Oncocytic papillary RCC

- It has a more apparent papillary architecture
- Presence of foamy macrophages in the fibrovascular core

Chromophobe RCC

- It displays more prominent cell membranes and has raisinoid or koilocytic nuclei
- Diffusely positive for CK7 and Hale colloidal iron stain
- Presence of abundant membrane-bound microvesicles by EM (see Table 39-2 for more information)

Oncocytic tumor, not otherwise specified or hybrid oncocytic tumor

- There are cases with histological and immunohistochemical features overlapping oncocytoma and chromophobe RCC
- These cases cannot be readily categorized into either oncocytoma or chromophobe RCC
- The term *oncocytic tumor, not otherwise specified* has been used for these difficult cases. However, it should be reserved for a very small subset of the most difficult cases, because this term may cause confusion for clinical management
- The other term *hybrid oncocytic tumor* is used by other pathologists for these difficult cases. We use the term *hybrid oncocytic tumor* exclusively for Birt-Hogg-Dube (BHD) patients

Clinical relevance (prognosis and treatment options)

- Benign with excellent prognosis
- Often treated with partial or radical nephrectomy. Active surveillance is also considered for biopsy-proven cases
- Rare cases of "renal oncocytoma with metastasis" usually turn out to be RCCs mimicking oncocytomas

RENAL MEDULLARY FIBROMA

Definition

- Benign stromal neoplasm arising from the renal medullary interstitial cells

Other term

- Renomedullary interstitial cell tumor

Pathogenesis

- Renomedullary interstitial cells have receptors for several vasoactive peptides; therefore, they are related to renin pathway and regulate the blood flow and pressure of the kidney
- This tumor is believed by some investigators to develop in response to hypertension
- However, most of these tumors are very small and incidental findings. There is insufficient clinical evidence that they are functional or responsible or the result of hypertension

Clinical features

- Most common renal tumors, found in autopsy series (10% to 40%)
- Nongrowing or slowing growing lesions
- Small typically <1 cm, well-circumscribed nodules
- Hardly any clinical significance or related to clinical symptoms

Gross pathology

- Small solid nodules, a few millimeters or 1 to 2 cm in size, with white or tan cut surface (Fig. 35-23)
- Located in the renal medullary portion (Fig. 35-24)

Histology

- Tumor is well circumscribed, composed of spindle cells of low cellularity (Fig. 35-25)
- Trapped renal tubules are occasionally seen (Fig. 35-26)

Immunohistochemistry

- Smooth muscle actin positive and COX 2 positive
- ER/PR, CD34, S100 negative
- Rarely necessary in clinical practice

Differential diagnosis

Angiomyolipoma

- Large medullary fibroma should be investigated further to exclude angiomyolipoma (AML)
- AML is more cellular than medullary fibroma
- Abnormal vessels and adipose tissue present
- AML positive for HMB45

Clinical relevance (prognosis and treatment options)

- Benign, no treatment necessary
- A very common renal tumor, but the least important clinically

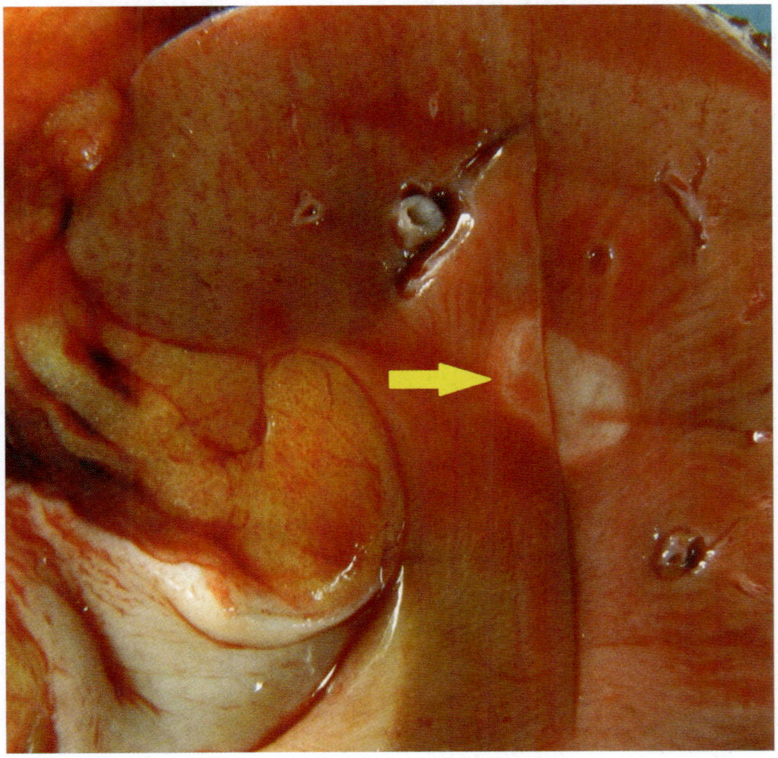

Figure 35-23.
Gross photo of a renal medullary fibroma indicated by arrow.

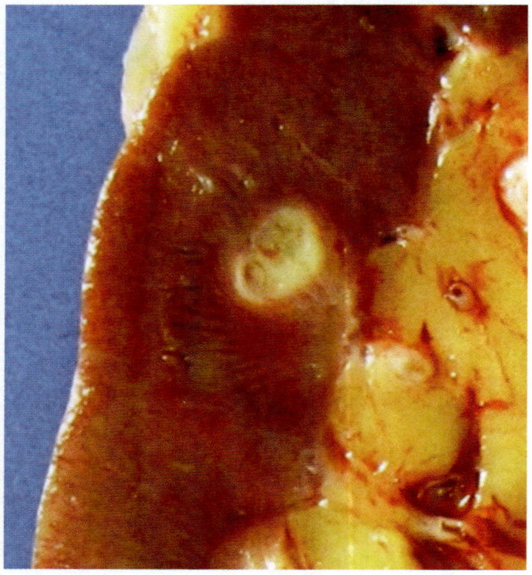

Figure 35-24.
Another case of renal medullary fibroma is a white-yellow mass located in the medulla.

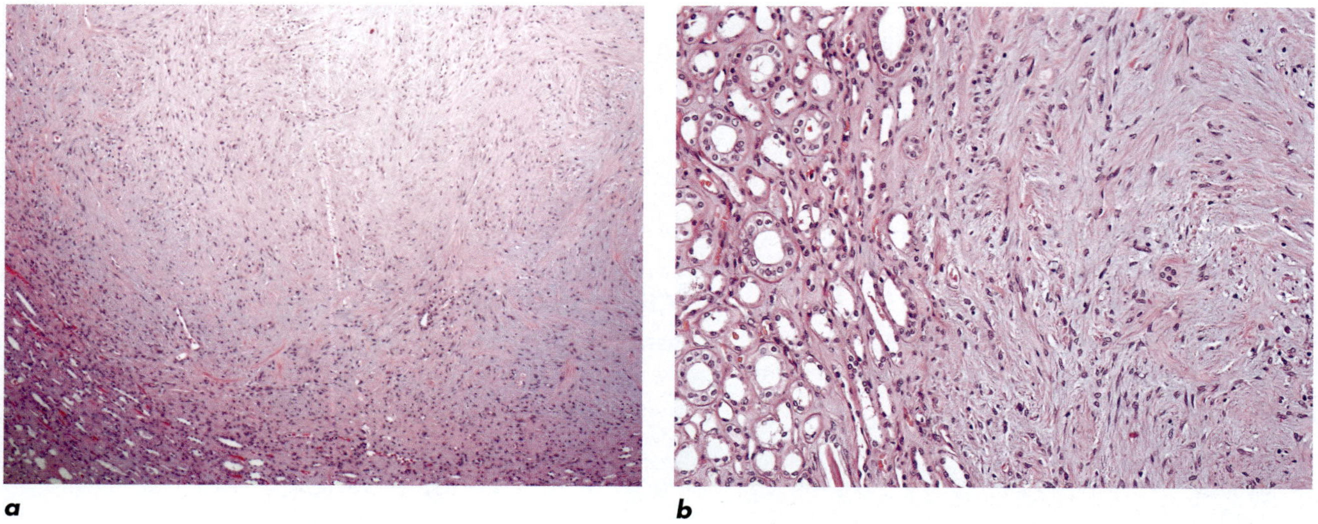

Figure 35-25.
Typical medullary fibroma with bland spindle cells of low cellularity (*a*). High magnification shows bland spindle cells and myxoid matrix (*b*).

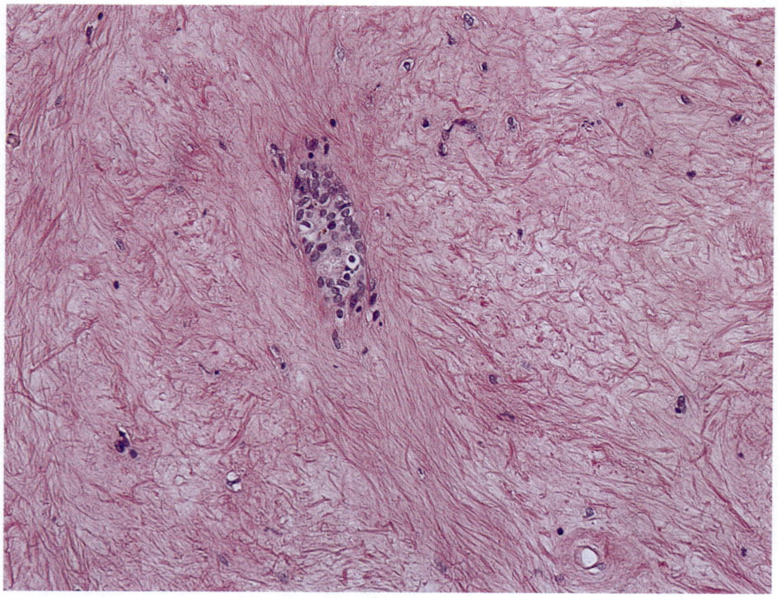

Figure 35-26.
Medullary fibroma showing scar-like appearance with trapped renal tubule.

RENAL ANGIOMYOLIPOMA

Definition

- A renal mesenchymal neoplasm composed of three components at a variable proportion: abnormal blood vessels, cells with smooth muscle features, and mature adipose tissue

Pathogenesis and epidemiology

- Angiomyolipoma (AML) is believed to be derived from perivascular epithelioid cells (PEC). Therefore, AML is also named perivascular epithelioid cell tumor (PECOMA), which may also develop in other organs such as liver
- AML accounts for 1% of all renal tumors in surgical specimens
- AML can be sporadic or familial if associated with tuberous sclerosis (TS)
- TS patients develop AML earlier, the mean age at diagnosis is 25 to 35 years for TS patients, while 40 to 45 years for non-TS patients
- The incidence of AML in non-TS is higher in females than in males, with a female to male ratio of 4:1
- Sporadic AMLs are four to five times more common than TS-associated AMLs

Clinical features

- Clinical presentations in patients with TS may be different from those without TS
- In TS patients, AMLs are usually asymptomatic and detected by imaging studies
- Patients without TS may present with renal mass lesions with typical symptoms of flank pain, hematuria, or palpable mass, which are similar to those of RCC
- One of the common clinical manifestations of AML is hemorrhage, because of the rupture of abnormal vessels in AML. Therefore, intra-abdominal bleeding could be an uncommon presentation initially or during observation follow-up

Gross pathology

- AMLs typically develop within the renal parenchyma, also it can be located on the renal capsule (Fig. 35-27)
- Tumors are typically well-circumscribed masses, with or without lobulation (Fig. 35-28). Sometimes, they may have subtly infiltrating edges
- Most AMLs are tan to white in color, although they can be slightly variable in color ranging from yellow to pink, depending on its lipid content (Figs. 35-27 and 35-28)
- AMLs are firm to rubbery in texture, epithelioid AMLs tend to be softer
- Hemorrhage and cystic changes are common (Fig. 35-29), necrosis is usually not seen

Histology

- AML is typically composed of three components (Fig. 35-30): vessels (angio), spindle cells (myo), and adipose tissue (lipo)
- Vessels typically are eccentric thick walled, which is the origin of bleeding (Fig. 35-31)

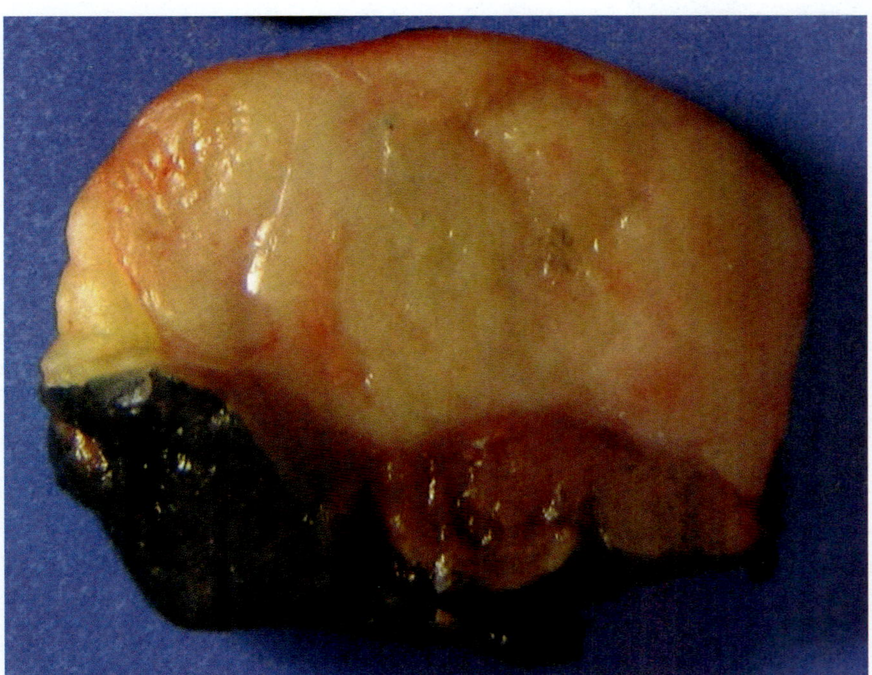

Figure 35-27.
Angiomyolipoma (AML) in a partial nephrectomy specimen demonstrates a tan-yellow homogenous cut surface.

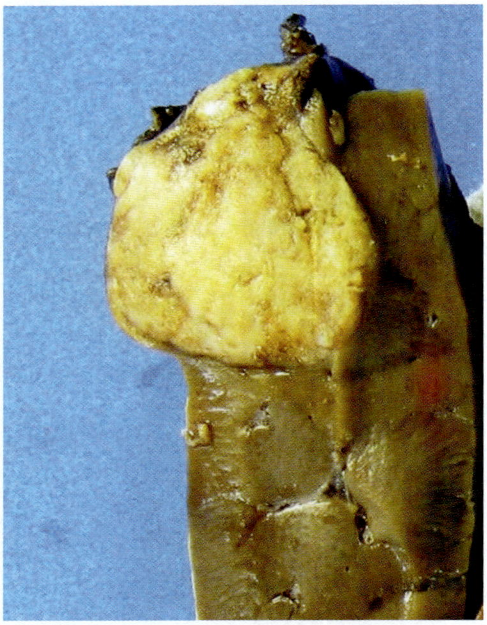

Figure 35-28.
Angiomyolipoma shows the yellow-white cut surface with focal hemorrhage.

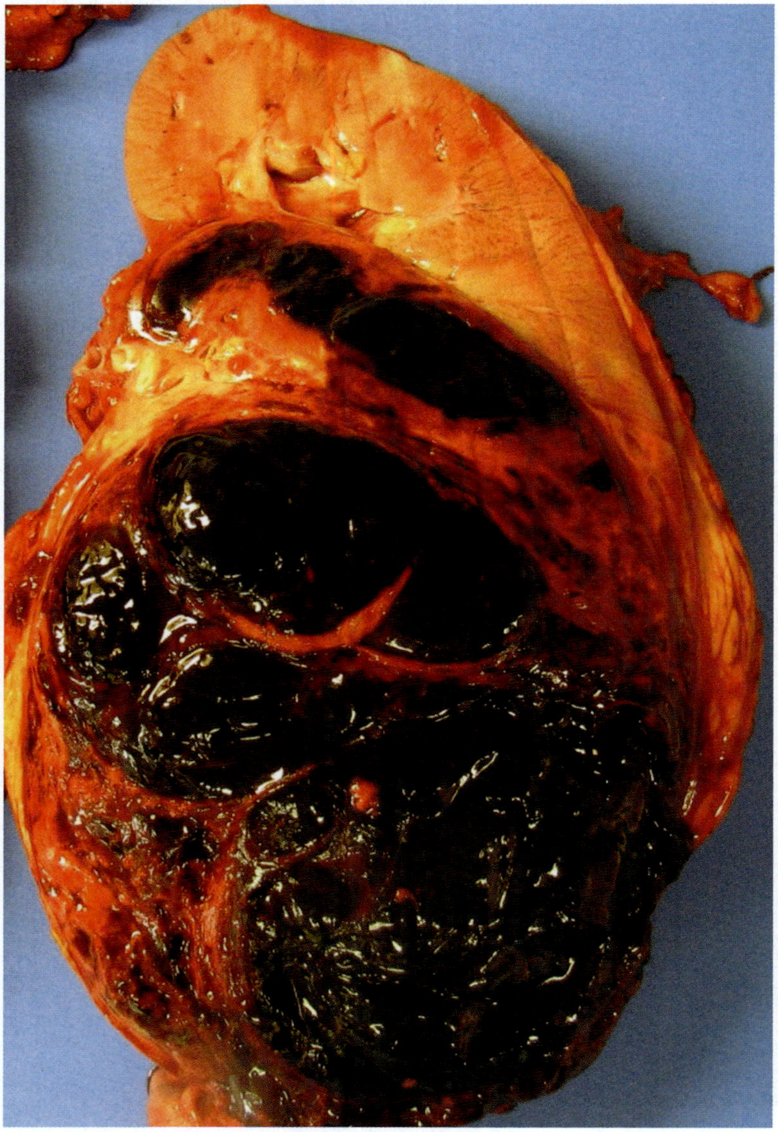

Figure 35-29.
A large renal angiomyolipoma showing extensive hemorrhage, which is a common complication of this tumor.

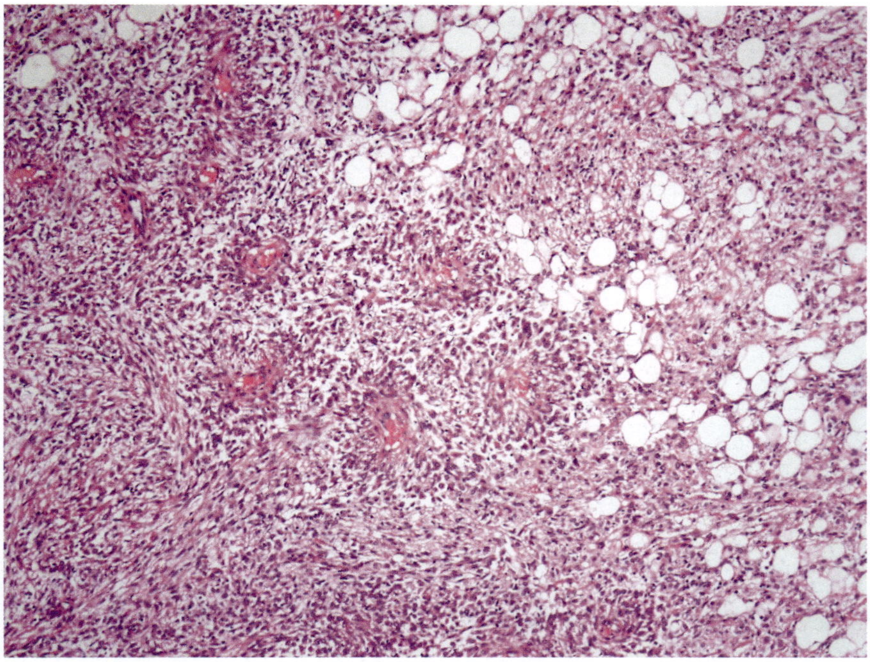

Figure 35-30.
Typical histology of renal angiomyolipoma with three components: blood vessels, spindle cells, and adipose tissue.

Figure 35-31.
Angiomyolipoma contains large thick-walled vessels surrounded by spindle cells and adipocytes (*a*). One of the abnormal vessels shows uneven thickness of the wall (*b*).

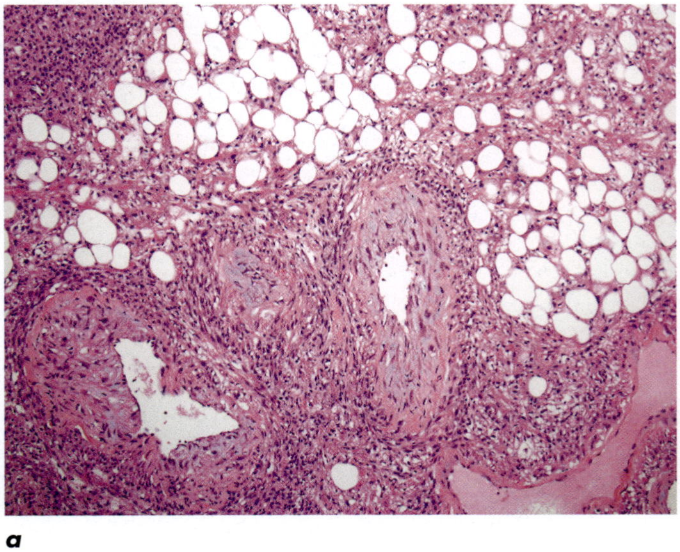

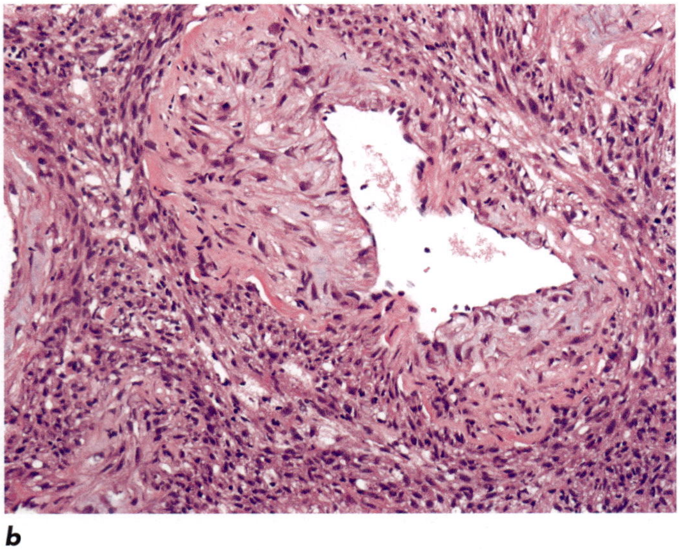

- Spindle tumor cells have the features of smooth muscle with blunt-end elongated nuclei (Figs. 35-31 to 35-34) and eosinophilic cytoplasm. However, most of these spindle cells are not mature looking. They range from mature-appearing smooth muscle cells, immature spindle cells, and epithelioid cells with or without clear cytoplasm to bizzard-looking cells with degenerative nuclear atypia
- Adipocytes, which are intermingled with spindle cells, are mature without cytological atypia (Fig. 35-32)
- Focal epithelial appearance can be seen (Fig. 35-33)
- Hyalinization or calcification could also be present (Fig. 35-34)
- The presence focal nuclear atypia or high cellularity of spindle cells is not associated with malignant behaviors. However, this tumor can be mistaken for RCCs or sarcomas
- Although renal AML was considered a hamartoma, it has been shown to be a neoplasm. A hamartoma is defined as an overgrowth of mature tissues normally present in the affected organ. However, the major component of AML are smooth muscle cells, which are abnormal with a high cellularity and sometimes atypia, rather than mature smooth muscle cells

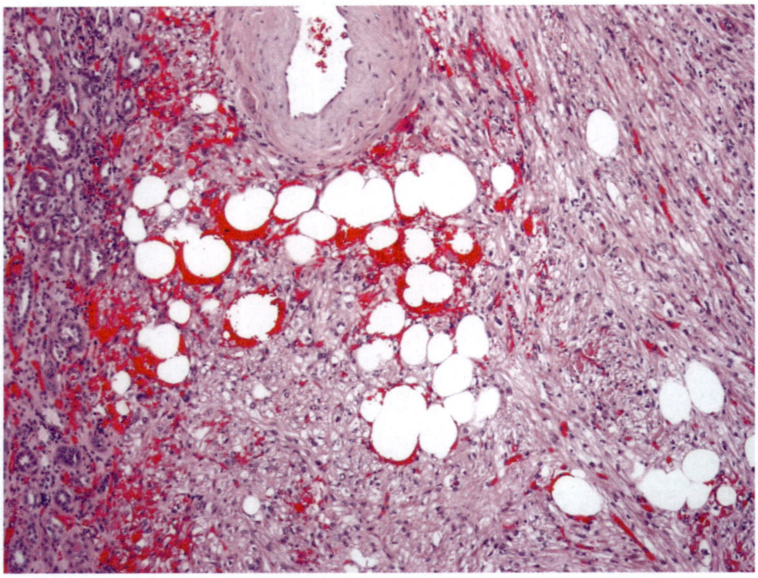

Figure 35-32.
Angiomyolipoma with focal hemorrhage.

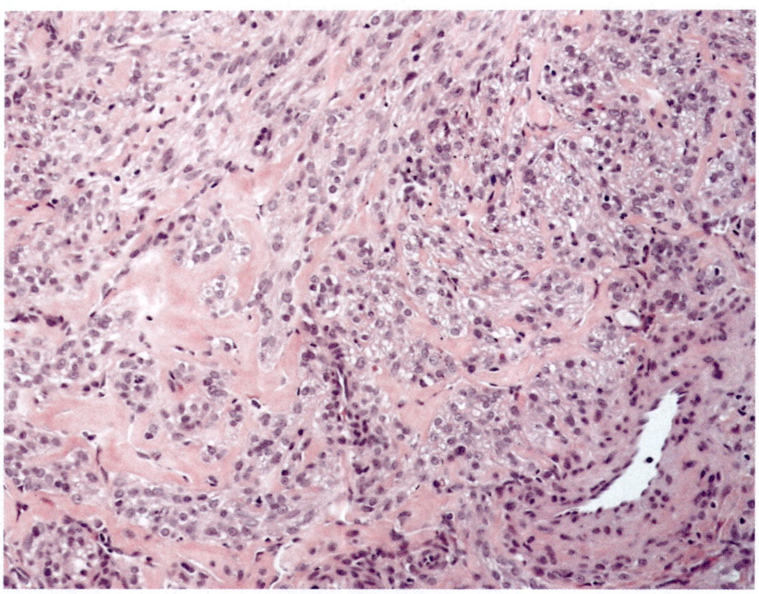

Figure 35-33.
Angiomyolipoma with increased cellularity and focal epithelioid changes, but not sufficient for epithelioid angiomyolipoma.

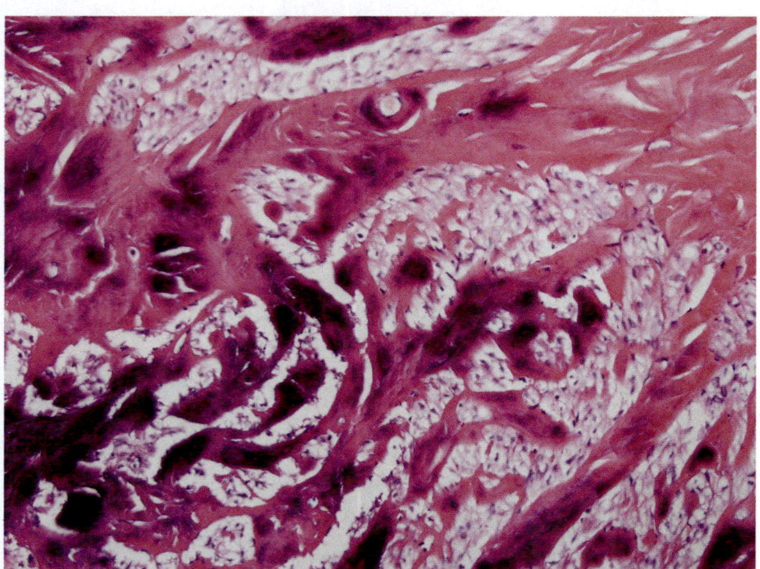

Figure 35-34.
Angiomyolipoma with an area of hyalinization and calcification.

Immunohistochemistry and special study

- HMB45 is positive in the tumor cells (Fig. 35-35)
- The HMB45 positivity can be very focal, multiple sections with immunostaining may be necessary for finding the HMB45 positive cells
- Smooth muscle markers such as smooth muscle actin are positive
- Keratins and other epithelial markers negative even in epithelioid AML variants

Figure 35-35.
Renal angiomyolipoma, with typical tricomponents (*a*). The spindle cells around a vessel (*b*). The tumor cells are positive for melan A (*c*) and HMB45 (*d*).

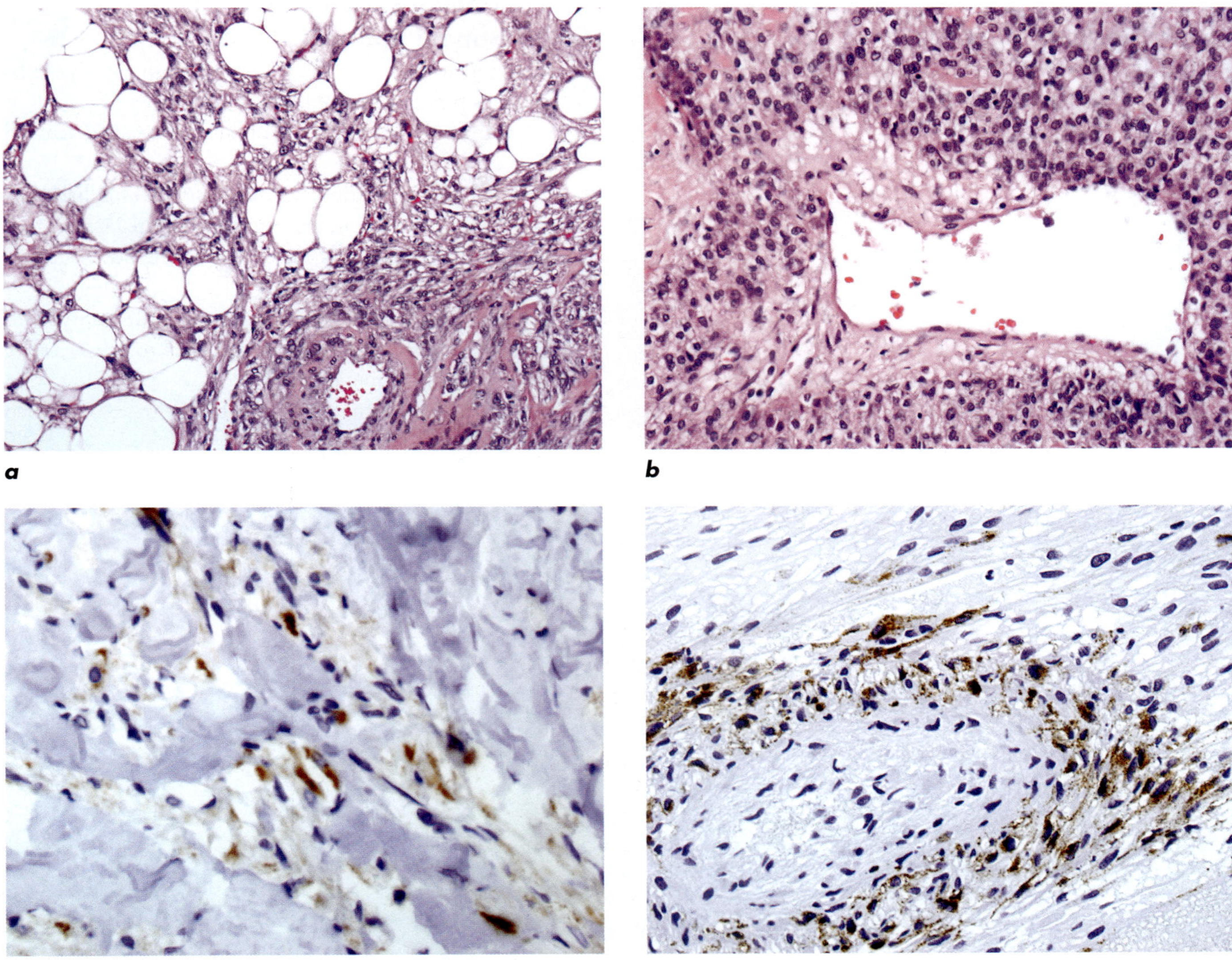

a b c d

Molecular diagnostics

- The molecular signature of AML is different from those of other renal neoplasms
- No molecular diagnostic markers have been used in clinical practice

Differential diagnosis

Renal cell carcinoma

- Clear cell RCCs typically have "chicken-wire" vascular patterns
- Papillary RCC is characterized by the presence of papillary configurations
- These features are not present in AMLs
- The eccentric thick-walled vessels typical of AML are not seen in RCC
- High-grade RCC shows much more prominent cytological atypia
- Renal cell markers such as CA9, AMACR, or keratin markers are positive in RCC, not in AML
- Chromophobe RCC is positive for C-kit, although a small subset of AML can also be positive for C-kit

Sarcoma particularly leiomyosarcoma

- Most leiomyosarcomas are typically located in the renal capsule unlike AML located in renal parenchyma
- Leiomyosarcoma typically have high cellularity, frequent mitotic activity along with cytological atypia
- While high cellularity and frequent mitoses are not common features of AML
- Furthermore, leiomyosarcoma are positive for smooth muscle markers such as smooth muscle actin, muscle-specific actin and desmin, but negative for HMB45

Myelolipoma

- Myelolipoma, located in adrenal not the kidney, is composed of adipose tissue and bone marrow elements. Spindle cells are not component of the tumor

Clinical relevance (prognosis and treatment options)

- The vast majority of renal AMLs are benign, which can be cured by surgical resection
- Large tumors may have the risk of hemorrhage as discussed earlier
- If a preoperative pathologic diagnosis is established, a small AML may be followed without immediate surgery. These small AML have a lower risk for hemorrhage and associated with malignancy
- Epithelioid AML is uncommon variant or subtype of renal AML, which may have the potential to be aggressive or even developing metastasis
- Occasionally, AML may be associated with RCC, which can also be life threatening

HISTOLOGICAL VARIANTS OF ANGIOMYOLIPOMA

Monomorphic (spindle cell) angiomyolipoma

- These tumors are usually small and composed of spindle cells in addition to the presence of blood vessels, but adipose tissue is not seen (Fig. 35-36*a*)
- Most of these tumors are found incidentally in the nephrectomy specimens performed for other purposes, therefore, with very limited clinical significance
- The confirmation of diagnosis is based on the HMB45 immunoreactivity of the spindle cells (Fig. 35-36*b*)

Epithelioid angiomyolipoma

- Epithelioid variant of renal AML is characterized by the presence of epithelioid cells in an AML (Fig. 35-37)
- In contrast to typical spindle cells appearance, these tumor cells may be round, ovoid, or pleomorphic in shape (Fig. 35-37*a* and *b*). Sometimes, they may have clear cytoplasm resembling RCC (Fig. 35-37*c*) or bubbling cytoplasm (Fig. 35-37*d*)
- Despite of their appearance, the epithelioid tumors cells are stromal cell in nature, they typically do not express keratins. They are positive for HMB45 and smooth muscle markers, similar to typical spindle cells in AML
- Epithelioid appearance can be observed in many of renal AMLs, ranging from a small cluster of epithelioid cells to extensive epithelioid cells. There is a lack of agreement on the definition of epithelioid AML quantitatively. Some investigators use 10%, while others use 50% to 90%
- There is also controversy on the behavior of epithelioid AML
- Some investigators believe that all epithelioid AMLs should be considered malignant or potentially malignant because of all the reported malignant AMLs often show epithelioid features
- Studies have shown that the majority of epithelioid AML are benign since malignant AMLs are very rare with only a handful cases reported
- Therefore, we believe that generally an epithelioid AML should be considered a benign tumor
- However, a pure epithelioid AML (which is rare) has a much higher risk to be malignant particularly if they are big (greater than 7 cm), associated with necrosis, significant cytological atypia and carcinoma-like growth patterns.

Angiomyolipoma with cytological atypia

- Sometimes cytological atypia can be seen in an AML (Fig. 35-38)
- The cytological atypia can be seen in spindle cells or epithelioid tumor cells
- Atypia is usually focal, not affecting the entire tumor
- Typically the atypical cells show degenerative atypia with smudged chromatin (Fig. 35-39)
- AML with focal cytological atypia does not correlate with an aggressive behavior; however, it might be mistaken for a malignant tumor

Figure 35-36.
Spindle cell angiomyolipoma composed of spindle cells only with no adipose tissue seen (*a*). HMB45 positivity (*b*) in the tumor cells confirms the diagnosis of angiomyolipoma.

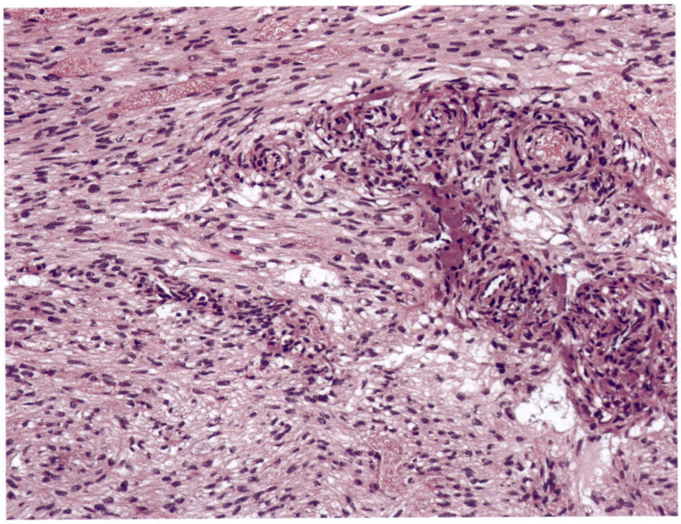

a

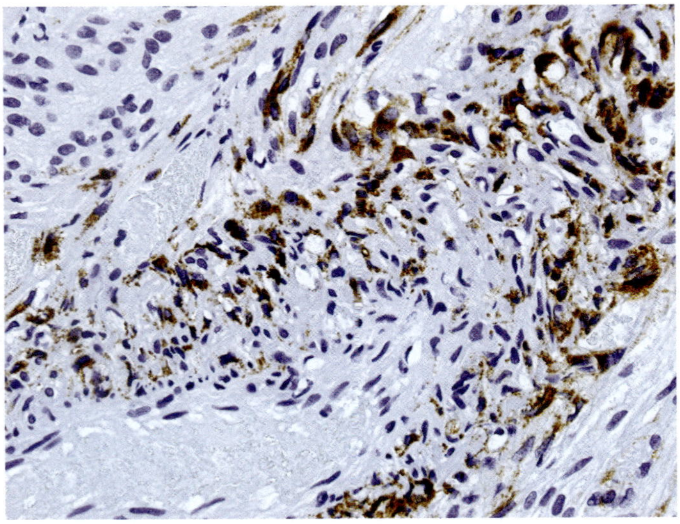

b

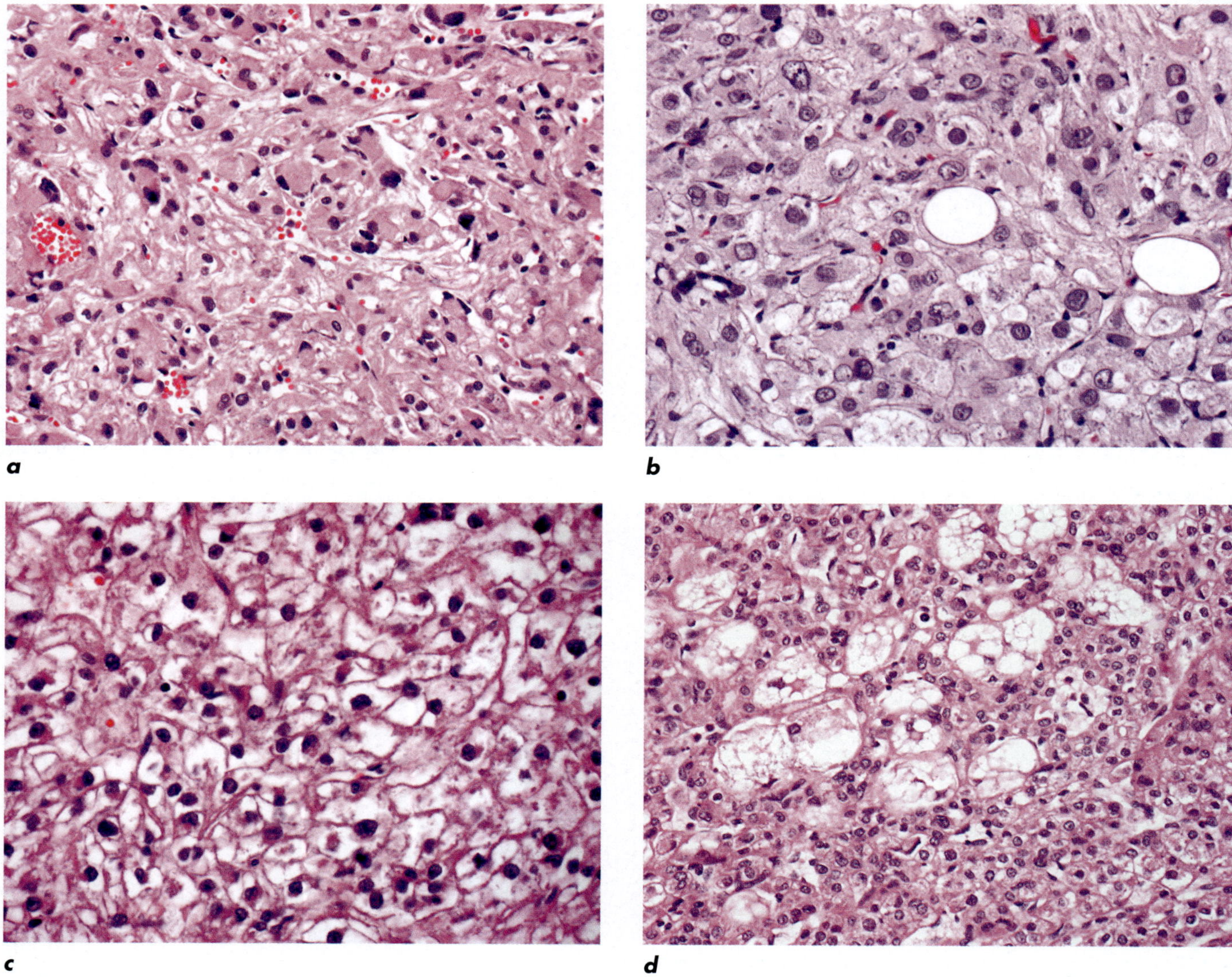

Figure 35-37.
Epithelioid angiomyolipoma (AML). Epithelioid AML cells with eosinophilic cytoplasm (*a*), epithelioid cells with atypia (*b*), clear cytoplasm (*c*), which can be easily confused with clear cell renal cell carcinoma, or bubbling cytoplasm with vacuoles mimicking lipoblasts (*d*).

Cystic angiomyolipoma

- In addition to the typical components of AML, this tumor contains cystic spaces
- Cysts are lined by benign cuboidal epithelial cells (Fig. 35-40)
- It is not clear that the cysts are actual neoplastic components of the lesions or entrapped renal tubules
- Nevertheless, the spindle cells show immunoreactivity for HMB45. The adipocytes may not be obvious

Malignant angiomyolipoma

- Malignant AMLs are very rare, probably represents malignant transformations of benign AML
- Coexisting clear cell RCC with benign AML (Fig. 35-41) is not a true malignant AML, which is more common than a malignant AML
- There are only a dozen of malignant AML cases reported in literature with sufficient documentation

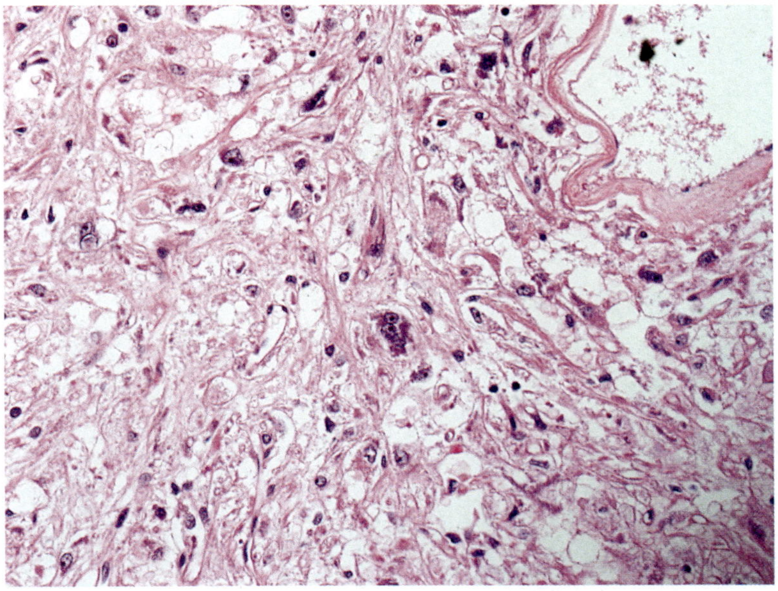

Figure 35-38.
Angiomyolipoma showing degenerative nuclear atypia of tumor cells with smudged chromatins.

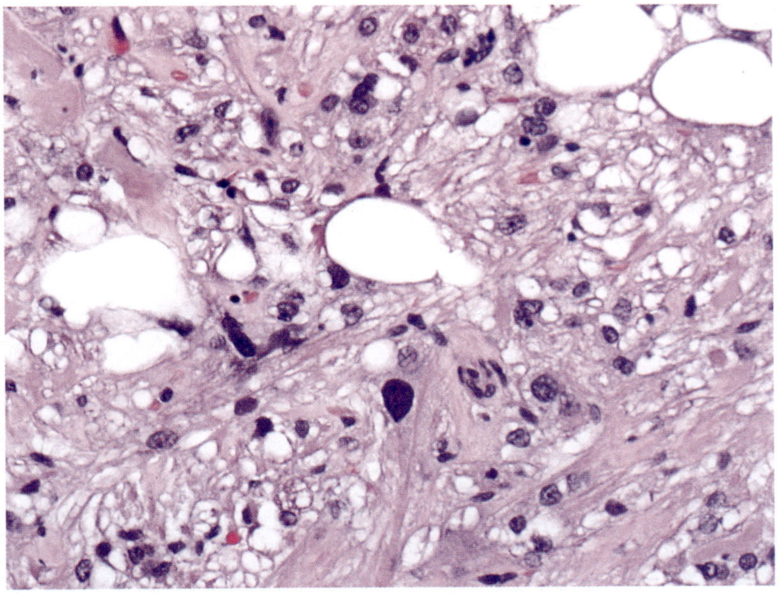

Figure 35-39.
Angiomyolipoma with atypical spindle cells.

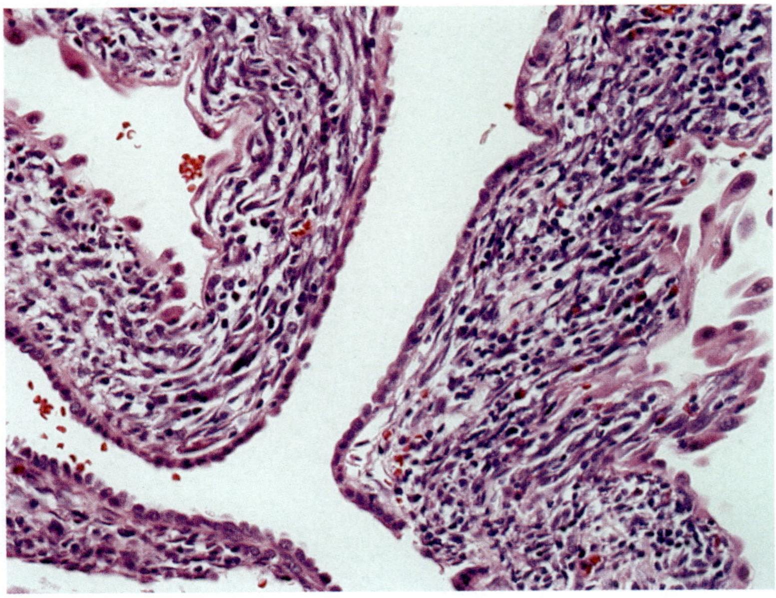

Figure 35-40.
Cystic angiomyolipoma containing cystic spaces lined by benign epithelial cells.

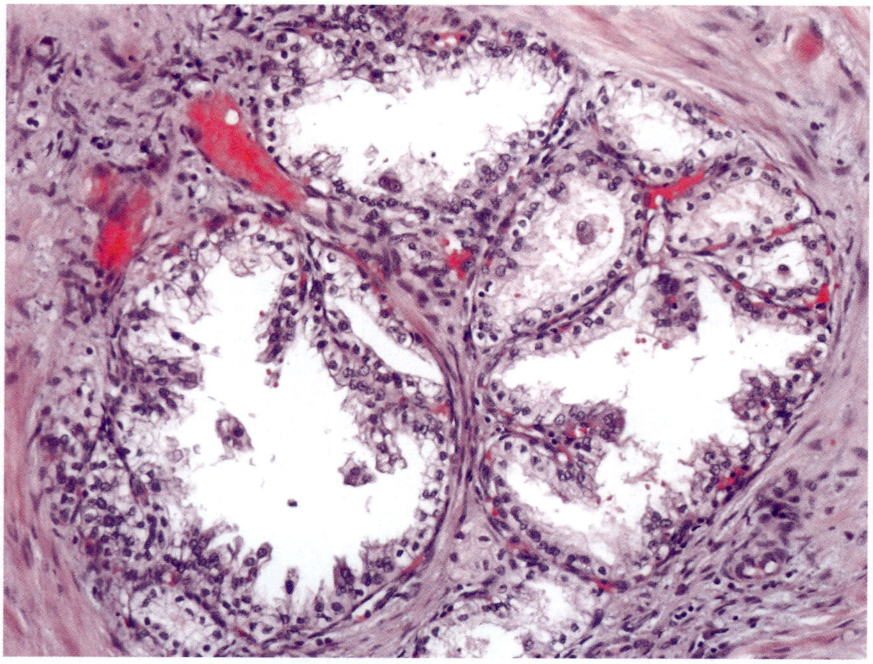

Figure 35-41.
Clear cell renal cell carcinoma associated with an angiomyolipoma. A classic clear cell renal cell carcinoma found adjacent to a benign renal angiomyolipoma.

- The definitive evidence of true malignancy is that these malignant tumors caused metastases and fatalities (Fig. 35-42)
- Sometimes, the cytological atypia can be very prominent in an AML but no evidence of metastasis after resection
- AML may occur in other locations such as the liver or even pelvic lymph nodes
- Therefore, the presence of benign-appearing AML component in the pelvic lymph nodes is not evidence of malignancy
- The morphological variants of AML are summarized in Table 35-1

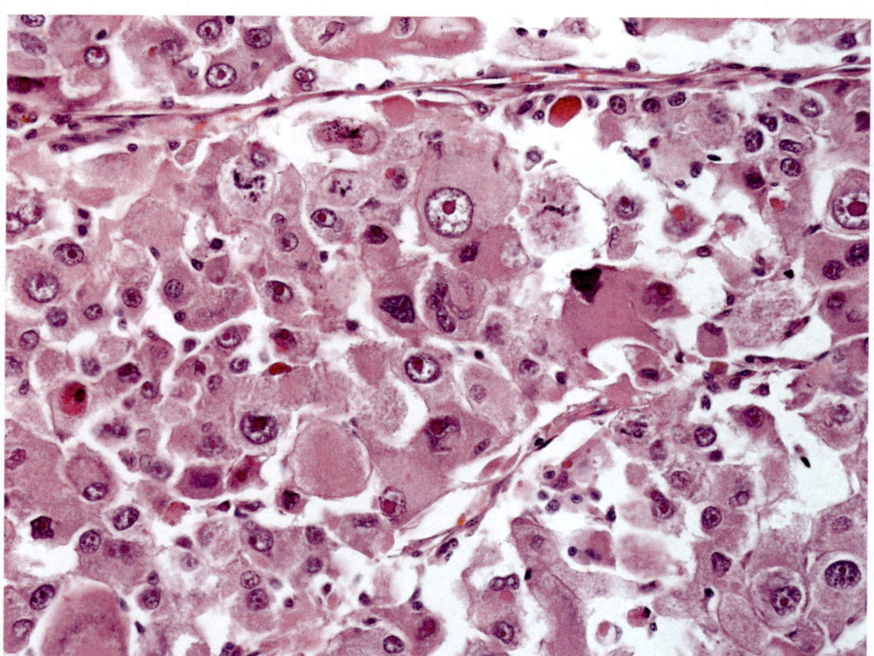

Figure 35-42.
Malignant angiomyolipoma. In addition to the typical AML component, the malignant component contains marked pleomorphic tumor cells with bizzard nuclei and numerous atypical mitotic figures. The patient with this tumor eventually died of lung metastasis shortly after diagnosis.

Table 35-1. Comparison of Angiomyolipoma (AML) Variants

	Component	*Behavior*
Typical AML	Vessels, spindle cells, and adipose tissue	Benign
Monomorphic AML	Spindle cells, no adipocytes	Benign
Cystic AML	Cystic lining similar to renal tubules	Benign
AML with atypia	Typical AML with focal degenerative atypia	Benign
Epithelioid AML	AML with epithelioid features at least 10% of the cells	Mostly benign, some cases may be aggressive
Malignant AML	Pleomorphic cells	Vary rare
AML associated with RCC	Coexisting of RCC and AML	Behavior depending on the coexisting RCC

AML, angiomyolipoma; RCC, renal cell carcinoma.

JUXTAGLOMERULAR CELL TUMOR

Definition

- A renal neoplasm derived from specialized smooth muscle cells that comprise the vasculature of the juxtaglomerular apparatus
- A benign renin-secreting tumor

Other term

- Reninoma

Pathogenesis

- It has a phenotype of juxtaglomerular apparatus

Clinical features

- A rare tumor with only fewer than 100 cases reported in literature
- Developing in younger individual with mean age 27 years
- Severe hypertension in a young patient, which is poorly controlled or difficult to control by medical treatment
- High serum renin and marked hypokalemia (effect by renin) are also present
- Imaging studies reveal the presence of a renal mass

Gross pathology

- Solitary, solid well-circumscribed mass, typically small, 2 to 3 cm in size
- Yellow to tan cut surface

Histology

- Juxtaglomerular cell tumor is composed of sheets of small polygonal or spindle cells, next to blood vessels (Fig. 35-43)
- Tumor cells have a well-defined cell border with clear or eosinophilic cytoplasm
- Tumor cells appear to be associated with vessels as hemangiopericytic patterns (Fig. 35-34)

Immunohistochemistry

- Renin positive
- Vimentin and CD34 positive (Fig. 35-34c)

Ultrastructure analysis

- Abundant rough endoplasmic reticulum, numerous peripherally located sharply angulated renin granules

Clinical relevance (prognosis and treatment options)

- Typically benign, no metastasis reported
- Surgical removal, particularly partial nephrectomy, is the treatment of choice

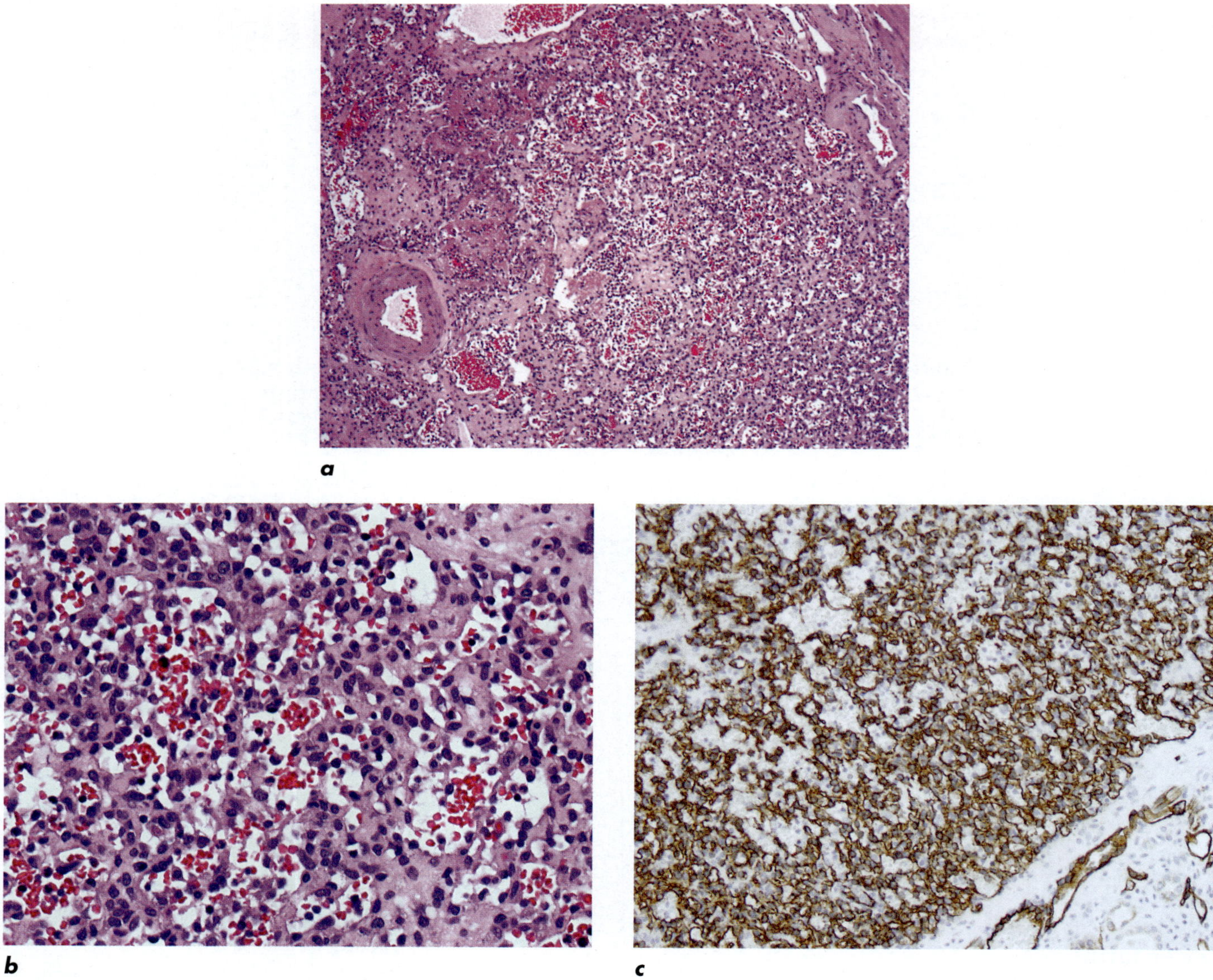

Figure 35-43.

Juxtaglomerular cell tumor from a patient with high serum renin level and hypertension. The tumor is composed of small polygonal cells closely associated with blood vessels (*a*). High magnification shows the cuboidal tumor cells in perivascular patterns (*b*), which is confirmed by positive CD34 immunostaining in tumor cells (*c*).

CHAPTER 36

Immunohistochemical Markers for Classification of Renal Neoplasms

Ximing J. Yang, Fan Lin, Liwei Jia

There are many different types of renal neoplastic lesions. A panel of immunohistochemical markers will be useful for an accurate classification. Only some of commonly used markers are discussed in this chapter and summarized in Table 36-1.

Table 36-1. Summary of Common Immunostaining Markers in Renal Epithelial Neoplasms

Antibody	*Clear cell RCC*	*Papillary RCC*	*Chromophobe RCC*	*Oncocytoma*	*MTSCC*	*Urothelial carcinoma*
EMA	+	+	+	+	+	+
CK7	−	+	+	−	+	+
CK20	−	−	−	−	−	+ or −
CK903	−	−	−	−	−	+
P63	−	−	−	−	−	+
CD10	+	+	− or +	− or +	−	−
KIM-1	+	+	−	−	N/A	−
PAX2/PAX8	+	+	+ or −	+	−	−
RCCMa	+	+	− or +	−	−	−
CD117	−	−	+	+	−	−
S100A1	+	+ or −	−	+	−	−
S100P	−	−	−	−	−	+
GATA3	−	−	−	−	−	+
GST-α	+	− or +	−	− or +	−	N/A
Vimentin	+	+ or −	−	−	−	−
TFE3[a]	−	−	−	−	−	−
AMACR (P504S)	− or +	+	−	−	+ or −	−
CAIX	+	+	−	−	N/A	+
UEA1	−	−	−	−	−	+

Note: +, usually greater than 70% of cases are positive; −, less than 5% of cases are positive; + or−, usually more than 50% of cases are positive; − or +, less than 50% of cases are positive.

AMACR, α-methylacyl-CoA racemase; CAIX, carbonic anhydrase 9; CK7, cytokeratin; CK20, cytokeratin 20; EMA, epithelial membrane antigen; KIM-1, kidney injury molecule; MTSCC, mucinous tubule and spindle cell carcinoma; N/A, data not available; PAX2/PAX8, paired box gene 2 or 8; UEA1, uroplakin.

[a]TFE3 antibody is positive (nuclear staining) in TFE3 translocation carcinoma, not in normal kidney tissue or other RCC.

EMA (EPITHELIAL MEMBRANE ANTIGEN)

- Nonspecific epithelial marker
- Positive in almost all renal cell neoplasms as well as urothelial neoplasm
- Has little value in classification of renal tumors

CK7 (CYTOKERATIN 7)

- Normally present in distal tubules
- Strongly positive in papillary RCC (Fig. 36-1*a*)
- High-grade papillary RCC tends to loss CK7, so that CK7 positivity can be focal
- Strongly positive in chromophobe RCC, but negative in oncocytoma
- Positive in tubulocystic RCC but may be focal
- Patchy positivity in oncocytic hybrid tumors of the Birt-Hogg-Dube (BHD) patients
- Major utility: determine chromophobe RCC and papillary RCC

Figure 36-1.
CK7 immunoreactivity in a papillary adenoma (*a*). CD10 positivity in a clear cell RCC (*b*). PAX8 nuclear staining in a clear cell RCC (*c*). C-kit immunoreactivity in a chromophobe RCC (*d*).

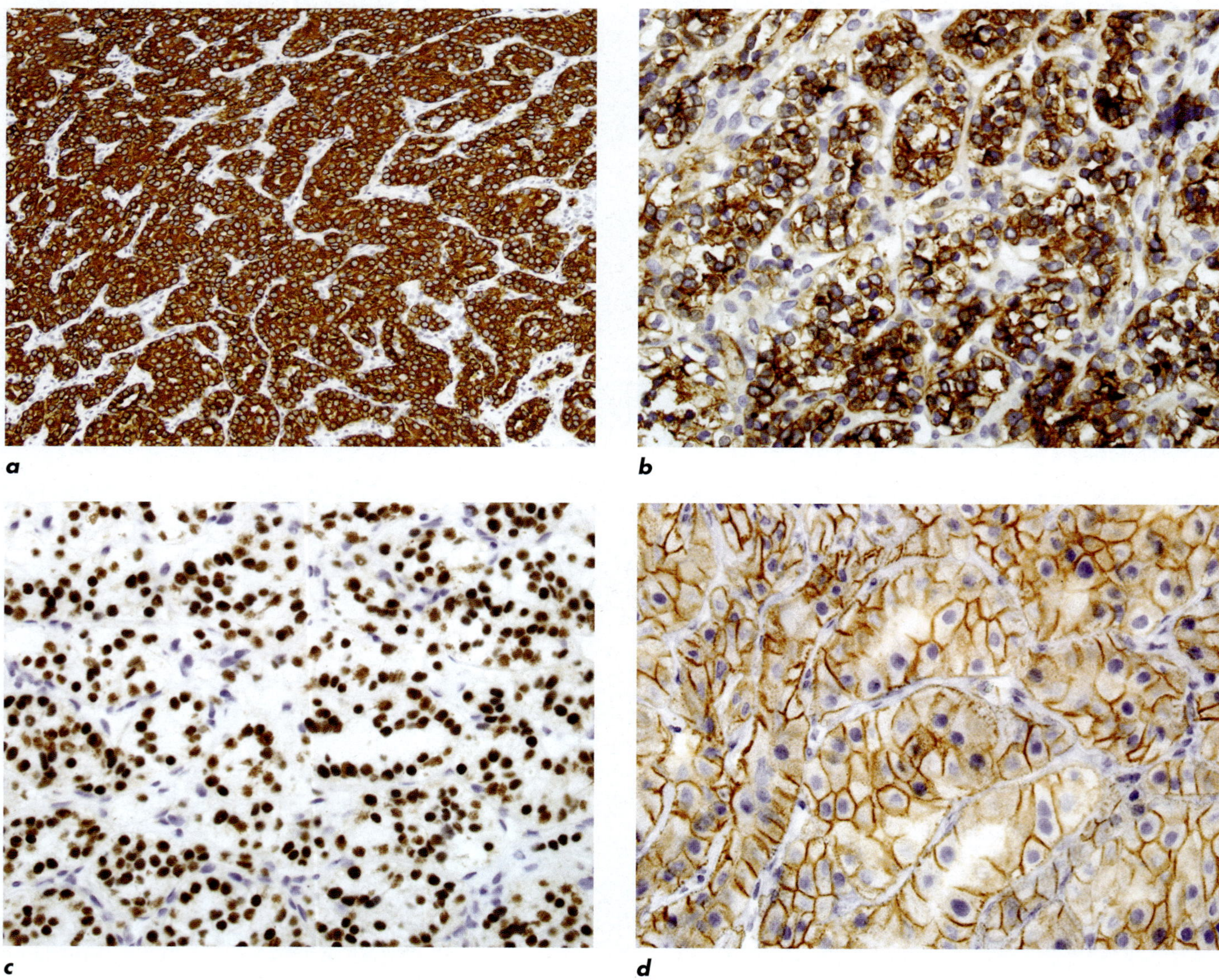

a *b* *c* *d*

CK20 (CYTOKERATIN 20)

- Normally present in the umbrella cells of the urothelium
- Diffusely positive in the majority of urothelial neoplasms
- Immunoreactivity for both CK20 and CK7 in a renal tumor is suggestive of urothelial carcinoma
- Variable in reactive urothelial lesions
- Negative in the majority of renal cell neoplasms including all common types of RCCs

CK903 (HIGH MOLECULAR WEIGHT CYTOKERATINS)

- Similar to (CK5/CK6)
- Normally positive in the urothelium
- Positive in urothelial carcinoma
- Negative in the majority of RCC, except collecting duct carcinoma

P63

- Similar to high molecular weight cytokeratins
- Normally present in the urothelium
- Nuclear staining without background problem
- Positive in urothelial carcinoma
- Positive in benign urothelial lesions
- Positive in squamous cell carcinoma
- Negative in different types of renal cell neoplasm
- Major utility: determine urothelial origin

CD10

- Normally present in renal tubules
- Higher positive rate in clear cell RCC (Fig. 36-1*b*) and papillary RCC
- Lower positive rate in chromophobe RCC and oncocytomas
- Negative in urothelial carcinoma
- Limited value in classification of renal cell neoplasms

KIM-1 (KIDNEY INJURY MOLECULE 1)

- Positive in clear cell RCC and papillary RCC
- Negative in urothelial carcinoma
- Negative in the vast majority of carcinoma of other organs
- One of the highly specific antibodies for RCC
- But this antibody is not commercially available yet

PAX2/PAX8 (PAIRED BOX GENE 2 OR 8)

- Normally present in the renal tubules
- Good nuclear staining
- Relatively specific renal marker, especially for males
- Also present in some tumors of female genital organs
- Positive for all types of renal cell neoplasms (Fig. 36-1*c*)
- Positive in male genital organs such as seminal vesicles, epididymis, and rete testis
- Positive in nephrogenic adenoma
- Negative or weak in urothelial carcinoma
- Major utility: determine the renal origin

RCCMa (RENAL CELL CARCINOMA MARKER)

- Positive in clear cell RCC and papillary RCC
- Lower positive rate for chromophobe RCC
- Negative for urothelial carcinoma
- Generally low specificity and low sensitivity for RCC (50% to 70%) limiting its value in classification of RCC

CD117 (C-KIT)

- Normally present in proximal renal tubules
- Positive for chromophobe RCC (Fig. 36-1*d*) and oncocytoma
- Negative or very low positive for other renal cell neoplasm
- Negative for the majority of sarcomatoid RCC
- Occasionally positive for papillary RCC, particularly oncocytic papillary RCC
- Occasionally positive for renal angiomyolipoma (10%)
- Major utility: determine or rule out chromophobe RCC and oncocytoma

S100A1

- Negative for chromophobe RCC
- Positive for oncocytoma
- Positive for clear cell RCC and papillary RCC
- Negative for urothelial carcinoma
- Majority utility: distinguish chromophobe RCC from oncocytoma

S100P

- Normally present in trophoblasts in the placenta (placental S100)
- Positive for urothelial carcinoma
- Sensitivity can be variable depending on the antibody
- Positive in benign reactive urothelial lesions
- Negative in all types of RCC
- Negative in the vast majority of carcinoma from other organs
- Major utility: determine the urothelial origin

VIMENTIN

- Positive in clear cell RCC (Fig. 36-2*a*) and papillary RCC
- Negative in chromophobe RCC and oncocytoma
- Negative for urothelial carcinoma
- Major utility: determine the nature of common RCC (clear cell RCC and papillary RCC)

GATA3

- Highly specific marker for urothelial carcinoma (Fig. 36-2*b*)
- Clear nuclear staining with no background
- Positive in breast adenocarcinoma
- Negative in the vast majority of carcinomas from other organs
- Major utility: determine the urothelial (or breast) origin

GST-α

- Normally present in renal tubules
- Positive in clear cell RCC
- Negative or weakly positive in other types of RCC
- Because of the unreliable antibodies, the application of this antibody has been replaced by CAIX antibody (see below)

AMACR (α-METHYLACYL-CoA RACEMASE, P504S)

- Normally present in the renal tubules
- Strongly positive in papillary RCC (almost 100% sensitive) (Fig. 36-2*c*)
- Low positive rate and weaker positivity in clear cell RCC
- Low positive in papillary carcinomas of other organs
- Positive in colonic adenocarcinoma
- Positive in prostatic adenocarcinoma
- Positive for tubulocystic carcinoma
- Positive for mucinous tubule and spindle cell carcinoma
- Negative for clear cell papillary RCC
- Not specific for determining the origin of a metastatic carcinoma
- Major utility: determine papillary RCC

CAIX OR CA9 (CARBONIC ANHYDRASE 9)

- Normally not present in the renal tubules
- Positive in clear cell RCC (box-shaped strong membrane staining) (Fig. 36-2*d*)
- Positive in clear cell papillary RCC (cup-shaped membrane staining)
- Negative or weakly staining in other types of RCC
- Positive in the areas around the necrosis
- Major utility: determine clear cell RCC

TFE3

- Normally not present in the renal tissue
- Positive in TFE3 translocation carcinoma (Fig. 36-2*e*)
- Negative for other types of RCC
- Nuclear staining
- This antibody is difficult to work with
- Cytoplasmic staining and/or any staining of nonneoplastic kidney tissues indicates the nonspecific staining
- Major utility: determine TFE3 translocation tumor

UEA1 (UROPLAKIN)

- Normally present in the urothelium
- Positive in urothelial carcinoma
- Positive in collecting duct carcinoma

HMB45

- Positive in melanoma
- Positive in angiomyolipoma (Fig. 36-2*f*)
- Major utility: diagnosis of angiomyolipoma and melanoma

Figure 36-2.
Vimentin immunoreactivity in a clear cell RCC (*a*). GATA3 nuclear immunoreactivity in an invasive high-grade urothelial carcinoma (*b*). AMACR strong positive in papillary RCC (*c*). CAIX (membrane) immunostaining in a clear cell RCC (*d*). TFE3 nuclear staining in a translocation carcinoma of the kidney (*e*). Focal HMB45 positive staining in a renal angiomyolipoma (*f*).

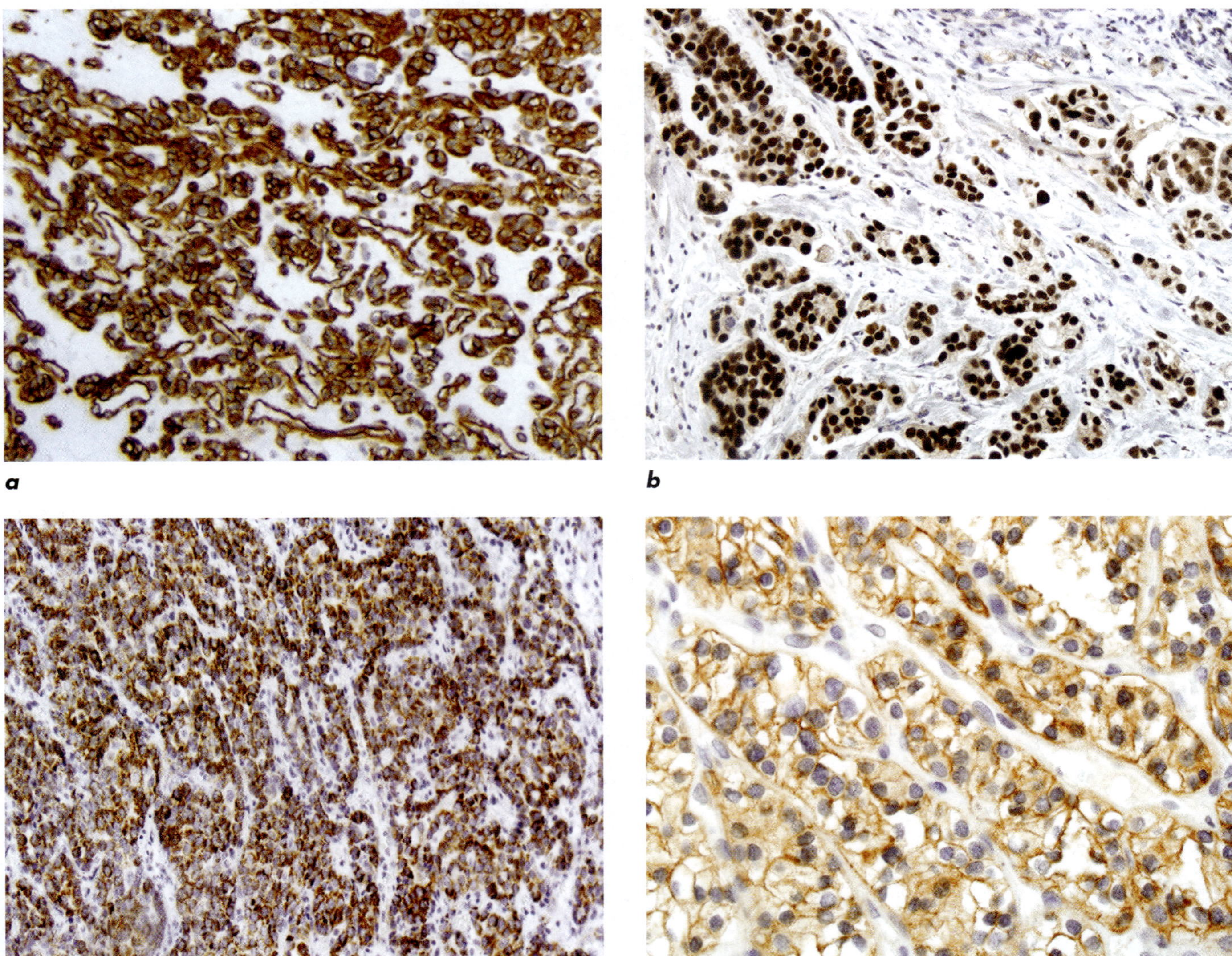

a *b* *c* *d*

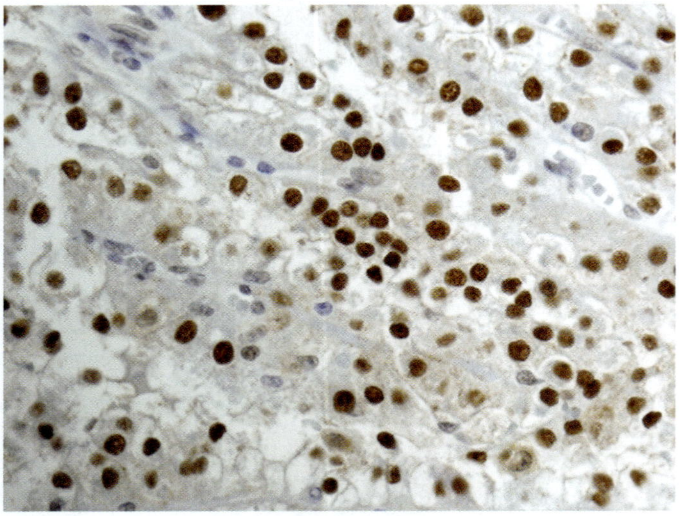

e

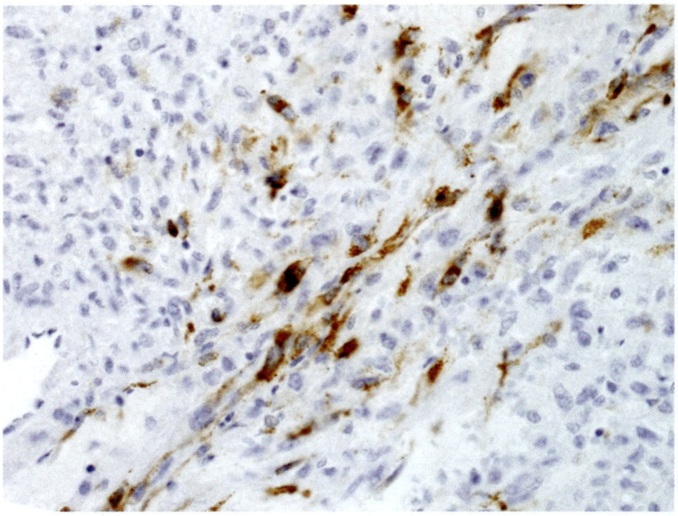

f

Figure 36-2.
(*Continued*)

CHAPTER 37

Pediatric Renal Diseases

Bing Zhu, Pauline M. Chou, Ximing J. Yang, Ondrej Hes

RENAL DYSPLASIA

Definition

- Congenital renal anomaly characterized by enlargement of kidney, cyst formation, and islands of immature mesenchyme present between cysts

Other terms

- Multicystic renal dysplasia
- Cystic renal dysplasia

Pathogenesis and epidemiology

- Most common renal cystic disease in children, affecting 1/1000 live birth
- Most cases are sporadic, familial cases have been seen
- Abnormal nephrogenesis caused by the failure of the ureteric bud to communicate with metanephric blastema

Clinical features

- Dysplasia develops in the fetal stage, sometimes can be detected before birth
- Neonatal unilateral or bilateral abdominal mass
- Fever and signs of infection because of the presence of pyelonephritis
- Often associated with malformation of other organs such as pulmonary hypoplasia, cardiac anomalies, thanatophoric dysplasia, pancreatic fibrosis, or intrahepatic biliary dysgenesis
- If blastema is present, the patient will be at a slightly higher risk for the development of Wilms tumor

Gross pathology

- The size of the affected kidney is variable, ranging from small to large
- The kidney is partially or completely replaced by multiple cysts
- The cysts are variable in size and shapes

Histology

- Disorganized primitive renal tubules and glomeruli distorted by cysts of various sizes (Fig. 37-1)
- Some immature collecting ducts lined by cuboidal epithelium tufting into the lumen (Fig. 37-2)
- Islands of undifferentiated mesenchyme, such as cartilage, can be seen in some cases (Fig. 37-3)
- The cysts are lined by flattened to cuboidal epithelium (Figs. 37-2*d* and 37-4)
- The dilated cystic ducts are cuffed by cellular spindle cell collars (Fig. 37-4)

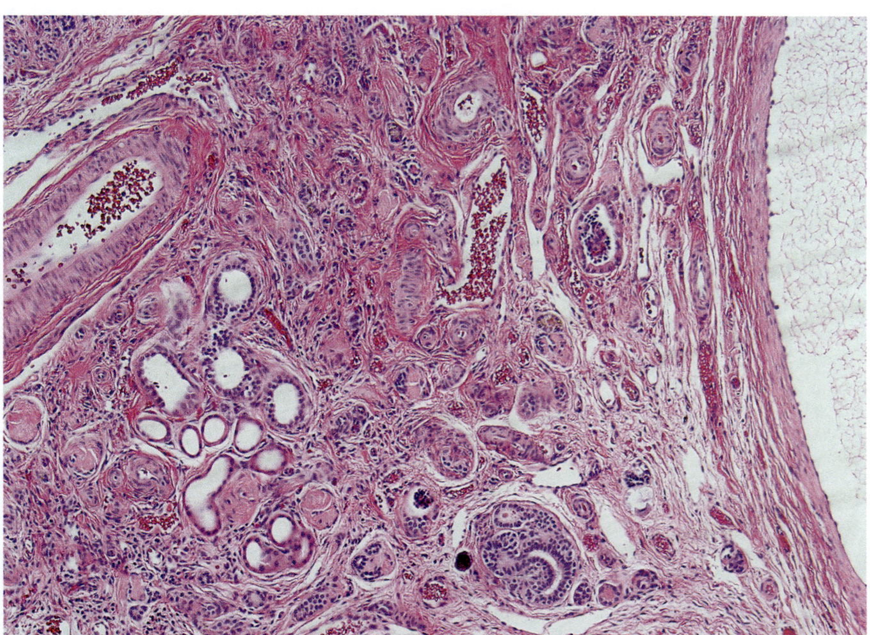

Figure 37-1.
Renal dysplasia is characterized by the presence of cysts with disorganized primitive renal tubules and glomeruli.

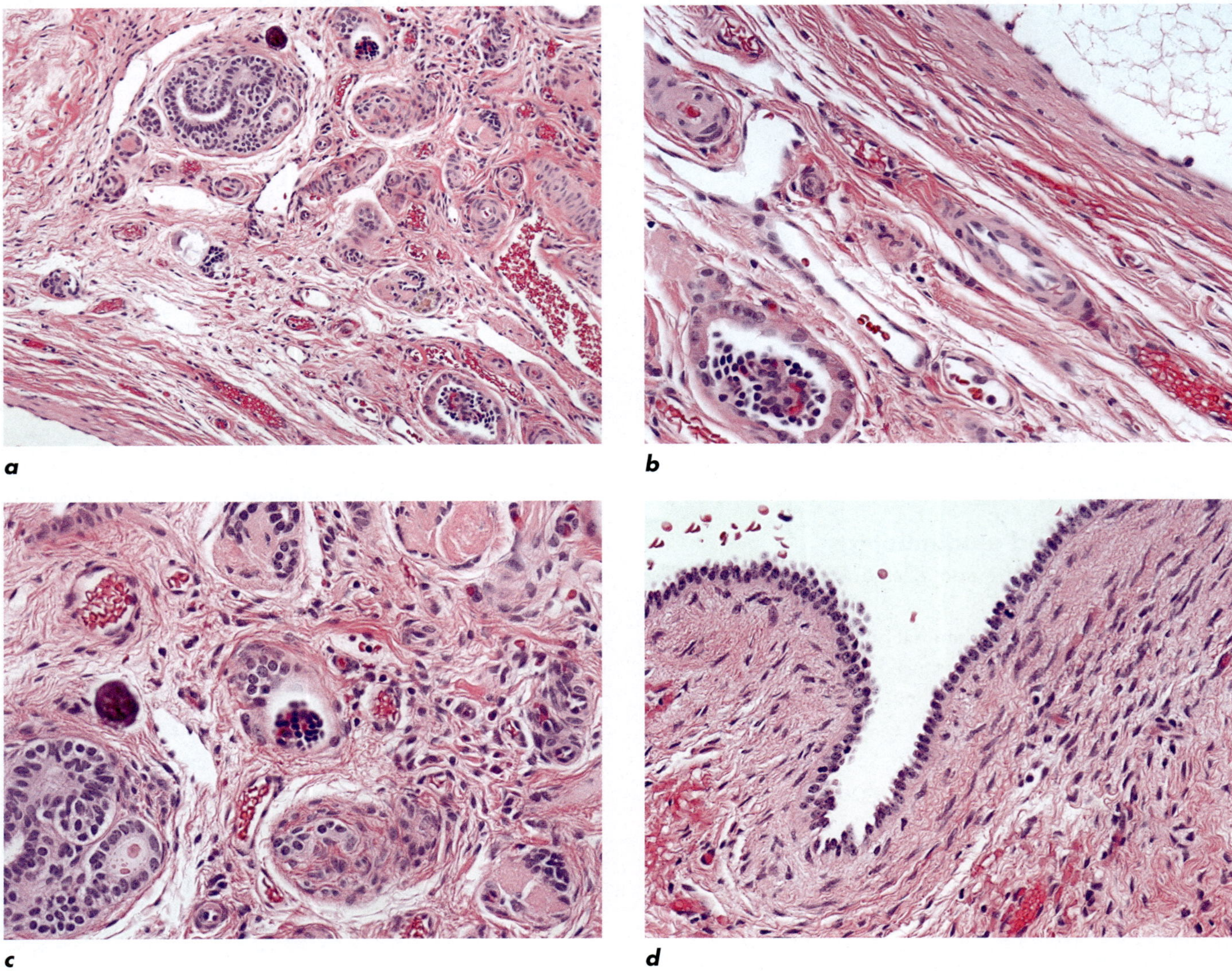

Figure 37-2.
Renal dysplasia. Immature glomeruli are surrounded by disorganized primitive tubules and microcalcification (*a*). High magnification shows a disorganized glomerulus inserted in a tubule (*b*); a poorly formed glomerulus is surrounded by abnormal immature tubules (*c*). Dilated cyst lined by cuboidal epithelial cells in renal dysplasia (*d*).

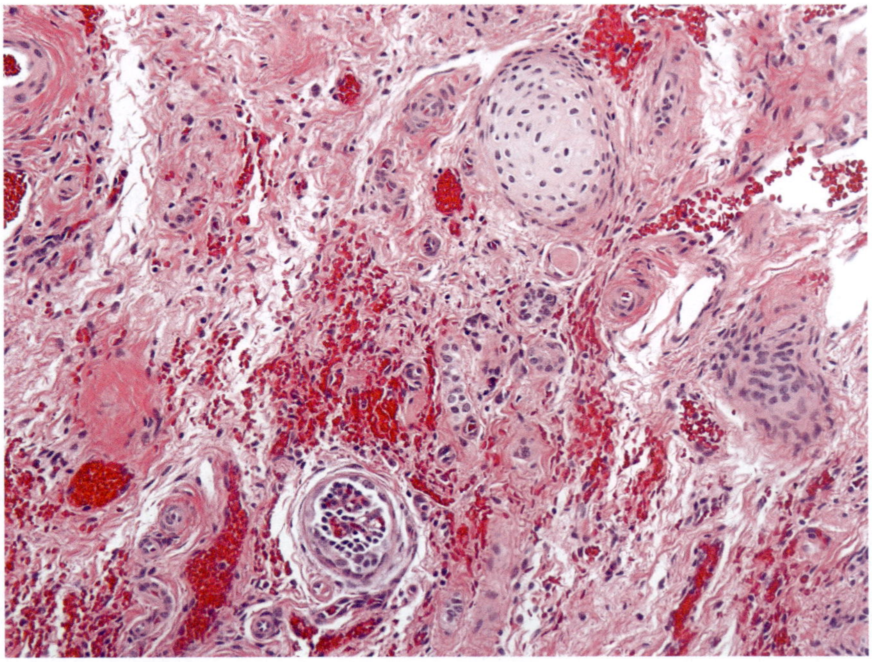

Figure 37-3.
Renal dysplasia with a characteristic cartilage island.

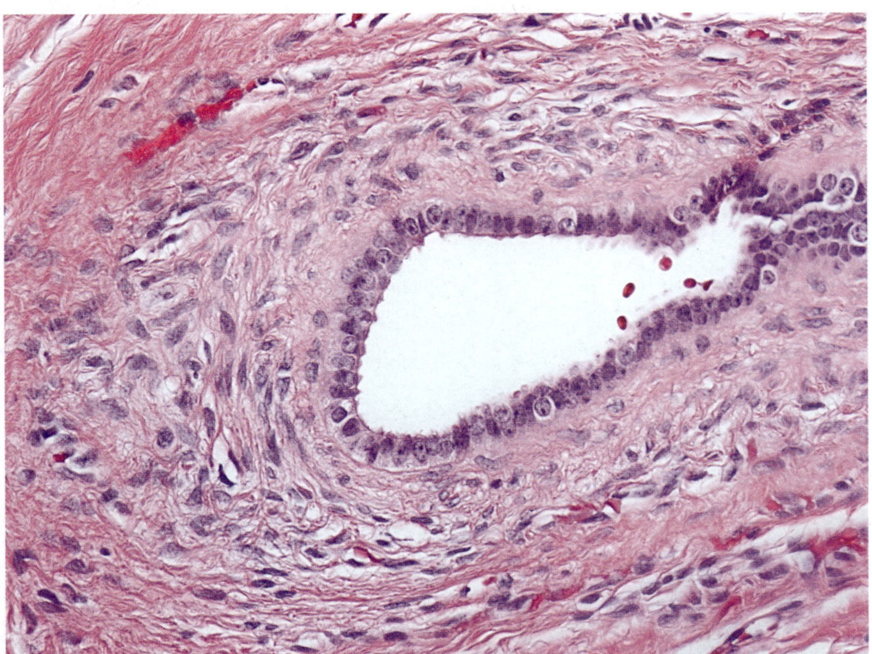

Figure 37-4.
Renal dysplasia with a dilated tubular structure with a characteristic spindle cell collarette.

Immunohistochemistry

- PAX2/PAX8 positive in tubular cells
- Galectin-3 and Bcl-2 positive in dysplastic epithelium
- Differential diagnosis with other cystic lesions is summarized in Table 37-1

Molecular analysis

- Mutation of *TCF2*
- Other genetic alterations such as PAX2 and uroplakins have been reported

Clinical relevance (prognosis and treatment options)

- Typically dysplasia involves only one kidney (80%)
- A child with one kidney involved by renal dysplasia may not have any symptoms or signs
- Bilateral renal dysplasia (20%) is often fatal and causes stillborn
- The patients who survive typically develop chronic renal failure in childhood and require renal transplants early in life

Table 37-1. Comparison of Cystic Kidney Lesions

	ADPCK	*ARPCK*	*Renal dysplasia*	*Cystic nephroma*	*Acquired renal cystic disease*
Genetic	Autosomal dominant	Autosomal recessive	Most sporadic	Sporadic	
Genes related	*PKD1, PKD2, PKD3*	*PKHD1*	*TCF2*	Not known[a]	Not known
Onset of disease	Adult	Before birth or neonatal	Before birth or neonatal	Adult	Adult
Size of kidney	Very large diffuse	Small diffuse	Variable	Demarcated cystic mass	Small
Laterality	Bilateral	Bilateral	Unilateral (80%)	Unilateral	Bilateral or unilateral
Distribution of cysts	Diffuse	Diffuse	Diffuse	Mass lesion	Variable
Size of cysts	Variable	Uniform	Variable	Variable in mass	Variable
Cyst characteristic	Numerous cysts with residual nephron between cysts	Cysts radially arranged perpendicular to renal capsule	Cysts with spindle cell collar	No renal tissue between cysts Ovarian type of stroma	Smaller number of cysts End-stage kidney disease
Cartilage	Absent	Absent	Present	Absent	Absent
Associated RCC	Rare	No	Uncommon	No	Common

ADPCK, autosomal dominant polycystic kidney; ARPCK, autosomal recessive polycystic kidney.

[a]Recently, cystic nephroma has been added to the constellation of tumors associated with heterozygous germline *DICER1* mutations that developed in children or young adults.

METANEPHRIC STROMAL TUMOR

Definition

- Benign spindle cell neoplasm of the kidney in children
- The tumor is composed of bland spindle cells that entrap kidney parenchymal tissue

Pathogenesis

- Unknown etiology
- Tumor occurs in infants with a mean age of 2 years
- Rarely develops before age 1

Clinical features

- Flank mass

Gross pathology

- No capsule, a poorly defined border
- Fibrous and firm lesion
- Mostly centrally located in the cortex, can involve medulla
- May be solid or contain small cysts

Histology

- Metanephric stromal tumor is composed of bland spindle cell proliferation with an infiltrating border (Fig. 37-5*a*)
- Individual renal tubules are often entrapped within the tumor (Fig. 37-5*b*)
- The tumor cells are bland with oval or short spindle-shaped nuclei. There are alternating hypercellular and hypocellular (myxoid or sclerotic) areas resulting in a nodular appearance. Mitoses can be seen (Fig. 37-6)
- Onion skin cuffing around the entrapped renal tubules similar to those of renal dysplasia is characteristic (Fig. 37-6*c*)
- Angiodysplasia: epithelioid transformation of smooth muscle cells of the entrapped blood vessels is a common finding (Fig. 37-6*d*).
- Juxtaglomerular cell hyperplasia associated with entrapped glomeruli could be seen (Fig. 37-7)
- Heterotopic elements such as glial (usually associated with epithelial differentiation), cartilaginous, or adipose tissue may be present

Immunohistochemistry

- Vimentin positive, S100 variably positive, and CD34 focally positive

Differential diagnosis

- See Table 37-2

Clinical relevance (prognosis and treatment options)

- Benign tumor. Surgical excision is the treatment of choice

Figure 37-5.
Metanephric stromal tumor displays an irregular infiltrative border (*a*) with individually entrapped tubules (*b*).

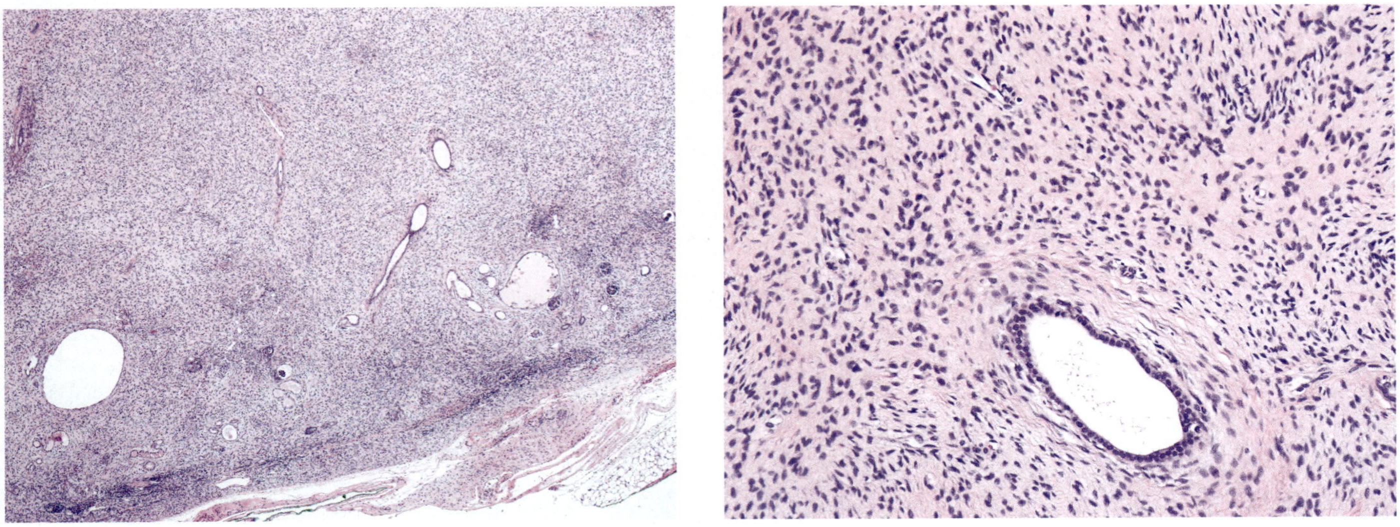

a b

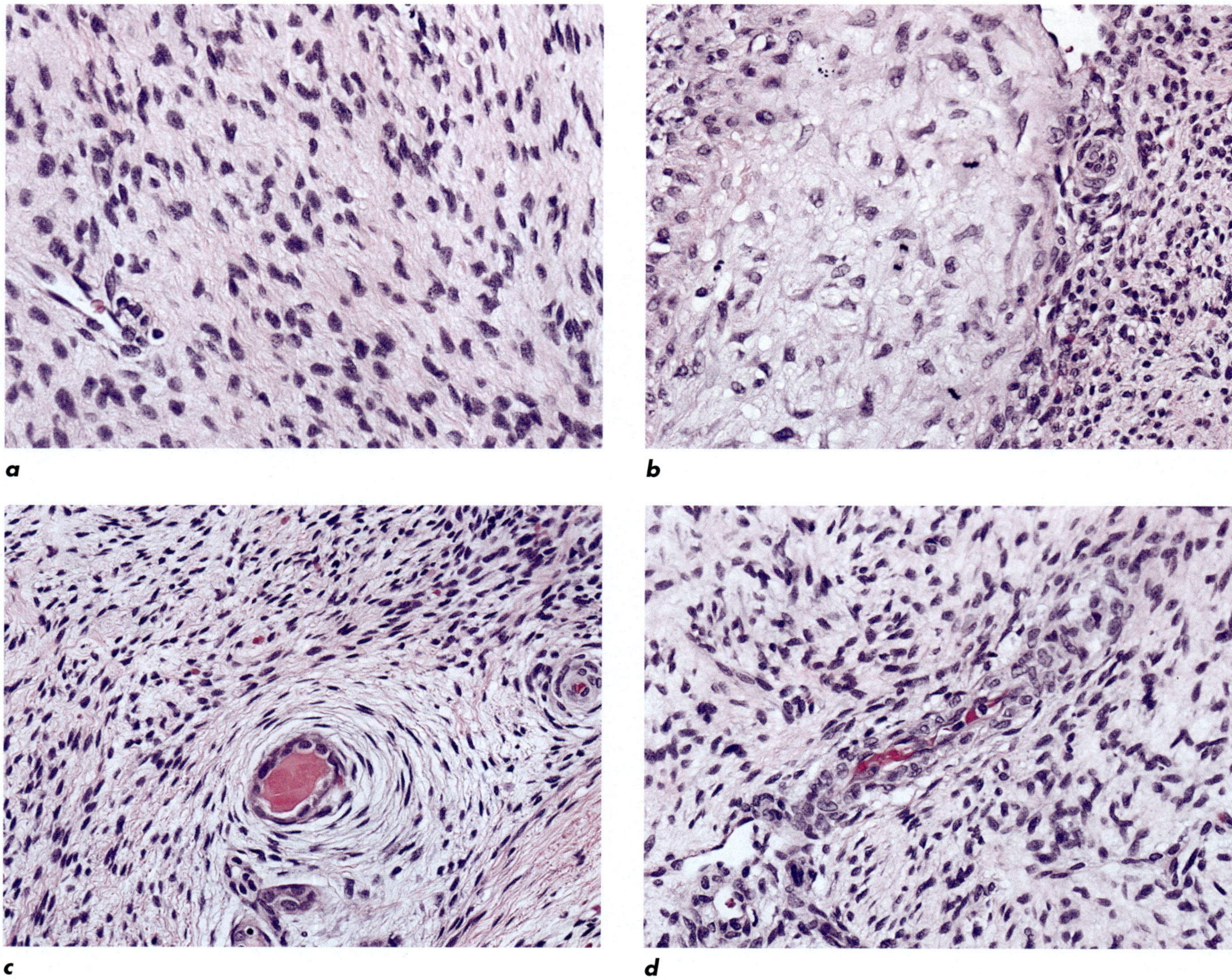

Figure 37-6.

Metanephric stromal tumor is composed of bland spindle cells with oval- or spindle-shaped nuclei. Nucleolus can hardly be seen (*a*). Hypercellular (*b*, right side) and hypocellular areas with frequent mitoses can be seen (*b*, left side). "Onion skinning" formation by concentric spindle cells around a tubule is characteristic (*c*). Angiodysplasia with epithelioid transformation of smooth muscle cells of an entrapped blood vessel is evident (*d*).

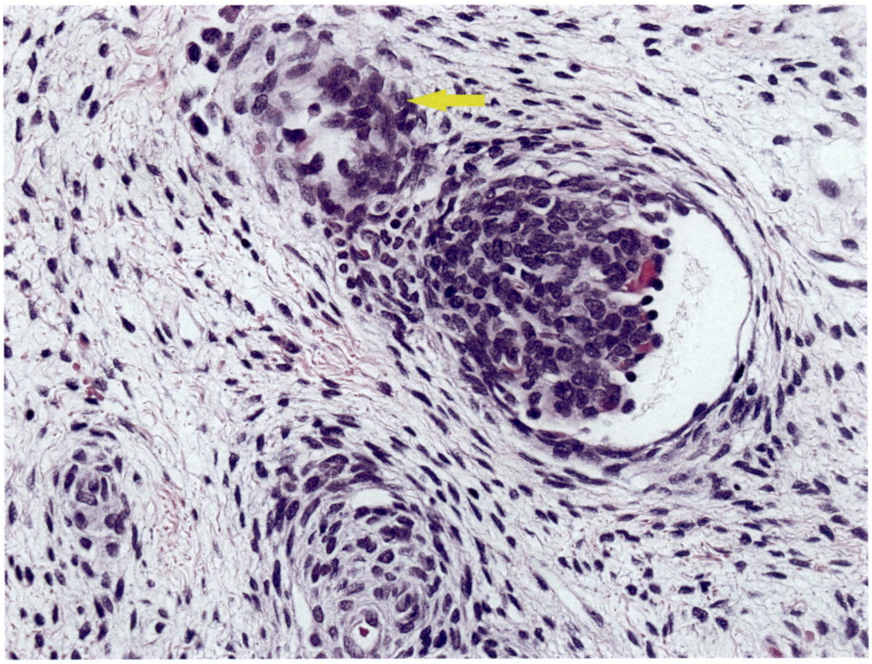

Figure 37-7.
Juxtaglomerular cell hyperplasia (arrow) adjacent to an entrapped glomerulus can be seen.

Table 37-2. Comparison of Benign Spindle Cell Renal Tumors in Children

	Congenital mesoblastic nephroma	*Metanephric stromal tumor*	*Metanephric adenofibroma*
Age	Before birth	Mean age = 2 years	Mean age = 14
Gross	Variably infiltrating border	Delicately infiltrative, fibrous lesions	Well defined
Spindle cells	Cellular	Hypo- and hypercellular areas	Hypo- and hypercellular areas
Epithelial components	Entrapped tubules in cluster	Entrapped tubules, single	Primitive tubules (as in metanephric adenoma)
Heterologous elements such as glia, cartilage	Absent	Possible	Absent
Onion skin cuffing around the tubules	No	Yes	No
Neoplastic epithelium	No	No	Yes
Mitosis	Frequent	Rare	Less frequent
Angiodysplasia	No	Yes	No
CD34	Negative	Positive	Negative

CONGENITAL MESOBLASTIC NEPHROMA

Definition

- Congenital low-grade myofibroblastic neoplasm affecting the renal medulla
- Subtypes include classical, cellular, and mixed

Other terms

- Fetal mesenchymal
- Leiomyomatous hamartoma

Pathogenesis

- Unknown
- It is a neoplasm not a hamartoma

Clinical features

- 2% to 4% of pediatric renal tumor
- 90% present in the first year of life
- Unilateral solitary abdominal mass
- May be associated with hypertension

Gross pathology

- Solitary, unilateral mass, 1 to 14 cm in size (Fig. 37-8)
- Classic type: mean 5 cm, variably circumscribed, white/yellow whorled mass near hilum; cellular type: mean 9 cm, cysts, hemorrhage, and necrosis common; and mixed type: mean 10 cm, cysts, hemorrhage, and necrosis in cellular areas

Histology

- Two histological types: classic and cellular types
- Classic type
  - Bland spindle cells in a variably collagenous stroma, resembling infantile fibromatosis or leiomyoma (Fig. 37-9)
  - Intersecting fascicles of fibroblastic cells (Fig. 37-10)
  - Clusters of entrapped renal tubules are characteristic (Fig. 37-9)
  - Cystic dilated tubules are surrounded by dense but bland spindle cells (Fig. 37-11)
- Cellular type
  - Resembles infantile fibrosarcoma
  - More densely cellular than classic type (Fig. 37-11)
  - Poorly formed fascicles and sheets
  - Monomorphous sheets of closely packed spindle cells
  - Increased mitoses and even focal necrosis (Fig. 37-12)
- Mixed type
  - Multiple foci
  - Classic type at the periphery of a cellular type

Immunohistochemistry

- Not particularly useful, the diagnosis being a combination of morphological findings and molecular studies
- Spindle cells are usually positive with vimentin and actin

Differential diagnosis

- Differential diagnoses from other pediatric spindle cell neoplastic lesions such as metanephric stromal tumor, metanephric adenofibroma as listed in Table 37-2, and clear cell sarcoma

Molecular analysis

- Classic and mixed
  - No recurrent genetic aberration identified
  - Usually diploid
  - Cases with trisomy 11, duplication of paternal Insulin Growth factor (IGF) 2 allele, and increased expression of IGF2 mRNA have been reported
- Cellular
  - Demonstrates a t(12;15)(p13;q25) (ETV6-NTRK3 translocation) similar to infantile fibrosarcoma

Clinical relevance (prognosis and treatment options)

- Excellent prognosis when completely excised, >95% event-free survival
- 5% to 10% cases have local recurrence and metastasis (usually to lung)
- Worse prognosis group: stage III cellular type in patients age 3 months or older correlates with local recurrence

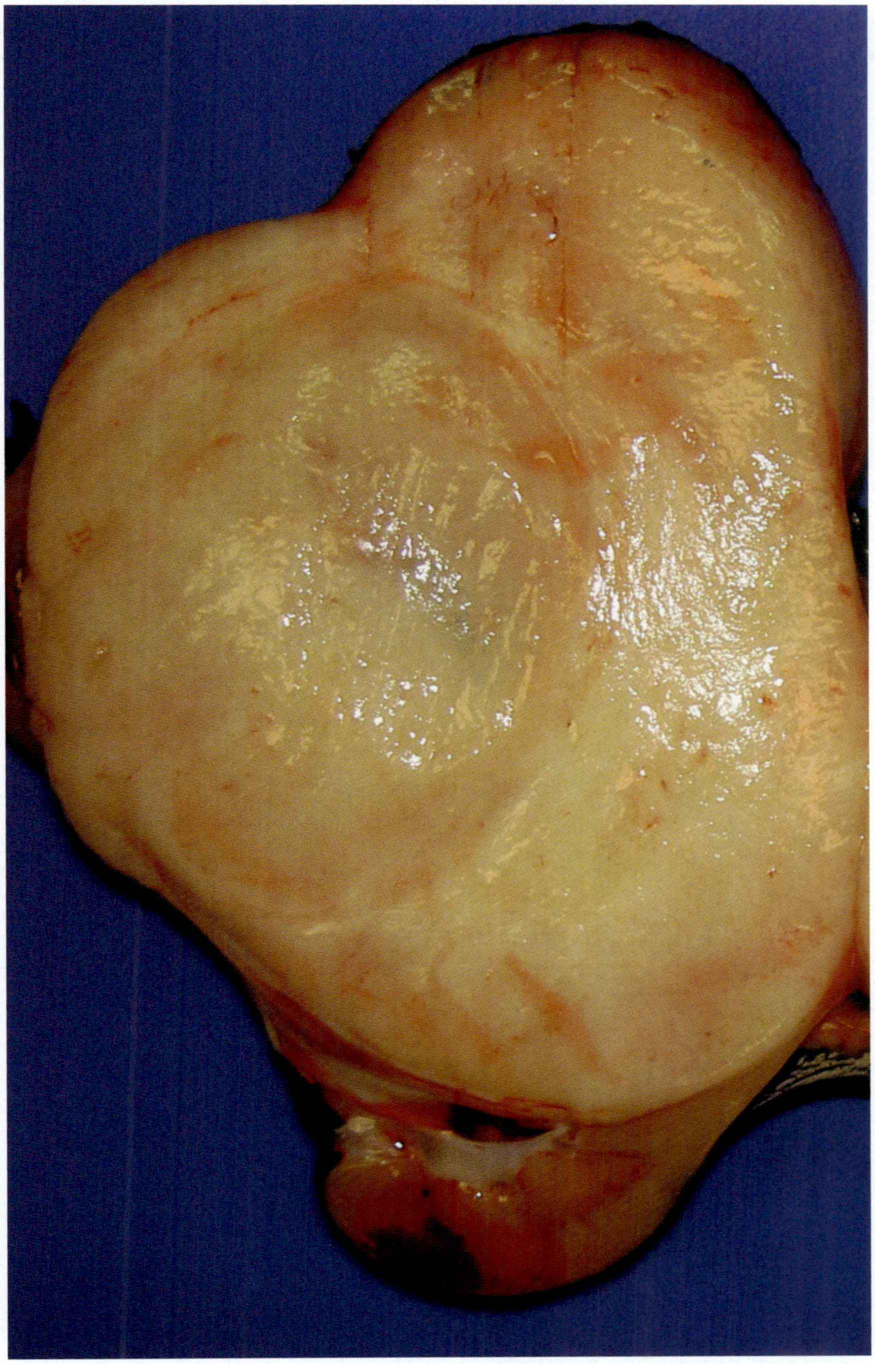

Figure 37-8.
Gross photo of congenital mesoblastic nephroma (CMN) in the upper pole, which is replacing the majority of the kidney. The tumor is well circumscribed with white-yellow cut surface.

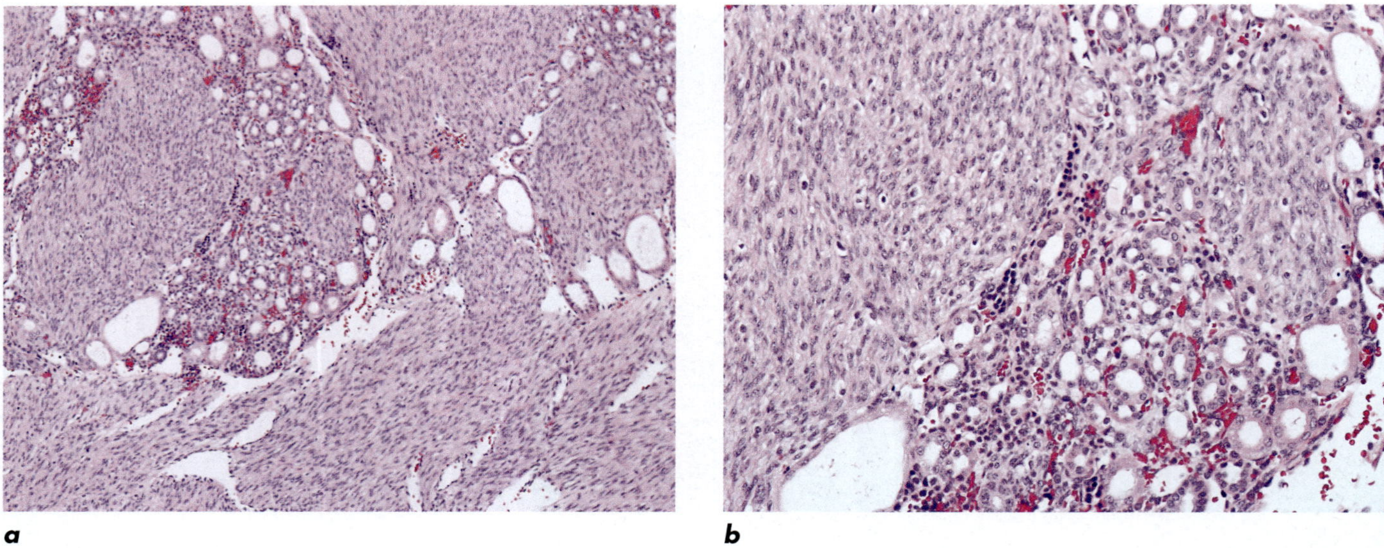

Figure 37-9.
The classic-type mesoblastic nephroma is composed of fascicles of spindle cells with clusters of entrapped renal tubules (*a*). High magnification shows the renal tubules are encased by cellular but bland spindle tumor cells (*b*).

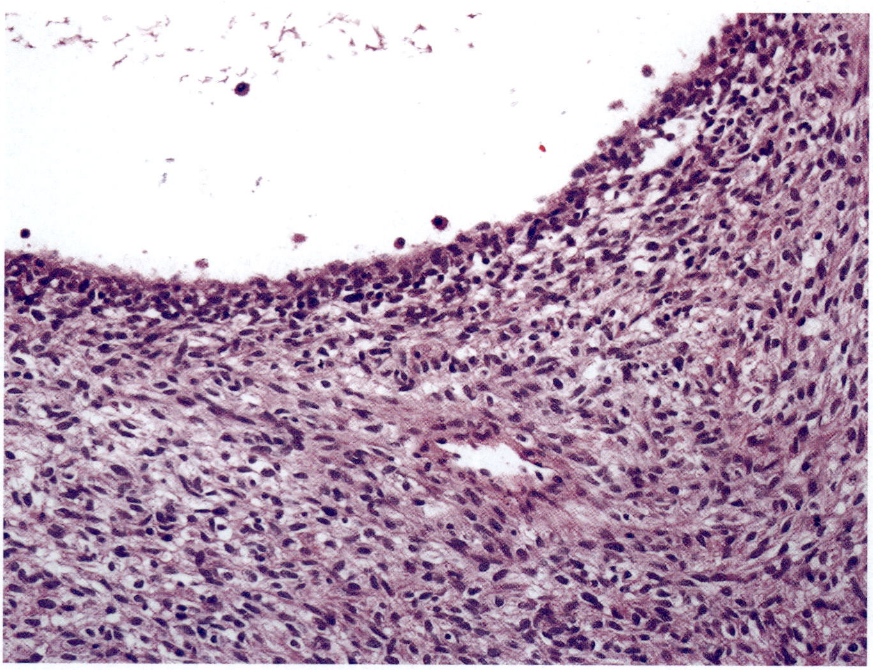

Figure 37-10.
Mesoblastic nephroma with cystic dilated tubule surrounded by neoplastic spindle cells.

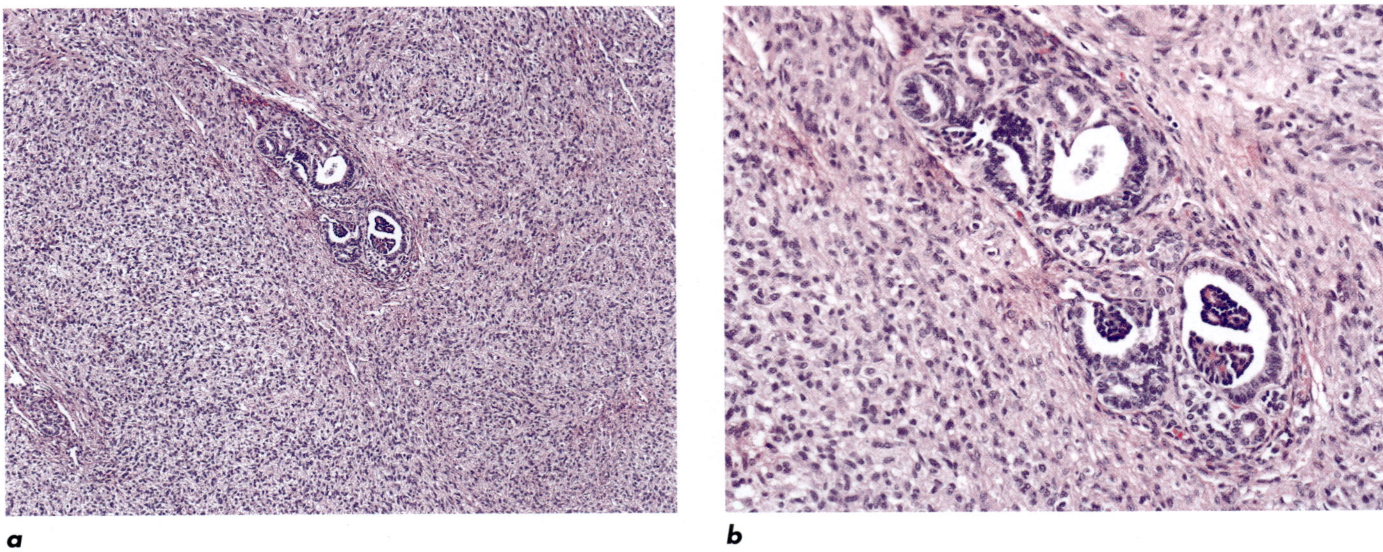

Figure 37-11.
Cellular-type CMN with increased cellularity and entrapped immature renal tubules (*a*). High magnification demonstrates fetal-type tubules (embryonal metaplastic tubules) surrounded by the spindle cells (*b*).

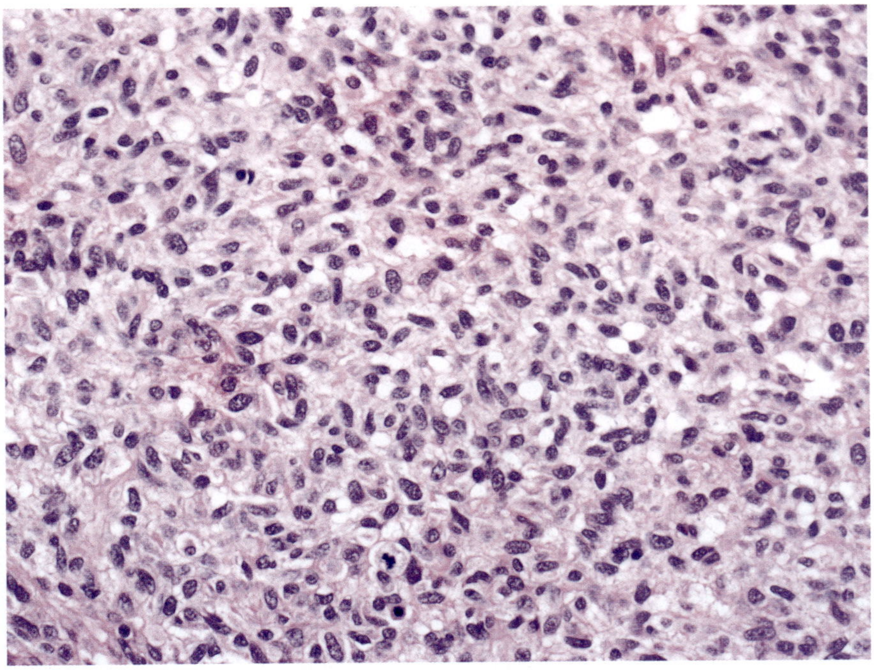

Figure 37-12.
Cellular CMN with higher cellularity and mitoses of spindle cells.

NEPHROGENIC RESTS

Definition

- Abnormally persistent foci of embryonal tissue seen beyond 36 weeks of gestation (after the period of normal nephrogenesis)
- Nephrogenic rests are capable of developing into Wilms tumor

Other term

- Nephroblastomatosis: multifocal or diffuse form of nephrogenic rests

Pathogenesis

- <1% in the kidneys of infants with no history of tumor
- Evidence of nephrogenic rests as a precursor lesion of Wilms tumor
  - Found microscopically adjacent to normal renal parenchyma of approximately one-third of patients with Wilms tumor
  - The primitive cells in nephrogenic rests resemble blastemal cells of Wilms tumor
- Nephrogenic rests can be divided into intralobar or perilobar type
- Perilobar nephrogenic rests (PLNR)
  - Seen in sporadic Wilms tumors
  - Located at the periphery of the renal lobule
  - Occurs bilateral and developed synchronously
  - Are associated with genetic/epigenetic dysregulation at 11p15, idiopathic hemihypertrophy and Beckwith-Wiedemann syndrome
  - Serves as a marker of loss of imprinting or loss of heterozygosity for *IGF2*
- Intralobar nephrogenic rests (ILNR)
  - In contrast located centrally within the renal lobule
  - Irregular borders
  - More often associated with early-onset, stromal predominant Wilms tumor; or Wilms tumor with divergent differentiation
  - Are more commonly associated with *WT1* mutations, Denys-Drash syndrome, and WAGR syndrome
- Combined nephroblastomatosis: lesions with both PLNR and ILNR

Clinical features

- No symptoms related directly to nephrogenic rests
- Generally, it is a microscopic finding unless it causes diffuse enlargement of the kidney
- May be associated with clinical implications for their genetic associations as well as for the risk of development of bilateral or metachronous Wilms tumor in the contralateral kidney

Gross pathology

- May not be apparent on gross examination or appear as small pale discoloration or nodules with foci of capsular thickening
- Rarely, massive renal enlargement present due to diffuse hyperplastic perilobar nephroblastomatosis

Histology

- Tightly packed nests or diffuse sheets of primitive but nonanaplastic blastema/primitive epithelial tubules with scant intervening stroma. The comparison of PLNR and ILNR is summarized in Table 37-3
- Perilobar nephrogenic rests
  - More common
  - Found in subcapsular peripheral locations (Fig. 37-13)
  - Well-demarcated margins
  - Composed of predominantly blastema and primitive tubules (Figs. 37-14)
  - Scant sclerotic stroma, often multiple
- Intralobar nephrogenic rests
  - Located deep within the lobule, often solitary (Fig. 37-15)
  - Have a more irregular and intermixed margin
  - Predominantly stroma
  - Blastema or tubules also present (Fig. 37-15)
- Possible fates of nephrogenic rests
  - Regression for most cases
  - Indolent without progression
  - Hyperplasia, proliferation of both blastemal and epithelial components (Fig. 37-16)
- When a Wilms tumor develops within a nephrogenic rest
  - Superimposed nodular growth of the proliferating component
  - Formation of a fibrous capsule around the tumor with peripheral compressed rest

Immunohistochemistry

- WT1 nuclear positivity

Clinical relevance (prognosis and treatment options)

- Risk appears highest for intralobar rests in patients under 1 year of age
- Conservative treatment

Table 37-3. Comparison of Perilobar and Intralobar Nephrogenic Rests

Nephrogenic rests types	*PLNR*	*ILNR*
Prevalence in all cases	More common (1%)	Less common (0.1%)
Prevalence in Wilms tumor cases	Similar, 25% to 80%	Similar, 15% to 75%
Location	Periphery of the lobe or subcapsular	Within the lobule
Margins	Sharply demarcated	Irregular
Blastemal component	Dominant	Present
Epithelial component	Dominant	Present
Stromal component	Present	Dominant
Risk for Wilms tumor	Yes	High

ILNR, intralobar nephrogenic rests; PLNR, perilobar nephrogenic rests.

Figure 37-13.
Perilobar nephrogenic rests in an infant are characterized by the presence of primitive tubules and blastemal cells in the subcapsular areas (*a*). High magnification shows the primitive tubules and blastemal components (*b*).

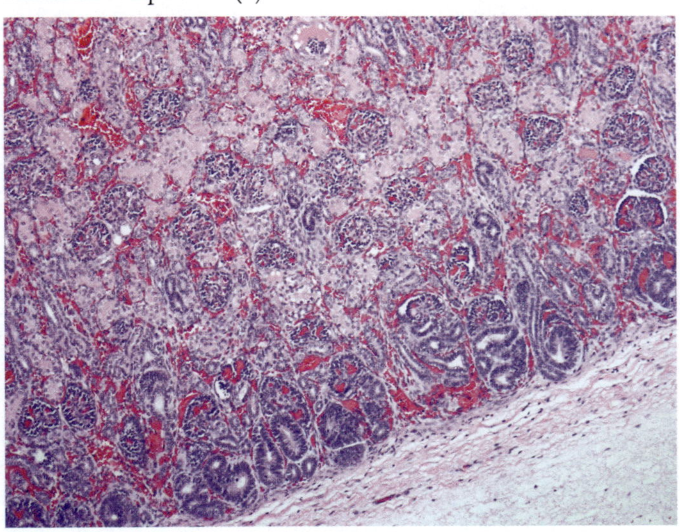

a

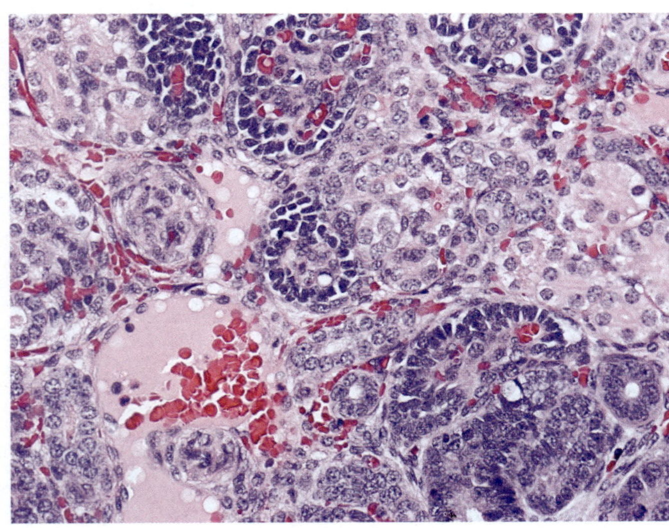

b

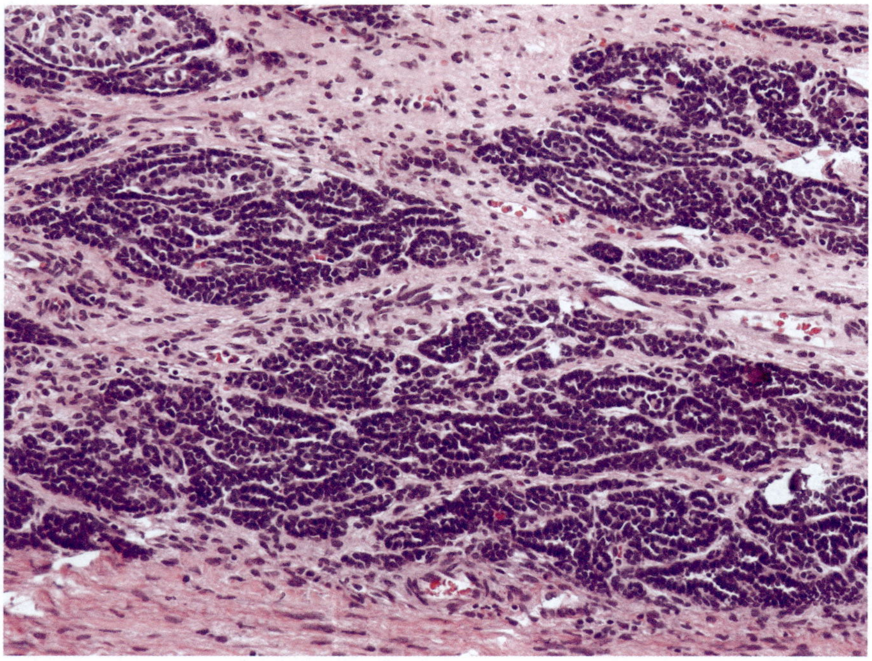

Figure 37-14.
Nephrogenic rests composed of mostly primitive tubules with minimal cytoplasm.

Figure 37-15.
Intralobar nephrogenic rests are characterized by the presence of primitive tubules and blastemal cells deep in the kidney parenchyma (*a*). High magnification shows the presence of primitive tubules along with blastemal cells with scant cytoplasm (*b*).

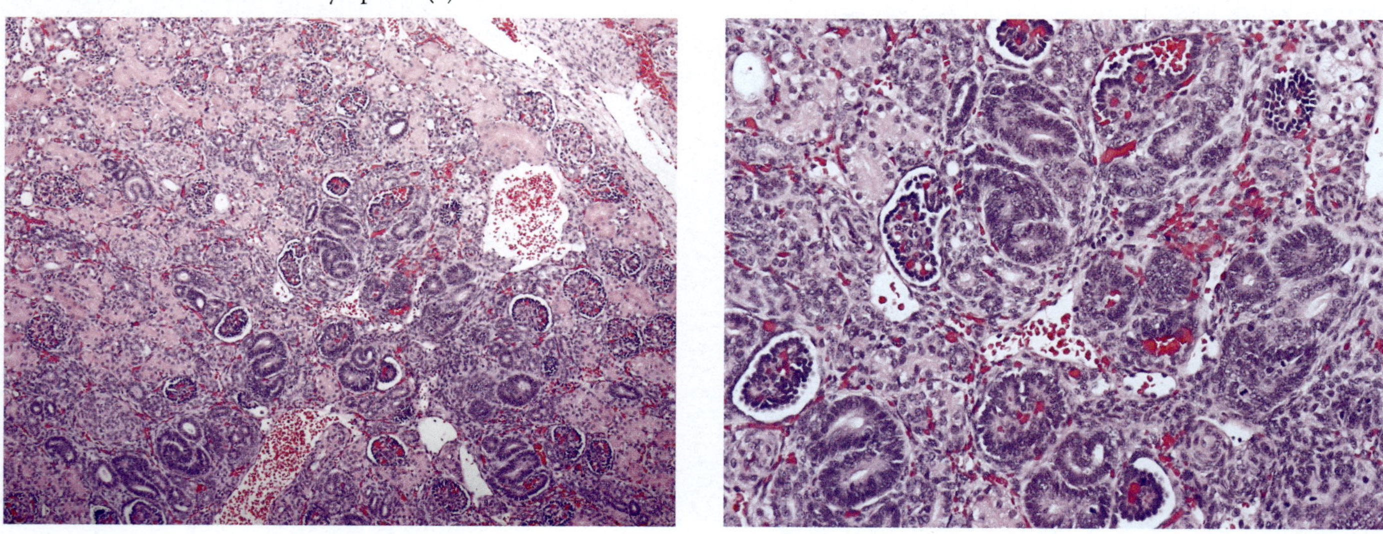

a **b**

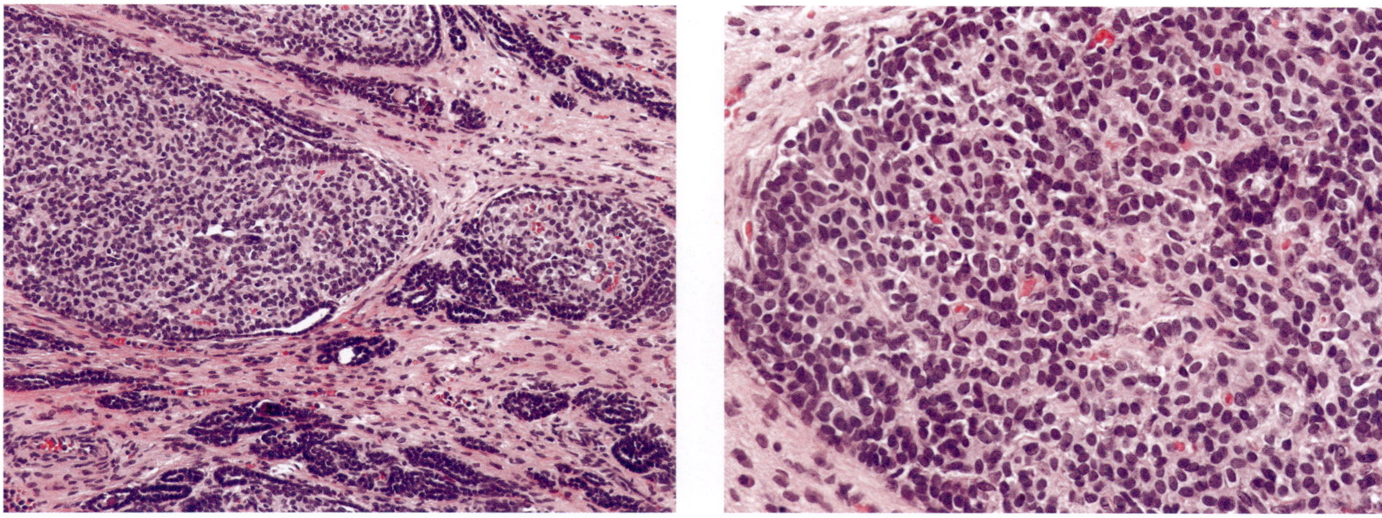

a b

Figure 37-16.
Hyperplasia of nephrogenic rests is composed of oval-shaped collection of blastemal cells (*a*) with increased proliferation (*b*).

WILMS TUMOR

Definition

- A malignant renal tumor composed of embryonal cells derived from nephrogenic blastema in children

Other term

- Nephroblastoma

Pathogenesis and epidemiology

- The tumor is believed to be derived from the primitive stem cells of the kidney
- It is the most common kidney malignancy in children
- Approximately 8% of all pediatric malignancies, 85% of all renal malignancies in childhood
- Adult cases of Wilms tumor (WT) as well as unusual locations (for example, inguinal canal) are well known, however, extremely rare

Clinical features

- Peak incidence: 2 to 3 years of age
- The most common clinical sign is palpable mass
- Typical signs of hematuria, back/flank pain, acute abdominal crisis, and hypertension are also common
- The most common metastatic sites are lymph nodes, lung, and liver
- 10% of WT are associated with specific syndromes
  - WAGR: WT, aniridia, GU malformations, and mental retardation
  - Denys-Drash syndrome: WT (90% risk), mesangial sclerosis, and pseudohermaphroditism
  - Beckwith-Wiedemann syndrome: WT, hemihypertrophy, macroglossia, omphalocele, and visceromegaly
- Familiar nephroblastoma (1% of patients with WT): most likely autosomal dominant trait with variable penetrance and expressivity
- Other conditions associated with higher incidence of WT
  - Frasier syndrome; Simpson-Golabi-Behmel syndrome; Klippel-Trenaunay syndrome; Bloom syndrome; Perlman syndrome; and Sotos syndrome
  - Renal and genital malformations; trisomy of chromosome 18; neurofibromatosis; and cerebral gigantism

Gross pathology

- Mostly solid soft mass, tumors are usually well demarcated
- Multicentric and/or bilateral cases are well known
- Pale, whitish, gray to tan cut surface (Fig. 37-17), cystic formations may be prominent
- Polypoid protrusions into the renal pelvis have been described
- Two main staging systems are now in use
  - COG (Children's Oncology Group)
  - Revised SIOP (International Society of Pediatric Oncology)
  - Both only applicable for primary nephrectomy cases, both for pretreated cases

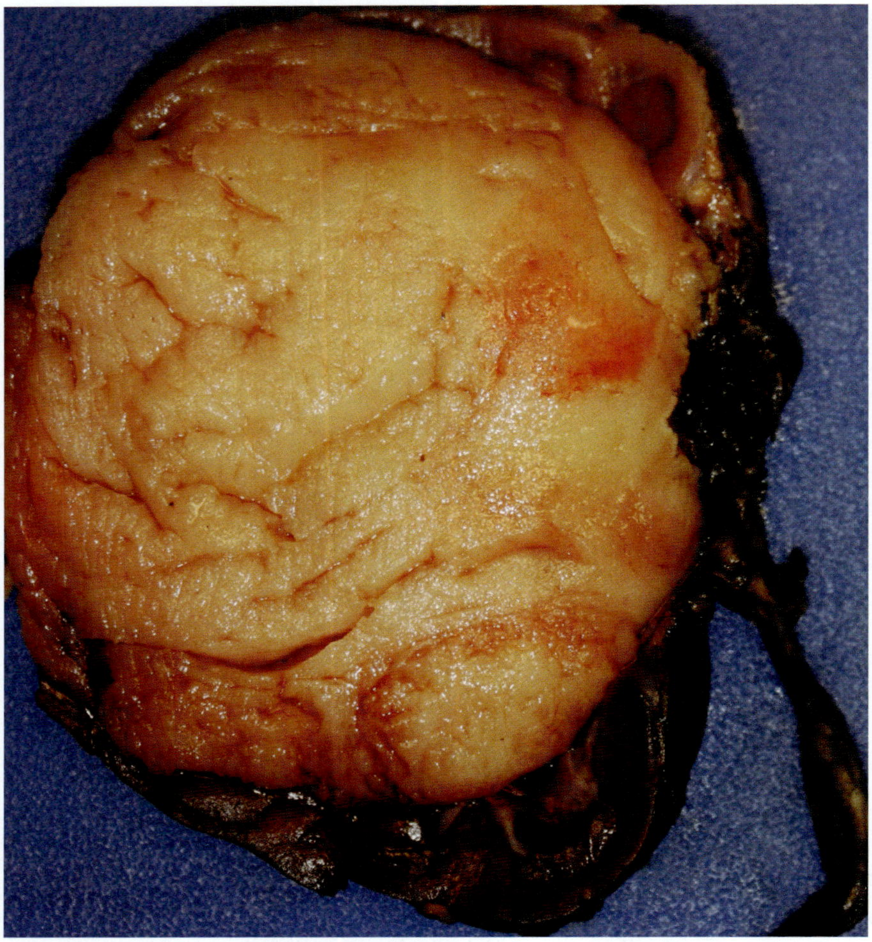

Figure 37-17.
A large Wilms tumor replacing most of the kidney with homogenous white-yellow cut surface.

Histology

- Tumor is well demarcated (Fig. 37-18)
- Architecture is variable, as well as cytological features. Both depend on degree of differentiation
- Differentiation toward epithelial and stromal lineages is frequently seen, even within the same tumor
- The most common pattern is the triphasic pattern (Fig. 37-19), which includes
  - Epithelial (Fig. 37-19*b*)
  - Undifferentiated blastema (Fig. 37-19*c*)
  - Stromal component (Fig. 37-19*d*)
- However, biphasic and monophasic patterns frequently occur (Figs. 37-20 and 37-21)
- Blastemal cells: small, primitive, with hyperchromatic nuclei, coarse chromatin, scant cytoplasm, and visible small nucleoli
- Epithelial cells: variable morphology, depending on differentiation. There is a continual spectrum of small primitive-looking cells to large, well-differentiated squamous cells or mucinous epithelium. Architecture of epithelial component varies from solid areas to pseudotubular or tubular/papillary areas
- Stromal cells: also variable, range from undifferentiated spindle cells, skeletal muscles, fibroblasts to cartilage or bone formations
- Presence of anaplasia is an important prognostic feature. Diffuse anaplasia is considered unfavorable histology with variable treatment regimen
- Anaplasia is defined as increased size of tumor nuclei (x3) with hyperchromasia and multipolar mitoses (Fig. 37-22)
- Specific group of so-called postchemotherapy WTs
  - Tumor frequently shows the following changes: necrosis, xanthogranulomatous areas, hemosiderin deposition, fibrosis, maturation of blastemal, epithelial, and stromal components
  - According to the morphology of postchemotherapy WTs, three prognostic groups are recognized: low, intermediate, and high risks

Immunohistochemistry

- Vimentin is constantly present in blastemal cells
- NSE, cytokeratins, and desmin are variably positive
- WT1 (for N-terminus region) shows nuclear positivity, but its reactivity is inconsistent; negativity does not exclude the diagnosis of WT

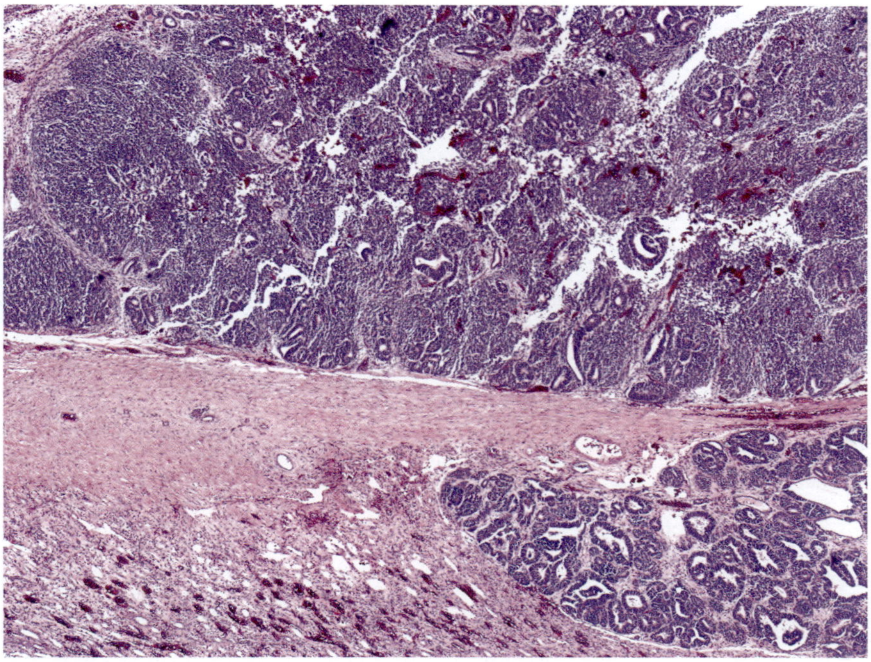

Figure 37-18.
Low magnification view of a Wilms tumor composed of primitive (blue areas, upper portion) cells, which are well demarcated from the nonneoplastic kidney.

Molecular genetics

- *WT1* gene alterations present in WAGR and Denys-Drash syndrome
- *WT1* mutations associated with prominent stroma and rhabdomyogenesis
- *WT2* gene alterations common in Beckwith-Wiedemann syndrome
- 33% to 50% of WT associated with loss of imprinting of *IGF2* and hypermethylation of *H19*-related genes
- WT with favorable histology but aggressive behavior have LOH (loss of heterozygosity) for 1p and 16q
- Familial WT: duplication at 2p24.3 including the *DDX1* and *MYCN* genes.

Differential diagnosis

Papillary RCC

- Prominently papillary or tubular patterns
- Foamy macrophages and hemosiderin are often present
- So-called solid variant of papillary RCC (PRCC)could be difficult to differentiate from well-differentiated epithelial WT
- PRCC tumors may occasionally have glomeruloid formations
- Blastemal or stromal component are rarely seen in PRCC, although sarcomatoid differentiation could be present
- PRCC is usually strongly diffusely positive for AMACR and CK 7, while in WT such positivity is not constant and if present, usually focal
- The presence of trisomy 7, 17 by FISH is diagnostic of PRCC

Metanephric adenoma

- Usually composed of small uniform epithelial cells arranged with low-grade nuclei
- Mitoses are exceptional in metanephric adenoma
- In some rare and unusual cases, it is extremely difficult to differentiate between metanephric adenoma and WT. Some authors speculate about "metastatic" MA as about extremely well-differentiated epithelial WTs

Immature teratoma

- The differential diagnosis can be sometimes difficult especially if there are immature neurotubes
- It is possible to find well-differentiated areas such as
  - Bronchial-like structures, composed of ciliated epithelium with cartilage and/or smooth muscles
  - Structures resembling gastric/colonic mucosa, etc.
  - In WT, it is possible to find anaplastic areas, or real renal blastema. Also, brisk mitotic activity favors diagnosis of WT

Treatment

- Surgery with/without subsequent adjuvant therapy (radio or combined chemotherapy)
- Preoperative chemotherapy followed by surgical resection has shown promising results

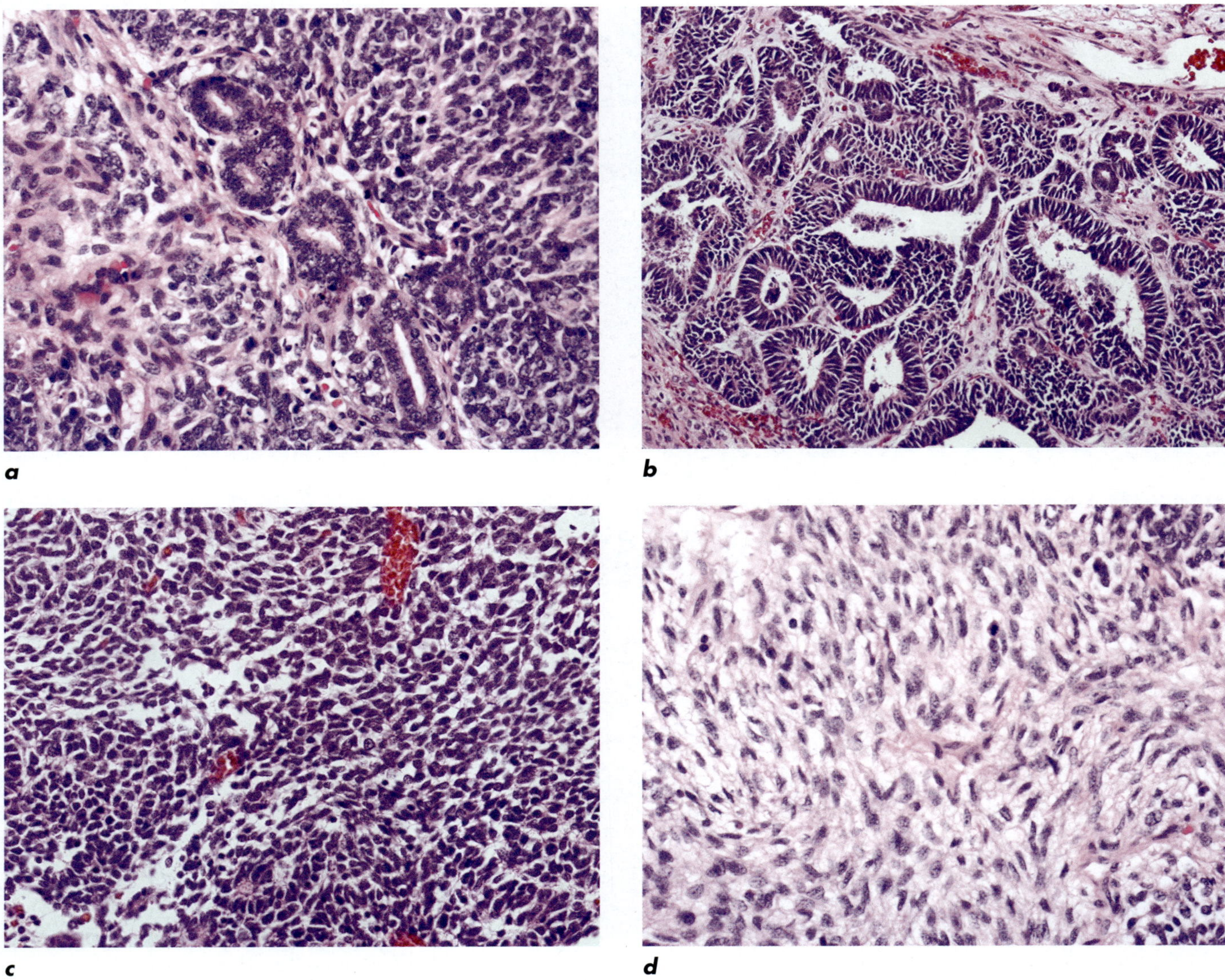

Figure 37-19.
Triphasic Wilms tumor is composed of stromal, epithelial, and blastemal components (*a*). High magnification shows the pseudostratified epithelial cells with high N/C ratio (*b*). Blastemal component is characterized by the presence of diffuse small primitive (blue) cells with scant cytoplasm (*c*). Stromal component is composed of spindle cells with mitotic activity (*d*).

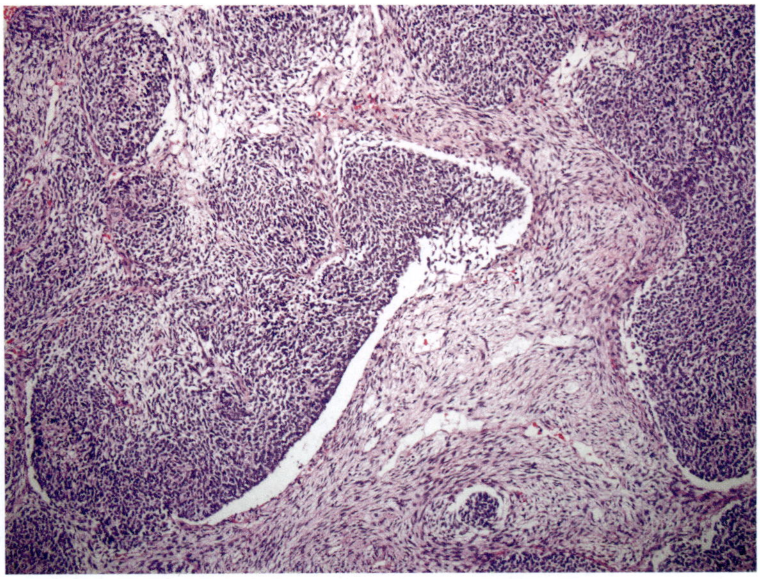

Figure 37-20.
Wilms tumor with both blastemal and stromal components.

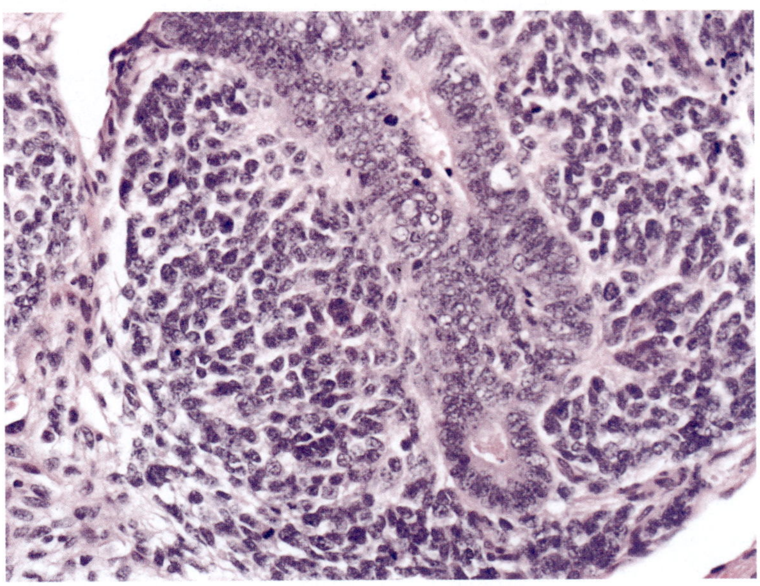

Figure 37-21.
Wilms tumor with both blastemal and epithelial components.

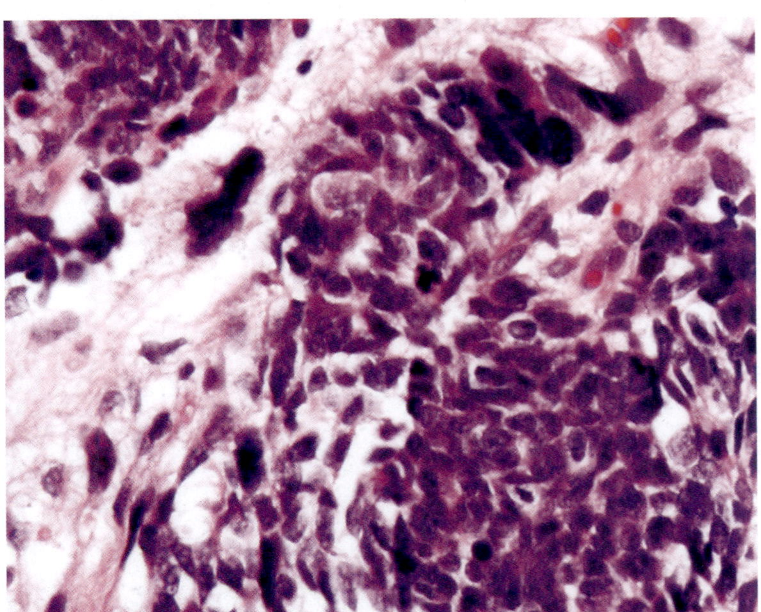

Figure 37-22.
Anaplastic Wilms tumor is characterized by the presence of increased size of tumor nuclei (x3) with hyperchromasia and multipolar mitoses.

CLEAR CELL SARCOMA OF THE KIDNEY

Definition

- Clear cell sarcoma of the kidney (CCSK) is a malignant pediatric tumor of the kidney, composed of tumor cells with clear cytoplasm and the propensity to metastasize to the bone

Other term

- Bone-metastasizing Wilms tumor (outdated)

Pathogenesis

- Uncertain
- The tumor is probably derived from the renal mesenchymal cell with neural features

Clinical features

- A large unilateral renal mass, typically not associated with other syndrome or renal dysplasia

Gross pathology

- A large renal mass, average = 11.3 cm, often distorting or replacing the kidney
- The renal medulla was the most common location initially
- Cut surface is tan-gray or white-yellow and mucoid (Fig. 37-23)
- Cystic changes, necrosis, or hemorrhage may be present

Histology

- Tumor cells may form variable patterns. The most common classic histologic pattern is characterized by cord cells arranged in cords, nests, or groups surrounded by thin fibrovascular septa (Figs. 37-24 and 37-25)
- Classically there are three components (Fig. 37-25)
  - Small round-to-oval (cord) cells with bland cytologic features
  - Branching vessels ("chicken-wire" pattern) accompanied by spindle (septal) cells along the fibrovascular septa
  - And intercellular mucoid (alcian-blue-positive) matrix
- Myxoid pattern (50%), sclerosing pattern (35%), and cellular pattern (26%) are also common and often present in mixed forms
- Increased mitosis and hypercellularity can be easily seen (Fig. 37-26)
- Other less common patterns including epithelioid, palisading, spindle cell, sinusoidal (pericytomatous), and storiform patterns
- Anaplasia defined similarly as in Wilms tumor (3 times enlarged nuclei and multipolar mitosis)is seen in 2-3% of primary or recurrent tumors, and associated with a more aggressive behavior
- The tumor is not associated with ILNR

Immunohistochemistry

- Anaplastic CCSK is p53 positive
- There are no specific diagnostic features by immunohistochemistry
- The tumor cells are vimentin positive and negative for epithelial markers

Clinical relevance (prognosis and treatment options)

- It is listed as a renal tumor with "unfavorable histology" in the National Wilms Tumor Study Group (NWTSG) clinical protocols although it is not a Wilms tumor
- Highly aggressive tumor with poor prognosis, 70% cases are stage II or III at the time of diagnosis
- Less than 5% of the CCSK cases develop distant metastasis at diagnosis
- The most common site of metastasis is pelvic lymph nodes (29% at presentation)
- There is a propensity to develop distant metastasis in the bone, followed by the lung, abdomen, brain, and liver and soft tissue
- Treatment includes nephrectomy if tumor is resectable, followed by chemotherapy
- With advances in chemotherapy, the 8-year survival rate for stages I-III CCSK is better than 80% in this country

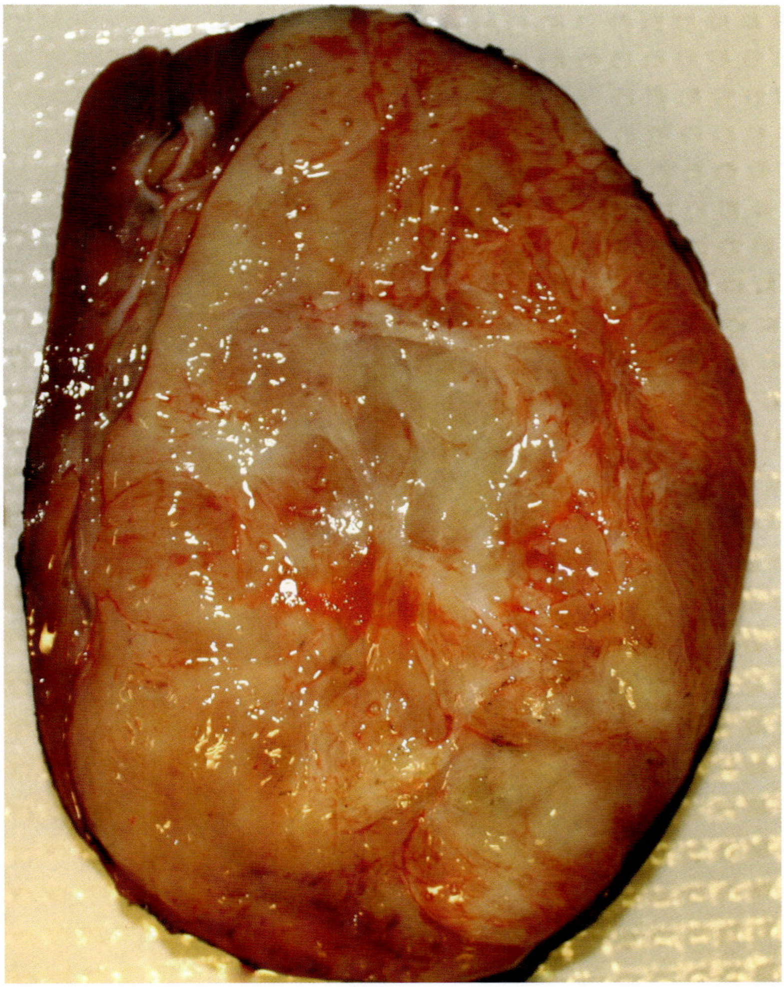

Figure 37-23.
Gross appearance of clear cell sarcoma of the kidney (CCSK). This tumor is large and replacing the entire kidney. Only a small rim of residual renal tissue can be seen on the left side. The cut surface is white-yellow with mucoid appearance.

Figure 37-24.
Clear cell sarcoma of the kidney (CCSK). Because of the low cellularity of the tumor, the H&E stained section has a very pale appearance (*a*). Typically, CCSK is composed of small tumor (cord) cell component with very bland cytological features. The spindle cells form septa with thin-vessels giving the "chicken-wire" appearance (*b*).

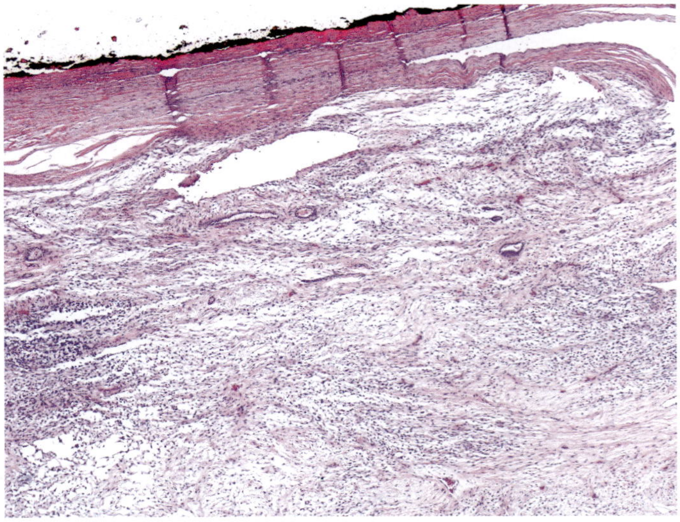

a

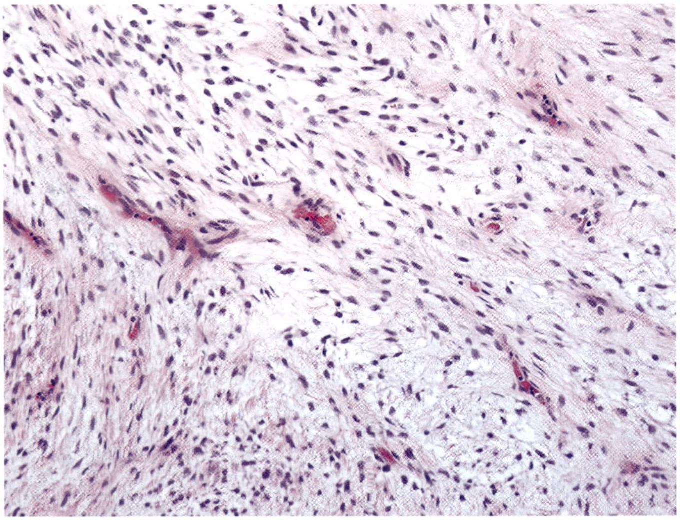

b

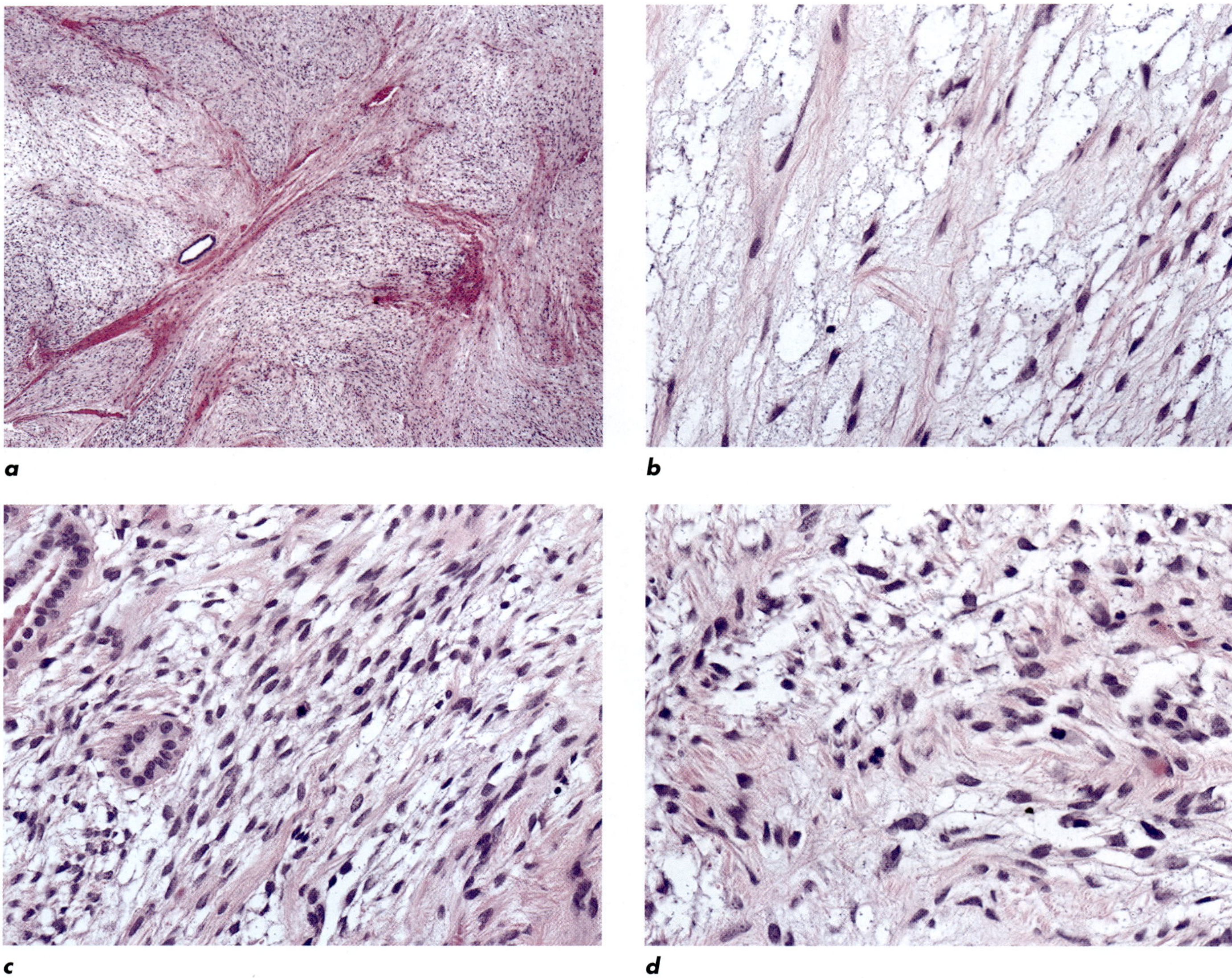

Figure 37-25.
Clear cell sarcoma of the kidney. At low magnification, CCSK is lobular with tumor cell lobules separated by fibrous septa, containing some renal tubules entrapped by the tumor cells (*a*). High magnification shows the bland spindle cells with mucoid component in a low cellular area (*b*). Mitotic figures of the tumor cells adjacent to entrapped tubules can be seen (*c*). Although the cellularity is generally low, mitotic figures are brisk in CCSK (*d*).

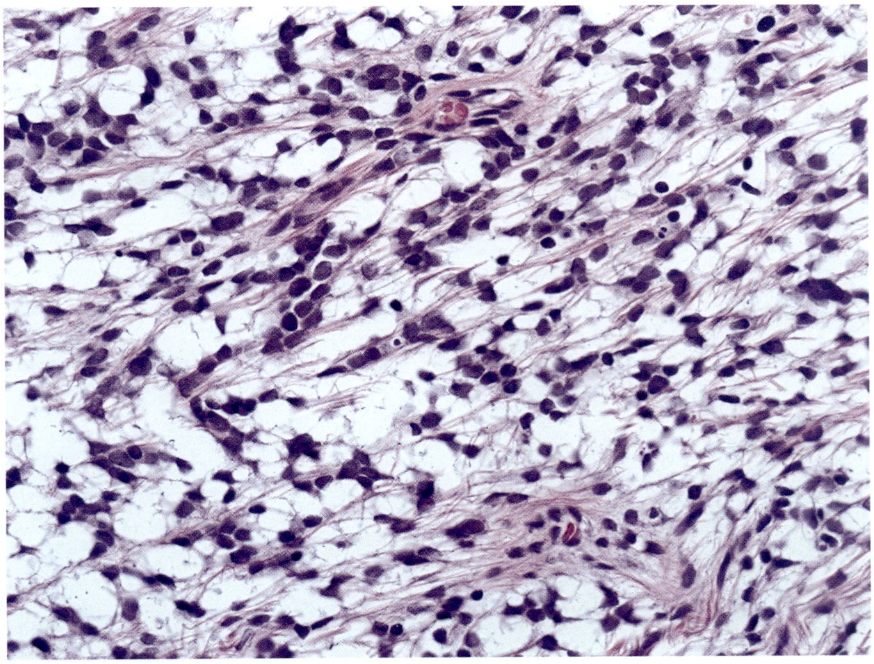

Figure 37-26.
Higher cellular area of CCSK.

MALIGNANT RHABDOID TUMOR

Definition

- A high-grade renal tumor composed of diffusely growing monomorphic tumor cells with vesicular nuclei, prominent nucleoli, and eosinophilic hyaline inclusions within cytoplasm

Pathogenesis

- Unclear, the most likely originated from primitive stem cells in the renal medulla

Clinical features

- Approximately 2% of pediatric renal tumors
- 80% of the patients are under age of 2 years
- Hematuria is the most common clinical feature
- Usually high-stage tumor at presentation, metastatic activity is common (brain, lung, liver, abdomen, bones)
- Rhabdoid tumors of the kidney are associated (about 15%) with primary embryonal cell tumors of midline brain posterior fossa (PNET-like, medulloblastoma-like tumors also called atypical teratoid/rhabdoid tumors, increasingly recognized as extrarenal rhabdoid tumors)
- High tumor stage and male sex are unfavorable prognostic features
- A familial *rhabdoid predisposition syndrome* has been described (patients harbor constitutional inactivation of *hSNF5/INI1*. They have renal rhabdoid tumors associated with similar extrarenal lesions

Gross pathology

- Large solid nonencapsulated mass with infiltrative borders
- Hemorrhage and necrosis are common
- Vascular invasion is common as well as extrarenal spread

Histology

- Diffuse growth pattern or sheets of polygonal cells with eccentric large prominent nuclei (Fig. 37-27)
- Infiltrative spread within renal parenchyma at the border of the tumor is common
- Nuclei are typically pleomorphic with vesicular chromatin, prominent nucleoli
- Hyaline, pink inclusions are located in cytoplasm of many cells. Globules are composed of intermediate filaments (Fig. 37-28)
- Mitotic activity is high, including atypical mitoses

Immunohistochemistry

- Vimentin and EMA strongly expressed; however, EMA positivity could be focal
- A variety of markers including cytokeratin, desmin and neural markers (NSE, S100), and CD99 as well as MUC1 could be positive
- Loss of nuclear staining for SNF5(INI1)/BAF47

Molecular genetics

- Biallelic alteration (deletion or mutation) of the *hSNF5/INI1* locus at chromosome 22q11.2

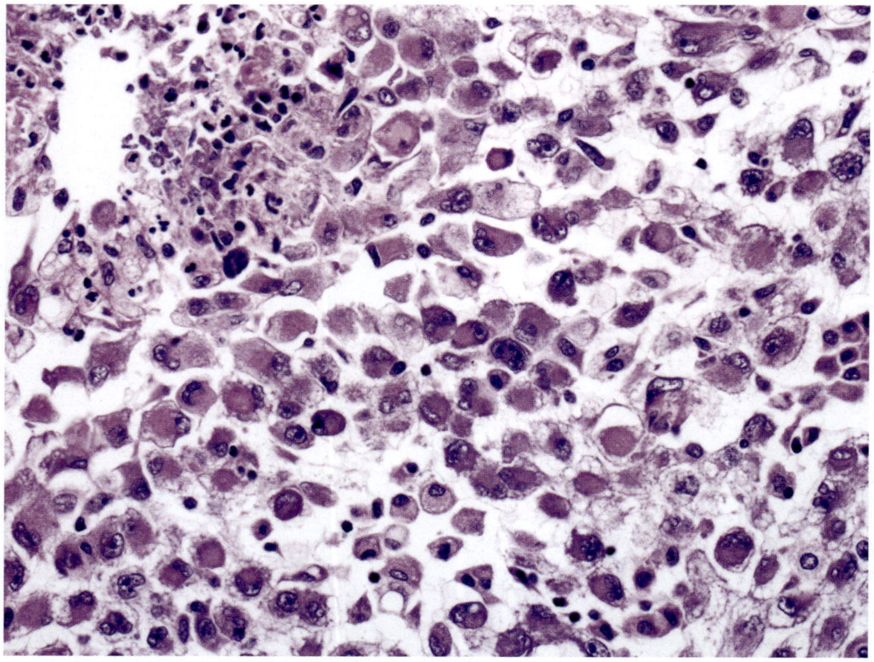

Figure 37-27.
Rhabdoid tumor is composed of large tumor cells in diffuse pattern. Focal necrosis can be seen on the left upper portion of the photo.

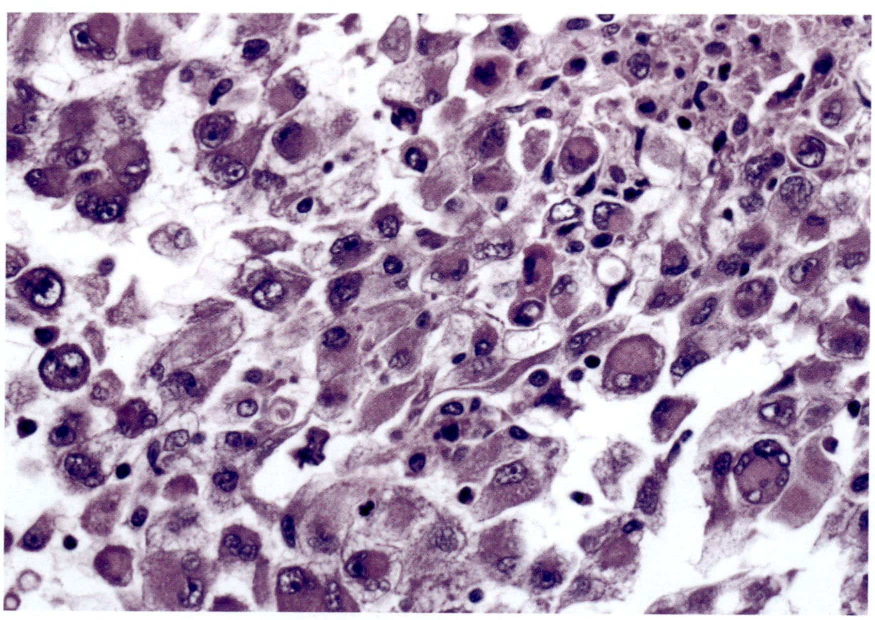

Figure 37-28.
Rhabdoid tumor exhibits the features of pleomorphic nuclei and prominent nucleoli, and its characteristic eosinophilic inclusions in the cytoplasm.

Differential diagnosis

Renal medullary carcinoma

- Usually in young adults, African-Americans with sickle cell trait
- Tumor cells are large, vesicular with variable glandular formation as opposed to the mostly solid appearance of rhabdoid tumor
- Renal medullary carcinoma (RMC) has prominent sclerosis with striking acute and chronic inflammatory cell component, and tumor necrosis

Metanephric nephroma (metanephric stromal tumor)

- Metanephric nephroma usually has "pushing" border in contrast to the infiltrating border of rhabdoid tumors
- Generally metanephric nephromas are composed of spindle cells lacking cytological atypia
- In cellular variant of metanephric nephromas, mitotic activity could be seen. However, necrosis and prominent nuclei are more commonly seen in rhabdoid tumors than in metanephric nephromas
- Immunohistochemical staining for SNF5 (INI1) is positive in metanephric nephromas, but negative in rhabdoid tumors

Clear cell RCC

- Although unusual, it is possible to find rhabdoid differentiation even in obviously typical clear cell RCC
- Consideration of age of the patient usually helps
- Adequate sampling of the entire tumor will show typical clear cell component

Treatment

- Surgery with subsequent chemotherapy
- Attempts with transplantations of autologous stem cells have been reported with some success
- Generally poor prognosis. According literature, 5-year survival ranged from 10% to 25%

CHAPTER 38

Renal Cell Carcinoma, Clear Cell Type

Ondrej Hes, Ximing J. Yang

Definition

- A malignant renal epithelial tumor composed of clear to eosinophilic cells in solid, alveolar, tubular, or focal papillary configuration
- This is the most common type of renal cell carcinoma (RCC), accounting for 50% to 70% of renal cancer cases

Other term

- Conventional renal cell carcinoma

Clinical features

- Typical signs of hematuria, back/flank pain, weight loss, and palpable mass are found in minor part of the cases
- With improved imaging methods, many cases can be detected early as an incidental finding
- Hematogenous metastases to distal organs may be the initial presentation
- Latent metastases may occur (even after 10 or more years of diagnosis and removal of the primary tumor)
- Usually metastases to the lung, liver, bone, soft tissue, or adrenals. But it is well known that clear cell RCC may metastasize to sites such as skin, or head and neck region

Gross pathology

- Mostly solid mass, low-stage tumors could be well demarcated
- Infiltrative borders are not uncommon, sometimes with small satellite tumors in adjacent kidney parenchyma
- Variably cystic, necrotic, and regressive changes in tumors are frequently noted, even in low-grade tumors
- Bright yellow to tan or brown cut surface, hemorrhage is common (Figs. 38-1*a* and 38-2*a*)
- High-grade tumors are often white with hemorrhage, necrosis or fibrosis giving a firmer consistency (Fig. 38-3)
- Multicentric and/or bilateral tumors are less common than solitary lesions

Histology

- Architecture is variable, mostly solid-alveolar pattern with delicate vascular "chicken-wire" network (Figs. 38-1*b* and 38-2)
- Cytological features are dependent on grade. Intratumoral variability of grade is nearly a constant finding (Figs. 38-4 to 38-6)
- When cysts are present, they are usually lined by the same type of clear tumor cells, as majority of the tumor mass (Fig. 38-7). Cells in low-grade clear cell RCC have mostly

Figure 38-1.
A small clear cell RCC with the typical bright yellow cut surface (*a*). Microscopically, the tumor cells have clear cytoplasm, rich vasculature, and a low Fuhrman grade (*b*).

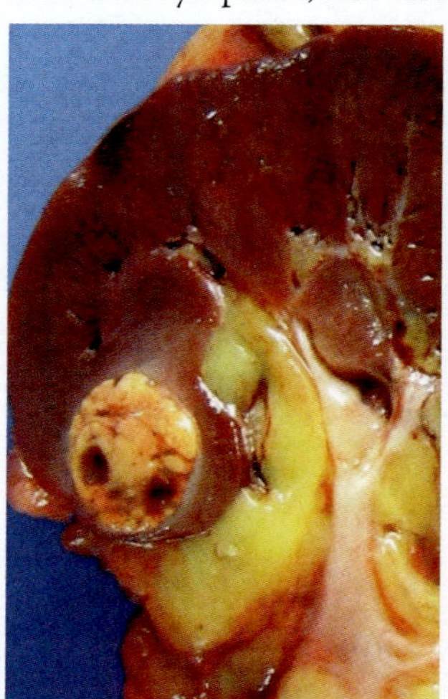

a

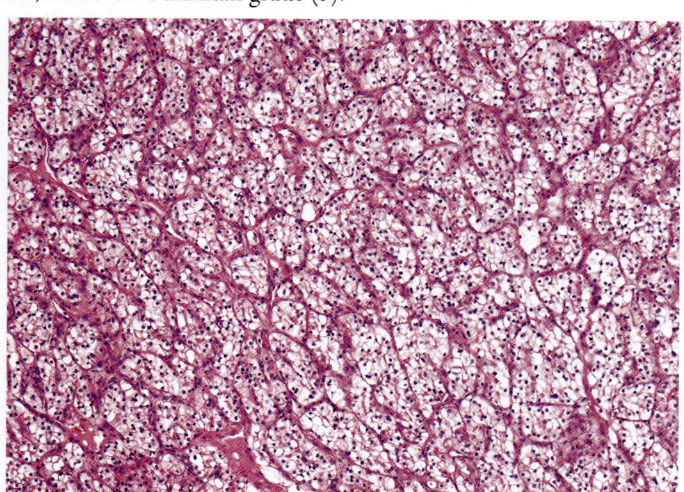

b

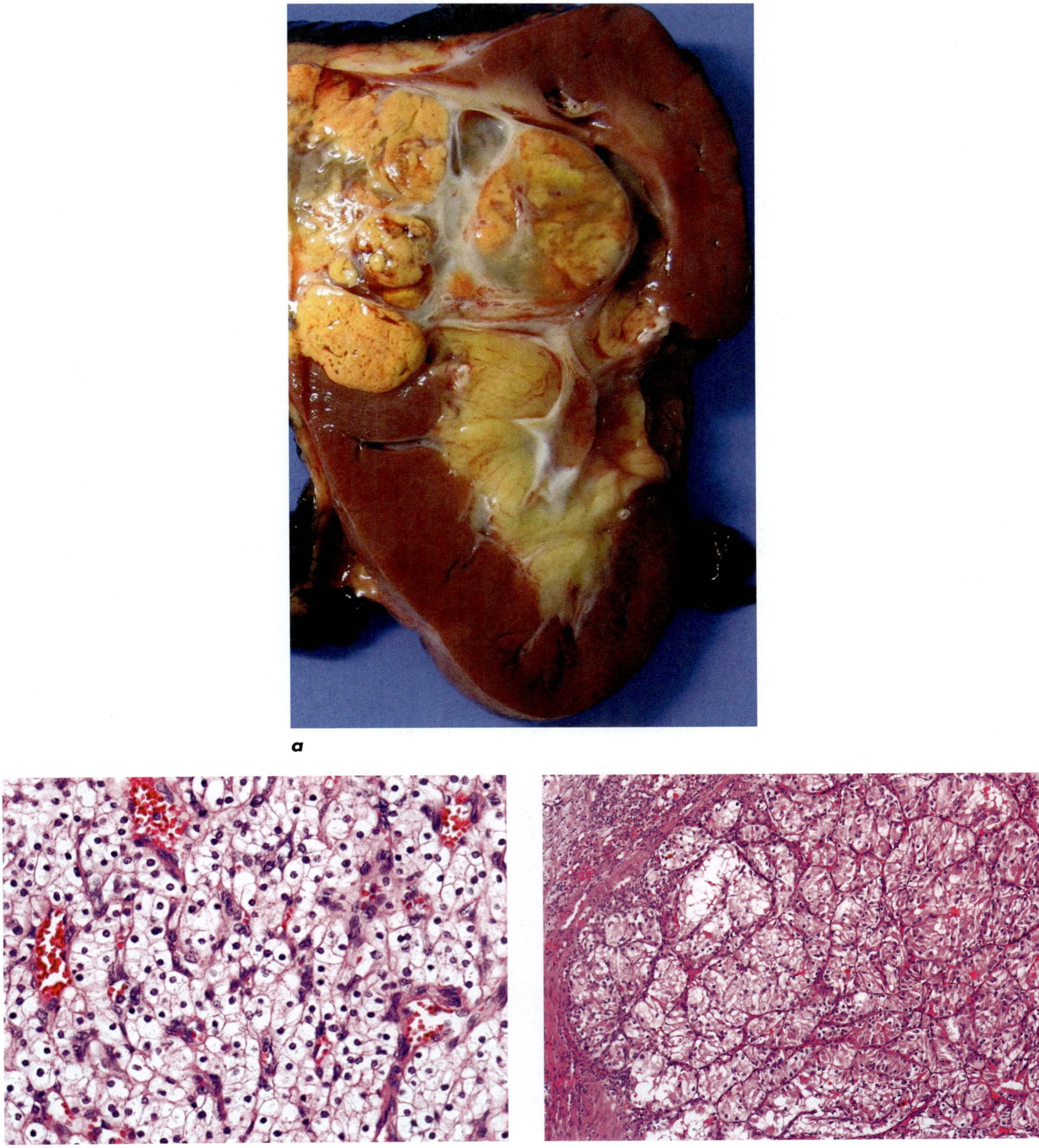

a

b **c**

Figure 38-2.
A large clear cell RCC is characterized by the presence of multilobular mass with bright yellow cut surface (*a*). Histological features are typical for clear cell RCC with complex "chicken-wire" vascular pattern (*b*). In another area of the tumor, the cells displaying more eosinophilic cytoplasm are still low grade (*c*).

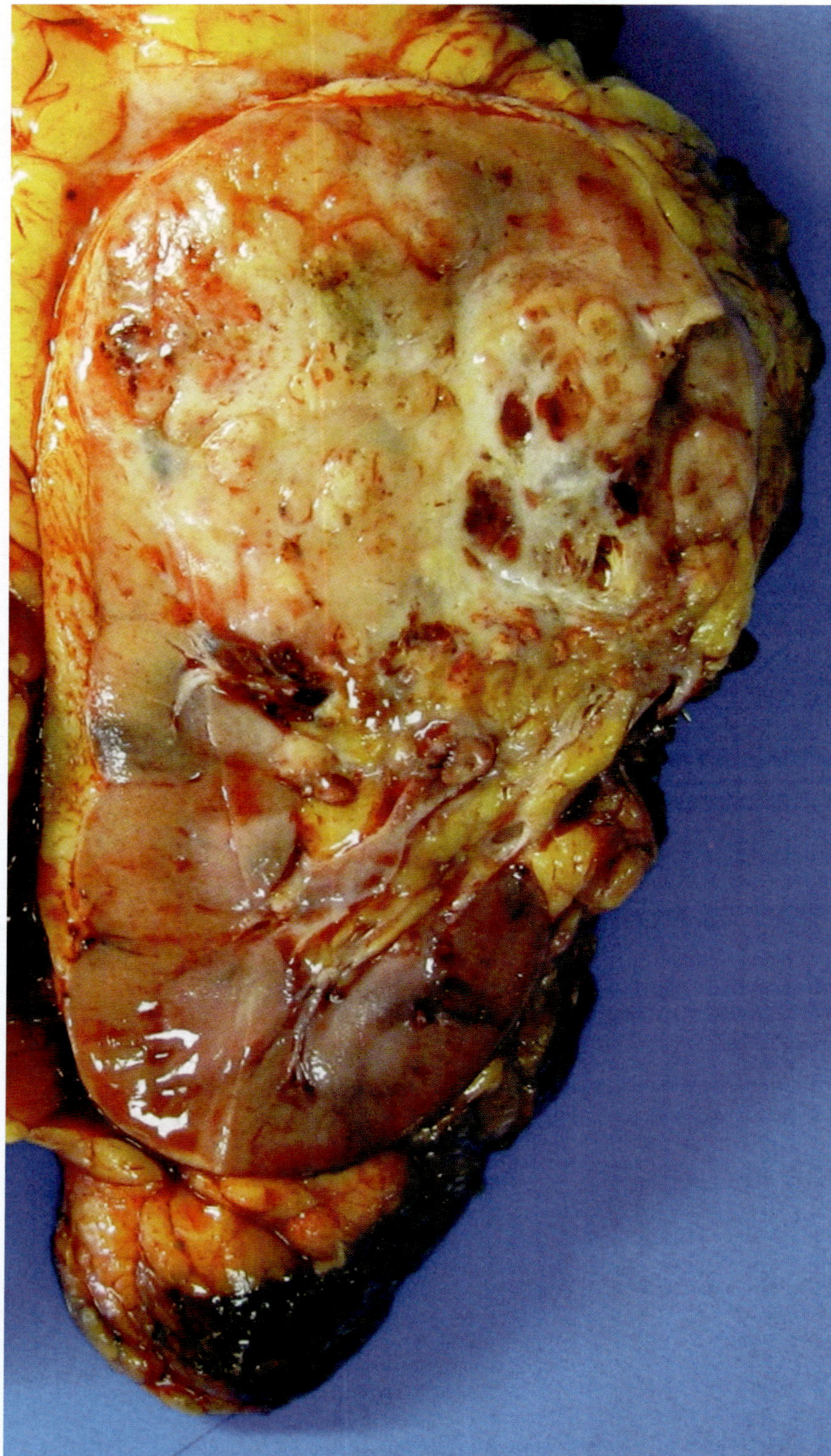

Figure 38-3.
A high-grade clear cell RCC replacing one half of the kidney. The cut surface of the tumor shows the large bright yellow mass with hemorrhage and areas of whitish areas, representing the high Fuhrman grade component.

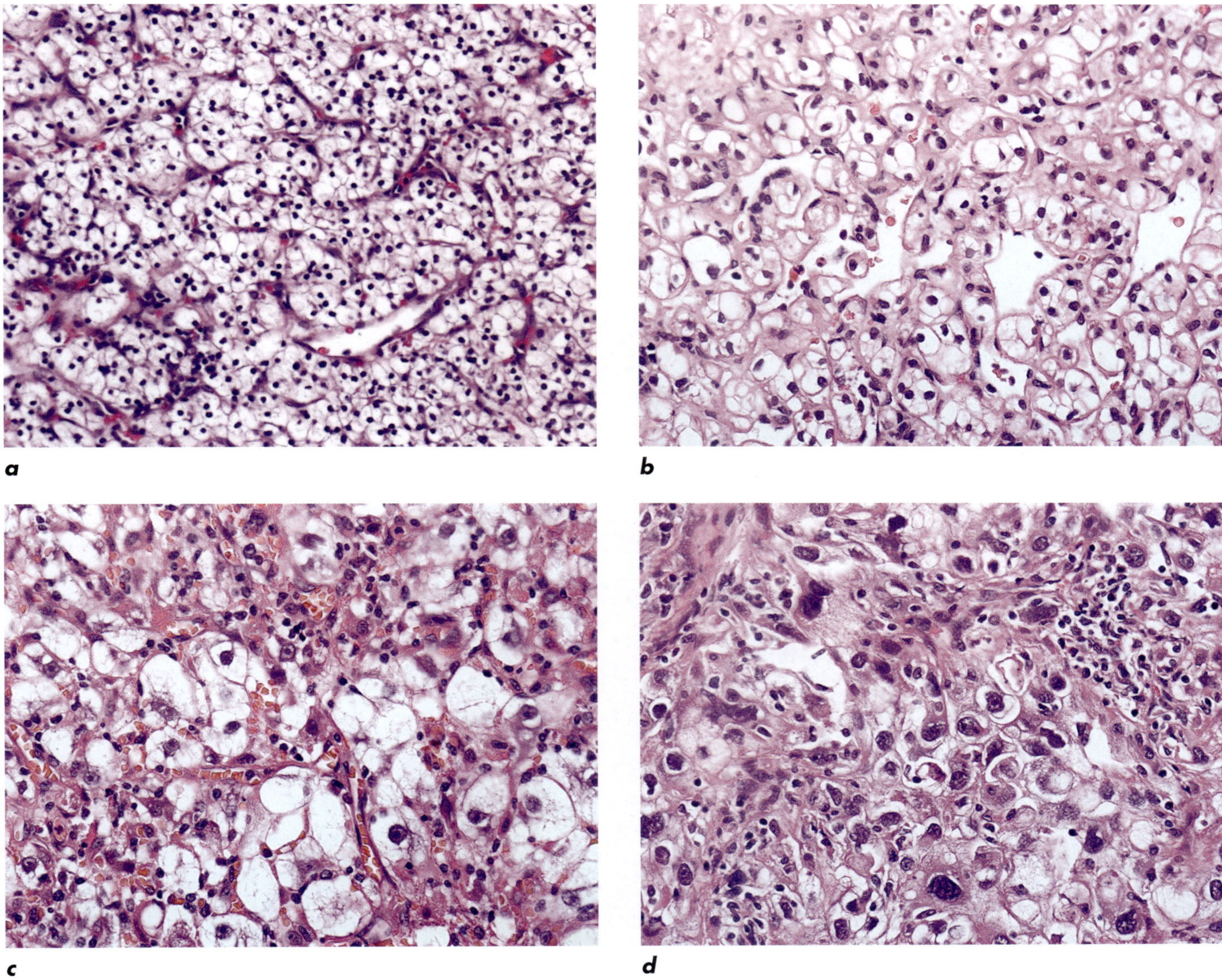

Figure 38-4.

Different Fuhrman grade components in a large tumor. Grade 1: tumor cells have no obvious nucleoli (*a*); Grade 2: tumor cells are slightly irregular in shape with nucleoli only seen at high magnification (*b*); Grade 3: Tumor cells are large with clear to eosinophilic cytoplasm and prominent nucleoli seen at low magnification (*c*); and Grade 4 with bizarre tumor cells with prominent nuclei (*d*).

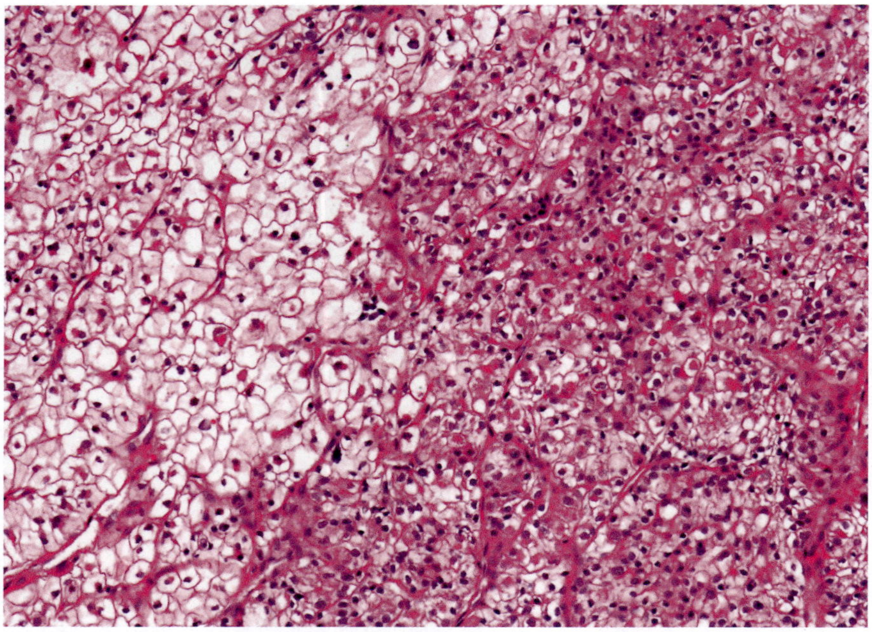

Figure 38-5.
Clear cell RCC with two Fuhrman grade components next to each other, the low-grade (G2) component on the left and higher grade (G3) component with more eosinophilic cytoplasm on the right.

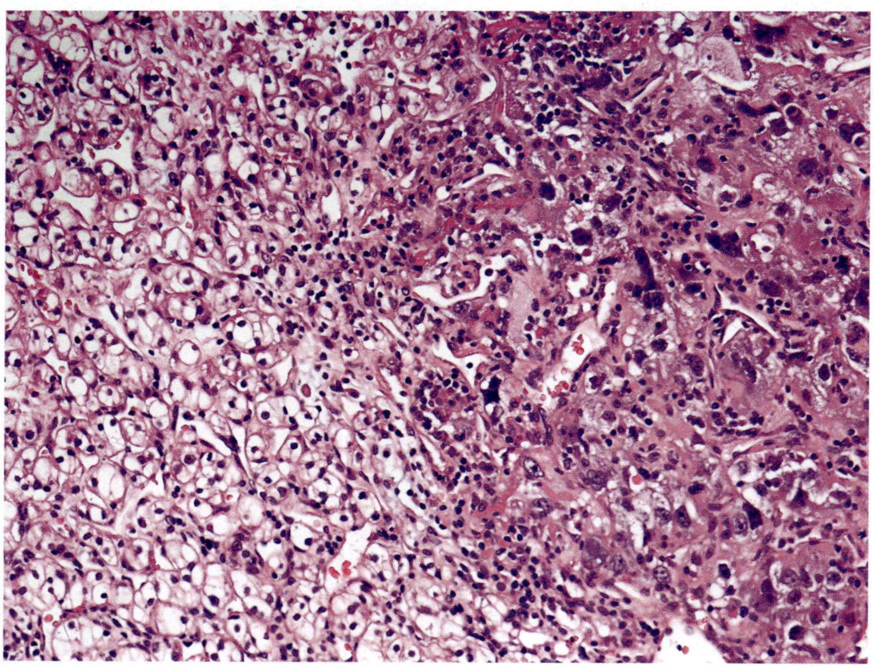

Figure 38-6.
Another case of clear cell RCC with the grade 2 component on the left and the grade 4 component on the right.

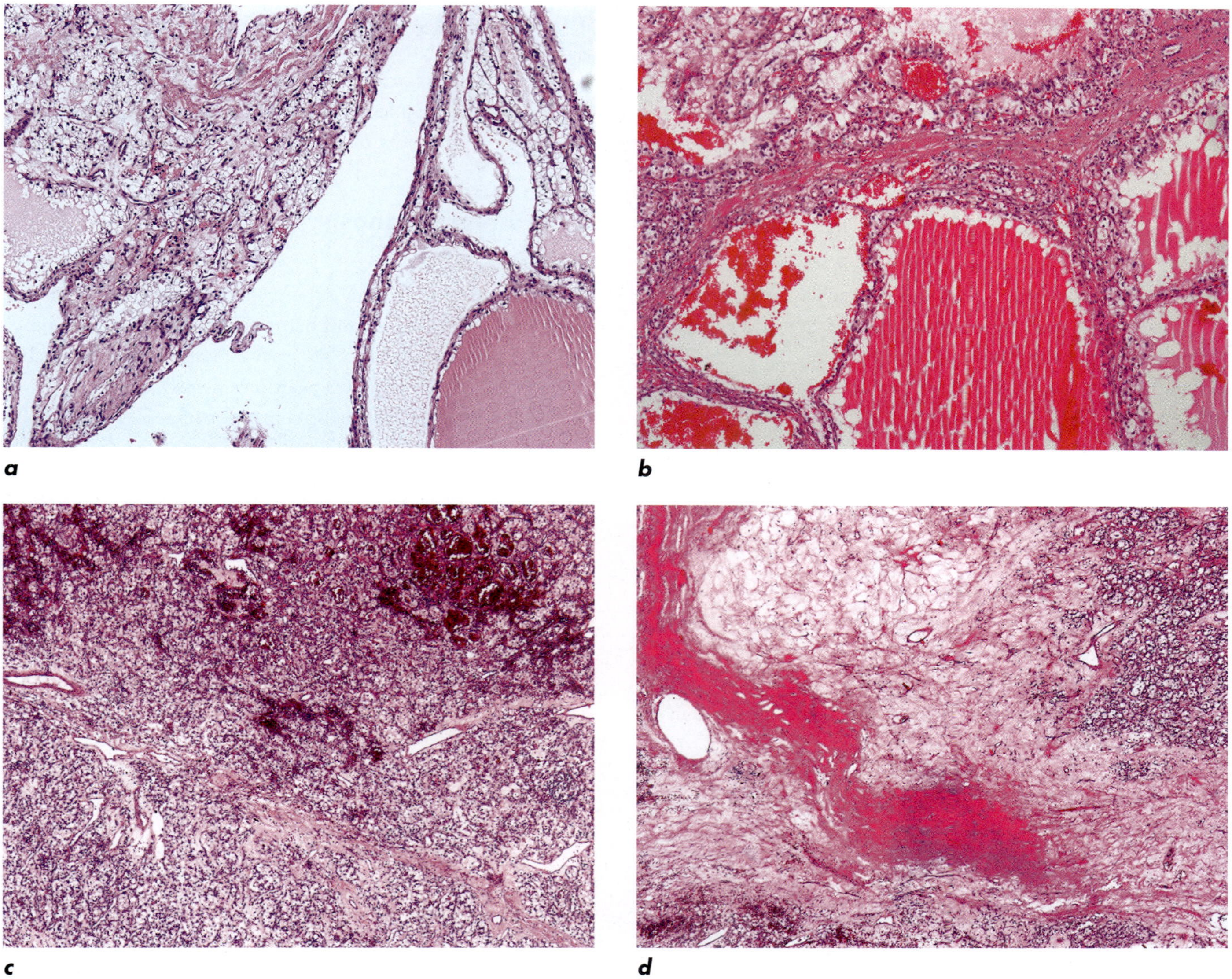

Figure 38-7.
Clear cell RCC with multiple cysts and solid areas (*a*); cystic structures containing dense eosinophilic material in the lumen (*b*); areas of hemorrhage (*c*); and area with degenerative changes (*d*).

clear voluminous cytoplasm with rounded nuclei. In high-grade areas, eosinophilic cytoplasm, rich with organelles, is common, nuclei tend to be irregular and polymorphic (Figs. 38-2*c* and 38-4*d*)

- So-called granular RCC is being considered part of the morphological spectrum of high-grade clear cell RCC (Figs. 38-5 and 38-6)
- Regressive areas composed of fibrotic tissues have very typical, well-preserved vasculature, which, in some areas, could resemble malignant vascular tumors such as angiosarcoma
- A particular attention should be paid to the renal vein involvement by the tumor (Fig. 38-8)
- Intratumorous granulomatous reaction can be occasionally seen (Fig. 38-9)
- Tubular, pseudotubular pattern is not uncommon, focal papillary configuration or pseudopapillary pattern could be seen. True papillae are rarely seen (Figs. 38-10 and 38-11)

Immunohistochemistry

- Vimentin, EMA, CA9 are positive; however, AE1-AE3 could be positive only focally
- RCC, PAX2, CD10 usually positive
- CK7 is usually negative, but can be focally positive in up to 25% of the cases
- AMACR is negative in the majority of cases, however, tumor cells with granular cytoplasm could be weakly positive
- Antimitochondrial antigen (MIA) can be weakly positive

Molecular genetics

- Up to 60% of the cases have *Von Hippel Lindau* (*VHL*) gene mutations or hypermethylated *VHL* promoter
- Chromosome 3p loss is a typical finding in clear cell RCC
- Trisomy/polysomy of chromosome 7 has been described

Differential diagnosis

Papillary RCC

- Prominent papillary or tubular patterns
- Foamy macrophages and hemosiderin are often present
- Some cases of papillary RCC may contain clear cell areas, but the rich "chicken-wire" vasculature is usually absent
- In difficult cases, analysis of chromosomes 7, 17, and Y (in males) will be helpful
- Immunohistochemically, the majority of papillary RCCs are diffusely positive for AMACR, vimentin, and CK7

Chromophobe RCC

- Composed of two types of cells: large pale cells and smaller eosinophilic cytoplasm. Perinuclear halo and raisinoid nuclei (see Chapter 39) are characteristic. Chromophobe RCC could be solid-alveolar, but tubular, adenomatoid and even microcystic variants have been published
- Immunohistochemically, ChRCC lacks diffuse vimentin positivity, mostly are CK7 at least focally and CD117 diffusely positive

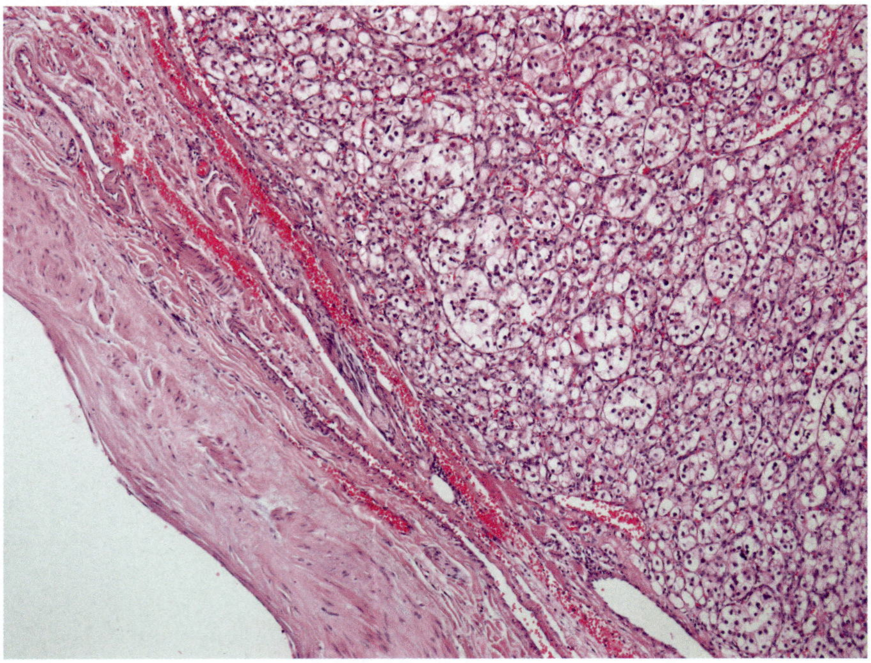

Figure 38-8.
Clear cell RCC involving the renal vein as a tumor thrombus.

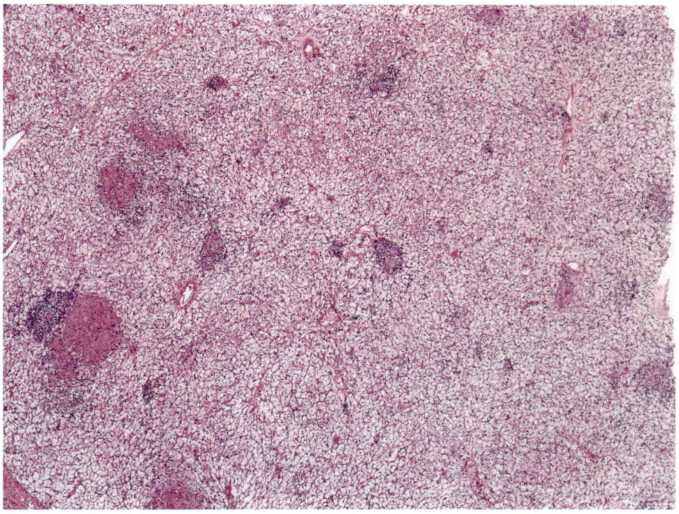

a

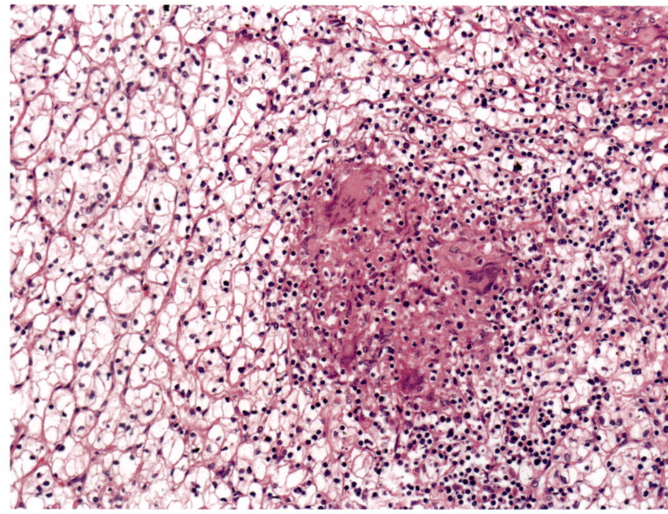

b

Figure 38-9.
Clear cell RCC with numerous granulomas (*a*). High magnification shows the granulomas consist of epithelioid histiocytes and multinuclear giant cells (*b*).

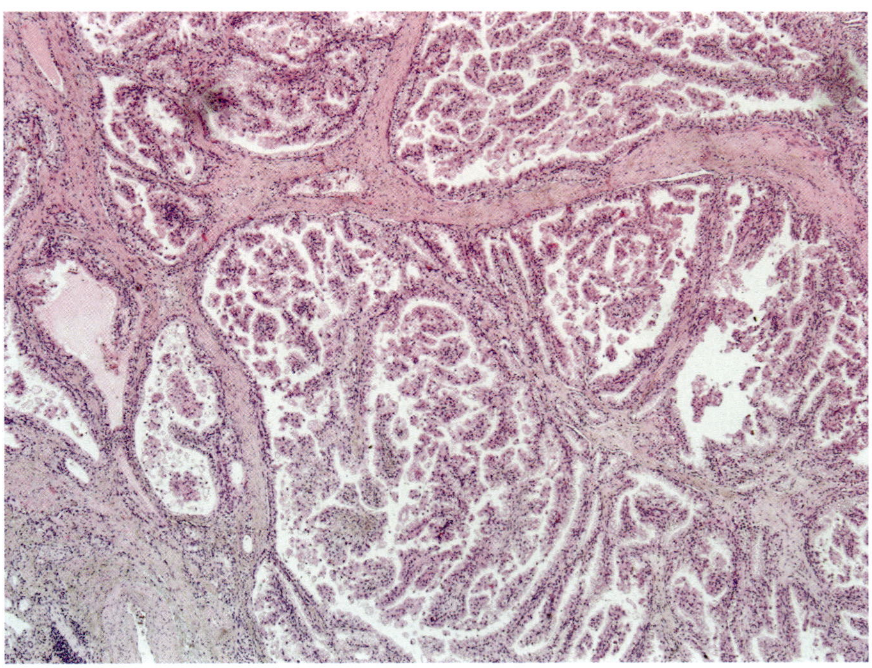

Figure 38-10.
Clear cell RCC with unusual papillary configuration, which should be distinguished from clear cell papillary RCC.

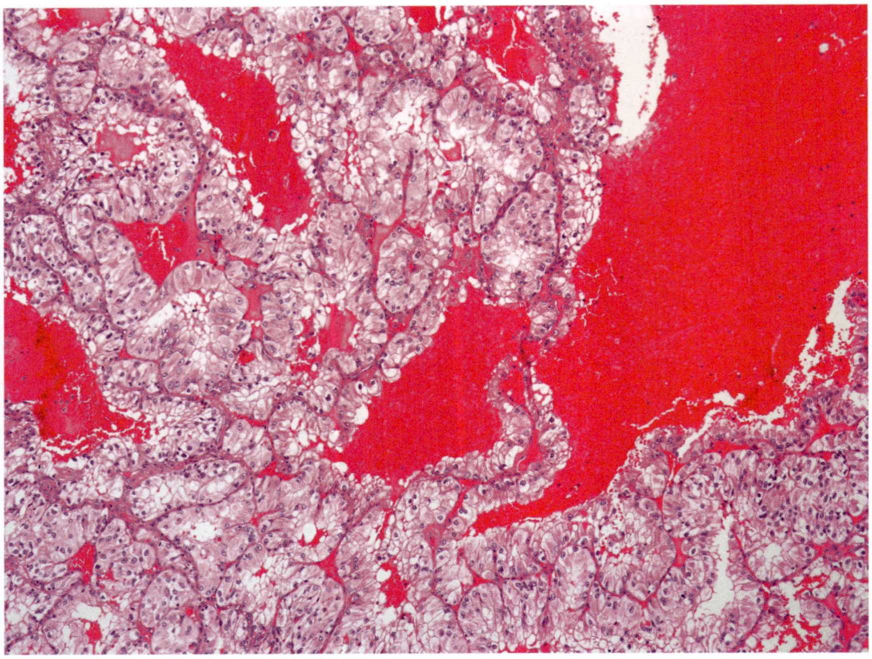

Figure 38-11.
A high-grade clear cell RCC with prominent papillary configurations.

Renal oncocytoma

- Clear cell RCC with granular cytoplasm could be morphologically similar to oncocytoma. High degree of nuclear atypia is not uncommon in some oncocytomas
- Sufficient sampling usually helps find more typical areas, where features typical for oncocytoma are obvious
- Immunohistochemical reaction to MIA (antimitochondrial antigen) could also help; however, so-called small cell variant of renal oncocytoma is weakly MIA positive with completely negative areas
- In granular variant of clear cell RCC, the MIA positivity could be strong, but not diffuse—there is patchy positivity
- Also, vimentin is mostly diffusely positive in clear cell RCC. In oncocytoma, the positivity with vimentin could be strong, but very focal

Clear cell papillary RCC

- Prominent papillary formations combined with solid-alevolar foci with low-grade clear cell population should rise suspicion for clear cell PRCC
- Prominent leiomyomatous stroma would be extremely unusual in clear cell RCC
- Immunohistochemically, clear cell papillary RCC is negative for vimentin and diffusely positive for CK7
- CD10, CA9 could be focally weakly positive

Epithelioid angiomyolipoma

- Composed of polymorphic epithelioid cells with prominent nuclear atypia
- The presence of any adipocytes, thick-walled, abortive vessels, information about tuberous sclerosis in patient should rise the suspicion for AML
- HMB45 and melan A are standard excellent markers for confirmation of AML diagnosis

Clinical relevance (prognosis and treatment options)

- Partial or radical nephrectomy
- Targeted therapies using antiangiogenic drugs have promising results. The most commonly involved pathways are HIF, mTOR, and VEGF
- Prognosis depends on stage and grade of the tumor, generally 5-year survival up to 75% of the patients, 10-year survival up to 62%
- Tumor stages: T1 (tumor ≤7 cm); T2 (tumor >7 cm but confined to the kidney); T3 (tumor invades main renal vein, renal sinus adipose tissue or perinephric tissue); and T4 (beyond Gerota fascia or involving ipsilateral adrenal)

CHAPTER 39

Renal Cell Carcinoma, Other Common Types

Ximing J. Yang, Huiying He, Fan Lin

MULTILOCULAR CYSTIC RENAL CELL CARCINOMA

Definition

- A variant of low-grade renal cell carcinoma composed of multilocular cysts lined by neoplastic cells with clear cytoplasm

Pathogenesis

- Possibly the early phase of clear cell RCC

Clinical features

- Most cases found incidentally by imaging studies as a complex cystic lesion but no solid areas

Gross pathology

- Solitary well-circumscribed cystic lesion (Fig. 39-1*a*) containing clear cystic fluid
- Cut surface of the tumor is typically multilocular with a smooth inner surface (Fig. 39-2*a*)

Histology

- A multilocular cystic mass separated by thin septa (Fig. 39-1*b*)
- Cysts are lined by single layer of epithelial cells with clear cytoplasm (Figs. 39-1*c* and 39-2*b*), with occasional stratification or tufting
- Fuhrman nuclear grade 1 (no nucleoli seen) (Figs. 39-2*b* and 39-3*a*)
- Fibrotic septa may contain small nests of clear cells (Fig. 39-3*a*), but solid areas of tumor cells are absent

Immunohistochemistry

- CA9 positive (Figs. 39-2*c* and 39-3*b*)
- Keratin markers positive, CK7 positive
- CD10 positive, PAX8 positive

Molecular analysis

- May have 3p deletion

Differential diagnosis

- *Cystic nephroma* has ovarian type of stoma (ER/PR positive) and lining epithelial cells have eosinophilic cytoplasm
- *Cystic clear cell RCC* has solid and cystic areas of tumor cells, which has higher metastatic potential

Clinical relevance (prognosis and treatment options)

- It may coexist with classic clear cell RCC, or progress to clear cell RCC if untreated
- Surgical treatment necessary since it may progress to full grown clear cell RCC
- Excellent prognosis, no evidence of metastasis after surgical removal

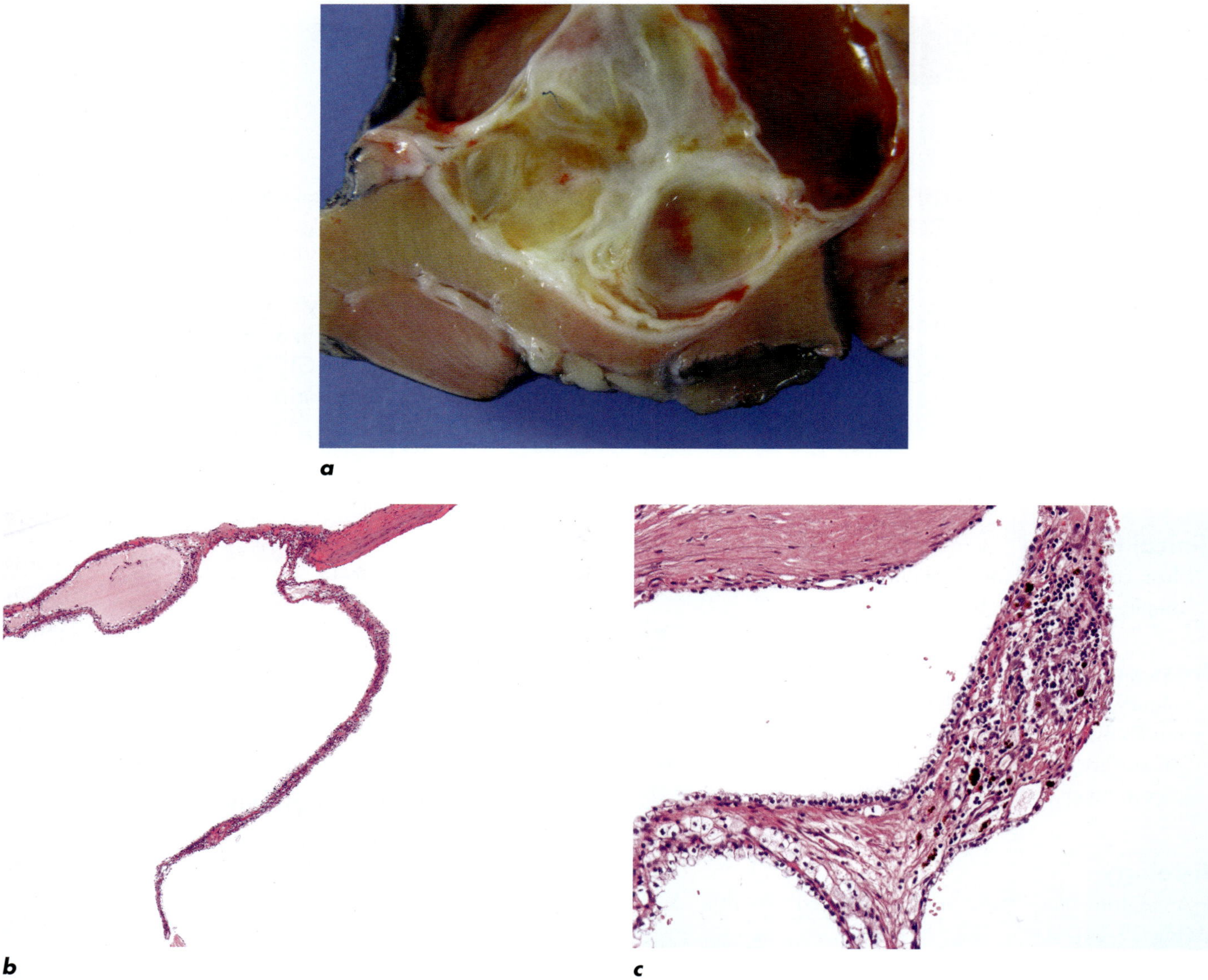

Figure 39-1.

Gross photo of multilocular cystic renal cell carcinoma (*a*). Microscopically, the tumor is composed of multilocular cyst separated by thin septa (*b*). High magnification shows lining tumor cells with clear cytoplasm with no nuclear atypia. Some small clusters of clear cells can be seen in the septa, but no solid area of tumor cells (*c*).

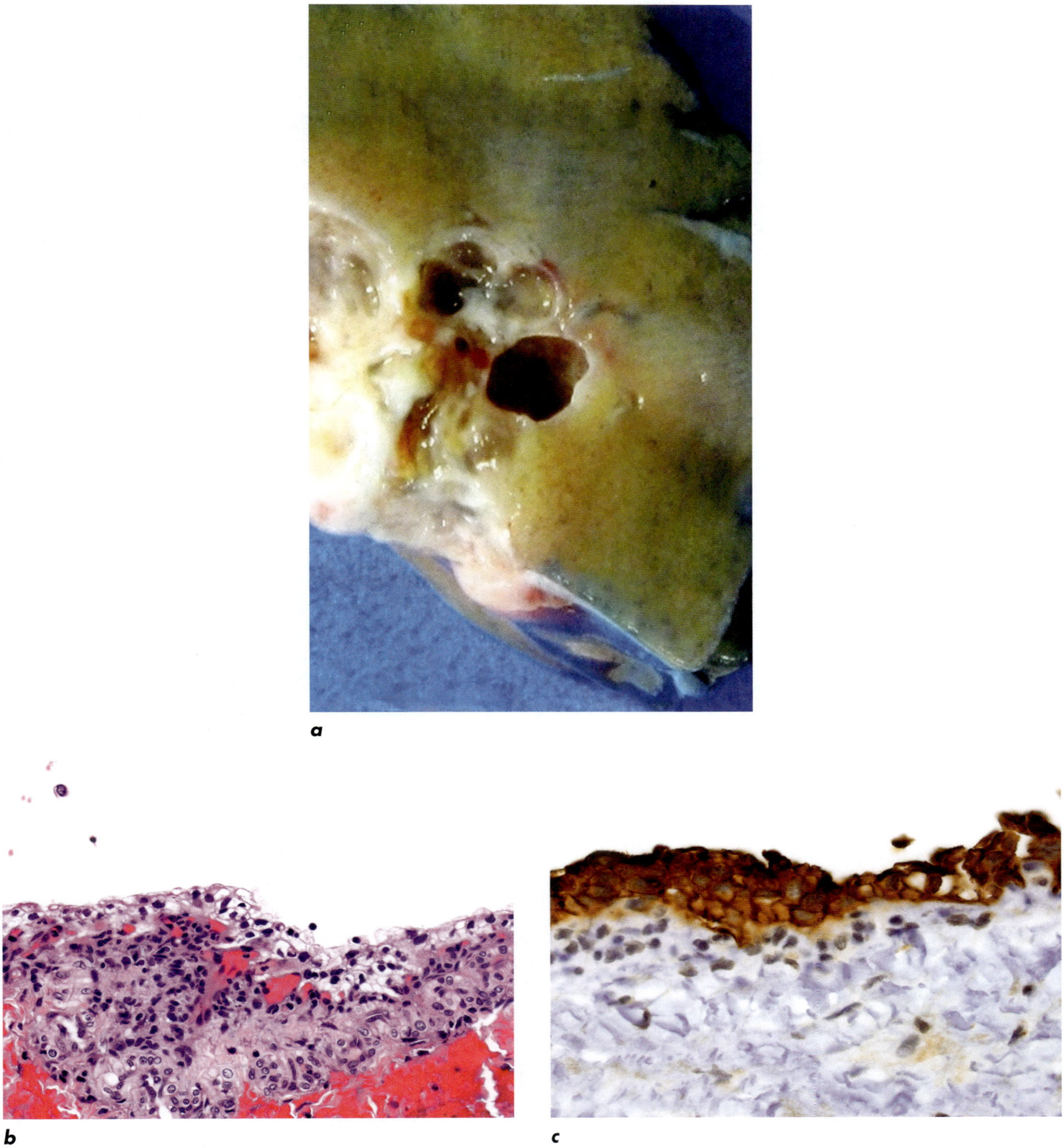

Figure 39-2.
Multilocular cystic RCC in a partial nephrectomy specimen (*a*). The cystic lining cells have clear cytoplasm with no obvious nucleoli seen (*b*) and they are positive for carbonic anhydrase (CA) 9 (*c*).

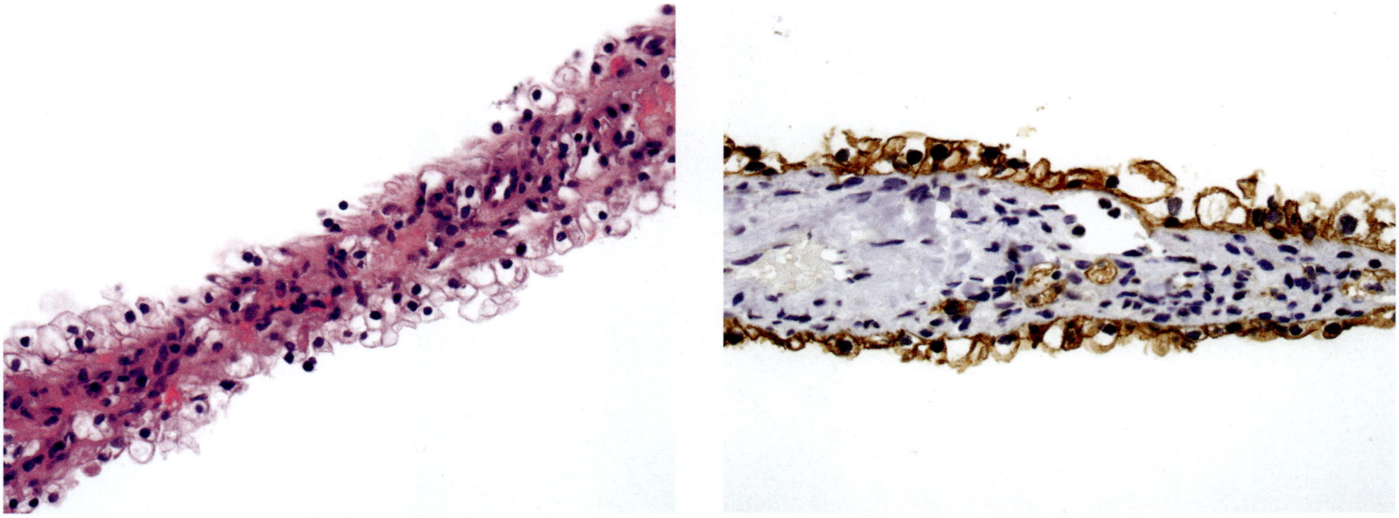

a *b*

Figure 39-3.
The septum of multilocular cystic RCC is lined by tumor cells with clear cytoplasm without atypia (*a*). The tumor cells demonstrate the membranous staining for CA9 (*b*).

PAPILLARY RENAL CELL CARCINOMA

Definition

- A malignant renal epithelial neoplasm with papillary architectures

Other term

- Chromophile renal cell carcinoma

Pathogenesis and epidemiology

- It is not derived from either proximal or distal tubular cells as generally believed
- It is most likely derived from multipotential stem cells
- The possible development sequence is from papillary adenoma to papillary renal cell carcinoma
- Second most common subtype of RCC, accounting for 10% to 15% of all RCCs
- Mean age 55 to 65 years and male to female ratio 3:1

Clinical features

- Signs and symptoms are not specific, such as flank mass, hematuria
- Radiographic features are not specific. Renal angiography studies show relative hypovascularity
- Hemorrhage is common in papillary RCC (PRCC)

Gross pathology

- Well circumscribed with no capsule (Fig. 39-4*a*)
- PRCC can be solitary or multiple (Figs. 39-5*a* and 39-6*a*). Bilateral and multifocal (papillary carcinomatosis) are more common in PRCCs than other subtypes of RCC. Small papillary adenomas (<5 mm) are often seen in the kidney harboring papillary RCC
- Wide range of color from white, yellow to light brown (Figs. 39-4*a*, 39-5*a*, 39-6*a*, 39-7*a*, and 39-8*a*)
- Hemorrhage is more common in PRCCs (Fig. 39-9*a*) than other renal tumors. Necrosis and cystic changes are also relatively frequent
- High-grade tumors, generally bigger than the low-grade ones, often have solid granular appearance of cut surfaces (Figs. 39-8*a* and 39-15*a*)
- Lymph node metastasis is more common than other type of RCC

Histology

- Both type 1 and type 2 PRCCs have papillary configurations
- Type 1: basophilic variant, scant cytoplasm, mostly low nuclear grade (Figs. 39-6 and 39-10)
- Type 2: eosinophilic variant, abundant eosinophilic cytoplasm, mostly high nuclear grade (Figs. 39-4, 39-5, and 39-11). Low-grade type 2 PRCCs are occasionally seen (Fig. 39-5)
- 20% to 30% of PRCCs contain both type 1 and type 2 components

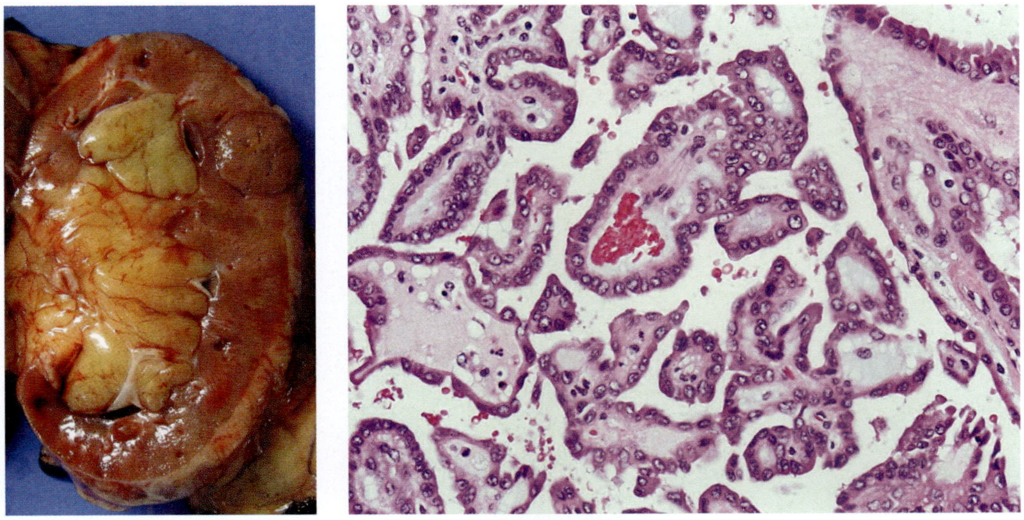

a b

Figure 39-4.
Gross photo of a papillary RCC shows a well-circumscribed mass in the cortex, which has almost the same color of the normal kidney parenchyma (*a*). Microscopically, this tumor is composed of tumor cells with eosinophilic cytoplasm (*b*) as a low-grade papillary RCC, type 2.

- Low (nuclear) grade PRCCs including Fuhrman grade 1 and grade 2 tumors are typically small in size, with an indolent behavior (Figs. 39-4 to 39-7)
- High (nuclear) grade tumors including Fuhrman grade 3 and grade 4 are less common and typically large in size, associated with an aggressive behavior (Figs. 39-8, 39-11, and 39-15)
- Hemorrhage and necrosis are commonly seen, which does not correlate with an aggressive behavior (Fig. 39-9)
- Foamy macrophages are often seen within the fibrovascular cores, more common in type 1 than in type 2, which may contribute to the bright yellow color of the tumor grossly (Figs. 39-5 and 39-7)
- Oncocytic papillary RCC (Figs. 39-12 and 39-13) can mimic a renal oncocytoma. The presence of macrophage in an oncocytic renal tumor is highly suggestive of papillary RCC
- Some unusual patterns including glomeruloid, tall columnar cell, or lipid-rich signet ring cell type (Fig. 39-14). Lymph node metastasis is more common in papillary RCC (Fig. 39-15) than in other types of RCC, while renal vein invasion is less common in papillary RCC (Fig. 39-16) than in clear cell RCC

Immunohistochemistry

- PAX2/PAX8 positive, vimentin positive
- AMACR positive (100%) (Fig. 39-13*d*)
- CK7 positive (Fig. 39-13*c*), type 1 is diffuse, and type 2 can be focal
- CD10, RCC, Ber-EP4 positive (50% to 70%)
- CA9 weakly positive or cytoplasmic positive
- C-kit negative (Fig. 39-13*d*), or weakly positive

Molecular analysis

- Trisomy 7, 17 are most common cytogenetic findings
- Familial PRCC may have *MET* mutation or fumarate hydratase gene alteration, the sporadic PRCCs have a very low rate of these gene mutations

Clinical relevance (prognosis and treatment options)

- For PRCC, the grading is the most important histological factor to predicate the prognosis
- Type 1 and type 2 are also important for prognosis predication (see Table 39-1 for summary)
- Papillary adenoma (low nuclear grade, <5 mm in size) is believed to be the precursor of PRCC
- Lymph node metastasis is more common than distant organ metastasis
- Treatment of choice is partial or radical nephrectomy
- No effective chemotherapy has been established so far although some clinical trials show promising results

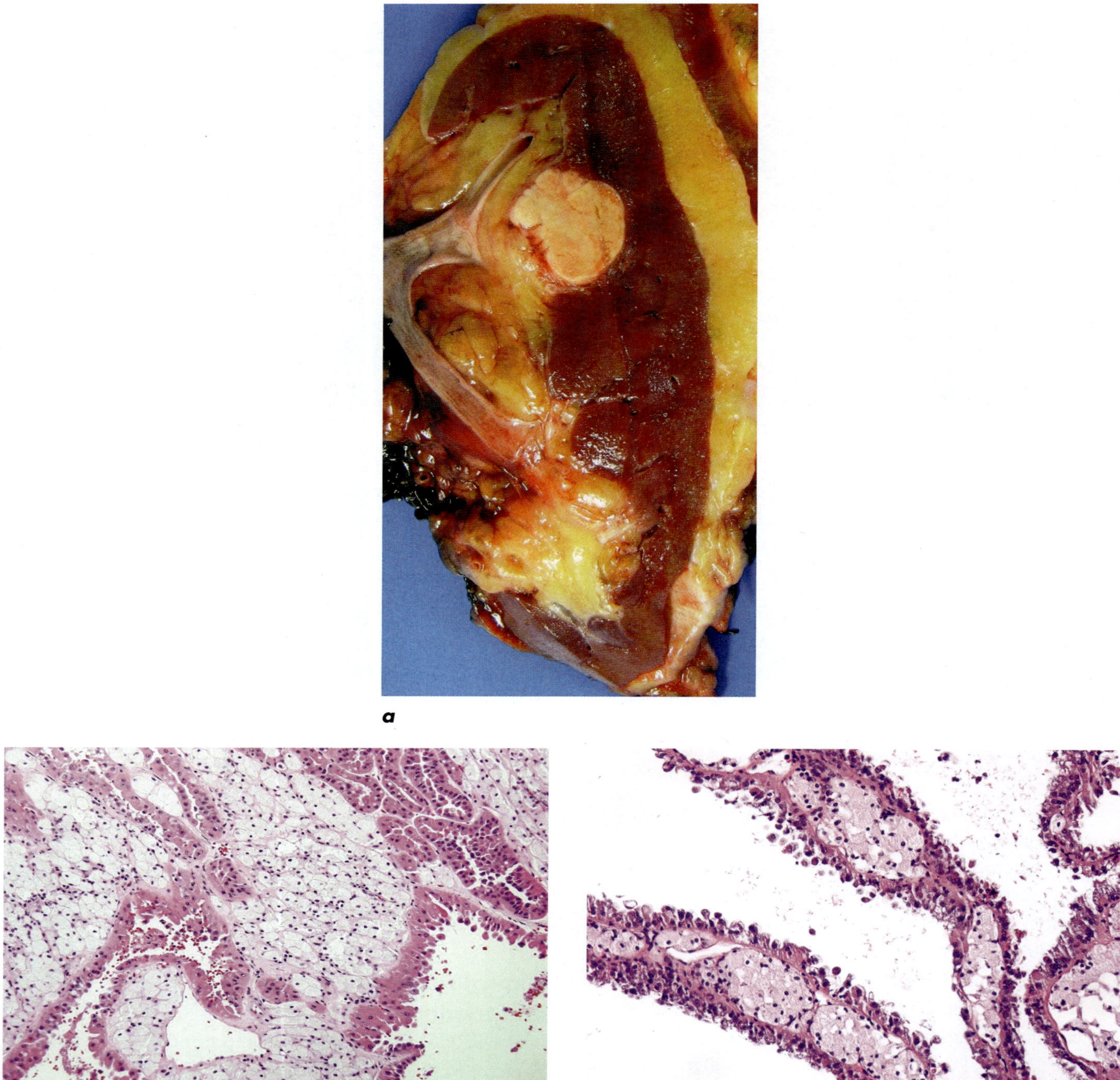

a b c

Figure 39-5.
This papillary RCC has a pale yellow cut surface, mimicking clear cell RCC (*a*). Microscopically, the tumor cells have eosinophilic cytoplasm (*b*) and numerous macrophages (*c*), as a low-grade, type 2, papillary RCC.

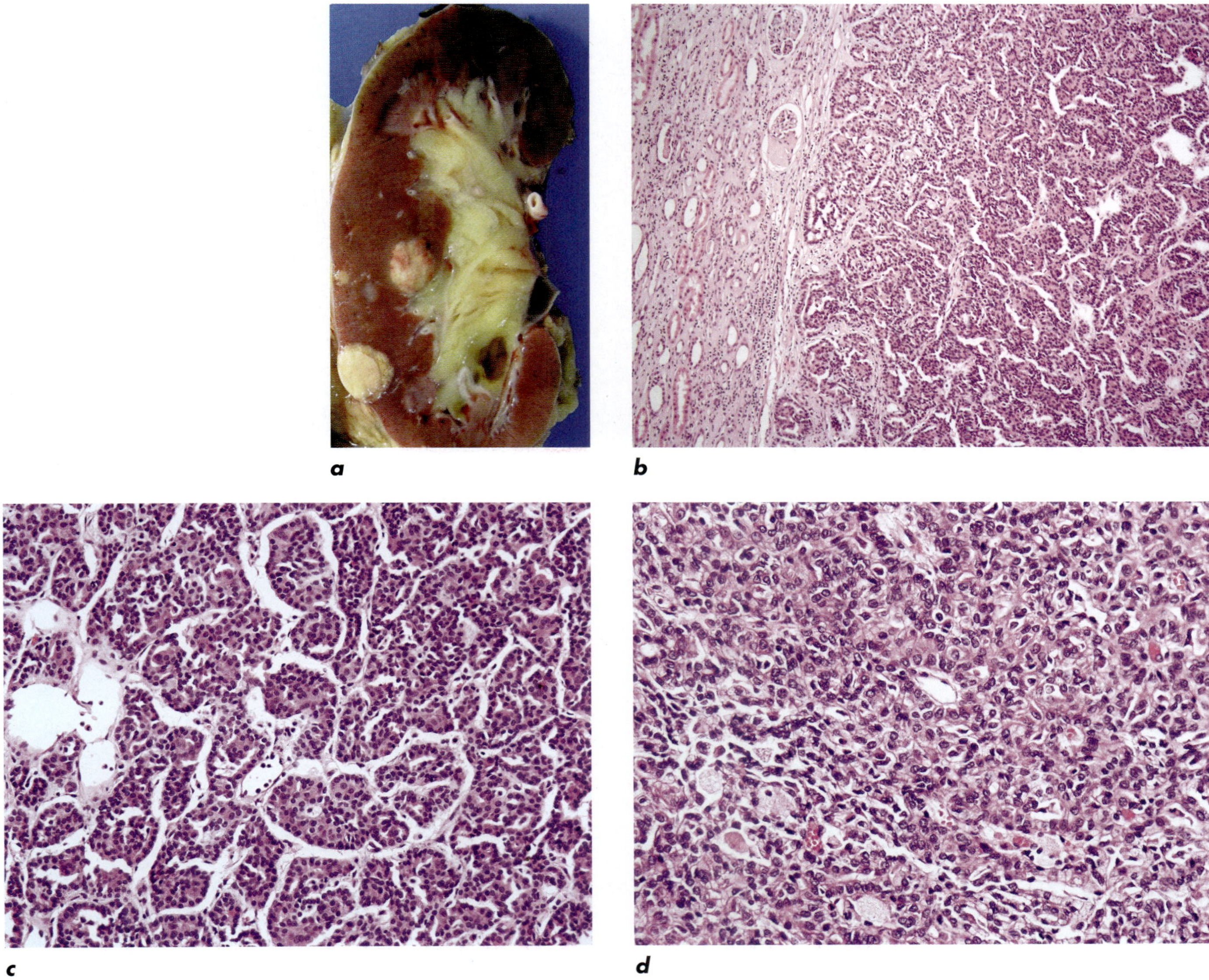

Figure 39-6.

Papillary carcinomatosis containing multiple nodules of papillary RCC and papillary adenomas (*a*). One of the papillary RCC nodules is composed of tumor cells forming tubular and papillary structures (*b*). High magnification shows tubular and papillary configurations (*c*) with low-grade tumor cells with small amount of cytoplasm (*d*).

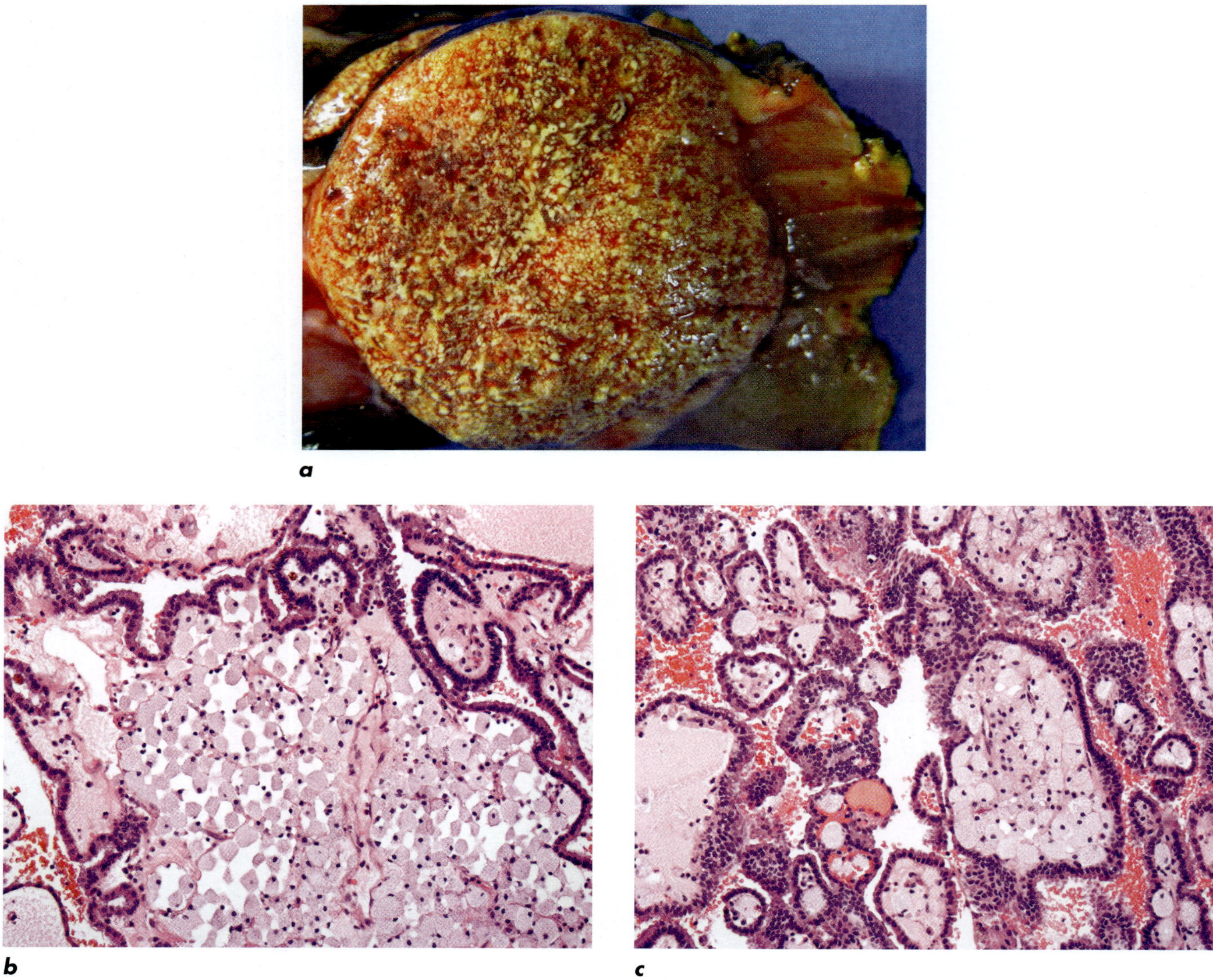

Figure 39-7.
Papillary RCC with a unique gross appearance with many yellow dots on the cut surface (*a*). This appearance is contributed by presence of a large number of foamy macrophages in the tumor (*b*), the tumor cells have moderate amount of eosinophilic cytoplasm, but somewhat between type 1 and type 2 (*c*).

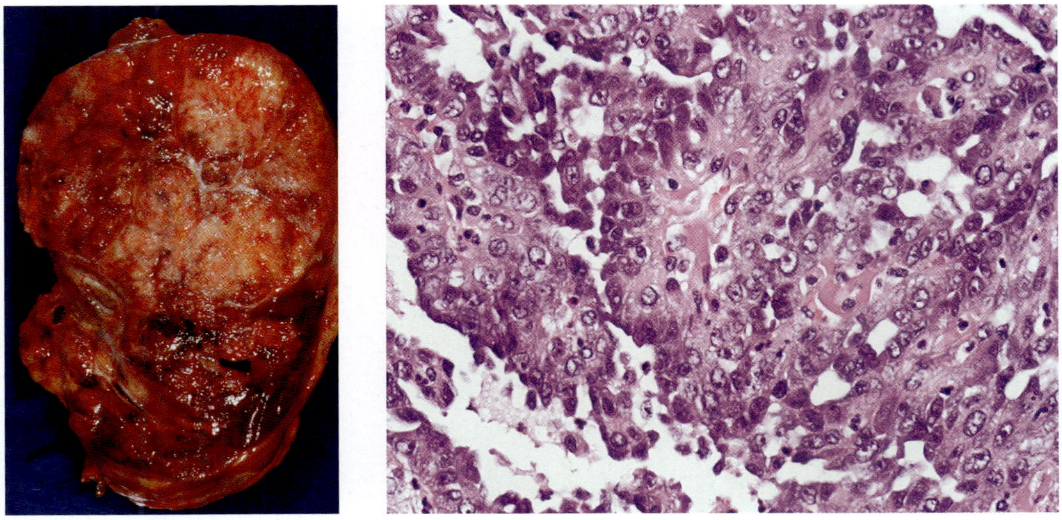

a b

Figure 39-8.
Gross photo of a high-grade papillary RCC type 2 displays a large mass in the upper pole with granular cut surface and focal hemorrhage (*a*). Microscopically, the tumor cells in papillary configuration have significant cytological atypia and prominent nucleoli (*b*).

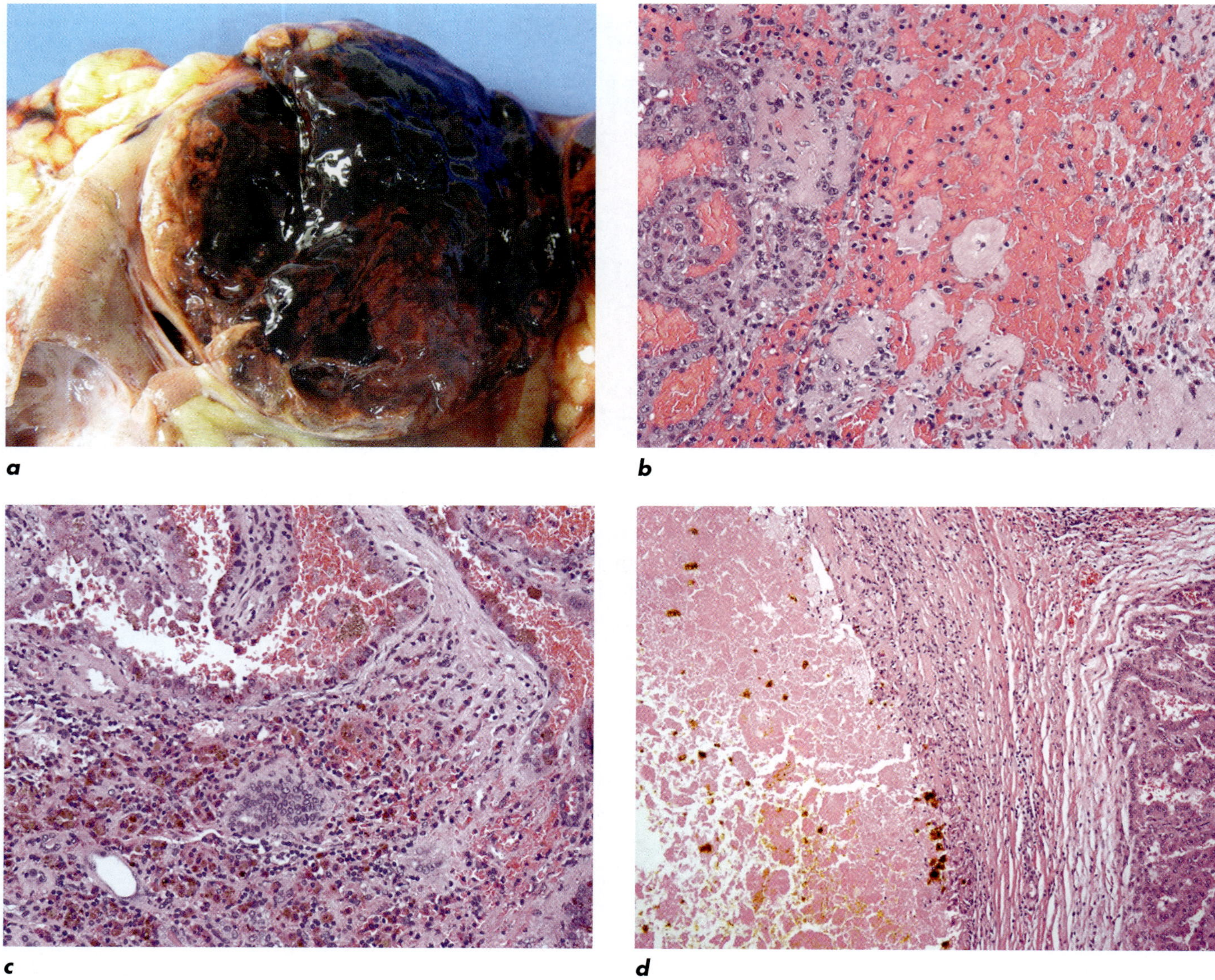

Figure 39-9.
Papillary RCC with extensive hemorrhage showing dark red cut surface (*a*). Microscopically, the tumor exhibits fresh (*b*) and old hemorrhage (*c*) as well as necrotic area adjacent to high-grade type 2 papillary RCC (*d*).

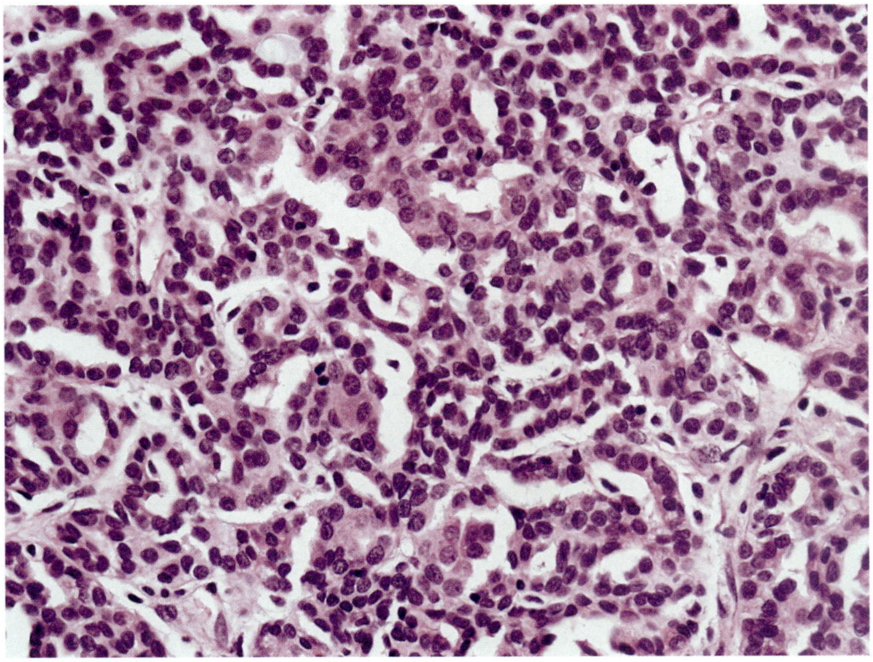

Figure 39-10.
Typical type 1 papillary RCC is characterized by the presence of tumor cells with scant cytoplasm, generally low nuclear grade.

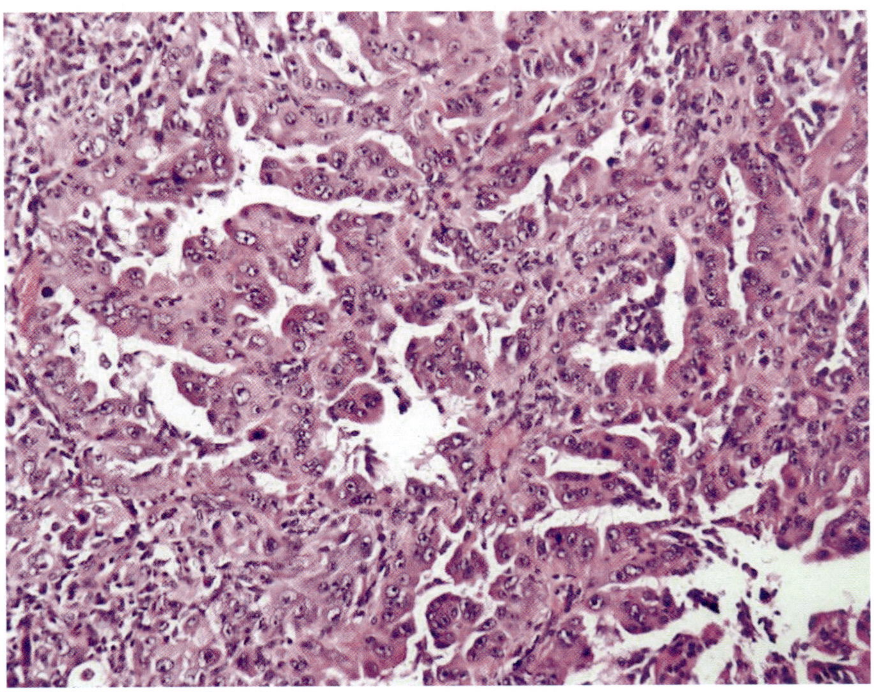

Figure 39-11.
Type 2 papillary RCC is characterized by the presence of tumor cells with eosinophilic cytoplasm, generally high nuclear grade.

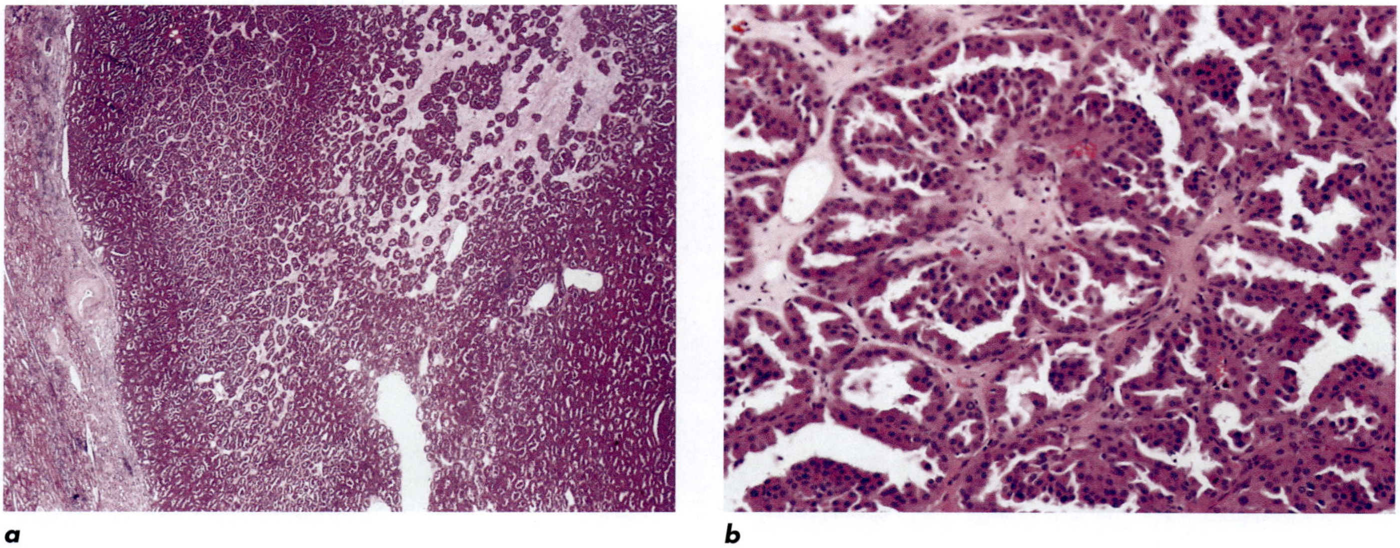

Figure 39-12.
Oncocytic papillary RCC consists of tubules formed by tumor cells with prominent eosinophilic cytoplasm, resembling oncocytoma (*a*). Subtle papillary or glomeruloid structures can be seen (*b*).

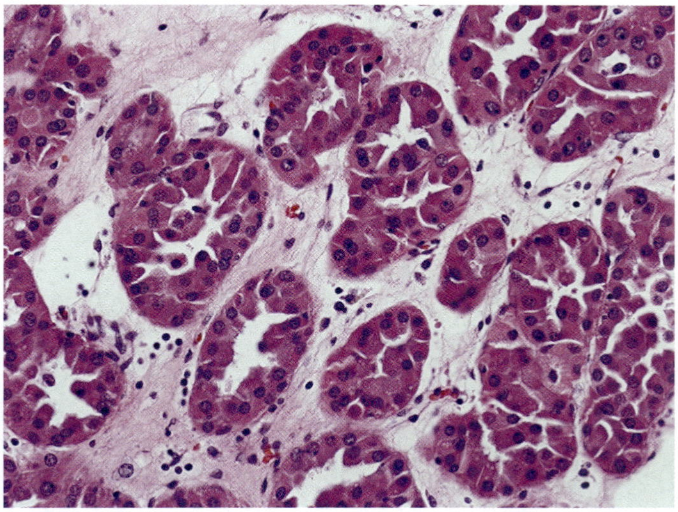

a

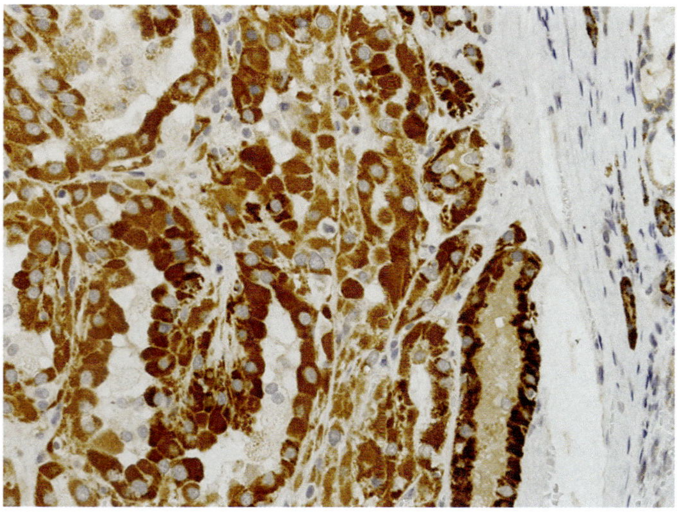

b

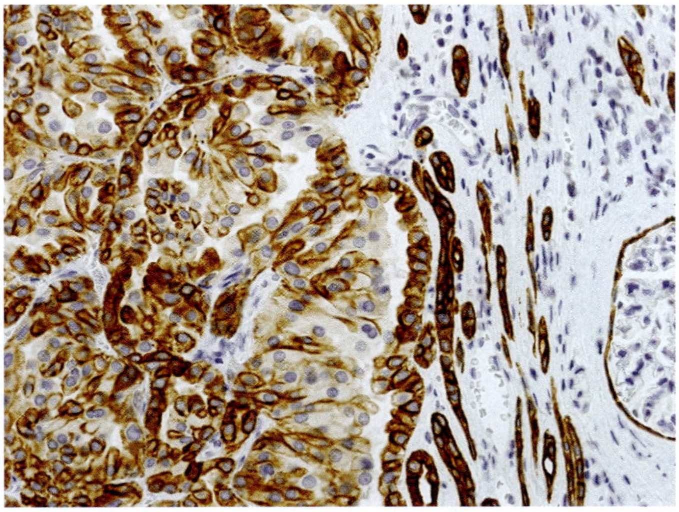

c

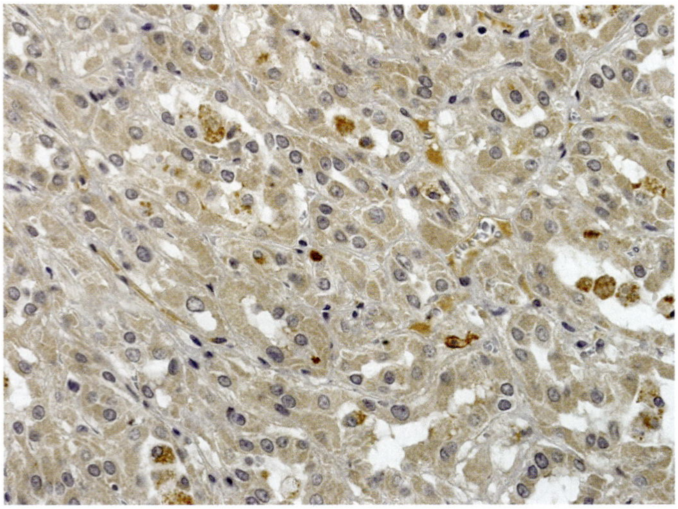

d

Figure 39-13.
Oncocytic papillary RCC composed of tumor cells with eosinophilic cytoplasm (*a*). By immunostaining, the tumor cells are strongly positive for AMACR (*b*), and CK7 (*c*), but negative for C-kit (*d*).

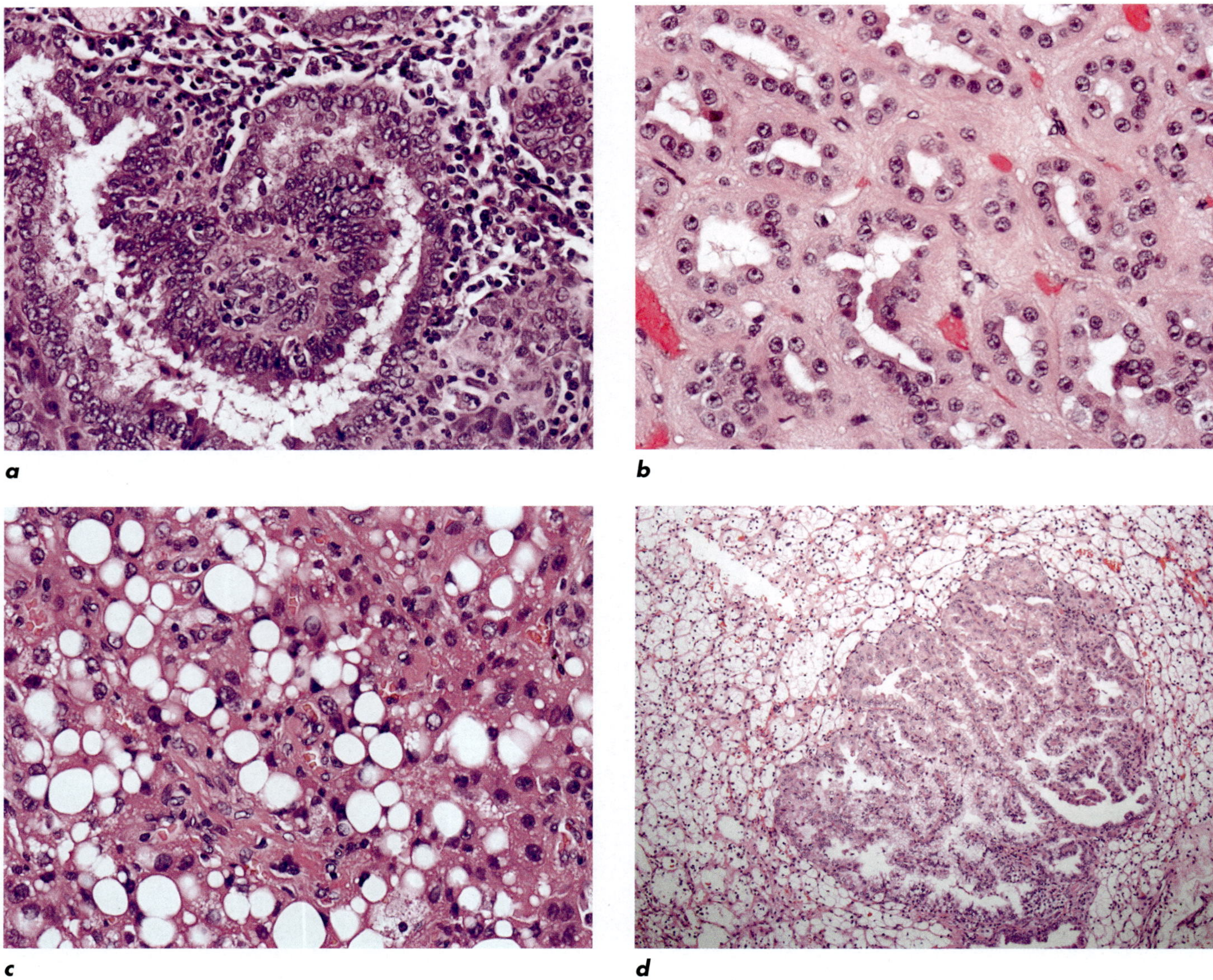

Figure 39-14.
Unusual patterns of papillary RCC. Papillary RCC with glomeruloid pattern (*a*, high grade), cribriform pattern (*b*, high grade), or lipid-rich appearance (*c*, low grade) and papillary RCC nodule surrounded by clear cell RCC (*d*).

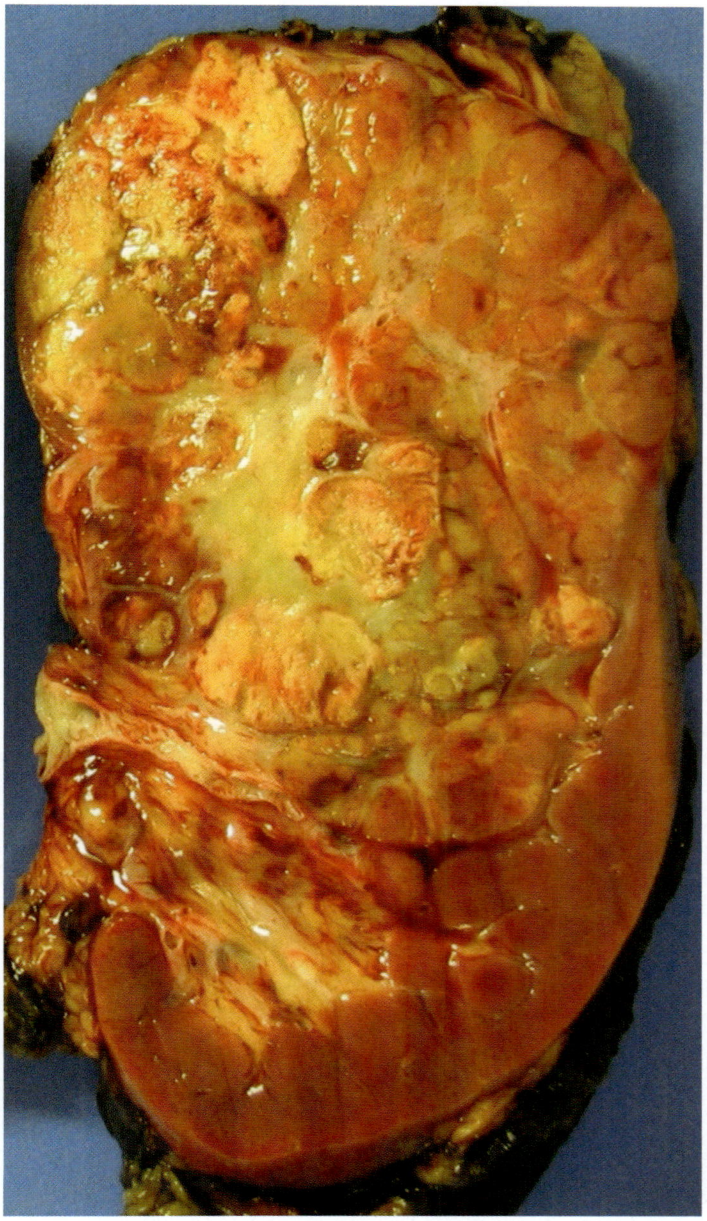

a

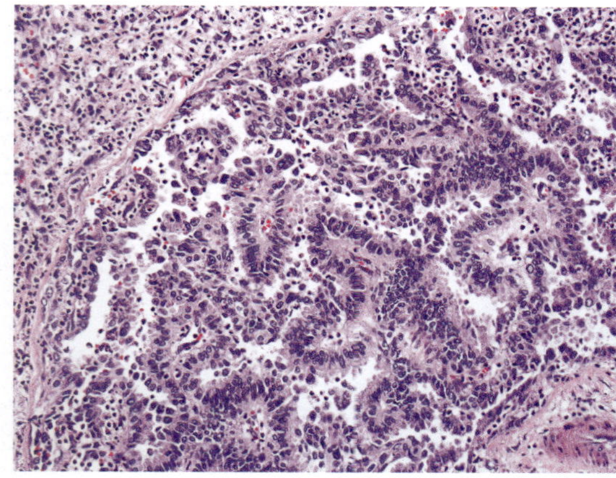

b

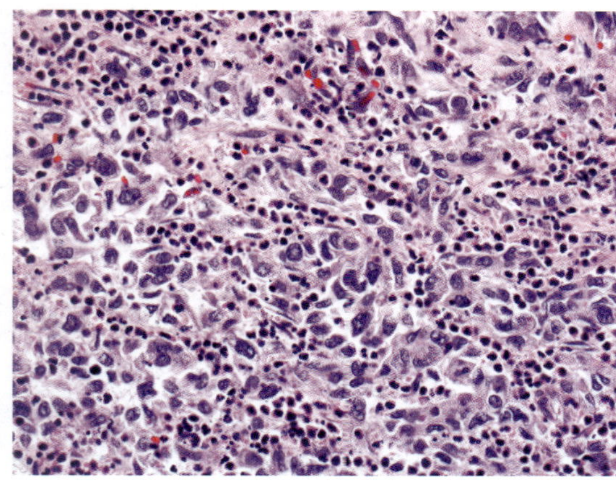

c

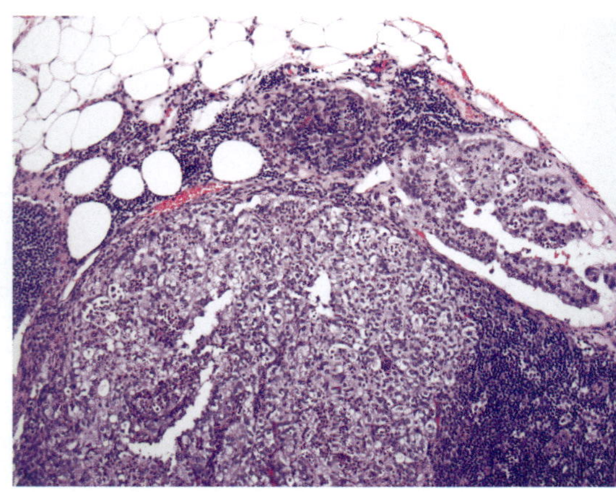

d

Figure 39-15.
A large high-grade papillary RCC replacing upper half of the kidney (*a*). The tumor cells are tall columnar with high nuclear grade (*b*). They display diffuse patterns in some areas (*c*) and develop metastasis to pelvic lymph nodes (*d*).

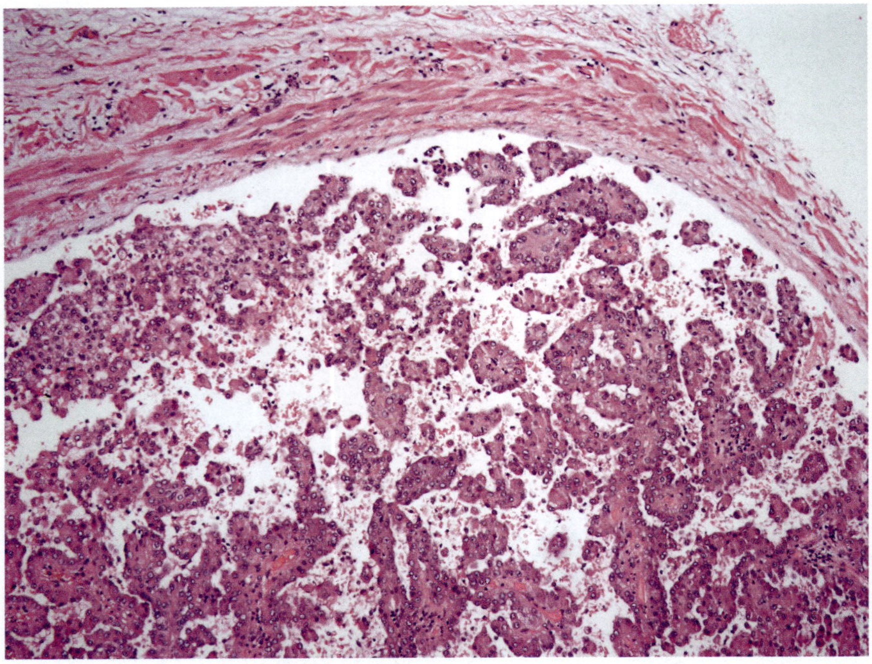

Figure 39-16.
High-grade type 2 papillary RCC invading the renal vein.

Table 39-1. Comparison of Grades and Types of Papillary RCC

Part A		
Grading	***Low grade***	***High grade***
Fuhrman nuclear grade	Grades 1 and 2	Grades 3 and 4
Size	Small	Large
Genetics	Low-grade different from high-grade PRCC	
Behavior	Indolent	Aggressive
Part B		
Type	***Type 1***	***Type 2***
Cytoplasm	Scant (appearing basophilic)	Abundant, eosinophilic
Macrophage	Common	Less common
Cell layer	Single	Single or pseudostratified
Nuclear grade	Often low grade	Often high grade Occasionally low grade
Behavior	Mostly indolent	Mostly aggressive

PRCC, papillary renal cell carcinoma.

CHROMOPHOBE RENAL CELL CARCINOMA

Definition

- A subtype of renal cell carcinoma is signified by large polygonal tumor cells with pale or eosinophilic cytoplasm and prominent cell membrane

Pathogenesis

- Unknown

Clinical features

- Third most common subtype of RCC, accounting 5% to 8% of all RCC
- Wide range of ages
- Most cases are asymptomatic
- Small set of chromophobe RCCs have an aggressive behavior

Gross pathology

- Well-circumscribed, nonencapsulated mass, with a noninfiltrating border (Fig. 39-17*a*)
- Tan to light brown in color (Fig. 39-18*a*)
- Hemorrhage and necrosis are uncommon (Fig. 39-18*b*)

Histology

- Classic type: large polygonal cells display pale cytoplasm with prominent cell membrane resembling the cell wall of plant cells. The cytoplasm is not optically clear, but containing fine granules (Fig. 39-17*b*)
- Eosinophilic type: large polygonal cells with prominent cell membrane, similar to classic type but containing more fine eosinophilic granules in cytoplasm (Fig. 39-17*c*)
- There is no clinical implication in dividing classic and eosinophilic types. Furthermore, in many cases, both classic and eosinophilic types are present (Fig. 39-17)
- Tumor cells form large nests or sheets, with very little stroma, not papillary patterns (Fig. 39-18)
- Wrinkled nuclei with raisinoid appearance is characteristic (Figs. 39-17*b* and 39-18*d*)
- Vessels within the tumor are delicate, sometimes hyalinized; resemble "chicken-wire" patterns in clear cell RCC (Fig. 39-19*a*)
- Sometimes nuclear atypia can be prominent similar to Fuhrman grade 3-4 (Fig. 39-19*b*). However, nuclear grading of chromophobe RCC is not correlated well with the clinical outcomes. Ultrastructurally, the tumor cells contain membrane-bound vesicles and variable number of mitochondria

Immunohistochemistry and histochemistry

- C-kit positive (Fig. 39-20)
- CK7 positive (Fig. 39-20*c*). Hale colloidal iron staining positive (blue) (Fig. 39-20*d*)
- Parvalbumin positive, vimentin negative

Differential diagnosis

- The main differential diagnosis is oncocytoma (see Table 39-2)
- Other tumors such as oncocytic papillary RCC, or high-grade clear cell RCC (see Table 39-3)

Molecular analysis

- The gene expression profiles of chromophobe RCCs and oncocytomas are very similar
- However, multiple chromosomal losses are seen in chromophobe RCC, including chromosomes 1, 2, 6, 10, 13, 17, occasionally 21 and Y. These chromosomal losses are uncommon in oncocytoma

Clinical relevance (prognosis and treatment options)

- Prognosis is better than other common subtypes of RCC with 5-year survival rate of approximately 90%
- Classic and eosinophilic types do not affect the prognosis
- Difficult to predicate the prognosis when sarcomatoid differentiation or metastasis is absent
- High nuclear grades have been reported to be associated with aggressive behavior but not on a consistent basis
- We typically report the Fuhrman grade of chromophobe RCC but also make a comment that the association of this grading with an aggressive behavior is not reliable
- No reliable chemotherapy is established. However, the C-kit positivity in chromophobe RCC indicates the potential for using tyrosine kinase inhibitors in therapy

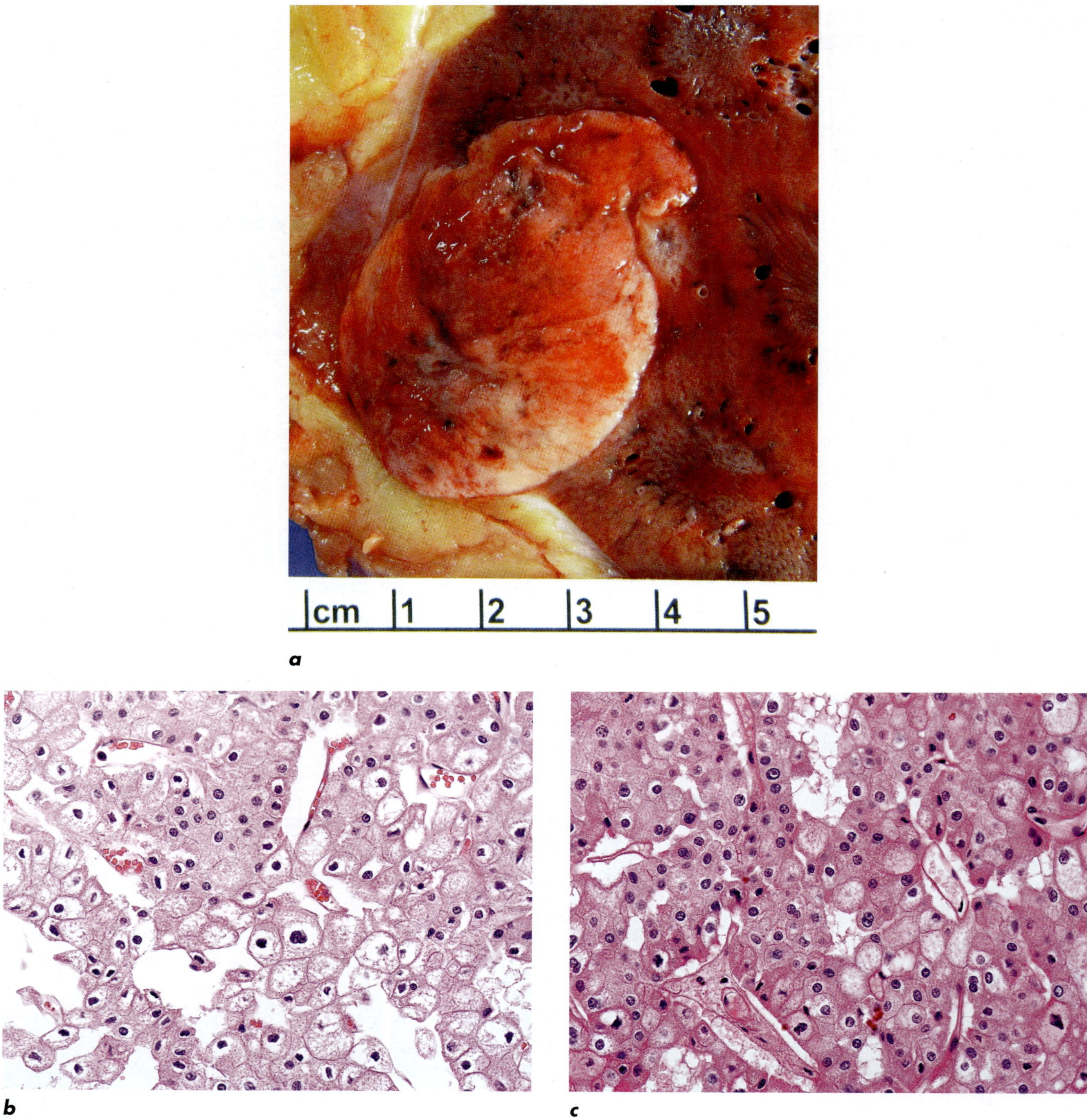

Figure 39-17.
Gross photo of a chromophobe RCC with a pink cut surface (*a*). Microscopically, the tumor is composed of classic chromophobe (pale stained) tumor cells with prominent cell membrane (*b*). The tumor cells have raisinoid nuclei. In another area, the tumor cells have more eosinophilic cytoplasm as well as the characteristic prominent cell membrane (*c*).

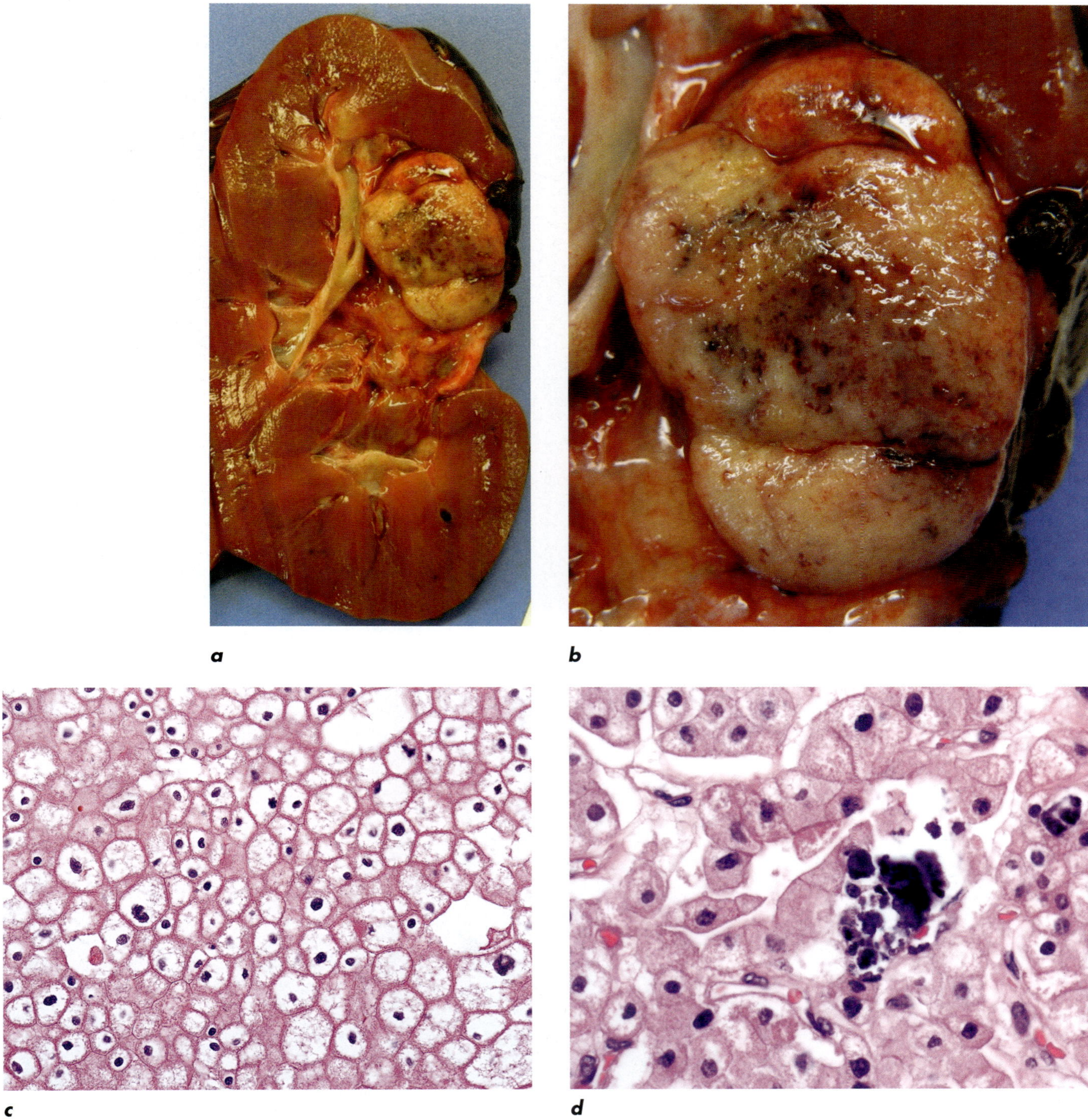

Figure 39-18.
Chromophobe RCC in a radical nephrectomy specimen (*a*). In close-up, the tumor is well circumscribed with tan fleshy and granular cut surface and focal spotty hemorrhage (*b*). The tumor cells show characteristics of chromophobe RCC (*c*). Another area of the tumor contains microcalcifications (*d*).

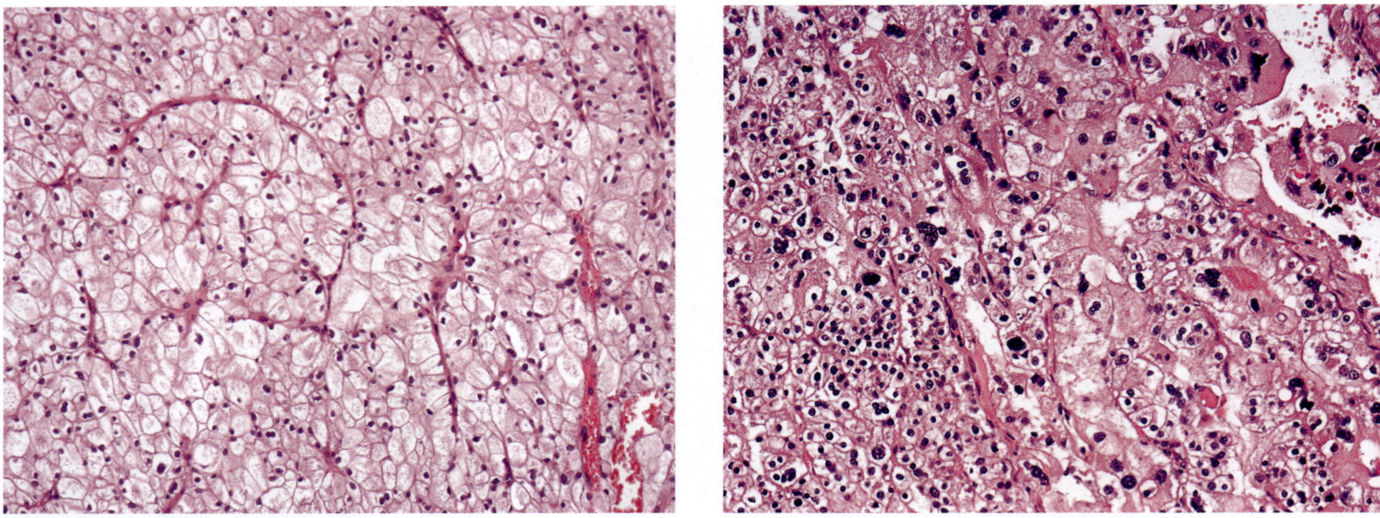

a b

Figure 39-19.
Chromophobe RCC showing "chicken-wire" vasculature resembling clear cell RCC (*a*). Chromophobe RCC showing prominent nuclear atypia in another area (*b*).

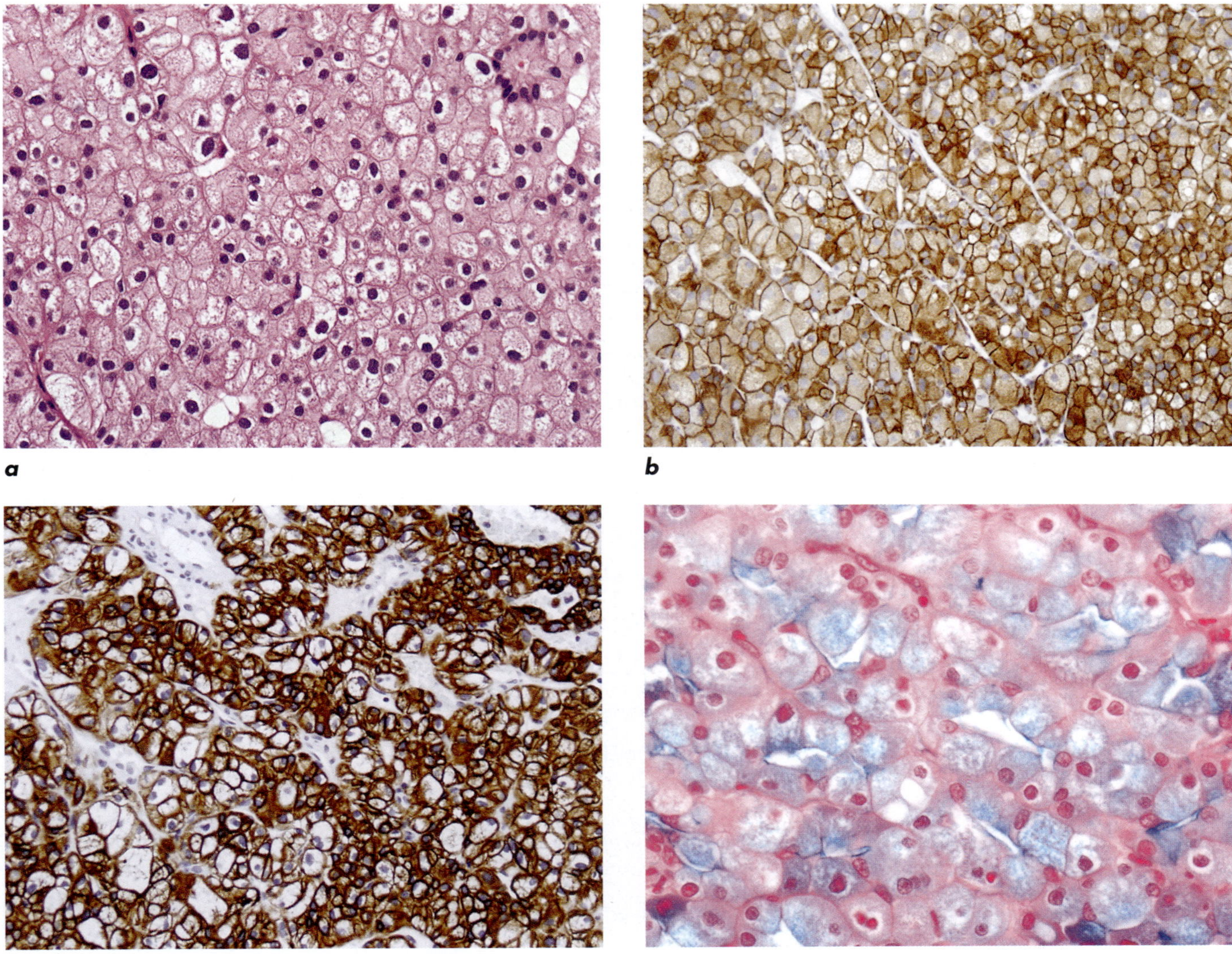

a b c d

Figure 39-20.
Chromophobe RCC with typical "plant-cell-wall-like" cell membrane (*a*). By immunostaining, the tumor cells demonstrate positive staining for C-kit (*b*, membranous), CK7 (*c*, diffuse), and Hale colloidal iron stains (*d*, blue).

Table 39-2. Comparison of Chromophobe RCC and Oncocytoma

Characteristics		*Chromophobe RCC*	*Oncocytoma*
Gross	Color of tumor cut surface	Pink to tan	Mahogany brown
	Central scar	Unlikely	Possible (20% to 30%)
	Multiple	Unlikely	Possible
Histochemistry	Hale colloidal iron	Positive	Negative or positive (luminal)
Immunohistochemistry	CK7	Positive	Negative
	Claudin 7	Positive	Negative
	PAX2	Positive or negative	Positive
	S100A	Negative	Positive
	Vimentin	Negative	Negative
	C-kit	Positive	Positive
	Ber-EP4 (EpCam)	Positive (diffusely)	Negative or focally positive
	CD15	Negative	Positive or negative
	Claudin 8	Positive (membranous)	Positive (cytoplasmic)
Prognosis		Low-grade malignancy	Benign
EM		Membrane-bound vesicles Mitochondria	Numerous Mitochondria
Cytogenetics		Chromosome losses on chromosomes 1, 2, 6, and 17 Chromosome gain on chromosome 18	Minimal chromosome changes

CK7, cytokeratin 7; PAX2, paired box gene 2; RCC, renal cell carcinoma; EM, electron microscopy.

Table 39-3. Comparison of Clear Cell RCC and Chromophobe RCC by Immunohistochemistry

Antibodies	*Clear cell RCC*	*Chromophobe RCC*
RCC	Positive	Negative
CAIX	Positive	Negative
Vimentin	Positive	Negative
KIM-1	Positive	Negative
CK7	Negative or focally positive	Positive
CD117	Negative	Positive
β-definsin-1	Negative	Positive

CAIX, carbonic anhydrase 9; CK7, cytokeratin 7; KIM-1, kidney injury molecule; RCC, renal cell carcinoma.

SARCOMATOID RENAL CELL CARCINOMA

Definition

- Sarcomatoid RCC, not an independent subtype of RCC, is characteristic by the presence of high-grade spindle cell sarcomatoid component in any subtypes of RCC

Other terms

- Sarcomatoid change in RCC, sarcomatoid differentiation of RCC, sarcomatoid transformation of RCC, or carcinosarcoma

Pathogenesis

- It is a dedifferentiation process or high-grade transformation of an RCC
- This phenomena may be seen in any subtype of renal cell carcinoma
- Therefore, sarcomatoid RCC is not a histological subtype, but it is typically coexisting with a low-grade RCC component (Table 39-4)

Clinical features

- Older patients, mean age = 60 years
- Large renal mass
- Often associated with locally advanced disease or distant metastasis at the time of diagnosis

Gross pathology

- Typically large mass, mean size greater than 10 cm
- Occurring within renal parenchyma, not centered in the peripheral region (Fig. 39-21*a*)
- Variable color and sizes of nodules, white or fleshy appearance is characteristic (Fig. 39-22*a*)
- Presence of low-grade RCC component, bright yellow (Fig. 39-22*a*, clear cell RCC), tan or brown (papillary or chromophobe) (Fig. 39-23*a*) nodules can be seen

Histology

- The presence of high-grade malignant (sarcomatoid) spindle cells, either focal or diffuse, is required for diagnosis (Fig. 39-21*c*)
- The sarcomatoid component demonstrates high cellularity; pleomorphism and increased mitoses (Figs. 39-22*c* and 39-23*c*)
- It is uncertain whether the percentage of sarcomatoid component is related to the degree of malignancy
- The highly pleomorphic nonspindle malignant cells may be present, but no consensus whether they should be considered sarcomatoid RCC
- We normally would not diagnose a sarcomatoid RCC if RCC is pleomorphic but still retains the features of a carcinoma. We only make a diagnosis of sarcomatoid RCC if the pleomorphic area cannot be distinguished from a high-grade sarcoma
- The lower grade component of clear cell RCC (Figs. 39-21*b* and 39-22*b*), papillary RCC, or chromophobe RCC (Fig. 39-23*b*) should be identified although extensive sampling
- In rare instance, other sarcomatoid components such as angiosarcoma, rhabdomyosarcoma, chondrosarcoma, or osteosarcoma can be seen
- Low-grade spindle cells seen in mucinous tubular and spindle cell carcinoma or clear cell RCC should not be considered *sarcomatoid* RCC
- Also, we suggest to avoid the term *spindle cell differentiation* in the diagnosis of RCC because it may cause confusion

Table 39-4. Progression from Low-Grade Renal Cell Carcinoma (RCC) to Sarcomatoid RCC

Low-grade component	*High-grade component*
Clear cell RCC →	Sarcomatoid RCC
Papillary RCC →	Sarcomatoid RCC
Chromophobe RCC →	Sarcomatoid RCC
Collecting duct carcinoma →	Sarcomatoid RCC
Other types RCC →	Sarcomatoid RCC

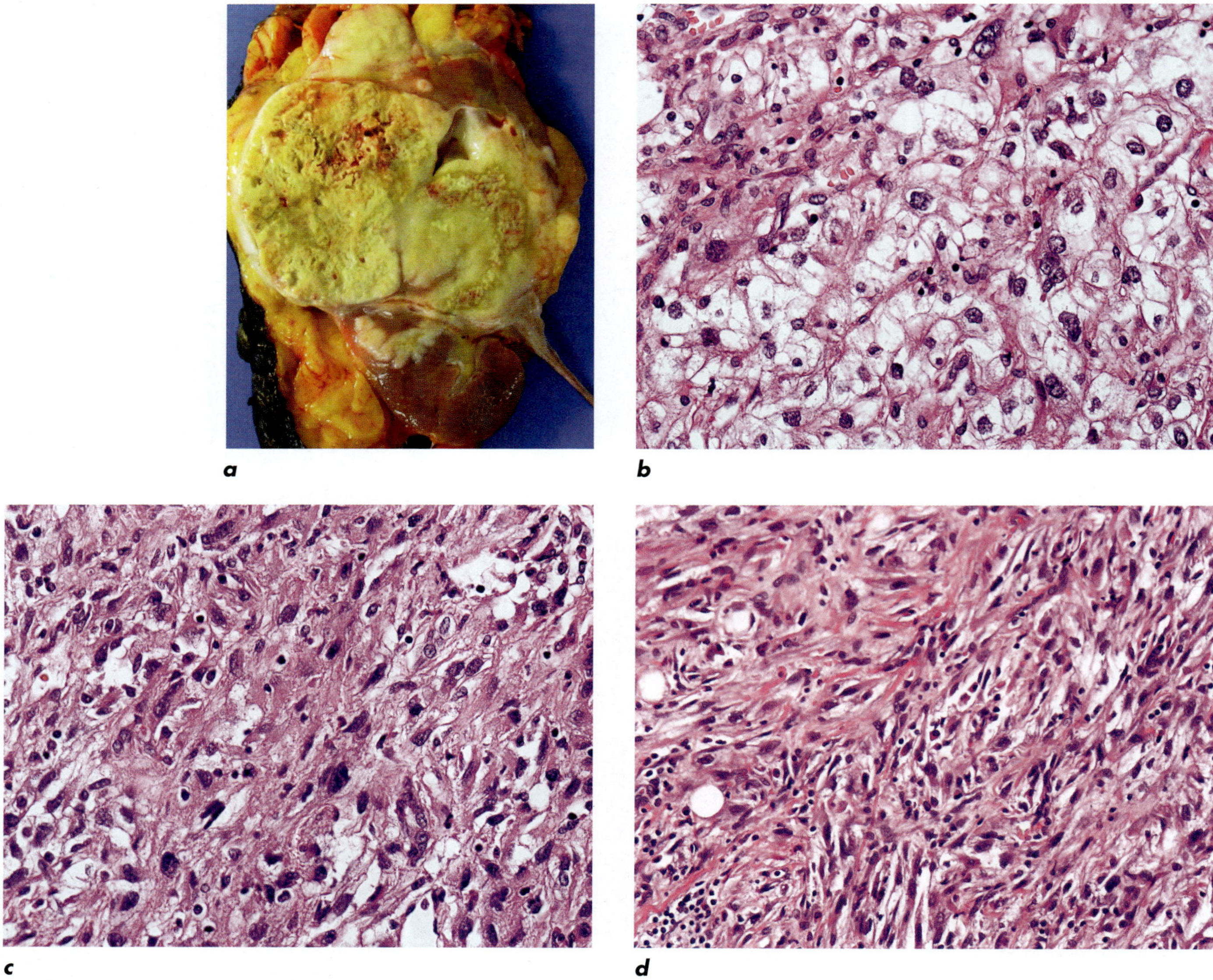

Figure 39-21.
Clear cell RCC with sarcomatoid differentiation. Grossly, the tumor is a large mass greater than 10 cm, replacing the most of kidney (*a*). Areas of clear cell RCC can be seen (*b*). In addition, areas of pleomorphic spindle tumor cells (*c* and *d*).

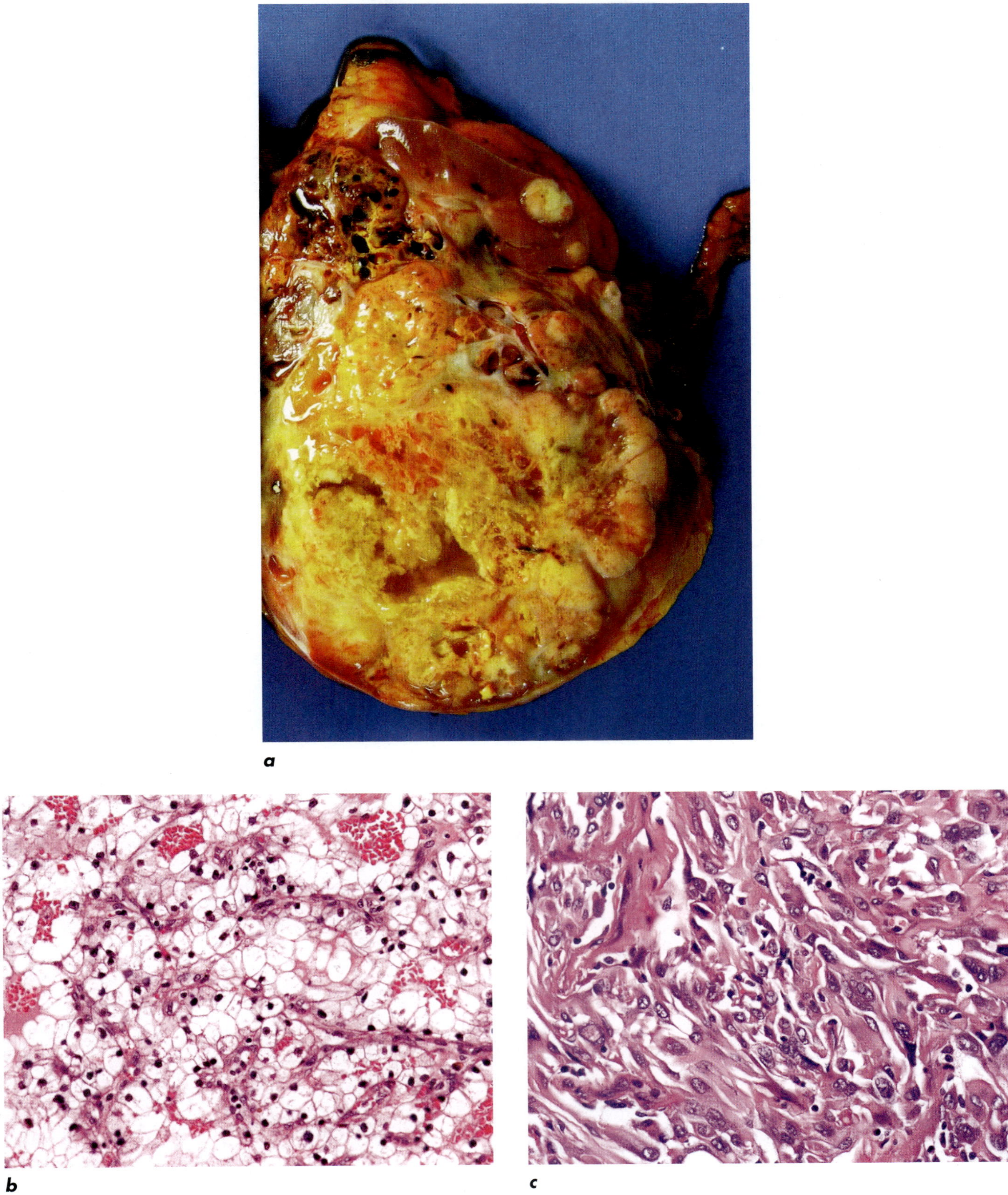

Figure 39-22.

A large sarcomatoid RCC replacing almost the entire kidney. The yellow areas represent clear cell component, while the white areas in the periphery represent the sarcomatoid component (*a*). High magnification shows the clear cell component (*b*) and high-grade spindle cell component (*c*).

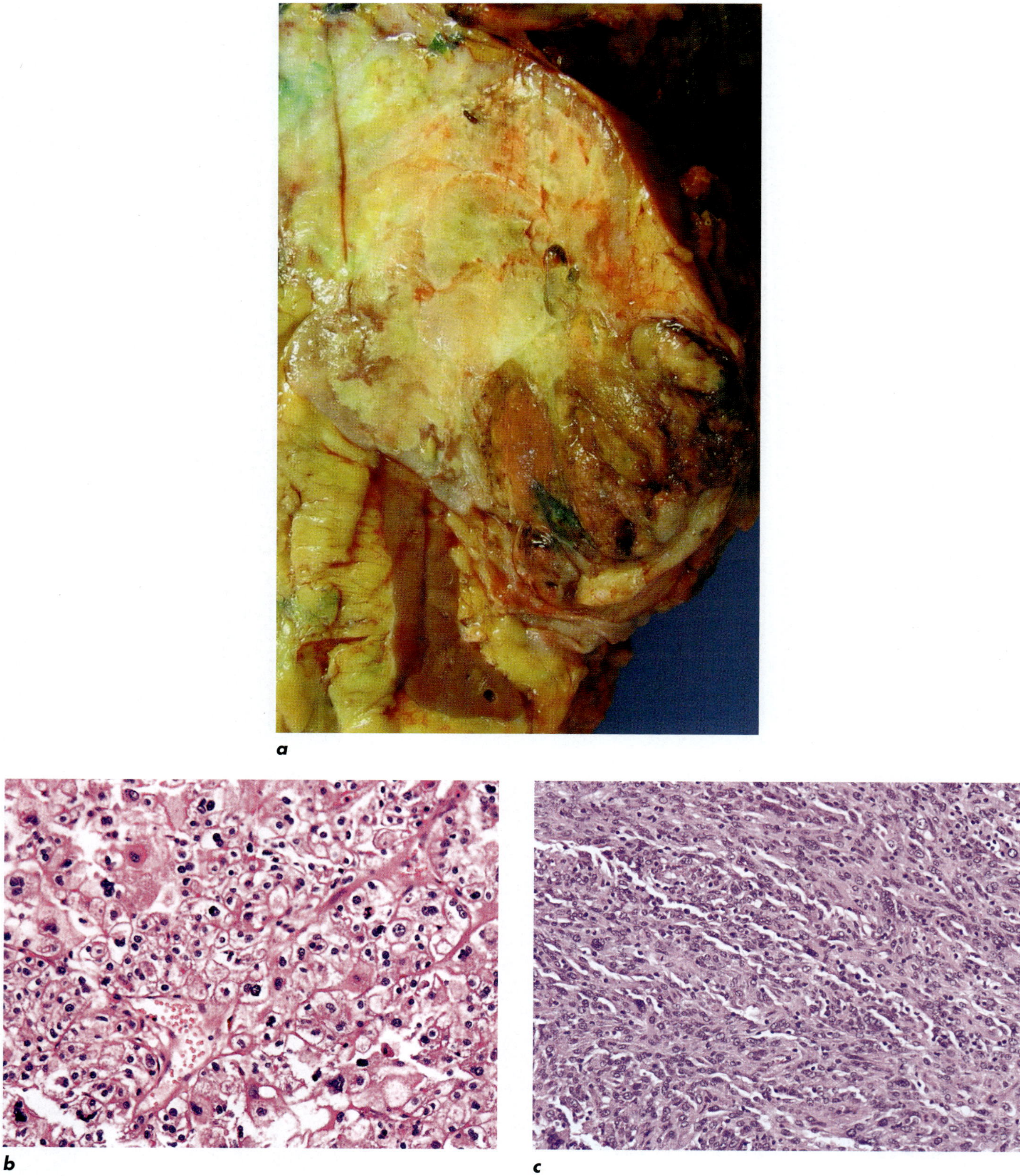

Figure 39-23.
Chromophobe RCC with sarcomatoid differentiation. A large tumor mass contains tan (chromophobe), white (sarcomatoid), and yellow (necrosis) areas (*a*). Microscopically, typical chromophobe RCC component (*b*) and sarcomatoid component can also be seen (*c*).

Immunohistochemistry

- Most of the sarcomatoid components are positive for PAX2/PAX8 (renal markers)
- Majority of cases are positive for epithelial markers such as AE1/AE3, Cam5.2, or EMA
- Vimentin positive in approximately 50% of cases
- Smooth muscle actin and desmin are rarely positive
- Subtype specific markers are variably positive in sarcomatoid components

Differential diagnosis

- The main differential diagnosis is sarcoma (see Table 39-5)
- In our experience, sarcomatoid RCC is 10 times more common than a true renal sarcoma
- We have seen many sarcomatoid RCCs were mistakenly diagnosed as a renal sarcoma because of insufficient sampling without including typical lower grade RCC components

Molecular analysis

- The genetic basis of sarcomatoid differentiation is not clear, although many of these tumors still retain the genotypes and phenotypes of the origin subtypes

Clinical relevance (prognosis and treatment options)

- We usually make a diagnosis of a sarcomatoid RCC in the following fashion: *renal cell carcinoma, clear cell type, Fuhrman grade 4, with sarcomatoid transformation (40%),* although the percentage of sarcomatoid component is not necessarily directly related to the tumor aggressiveness
- Most patients have stage 3 or 4 disease. Metastasis is most commonly seen in the lung
- Prognosis is very poor and patients die within a couple of years after diagnosis without an effective treatment
- Metastasis in other organ should be distinguished from sarcoma
- Some clinical trials are currently available for sarcomatoid RCC, although the effects of these experimental treatments are not conclusive

Table 39-5. Comparison of Sarcomatoid RCC with Renal Sarcoma

	Sarcomatoid RCC	*Renal sarcoma*
Location	Mostly in the renal parenchyma	Mostly in the renal capsule or perirenal areas
Gross pathology	Variable colors Flashy, yellow, tan nodules	Uniform flashy appearance
Size	>10 cm	Variable
Low-grade RCC	Present	Not present
Keratin markers	Positive	Negative
MSA, desmin	Negative	Positive
Metastasis at diagnosis	Common	Less common
Prognosis	Very poor	Poor

RCC, renal cell carcinoma; MSA, muscle specific actin

METASTATIC RENAL CELL CARCINOMA

Definition

- Renal cell carcinoma metastasizing to other organs

Pathogenesis

- RCC has a great propensity to metastasize to other distant organs
- Any subtypes of RCC may develop metastasis; however, the majority of the metastatic RCCs are clear cell types. Both high-grade and low-grade clear cell RCCs can develop metastases
- Renal vein invasion is the prelude of RCC metastasis
- A high-grade papillary RCC has the tendency to develop lymph node metastasis initially

Clinical features

- Clear cell RCC is responsible for the vast majority of metastatic RCC in distal organs
- The common sites of metastatic RCC is the lung and bone
- Metastatic RCC may be present as the initial finding before the primary renal carcinoma is noticed
- Clear cell RCC may develop early metastasis when the primary tumor is small and difficult to detect, which may present as so-called "metastatic carcinoma of unknown primary" when the renal tumor is not recognized . This situation rarely happens in papillary or chromophobe RCCs
- Metastatic RCC may also develop as an indolent disease, many years after the primary RCC was diagnosed. We have seen cases of metastatic RCC occurred 10 to 15 years after nephrectomy.

Gross pathology

- Well-circumscribed mass (Fig. 39-24*a*)
- The clear cell RCC may show typical bright yellow appearance (Fig. 39-24*a*)
- High-grade clear cell RCC, sarcomatoid, or other types of RCC will have a variable appearance (Figs. 39-25*a* and 39-26*a*)
- The clear cell RCC may show typical bright yellow appearance (Fig. 39-24*a*)

Histology

- In most cases of metastatic RCC, the typical features of clear cell, papillary, or chromophobe RCC (Figs. 39-24 to 39-27) can be identified with confidence
- While unusual type of RCC such as collecting duct RCC, unclassified or translocation RCC (Fig. 39-28), the diagnosis of metastatic tumors may be difficult without a history
- Application of immunohistochemical markers and comparison with the primary tumor of the same patient may be necessary for confirmation

Immunohistochemistry

- A typical RCC panel, which includes PAX2/8 (Fig. 39-27*b*), CD10 (Fig. 39-24*c*), CA9 (Fig. 39-27*d*), AMACR, CK7, C-kit, and vimentin (Fig. 39-24*b*) can be helpful for establishing a diagnosis and possible classification
- TFE3 immunostaining can be used if translocation carcinoma is suspected (high grade, clear cells with papillary configurations (Fig. 39-28*c*)

Molecular analysis

- It is promising, but not currently available for clinical practice. More validation tests are necessary

Clinical relevance (prognosis and treatment options)

- The prognosis of metastatic RCC is depending on the histological grade, type, and stage of the tumor
- However, the grade of metastatic RCC may be more important than the stage in this situation, since a patient with low-grade metastatic RCC (high stage) can have a good prognosis after the complete resection of a solitary metastatic tumor
- The diagnosis of metastatic RCC should include histological subtype and Fuhrman grade if possible

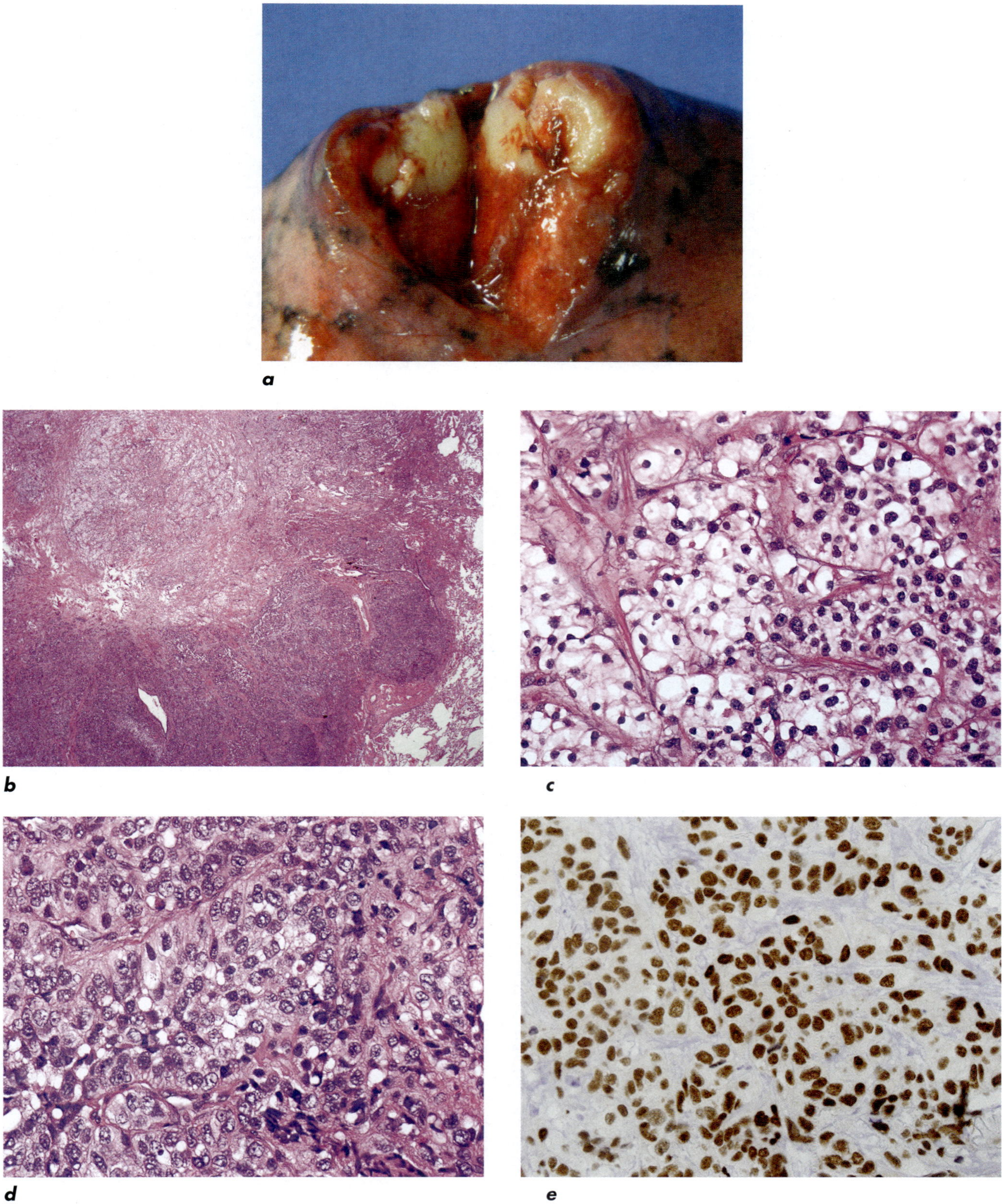

Figure 39-24.
Metastatic clear cell RCC in a wedge lung resection specimen with bright yellow cut surface (*a*). Low magnification shows a lobulated mass in the lung (*b*). Some areas show typical clear cell RCC (*c*), while other areas show no obvious features suggestive of RCC (*d*). By immunohistochemistry, the tumor cells are positive for PAX8 (*e*), CA9 (*f*), and vimentin (*g*), confirming the diagnosis.

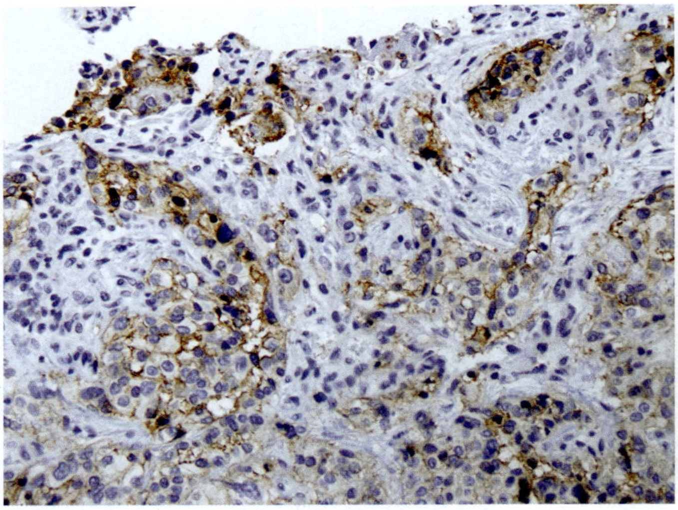

f

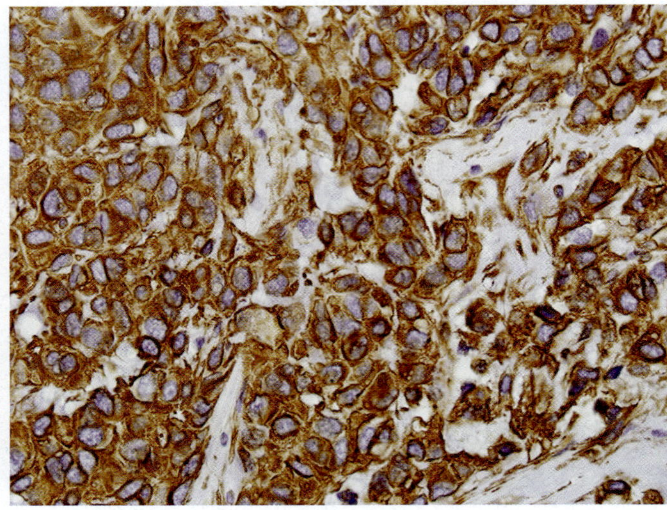

g

Figure 39-24.
(Continued)

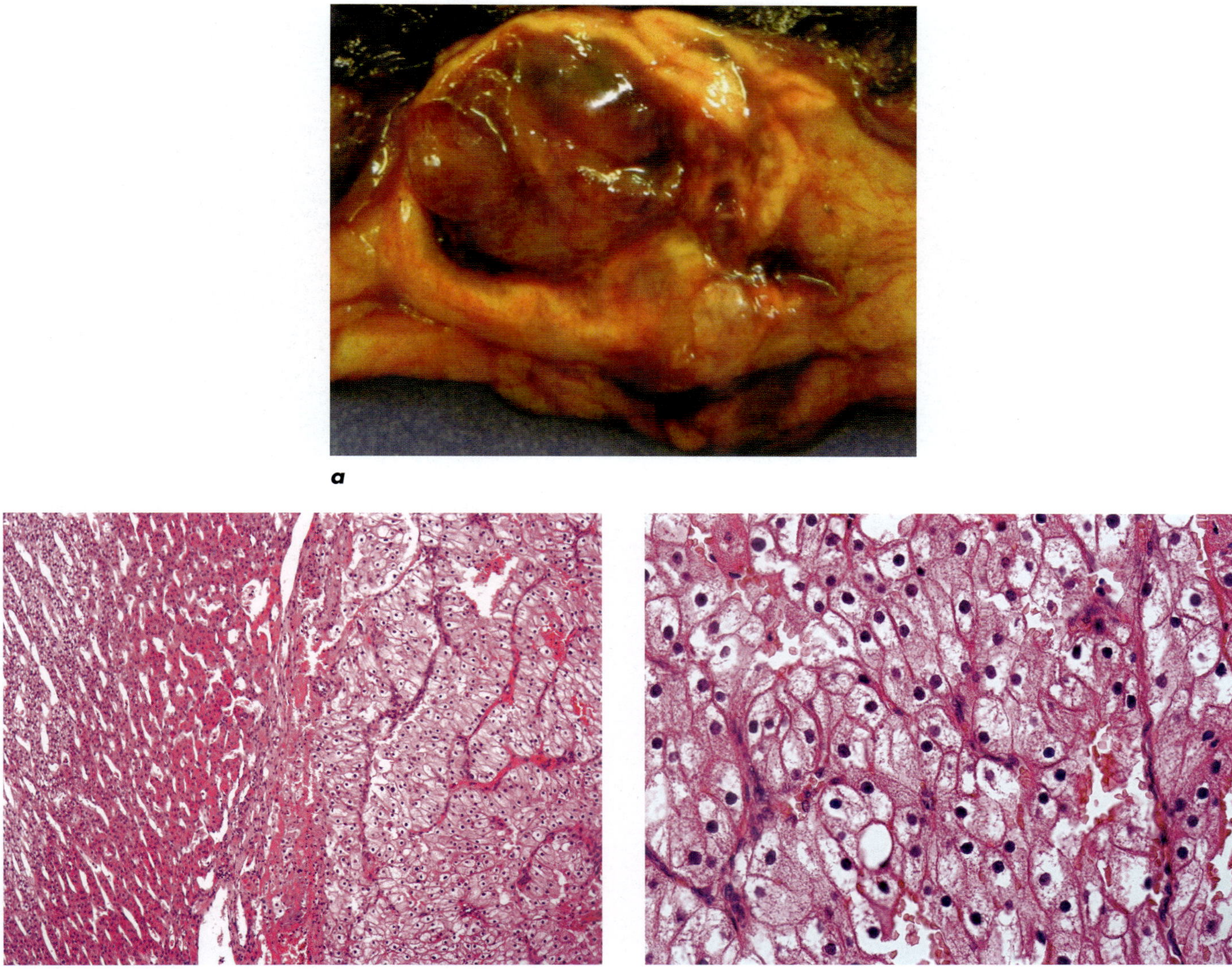

a

b

c

Figure 39-25.

Metastatic chromophobe RCC in the adrenal. The gross photo demonstrates a brown mass in the yellow background of adrenal cortical tissue (*a*). Microscopically, the presence of chromophobe RCC (*b*, right side) can be appreciated adjacent to the adrenal tissue (*b*, left side). High magnification confirms the typical chromophobe RCC with prominent cell membrane and fine cytoplasmic granules (*c*).

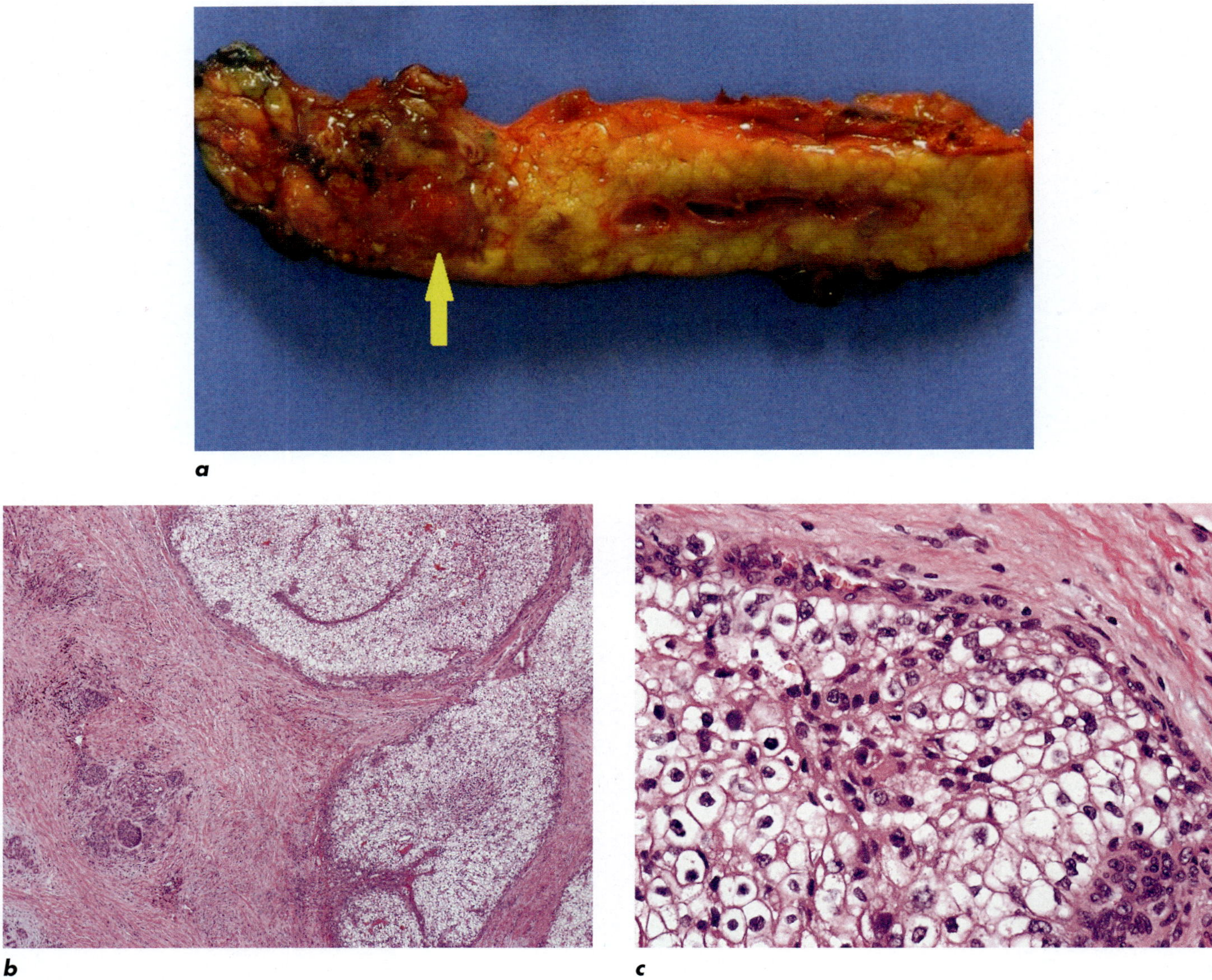

Figure 39-26.
Metastatic clear cell RCC in the pancreatic head indicated by an arrow (*a*). Microscopically, tumor nodules are present in the fibrotic background adjacent to residual pancreatic tissue (*b*). High magnification confirms the diagnosis of clear cell RCC , Fuhrman grade 3 (*c*).

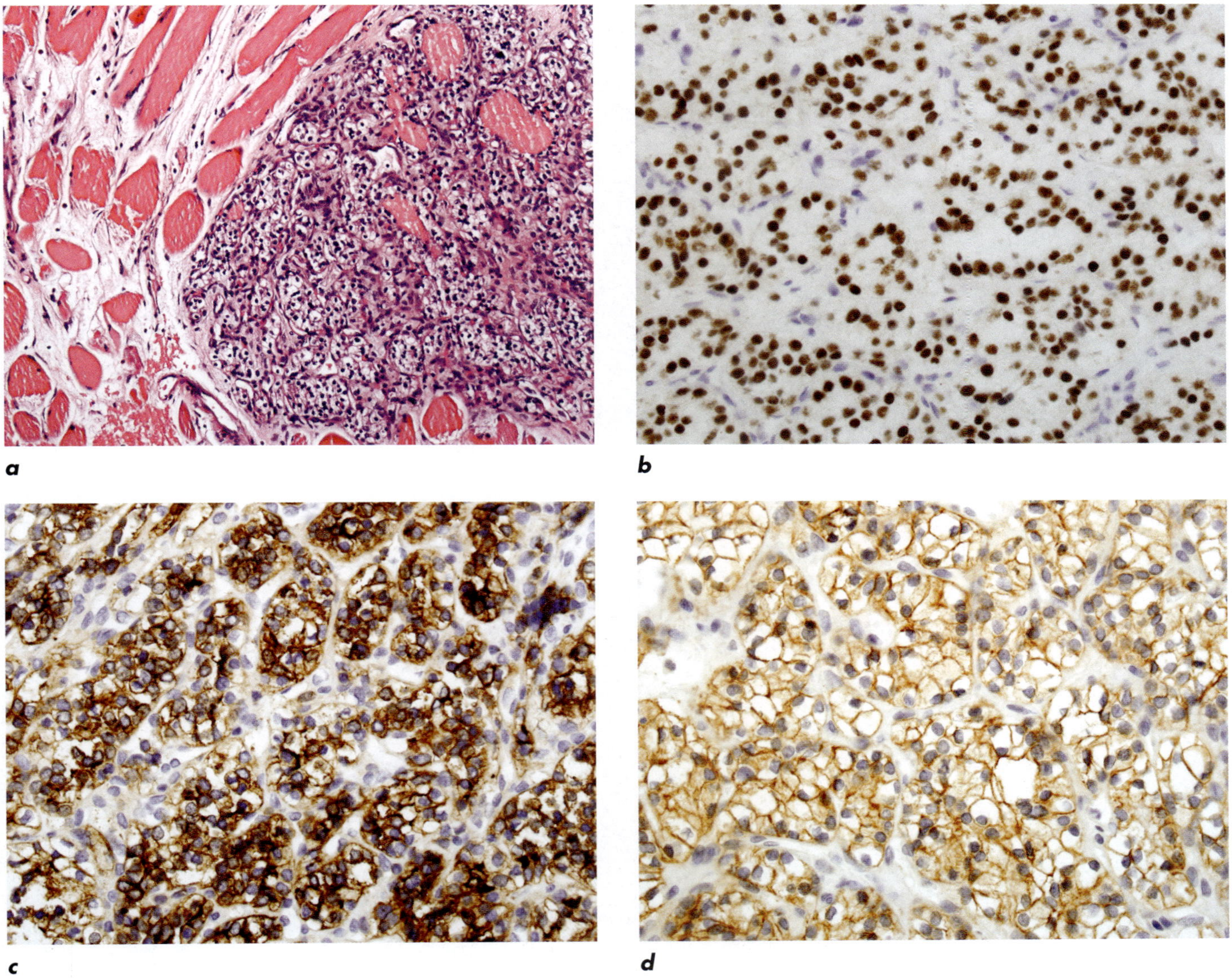

Figure 39-27.
Metastatic clear cell RCC in epidural space surrounded by the skeletal muscle (*a*). By immunostaining, the tumor cells are positive for PAX8 (*b*), CD10 (*c*), and CA9 (*d*), confirming the diagnosis.

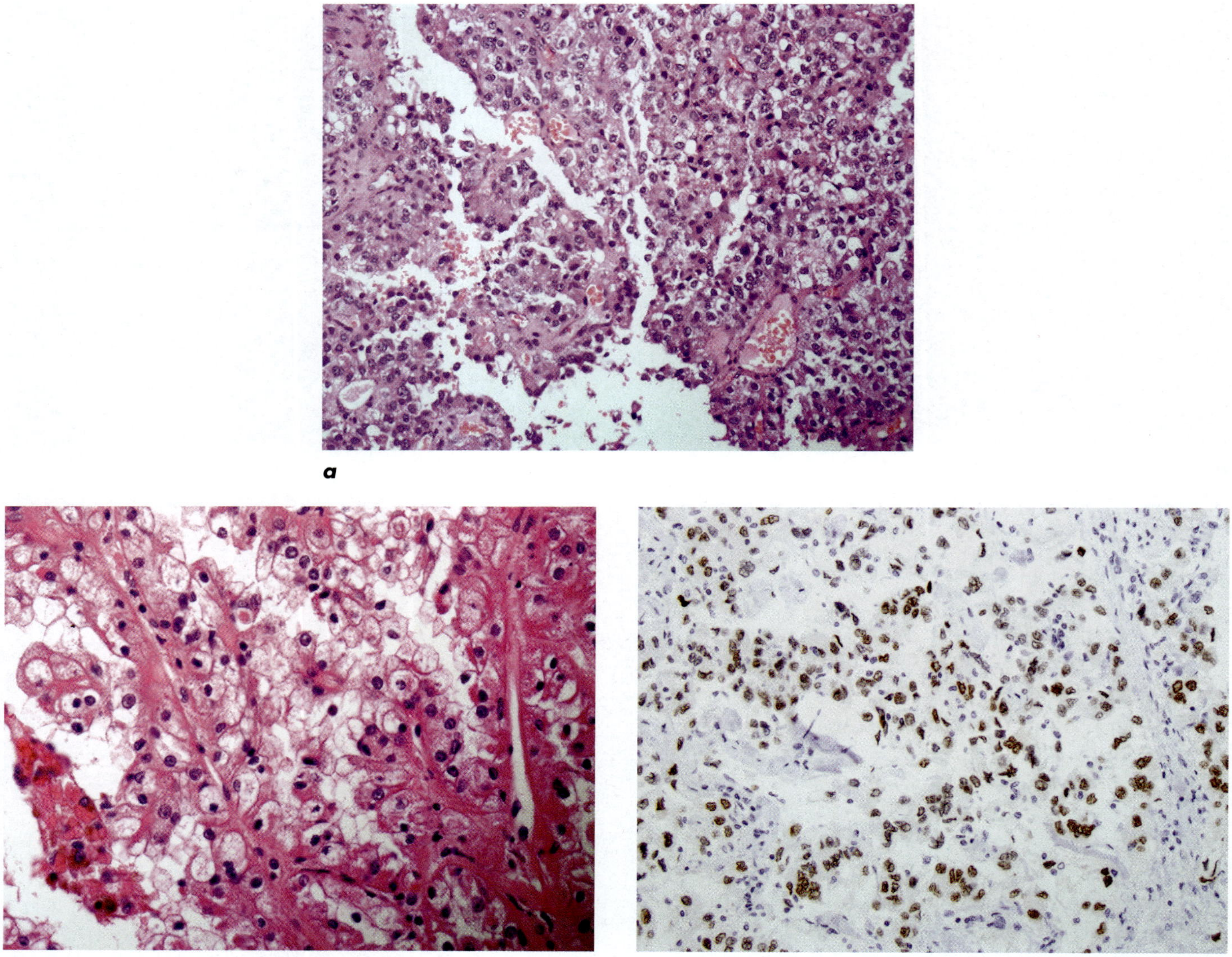

a

b

c

Figure 39-28.

Metastatic TFE3 translocation renal cell carcinoma to the vulva shows papillary configuration (*a*). Some area displays typical features of papillary configuration formed by tumor cells with clear cytoplasm (*b*). The diagnosis of TFE3 translocation carcinoma is confirmed by the positive TFE3 nuclear staining (*c*).

CHAPTER 40

Uncommon Malignant Neoplasms of the Kidney

Ximing J. Yang, Ondrej Hes, Liwei Jia, Bing Zhu, Bin Tean Teh, Minghao Zhong, William Laskin, Lauie Eisengart

MUCINOUS TUBULAR AND SPINDLE CELL CARCINOMA

Definition

- A renal epithelial neoplasm composed of rounded epithelial cells forming tubules and blending with linear arrays of spindle cells in a fibrotic or myxoid background

Clinical features

- Usually asymptomatic, majority diagnosed incidentally
- Female predominance (ratio M:F = 1:4), age range 17 to 82 years
- Documented relation to nephrolithiasis

Gross pathology

- Well circumscribed, occasionally encapsulated solid mass
- Variable color: from yellow, tan to whitish on cut surface (Fig. 40-1*a*)
- Hemorrhage and necrosis are very uncommon (Fig. 40-2*a*)
- Size range 2 to 18 cm

Histology

- There are three histological components: mucinous stroma, epithelioid cells forming tubules, and spindle cells (Figs. 40-1 and 40-2)
- Only a small amount of mucinous material can be seen between tumor cells (Fig. 40-2*c*). In addition, stroma can be edematous, hypocellular, with a variable amount of mucin or myxoid changes (Fig. 40-1*d*)
- Lymphocytic infiltrate present within stroma (Fig. 40-1*c*)
- Areas composed of narrow elongated, sometimes branching tubules, lined by cuboidal to low-columnar cells with pale eosinophilic cytoplasm and small round nuclei (Figs. 40-1*b* and 40-2*b*). Tubular structures gradually transform to curvilinear thin trabecular arrays of low-grade spindle cells. Nuclei of both tubular cells and spindle cells are small and round with small inconspicuous nucleoli
- Areas of tumor may histologically resemble clear cell renal cell carcinoma (RCC) (Figs. 40-3*a* and 40-4), papillary RCC (PRCC) (Fig. 40-3*b*), oncocytoma (Fig. 40-3*c*), or leiomyoma (Fig. 40-3*d*)
- Occasionally, tumor cells form glomeruloid structures (Fig. 40-5)
- Sometimes, tumor cells have high-grade nuclear features (Fig. 40-6)
- Sarcomatoid differentiation is extremely rare in this subtype

Immunohistochemistry

- AMACR positivity usually strong and diffuse
- CK7 usually positive
- Vimentin staining is variable ranging from focally strong to completely negative reactivity
- NSE, synaptophysin, and chromogranin are frequently expressed by neoplastic cells
- CD10 invariably positive, but usually focal

Molecular diagnostics

- Variable chromosomal numerical aberrations
- Polysomy of chromosomes 7 and 17 was reported by one study
- Multiple genetic alterations involving chromosomes 1, 4, 6, 8, 9, 13, 14, 15, 18, 22 have been published

Main differential diagnosis

Papillary cell carcinoma

- Although papillae may occasionally be seen, the presence of extensive papillary architecture is not a typical feature of mucinous tubular and spindle cell carcinoma (MTSCC)
- Presence of prominent necrosis, hemorrhage, foamy cells, hemosiderin-laden macrophages (siderophages), and cholesterol clefts is unusual for MTSCC
- Myxoid stroma is not typical of PRCC. The value of immunohistochemistry or molecular genetic testing is limited

Angiomyolipoma

- Although examples of MTSCC with prominent spindle cell component may potentially mimic angiomyolipoma, the latter lacks a tubular epithelial component
- Immunohistochemical reaction with HMB45 and absence of CK7 reactivity in angiomyolipoma easily resolve the problem

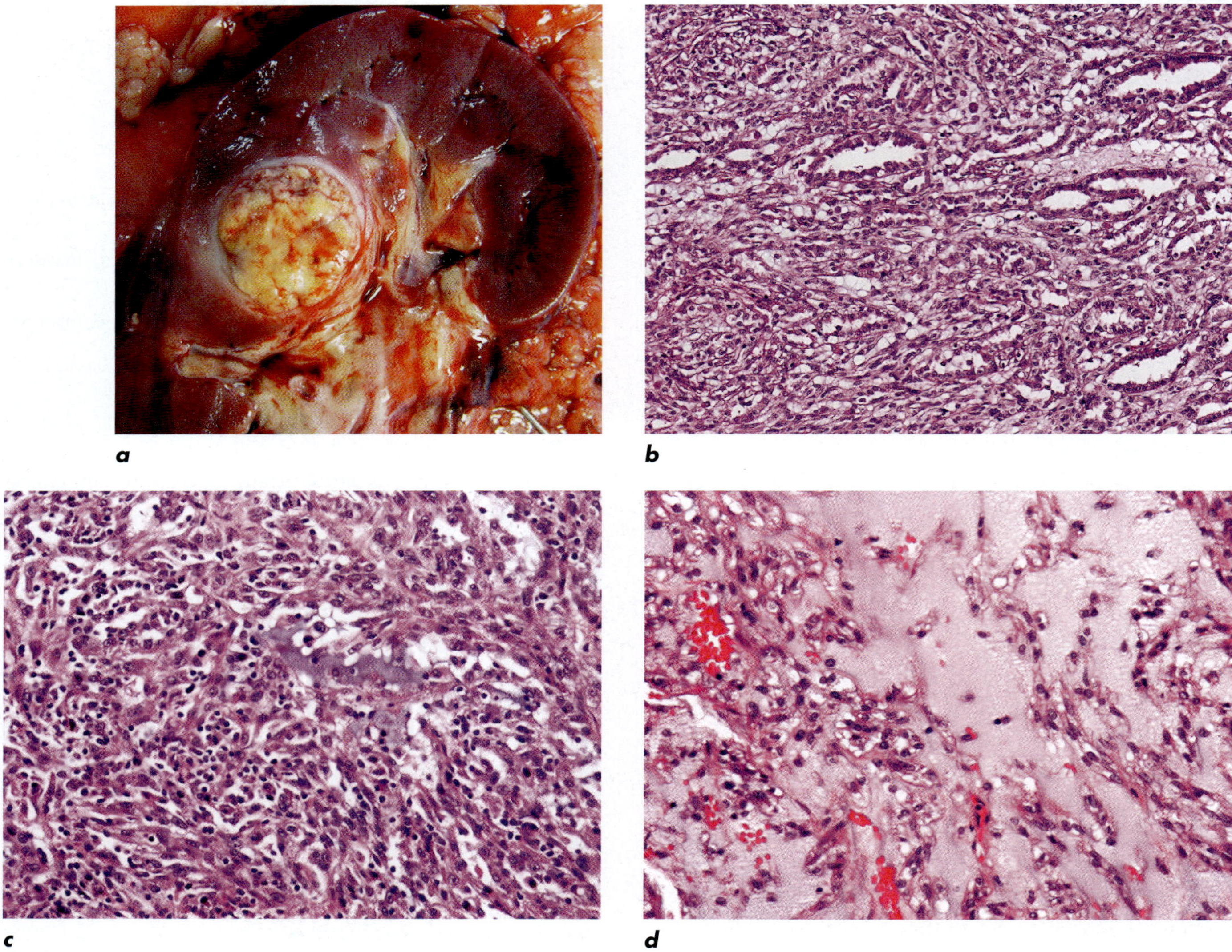

Figure 40-1.
Mucinous tubular and spindle cell carcinoma is an encapsulated tumor with yellow-tan cut surface (*a*). Microscopically, the tumor consists of epithelial cells with tubular structures (*b*) and spindle cells (*c*) within a mucinous background (*d*).

Clear cell RCC

- Clear cell RCC has an intricate vascular network, which is absent in MTSCC
- Despite the occasional presence of clear cell areas, MTSCC does not grow in a predominant nested pattern
- Clear cell RCC does not demonstrate low-grade spindle cell areas admixed with tubular structures

Clinical relevance (prognosis and treatment options)

- Majority of the tumors behave in an indolent manner
- Rare cases with lymph node metastasis exhibiting aggressive clinical course have been reported
- Sarcomatoid differentiation is extremely rare event in MTSCC
- Often treated with nephron-sparing or radical surgery

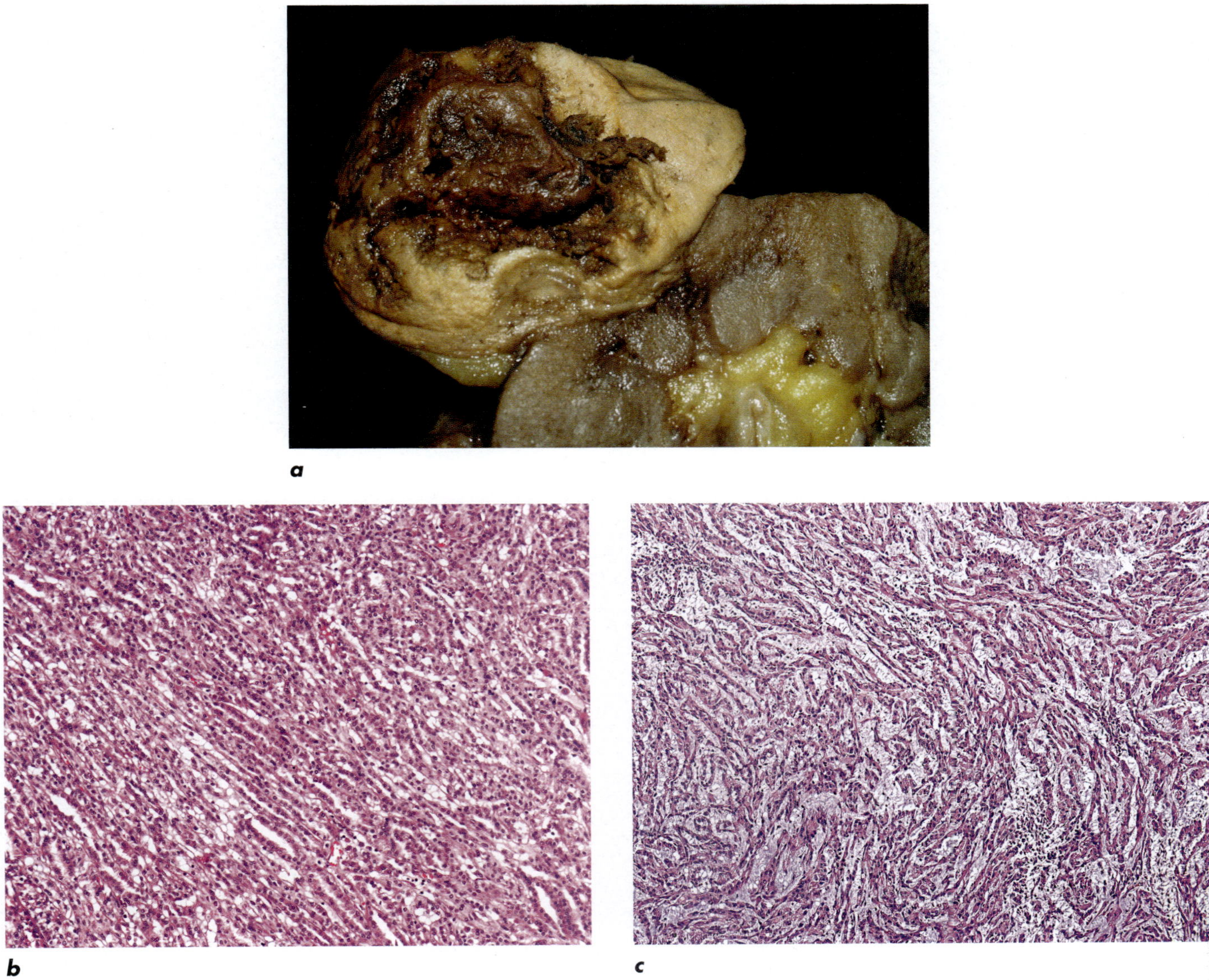

Figure 40-2.
Mucinous tubular and spindle cell carcinoma. Grossly the tumor is well-circumscribed with cystic changes in the center (*a*). Typical histological features of this tumor include low-grade tubular epithelial cells (*b*), and interconnecting spindle cells within a mucinous background (*c*).

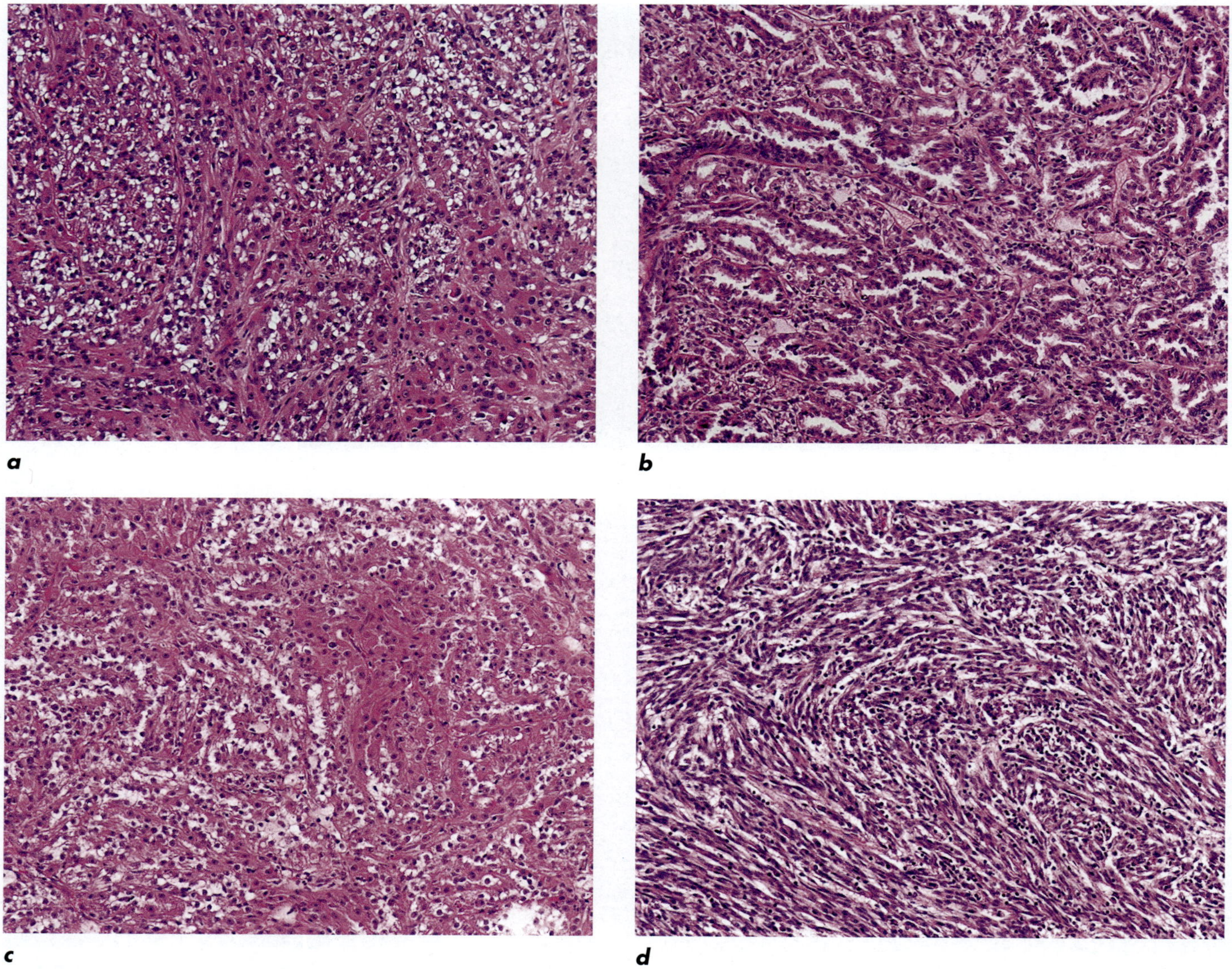

Figure 40-3.

Histological variations of mucinous tubular and spindle cell carcinoma: tumor cells with clear cytoplasm, mimicking a clear cell RCC (*a*); papillary structures, mimicking a papillary RCC (*b*); prominent oncocytic changes, mimicking an oncocytoma (*c*); and prominent spindle cell component, importing the appearance of a leiomyoma (*d*).

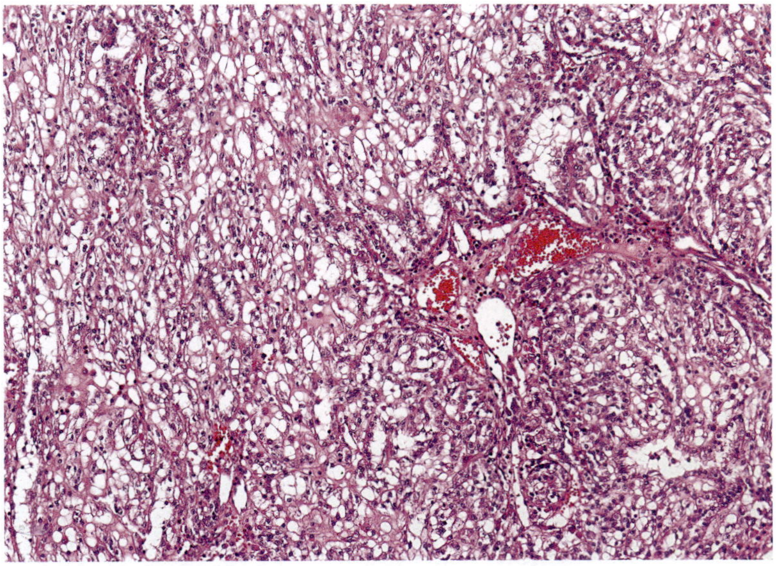

Figure 40-4.
Mucinous tubular and spindle cell carcinoma with a haphazard arrangement of both key proliferating elements.

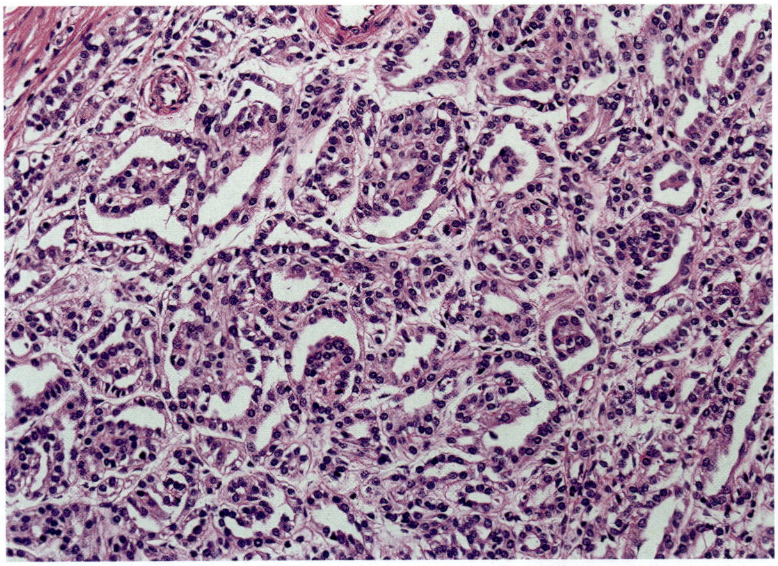

Figure 40-5.
Mucinous tubular and spindle cell carcinoma with glomeruloid structures.

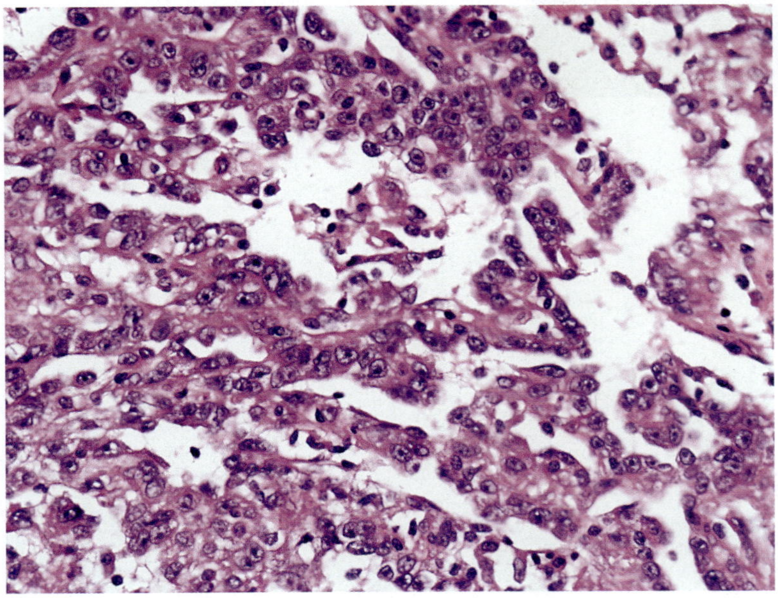

Figure 40-6.
Mucinous tubular and spindle cell carcinoma cells with high-grade nuclei possessing prominent nucleoli.

TUBULOCYSTIC CARCINOMA

Definition

- A morphologic variant of RCC characterized by the presence of a unique tubular and cystic architecture

Other term

- Low-grade collecting duct carcinoma (obsolete term)

Clinical features

- Tubulocystic carcinoma of the kidney is a rare epithelial renal neoplasm, with only less than 100 cases reported
- It predilects in patients in the fourth through ninth decades of life, ranging in age from 30 to 80 (mean = 57.2) years
- This tumor shows a striking male predilection with a male to female ratio of 7:1
- Most cases were discovered incidentally
- Less commonly, it may present with nonspecific abdominal pain, distention, or gross hematuria
- By imaging studies, the tumor appears cystic with thick septa and interspersed solid foci (Fig. 40-7)

Gross pathology

- Tubulocystic carcinoma typically presents as a solitary well-circumscribed nonencapsulated mass
- The majority of the tumors involve the renal cortex or both the cortex and medulla, but generally not the medulla exclusively
- In our experience, roughly 30% of the cases are associated with papillary adenomas or PRCC of the kidney
- Tubulocystic carcinoma is grossly characterized by a mass with multilocular cystic spaces filled with serous fluid, which imparts a sponge-like or "Swiss-cheese" appearance (Fig. 40-8)

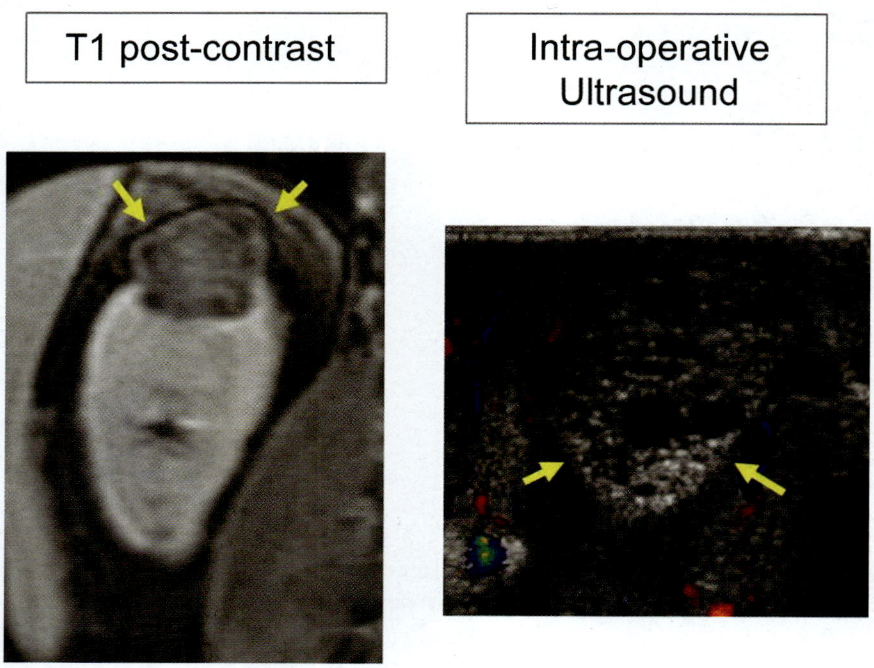

Figure 40-7.
Radiological images of tubulocystic carcinoma. CT image shows a well-defined multicystic lesion (left). Ultrasound image also demonstrates multiple cystic spaces (right). (Courtesy of Dr. David Casalino.)

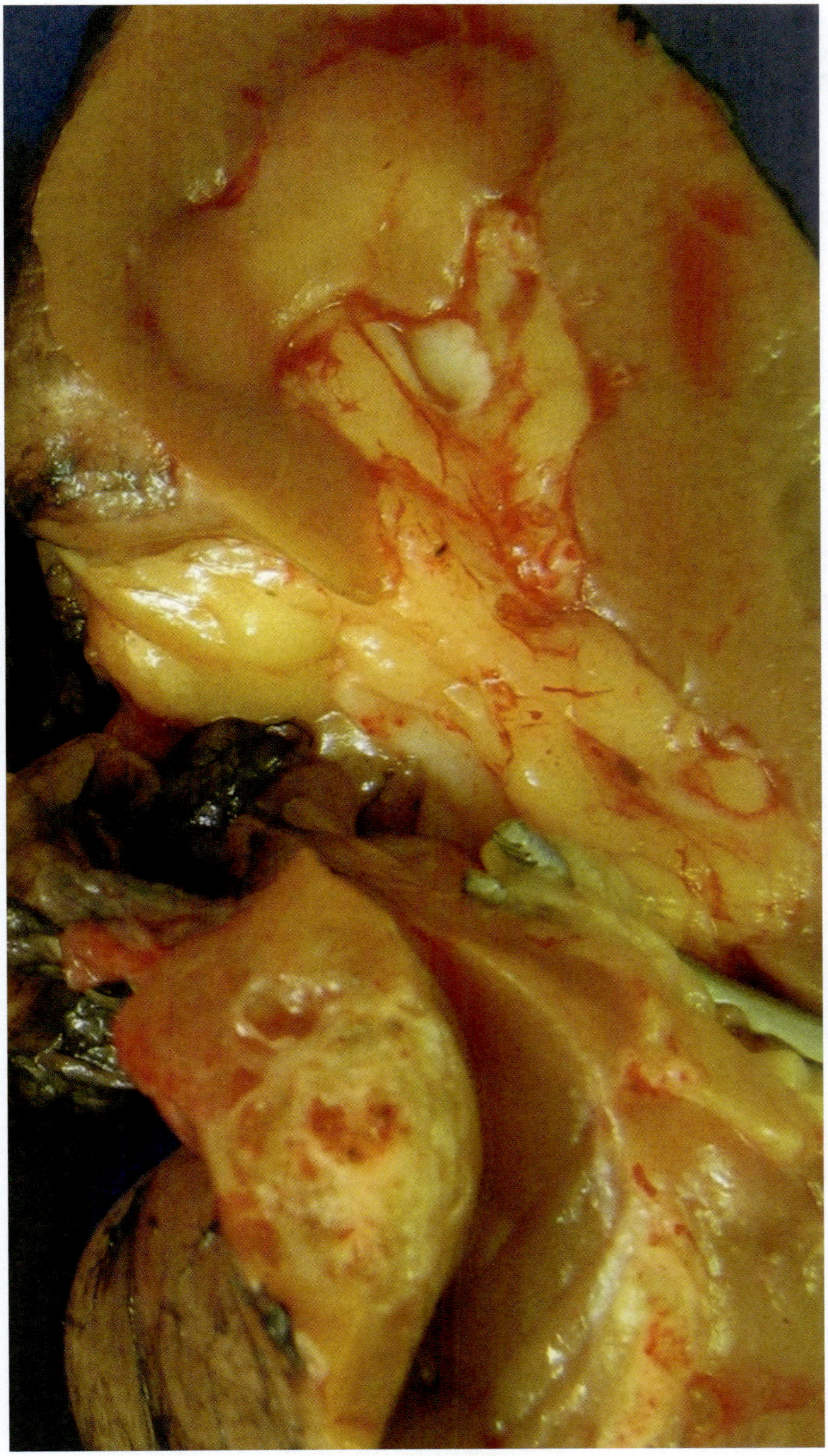

Figure 40-8.
Gross photograph of tubulocystic carcinoma demonstrates a mass with solid and cystic appearance.

Histology

- The tumors are composed of closely packed tubules and cysts separated by thin fibrous septa devoid of ovarian-type stroma (Fig. 40-9)
- The cysts range in size from 0.05 to 2 mm, but can be as large as 1 cm (Fig. 40-10)
- A single layer of large, polygonal tumor cells with eosinophilic cytoplasm and prominent nucleoli lines the cysts (Fig. 40-11)
- A hobnail morphology of the lining tumor cells is a common finding (Fig. 40-12)
- Because of the prominent nucleoli, the majority of cases would be graded as Fuhrman nuclear grade 3 (Fig. 40-12)
- Mitoses are rare or absent
- Areas of papillary architecture or solid growth are not identified unless the tumor is associated with papillary neoplasms, an occurrence reported in 30% of cases (Figs. 40-13 and 40-14)

Immunohistochemistry

- AMACR positivity usually strong and diffuse (Fig. 40-15)
- CK7 positive, but may be weak or heterogeneous (Fig. 40-15)
- The immunoprofile of tubulocystic carcinoma is similar to that of PRCC
- CD10 positive, PAX2 or PAX8 positive

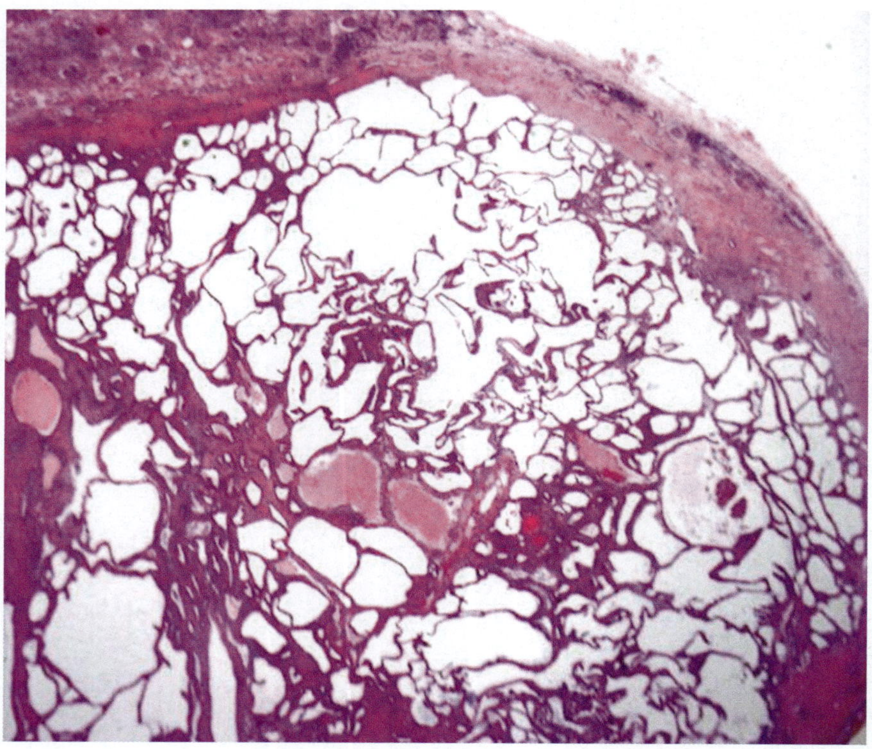

Figure 40-9.
Tubulocystic carcinoma is composed of dilated cystic structures of varying sizes.

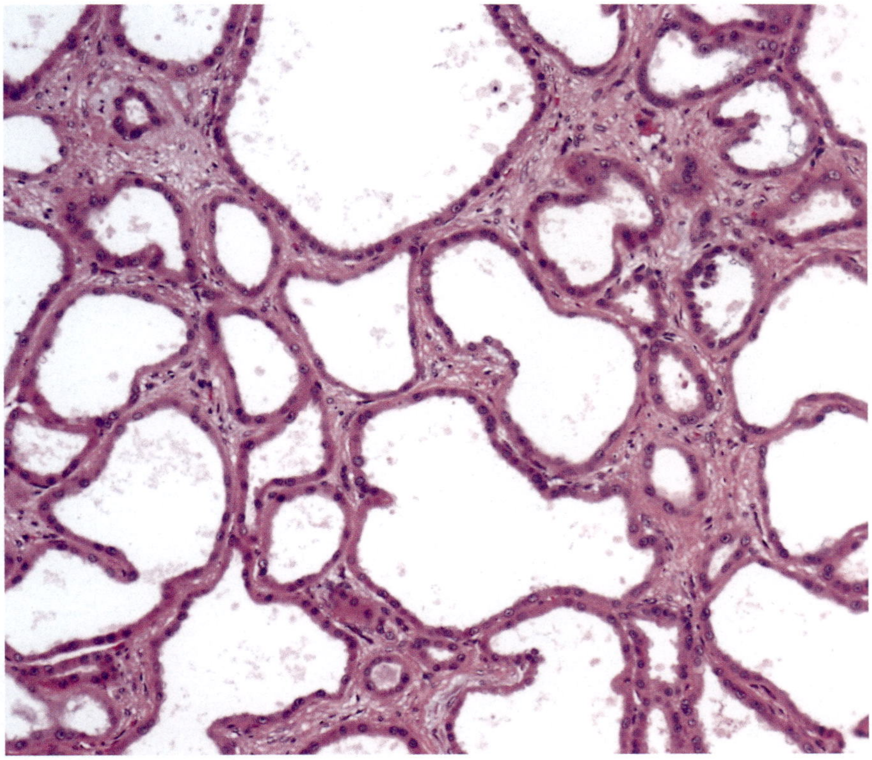

Figure 40-10.
Tubulocystic carcinoma with cystic spaces lined by tumor cells with eosinophilic cytoplasm and separated by thin fibrotic septa.

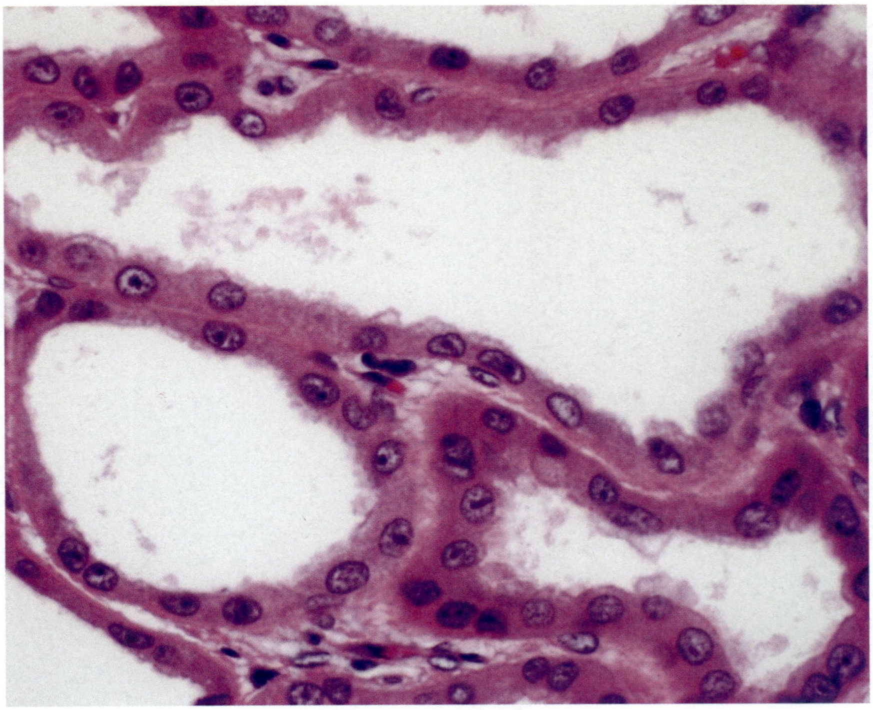

Figure 40-11.
High magnification of tubulocystic carcinoma shows lining tumor cells with prominent nucleoli and abundant brightly eosinophilic cytoplasm.

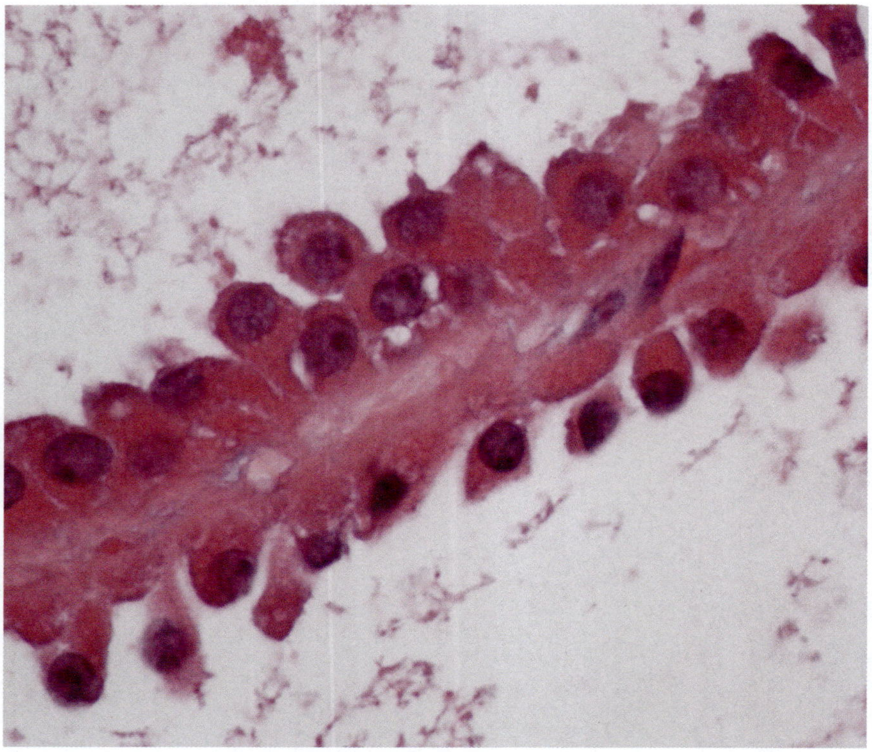

Figure 40-12.
Typical hobnail appearance of tubulocystic carcinoma cells.

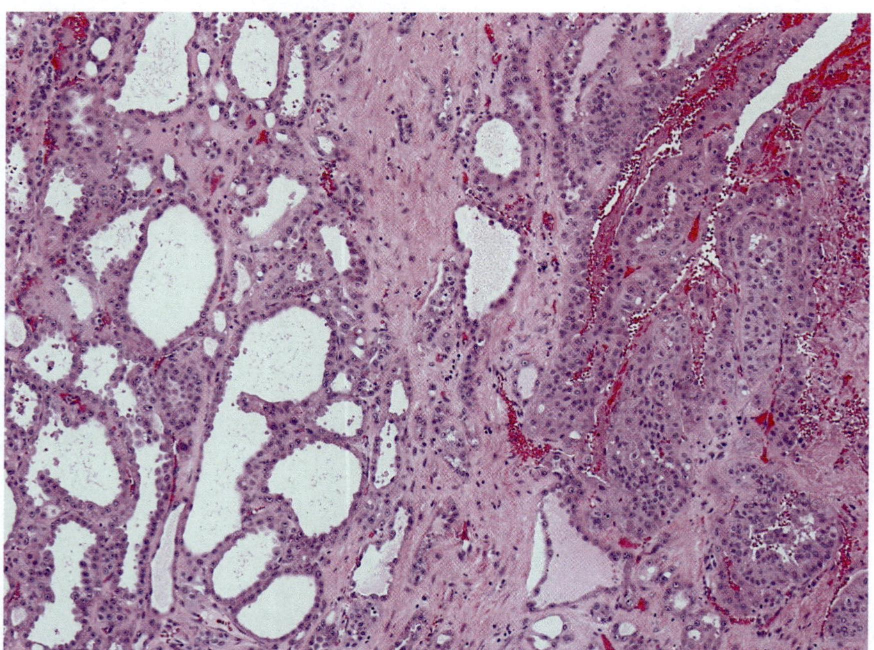

Figure 40-13.
Tubulocystic carcinoma (left) coexisting with high-grade type 2 papillary RCC (right side).

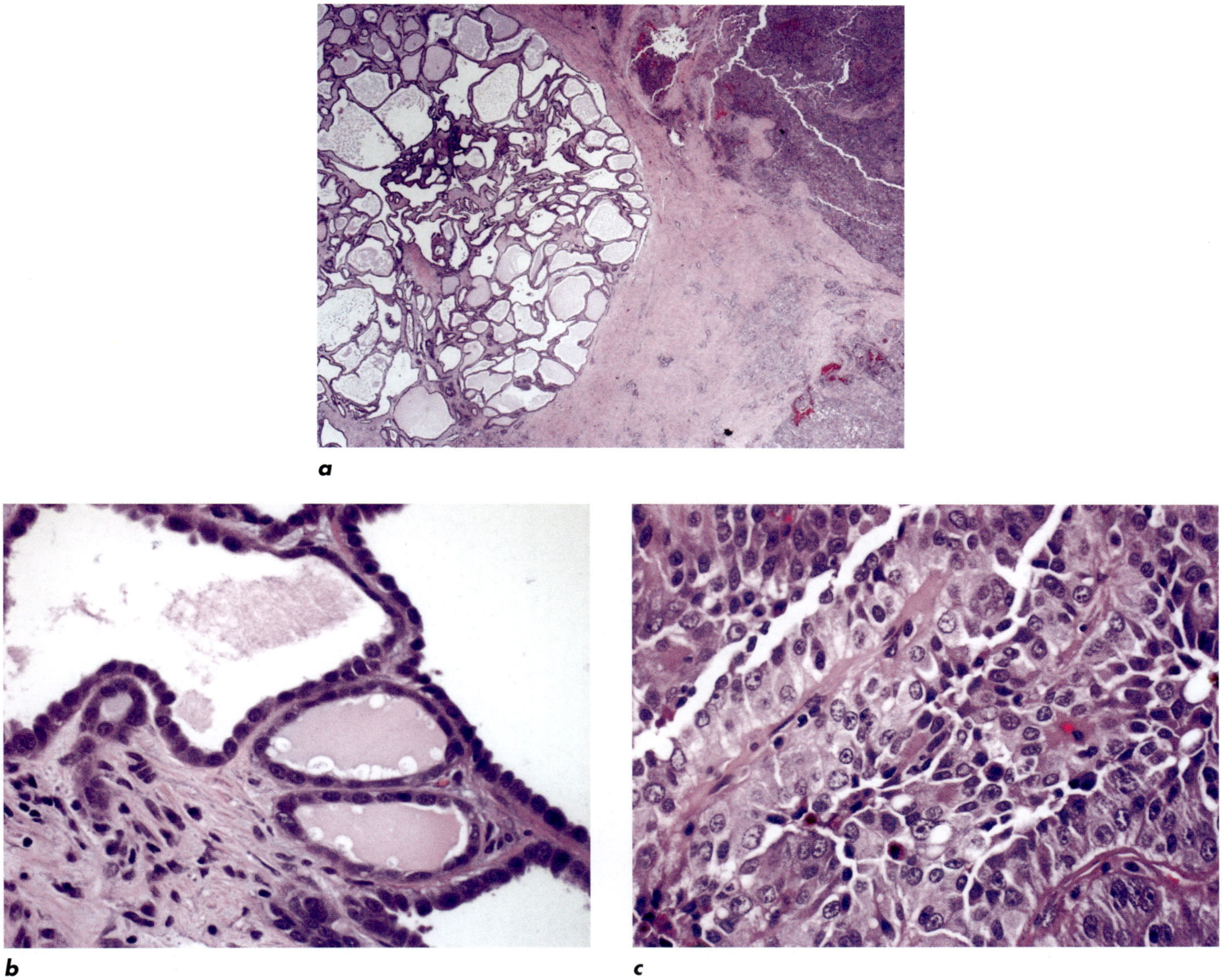

Figure 40-14.
Tubulocystic carcinoma (left) and high-grade papillary RCC (right) in another case (*a*). High magnification confirms the histological features of tubulocystic carcinoma (*b*) and high-grade type 2 papillary RCC (*c*).

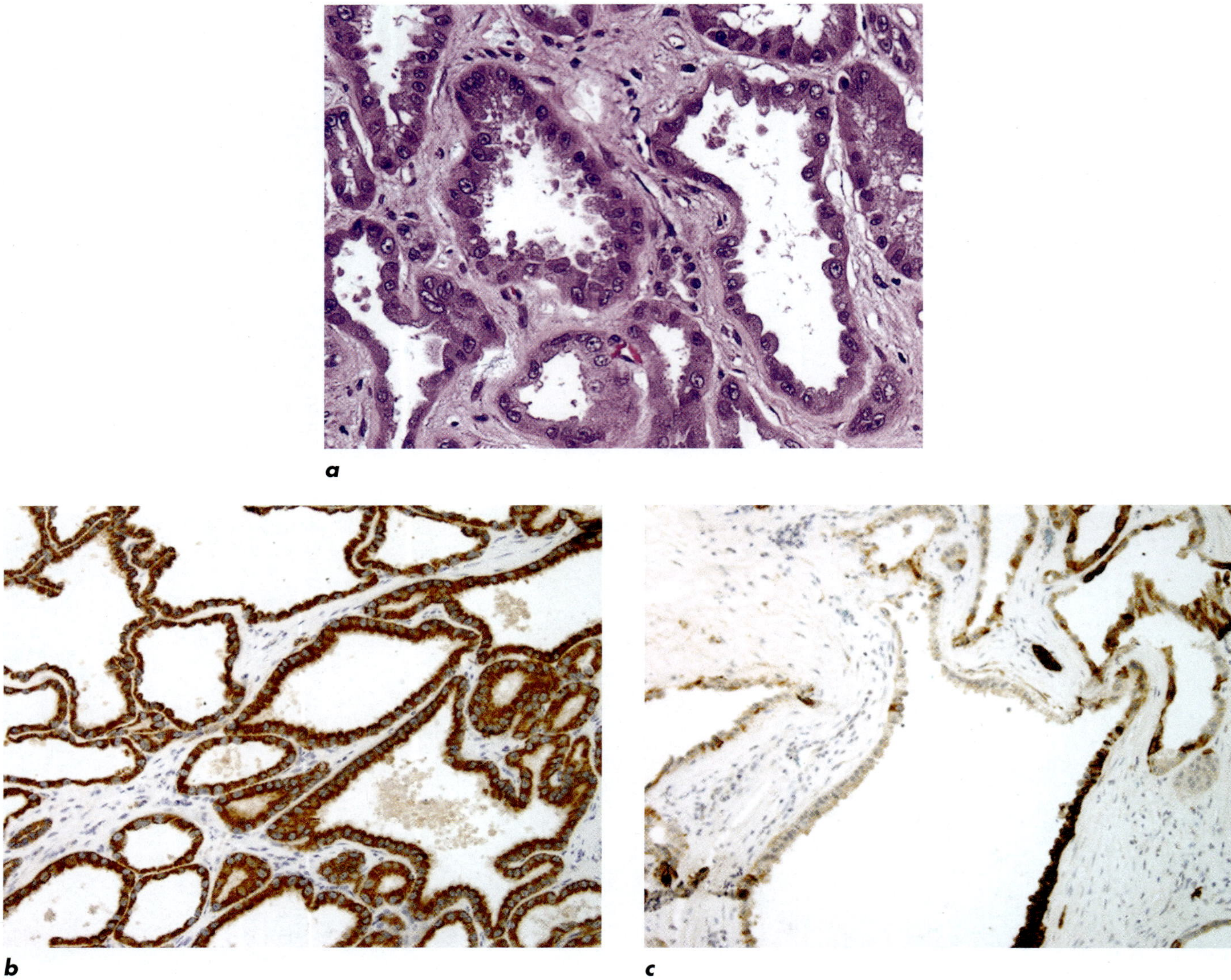

Figure 40-15.
Tubulocystic carcinoma cells (*a*) with diffuse immunoreactivity for AMACR (*b*) and focal immunoreactivity for CK7 (*c*).

Molecular diagnostics

- This tumor is similar to PRCC by gene expression microarray clustering analysis
- Gains of chromosome 17p and 17q (trisomy 17), typical for PRCCs, can be seen. However, trisomy 7, also characteristic of PRCC, is less common

Clinical relevance (prognosis and treatment options)

- Treatment of choice is surgical resection
- Most cases have a good to fair prognosis despite the high-grade appearance of the nuclei
- Metastasis can be seen in a small percentage of cases (Fig. 40-16)
- However, tumors associated with high-grade papillary RCC tend to act more aggressively

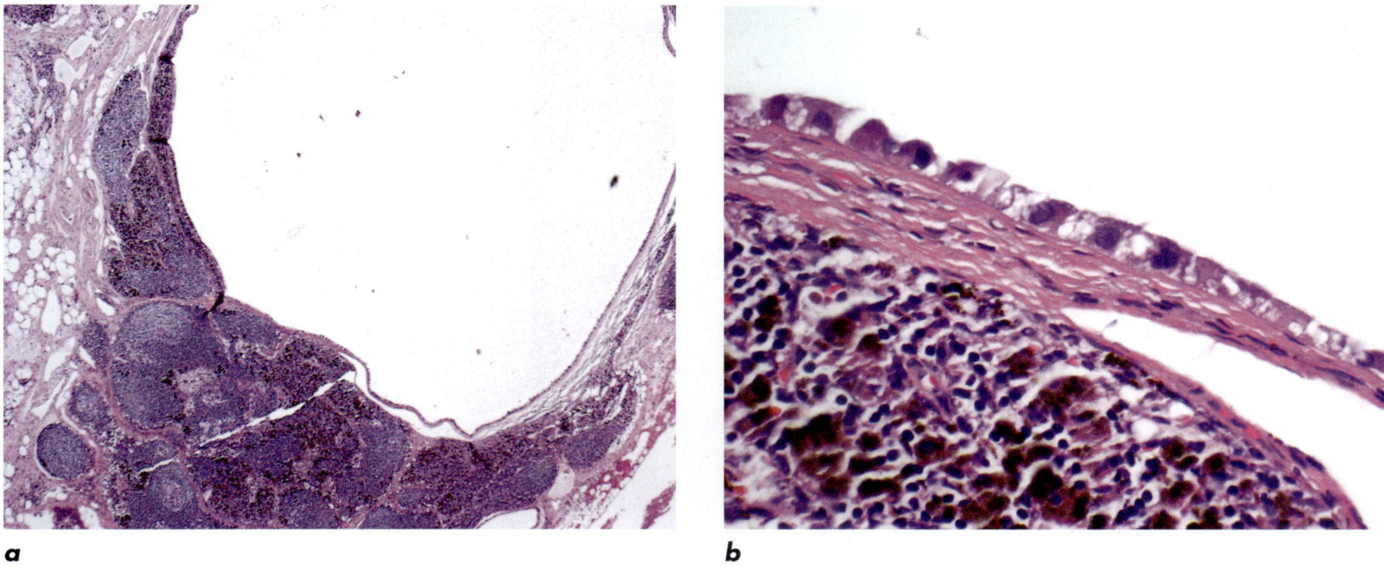

Figure 40-16.
Metastatic tubulocystic carcinoma in the pelvis lymph node (*a*). High magnification shows the tumor cells with prominent nucleoli and eosinophilic cytoplasm lining the cystic structure (*b*).

COLLECTING DUCT CARCINOMA

Definition

- Collecting duct carcinoma (CDC) is defined as a carcinoma with morphological features resembling the collecting duct of Bellini (which is the large collecting duct at the most distal portion of the collecting system and empties into the calyx)
- Because of the lack of strict histological criteria for diagnosing this tumor, an undisclosed number of renal carcinomas composed of cuboidal cells have been classified as CDC
- However, generally speaking, we prefer to define this entity as a high-grade carcinoma composed primarily of tubular structures, which morphologically resemble collecting ducts

Other term

- Collecting duct carcinoma of Bellini

Pathogenesis

- The tumor is believed to arise from lower collecting ducts

Clinical features

- Uncommon, contributing to less than 1% of all renal carcinomas
- Slight male predilection (M:F = 2:1), wide age range (13 to 83 years)
- Most tumors present with symptoms such as hematuria, pain, palpable mass, or weight loss
- Usually high-stage tumor at presentation with metastatic spread to lymph nodes, lung, bones
- Right kidney predilection

Gross pathology

- Solid mass located in medulla. However, large tumors often involve both medulla and cortex, making the determination of site of origin difficult (Fig. 40-17*a*)
- Gray to tan-white cut surface
- Focal cystic changes, hemorrhage, and necrosis can be observed
- Invasions of perinephric fat, renal sinus, and renal pelvis by the tumor are frequent findings

Histology

- Histological spectrum of the tumor is broad
- Predominant growth pattern is tubular or papillary with infiltrating angulated glands and solid cords (Fig. 40-17*b* and *c*). True papillae are invariably present
- Focal mucin production is common (Fig. 40-18)
- Desmoplastic stroma is a key histological feature. Quality of the stroma varies from loosely to densely collagenous (Fig. 40-19)
- Inflammatory infiltrate with numerous neutrophils is a nearly constant finding
- Tumor cells typically have eosinophilic cytoplasm, highly pleomorphic nuclei, and high mitotic activity (Figs. 40-19 and 40-20)
- Hobnail cells are frequently present

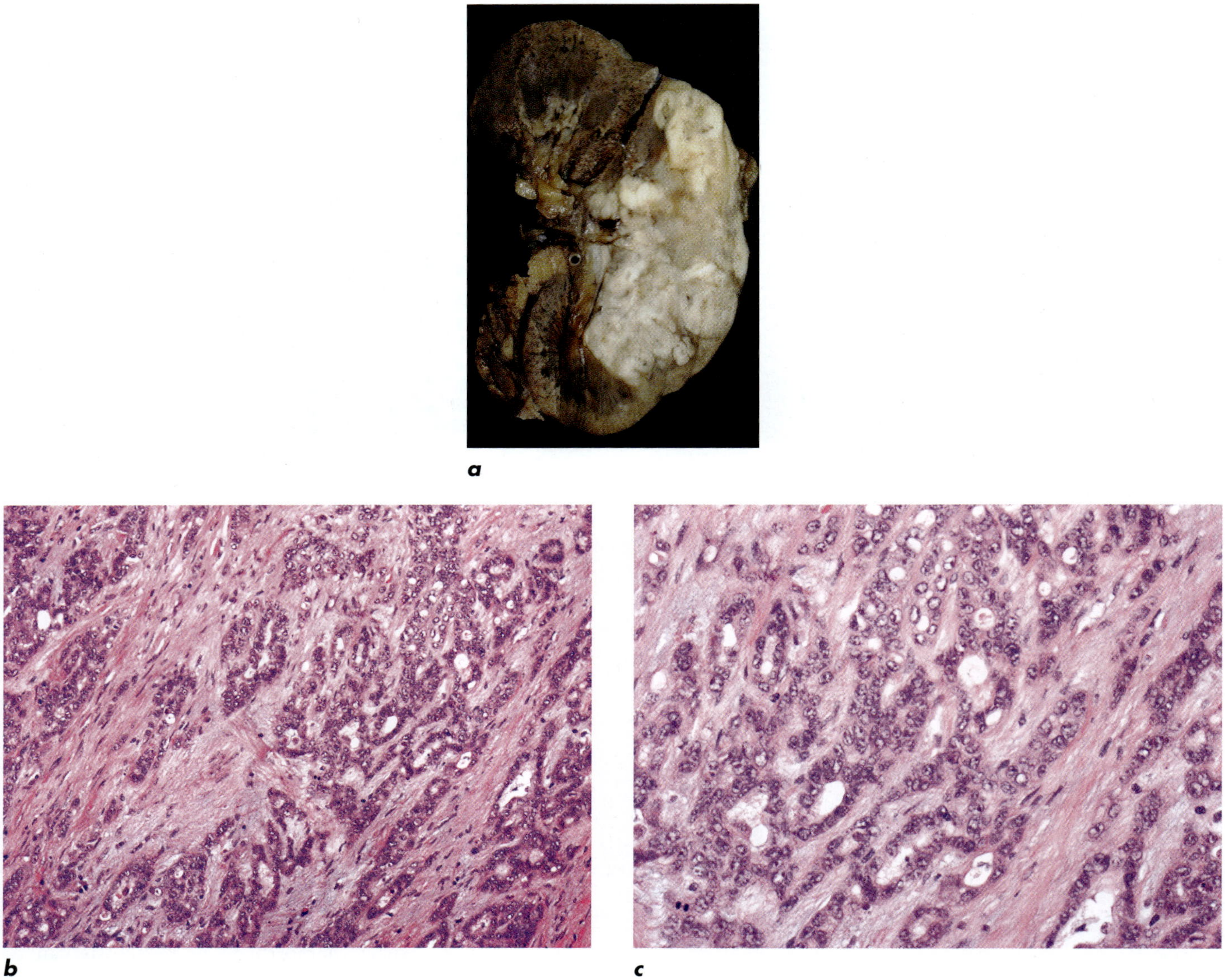

Figure 40-17.

A large collecting duct carcinoma replacing the majority of the kidney. The cut surface of this tumor is white (postfixation) with infiltrating borders (*a*). The tumor is composed of cuboidal tumor cells forming tubular structures resembling collecting ducts (*b*). Desmoplastic stroma is characteristic. High magnification shows the presence of nuclear pleomorphism and prominent nucleoli (*c*).

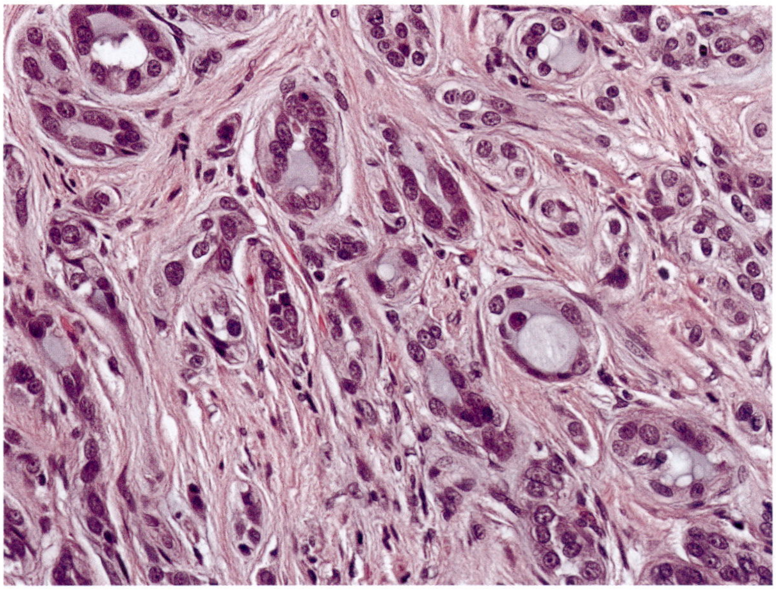

Figure 40-18.
Collecting duct carcinoma is characterized by the presence of high nuclear grade, cuboidal tumor cells forming glandular structures, and a prominent desmoplastic stroma.

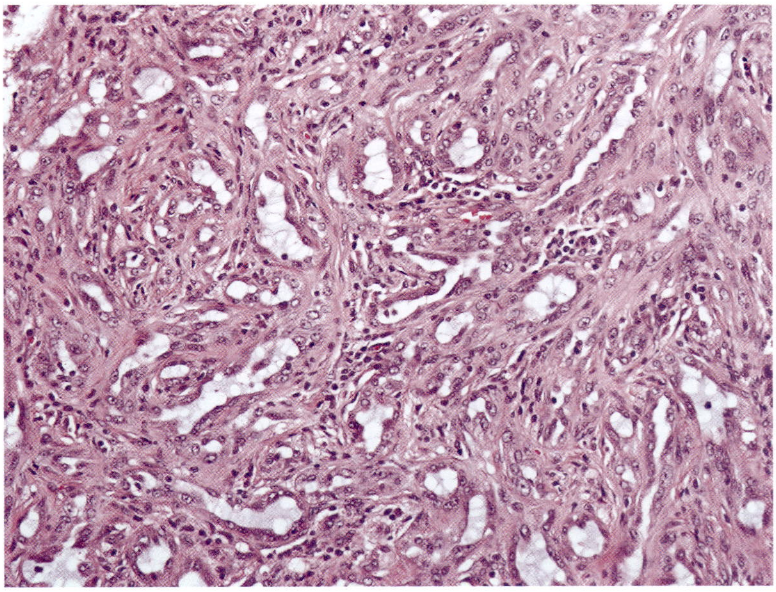

Figure 40-19.
Collecting duct carcinoma with high-grade tumor cells forming small, irregular tubules containing blue intraluminal secretions.

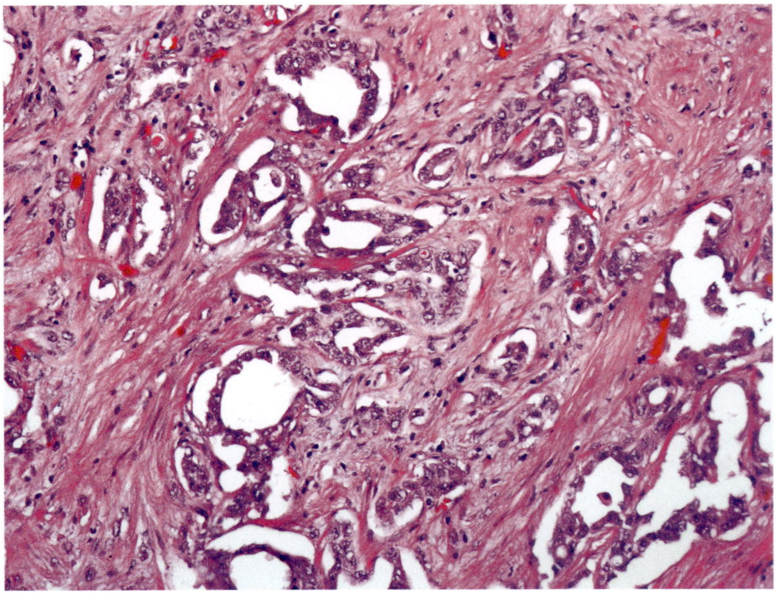

Figure 40-20.
Collecting duct carcinoma featuring poorly formed tubules and a desmoplastic stroma.

Immunohistochemistry

- Ulex europaeus, CK7 and HMCK are almost always positive
- AMACR, p63, CD10, Ksp-cadherin are negative
- Vimentin variably positive

Molecular genetics

- Only a few cases have been analyzed with inconsistent results, which may be explained by contamination with other subtypes of renal tumors
- LOH was identified in 1q, 6p, 8p, 13q, 21q, and chromosomal 3p losses have been described
- Monosomy of chromosomes 1, 6, 14, 15, 22 has been reported
- Her2/neu amplification has been noted in CDC
- Association with BK polyoma virus positivity, confirmed by immunohistochemistry, has been described in transplanted patients

Differential diagnosis

Papillary RCC

- PRCC is usually circumscribed, but high-grade ones have an infiltrative border
- Papillary architecture is usually more prominent in PRCC, although solid and tubular variants exist. In addition, the cells comprising these tumors are typically less pleomorphic than CDC
- Stromal mucinous material is not characteristic of PRCC
- Papillary cores usually contain foam cells
- PRCC is positive for AMACR, CK7, and vimentin
- Analysis of chromosomes 7 and 17 trisomy/polysomy (loss of Y in males) may be helpful, since these genetic aberrations are typical for PRCC, not for CDC

Urothelial carcinoma

- Majority of urothelial carcinoma (UC) are limited to the renal pelvis, but larger tumors may extend into the medulla and cortex or grow along collecting ducts
- Microscopically, invasive UC mimics CDC by its solid tubular growth pattern, but UC shows characteristic in situ component or papillary architectures in the renal pelvis
- Squamous and glandular differentiation favors diagnosis of UC
- Immunohistochemical profile of CDC and TCC shows overlaps with expression of CK7 and CK20, HMCK, ULEX-1, as well as PAX8. However, p63, Gata3, and S100p are more commonly expressed in UC

Clinical relevance (prognosis and treatment options)

- Surgery is the major treatment choice
- Experience with chemotherapy is limited
- May not respond well to any current therapy
- Poor prognosis, 50% of the patients die of disease within 2 years

RENAL MEDULLARY CARCINOMA

Definition

- A highly malignant renal epithelial carcinoma in patients with sickle cell trait or other hemoglobinopathies

Pathogenesis

- The majority of patients have sickle cell trait
- Rarely patients with other hemoglobin diseases such as SC and SS diseases have been described
- One hypothesis is that susceptible red blood cells sickle and clot in the oxygen-poor circulation of the renal medulla, which induces renal papillary necrosis.
- In this long-standing ischemic environment, hypoxia induces elaboration of growth factors during the reparative process that promotes neoplastic transformation
- Renal medullary carcinoma may be considered a special form of CDC, while other carcinomas formerly considered variants of CDCs are now classified as separate entities (Table 40-1)
- In the cases morphologically resembling medullary carcinoma, but with no hemoglobinopathy, we prefer the term *medullary-like carcinoma*

Clinical features

- Uncommon type of tumor with only approximately 100 cases reported in the English literature
- Typically African males with sickle cell trait
- Presents with hematuria and large renal mass
- Often evidence of distant metastases at the time of diagnosis

Gross pathology

- Bulky infiltrating mass with central location close to the renal pelvis (Fig. 40-21)
- Necrosis, fibrosis, and focal hemorrhage commonly identified
- Cut surface shows an ill-defined white, yellow tumor mass resembling brain tissue

Histology

- Highly infiltrative tumor with epithelial clusters surrounding or encasing glomeruli (Figs. 40-22 and 40-23)
- Tumor cells with deeply eosinophilic cytoplasm and large pleomorphic nuclei (Fig. 40-24) grow in syncytial pattern and exhibit high mitotic counts and foci of necrosis (Figs. 40-25 and 40-26)
- Tumor cells with rhabdoid features are often encountered
- Presence of desmoplastic stroma and infiltrating neutrophils are common (Fig. 40-25)
- Presence of characteristic sickling red cells in the vasa recta of the medulla can be seen in the majority of cases (Figs. 40-26 to 40-28)
- Morphologically, medullary carcinoma shows a closer resemblance of UC or CDC than typical RCCs
- Metastases to lymph node (Fig. 40-29) or distant organs are commonly present

Immunohistochemistry

- Topoisomerase II (Top2) staining increased
- INI-I (SNF5) is negative in almost all the medullary carcinoma cases tested while INI-1 is negative in only 15% of CDC and positive in most RCC studied
- OCT-4 immunoreactivity in the majority of cases (70%)

Table 40-1. Evolving Concept of Collecting Duct Carcinoma

Old terms	*New preferred diagnostic terms*
Low-grade collecting carcinoma	Mucinous tubular and spindle cell carcinoma
	Tubulocystic carcinoma
High-grade collecting duct carcinoma	Medullary carcinoma (sickle cell trait or other hemoglobin abnormalities)
	Medullary-like carcinoma (without hemoglobin abnormalities)
	High-grade papillary RCC
	Collecting duct carcinoma (high grade)

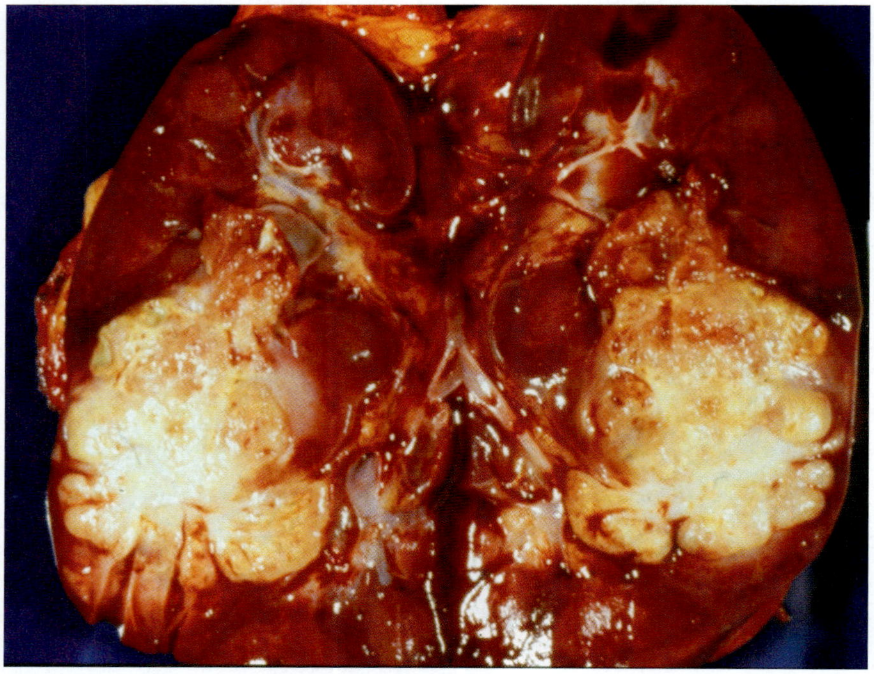

Figure 40-21.
Gross photo of renal medullary carcinoma from a 20-year Black man. The tumor is large, soft, white-yellow, and centered around the medulla and renal pelvis.

Differential diagnosis

Collecting duct carcinoma

- Older patients
- No evidence of hemoglobinopathy
- Immunoprofile: a combination of positive vimentin, strong PAX8, focal or absent p63, absence of INI-1, and presence of OCT-4 would favor the medullary carcinoma over CDC

Molecular analysis

- The tumor clusters with UC rather than conventional RCCs by gene expression profiling
- VCL-ALK translocation has recently been reported in a subset of renal cell neoplasms with features of medullary carcinoma in patients with sickle cell trait

Clinical relevance (prognosis and treatment options)

- Very aggressive tumor, no cure is currently available
- We do not make a diagnosis of medullary carcinoma in a patient without hemoglobinopathy. In that situation, we use the term *medullary-like carcinoma*
- Many cases have metastases at the time of diagnosis
- Average survival without treatment is a couple of months
- With advanced chemotherapy including Topo2 inhibitors, the survival has been prolonged

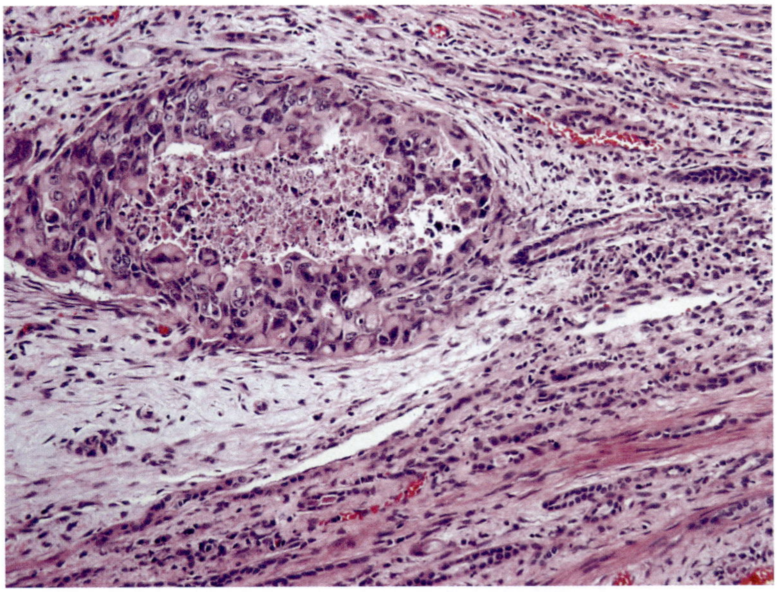

Figure 40-22.
Tumor cells forming a gland with comedo necrosis. Characteristic stromal features observed in medullary carcinoma including desmoplastic reaction and inflammation.

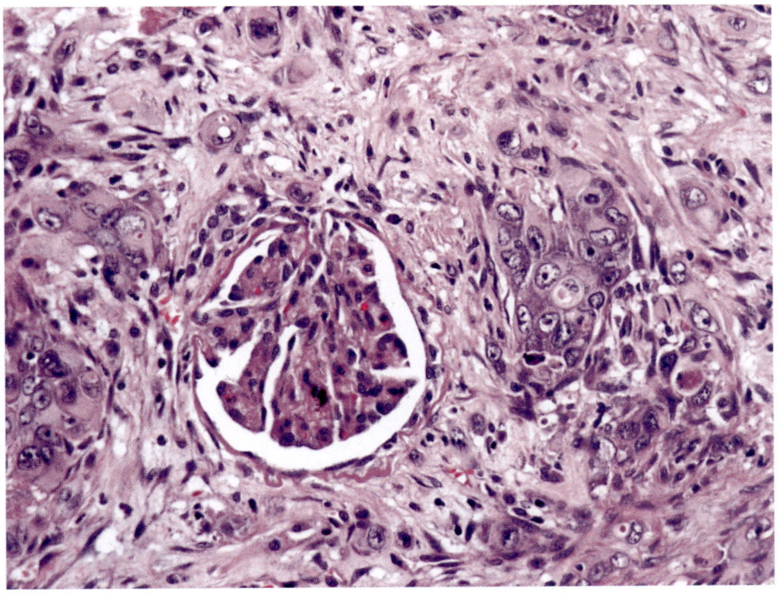

Figure 40-23.
Medullary carcinoma entrapping a glomerulus. Intracellular lumen can be seen in some tumor cells.

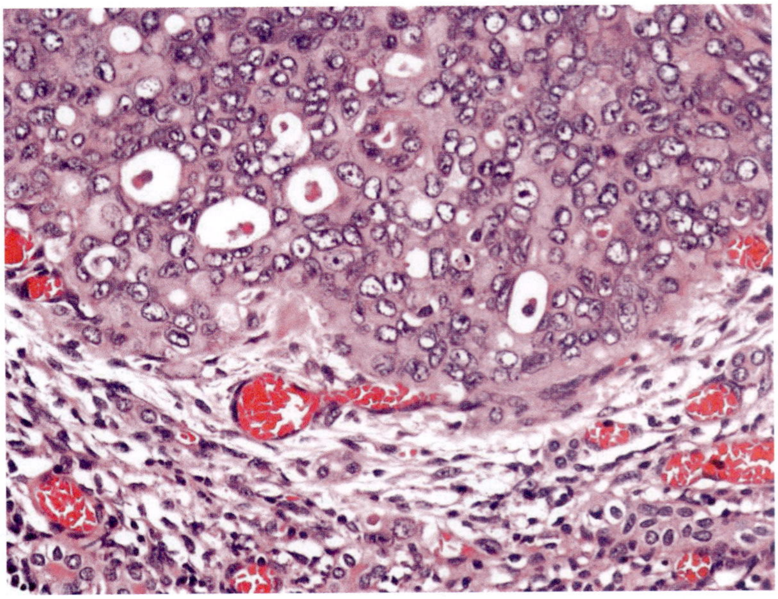

Figure 40-24.
Renal medullary carcinoma composed of large pleomorphic tumor cells forming a large cribriform nest.

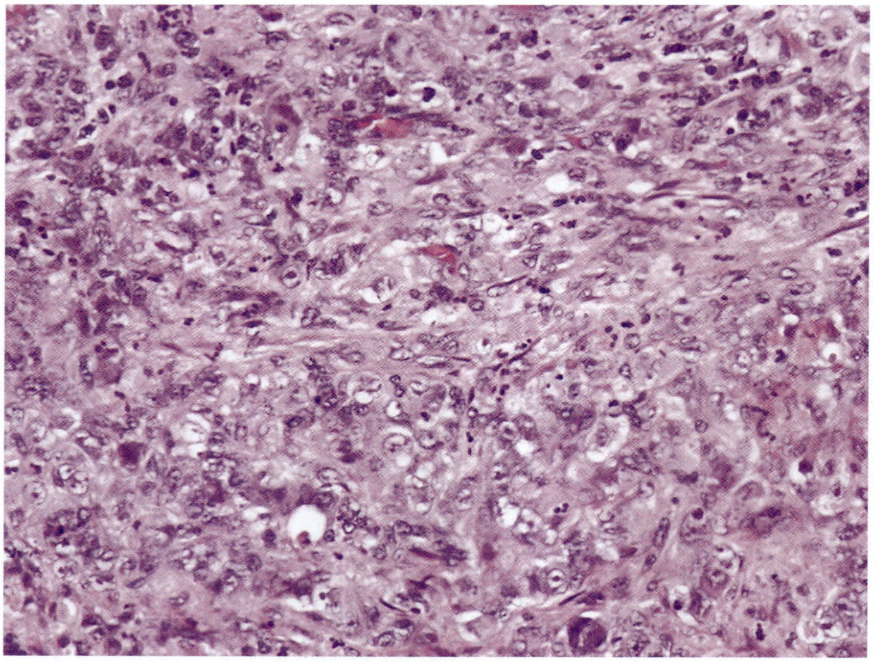

Figure 40-25.
Medullary carcinoma with tumor cells arranged in solid and syncytial patterns, and associated with a neutrophilic infiltrate.

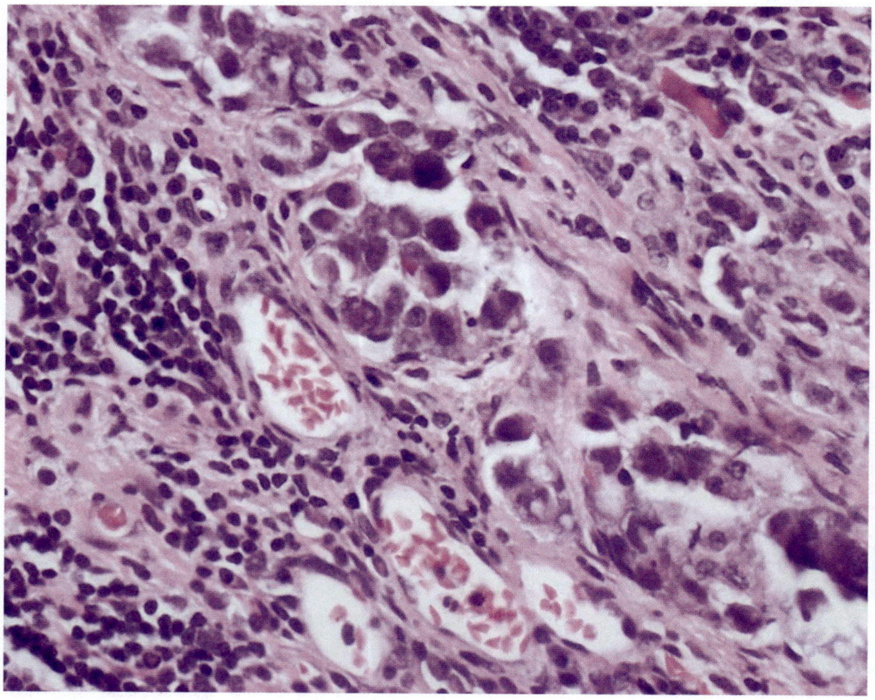

Figure 40-26.
Medullary carcinoma with highly pleomorphic cells adjacent to capillaries containing sickling red cells.

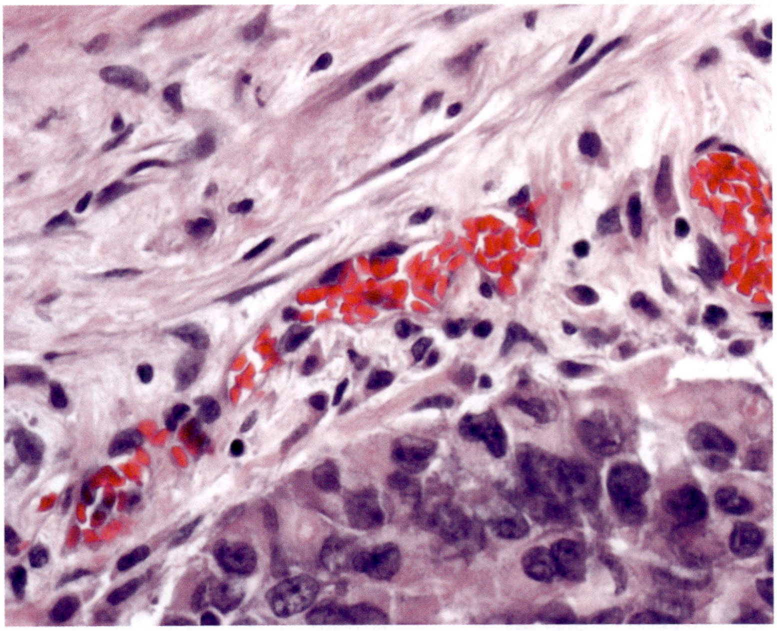

Figure 40-27.
A nest of large tumor cells with intracellular lumens adjacent to a focus of sickling red cells in medullary carcinoma.

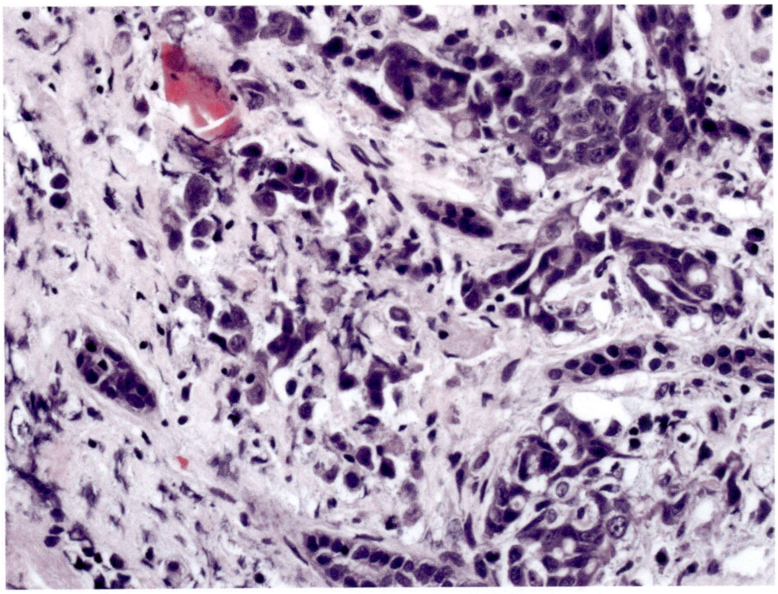

Figure 40-28.
Medullary carcinoma in a needle biopsy specimen features pleomorphic tumor cells forming small tubular structures within a marked desmoplastic and inflammatory stroma. Occasionally, intracellular lumen can be seen.

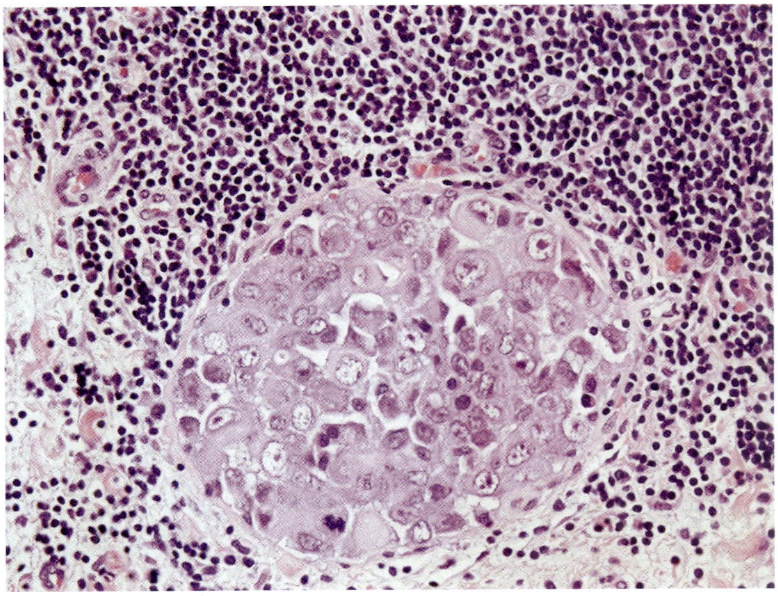

Figure 40-29.
Metastatic medullary carcinoma metastatic to the pelvic lymph node.

CLEAR CELL PAPILLARY RENAL CELL CARCINOMA

Definition

- A low-grade RCC composed of tumor cells with clear cytoplasm in a papillary configuration

Other terms

- Clear cell tubular papillary carcinoma, clear cell tubulo-papillary carcinoma

Clinical features

- Most patients are asymptomatic and the tumor is discovered incidentally by imaging studies. Some patients may present with typical symptoms of conventional RCC, such as flank pain or hematuria
- This tumor may be associated with end-stage kidney disease
- The tumor incidence in routine radical and partial nephrectomy specimens is approximately 3%. In the past, most of these cases were probably misclassified as conventional clear cell RCC
- Metastasis is extremely rare

Gross pathology

- Solid, well-circumscribed nonencapsulated mass (Fig. 40-30*a*)
- Fleshy, salmon-color, or tan cut surface, but not the typical bright yellow appearance of clear cell RCC (Figs. 40-31*a* and 40-32*a*)
- Cystic degenerative change can be seen (Fig. 40-31*a*), but hemorrhage and necrosis are uncommon

Histology

- Tumor cells are arranged in branching tubules or papillary configurations with intraluminal infoldings (Figs. 40-30*b*, 40-31*b*, and 40-32*b*)
- Tumor cells have prominent clear cytoplasm and low (Fuhrman 1 or 2) nuclear grade nuclei (Figs. 40-31*c* and 40-32*c*)
- Apical nuclear location with a "piano-key" appearance (nuclei pulling away from the basement membrane) (Figs. 40-30*c* and 40-32*c*)

Immunohistochemistry (Fig. 40-33)

- CK7 strongly and diffusely positive
- CA9 positive with cup-shaped membranous staining (missing luminal staining) (Fig. 40-33*d*)
- AMACR negative

Molecular genetics

- Lack of *VHL* gene mutations

Differential diagnosis (see Table 40-2)

TFE3 translocation carcinoma

- This is a high-grade tumor with aggressive behavior
- TFE3 immunostaining or FISH is necessary for confirmation of the diagnosis
- Tumor often shows focal or absent keratin immunoreactivity

Clear cell RCC

- Tumor cells lack typical "piano-key" appearance
- Immunostaining profile is different
- CA9 in clear cell RCC is box-shaped (circumferential membranous), and not cup-shaped

Clinical relevance (prognosis and treatment options)

- Surgery, particularly partial nephrectomy
- Good prognosis. No metastases have been documented to date, raising the question of whether this is truly a malignant neoplasm

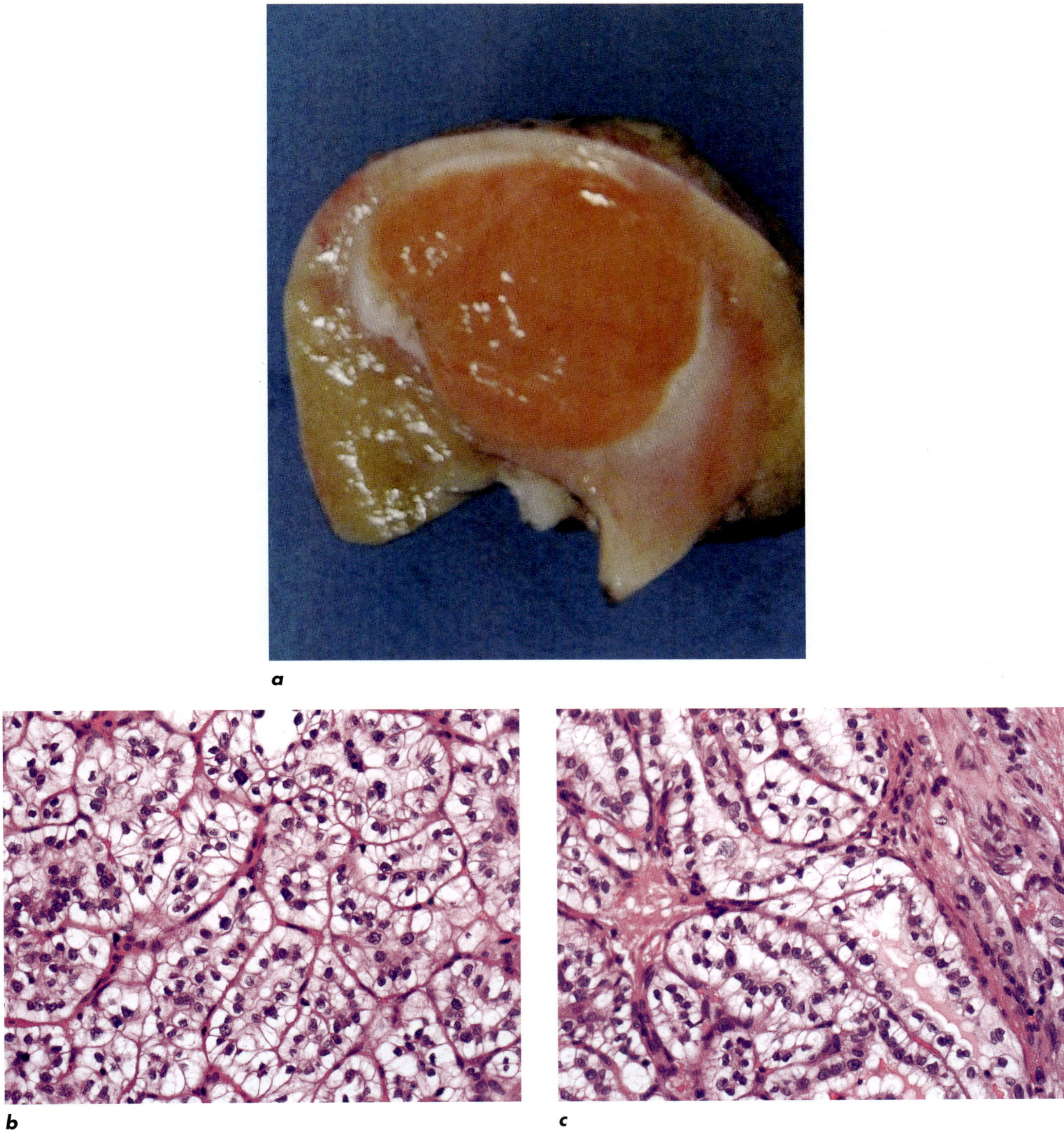

Figure 40-30.

Clear cell papillary renal cell carcinoma. A well-defined solid mass with salmon-colored cut surface in a partial nephrectomy specimen (*a*). Microscopically, the tumor is composed of low-grade tumor cells with clear cytoplasm forming tubules (*b*). The characteristic feature is the luminal position of tumor cell nuclei, giving the "piano-key" appearance to the cell (*c*).

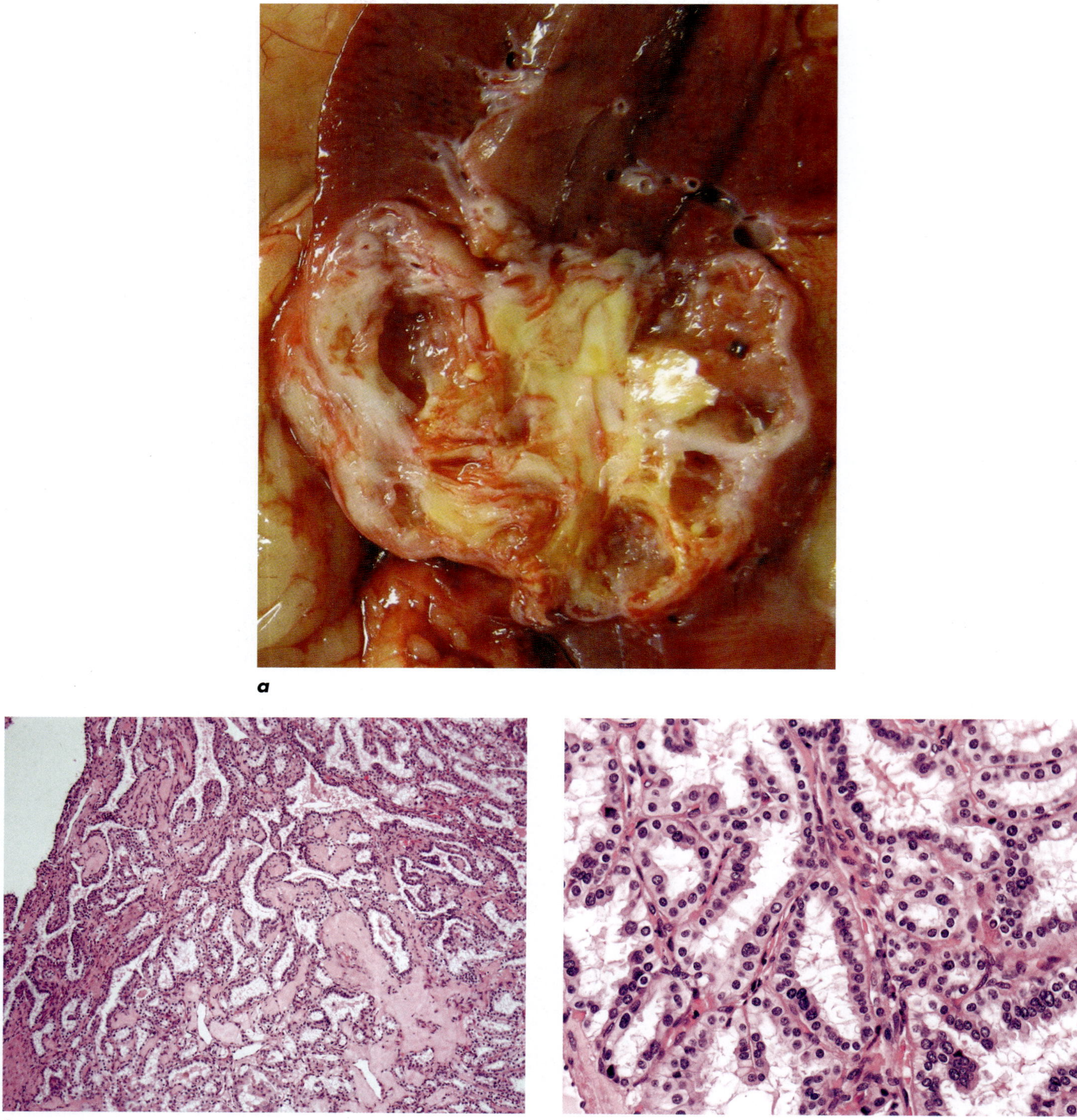

a b c

Figure 40-31.
Clear cell papillary RCC with cystic appearance (*a*). The tumor cells form papillary and tubular structures (*b*) with cuboidal or columnar cells with clear cytoplasm and low-grade nuclei (*c*).

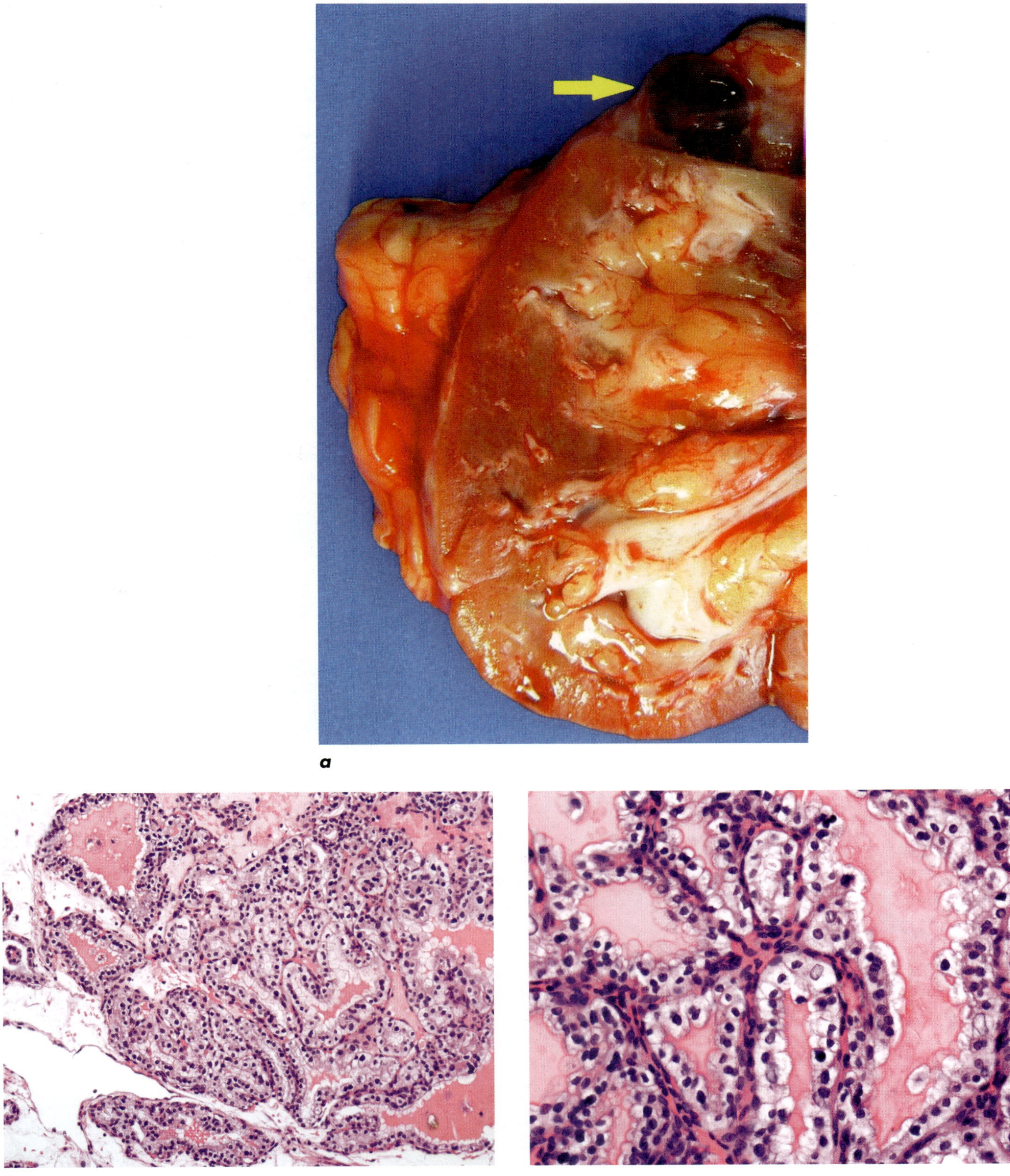

Figure 40-32.
Clear cell papillary RCC presents as a dark beefy red mass (arrow) located in the upper pole in a nephrectomy specimen (*a*). Microscopically, tumor cells are arranged in the typical tubular and papillary configuration (*b*) and possess low-grade clear cells (*c*).

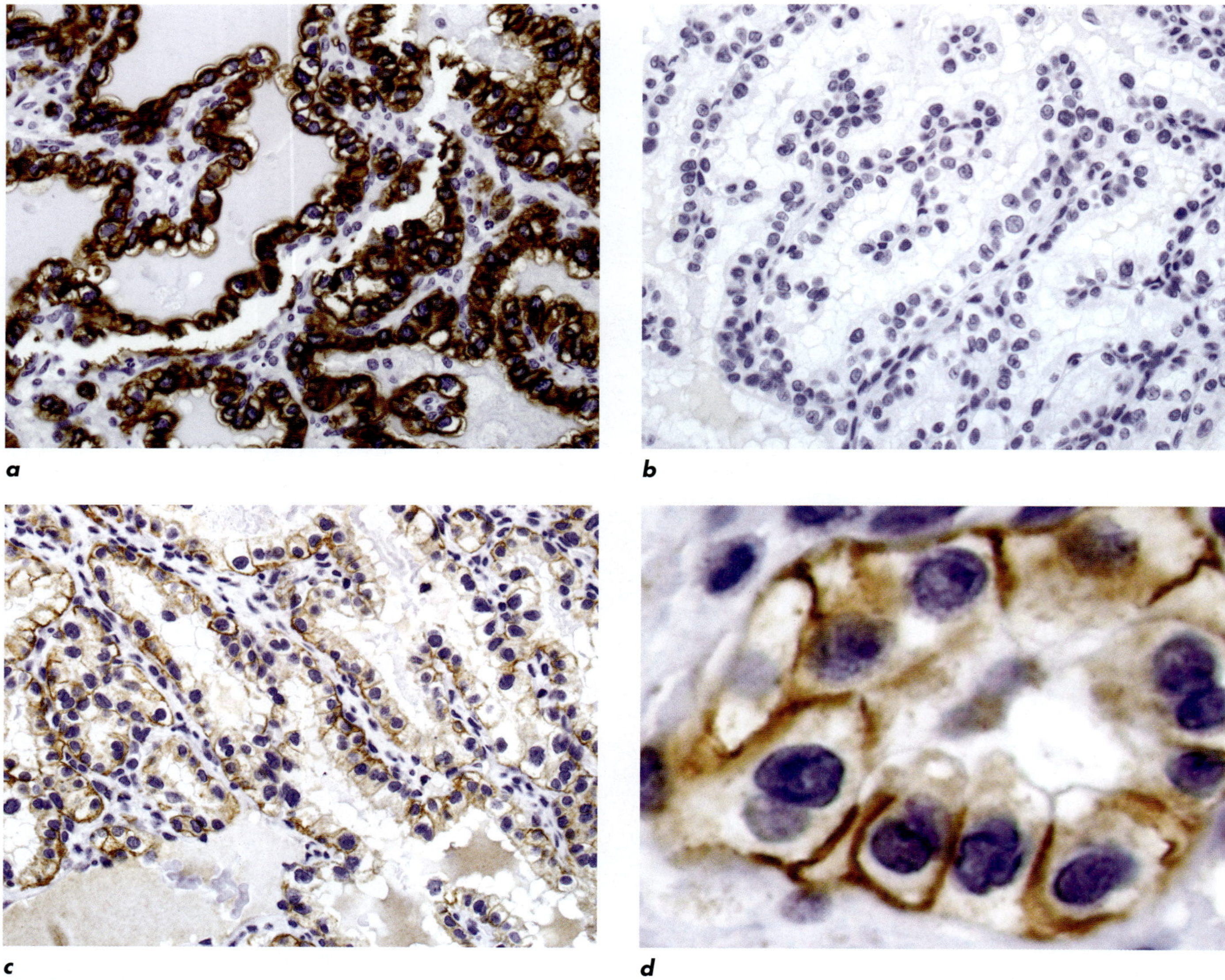

Figure 40-33.
Clear cell papillary RCC immunohistochemical profile. The tumor cells are positive for CK7 (*a*), negative for AMACR (*b*). The unique pattern of CA9 positivity (*c*) is the characteristic "cup-shaped" (missing luminal side staining) CA9 membranous staining (*d*).

Table 40-2. Comparison of Subtypes of RCC with Clear Cytoplasm

RCC types	*Clear cell papillary RCC*	*Clear cell RCC*	*Papillary RCC*	*TFE3 translocation carcinoma*
Gross	White to tan	Bright yellow	Variable	Variable
Architecture	Papillary tubular	Sheets, nests, or alveoli	Papillary or solid	Papillary and glandular
Cytoplasm	Clear	Clear or granular	Basophilic or eosinophilic	Clear or amphophilic
Nuclear grade	low	Low to high	Low to high	High
Vascular pattern	Fibrovascular core	Chicken wire, surrounds nests of cells	Fibrovascular core	Fibrovascular core
Behavior	Indolent	Indolent to aggressive	Indolent to aggressive	Aggressive
CK7	Positive	Negative	Positive	Negative
CA9	Positive	Positive	Negative	Negative
AMACR	Negative	Negative/positive	Positive	Negative
TFE3	Negative	Negative	Negative	Positive

AMACR, α-methylacyl-CoA racemase; CA9, carbonic anhydrase 9; CK7, cytokeratin 7; RCC, renal cell carcinoma.

RENAL ANGIOMYOMATOUS TUMOR

Definition

- Renal angiomyomatous tumor (RAT) is a low-grade RCC composed of clear to basophilic cells in papillary or tubular configuration and a prominent leiomyomatous stromal component

Pathogenesis

- Very rare neoplasm, with less than 50 cases reported in the literature
- There are many similarities between RAT and clear cell PRCC, except for the prominent leiomyomatous stroma in the former. Therefore, RAT may possibly represent a histological variant of clear cell PRCC

Clinical features

- Most tumors are detected incidentally
- Limited studies suggest an association of this neoplasm with tuberous sclerosis complex

Gross pathology

- Solid, well-demarcated mass often surrounded by a thick whitish capsule (Fig. 40-34)
- Cystic changes and septation could be present (Fig. 40-35*a*)
- Tan to brown cut surface (Fig. 40-36*a*)

Histology

- Haphazardly arranged fascicles of cytologically bland smooth muscle form pseudocapsule, and intermingled with neoplastic epithelial cells (Fig. 40-35)
- Epithelial tumor cells typically have clear voluminous cytoplasm with low-grade nuclei and are arranged in papillary and tubular profiles (Figs. 40-35*c* and 40-36*b*).
- Convoluted tubules, papillary structures, and prominent fibromuscular stroma generate a resemblance of prostatic parenchyma (Figs. 40-36*c* and 40-37*a*)
- Clear cells have blister-like snouts at their apical poles, forming "shark-smile" appearance (Fig. 40-37*b* and *c*)
- Each tubule is surrounded by fine capillary network, as are normal renal cortical tubules (Fig. 40-37*d*)

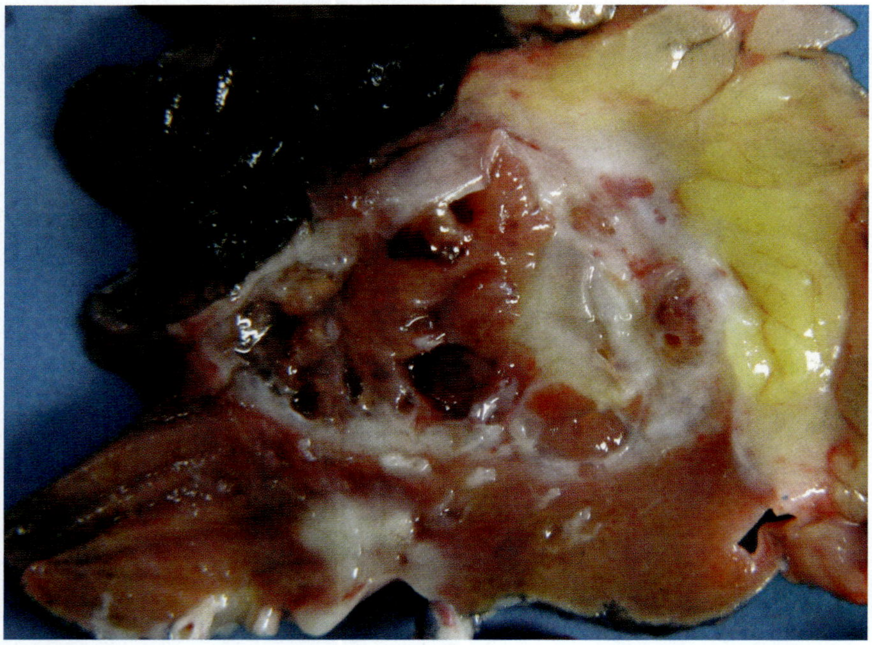

Figure 40-34. Renal angiomyomatous tumor (RAT) in a partial nephrectomy shows a salmon-colored mass with white septa traversing the lesion.

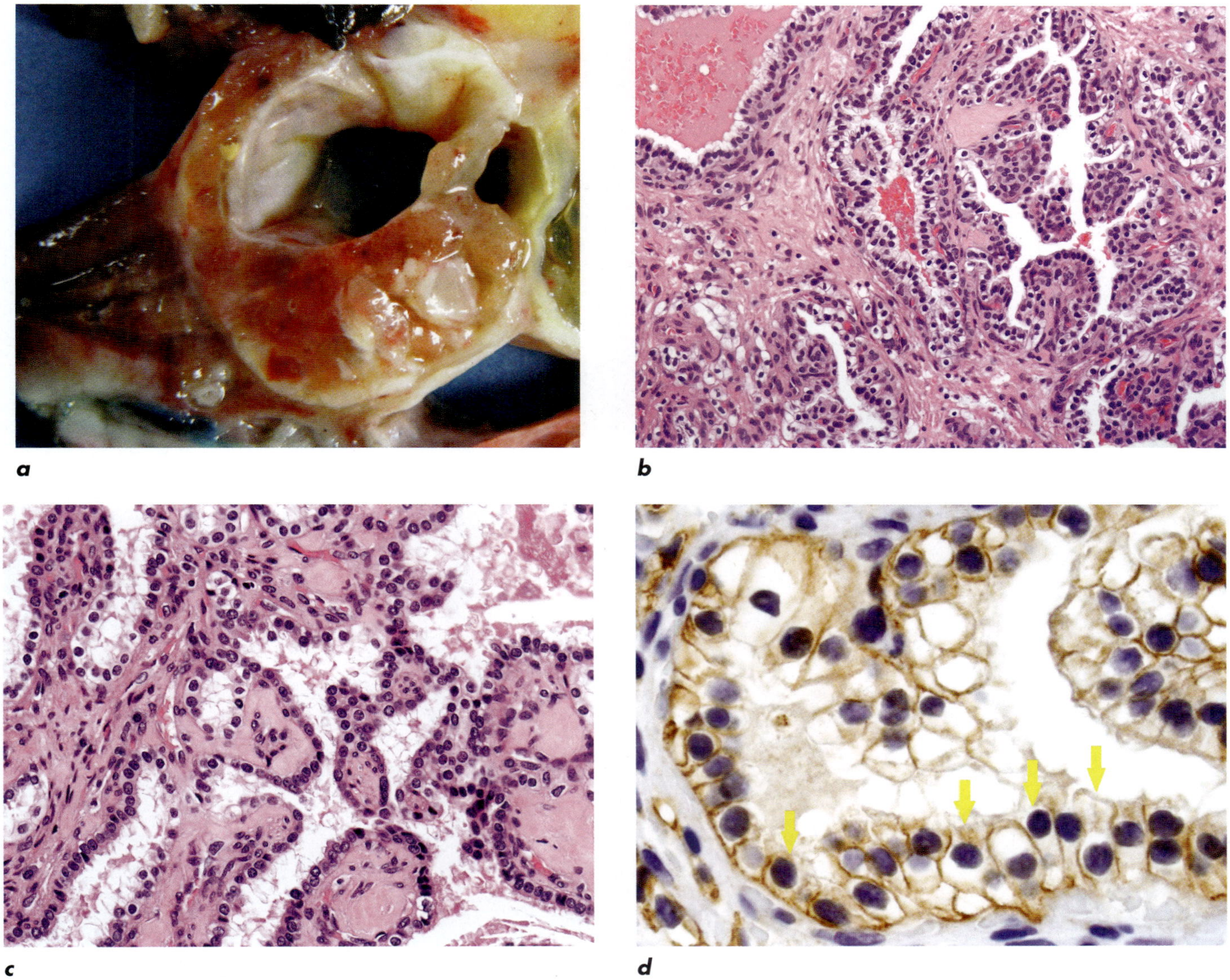

Figure 40-35.
Renal angiomyomatous tumor with a dark red thyroid-like cut surface and with multiple cysts (*a*). Microscopically, the tumor is composed of low-grade clear cells in papillary configurations and a characteristic angiomyomatous stroma (*b*). The tumor shows prominent angiomyomatous stroma (*c*) and characteristic "cup-shaped" CA9 staining (*d*, arrows).

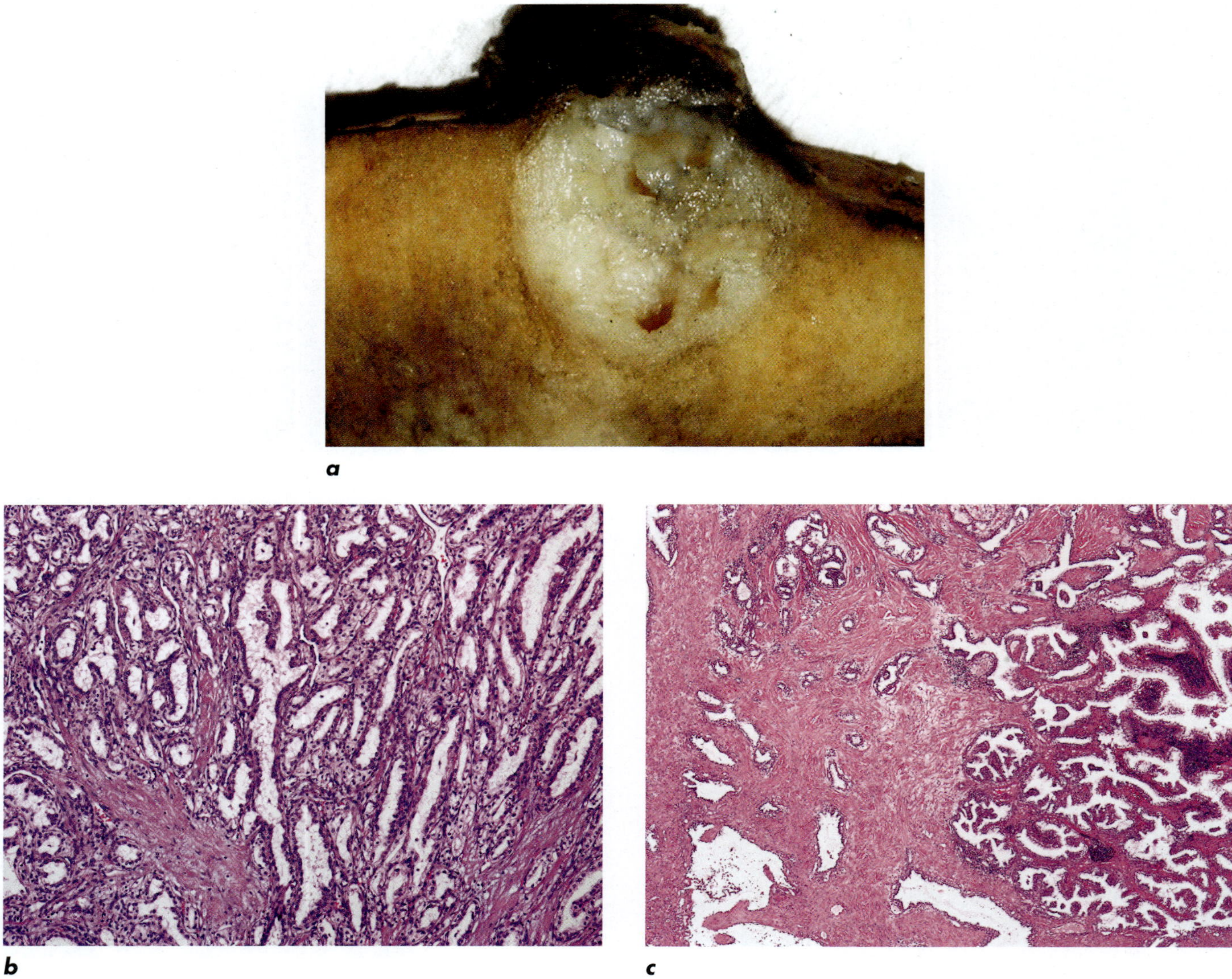

Figure 40-36.
Renal angiomyomatous tumor showing a white-tan cut surface with solid and cystic areas (*a*). Microscopically, the tumor is composed of clear cells arranged in a tubular and papillary pattern (*b*) and prominent angiomyomatous stroma, with the presence of convoluted glands results in a "prostate-like" appearance (*c*).

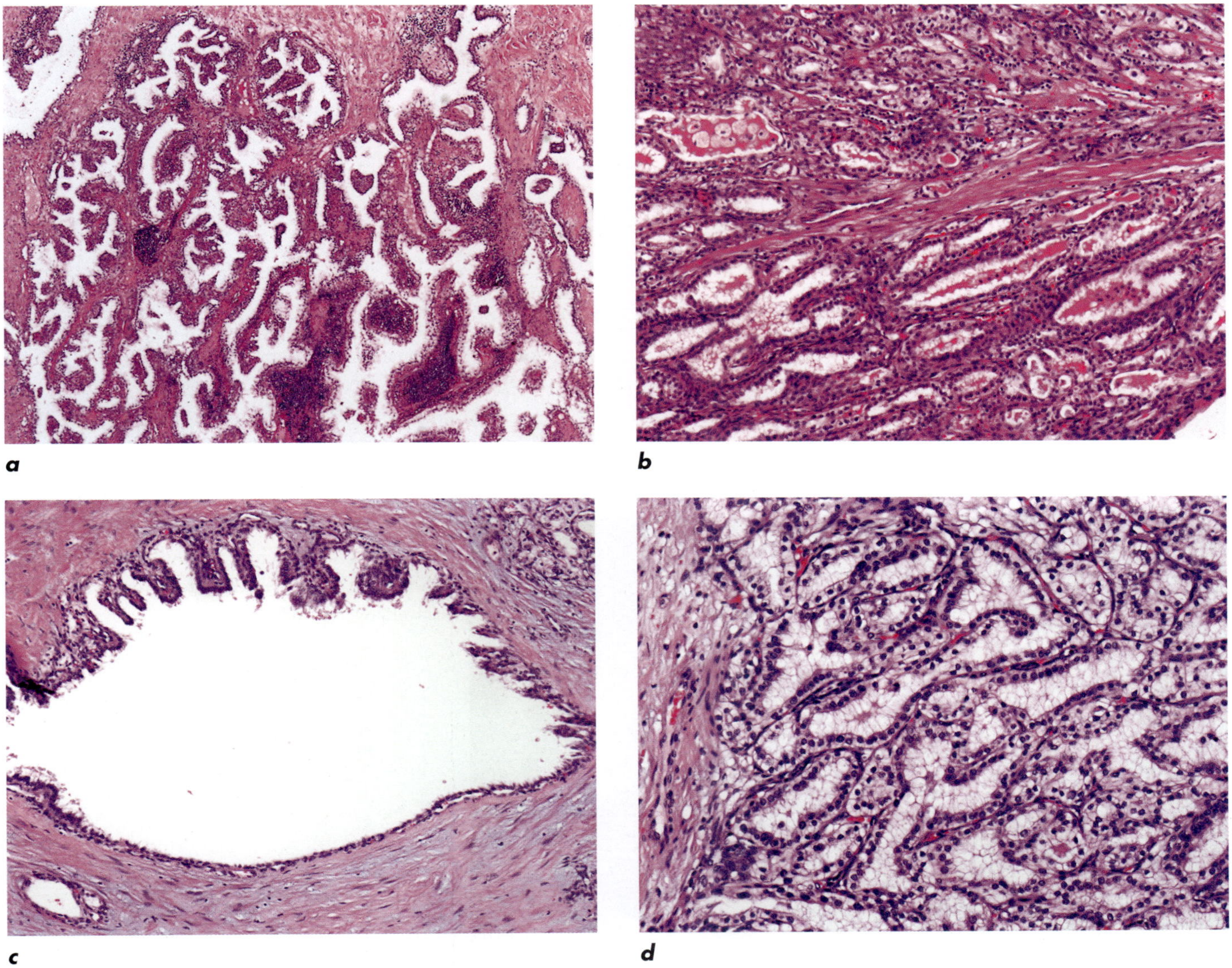

Figure 40-37.
Various patterns observed in renal angiomyomatous tumor: prostate-like pattern (*a*), tubular structures with clear cells with a "smiling shark mouth" appearance (*b*), prominent fibromuscular stroma and cystic dilated glands with intracystic projections (*c*), and tubular papillary features similar to those of clear cell papillary RCC (*d*).

Immunohistochemistry

- Similar to clear cell PRCC, with "cup-shaped" CA9 positivity (Fig. 40-35*d*)
- CK7 positive
- AMACR negative and vimentin variably positive

Molecular genetics

- Most cases lack of *VHL* gene mutations (LOH3p)
- Lack of trisomy 7 and 17

Differential diagnosis

- List of entities with pathological features that overlap with those in clear cell PRCC (Table 40-2)

Clinical relevance (prognosis and treatment options)

- Surgery with excellent prognosis
- No reported case with metastatic spread after partial or radical nephrectomy

RENAL CELL CARCINOMA WITH LEIOMYOMATOUS STROMA

Definition

- A low-grade RCC composed mostly of clear cells arranged in solid and/or papillary and tubular growth patterns with a prominent leiomyomatous stroma
- A subset of this tumor probably represents a low-grade variant of clear cell RCC

Clinical features

- Mostly an incidental finding, no specific clinical presentation
- Very rare neoplasms, with such tumors are probably underrecognized
- No reported case to date with metastatic spread
- Studies suggest an association with tuberous sclerosis complex
- One reported case associated with large angiomyolipoma

Gross pathology

- Solid, well-demarcated mass, sometimes with a thick whitish pseudocapsule
- Whitish, tan to brown cut surface with whitish septa identified. Consistency depends on amount of stroma (Fig. 40-38)
- Regressive changes and hemorrhagic foci are less often encountered than in clear cell RCC

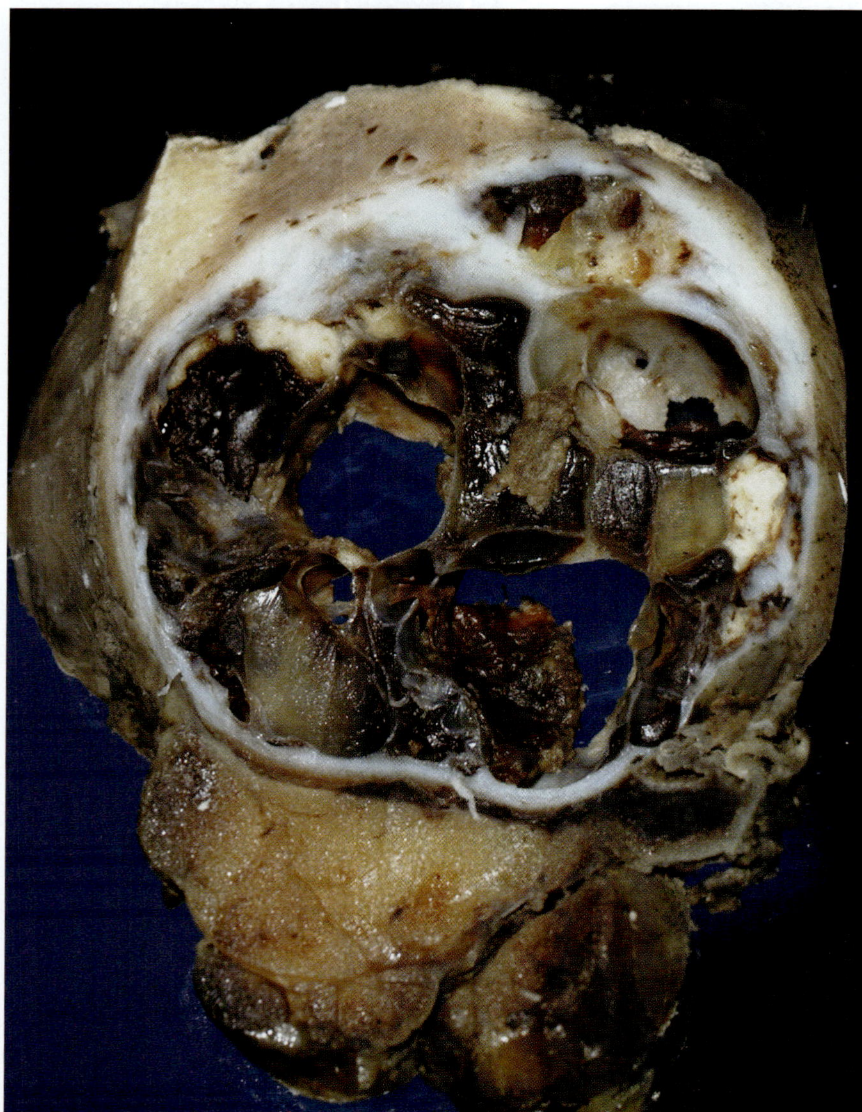

Figure 40-38.
RCC (RAT-like) with angiomyomatous stroma shows cystic spaces and white fibrous bands traversing the tumor.

Histology

- Presence of leiomyomatous stroma is characteristic, which is intermingled with the epithelial component (Fig. 40-39). Histological picture is variable with features shared by both clear cell RCC and clear cell PRCC
- Low-grade clear cells form papillae, tubules, and solid alveolar nests
- Tumor cells have voluminous clear cytoplasm with nuclei basally positioned (Fig. 40-40) similar to clear cell RCC, but different from the luminal location seen in clear cell PRCC
- Focally, clear cells forming tubules have blister-like snouts in the apical pole ("shark-smile" appearance), reminiscent of RAT
- Fine capillary network surrounding tumor cells, typical of clear cell RCC, is often seen

Immunohistochemistry

- Variable immunoprofiles
- CK7 usually positive with a minority of the cases negative
- AMACR variably positive
- Vimentin variably positive
- CD9 positivity (box-shaped) seen in most cases

Molecular genetics

- *VHL* gene mutations (3p), and methylation of *VHL* promoter variably found in some cases
- Polysomy of chromosomes 7 and/or 17 reportedly identified in other cases

Clinical relevance (prognosis and treatment options)

- This tumor may represent a histological variant of low-grade clear cell RCC
- The metastatic potential of this tumor exists, but it is low
- Surgical removal associated with a good prognosis

Figure 40-39.
Microscopically, RAT-like RCC is composed of large nests of tumor cells and prominent angiomyomatous stroma (*a*). High magnification shows the histological features of typical clear cell RCC (*b*).

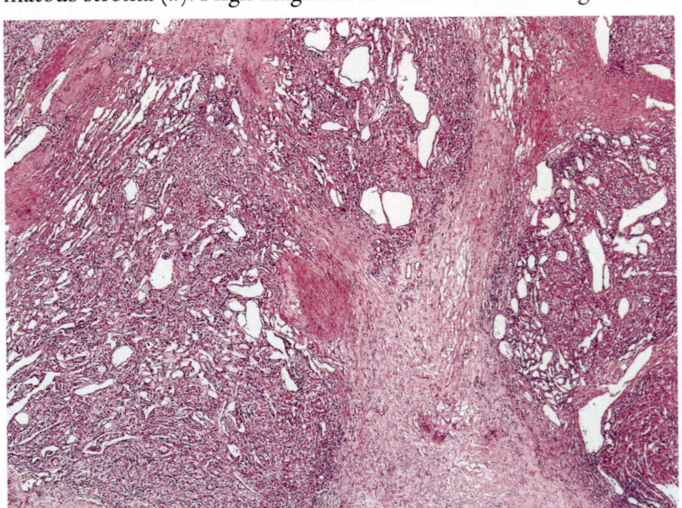

a

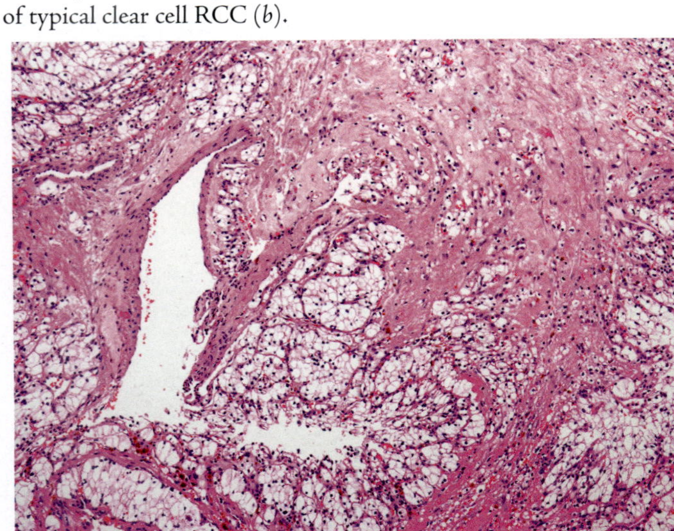

b

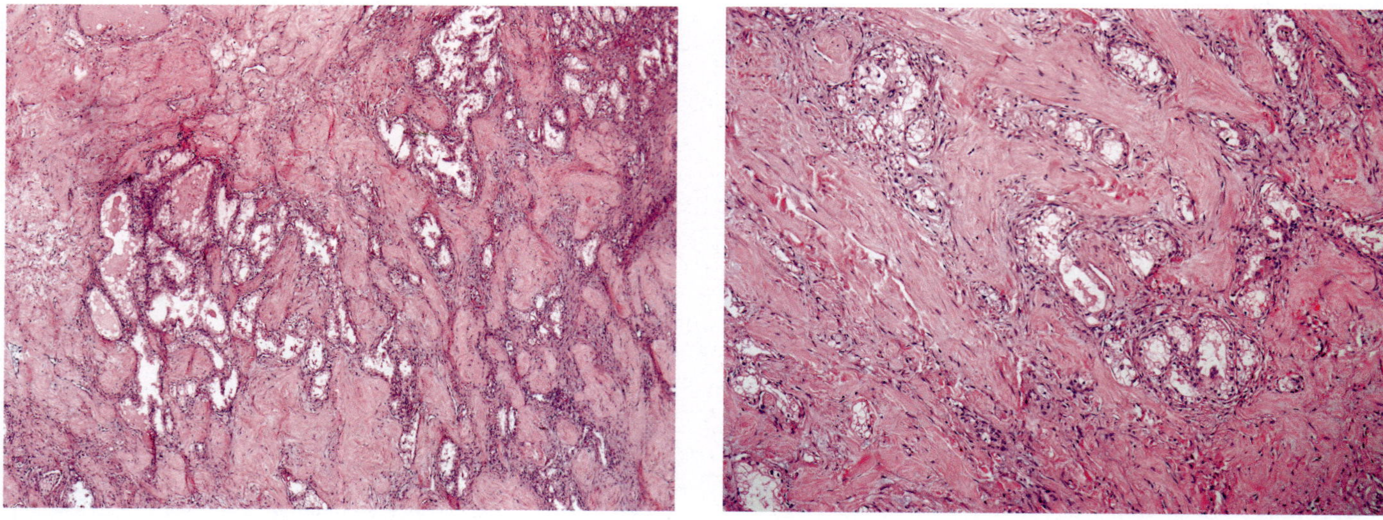

a b

Figure 40-40.
RCC with RAT-like stroma. Large nests of tumor cells with clear cytoplasm and prominent leiomyomatous stromal component are seen (*a*). High magnification shows low-grade tumor cells in a prominent fibromuscular stroma (*b*).

HYBRID ONCOCYTIC TUMOR IN BIRT-HOGG-DUBE PATIENTS

Definition

- Renal cell neoplasms developing in a patient with Birt-Hogg-Dube (BHD) syndrome and demonstrating histological features shared by both renal oncocytoma and chromophobe RCC
- Some investigators also use this term to describe any oncocytic renal cell neoplasm with characteristics of both renal oncocytoma and chromophobe RCC
- In this chapter, we are focusing only the hybrid tumors in BHD patients

Pathogenesis and epidemiology

- BHD is a rare autosomal dominant disorder with an incidence of 1:36,000 to 1:45,000
- In the initial report, hybrid oncocytic tumors accounted for approximately 50% of the renal tumors occurring in the BHD patients

Clinical features

- BHD patients can present with cutaneous lesions (such as fibrofolliculomas, trichodiscomas, and angiofibromas), kidney masses, or spontaneous pneumothorax due to ruptured pulmonary cysts
- In most cases, skins lesions are identified first
- Hybrid oncocytic tumors of the kidney in BHD patients are found mostly by radiographic imaging studies before they cause symptoms
- BHD patients may first present with renal masses, and have clinical symptoms and signs attributed to conventional RCC, including flank pain, palpable mass, and hematuria

Gross pathology

- Well-circumscribed, solid, nonencapsulated mass (Fig. 40-41*a*)
- The cut surface is pale-tan to light brown (Fig. 40-42*a*)
- Multiple renal lesions can occur

Histology

- Hybrid tumor cells grow in a diffuse pattern, similar to that of chromophobe RCC
- The tumor cells show prominent cell membranes (like chromophobe RCC) and dense eosinophilic cytoplasm (like oncocytoma) (Fig. 40-41*b*)
- In addition, hybrid tumors contain scattered epithelial cells with clear cytoplasm and nuclei with regular contours (Figs. 40-41*b* and 40-42*b*). These elements contribute to 5% to 50% of the tumor cell population (Fig. 40-43)
- The tumor cells are typically of low nuclear grade
- Ultrastructurally, hybrid tumor cells contain small membrane-bound microvesicles (like chromophobe RCC) and abundant mitochondria (like oncocytoma)

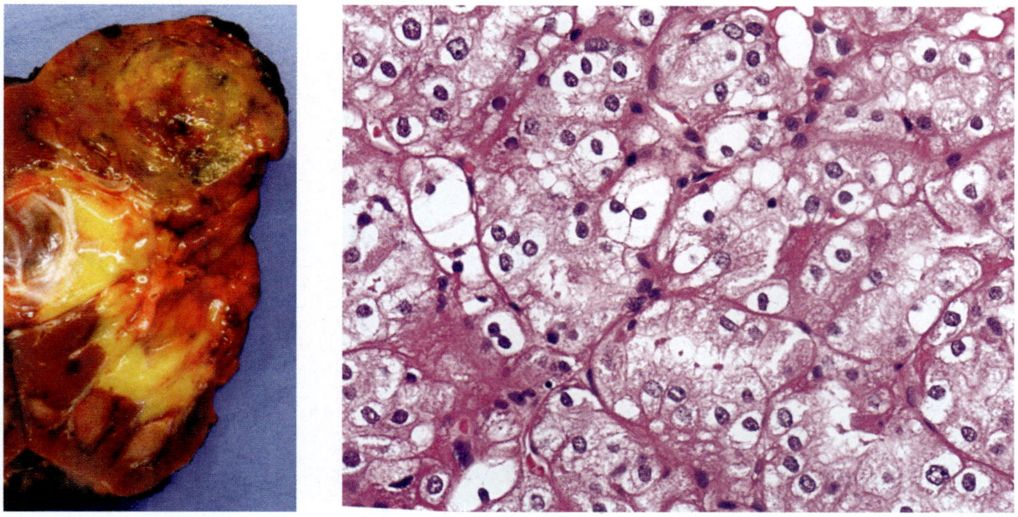

a *b*

Figure 40-41.
An oncocytic hybrid tumor of the kidney in a patient with Birt-Hogg-Dube syndrome. The mass is located in the upper pole and well circumscribed with tan-brown cut surface (*a*). Microscopically, this hybrid tumor is characterized by the presence of large polygonal tumor cells with abundant eosinophilic cytoplasm intermingled with small clusters of cells with clear cytoplasm (*b*).

Immunohistochemistry and special study

- Hybrid tumor cells are positive for C-kit (like chromophobe RCC and oncocytoma)
- Patchy CK7 positivity in hybrid tumor is characteristic (Fig. 40-42*c*) (typically oncocytoma is negative for CK7, while chromophobe RCC is positive for CK7)

Molecular diagnostics

- By molecular clustering analysis, hybrid tumors cluster between typical chromophobe RCCs and renal oncocytomas
- The most prominent molecular feature of hybrid tumors is the high level of expression of genes associated with mitochondria and oxidative phosphorylation
- Comparative genomic microarray analysis shows minimal chromosomal loss (like oncocytomas, but different from chromophobe RCCs, which usually harbors numerous chromosomal losses)

Main differential diagnosis (see Table 40-3)

Oncocytic papillary RCC

- Tumor is composed of cells with eosinophilic granular cytoplasm
- Papillary structures are subtle
- Occasional foamy macrophage can be seen
- This tumor is positive for CK7 and AMACR, but negative for C-kit

Metastatic oncocytic tumors from the thyroid

- Malignant oncocytic tumors such as Hurthle cell carcinoma of the thyroid can metastasize to the kidney
- However, as oncocytic epithelial tumors can develop in other organs in the BHD patients, especially the parotid, caution should be exercised when making a diagnosis of primary hybrid tumor without excluding tumors from elsewhere.

Oncocytoma

- When multiple oncocytic tumors are encountered in a kidney from a relative young patient, clinical evaluation, genetic testing for BHD mutation, and a complete evaluation of all renal tumors are warranted
- The presence of clusters of clear cells in an oncocytic renal tumor with shared features of oncocytoma and chromophobe RCC should raise the possibility of a hybrid oncocytic tumor in a BHD patient
- Genetic testing to confirm the diagnosis of BHD syndrome is necessary

Clinical relevance (prognosis and treatment options)

- The diagnosis of BHD will benefit clinical management of the these patients and should promote genetic testing of their direct family members because of its autosomal dominant inheritance

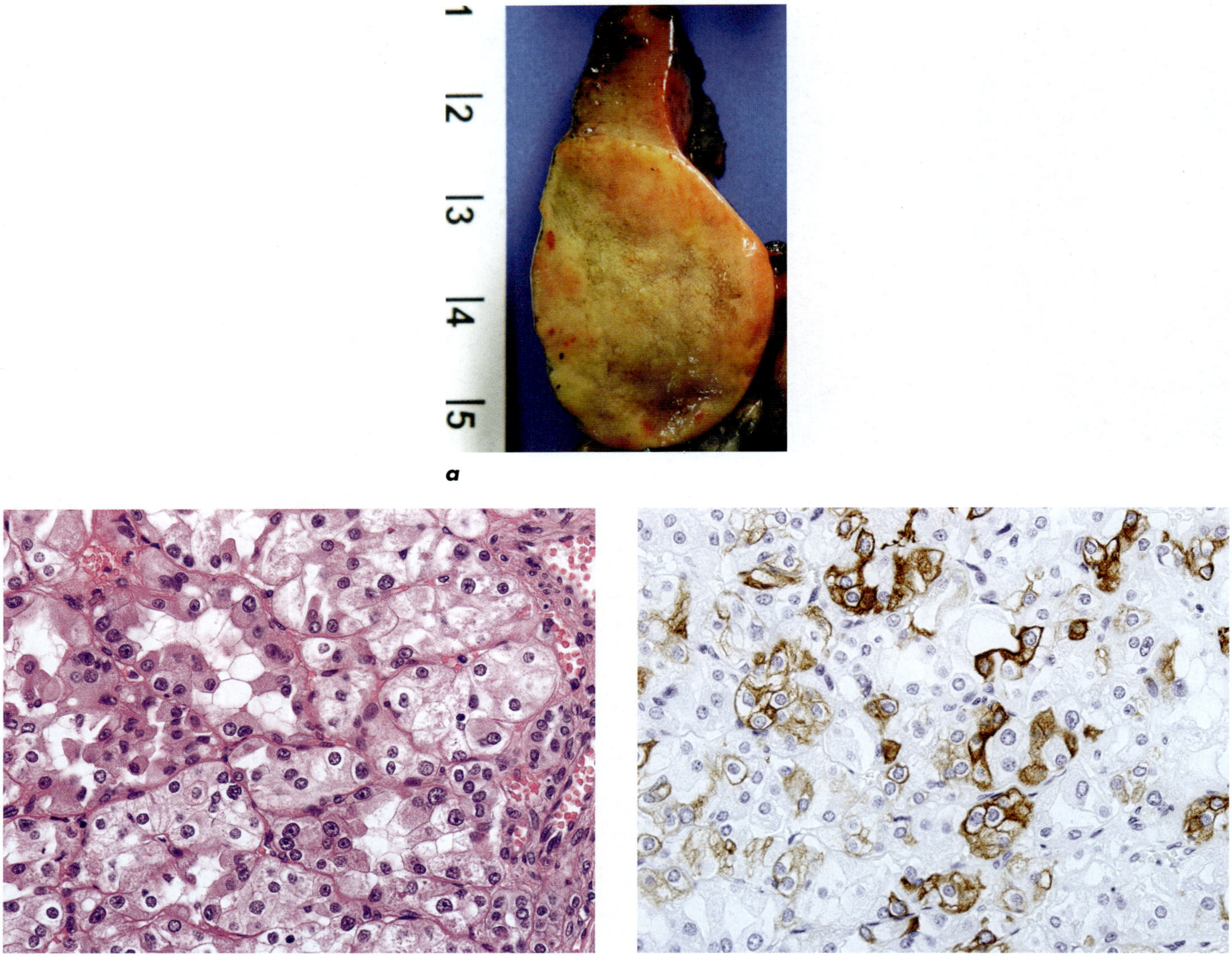

a

b

c

Figure 40-42.
Oncocytic hybrid tumor in a BHD patient appears slightly different from an oncocytoma (brown) or chromophobe (light brown) (*a*). The tumor cells share histological features with both oncocytoma and chromophobe RCC with clusters of clear cells (*b*). Focal CK7 immunoreactivity can be identified in this tumor (*c*).

- Surgical treatment is the curative for solitary hybrid tumors. However, if tumors are multiple, clinical management is challenging
- Tumors are typically slow growing and allow for multiple local resections of larger tumors and close follow-up rather than radical nephrectomy as the initial surgical intervention
- It is not known whether hybrid oncocytic tumors in BHD patients can metastasize. We have not seen a metastatic hybrid tumor in the limited number of BHD patients with hybrid tumors encountered in practice or in cases reported in the literature
- Therefore, the hybrid tumor is considered a very low-grade neoplasm
- Furthermore, some investigators speculate that almost all the renal tumors in BHD patients are hybrid tumors even when they contain a significant population of tumor cells with clear cytoplasm. Further studies are necessary to substantiate this possibility

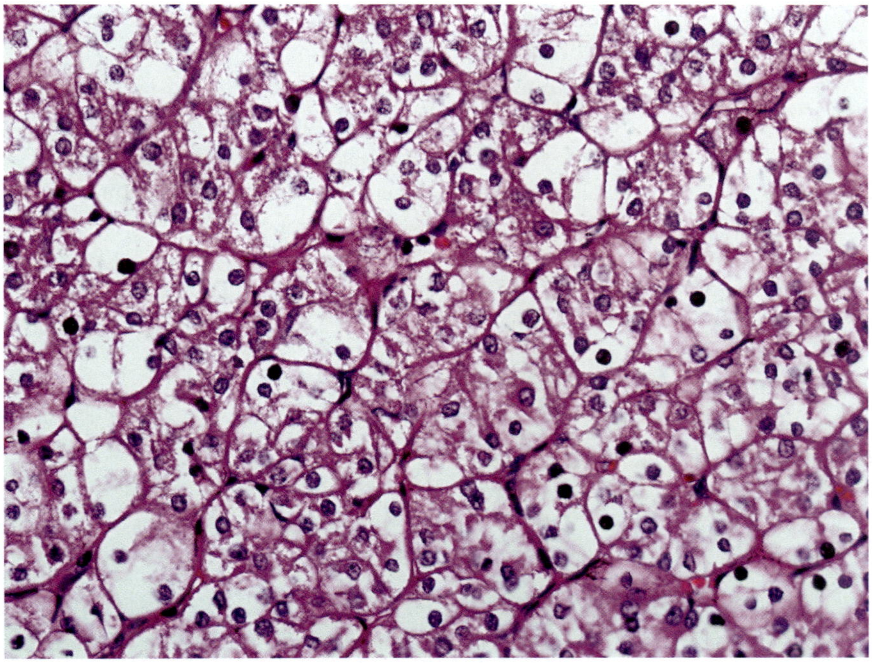

Figure 40-43.
BHD-associated hybrid tumor significant population of clear cells, which may lead to a misdiagnosis of clear cell RCC.

Table 40-3. Comparison of Oncocytic Hybrid Tumor with Oncocytoma and Chromophobe RCC

	Oncocytoma	*Oncocytic hybrid tumor in BHD syndrome*	*Chromophobe RCC*
Gross color	Brown	Yellow-tan	Light brown
Multifocality	Single or multiple	Multiple	Solitary
Cytoplasmic characteristrics	Eosinophilic	Eosinophilic and chromophobic	Chromophobic or eosinophilic
Clear cell cluster	No	Yes	No
CK7 immunoreactivity	Negative	Focally positive	Diffusely positive
Cytogenetic changes	Minimal	Minimal	Multiple chromosomal deletions
Biological behavior	Benign	Probably very low grade Multiple tumors lead to parenchymal loss	Low grade

BHD syndrome, Birt-Hogg-Dube syndrome; CK7, cytokeratin 7; RCC, renal cell carcinoma.

ACQUIRED CYSTIC DISEASE–ASSOCIATED RENAL CELL CARCINOMA

Definition

- RCC that develops in the background of acquired cystic renal disease and displays a relatively specific histological features

Pathogenesis

- Acquired cystic disease of the kidney (ACD, ACDK, or ACKD)–associated RCC is found exclusively in an end-stage kidney disease background
- It is believed to be the most common type of RCC in end-stage kidneys

Clinical features

- ACD-associated RCC frequently occurs in patients receiving hemodialysis of more than 10 years
- The incidence increases with the duration of the hemodialysis
- Majority of the cases are discovered incidentally during routine follow-up of patients on dialysis

Gross pathology

- The background of multiple cysts in an atrophic kidney
- ACD-associated RCC can be solitary or multiple, unilateral or bilateral
- The masses are well circumscribed with tan to brown or gray cut surfaces (Fig. 40-44*a*)
- Necrosis, hemorrhage, and calcification are occasionally present

Histology

- The background ACD kidney demonstrates numerous cysts displacing most of the renal tissue. The cystic lining is flat epithelium with eosinophilic cytoplasm (Fig. 40-45)
- The architecture of the tumor is variable, including cribriform, solid, solid-alveolar, microcystic, or even macrocystic growth patterns (Figs. 40-44 and 40-46)
- Two most common histological patterns are papillary (Figs. 40-47 and 40-48) and tubulocystic (Fig. 40-49)
- Tumors cells are large with eosinophilic granular or oncocytic cytoplasm with large nuclei and prominent nucleoli (Figs. 40-44 and 40-47). Small foci with clear cell morphology may occur (Fig. 40-44*e*)
- Intracytoplasmic lumina are frequently present and impart a sieve-like or cribriform architecture. Other patterns such as spindle cells or signet-ring cells have been observed (Fig. 40-50)
- Intratumoral oxalate crystals are believed to be specific for ACD-associated carcinoma, but these crystals can also be seen in the benign cystically dilated tubules in ACD (Fig. 40-46). The crystals can be abundant in some cases, but only scattered in others
- Rarely, sarcomatoid transformation differentiation has been reported in ACR-associated RCC

Immunohistochemistry

- Neoplastic cells are positive for AMACR
- Positivity for CD10, CD57, and vinculin
- Mostly negative for CK7 and high molecular weight cytokeratin

Molecular genetics

- ACD-associated RCC usually lacks trisomy of chromosomes 7 and 17. However, gains in these chromosomes have been observed
- Gains of chromosomes 1, 2, 3, 6, 10, and Y were also reported
- Numerical abnormalities of chromosomes 3 and 16, irrespective of gain or loss, were also reported

Differential diagnosis

Papillary RCC

- PRCC usually lacks oxalate crystals or intracytoplasmic lumina
- PRCC often show nuclear grooving, which is absent in ACD-associated RCC
- Foamy macrophages seen in PRCC are uncommon in ACD-associated RCC
- Immunohistochemical profiles of PRCC and ACD-associated RCC are similar, which raises the possibility that some of ACD-associated RCCs may be related to PRCC

Clear cell papillary RCC

- Composed of low-grade tumor cells, arranged in papillary, or stellate-shaped tubular profiles
- All tubular structures are rimmed by fine capillary network
- Tumor cells are positive for CK7 and CA9, but negative for AMACR
- Clear cell PRCC usually lacks oxalate crystals except when this tumor develops in the setting of end-stage kidney disease

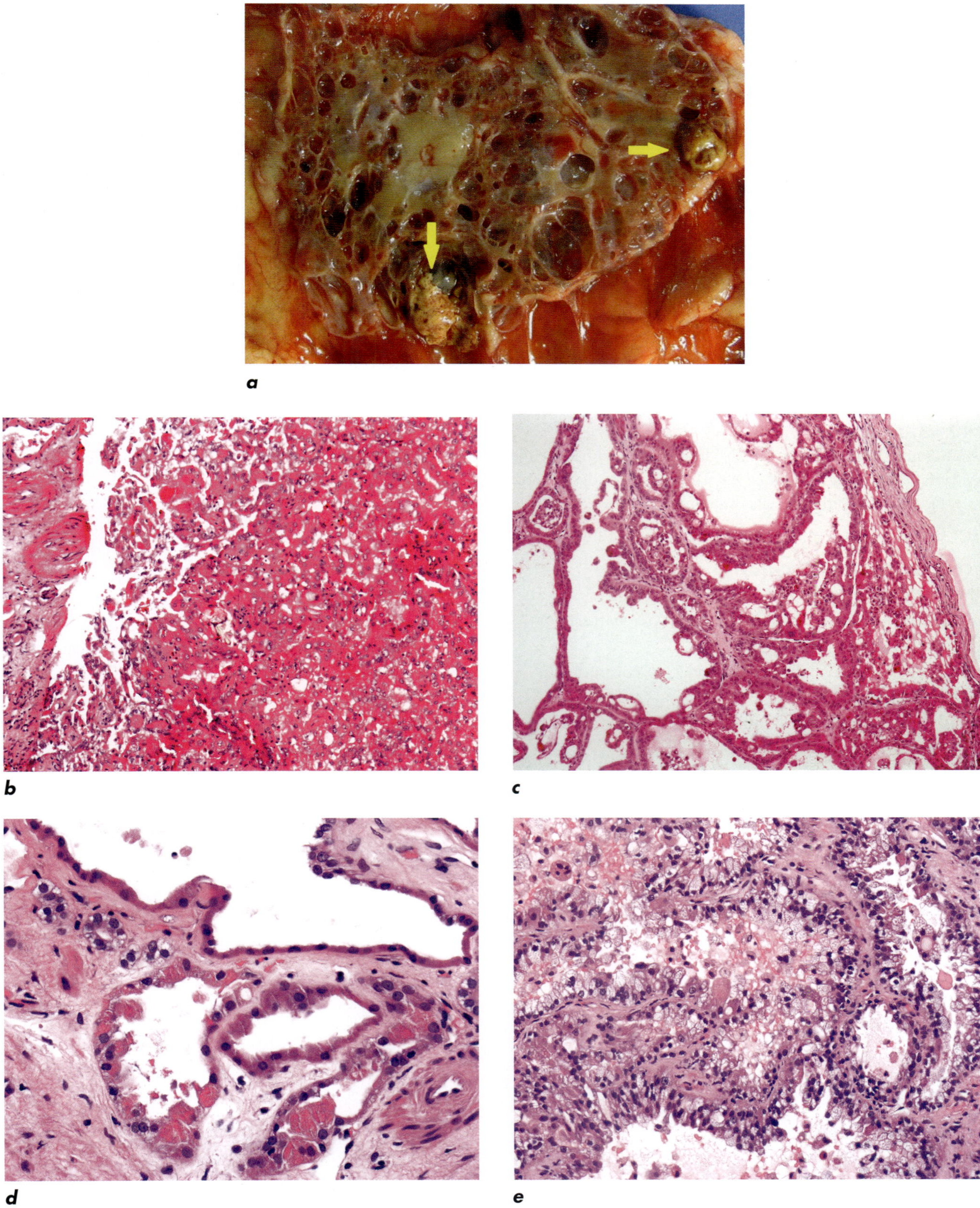

Figure 40-44.
Acquired cystic disease (ACD)–associated RCC includes two masses (*a*, arrows) in the background of an acquired cystic kidney disease. The common architectural patterns of ACD-associated RCC shown here are papillary (*b*), tubular with cribriform nests (*c*), and tubulocystic (*d*). The tumor cells are characterized by the bright eosinophilic or clear cytoplasm (*e*).

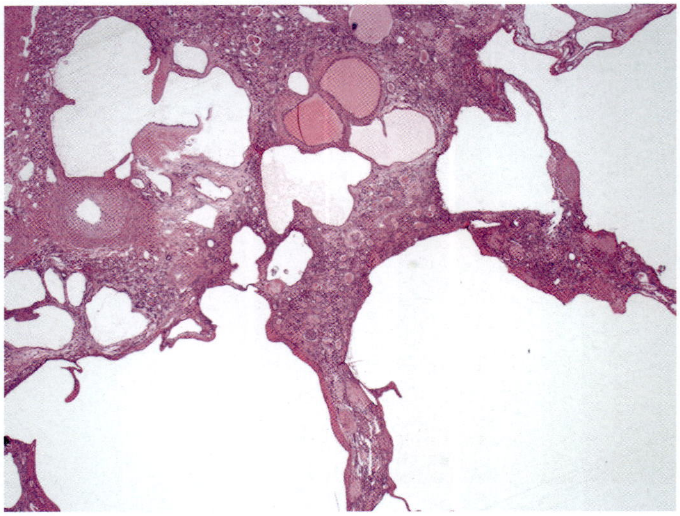

a

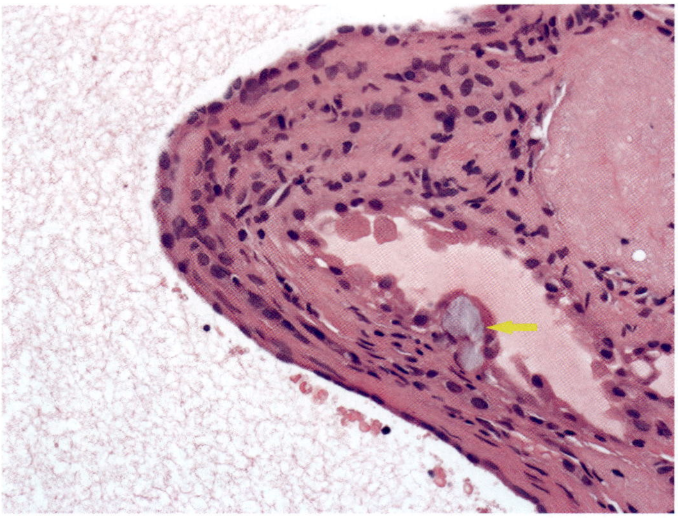

b

Figure 40-45.
Background acquired cystic disease (ACD) from the same specimen in Fig. 40-44 containing numerous cysts throughout the kidney (*a*). The cysts and adjacent atrophic renal tubules are lined by flat or cuboidal epithelial cells containing calcium oxalate crystals (*b*).

Clear cell renal cell carcinoma with granular cytoplasm

- Lack of typical cribriform/sieve-like growth pattern of ACD-associated RCC
- Intratumoral oxalate crystals are very uncommon in conventional clear cell RCC
- Up to 60% of the cases have mutation in *VHL* gene and vast majority demonstrates LOH of 3p

Clinical relevance (prognosis and treatment options)

- Treatment of choice is surgical resection
- Most tumors are low grade, low stage, nonaggressive with good prognosis
- A small subset of large tumors may exhibit aggressive clinical behavior
- Sarcomatoid differentiation is also documented in the literature

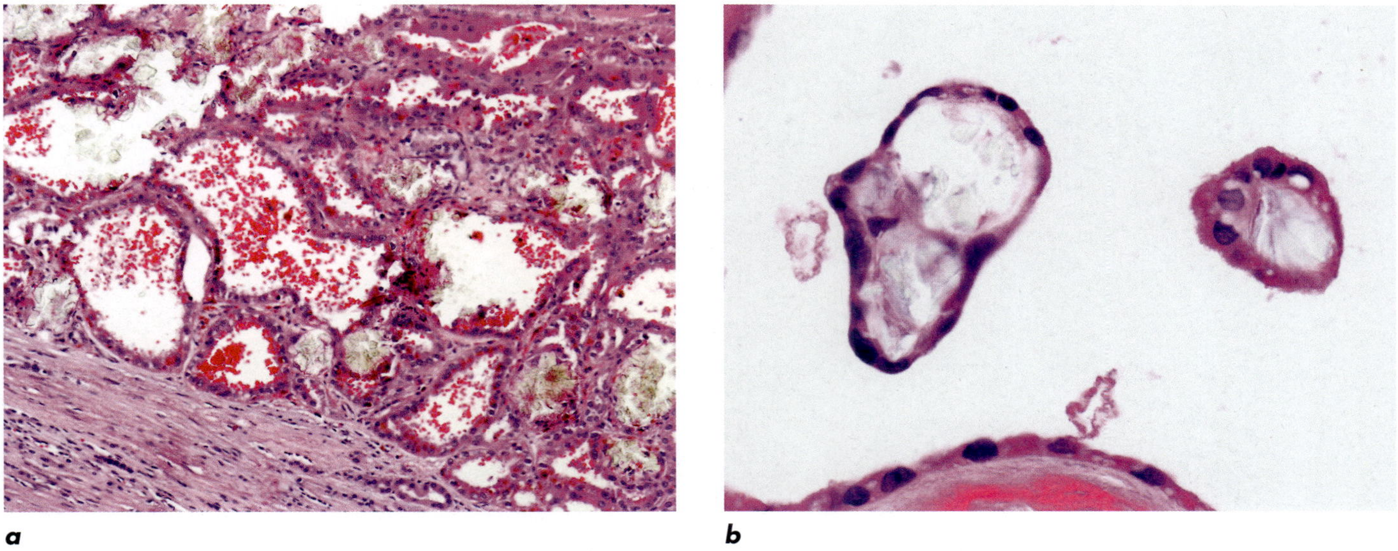

Figure 40-46.
Calcium oxalate crystals within RCC associated with ACD (*a*) and in benign cyst in ACD (*b*).

Figure 40-47.
ACD-associated RCC with well-developed papillary structures (*a*) and cribriform nests (*b*).

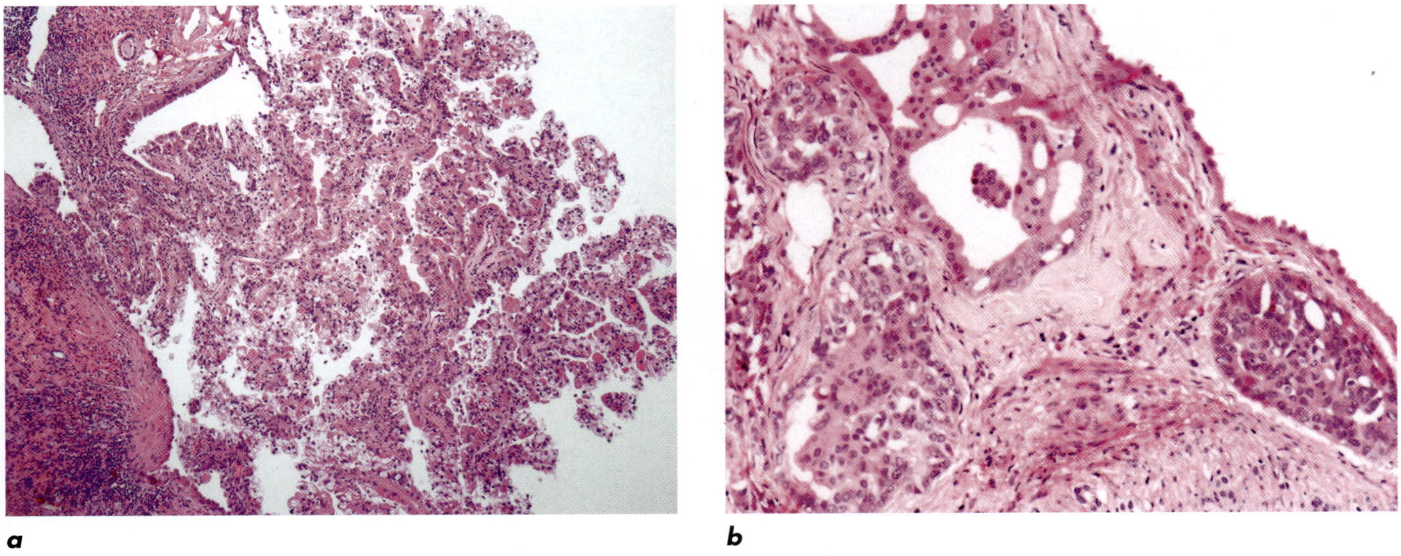

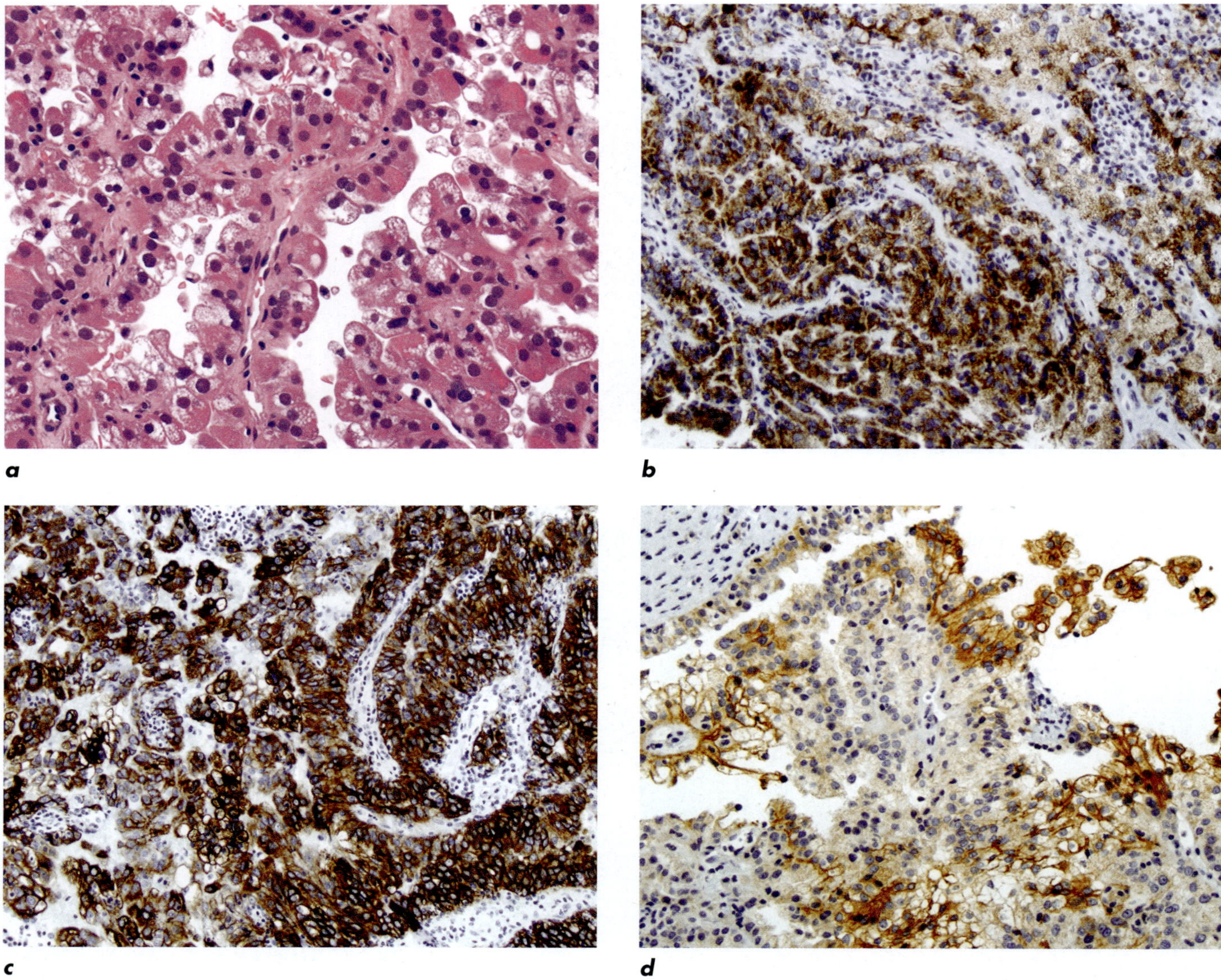

Figure 40-48.
ACD-associated RCC with papillary structures (*a*) is composed of tumor cells positive for AMACR (*b*), CK7 (*c*), and focally positive for CA9 (*d*).

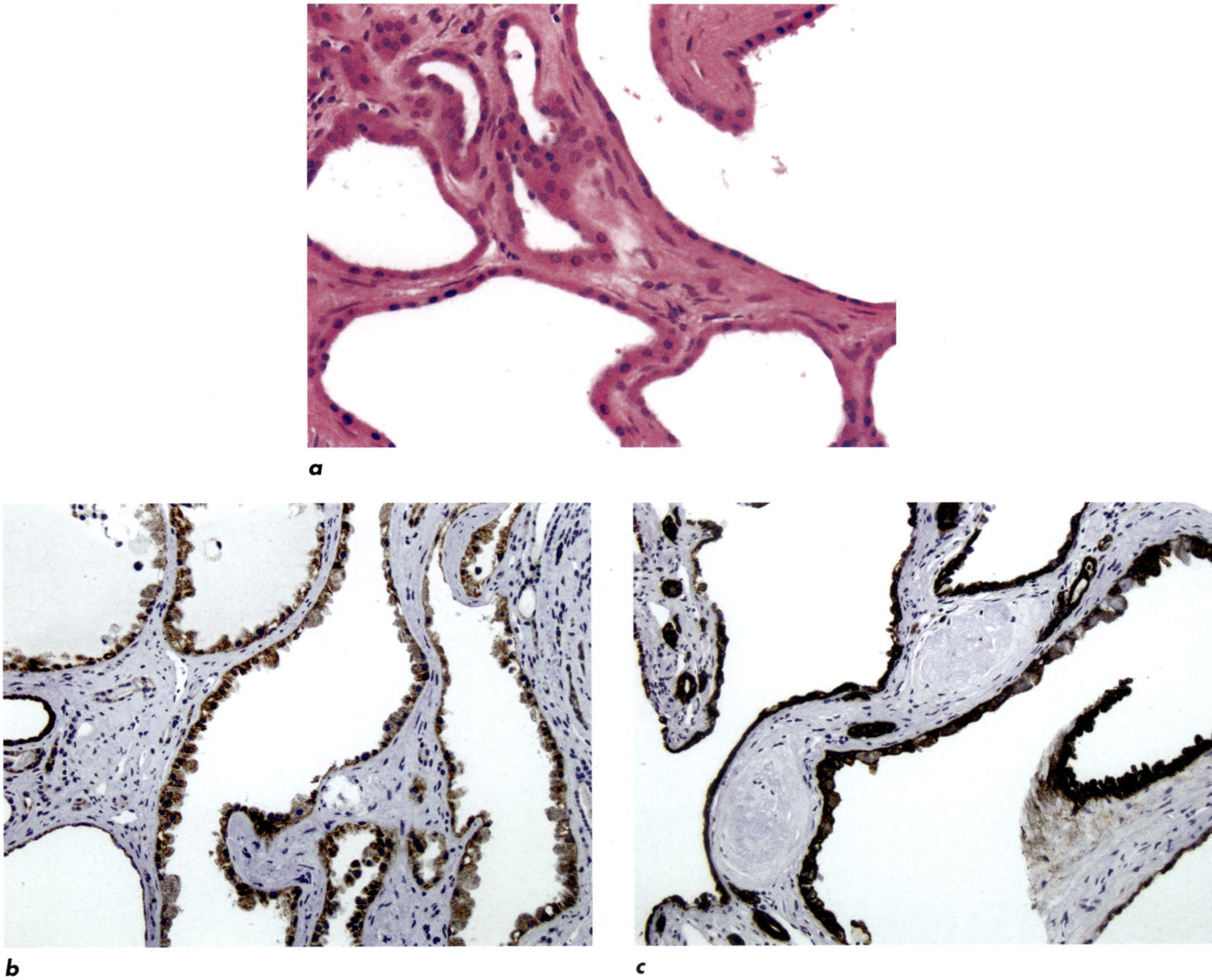

Figure 40-49.
ACD-associated RCC with tubulocystic pattern (*a*), reminiscent of tubulocystic carcinoma, is composed of tumor cells positive for AMACR (*b*) and CK7 (*c*).

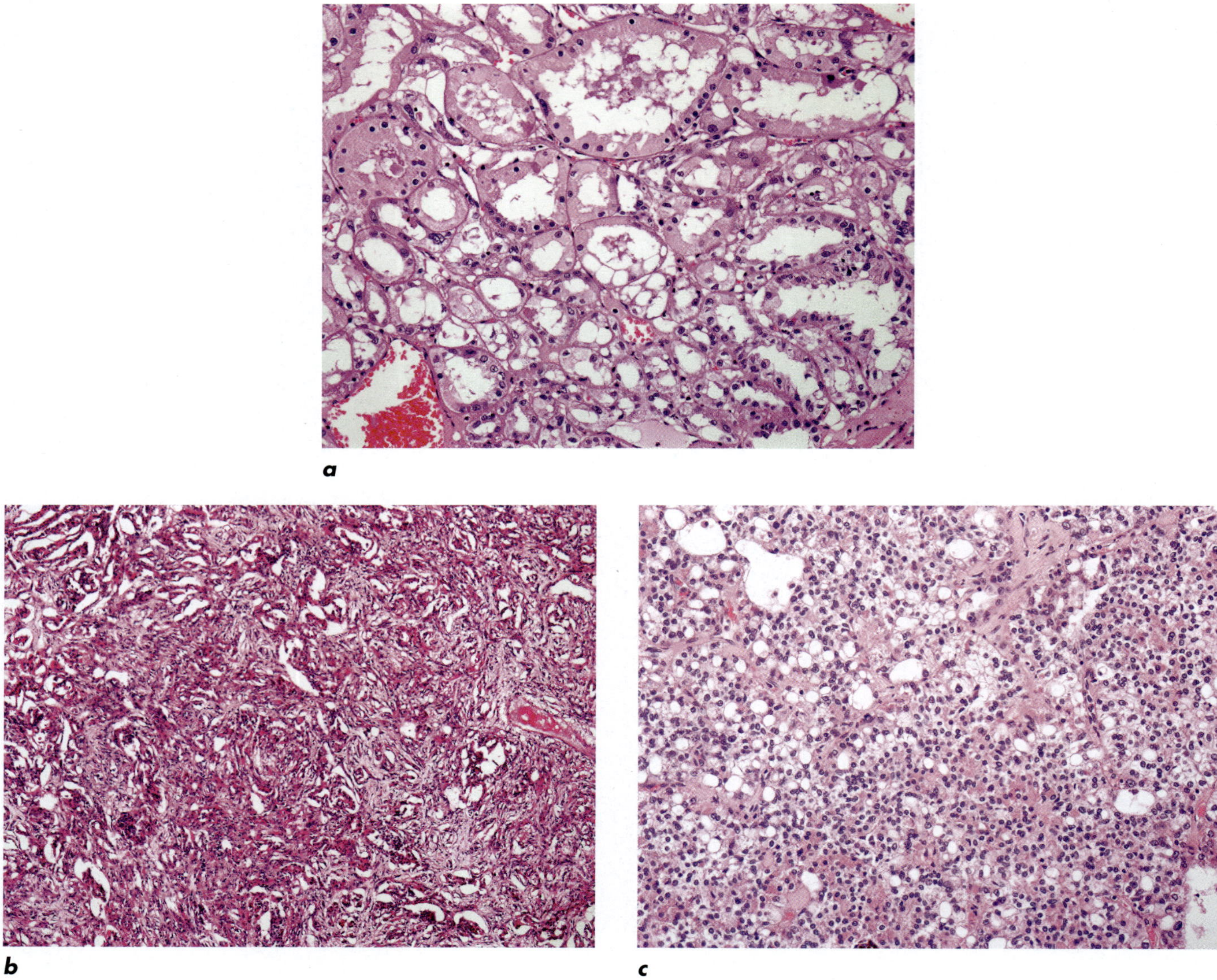

Figure 40-50.
ACD-associated RCC with less common architectural patterns, including oncocytic tubules (*a*), tubular cells with spindle cell appearance (*b*), and tumor cells with intracellular lumens resembling signet ring cells (*c*).

THYROID-LIKE FOLLICULAR CARCINOMA

Definition

- RCC with prominent proteinous fluid present within glandular structures resembling thyroid glands

Clinical features

- Thyroid-like follicular carcinoma of the kidney is very rare variant of epithelial neoplasm with less than 15 cases reported
- Patient's age range is 29 to 83 years
- This tumor arises more frequently in females (F:M = 8:5)
- Majority of the cases are discovered incidentally. Less commonly, it may be present with abdominal or flank pain, weight loss, or gross hematuria

Gross pathology

- Thyroid-like follicular carcinomas are well circumscribed, typically nonencapsulated masses with tan to brown spongy cut surface
- Majority of the cases are located in the cortex of the kidney

Histology

- The tumor consists of variably sized tubular structures resembling *thyroidization* in the end-stage renal disease (Figs. 40-51 and 40-52)
- Small to large tubular structures are filled with colloid-like material as seen in end-stage kidney, and reminiscent of thyroid follicles (Figs. 40-52 and 40-53)
- Solid areas can be present
- Cuboidal and low columnar tumor cells lining the tubules have eosinophilic to amphophilic cytoplasm (Fig. 40-53)
- Occasionally, flat tumor cells comprise a substantial portion of the tumor
- Characteristic nuclear features of papillary thyroid carcinoma such as "orphan Annie eyes," and nuclear grooves are absent
- No bona fide papillary structures, clear cell areas, or spindle cell areas have been reported
- When clear cell and thyroid-like components coexist, the diagnosis of clear cell RCC should be considered (Fig. 40-54)
- Prominent lymphoid infiltrate can be present

Immunohistochemistry

- Due to the paucity of reported cases, immunohistochemical results are not consistent
- CK7 and vimentin variably positive. Keratin AE1/AE3 positive, EMA positive
- E-cadherin positive
- AMACR, thyroglobulin, TTF1, HBME-1, CD10 negative

Molecular genetics

- Very limited studies reported chromosomal gains of 7q36, 8q24, 12, 16, 17p11-q11, 17q24, 19q, 20q13, 21q22.3, and Xp and losses of 1p36, 3, and 9q21-33

Figure 40-51.
Thyroid-like RCC is composed of dilated neoplastic tubules containing colloid-like material (*a*), resembling thyroidization of tubules in an end-stage kidney or glands with colloid-like material (*b*).

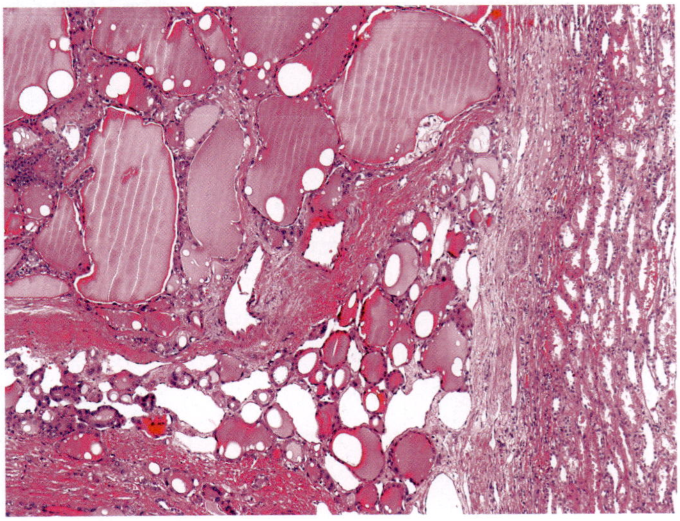

a

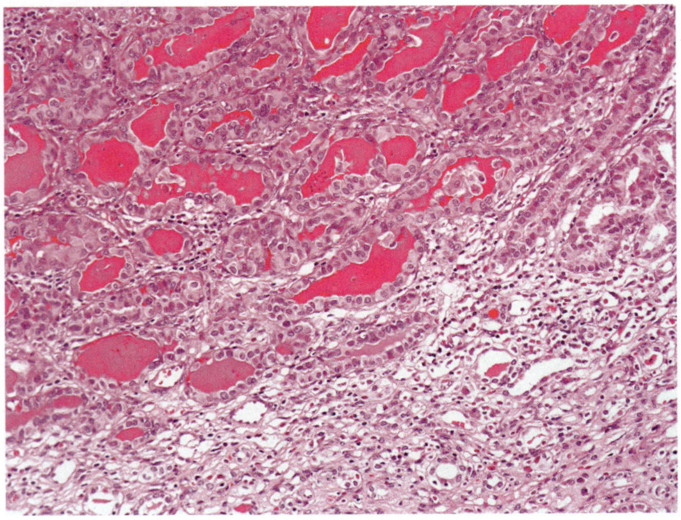

b

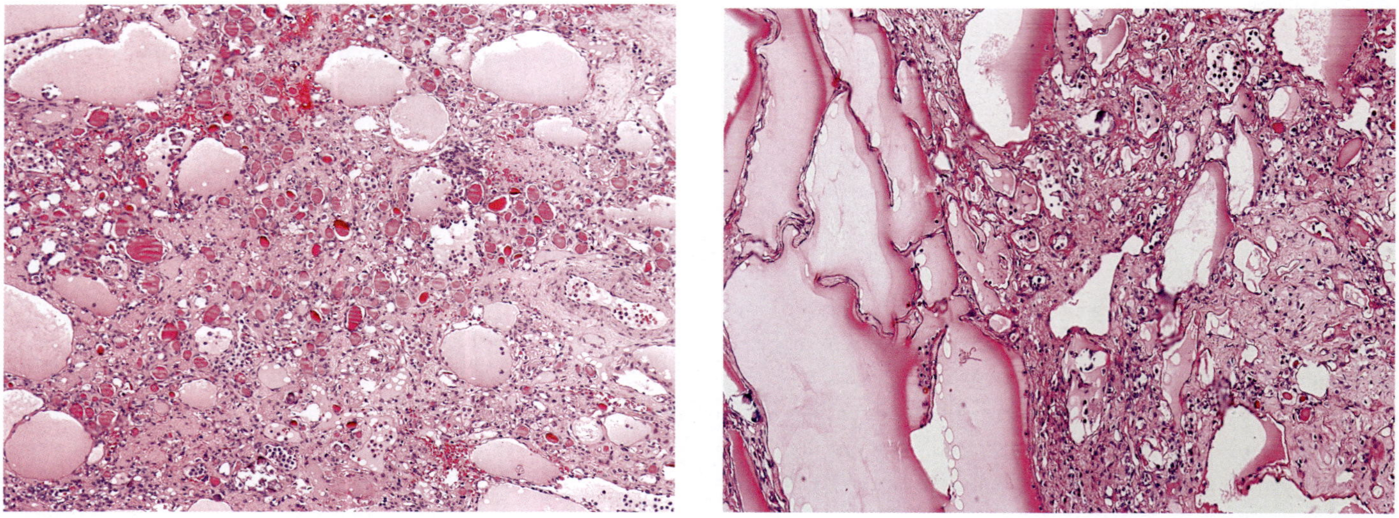

a b

Figure 40-52.
Thyroid-like RCC with atrophic glands resembling dilated renal tubules in end-stage kidney disease (*a*). Tumor cells lining the thyroid-like glandular structures (*b*).

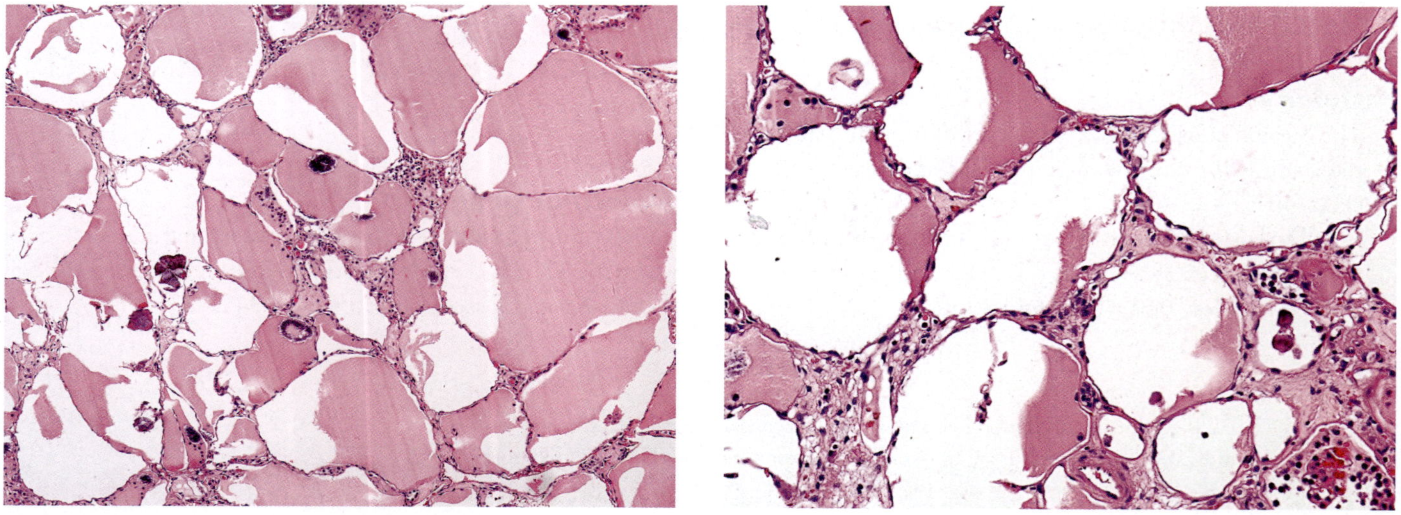

a b

Figure 40-53.
Thyroid-like RCC is composed of dilated tubules filled with colloid-like fluids (*a*). Tumor cells lining the dilated tubular structures are flat or cuboidal (*b*).

Main differential diagnosis

Metastatic thyroid carcinoma

- Typical papillary thyroid carcinoma exhibits nuclear grooving and chromatin clearing (Fig. 40-55)
- Negative immunohistochemical stains with thyroid markers such as TTF1, thyroglobulin, and CD56 are helpful in excluding thyroid carcinoma
- Follicular thyroid carcinoma more commonly metastasizes to visceral organs due to hematogenous spread

Thyroidization in end-stage kidney disease

- Usually this process is not a well-circumscribed mass
- Sclerotic glomeruli are admixed with clusters of dilated tubules filled with eosinophilic casts

Renal teratoma with thyroid glands

- Extremely rare
- Can be primary or secondary
- Careful examination looking for other teratomatous components is necessary

Clinical relevance (prognosis and treatment options)

- Treatment of choice is surgical resection
- Most cases are low grade with a good prognosis
- Metastasis is infrequent, but three cases with lymph node metastases and distant metastases to lung have been reported

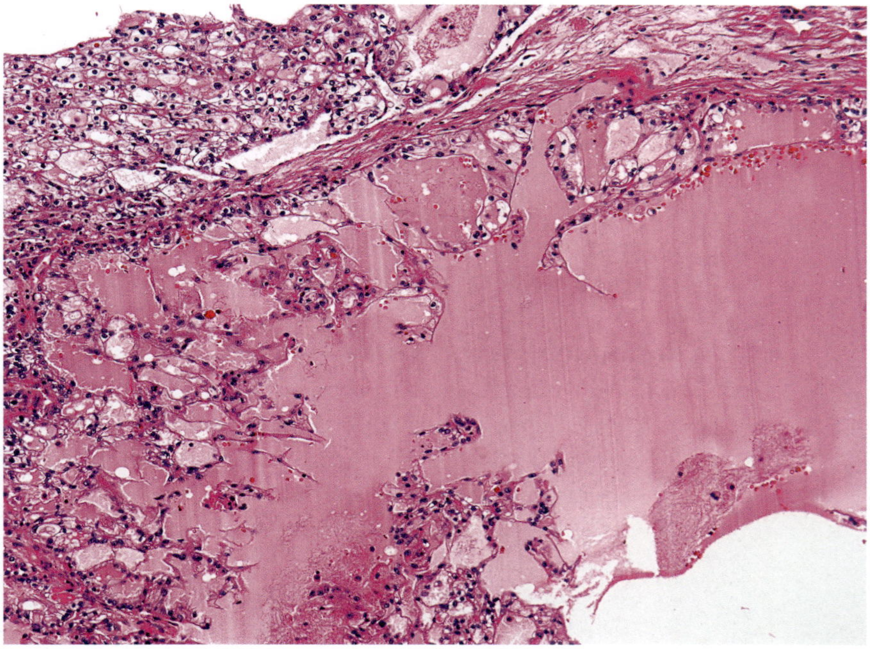

Figure 40-54.
This tumor features both a thyroid-like component and a clear cell RCC element; such a tumor should be diagnosed as clear cell RCC.

Figure 40-55.
Papillary carcinoma of the thyroid metastatic to the kidney, mimicking thyroid-like RCC or papillary RCC (*a*). Metastatic papillary carcinoma of the thyroid in the kidney composed of distinct papillary structures (*b*).

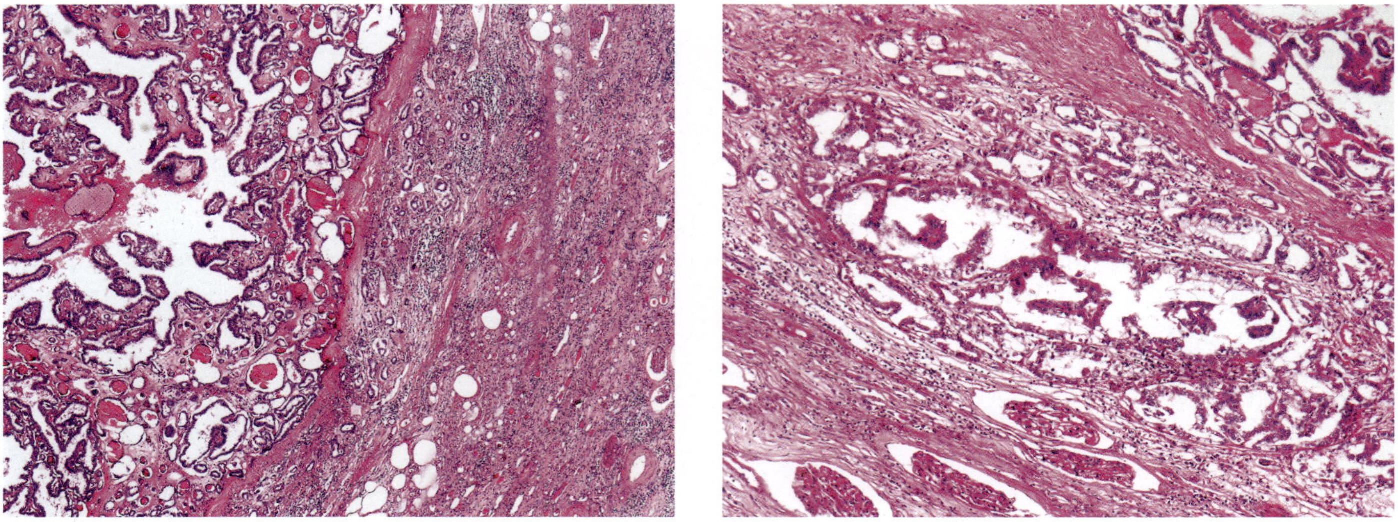

a **b**

RENAL CELL CARCINOMA ASSOCIATED WITH XP11.2 TRANSLOCATION AND *TFE3*-GENE FUSION

Definition

- Distinct subtype of RCC defined by chromosomal translocations involving a breakpoint at Xp11.2 and resulting in *TFE3* fusion genes

Other terms

- *MiTF/TFE* family translocation carcinoma
- Xp11.2 translocation renal cell carcinoma

Pathogenesis

- Translocations of *TFE3* gene on Xp11.2 with several other partner genes
    - *ASPL-TFE3*, t(X;17) (p11.2; q25)
    - *PRCC-TFE3*, t(X; 1)(p11.2; q21)
    - *PSF-TFE3*, t(X; 1)(p11.2; q34)
    - *NonO-TFE3*, inv(X)(p11.2; q12)
    - *CLTC-TFE3*, t(X; 17)(p11.2; q23)
    - In addition, three novel translocations have been reported, but the fusion gene partners have not be well defined: (1) t(X;10)(p11;q23), (2) t(X;3)(p11;q23), and (3) t(X;19)(p11;q13)

Clinical features

- Initially reported in children
- An increasing number of cases have been documented in adults, especially in young adults
- A subset of patients with prior exposure to chemotherapy

Gross pathology

- The tumor is solid and well circumscribed, consisting of a single or multiple interconnected nodules (Fig. 40-56)
- Tan-yellow, fleshy, or white cut surface. Foci of necrosis, hemorrhage, or cystic degenerative changes are occasionally identified (Figs. 40-56 and 40-57)
- Although the tumor does not have specific gross characteristics, its cut surface is significantly different from the bright yellow appearance indicative of clear cell RCC

Histology

- Typically papillary, solid nested, or tubular growth patterns are observed (Figs. 40-56*c* and 40-57*b*)
- Large tumor cells with abundant clear or eosinophilic cytoplasm and distinct borders (Figs. 40-56*d* and 40-57*c*)
- Psammoma bodies (Fig. 40-56*c*) or melanin pigment may be seen in some cases
- IHC or FISH analysis is necessary for confirmation, especially in a metastatic tumor suspicious from translocation carcinoma of the kidney (Fig. 40-58)

Immunohistochemistry

- TFE3 immunostaining shows strong nuclear positivity (Figs. 40-56*e* and 40-57*f*). Weak nuclear or cytoplasmic staining is considered negative staining. No background staining in renal tubules is expected
- Cathepsin K is another sensitive and specific marker of these neoplasms
- Only 50% of cases are positive for epithelial markers such as AE1/AE3, and the staining is typically weak. PAX8 can be completely negative
- Melanocytic markers occasionally positive. Such tumors are best classified as *TFE3* translocation carcinoma with melanocytic differentiation. CA9 (for clear cell RCC) and AMACR (for PRCC) should be negative (Figs. 40-56 and 40-58)

Molecular analysis

- Break-point FISH analysis can be used to identify the TFE3 translations

Clinical relevance (prognosis and treatment options)

- Aggressive in the majority of cases in adults and children with metastases
- Based on some reports, children without metastasis have a favorable course
- No effective chemotherapy has been established

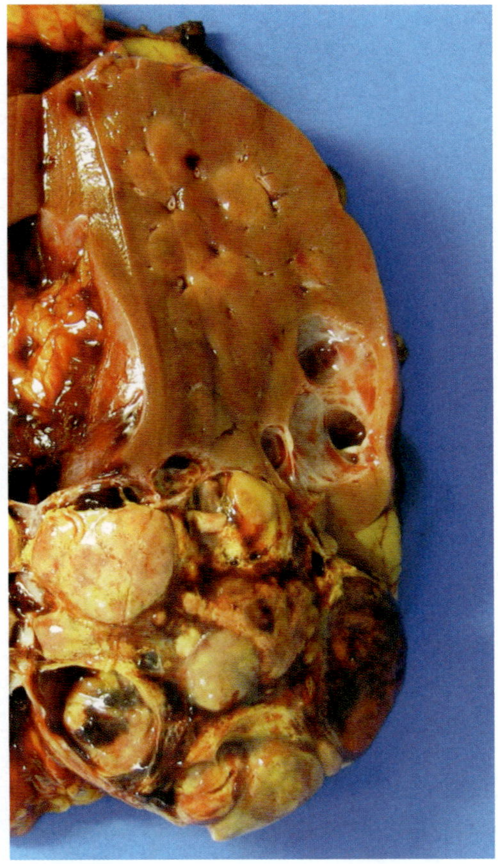

a

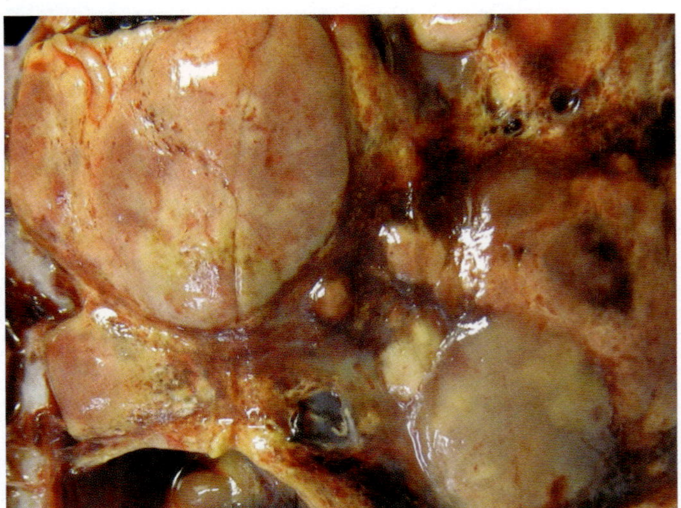

b

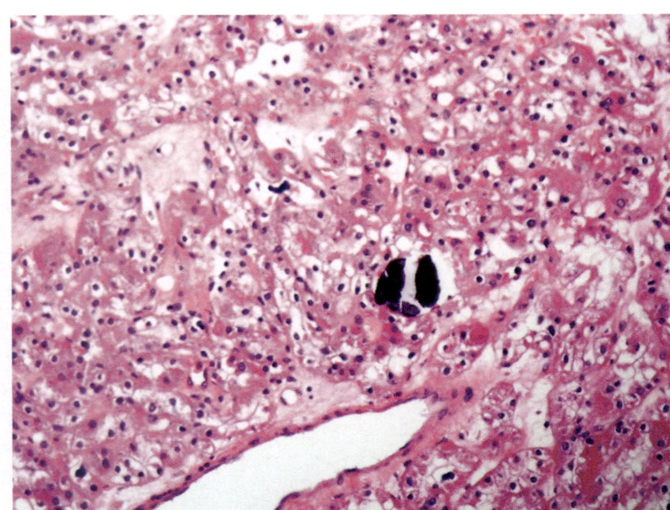

c

Figure 40-56.
A large TFE3 translocation carcinoma consisting of multiple yellow, tan, and fleshy nodules (*a*). Close-up shows the pink nodules with yellow puncta (*b*). Microscopically, the tumor is composed of clear cells in papillary configurations with occasional microcalcifications (*c*). High magnification shows large tumor cells with abundant clear cytoplasm (*d*). By immunohistochemistry, the tumor cells are positive for TFE3 (*e*, nuclear staining), but negative for AMACR (*f*) and CA9 (*g*).

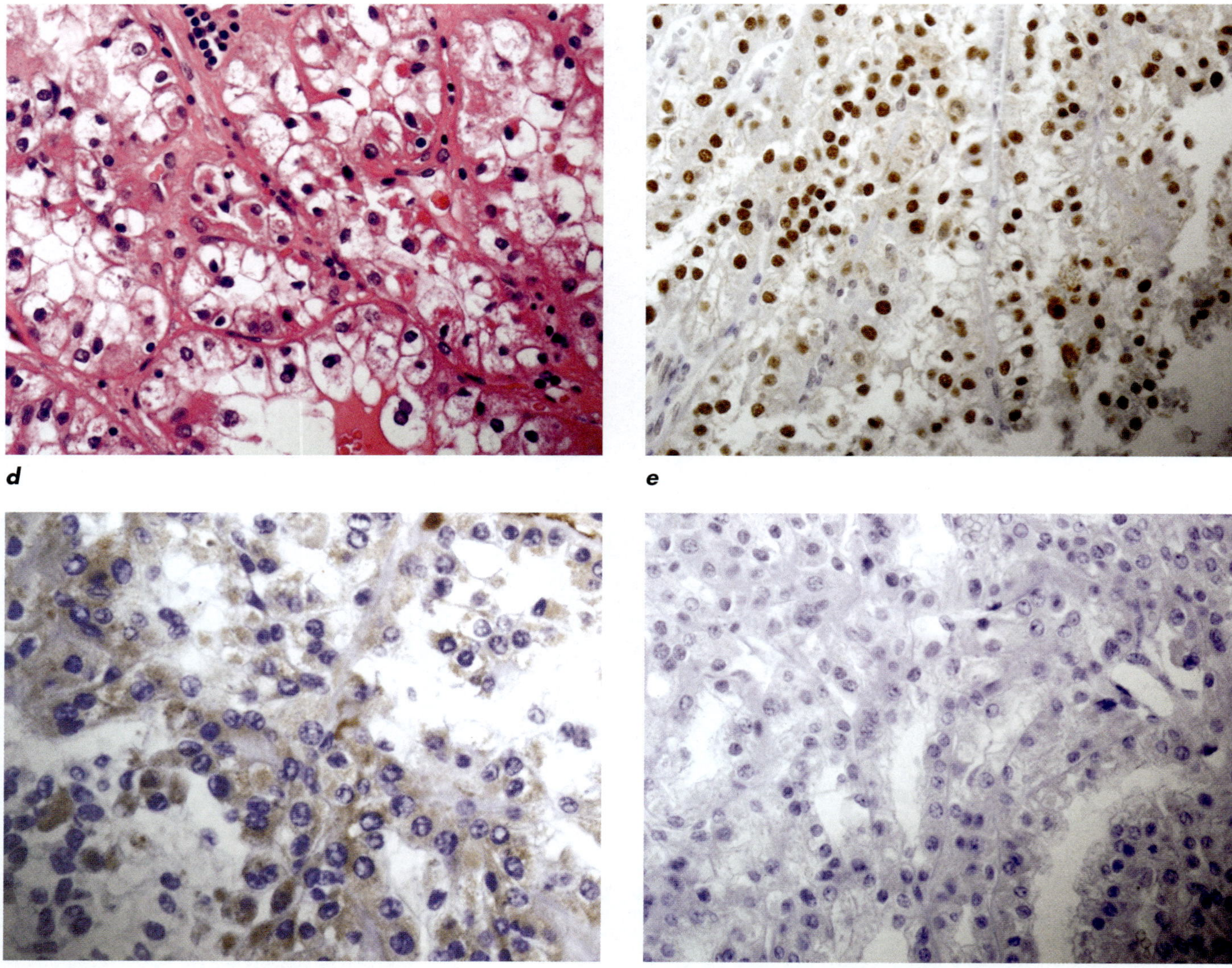

d e f g

Figure 40-56.
(Continued)

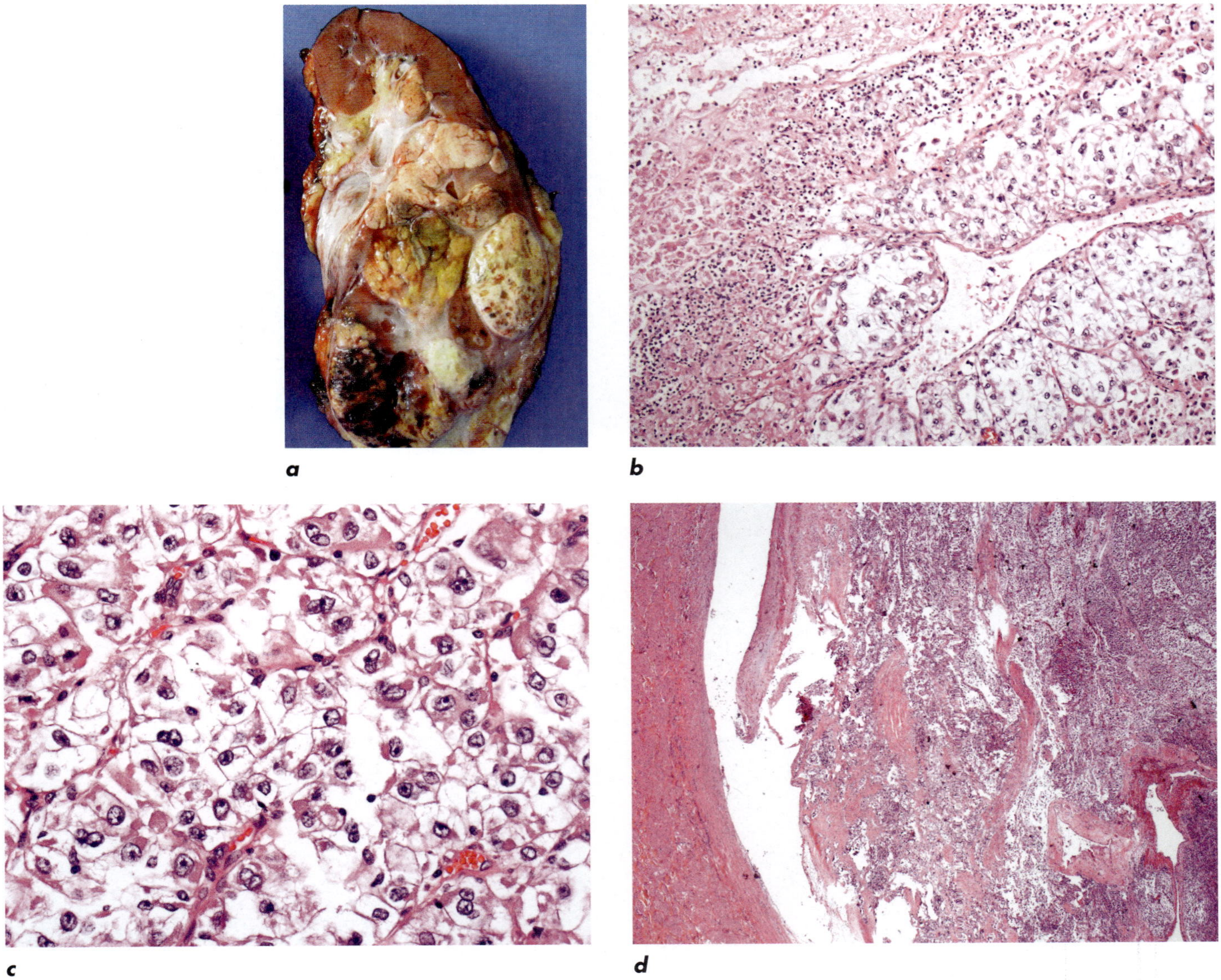

Figure 40-57.
TFE3 translocation carcinoma composed of multiple yellow-tan nodules exhibiting focal hemorrhage and necrosis (*a*). Tumor cells form large nests associated with necrosis (*b*). High magnification shows tumor cells with clear cytoplasm, a high N/C ratio, and marked cytological atypia (*c*). Tumor cells invade the renal vein (*d*) and perinephric fat (*e*) and demonstrate the characteristic TFE3 nuclear staining (*f*).

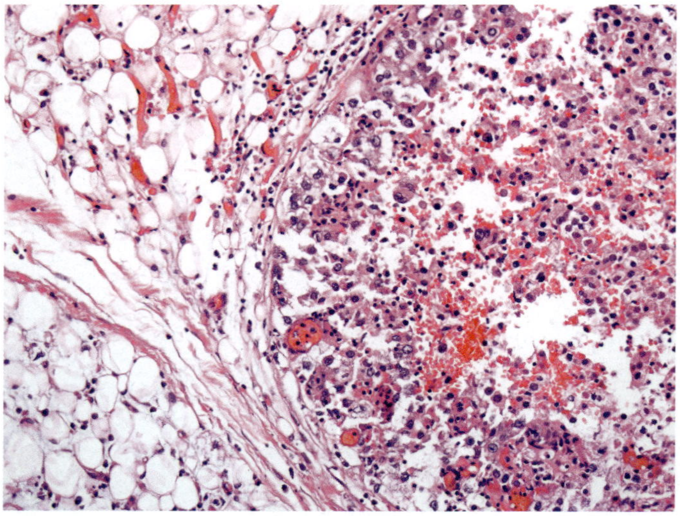

e

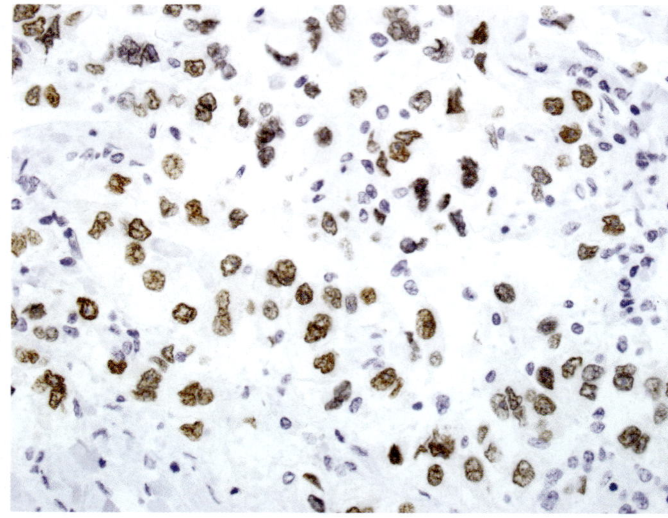

f

Figure 40-57.
(Continued)

Figure 40-58.
TFE3 translocation carcinoma metastatic to the lung is a white-tan mass (*a*). The tumor is composed of columnar cells in a papillary configuration (*b*), mimicking adenocarcinoma of the lung. Tumor cells are positive for TFE3 (*c*), and negative for AMACR (*d*), CA9 (*e*), and TTF1 (*f*), confirming the diagnosis.

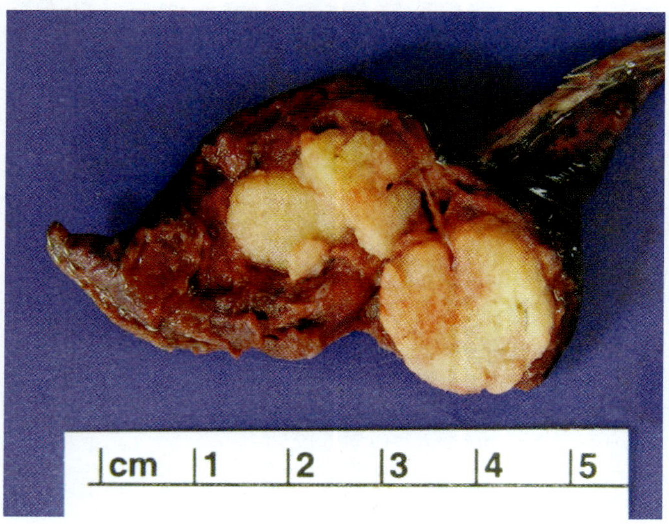

a

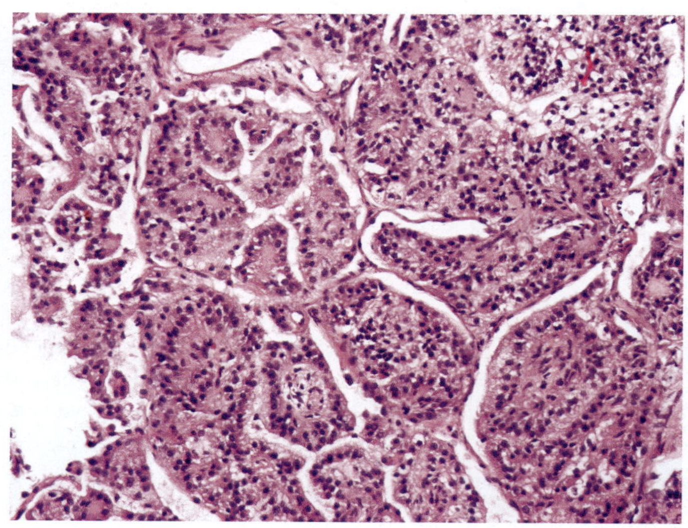

b

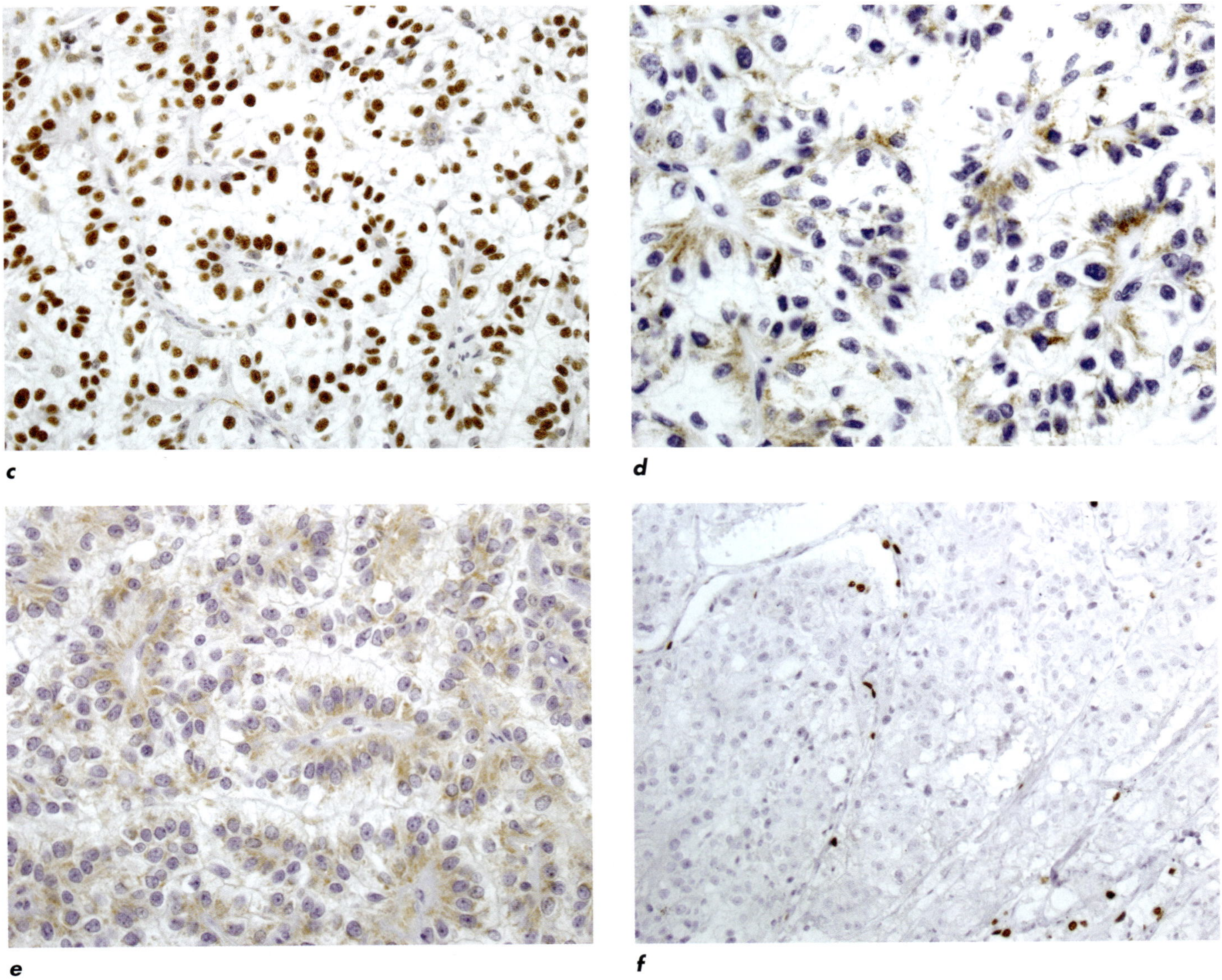

Figure 40-58.
(Continued)

RENAL CELL CARCINOMA, UNCLASSIFIED

Definition

- A group of RCCs with morphological features that do not fit any of the known RCC subtypes defined by the current WHO classification
- The definition is vague, resulting in the potential classification of any renal tumor unfamiliar to the diagnosing pathologist as an unclassified RCC
- The frivolous use of this diagnosis provides limited information for clinical management
- We typically reserve this diagnostic category for a small subset of high-grade RCC, which does not meet the established pathologic criteria for any of the known RCC subtypes

Pathogenesis

- It is a diagnostic term of exclusion and not a true pathologic entity

Clinical features

- Not specific, mostly depending on the definition and experience of each institution or individual. This diagnosis may account for 1% to 5% of RCCs diagnosed in practice

Gross pathology

- Usually a large mass with a white to tan cut surface (Fig. 40-59)

Histology

- Typically, a poorly differentiated tumor, which does not have any characteristic histological features for unequivocal classification (Figs. 40-60 and 40-61)
- A tumor with mixed features of different types of carcinomas such as components of clear cell, collecting duct, and urothelial carcinomas within the same tumor can be classified as such
- To render this diagnosis, a careful work-up using immunomarkers is necessary to exclude potential specific subtypes
- No evidence of sickled red blood cells

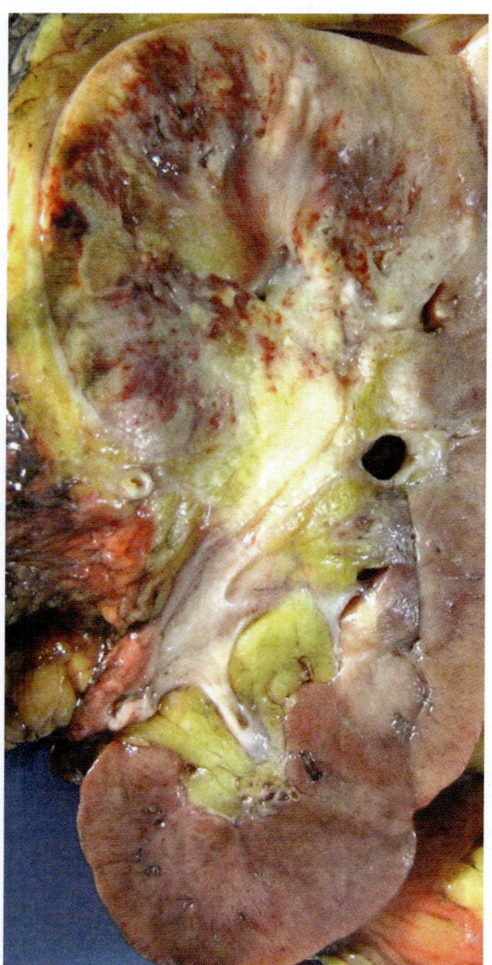

Figure 40-59.
Unclassified carcinoma of the kidney with poorly defined borders located in the cortex and medulla of the upper pole.

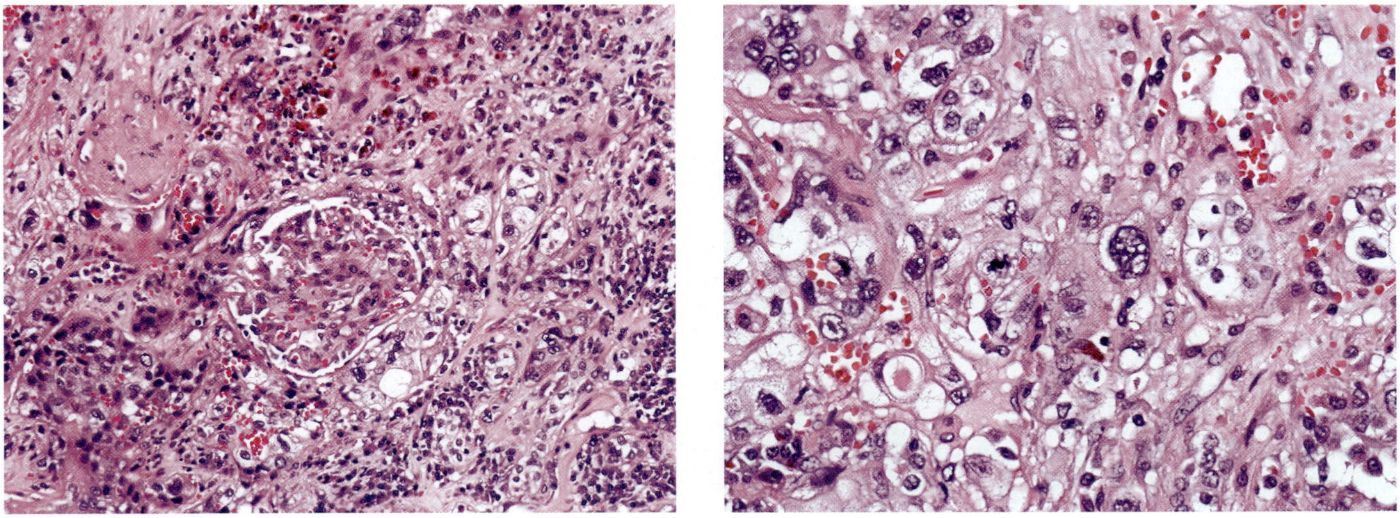

a b

Figure 40-60.
Unclassified carcinoma of the kidney exhibiting diffusely infiltrative high-grade tumor cells encasing a glomerulus, but showing no special architectural patterns (*a*). High magnification shows tumor cells with eosinophilic to clear cytoplasm and marked cytological atypia forming solid sheets and cords (*b*).

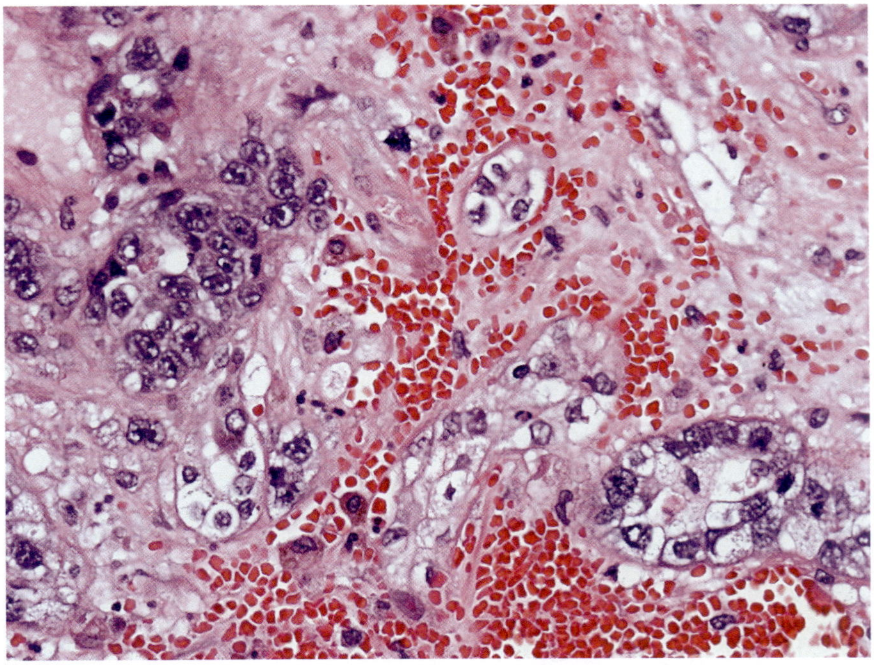

Figure 40-61.
Tumor cells of an unclassified carcinoma display marked pleomorphism and associated with hemorrhage. Note the presence of normal-appearing red cells.

Immunohistochemistry

- Does not fit any defined RCC subtypes

Clinical relevance (prognosis and treatment options)

- If this diagnosis is restricted to very poorly differentiated renal tumors, the prognosis is very poor
- If it is used too frequently, particularly with low-grade tumors, this diagnosis will pose challenges for clinical colleagues on proper management of the patient carrying such a diagnosis

RENAL PARAGANGLIOMA OF THE KIDNEY

Definition

- Primary paraganglioma is a neoplasm of paraganglia, which are aggregates of cells derived from the neural crest and associated with the autonomic nervous system

Other terms

- Pheochromocytoma of the kidney, extra-adrenal pheochromocytoma

Pathogenesis and epidemiology

- It is very rare, only less than 10 cases reported in the literature
- Most of reported cases are malignant

Clinical features

- Renal mass and possible hematuria
- Other symptoms such as hypertension, headache, and palpation related to the catecholamine released by the tumor
- Asymptomatic tumors are incidentally identified by imaging studies for other conditions

Gross pathology

- Well-delineated mass without a capsule
- Fleshy or tan cut surface, but not the bright yellow color typical of clear cell RCC

Histology

- Paraganglioma is signified by the presence of variably sized nests of tumor cells as well as more characteristic small rounded cell balls known as *Zellballen* surrounded by thin fibrovascular septa (Fig. 40-62)
- Large tumor cells with abundant eosinophilic, amphophilic, or pale cytoplasm (Fig. 40-63)
- Nuclear atypia can be seen, but mostly degenerative in nature. Intranuclear inclusions are common
- Some renal tubules trapped in the tumor can be mistaken for glandular differentiation (Fig. 40-64*a*)
- Prediction of malignant behavior from histological features alone is far from reliable, but large size, mitotic activity, necrosis, invasion are features often associated with more aggressive clinical behavior

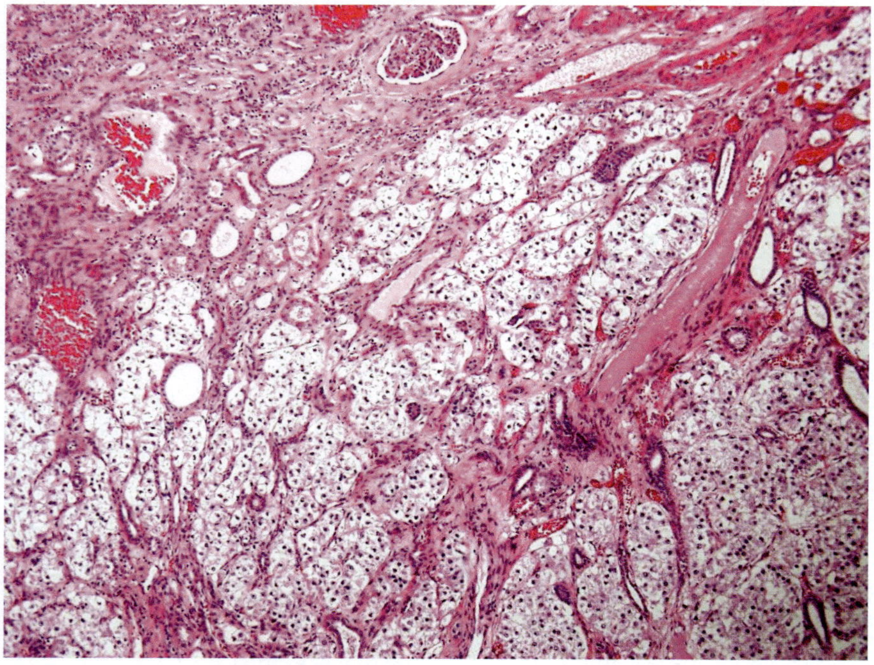

Figure 40-62.
A primary renal paraganglioma of a 20-year-old man composed of islands of epithelioid tumor cells infiltrating the renal parenchyma and mimicking renal cell carcinoma.

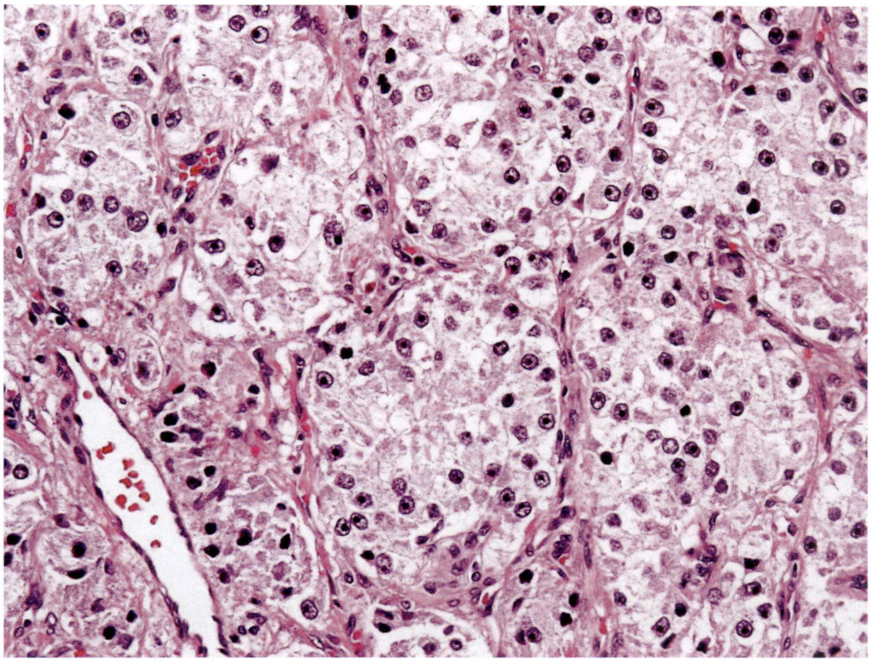

Figure 40-63.
Renal paraganglioma displays the typical nested and Zellballen pattern. Tumor cells have prominent nucleoli and abundant pale to lightly eosinophilic granular cytoplasm.

Immunohistochemistry

- Positive for neuroendocrine markers (chromogranin, synaptophysin or NSE) (Fig. 40-64*c*) and Gata-3
- Sustentacular cells (scattered supporting dendritic cells) positive for S100 (Fig. 40-64*d*)
- Negative for keratin markers (AE1/AE3, CAM5.2) (Fig. 40-64*b*), renal marker (PAX8), and renal carcinoma markers (AMACR, CA9)

Differential diagnosis

Renal cell carcinoma, particularly clear cell RCC

- In clear cell RCC, Zellballen nests are not identified
- RCC shows true nuclear atypia with abnormal chromatin patterns and nucleolar prominence
- Clear cell RCC displays a chicken-wire vasculature particularly low-grade tumors
- Immunohistochemistry of RCC is different from paraganglioma (positivity of renal cell markers and keratin markers)

Clinical relevance (prognosis and treatment options)

- Renal paraganglioma is so rare in the kidney that it is often not included in differential diagnosis of a renal tumor. If there is a doubt by histological examination, immunostains are helpful
- Extra-adrenal paraganglioma is more likely to be malignant than the adrenal pheochromocytoma, but still less aggressive than high-grade RCC. In addition, Renal paraganglioma is unlikely to respond the chemotherapies designed for high-grade RCC. However, it may respond better to radiation

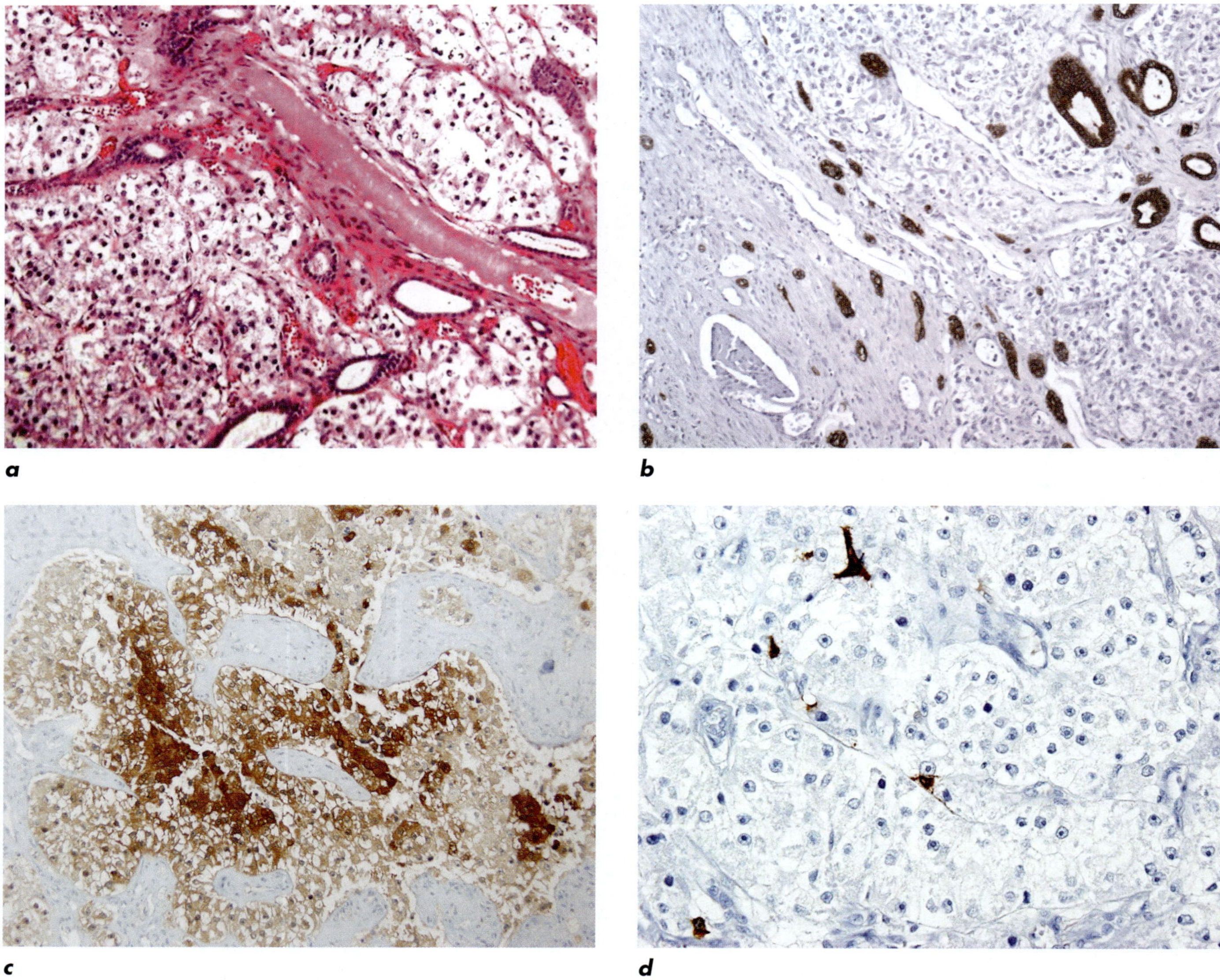

Figure 40-64.

Paraganglioma entrapping renal tubules (*a*). Tumor cells are negative for keratin AE1/AE3 (*b*) (residual renal tubules are positive), but positive for synaptophysin (*c*). Dendritic sustentacular cells surrounding the tumor nests are highlighted by S100 staining (*d*).

RENAL CARCINOID TUMOR

Definition

- Neuroendocrine neoplasm arising in the kidney

Other terms

- Well-differentiated neuroendocrine carcinoma
- Neuroendocrine tumor

Pathogenesis

- Primary carcinoid tumors of the kidney are rare; secondary carcinoid tumors are metastatic from other organs, such as the small bowel and colon

Clinical features

- Flank pain, mass, and hematuria
- May be associated with carcinoid syndrome, such as flushing, perfuse sweating, and diarrhea

Gross pathology

- Typically, a variably sized solitary solid well-circumscribed mass
- Homogenous white to yellow-tan cut surface
- Secondary carcinoid tumors are often multifocal

Histology

- Tumor cells, regular in size and shape, form corded, ribbon-like, or trabecular patterns (Figs. 40-65 and 40-66)
- Chromatin is fine and evenly dispersed, which results in the characteristic "salt-and-pepper" appearance typical of neuroendocrine cells (Fig. 40-67*a*)
- Mitotic counts should be ≤2/10 high-power fields in a typical carcinoid tumor
- Tumor may invade renal capsule or renal vein

Immunohistochemistry

- Neuroendocrine markers, such as synaptophysin and chromogranin, are positive (Fig. 40-67). Keratins Cam5.2 and AE1/AE3 as well as vimentin are positive

Clinical relevance (prognosis and treatment options)

- Generally, a low-grade malignancy
- Surgical removal is the treatment of choice
- However, metastatic carcinoid tumors are difficult to treat

Figure 40-65.
Carcinoid tumor of the kidney as a well-circumscribed lesion (*a*). This tumor, similar to carcinoid of other organs, is characterized by the presence of large insular nests of neuroendocrine tumor cells (*b*).

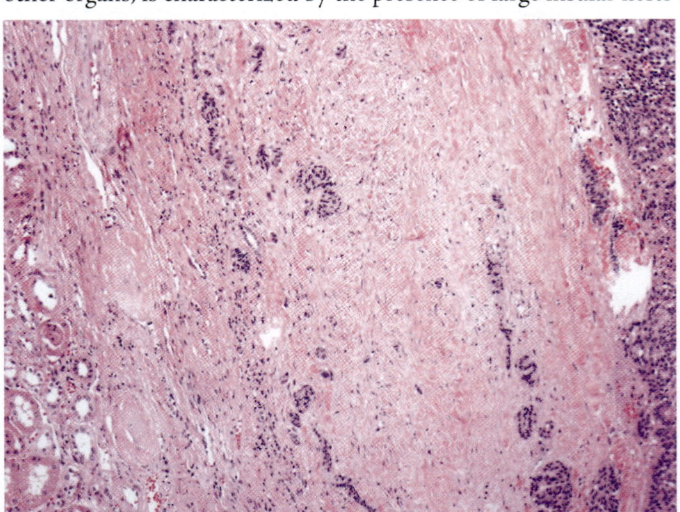

a

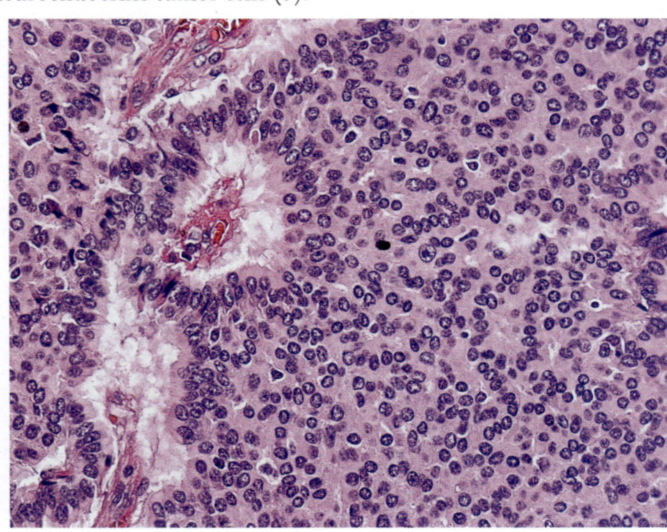

b

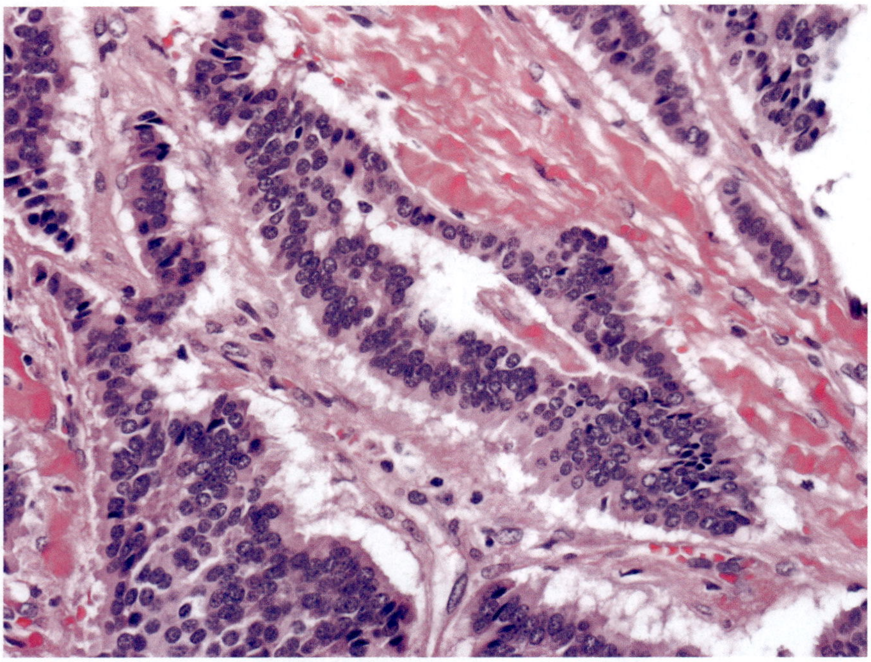

Figure 40-66.
Carcinoid tumor cells are regular in size and shape, forming acinar or glandular structures. Note characteristic "salt-and-pepper" chromatin pattern.

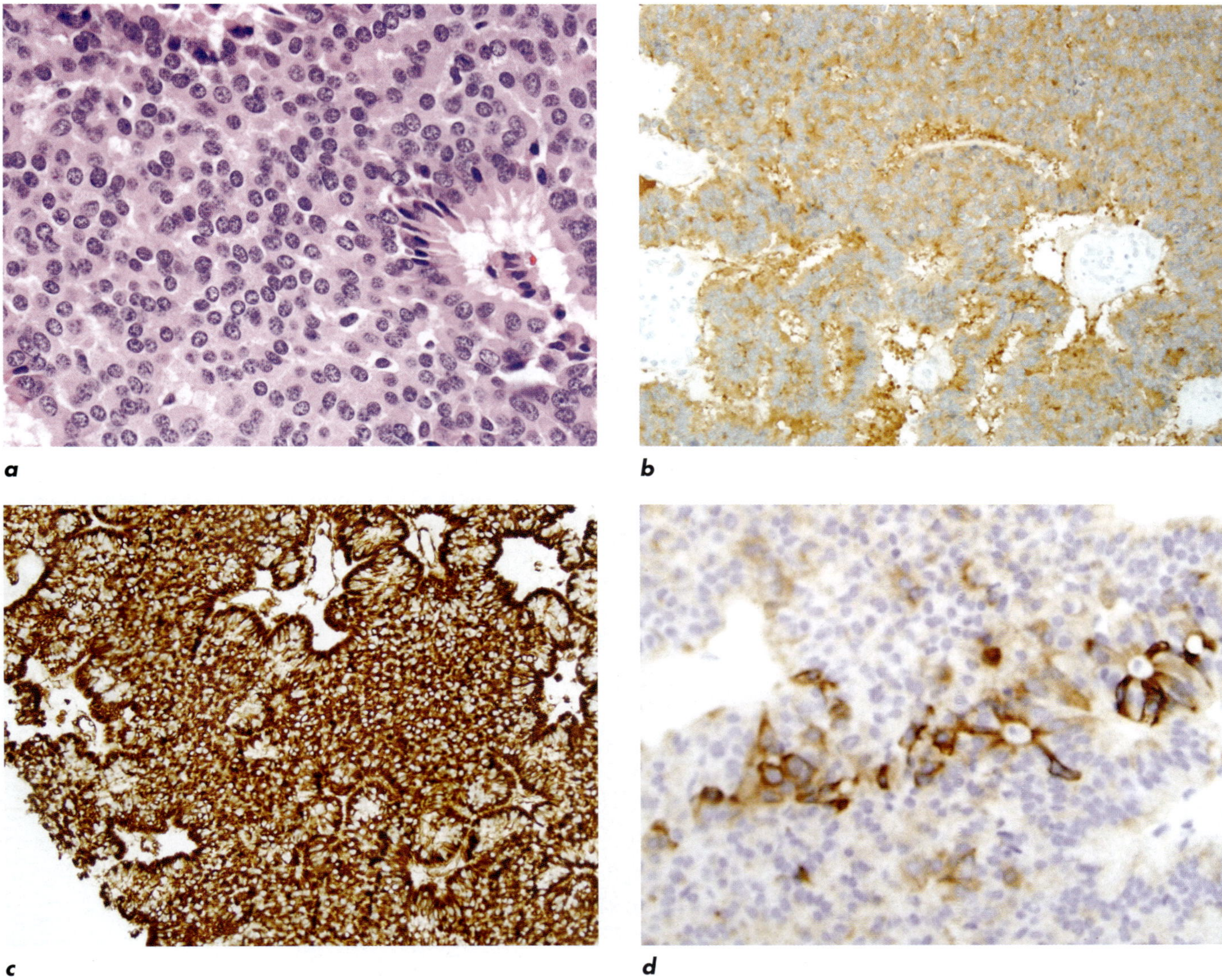

Figure 40-67.
High magnification of a carcinoid shows the typical "salt-and-pepper" chromatin pattern characteristic of a neuroendocrine cell, and low mitotic activity (*a*). The tumor cells are positive for synaptophysin (*b*) and vimentin (*c*), and focally positive for keratin AE1/AE3 (*d*).

PRIMITIVE NEUROECTODERMAL TUMOR/EWING SARCOMA OF THE KIDNEY

Definition

- Primary malignant neoplasm composed of small primitive epithelioid cells exhibiting neuronal differentiation
- This tumor harbors characteristic chromosomal translocations
- Primitive neuroectodermal tumor (PNET) and Ewing sarcoma are now considered to be the same entity. The old literature defined PNET as a primitive sarcoma exhibiting neural differentiation and Ewing sarcoma as an undifferentiated small cell sarcoma

Other term

- Soft tissue Ewing sarcoma

Pathogenesis

- This neoplasm is possibly derived from mesenchymal stem cells

Clinical features

- PNET/Ewing sarcoma often affect children and young adults with a wide age range from 5 to 70 (mean = 18) years
- Flank pain, abdominal mass, and/or hematuria

Gross pathology

- Usually a large mass in the kidney with fleshy, tan-white, homogenous encephaliod (medullary) cut surface (Fig. 40-68*a*)
- Hemorrhage and necrosis are commonly seen, cystic change is occasionally present

Histology

- Lobular or sheet-like growth patterns (Fig. 40-68*b*)
- Tumor is composed of small, uniform round, or oval cells (Fig. 40-69)
- Tumor cells are primitive with scant somewhat vacuolated (glycogen-rich) cytoplasm, with ill-defined cell borders (small blue round cells) (Figs. 40-69 and 40-70)
- As initially defined (but no longer used in clinical practice), tumor cells in PNET form Homer-Wright pseudorosettes indicating neuronal differentiation (Fig. 40-71), whereas no light microscopic evidence of neuronal differentiation is evident in Ewing sarcoma
- No tubular or glomeruloid formation
- Azzopardi phenomenon: basophilic material (DNA) released by crushed malignant small cells adherent to elastic connective tissue of vessels (Fig. 40-72)

Figure 40-68.
Gross photo of PNET/Ewing sarcoma of the kidney shows a poorly defined medullary mass destroying most of the kidney (*a*). Microscopically, the tumor displays an infiltrating border (*b*).

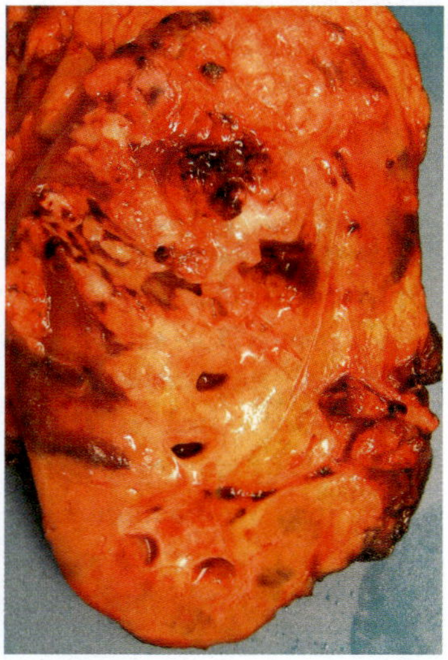

a

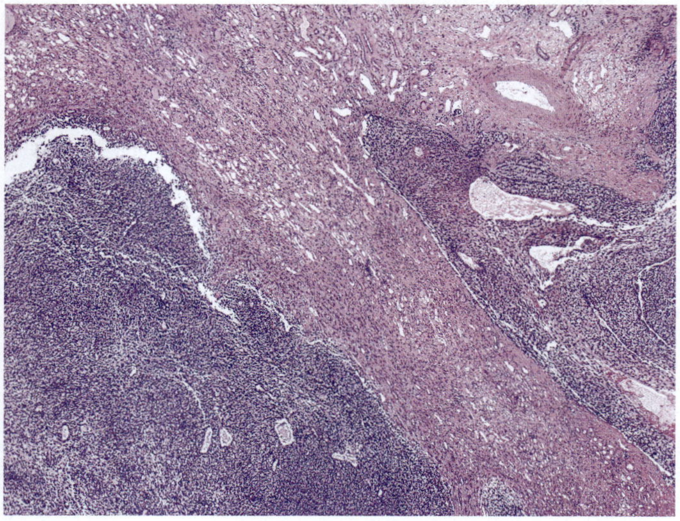

b

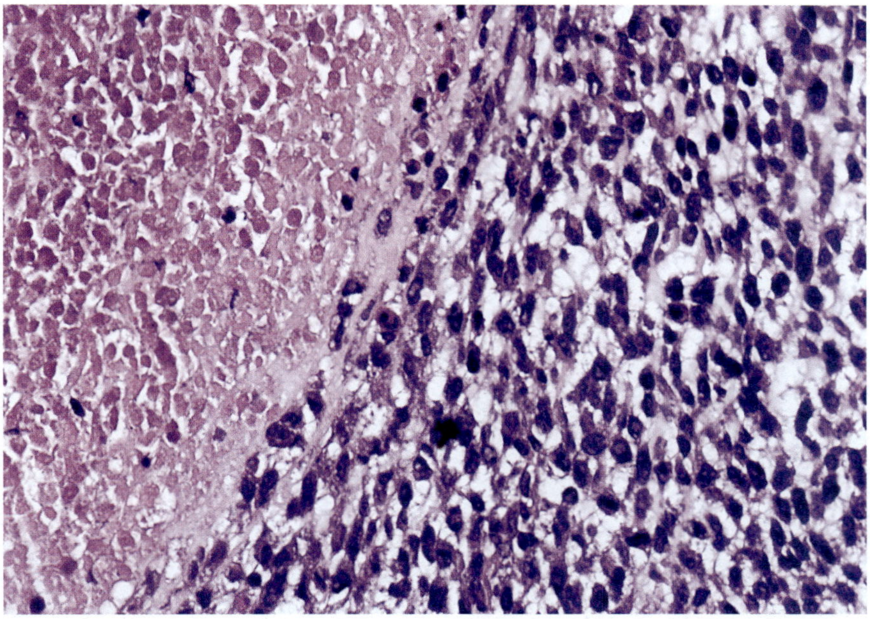

Figure 40-69.
PNET/Ewing sarcoma is composed of small cells with scant cytoplasm (small blue round cells) in diffuse growth patterns. Mitoses are frequent and necrosis is seen on the left.

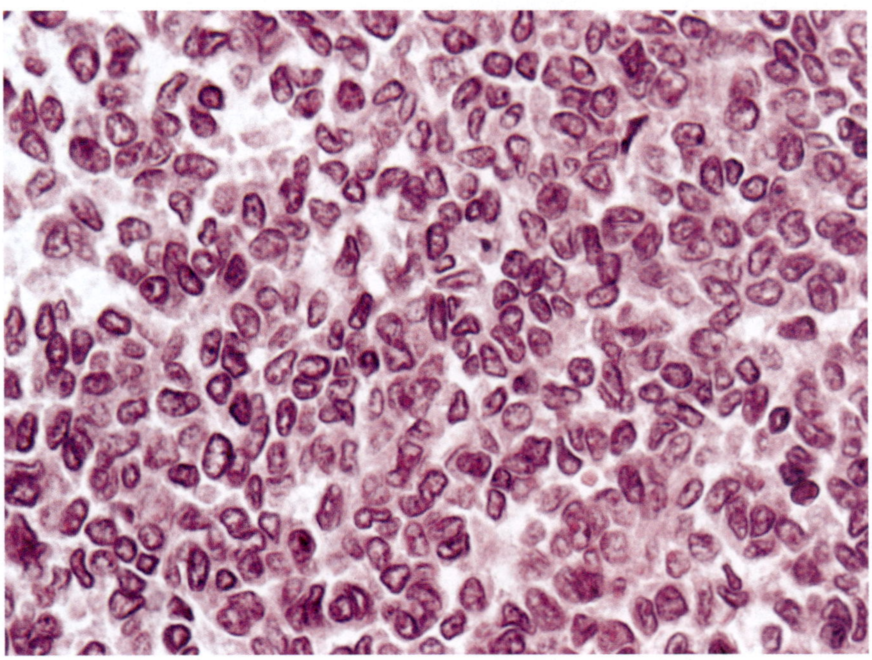

Figure 40-70.
PNET/Ewing sarcoma with a high density of small round cells with scant cytoplasm (high N/C ratio) and irregular-shaped nuclei.

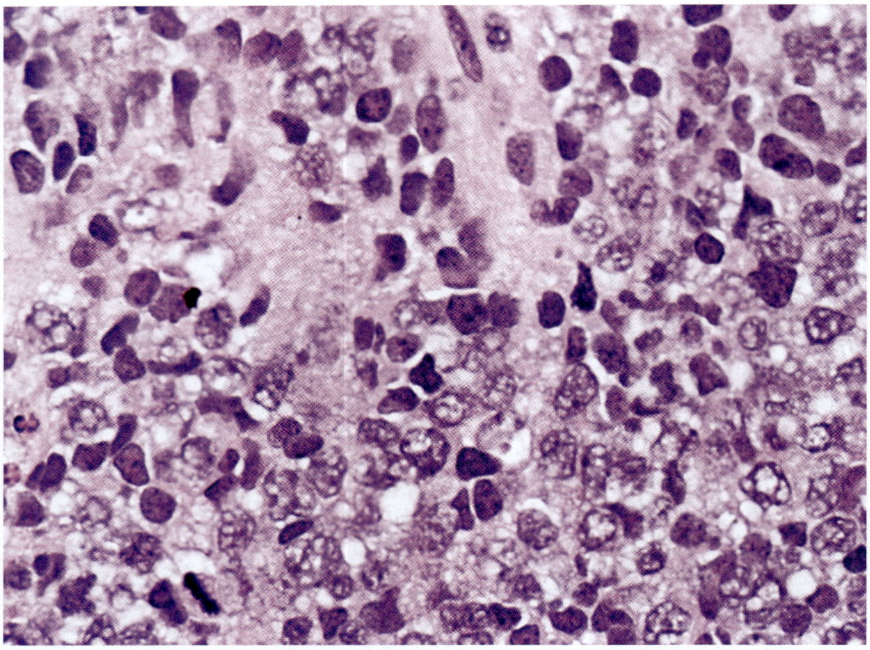

Figure 40-71.
Rosette-like structures (Homer-Wright pseudorosettes) seen in PNET/Ewing sarcoma indicating neuronal differentiation.

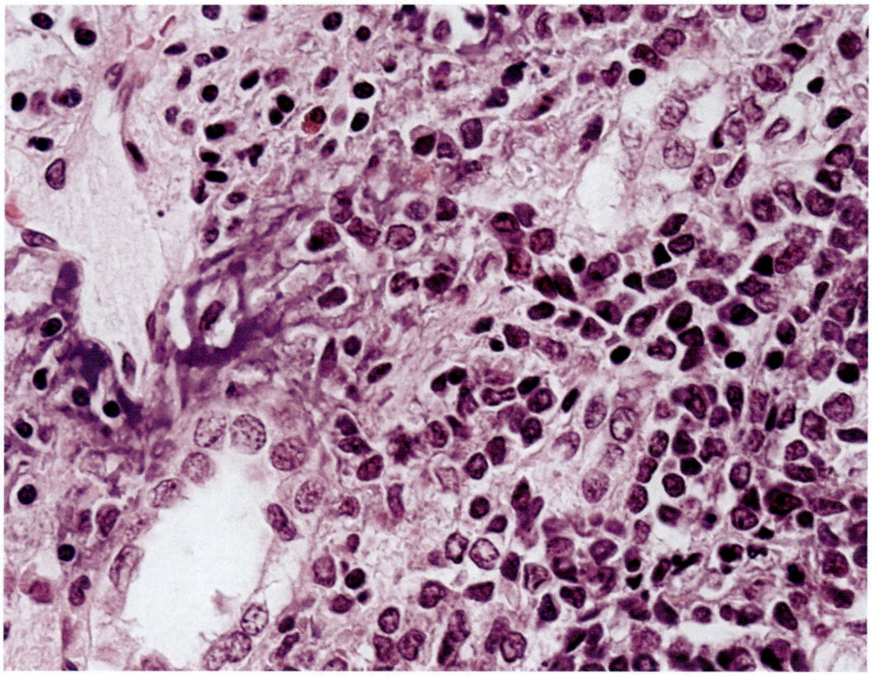

Figure 40-72.
PNET/Ewing sarcoma with basophilic DNA material seen around a blood vessel (Azzopardi phenomenon) on the left.

Immunohistochemistry and electron microscopy

- CD99 positive (membrane staining) (Fig. 40-73)
- FLI1 (Fig. 40-73*c*) and ERG (nuclear staining) positive
- Neuron-specific enolase and vimentin positive
- PAS positive (diastase sensitive) due to glycogen deposition (Fig. 40-73*d*)
- EM demonstrates intracytoplasmic neuroendocrine granules in tumor cells
- Keratin(s) positive in approximately 20% of the cases

Differential diagnosis

- See Table 40-4

Molecular analysis

- The presence of t(11;22) (q24;q12) (*EWS/FLI1*) translocation is found in the majority (85% to 90%) of cases. *EWS* gene (and less often *FLI5* gene) is translocated to other partners in the remaining cases
- Diagnosis can be established with PCR-based tests for *EWS/FLI1* translocation or "break-point" FISH to detect *EWS* translocation

Clinical relevance (prognosis and treatment options)

- Chemotherapy and surgery with or without radiation
- A very aggressive tumor without treatment
- With modern therapies, the 5-year survival rate has improved

Figure 40-73.
PNET/Ewing sarcoma cells (*a*) are positive for CD99 (*b*) and FLI1 (*c*), and demonstrate introcytoplasmic glycogen granules with PAS staining (*d*).

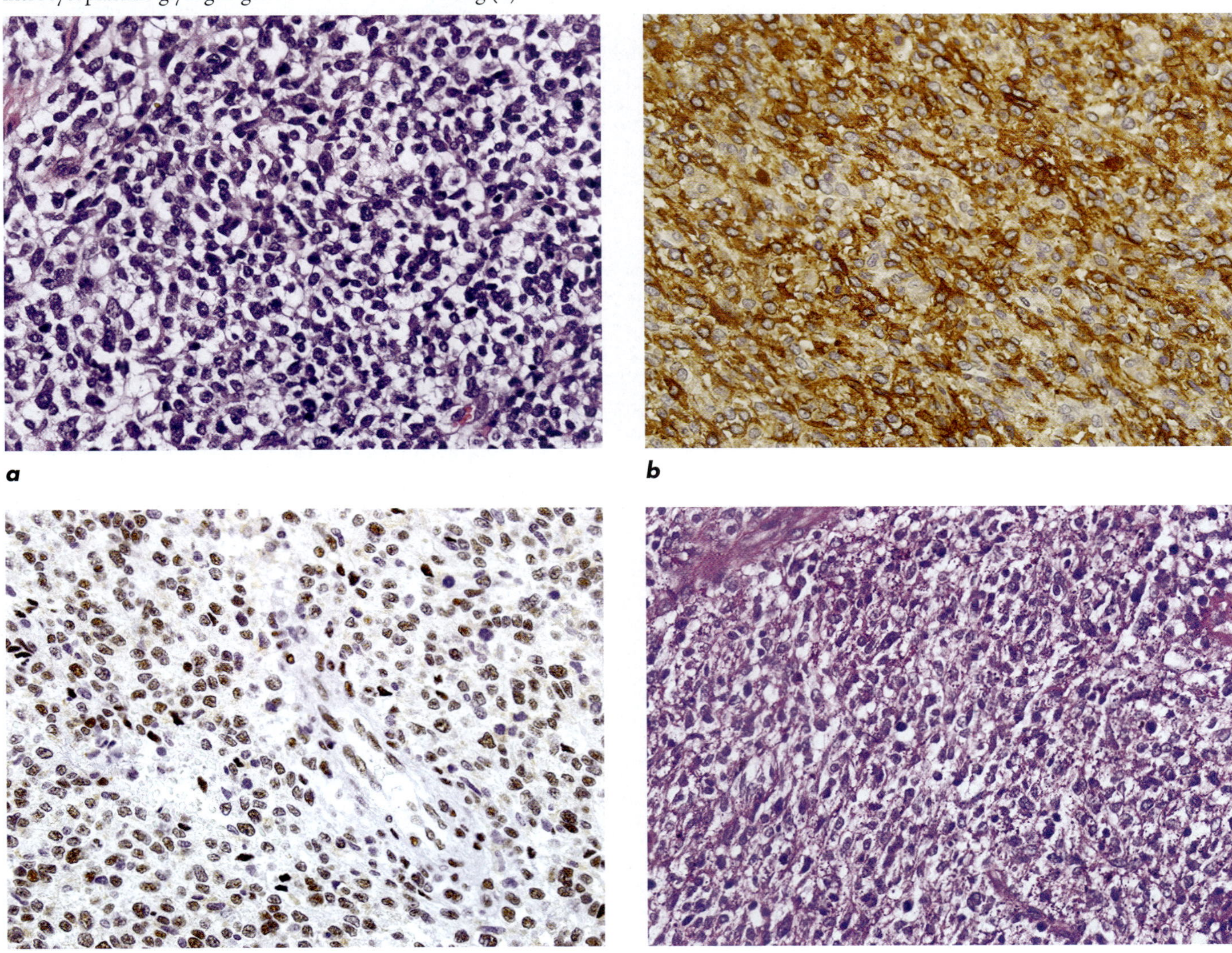

Table 40-4. Differential Diagnosis of Small Blue Cell Tumors in the Kidney

Kidney tumor	*Age*	*Incidence (kidney)*	*Special histology*	*IHC*
Wilms tumor	Young age (<5 years)	Most common tumor in children	Triphasic pattern	WT1+
Clear cell sarcoma	Young age (<5 years)	Relatively common	Vascular pattern	NGFR+
Neuroblastoma	Young age (<5 years)	Common in adrenal	Homer-Wright pseudorosettes	Neuronal markers + CD99– PAS–
PNET/Ewing sarcoma	Young adults	Rare in kidney	Homer-Wright rosettes (uncommon)	CD99+ FLI1+ PAS+
Lymphoma	Children and adults	uncommon	Diffuse pattern	CD45+ CD20+ or CD3+
Small cell carcinoma	Older adults	Uncommon in kidney	Islands, nests, and nuclear molding	TTF1+ (50%) Neuronal markers +
Synovial sarcoma (poorly differentiated)	Older adults	Rare in kidney	Hemangiopericytoma-like pattern, cellular overlap	Keratin 7 and 19+ Bcl-2+ CD34–

METASTATIC MALIGNANCY TO A RENAL CELL NEOPLASM

Definition

- A malignant tumor from an organ outside the kidney metastasizing to a renal cell neoplasm

Pathogenesis

- Because of the rich vascularity of some renal neoplasms, malignant cells that migrate from other organs can implant and grow in the environment of the renal neoplasm
- The most common renal cell neoplasm acting as a recipient for a metastasis is clear cell RCC. Other renal tumors such as PRCC or oncocytoma can also act as an acceptable recipient

Clinical features

- A very rare event with only a few case reports in the literature
- A history of a known primary carcinoma, commonly lung, breast, or colon
- The presence of renal mass(es)

Gross pathology

- The renal mass tends to be large, and mostly solitary, occasionally multiple
- The cut surface shows typical background of a renal neoplasm (ie, bright yellow mass for a clear cell RCC)
- Within the main tumor mass, there are discrete white or fleshy nodules (metastatic carcinoma) (Fig. 40-74)

Histology

- Two distinct populations of the tumor cells can be identified (Fig. 40-75)
- Recipient tumor: clear cell RCC or other type of renal cell neoplasm is the predominant component, usually low grade (Fig. 40-75)
- Metastatic tumor: nodules of high grade (donor) can be easily distinguished from typical clear cell RCC (Fig. 40-75)
- Vascular permeation by high-grade metastatic component may be present
- Previous history and pathology reports should be available for review

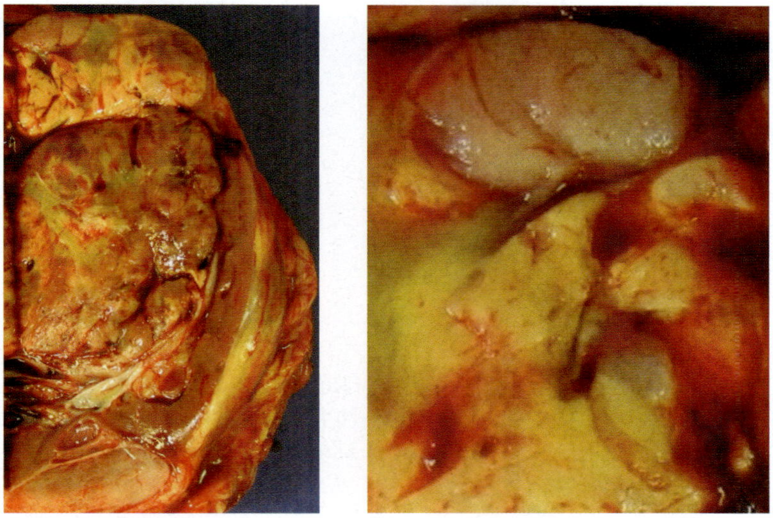

a b

Figure 40-74.
Metastatic breast carcinoma to a large clear cell RCC (*a*). Close-up shows the presence of bright yellow RCC area (left) and white-tan nodule of breast carcinoma (right) (*b*).

Figure 40-75.
Microscopically, two components are seen: islands of breast adenocarcinoma cells with eosinophilic cytoplasm embedded in a clear cell RCC (*a*). Higher magnification shows the cytological difference between the high-grade breast carcinoma (middle) and the low-grade clear cell RCC in surrounding areas (*b*).

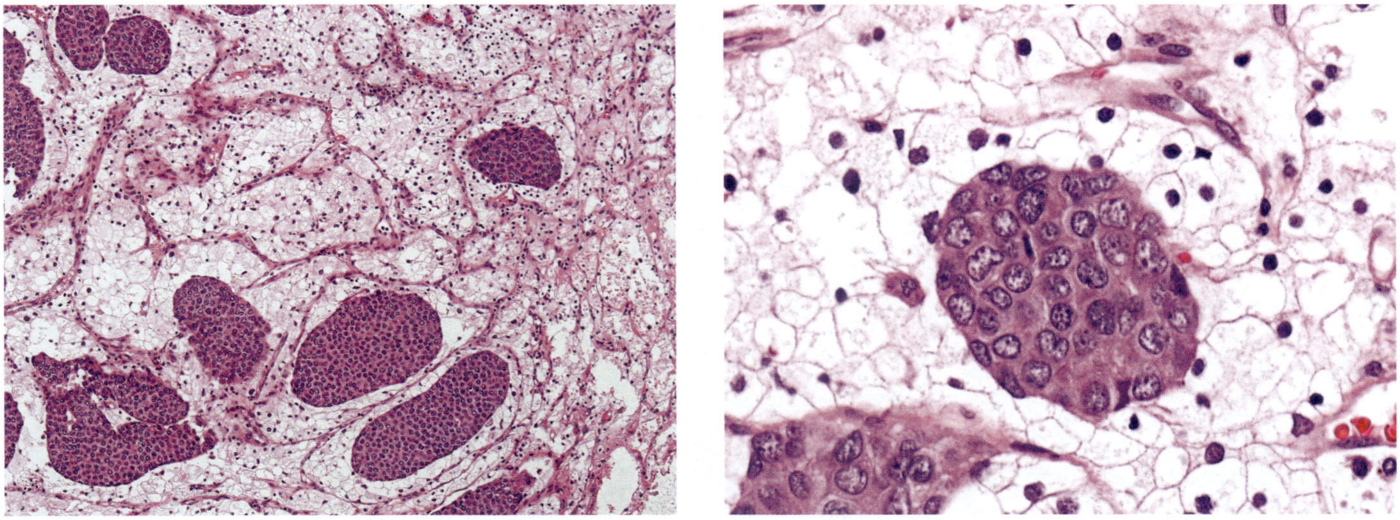

a b

Immunohistochemistry

- Metastatic tumor and recipient renal tumor have different immunoprofiles
- Clear cell RCC component: positive for CA9, vimentin, and PAX8
- Donor tumor negative for RCC markers but positive for other specific markers such as ER/PR for breast cancer (Fig. 40-76)

Clinical relevance (prognosis and treatment options)

- The donor tumor is often higher grade than recipient RCC
- The prognosis is mostly dependent on the metastatic donor tumor

Figure 40-76.
Clusters of metastatic breast carcinoma cells surrounded by clear cell RCC (*a*). The breast carcinoma cells are positive for ER, while RCC cells are negative (*b*). The clear cell RCC cells are positive for CA9 (*c*) and vimentin (*d*), while breast carcinoma components are negative for CA9 (*c*) and vimentin (*d*).

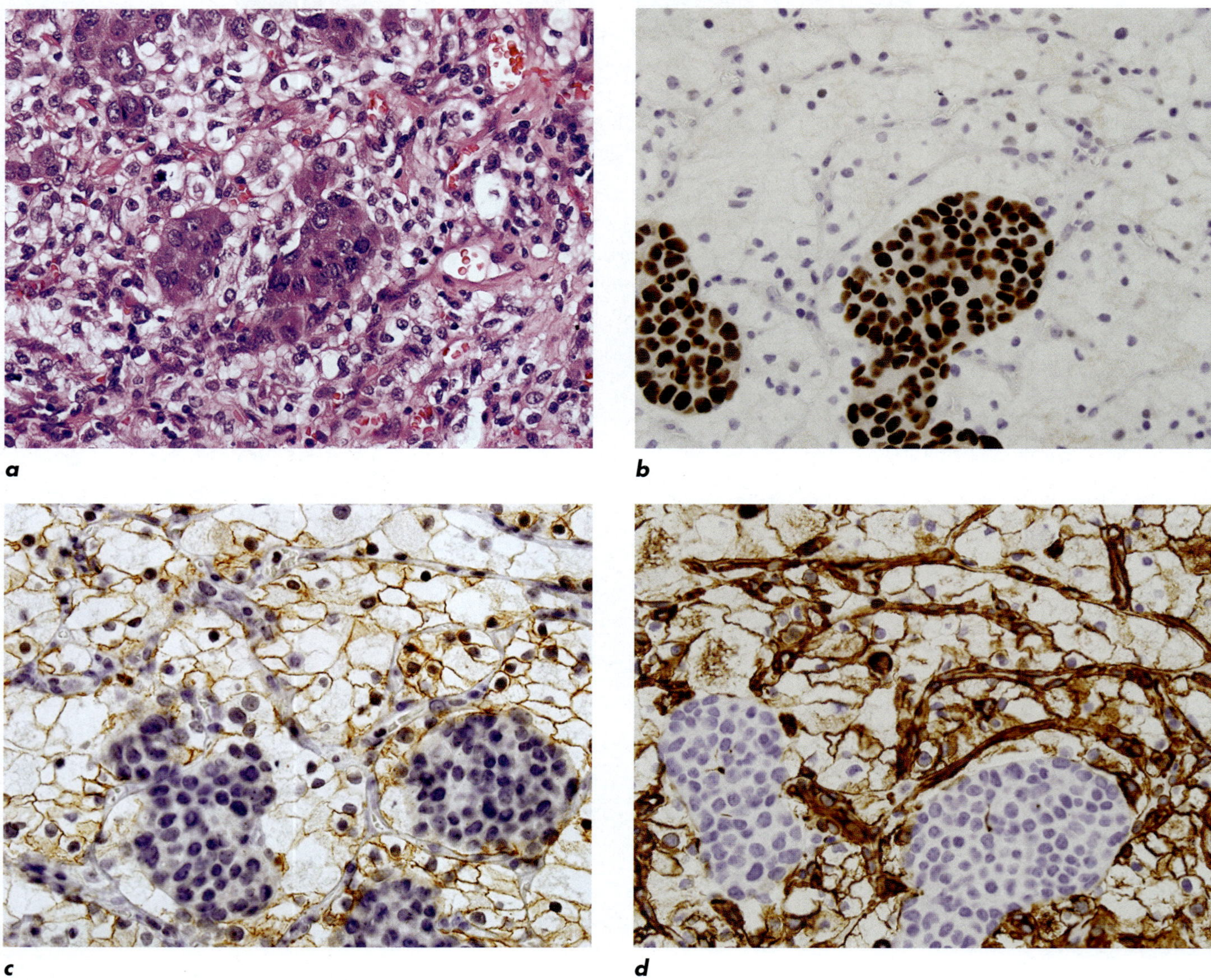

LYMPHOMA OF THE KIDNEY

Definition

- Primary renal lymphoma is a lymphoma presenting in the kidney without systemic involvement. This phenomenon is very rare with only about 100 cases reported in the literature
- Secondary renal involvement by a systemic lymphoma is relatively common

Clinical features

- Flank pain, mass, fever, and weight loss
- Hematuria
- Renal failure may present if lymphoma extensively involves the kidney

Gross pathology

- Single or multiple nodule(s) in the kidney
- Sometimes, the kidney shows diffuse renal enlargement, particular secondary renal lymphoma
- Cut surface is white homogenous
- Hemorrhage and necrosis may be present

Histology

- Both Hodgkin and non-Hodgkin lymphomas can be seen in the kidney
- Three patterns have been recognized
  - Diffuse infiltration
  - Formation of tumor nodules
  - Intravascular form is the rarest
- Most common type of renal lymphoma is diffuse large B-cell lymphoma (Fig. 40-77)

Immunohistochemistry

- Large B-cell lymphoma: tumor cells positive for B-cell markers such as CD20, CD79a, and PAX5 (Fig. 40-77*c*)
- Renal and RCC markers negative
- Keratin markers negative (rarely positive in anaplastic large cell lymphoma)

Clinical relevance (prognosis and treatment options)

- Secondary lymphoma indicates advanced disease with systemic involvement (Stage IV disease)
- Typically poor prognosis and patients require systemic chemotherapy
- Effectiveness of nephrectomy for renal lymphoma is not known
- Distinction from other renal neoplasms is important for treatment purpose

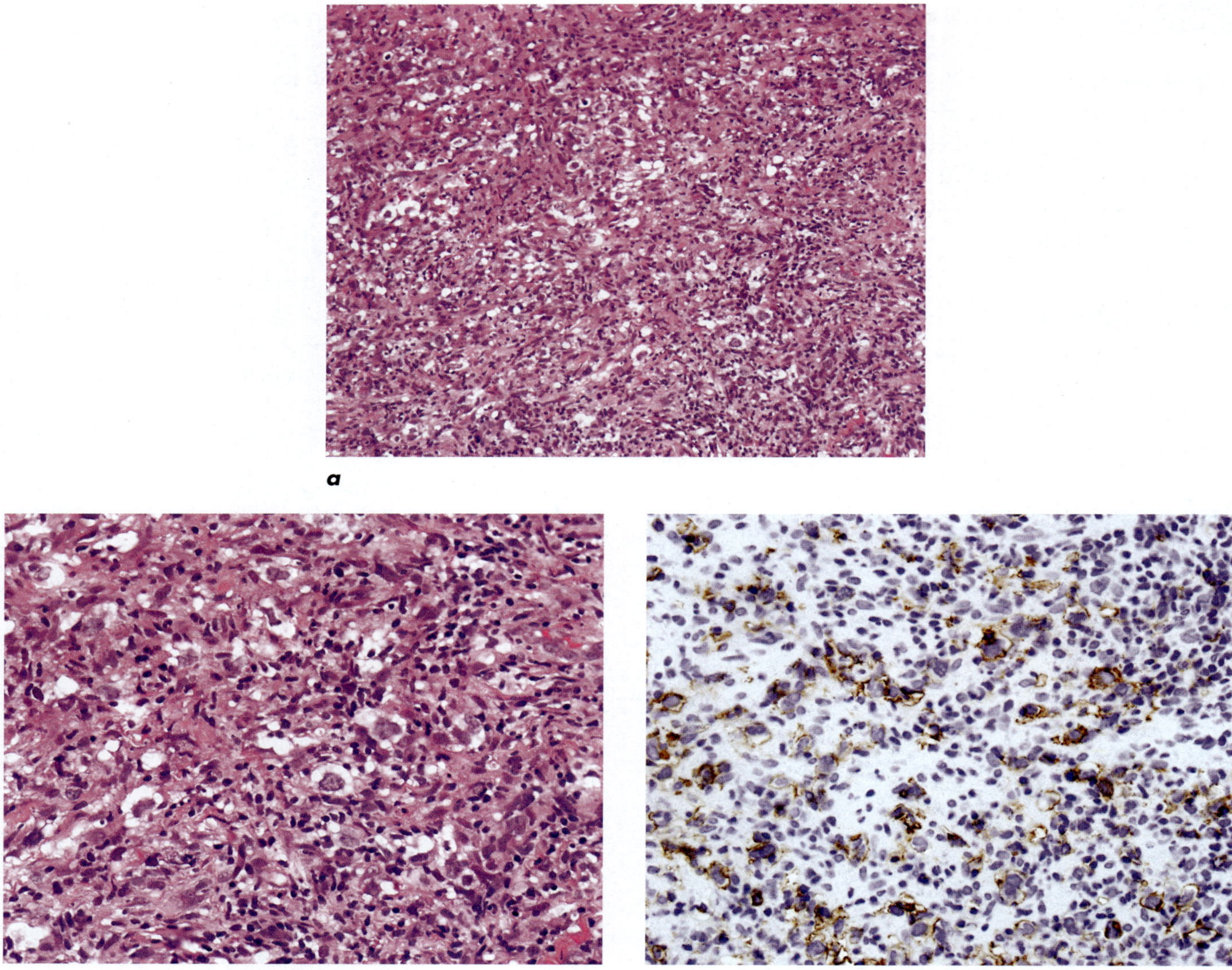

a

b

c

Figure 40-77.

Large diffuse B-cell lymphoma in the kidney. Malignant lymphocytes form a tumor nodule in which no renal tubules are seen (*a*). High magnification shows discohesive large malignant cells with atypical nuclei and moderate amount of clear cytoplasm in a background of small lymphocytes and histiocytes (*b*). Immunostaining for CD20 highlights the large tumor cells (*c*).

CHAPTER 41

Perirenal Neoplasms and Tumor-Like Lesions

Ximing J. Yang, Sanjiv V. Prabhu

HETEROTOPIC PANCREAS

Definition

- Presence of pancreatic tissue outside the pancreas, lacking an anatomic or vascular communication with the normal pancreas
- Most common locations are in the gastrointestinal tract, including stomach, small intestine, and colon. Occasionally, it can be seen in esophagus, gallbladder, spleen
- Rarely, it can be found in the area in or near the kidney or adrenal

Other terms

- Ectopic pancreas, accessory pancreas, aberrant pancreas

Pathogenesis

- Likely caused by the misplacement of pancreatic tissue during fetal development
- It may also develop as a metaplastic process, although it appears to be unlikely
- It is a relatively frequent finding in autopsy, present in at least 2% of autopsy cases by careful examination, based on some reports

Clinical features

- Mostly an incidental finding
- The vast majority of cases are asymptomatic
- Symptoms, if present, are related to the location and size of the lesion
- Pain may be related to the inflammation caused by pancreatic secretions
- Occasionally, intestinal or biliary obstruction may be seen if the lesion compresses adjacent organs
- Rare cases of pancreatitis and pseudocysts have been reported
- May be detected by imaging studies or laparotomy

Gross pathology

- White to yellow spots or well-circumscribed nodules similar to the color and texture of the pancreas
- Typically small ranging from microscopic foci (<1 mm, not grossly identifiable) to a few millimeters in size; rare cases up to a few centimeters in size have been reported

Histology

- Well-formed glandular structures surrounded by adipose tissue (Fig. 41-1)
- Heterotopic pancreatic tissue can be divided into three types
  - Ducts and acini, similar to normal pancreas (Fig. 41-2)
  - Ducts only
  - Acini only (Fig. 41-3)
- Islets can be seen (Fig. 41-3); however, they may be difficult to be identified in limited sampling

Immunohistochemistry

- Usually not necessary

Clinical relevance (prognosis and treatment options)

- Benign condition, no treatment unless symptomatic or suspicious for malignancy
- The possibility of malignant transformation of heterotopic pancreas to carcinoma exists

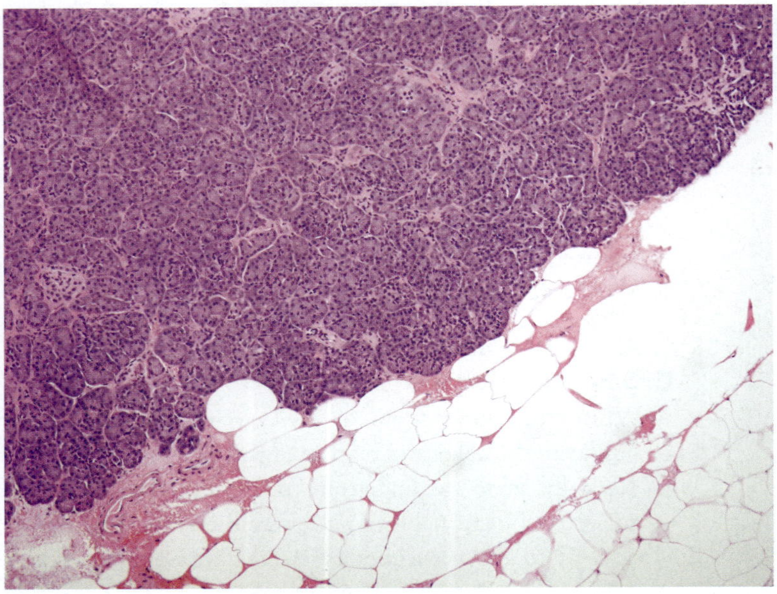

Figure 41-1.
A case of heterotopic pancreas was found in the area of the adrenal during radical nephrectomy for a renal cell carcinoma. A small 3-mm nodule of pancreatic tissue is surrounded by adipose tissue.

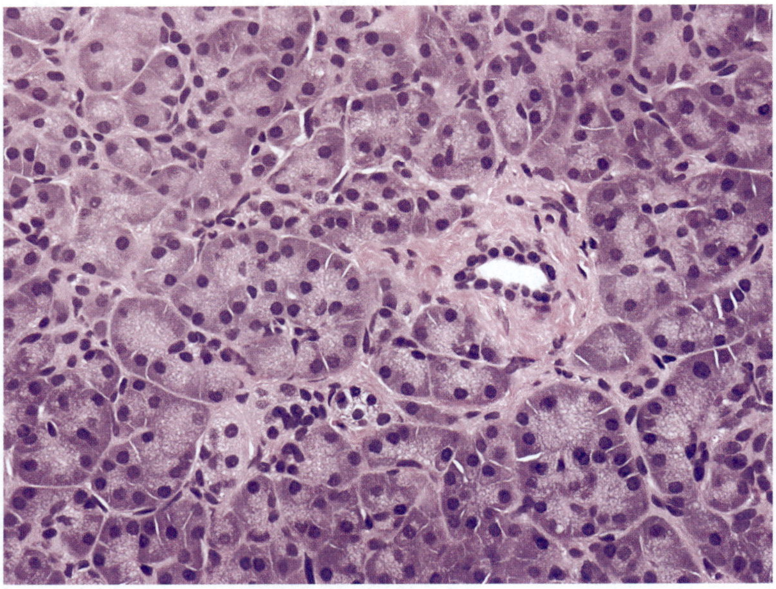

Figure 41-2.
The heterotopic pancreatic tissue is well organized with a small duct in the center, surrounded by serous acini.

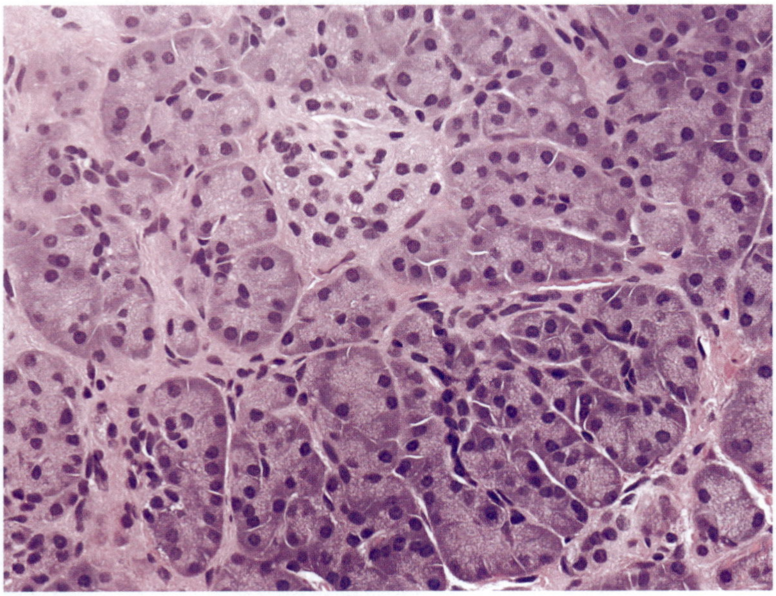

Figure 41-3.
An islet can be seen in the middle surrounded by acini in this heterotopic pancreas.

GASTROINTESTINAL STROMAL TUMOR (GIST)

Definition

- A mesenchymal neoplasm arising from interstitial cells of Cajal in the gastrointestinal tract
- A malignant GIST may involve or be attached to a GU organ by direct extension or metastasis; therefore, familiarity with this tumor is important for pathologists and urologists dealing with genitourinary organs

Pathogenesis

- This tumor is believed to arise from interstitial cells of Cajal in the GI tract
- The cells of Cajal play a role of gut pacemaker to regulate peristalsis
- The development of GIST is related to activating mutations of C-kit
- 20% to 30% of GISTs are malignant
- GISTs are mainly seen in the stomach (60%), small bowel (35%), and colon (5%)

Clinical features

- Abdominal pain, with possible gastrointestinal obstruction
- Palpable mass
- May be asymptomatic if small

Gross pathology

- A firm nodule or a large mass attached to the kidney, ureter, or bladder
- The tumor is typically softer and more homogenous than a leiomyoma (Fig. 41-4)
- Hemorrhage and necrosis may be seen, particularly in the malignant GIST

Histology

- Tumor is composed of neoplastic spindle cells of various patterns
- GISTs can be divided into four subtypes: spindle cell type and epithelioid type; benign and malignant (Figs. 41-5 to 41-8, Table 41-1)
- The neoplastic spindle cells appear similar to smooth muscle tumor cells
- Epithelioid GIST is composed of short spindle or round cells. Mitotic figures can be seen (Fig. 41-5)
- Malignant potential of GISTs (Figs. 41-6 and 41-8) can be predicted from the size and mitotic activity of the tumor (Table 41-2)

Immunohistochemistry

- C-kit (CD117) positive in greater than 90% of cases (Fig. 41-7), diffuse and mostly membranous
- DOG-1 positive in greater than 90%, and CD34 positive in greater than 70% of cases
- Smooth muscle actin (SMA) negative

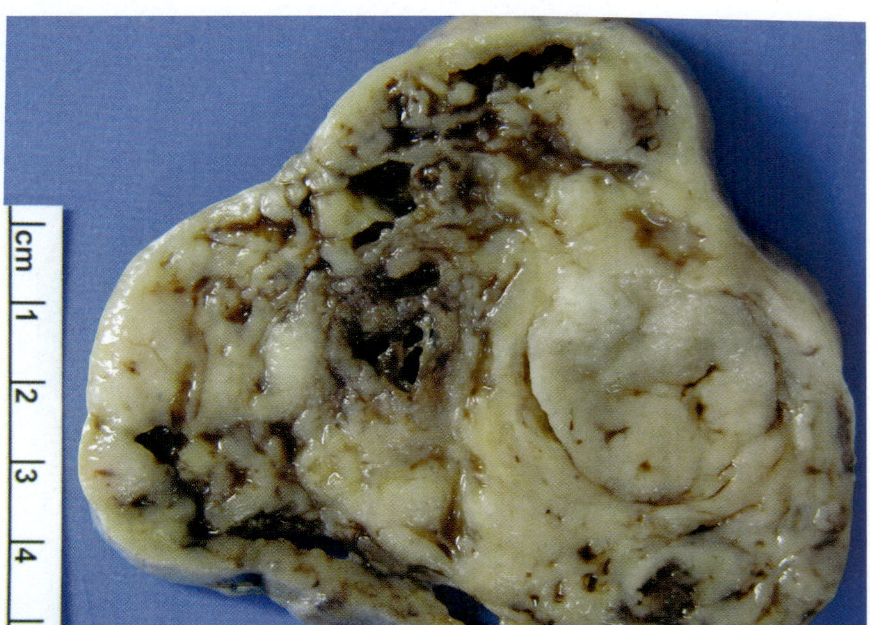

Figure 41-4.
Gross photo of a GIST, after formalin fixation, greater than 5 cm (one of those with high risk factors). The cut surface is white with focal degenerative changes. The tumor is softer than a leiomyoma.

Table 41-1. Subtypes of Gastrointestinal Stromal Tumor (GIST)

	Benign	*Malignant*
Spindle cell	*Benign cellular spindle cell GIST* Bland spindle cells with pale to eosinophilic fibrillar cytoplasm Cells in whorls or short intersecting fascicles Prominent nuclear palisading, extensive stromal hyalinization	*Malignant spindle cell GIST (sarcoma)* Spindle cells of high cellularity
Epithelioid	*Benign epithelioid GIST* Bland epithelioid cells	*Malignant epithelioid GIST* Epithelioid cells with high N/C ratio and pleomorphic

N/C ratio, nuclear/cytoplasmic ratio.

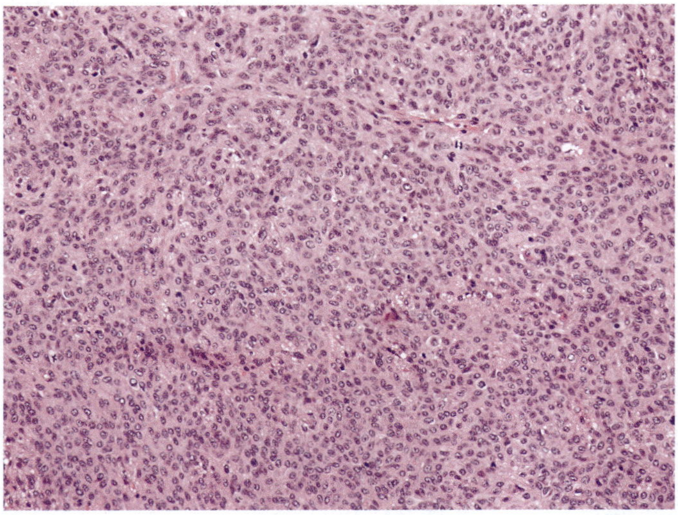

a

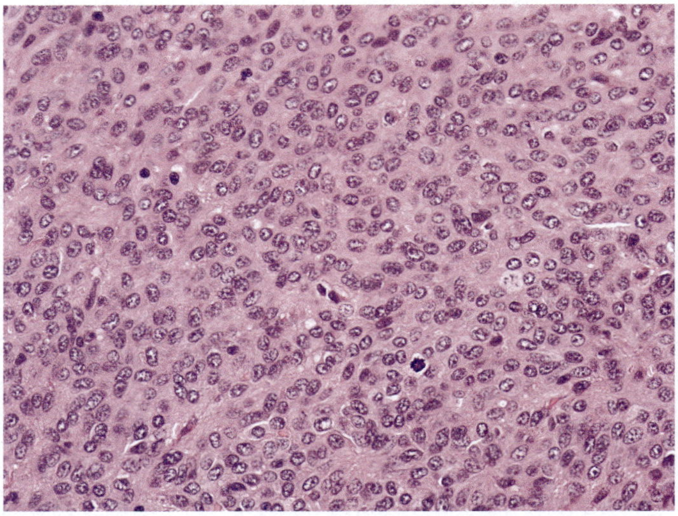

b

Figure 41-5.
Epithelioid GIST composed of short spindle cells (*a*). High magnification shows short spindle cells with epithelioid appearance with occasional mitotic figures seen (*b*).

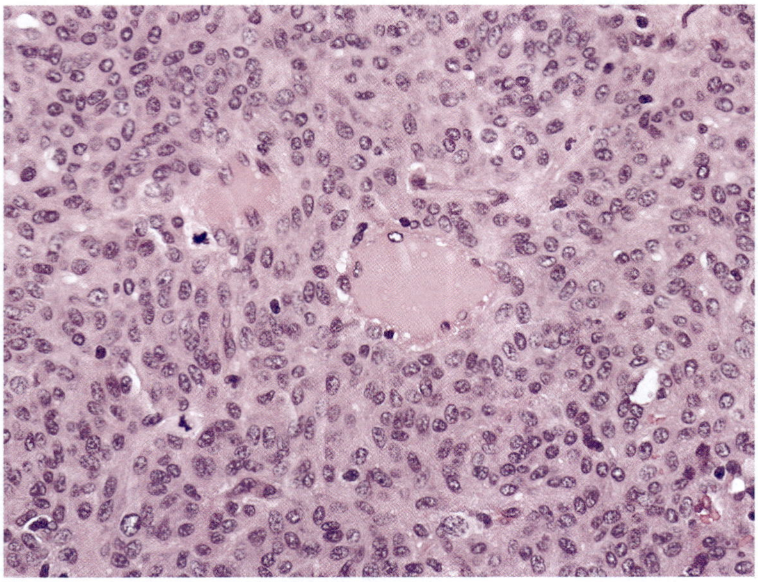

Figure 41-6.
Malignant GIST with two mitotic figures seen in one high power field (another high risk factor).

Table 41-2. Prediction of Aggressiveness of GIST

Group	*Size (cm)*	*Mitotic counts (per 50 HPF)*
Very low risk	<2	<5
Low risk	2 to 5	<5
Intermediate risk	<5	5 to 10
	5 to 10	<5
High risk	>5	>5
	>10	Any
	Any	>10

HPF, high-power field.

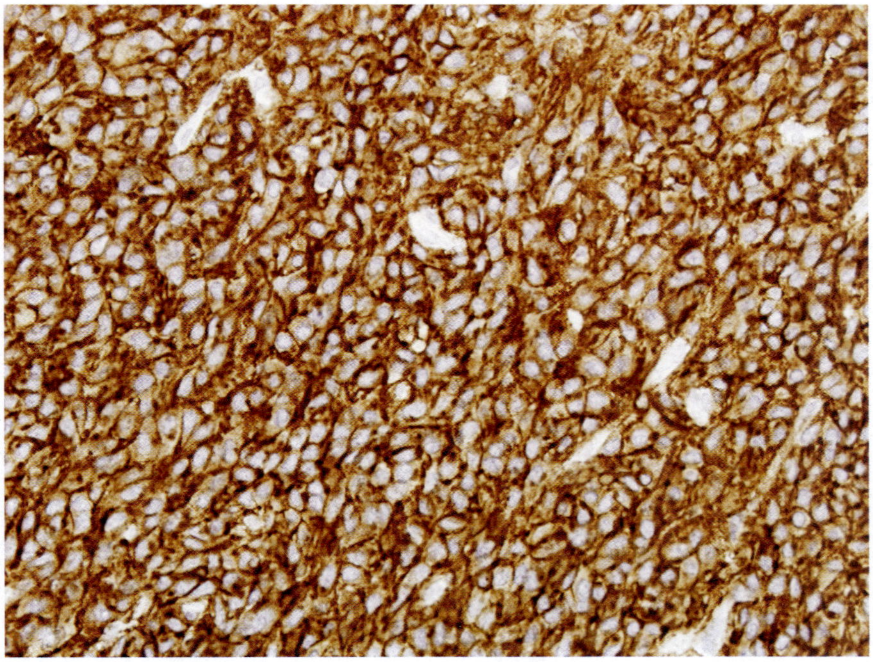

Figure 41-7.
C-kit immunostaining shows the GIST tumor cells are strongly positive for C-kit (membrane staining).

Differential diagnosis

Leiomyoma

- Since the interstitial cell of Cajal is considered to be a special type of smooth muscle cell, the distinction between leiomyoma and GIST can be difficult based on morphology alone
- Leiomyoma cells tend to have more eosinophilic cytoplasm
- Limited mitotic count
- SMA and desmin positive, C-kit (CD-117) and DOG-1 negative

Peripheral nerve sheath tumor

- More pointed nuclei
- C-kit (CD117) and DOG-1 negative
- S100 positive

Spindle cell sarcoma including leiomyosarcoma

- More pleomorphic, more elongated spindle cells (Fig. 41-8)
- Higher mitotic counts
- >5 mitoses per high power field for nonuterine leiomyosarcoma
- >10 mitoses per high power field for uterine leiomyosarcoma
- SMA and desmin positive, C-kit (CD117) and DOG-1 negative

Molecular analysis

- The majority (85%) of GISTs have either C-kit mutations or mutations of platelet-derived growth factor receptor-α (PDGFRA)
- PDGFRA is also a tyrosine kinase; tumors with mutated PDGFRA often have epithelioid morphology
- 10% to 15% of GISTs lack mutations of kit or PDGFRA

Clinical relevance (prognosis and treatment options)

- Important to know the location of the tumor, since uterine leiomyosarcoma, soft tissue leiomyosarcoma, and GISTs use different mitotic cutoffs for their diagnostic criteria
- Prognosis of a GIST is related to the tumor size and its mitotic activity
- Complete surgical excision is indicated
- Specific targeted therapy using tyrosine kinase inhibitors for C-kit or other tyrosine kinases such as imatinib mesylate or sunitinib malate is effective in most cases with C-kit mutations

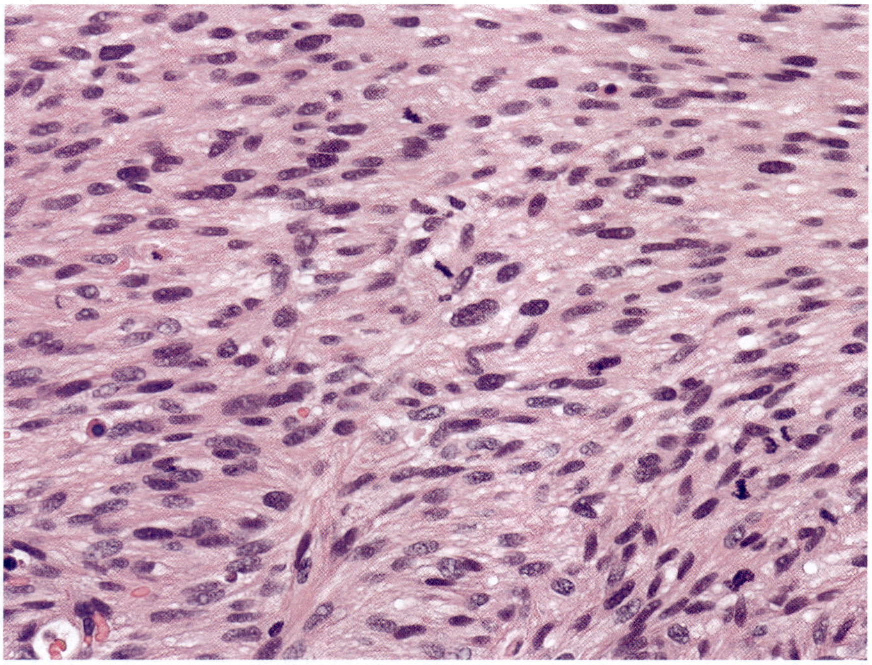

Figure 41-8.
Leiomyosarcoma with numerous mitotic figures in one high power field, which is histologically similar to a malignant GIST in Fig. 41-6. However, leiomyosarcoma is composed of longer spindle cells.

LEIOMYOSARCOMA

Definition

- Malignant mesenchymal neoplasm with smooth muscle differentiation

Clinical features

- Leiomyosarcoma is the most common sarcoma of the kidney accounting for more than half of the renal sarcoma cases
- The tumor more likely arises from the renal capsule than renal parenchyma
- The tumor may also arise in the renal vein, or smooth muscle of the renal pelvis. Patients usually present with flank pain and a mass
- Hematuria may be present if the tumor involves renal parenchyma or pelvis

Gross pathology

- Large mass lesions
- It may involve both renal capsule and parenchyma, so that the origin of the tumor can be difficult to determine. Or it may also involve the renal pelvis mimicking a urothelial tumor
- Cut surface is solid gray-white. Hemorrhage and necrosis are common findings (Fig. 41-9)

Histology

- Tumor may involve renal parenchyma, renal pelvis, or perirenal tissue (Fig. 41-10)
- The tumor is composed of spindle cells with some of the following features (Fig. 41-9*b*)
    - High cellularity
    - Mitotic activity
    - Cytological atypia
- The tumor cells may form fascicular or haphazard growth patterns (Fig. 41-10*b*)
- Other features including necrosis and hemorrhage (Fig. 41-10*c*)
- Invasion of the perinephric adipose tissue or adjacent organs
- Low-grade tumor cells resemble smooth muscle with cigar-shaped nuclei
- High-grade tumor cells are pleomorphic

Immunohistochemistry

- Smooth muscle markers such as smooth muscle actin or muscle specific actin are positive (Fig. 41-10*d*)
- Keratins are negative

Figure 41-9.
Leiomyosarcoma involving renal vein and ureter (*a*). The tumor is composed of malignant smooth muscle cells (*b*).

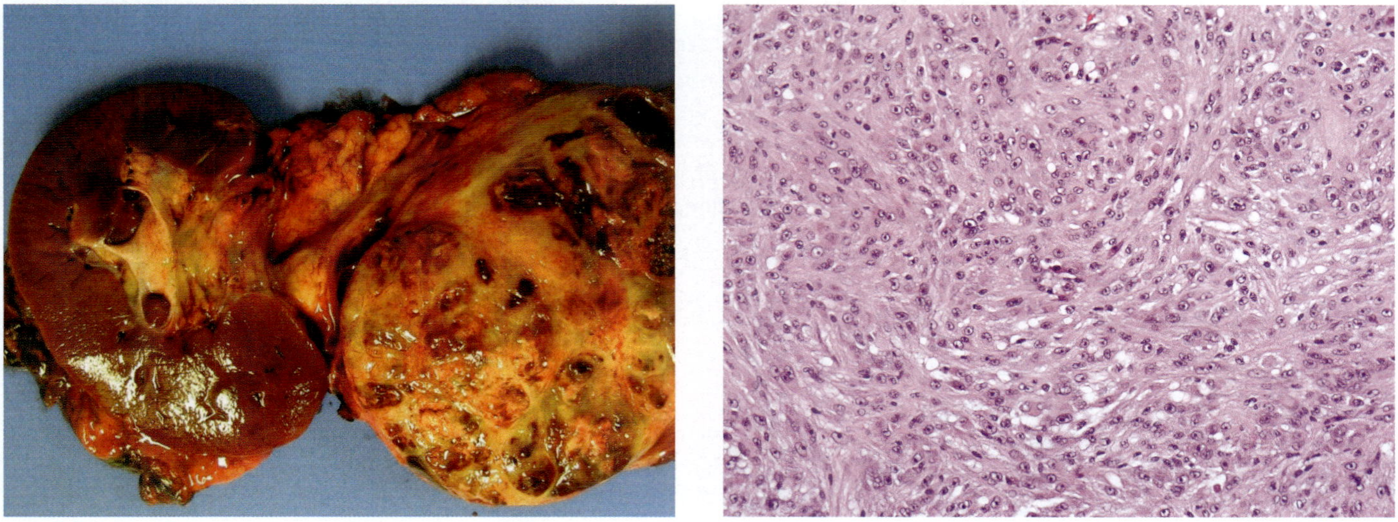

a *b*

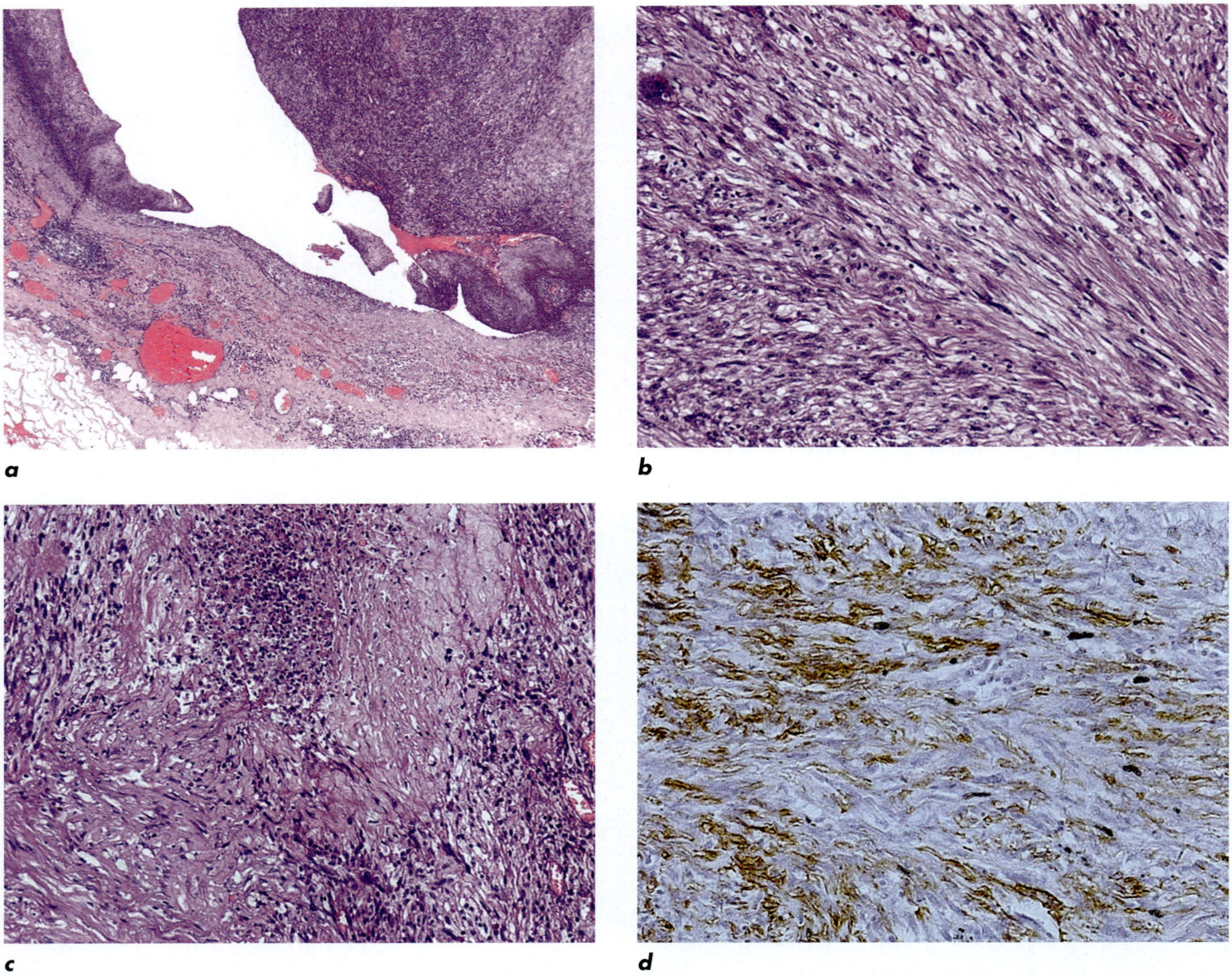

Figure 41-10.
Leiomyosarcoma involving renal pelvis (*a*). The tumor is composed of spindle cells in fascicles with high cellularity, nuclear atypia (*b*), and areas of necrosis (*c*). The tumor cells are positive for smooth muscle actin (*d*).

Differential diagnosis

Sarcomatoid RCC

- Associated with low-grade RCC components
- Most sarcomatoid RCCs are located in the parenchyma
- Keratin immunostains are usually positive in the malignant spindle cells

Other sarcomas

- Lack of smooth muscle differentiation
- Other cell differentiation is evident such as neuronal or lipocytic
- Generally need immunostaining for confirmation

Clinical relevance (prognosis and treatment options)

- The tumor is aggressive with a poor survival rate
- Complete surgical resection is the treatment of choice
- Chemotherapy and radiation have a limited effectiveness

LIPOSARCOMA

Definition

- Malignant mesenchymal neoplasm with lipocytic differentiation
- Renal liposarcoma usually develops in the perinephric adipose tissue

Clinical features

- Flank pain and mass, and, uncommonly, hematuria
- Typically occurs in older patients

Gross pathology

- Lobular mass with white-yellow cut surface
- Retroperitoneal liposarcoma may encase the kidney

Histology

- Low-grade liposarcoma shows the characteristic "chicken-wire" vasculature (Fig. 41-11*a*)
- The diagnosis of liposarcoma requires the presence of significant nuclear atypia of lipocytes
- Atypical lipocytes and lipoblasts with vacuolated cytoplasm are identified (Fig. 41-11*b*)
- Necrosis and hemorrhage can be seen (Fig. 41-12)
- Dedifferentiation is characterized by the presence of high-grade sarcomatous component (Fig. 41-13), morphologically similar to malignant fibrous histiocytoma

Clinical relevance (prognosis and treatment options)

- Treatment of choice is complete surgical resection

Figure 41-11.
Low-grade liposarcoma displays the typical "chicken-wire" vasculature (*a*). The presence of nuclear atypia of lipocytes is diagnostic of liposarcoma. Lipoblasts are often seen (*b*).

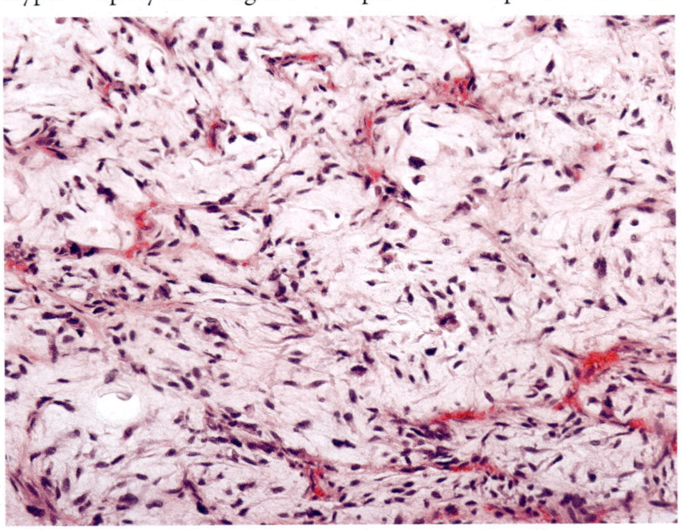

a

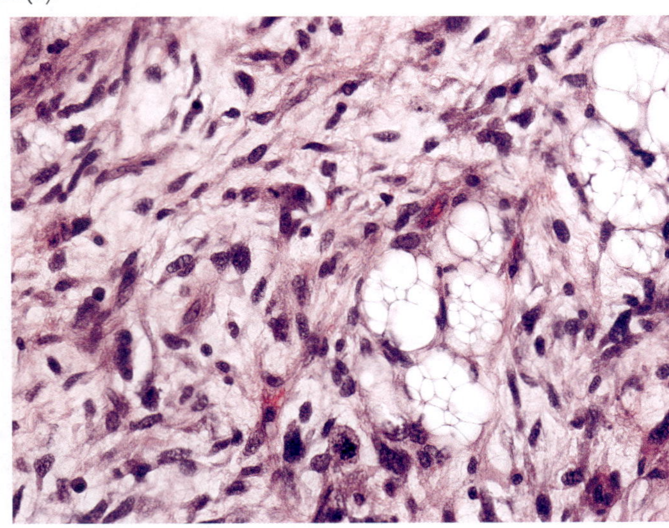

b

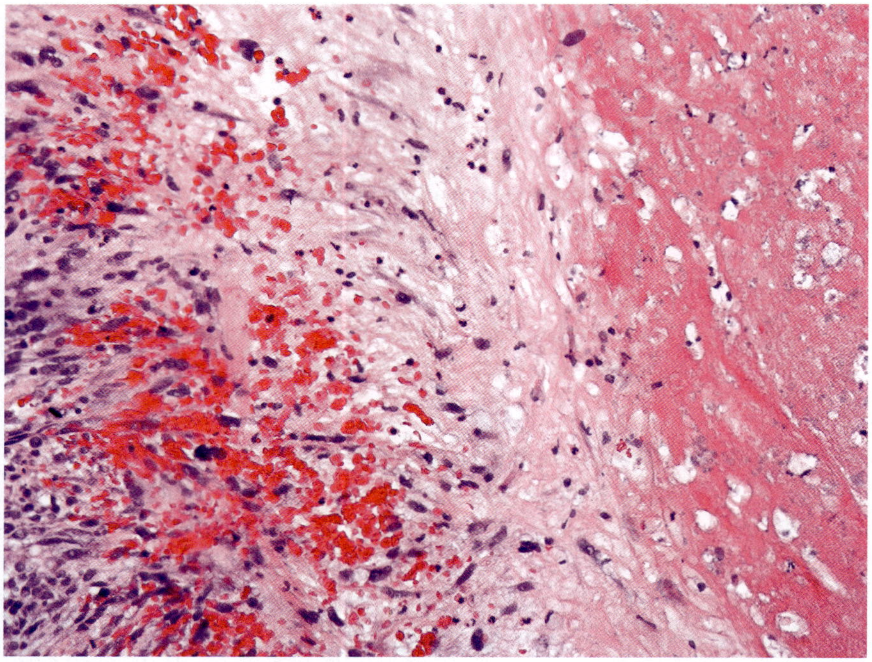

Figure 41-12.
Hemorrhage and necrosis in liposarcoma.

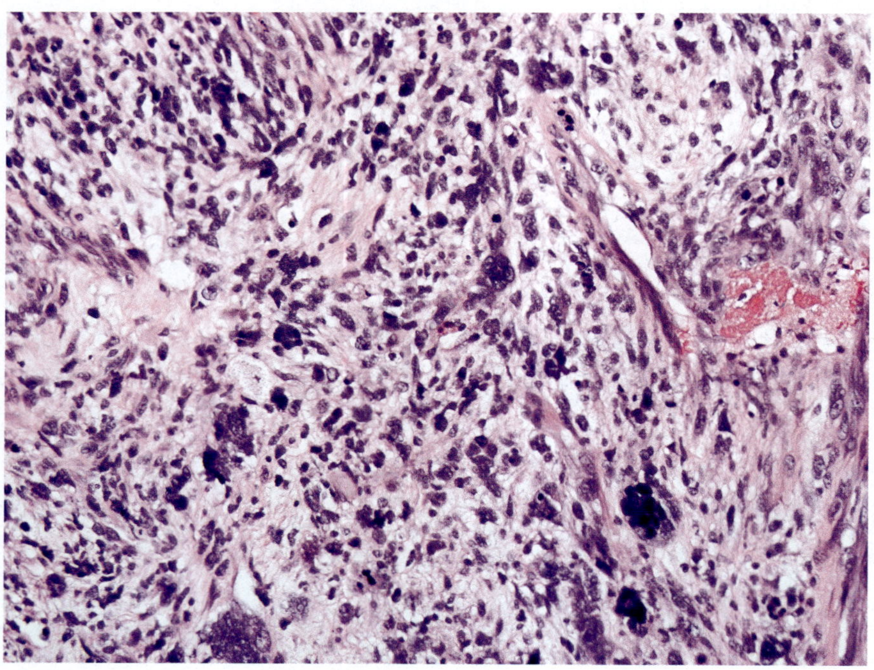

Figure 41-13.
Dedifferentiated liposarcoma is characterized by the presence of high-grade pleomorphic sarcoma in addition to typical low-grade liposarcoma.

SECTION 5
The Renal Pelvis and Ureter

CHAPTER 42 Benign Conditions of the Upper Urinary Tract

RENAL CALCULUS

Definition
- A solid concentration or aggregation of crystals formed in the kidney
- In the vast majority of cases, the stone is actually located in the renal pelvis, or calyces, rather than in the renal parenchyma
- The similar calculi can be seen in the ureter (ureterolithiasis) or bladder (cystolithiasis)

Other terms
- Kidney stone, nephrolithiasis

Pathogenesis
- When urine becomes supersaturated, a crystal seed will be formed as a nucleation
- Chemical deposits from soluble urine (solution) to insoluble material (stones). Different types of stones are summarized in Table 42-1
- PhH changes in urine are important for stone formation
- Absence or lack of sufficient stone formation inhibitors such as citrate contributes to stone formation

Clinical features
- Small calculi will pass through with urine
- Stones larger than 1 to 3 mm may be lodged in the renal pelvis

Table 42-1. Comparison of Different Types of Renal Calculi

Type of calculi	*Frequency*	*Circumstance*
Calcium oxalate	80%	Urine is acid Patients with renal failure
Ammonium magnesium phosphate (struvite)	10% to 15%	Infection
Uric acid	5% to 10%	Urine is acid In patients with gout
Calcium phosphate	Uncommon	Urine is alkaline
Cystine	Rare	Associated with genetic disorders

- If calculi cause urinary obstruction, hydronephrosis will develop
- Infection can be associated with formation of renal calculi
- Typical presentation includes pain (renal colic) with nausea, vomiting, and fever
- Blood or pus in urine
- Imaging studies are diagnostic
- Laboratory test: urine microscopic examination shows the presence of blood cells, crystals, or casts
- Positive culture if infection is associated with a calculus

Gross pathology

- Calculi can be small round and/or large irregular or staghorn shaped (Figs. 42-1 to 42-3)
- The kidney generally shows hydronephrosis if calculi are large and obstructive (Figs. 42-1 and 42-3) and cortical atrophy (Fig. 42-2)

Histology

- Calculi can be subjected to chemical analysis rather than histological analysis
- Chronic pyelonephritis is usually present (Fig. 42-4)
- Calcium oxalate crystals may be seen in the kidney
- Other material will be dissolved during tissue processing
- Reactive urothelial atypia can be prominent in the case with renal calculi (Fig. 42-5)

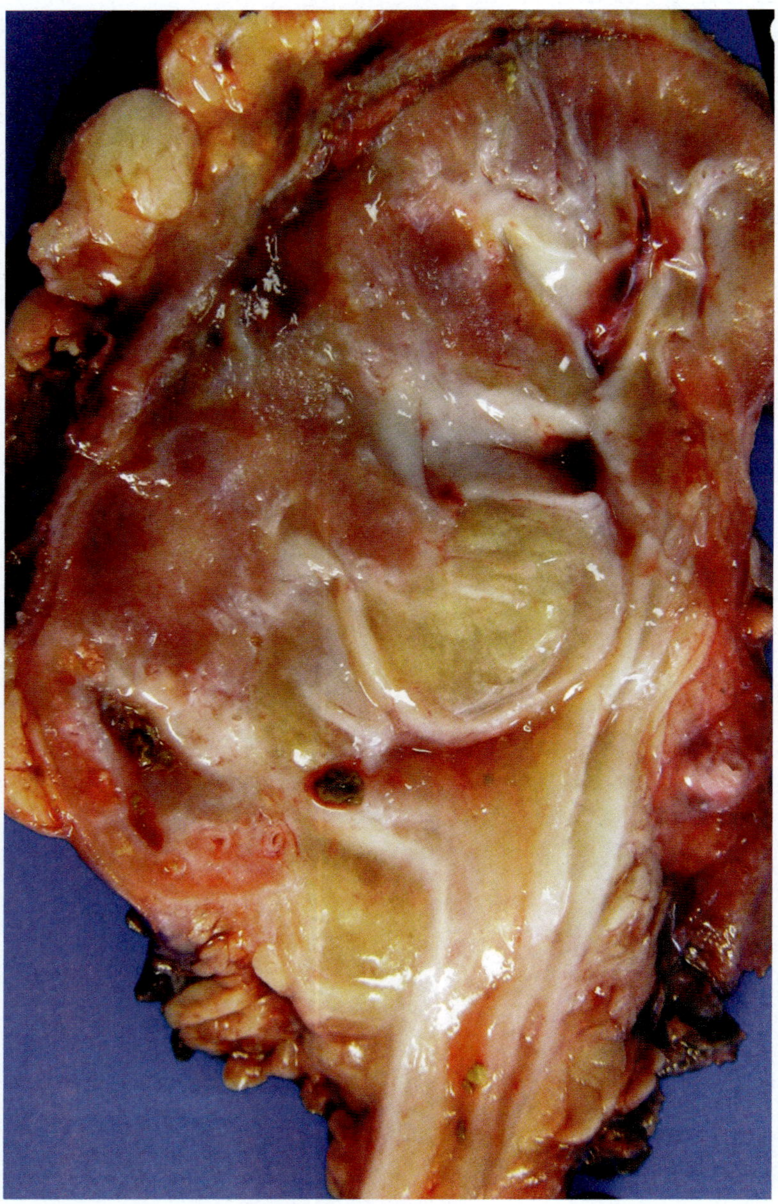

Figure 42-1.
Two small kidney calculi are located in the renal calyces. Hydronephrosis and thickening renal pelvic urothelial mucosa can be seen.

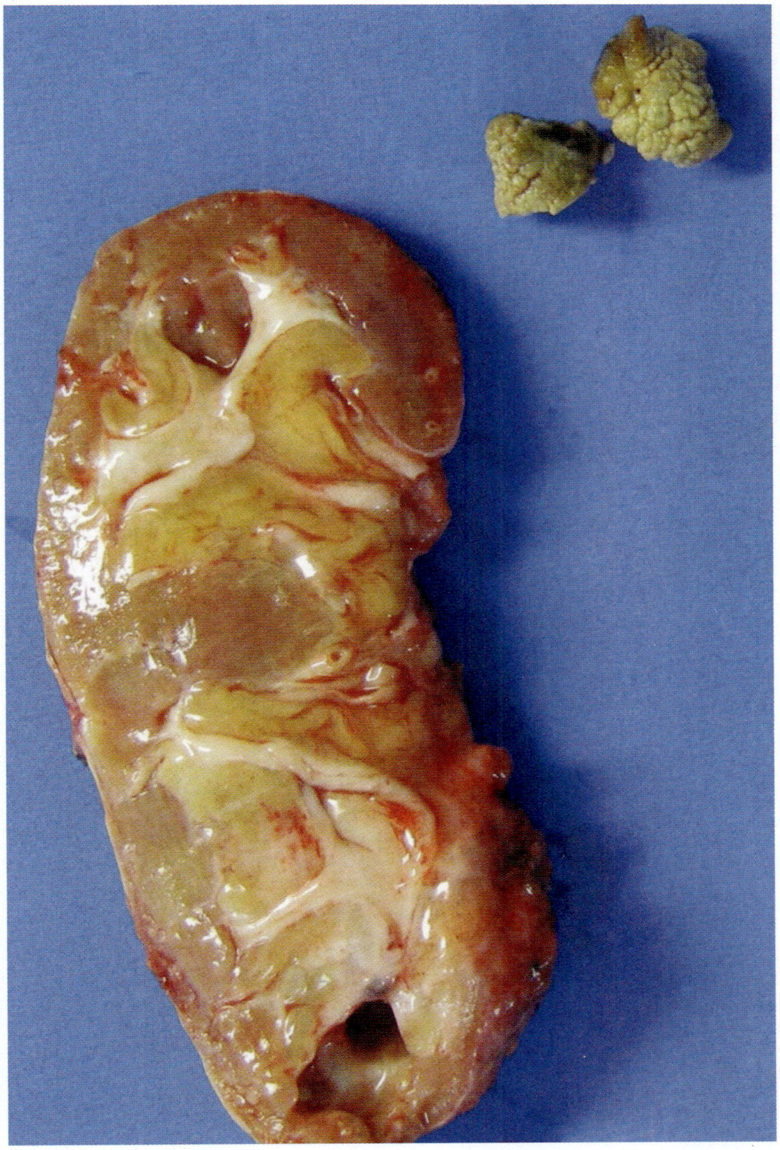

Figure 42-2.
Two large calculi, which were located in the dilated renal calyces, are displayed.

Clinical relevance (prognosis and treatment options)

- Medical treatment: alkalization of urine and diuretics
- Removal of calculi by extracorporeal shock wave lithotripsy or ureteroscopic surgery
- Stones may be associated with infection or neoplastic conditions
- Nephrectomy may be necessary to control those more serious conditions

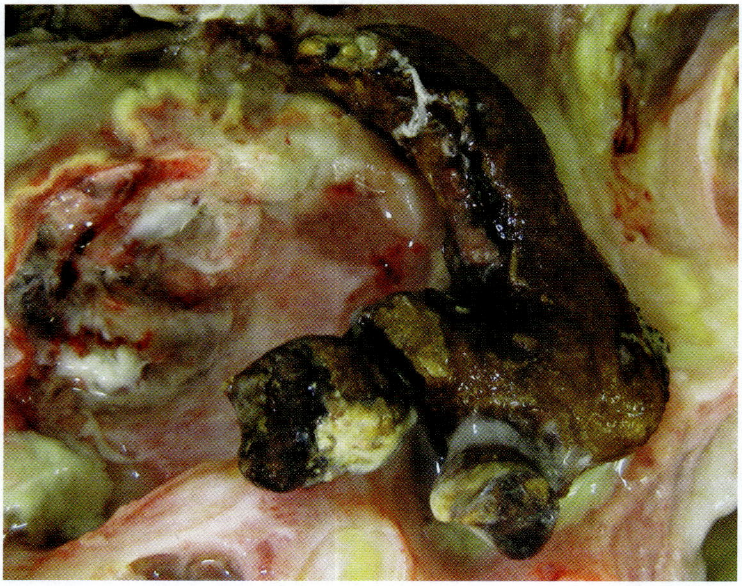

Figure 42-3.
A large staghorn calculus located in the dilated renal pelvis with associated pus (left). Inflammatory exudate can be seen on the surface of dilated renal pelvis.

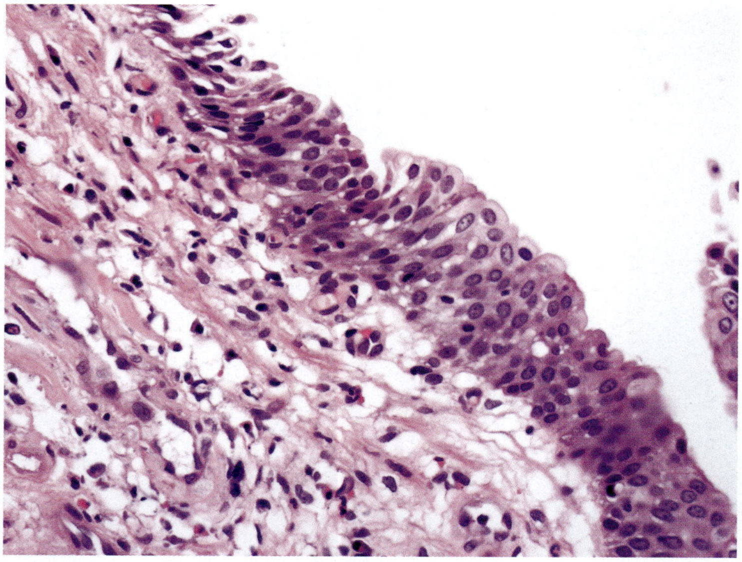

Figure 42-4.
Chronic inflammation of the renal pelvis and reactive urothelium associated with a calculus.

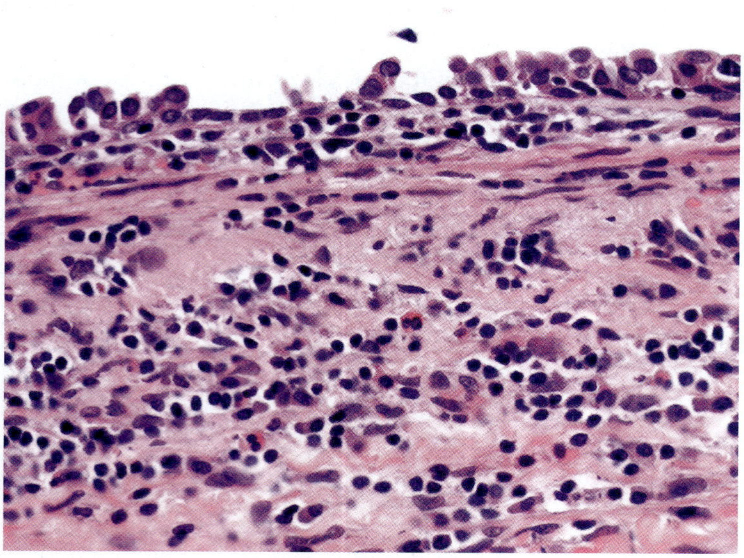

Figure 42-5.
Chronic pyelonephritis and reactive urothelial changes associated with calculus.

HYDRONEPHROSIS

Definition

- Hydronephrosis literally means "water kidney"
- A pathologic condition of dilation and distension of the renal pelvis and calyces caused by downstream urinary obstruction

Pathogenesis

- Obstruction may occur anywhere in the urinary tract, from the urethral meatus to the renal pelvis and calyces
- The common causes for the upper tract obstruction are stones, tumors, inflammation, scarring or an overlying vessel
- The most common obstruction site is the ureteropelvic junction (UPJ)

Clinical features

- Unilateral or bilateral, depending on the location of obstruction
- Obstruction can be complete or partial
- Imaging studies such as an intravenous urogram, retrograde pyelography, ultrasound, MRI, and CT can provide diagnostic information
- Renal function is often retained

Gross pathology

- Dilated renal pelvis (Fig. 42-6)
- Renal parenchyma is compressed (Figs. 42-6 and 42-7*a*) by the pressure from accumulated urine
- Stone, tumor may be identified

Histology

- Urothelium covering dilated renal pelvis and calyces (Fig. 42-7*b*)
- Urothelial surface intact or denuded
- Chronic inflammation of lining urothelium is common regardless of the cause (Figs. 42-8 and 42-9)
- Renal parenchyma is compressed but mostly normal or atrophic (Fig. 42-9*b*)

Clinical relevance (prognosis and treatment options)

- The prognosis of hydronephrosis is variable, depending on the causes
- Generally speaking, unilateral hydronephrosis has a better prognosis if the obstruction cause can be removed surgically
- The key for treatment is to remove the cause of obstruction such as a tumor, a stone, or BPH
- Drainage of the urine with a catheter can achieve temporary relief

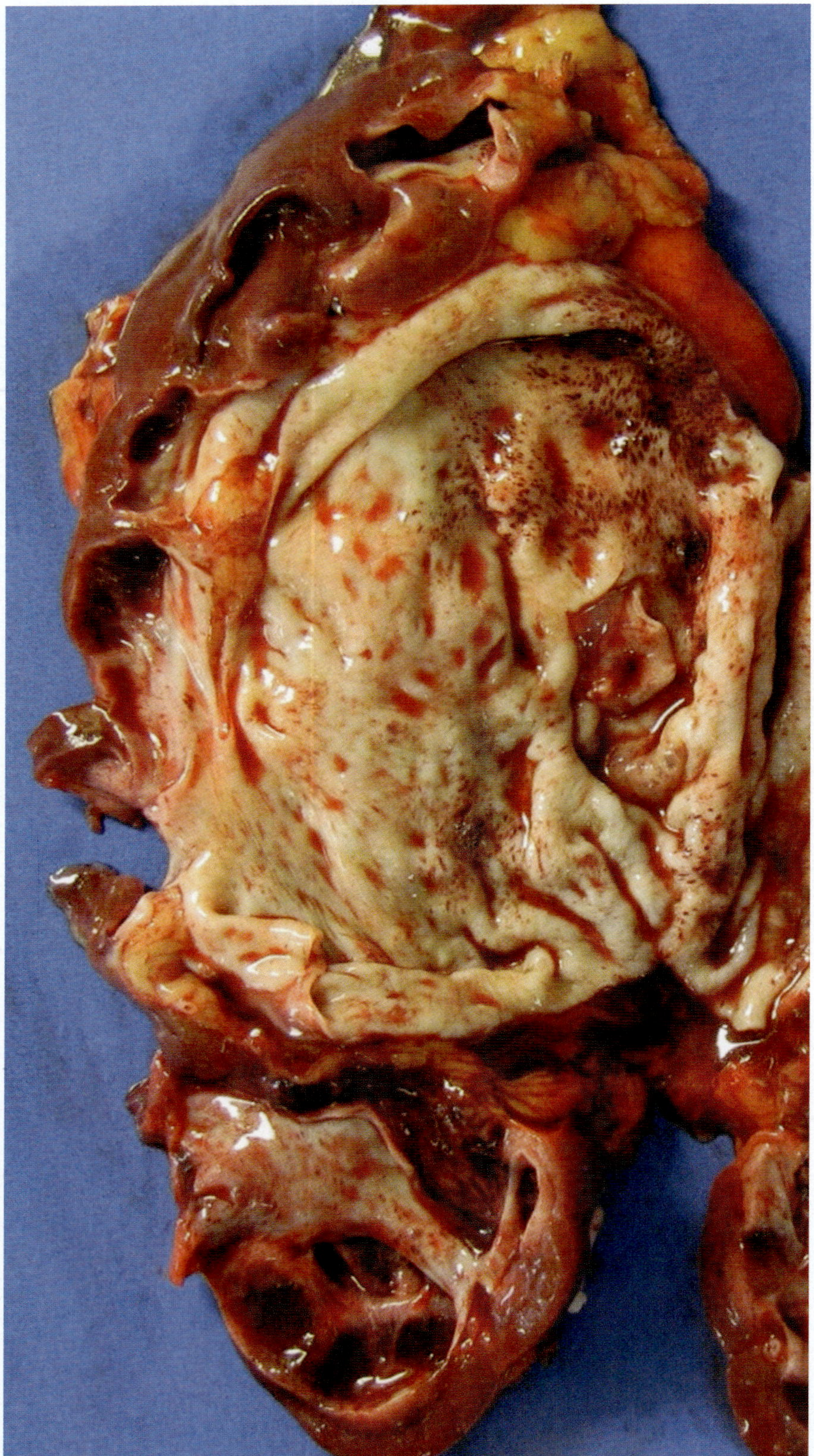

Figure 42-6.
Hydronephrosis with severely dilated renal pelvis. The kidney parenchyma is distorted and atrophic.

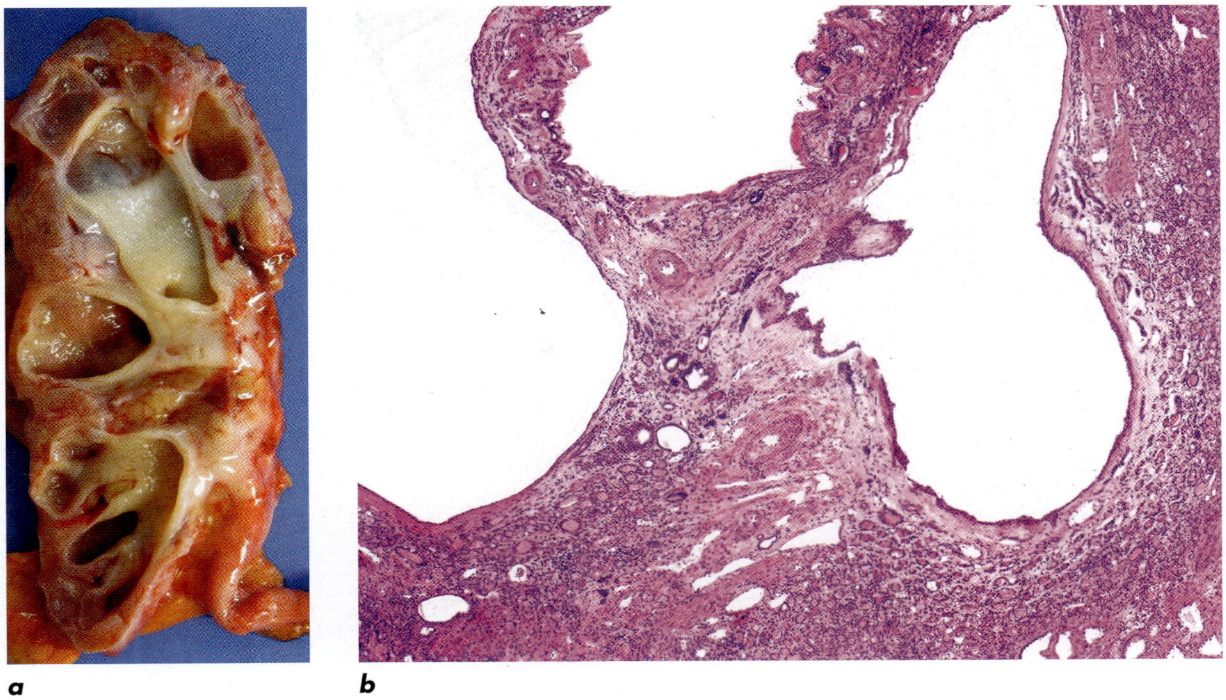

Figure 42-7.
Hydronephrosis shows severely dilated renal pelvis. The urothelial mucosa is thickened and the renal parenchyma is atrophic (*a*). Microscopically, the dilated pelvis/calyces compressing the renal cortex (*b*).

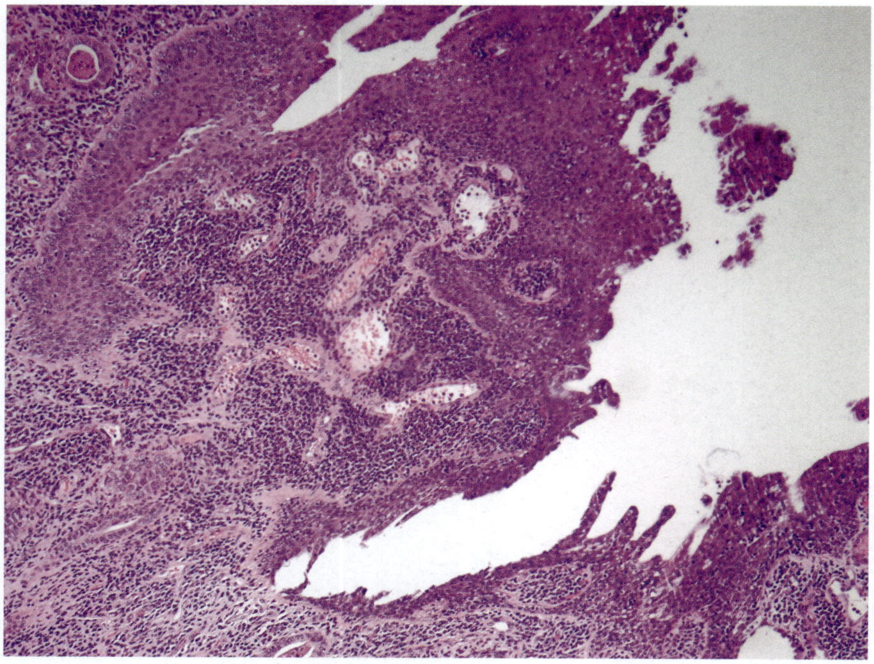

Figure 42-8.
Hydronephrosis associated with severe chronic pyelonephritis.

Figure 42-9.
Hydronephrosis associated with chronic pyelonephritis involving both renal pelvis (*a*) and renal cortex, which is showing features of glomerulosclerosis (*b*).

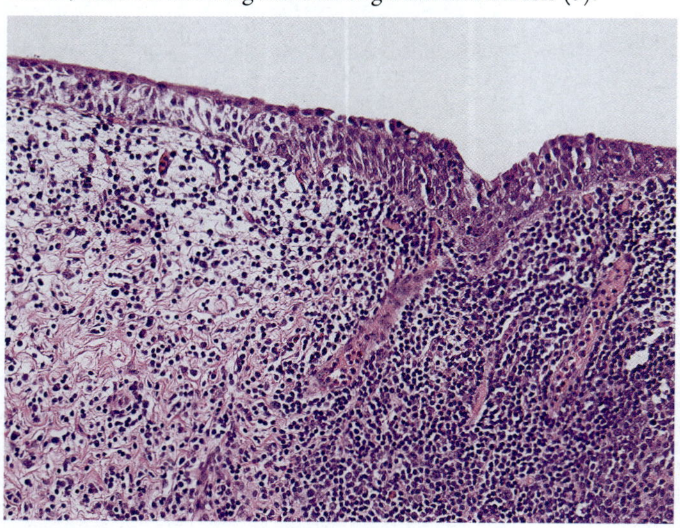

a

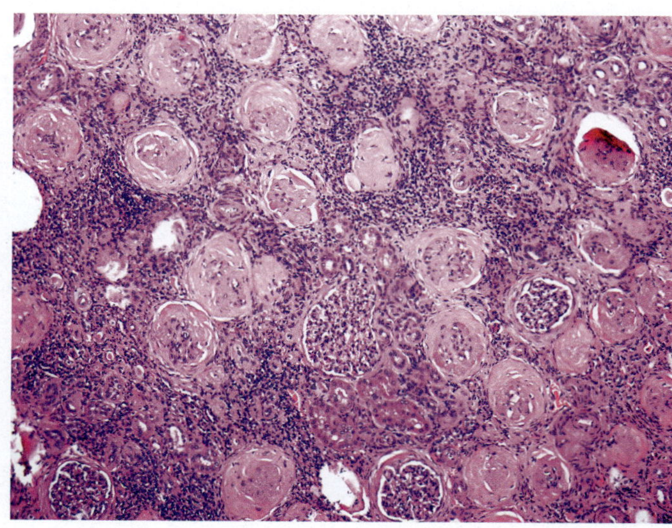

b

REACTIVE UROTHELIAL CHANGES OF UPPER URINARY TRACT

Definition

- Almost all the reactive changes of urothelium present in the bladder can be seen in the upper urinary tract. Only a few common lesions will be discussed in this chapter

Pathogenesis

- These lesions are reactive in nature, they develop in response to chronic or acute stimuli to urothelium

Clinical features

- Most of the patients with these reactive lesions may be asymptomatic
- Some patients may have symptoms associated with carcinoma, stones, or other more severe pathological conditions
- Other nonspecific symptoms include hematuria, pain, or infection

Gross pathology

- Mostly not grossly visible
- Or small granular, papillary, or dome-shaped lesions

Histology

Intestinal metaplasia

- Benign glandular structures undergoing colonic metaplasia in urothelium (Fig. 42-10)
- May or may not be associated with chronic inflammation
- It may be a precursor lesion for adenocarcinoma

Florid von Brunn nests

- Von Brunn nests are reactive urothelial cells residing in a confined nest (Fig. 42-11)
- Florid von Brunn nests are characterized by the presence of numerous benign solid nests of urothelial cells in lamina propria of renal pelvis or ureter. The cells have minimal cytological atypia

Nephrogenic adenoma

- Small clusters of glandular epithelial cells present (Fig. 42-12)
- It is a benign reactive change in response to urothelial injury such as stone, catheterization, or prior biopsy
- In most cases, these glandular epithelial cells represent implanted renal tubules

Clinical relevance (prognosis and treatment options)

- Benign reactive conditions
- No treatment unless it is symptomatic
- Histologically, these reactive lesions should not be confused with neoplastic conditions

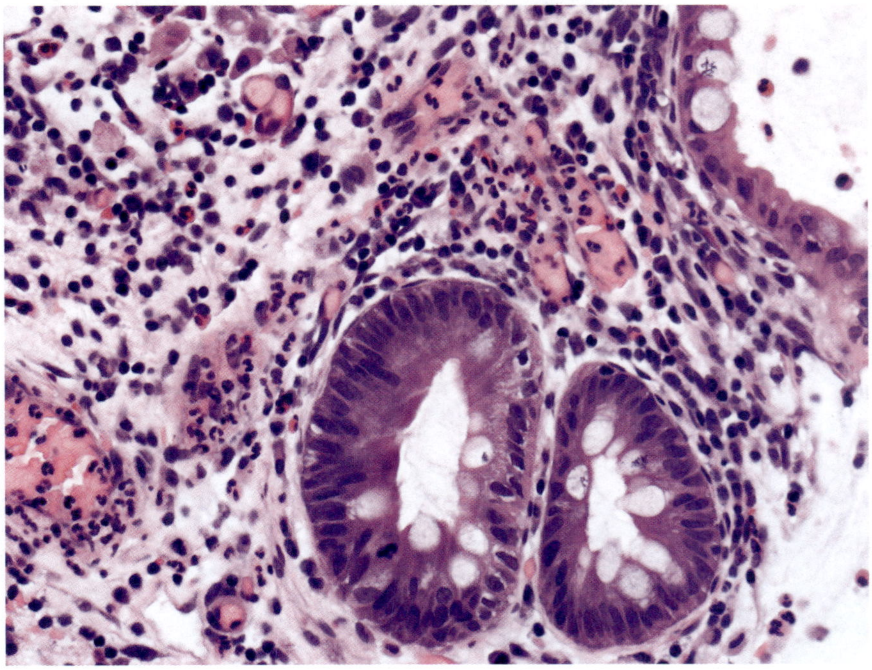

Figure 42-10.
Colonic metaplasia present in the renal pelvis, associated chronic inflammation is apparent.

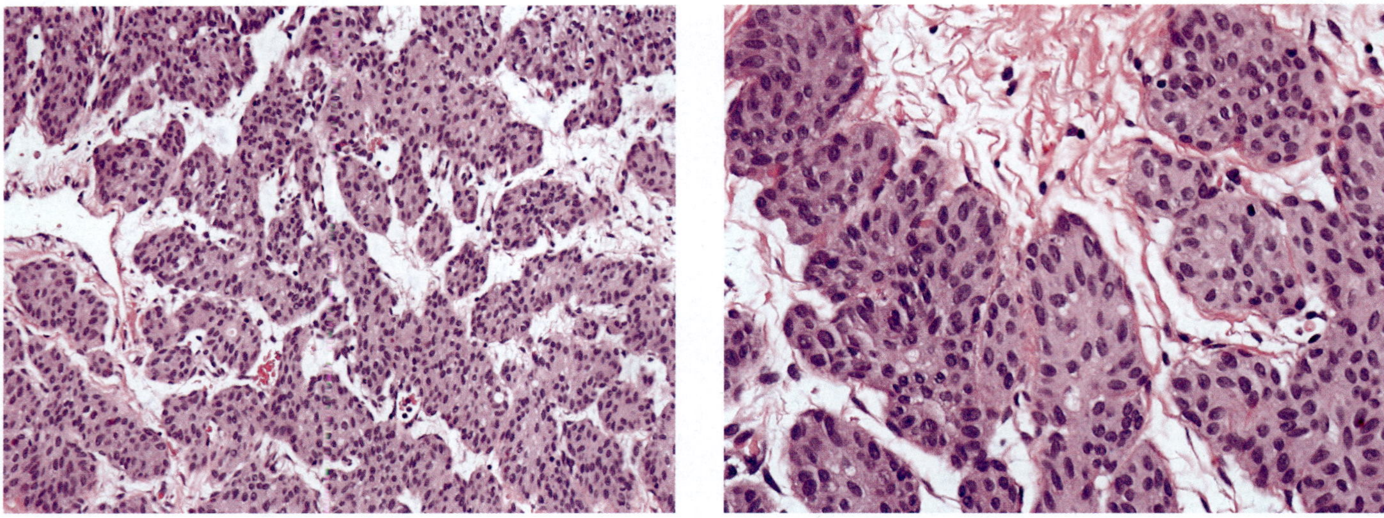

a b

Figure 42-11.
Florid von Brunn nests present in the lamina propria of renal pelvis. The solid nests of benign urothelial cells are separated by edematous stroma (*a*). High magnification shows the urothelial cells with bland cytological features and nuclear groove. No mitosis or obvious nuclear atypia is seen (*b*).

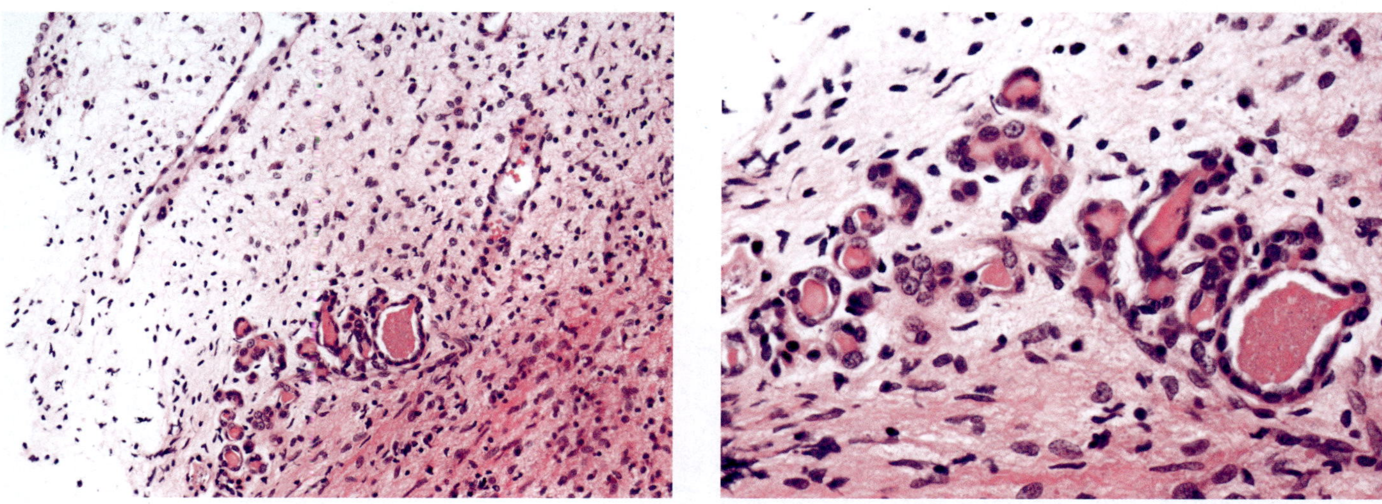

a b

Figure 42-12.
Nephrogenic adenoma of renal pelvis is characterized by the presence of small cluster of glandular structures in the lamina propria (*a*). High magnification shows the glandular structures are lined by a single layer of cuboidal epithelial cells with pink secretion in the lumen (*b*) (which may be considered mesonephric remnants).

INVERTED PAPILLOMA

Definition

- Inverted papilloma of the renal pelvis is characterized by the presence of islands of benign neoplastic urothelial cells in a predominantly inverted (endophytic) fashion

Clinical features

- Hematuria
- Small lesions in the renal pelvis or ureter

Gross pathology

- Dome-shaped or flat lesions in the renal pelvis or ureter
- Typically smaller than 3 cm

Histology

- Predominantly endophytic growth patterns (Fig. 42-13)
- Islands of urothelial nests separated by fibrovascular septa or cores (Fig. 42-13) with peripheral palisading (Fig. 42-14)
- No significant cytological atypia

Clinical relevance (prognosis and treatment options)

- Local resection if symptomatic
- No radical resection such as nephrectomy is indicated
- Although the lesion is benign, it may recur in a small subset of cases

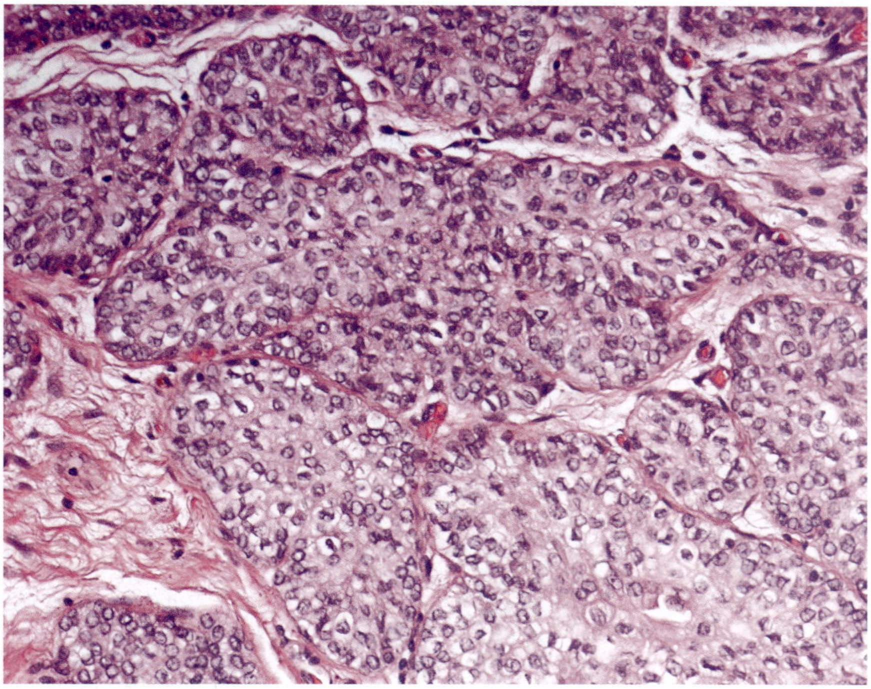

Figure 42-13.
Inverted papilloma. The islands of tumor cells have smooth borders separated by thin fibrovascular cores, which gives the appearance of "jigsaw puzzle." No obvious cytological atypia is seen.

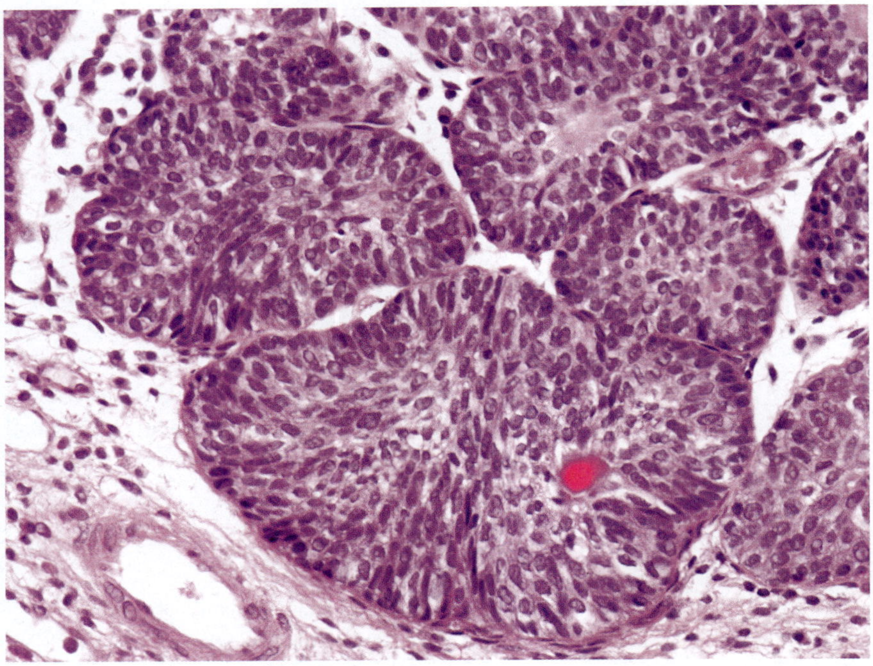

Figure 42-14.
Inverted papilloma consisting of large nests of tumor cells in the lamina propria with peripheral palisading and occasional spindle appearance.

MUCINOUS CYSTADENOMA OF THE RENAL PELVIS

Definition

- A benign mucinous neoplasm develops in the renal pelvis, growing along the urothelial lining without invasion

Pathogenesis

- Neoplastic transformation may be related to the presence of intestinal metaplasia of the urothelium

Clinical features

- Urinary obstruction symptoms, which may be associated with signs of infection
- Mucinous material in urine
- Imaging studies showing the hydronephrosis
- Negative urine cytology, but benign neoplastic glandular cells may be seen in urine

Gross pathology

- Dilated renal pelvis and calyces, similar hydronephrosis caused by the pyelonephritis (Fig. 42-15)
- Mucinous material on the surface urothelium (Fig. 42-15)

Histology

- Hydronephrosis containing large amount of mucinous material. The urothelial lining may be denuded (Fig. 42-16*a* and 42-16*b*)
- Pseudostratified tall columnar cells similar to tubular adenoma of the colon, replacing the urothelial lining. (Fig. 42-16*c*)

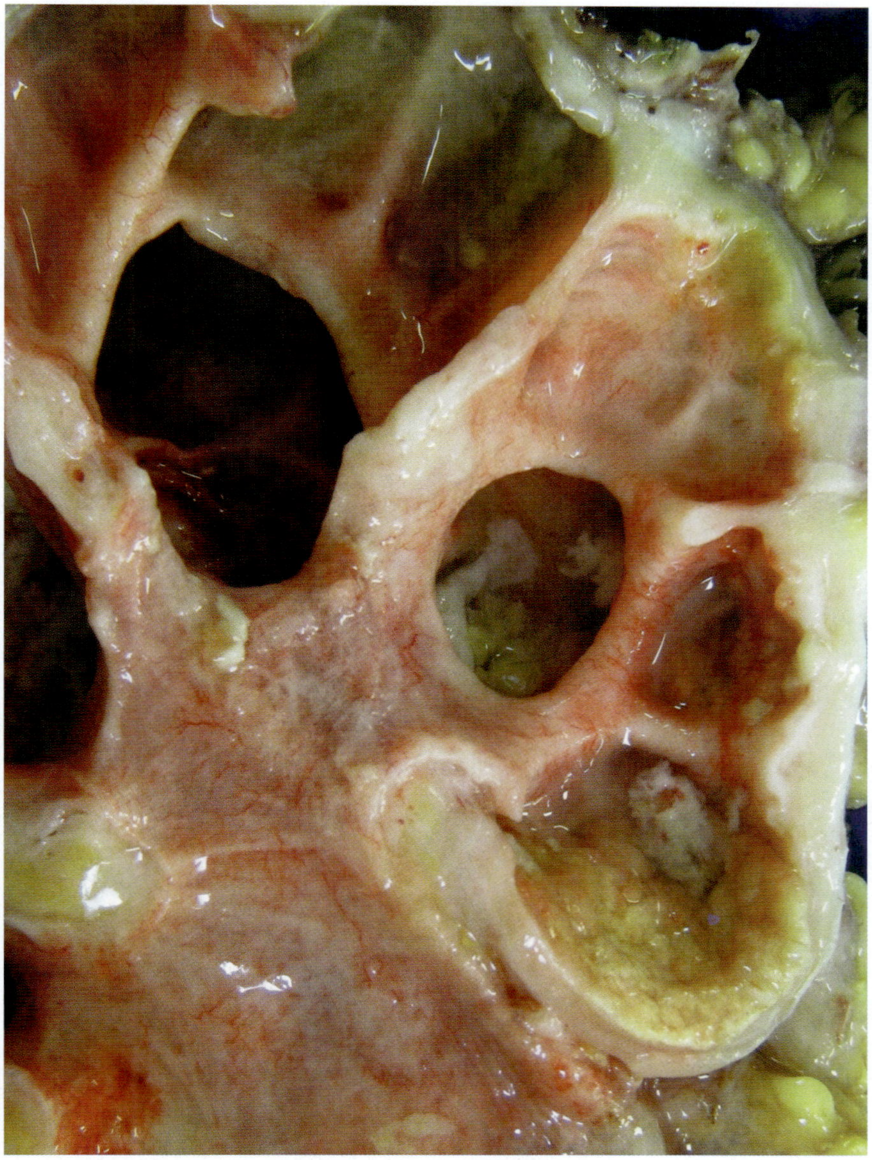

Figure 42-15.
Mucinous cystadenoma of the renal pelvis demonstrates dilated renal pelvis with a smooth surface and partially covered with mucinous material.

- Secondary chronic inflammation with numerous mucin-laden macrophages (Fig. 42-16*d*)
- Tumor cells are confined within the basement membrane, but may possibly spread to the urothelial lining of renal calyces or ureter
- Invasive adenocarcinoma can develop in the background of adenomatous neoplasms. Ample sampling and careful examination are warranted to exclude the presence of carcinoma

Immunohistochemistry

- CK20 and CK7 positive, and CDX2 positive
- P53 negative

Clinical relevance (prognosis and treatment options)

- Neoplastic lesion will lead to loss of renal function and requires nephrectomy
- Benign condition with a good prognosis after surgery
- Malignant transformation to mucinous carcinoma has been reported, but is extremely rare

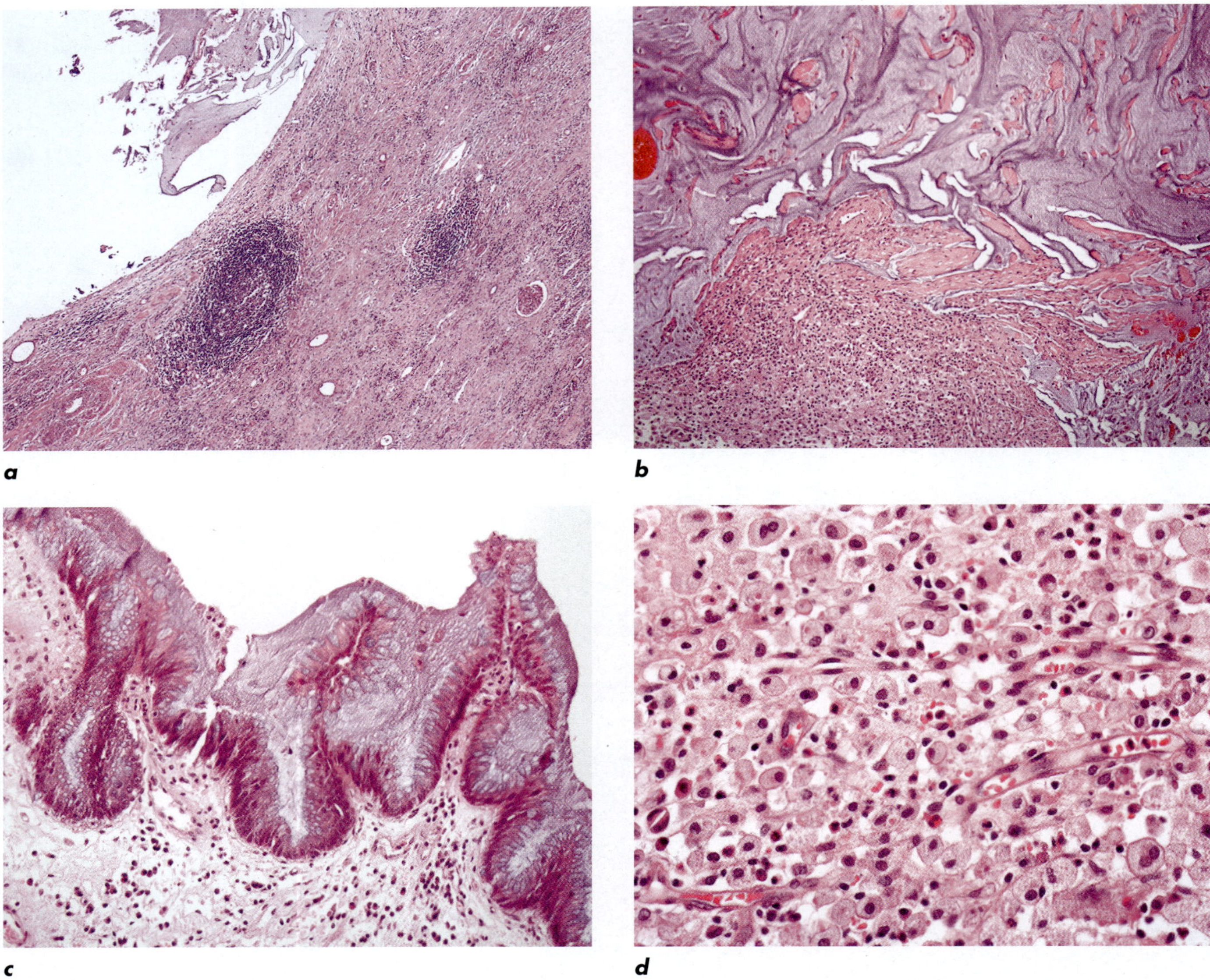

Figure 42-16.
Microscopically, mucinous cystadenoma of the renal pelvis shows the renal pelvic mucosa partially denuded with chronic inflammation (*a*) and acellular mucinous material on the surface (*b*). The lining columnar cells show dysplastic changes similar to a tubular adenoma of the colon, which is diagnostic (*c*). A large number of mucin-laden macrophages (mucinophages) are present (*d*).

CHAPTER 43

Malignant Neoplasms of the Upper Urinary Tract

UROTHELIAL CARCINOMA IN SITU

Definition

- High-grade noninvasive, urothelial carcinoma develops in the upper urinary tract including renal pelvis, calyces, or ureter

Other terms

- Transitional cell carcinoma, high-grade urothelial dysplasia, or severe urothelial dysplasia

Clinical features

- Hematuria, positive cytology
- May be detected by imaging studies as an incidental finding

Gross pathology

- Ureteroscopic findings are negative for a mass lesion
- Urothelial carcinoma in situ (CIS) is an erythematous flat lesion, although the change is nonspecific

Histology

- Flat lesion without papillary configuration
- Tumor cells present within the basement membrane, no invasion can be identified (Fig. 43-1)
- Tumor cells with high-grade cytology, including hyperchromasia, a high N/C ratio, prominent nuclear enlargement, which is four times greater than the diameter of a small lymphocyte (Fig. 43-2)
- Diagnosis of CIS is based on cytologic features, not full thickness involvement
- Tumor cells may involve von Brunn nests (Fig. 43-3) or a pagetoid spread

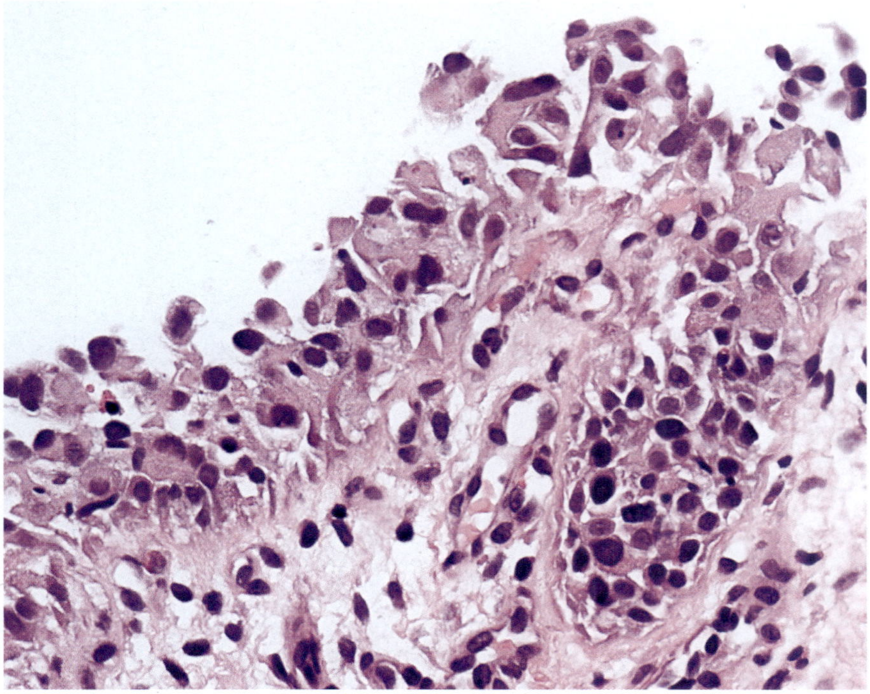

Figure 43-1.
Urothelial carcinoma in situ (CIS) of the renal pelvis is characterized by the presence of highly atypical urothelial carcinoma cells confined within the urothelium.

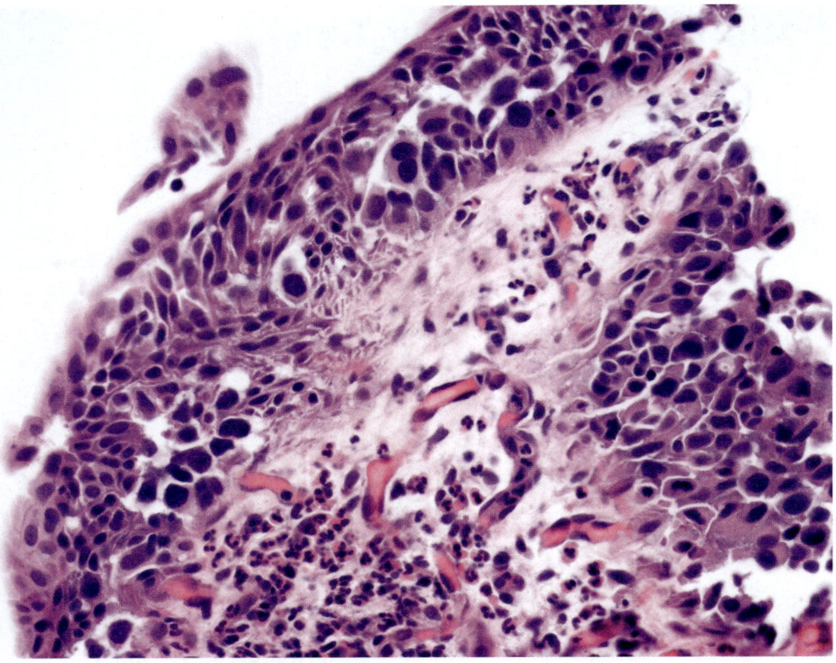

Figure 43-2.
Urothelial CIS with tumor cells showing hyperchromatic nuclei in pagetoid spread.

Figure 43-3.
Urothelial carcinoma in situ of the renal pelvis involving the surface urothelium and a von Brunn nest (*a*). High magnification shows that some of the cells in this von Brunn nest are magnificent (*b*).

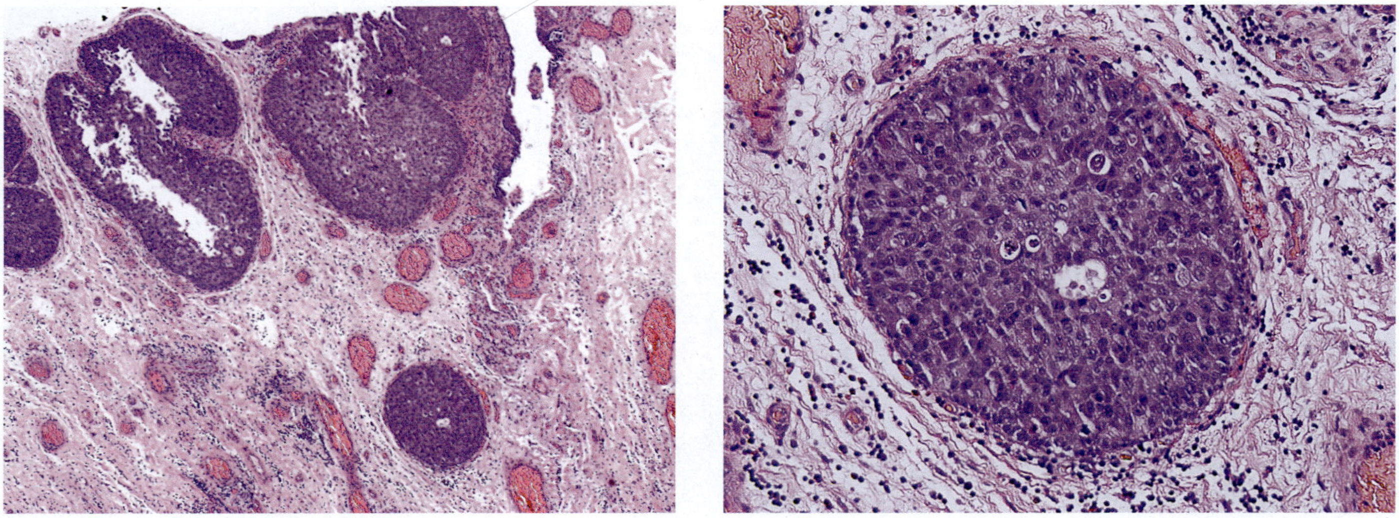

a **b**

- Tumor cells of the renal pelvis may also involve renal tubules (Fig. 43-4) and/or renal stroma
- Sometimes, papillary urothelial carcinoma and urothelial carcinoma in situ can coexist
- Because the biopsy material can be very small, caution in diagnosis of malignancy is warranted

Immunohistochemistry

- CIS positive for p53 and diffusely positive for CK20
- Ki67 proliferative activity high, and CD44 negative

Clinical relevance (prognosis and treatment options)

- Possible local treatment with BCG for CIS of the upper GU tract
- Nephrectomy with ureterectomy is an option for definitive treatment

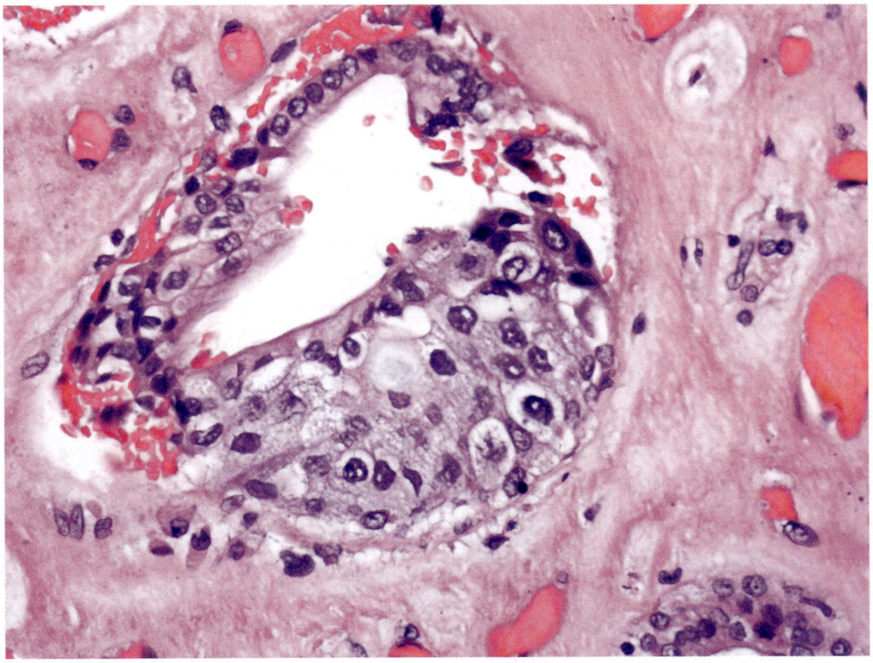

Figure 43-4.
Urothelial carcinoma in situ of the renal pelvis involving a renal collecting duct.

NONINVASIVE LOW-GRADE PAPILLARY UROTHELIAL CARCINOMA

Definition

- Low-grade papillary urothelial carcinoma without invasion develops in the renal pelvis, calyces, or ureter

Other terms

- Low-grade transitional cell carcinoma, grade I transitional cell carcinoma

Pathogenesis

- Typically, low-grade noninvasive papillary urothelial carcinoma is the early phase of cancer, which may progress to invasive and/or high-grade urothelial carcinoma if untreated
- It can also coexist with urothelial carcinoma of the lower urinary tract. The upper tract tumors more frequently involve the lower tract, while the lower tract tumors infrequently involve the upper tract
- The molecular, biological, and biochemical evidences suggest that the coexisting lower tract urothelial carcinoma in this situation is most likely caused by the seeding of the upper tract tumor
- The field effect (multifocal origin of the upper and low tract tumors) is possible, but less common

Clinical features

- Hematuria
- Positive or atypical cytology and negative bladder findings by cystoscopic examination
- Imaging or ureteroscopic studies may show mass lesions
- Obstruction and hydronephrosis may be present

Gross pathology

- Ranging from small granular lesions, papillary lesions to polypoid masses (Fig. 43-5)
- Typically the mass does not involve renal parenchyma

Histology

- Papillary configurations with the presence of branching papilla (Figs. 43-5*b*, 43-6, and 43-7)
- Large nests of cells with fibrovascular cores (inverted growth patterns) (Fig. 43-5*c*)
- Multilayered low-grade tumor cells covering the papilla have cytological features such as low N/C ratio and mild atypia (Figs. 43-6 and 43-7*b*)
- In a small biopsy specimen, the diagnosis can be difficult (Fig. 43-8)

Immunohistochemistry

- CK20 positive, but limited value

Molecular analysis

- Similar to bladder urothelial carcinoma
- Some genetic differences between the upper tract and low tract urothelial carcinomas have been reported in the literature
- However, the differences may be created by the presence of different stromal components in the specimens rather than a true biological significance
- So far there is no convincing evidence that the upper tract urothelial carcinoma is genetically or biochemically different from bladder urothelial carcinoma, although the former is biologically more aggressive

Clinical relevance (prognosis and treatment options)

- The upper tract urothelial carcinomas are generally considered more aggressive than the low tract ones, probably because of the anatomic location with thin walls of the renal pelvis and ureter, which provides little protection from tumor invasion
- In the upper urinary tract, muscle invasion is not the only indication for a radical resection, because of the aggressive nature of the disease
- Reactive changes have to be considered in differential diagnosis, particularly in a patient with a history of renal calculi or catheters
- The diagnosis is challenging for the following reasons:
    - The limited specimen
    - Low-grade nature of the tumor, difficult to distinguish from reactive changes
    - Muscularis propria invasion may not be required for a radical surgery such as nephrectomy or ureterectomy
    - CIS, noninvasive low-grade and invasive high-grade tumors can all be considered for surgical candidates
- Segmental resections of the ureter have been attempted in some cases of small ureteral tumors with success
- Local treatments such as BCG and segmental resection of the ureter can be options but success rates are uncertain
- Therefore, the diagnosis of upper tract carcinoma should be cautiously, because of the possible consequence of major surgical procedures
- Similar to bladder cancer, stages T1a (noninvasive) and Tis (carcinoma in situ)

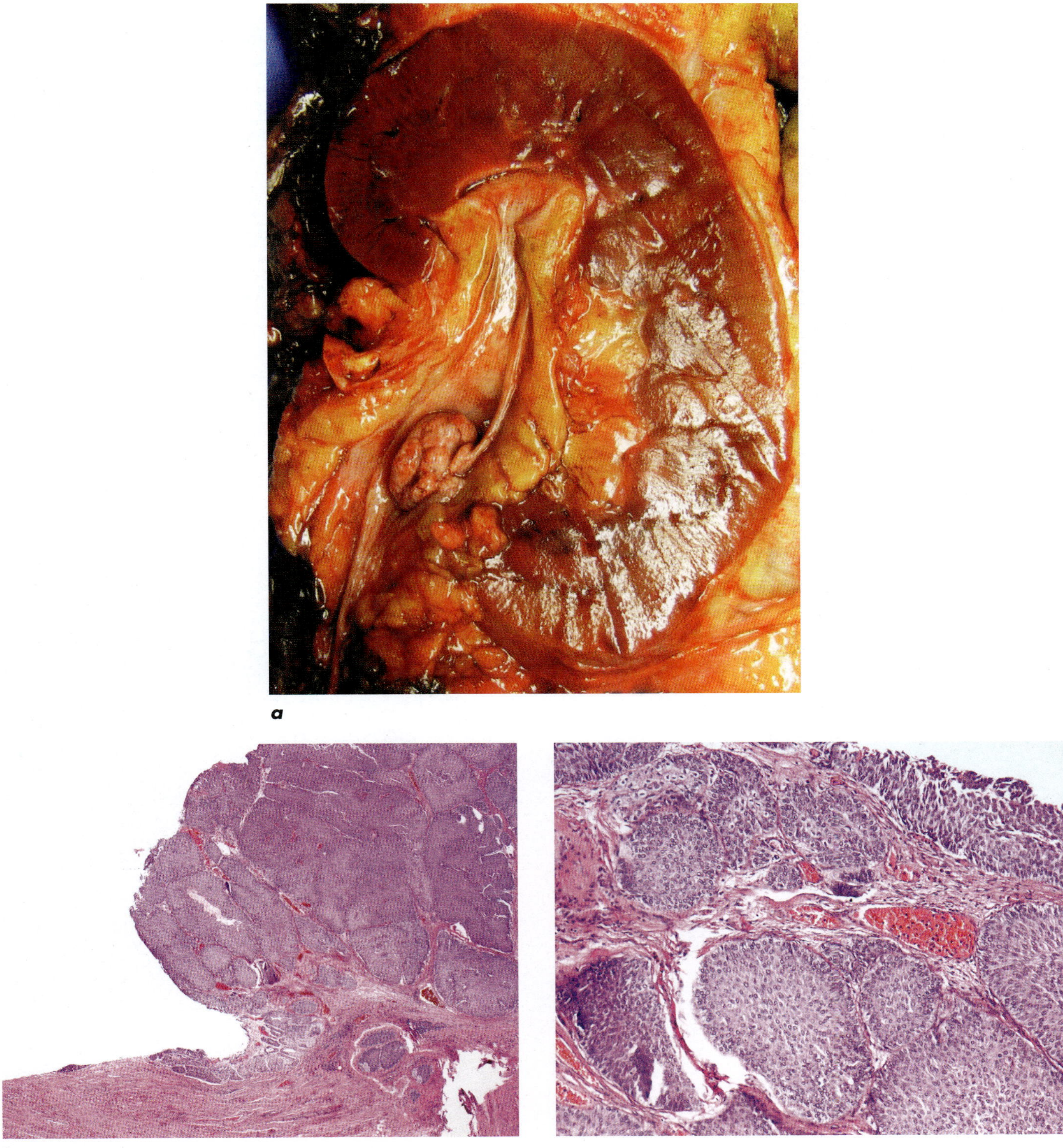

Figure 43-5.
Papillary urothelial carcinoma in the ureter-pelvic junction (UPJ) as a papillary mass growing in the lumen (*a*). Microscopically, the tumor is composed of large nests of tumor cells with both exophytic (papillary) and endophytic (inverted) growth patterns (*b*). The tumor cells are low-grade with no invasion seen (*c*).

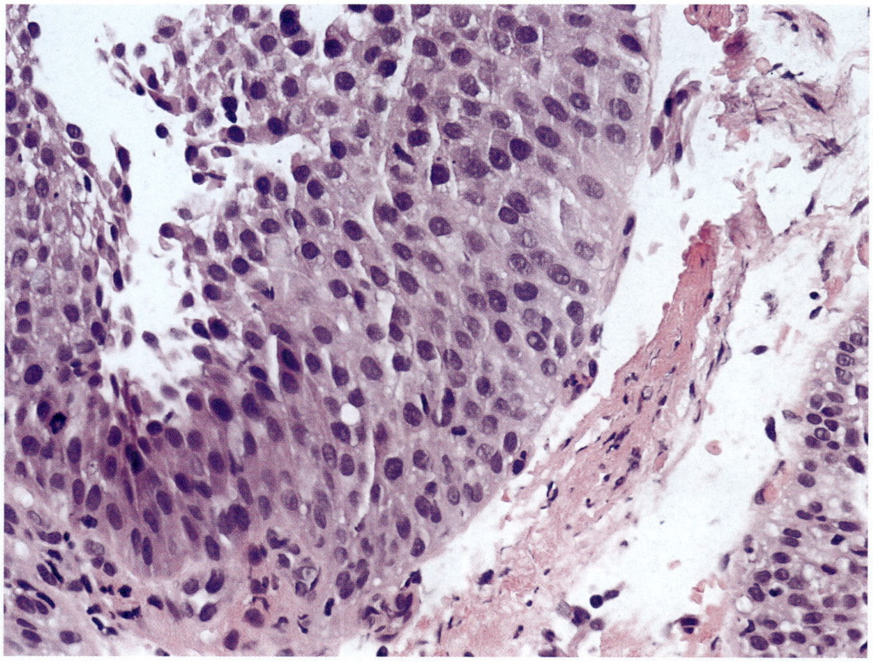

Figure 43-6.
Low-grade urothelial carcinoma of the renal pelvis in a biopsy specimen. The tumor cells form thickened layers with mild cytological atypia. The presence of fibrovascular cores that separate the tumor cell nests can be appreciated.

Figure 43-7.
Low-grade urothelial carcinoma in a ureteral biopsy containing small fragments of papillary urothelial carcinoma (*a*). Branching papilla are covered by tumor cells with mild to moderate cytological atypia (*b*).

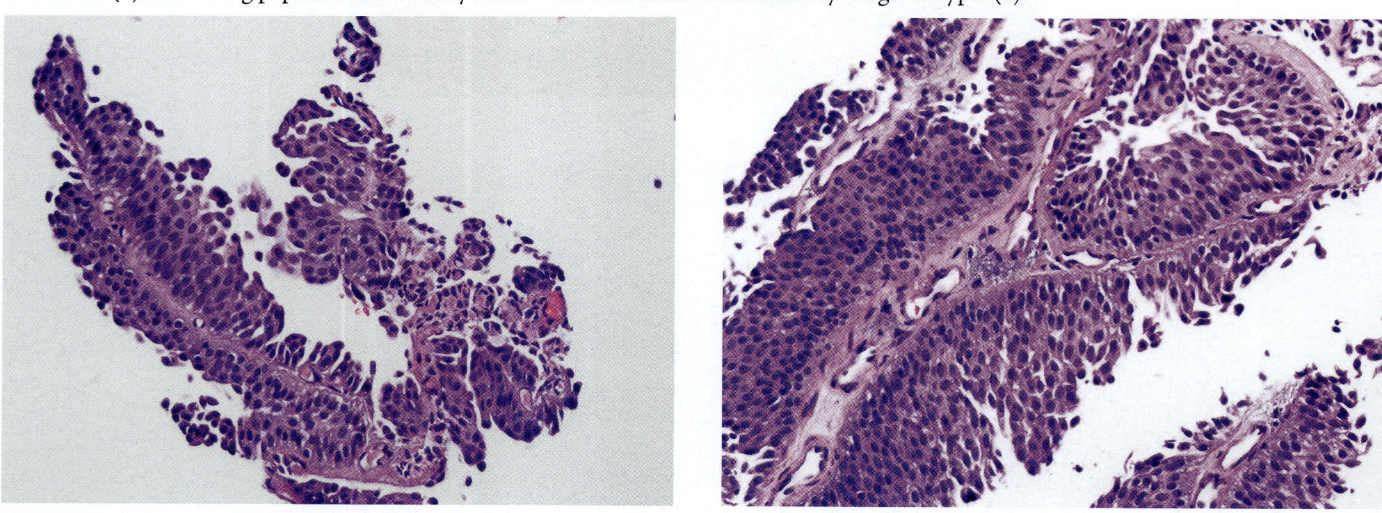

a **b**

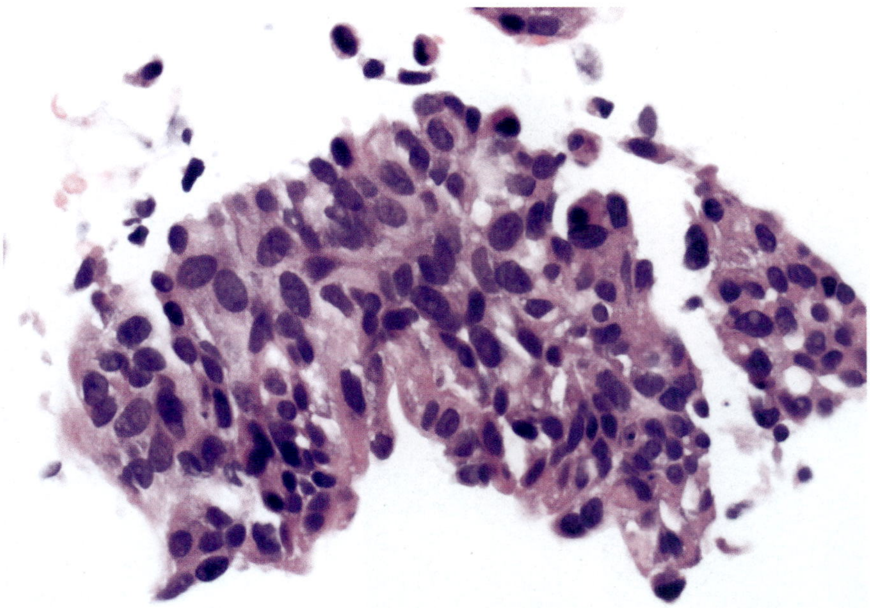

Figure 43-8.
A small detached fragment of urothelial cells in a ureteral biopsy displays moderate cytological atypia but without fibrovascular cores. This case was reported as *suspicious for urothelial carcinoma* because of the limited specimen. Rebiopsy confirms the presence of urothelial carcinoma.

INVASIVE UROTHELIAL CARCINOMA

Definition

- Urothelial carcinoma invading the renal pelvis, calyces, or ureter

Other term

- Invasive transitional cell carcinoma

Pathogenesis

- Invasive urothelial carcinoma may arise in the background of low-grade or high-grade noninvasive papillary UC or from urothelial CIS (high grade)

Clinical features

- Hematuria and positive urine cytology
- Cystoscopy of the bladder is negative
- Cystoscopy is positive for tumor if bladder cancer is also present
- Ureteroscopy may be positive for papillary or flat lesions
- Early invasive tumors show a filling defect in retrograde image studies
- Late stage and invasive tumors show large mass lesions by imaging studies, which are often indistinguishable from renal cell carcinoma
- It is important to establish preoperative diagnosis of the upper tract urothelial carcinoma
- Because of the major implication in choosing different surgical procedures, intraoperative frozen section diagnosis to distinguish a urothelial carcinoma from a renal cell carcinoma is not accurate and should be avoided if possible

Gross pathology

- Three types of macroscopic appearance are observed
  1. Exophytic growth, single or multiple, in the renal pelvis or ureter (Fig. 43-9*a*), because of the limited space for growth, the tumor is often smaller, and less-developed papillary appearance
  2. Endophytic growth, the mucosal surface is flat or granular with most tumor cells invading lamina propria or deeper (Figs. 43-9*a* and 43-10*a*)
  3. Large masses, resembling renal cell carcinoma, involving renal parenchyma (Fig. 43-11*a*)
- Hydronephrosis may be seen if the tumor obstructs the urinary flow
- Advanced tumors with invasion show mass lesions with poorly defined and infiltrative borders (Figs. 43-11*a* and 43-12*a*)
- A tumor may be present in the renal parenchyma, without an obvious renal pelvic papillary lesion (Fig. 43-10*a*)

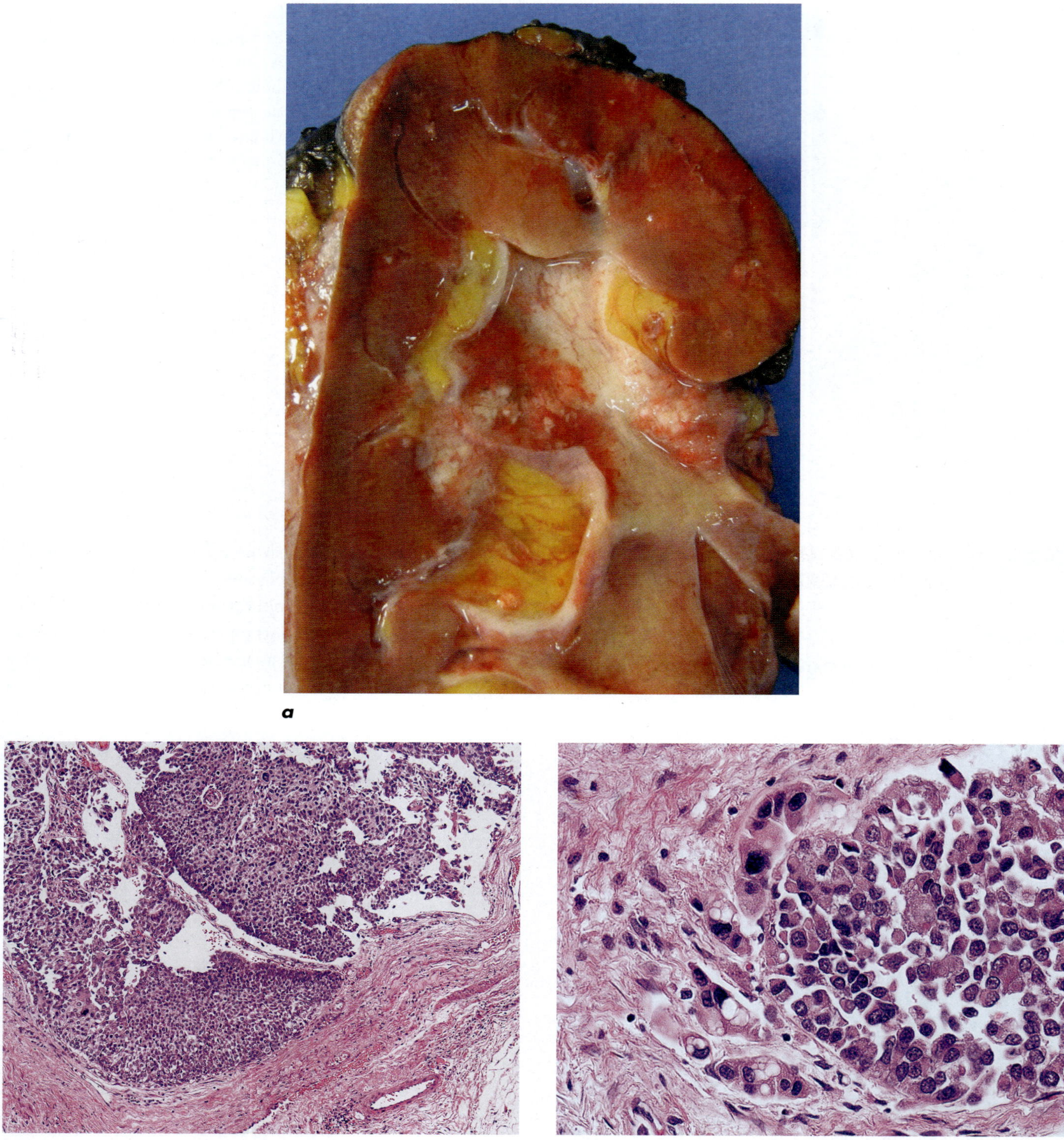

a b c

Figure 43-9.

Invasive urothelial carcinoma of the pelvis appears to be granular and small papillary lesions in the dilated renal pelvis (*a*). Microscopically, the tumor cells form large nests separated by fibrovascular cores (*b*). Focal high-grade tumor cells are seen invading lamina propria (*c*).

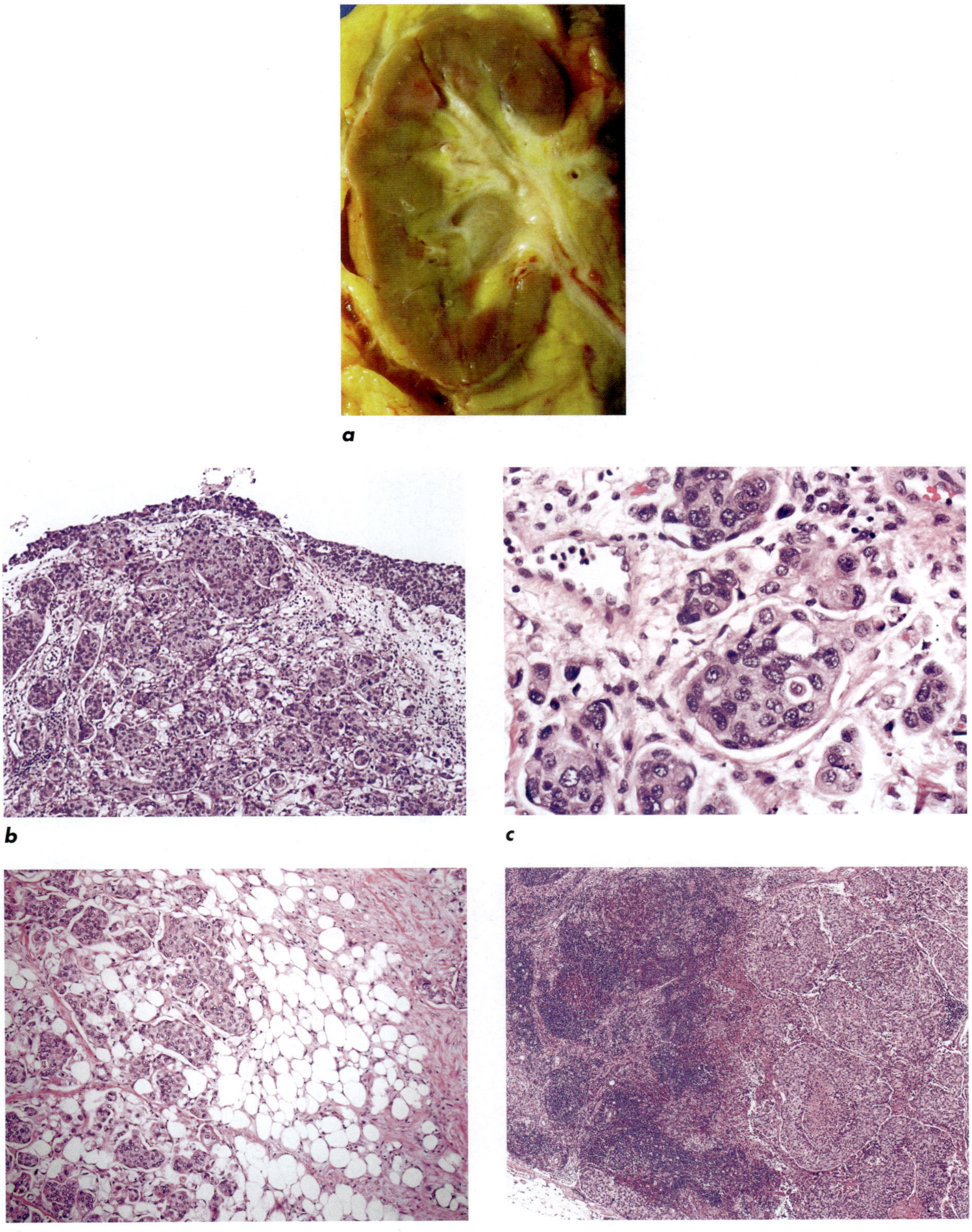

Figure 43-10.
High-grade invasive urothelial carcinoma of the renal pelvis with thickened flat urothelial mucosa and a deeply invasive lesion (*a*). Microscopically, the surface urothelium is involved by the tumor cells and invasive nests of the urothelial carcinoma can be seen (*b*). High magnification shows the pleomorphic tumor cells with micropapillary patterns (*c*). The tumor cells invade perinephric adipose tissue (*d*) and metastasize to a pelvic lymph node (*e*).

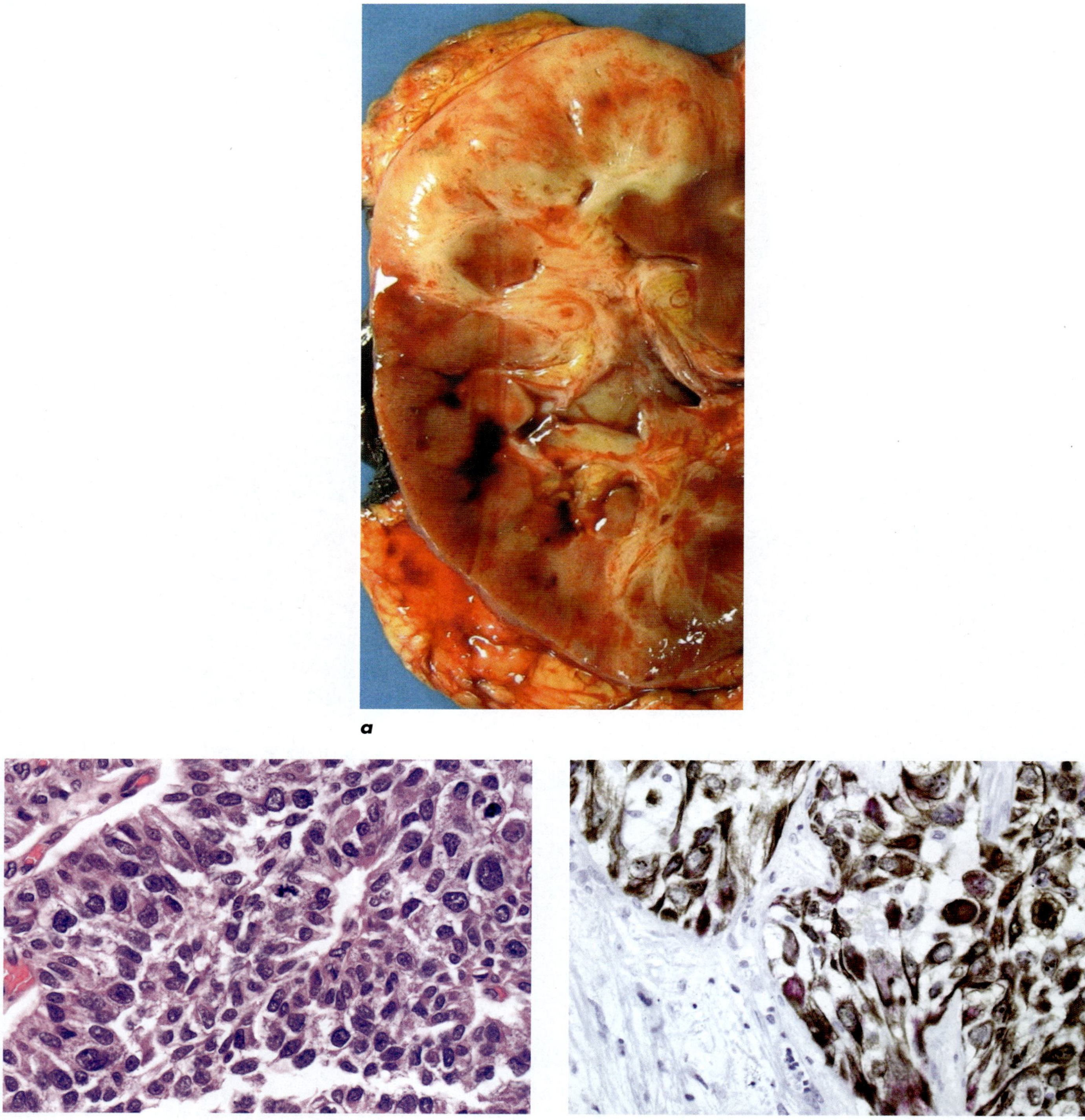

Figure 43-11.
High-grade invasive urothelial carcinoma. A large mass with poorly defined borders involving renal cortex, medulla, and pelvis (*a*), mimicking an RCC. Microscopically, the tumor cells are pleomorphic (*b*) and positive for HMWCK and p63, and weakly positive for AMACR, which is typical for urothelial carcinoma (*c*).

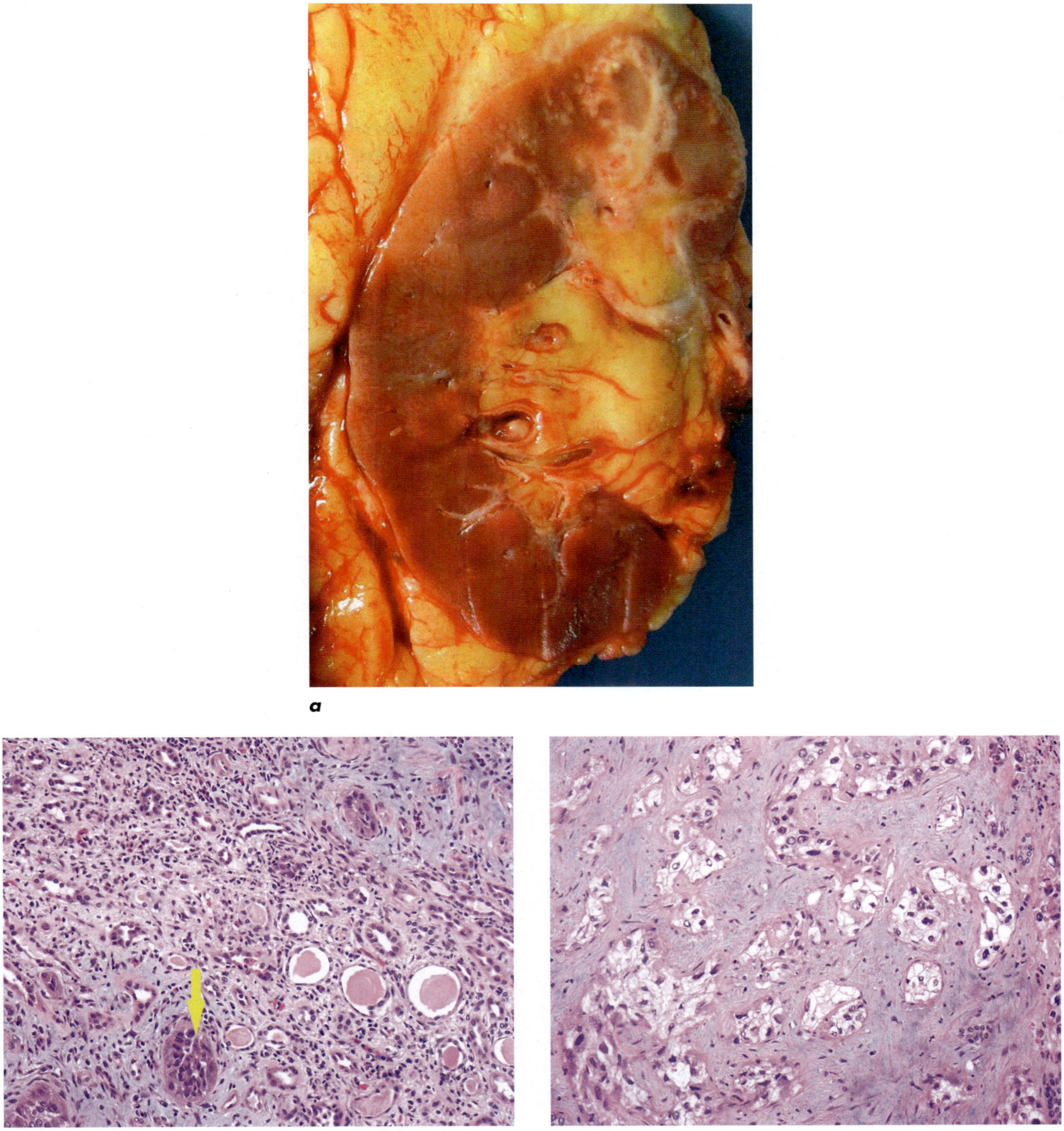

a

b

c

Figure 43-12.

High-grade invasive urothelial carcinoma grossly involves renal parenchyma and pelvis as a large mass (*a*). Microscopically, the tumor involving renal tubules (*b*, arrow) and invading renal parenchyma (*c*).

Histology

- Tumor cells form large irregular islands or smaller nests (Fig. 43-9). The pleomorphism can be prominent in urothelial carcinoma (Fig. 43-11*b*)
- The typical feature of urothelial cells with high-grade and low-grade nuclei intermingled together (Fig. 43-9*b*) is different from that of RCC, which shows areas of higher or lower nuclear grade
- Desmoplastic reaction can be seen (Fig. 43-11)
- The presence of exophytic tumor or urothelial carcinoma in situ will help confirm the diagnosis
- Glandular differentiation may be occasionally seen in urothelial carcinoma, which can be confused with RCC
- Squamous differentiation may also be seen, which is very rare in RCC
- Tumor cells may have retrograde extension to renal tubules and invade renal parenchyma (Fig. 43-12)
- Invasion of lamina propria, muscularis propria, or adipose tissue is present focally or extensively (Figs. 43-10 and 43-13)
- Lymph node metastasis can be seen (Fig. 43-10*e*)

Immunohistochemistry

- GATA3 positive, S100P positive, P63 positive, and HMWCK positive (Fig. 43-11*c*)
- AMACR negative or weakly positive, PAX2/PAX8 negative, and other RCC markers negative

Differential diagnosis

- The main differential diagnosis is renal cell carcinoma (see Table 43-1)

Molecular analysis

- Chromosome changes in upper tract urothelial carcinoma similar to those of the bladder

Clinical relevance (prognosis and treatment options)

- Because of high risk of coexisting a lower tract urothelial carcinoma, cystoscopy is necessary for any patients with upper tract urothelial carcinoma before and after nephrectomy
- The treatment of choice for upper tract urothelial carcinoma is radical nephrectomy, ureterectomy, and resection of bladder cuff, which is significantly different from the surgical procedure of partial or radical nephrectomy for a renal cell carcinoma
- Segmental resection of the ureter has been tried in some cases. However, the benefits of a local resection have not been confirmed for invasive urothelial carcinoma of the ureter
- It is recommended that the diagnosis of urothelial carcinoma is established preoperatively by biopsy with confirmation with immunostains
- Sometimes, particularly early noninvasive lesion only involving pelvic mucosa, the diagnosis of urothelial carcinoma can be made intraoperatively
- On the other hand, smaller RCC in the renal parenchyma without invading renal pelvis can also be easily diagnosed and distinguished from urothelial carcinoma by gross and microscopic examination intraoperatively
- However, if the tumor is large, it may be difficult to distinguish between urothelial carcinoma from a high-grade RCC even for the most experienced pathologists on frozen section

Figure 43-13.
Urothelial carcinoma of the renal pelvis appears to be composed predominantly of large nests of low-grade tumor cells (*a*). Higher magnification demonstrates the presence of focal high-grade tumor cells invading lamina propria (*b*, arrows).

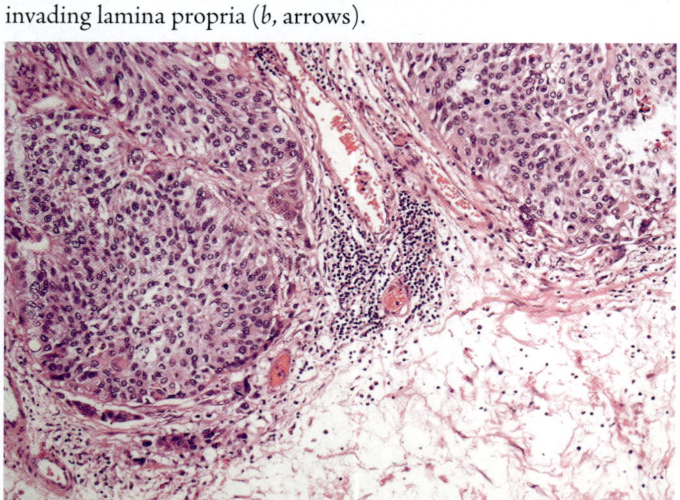

a

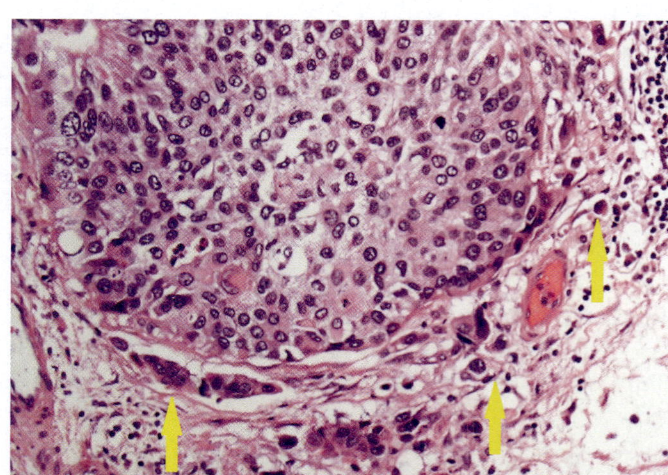

b

Table 43-1. Comparison of Urothelial Carcinoma and Renal Cell Carcinoma

	Invasive UC	*RCC*
Location	Pelvis centered May extend to medulla and cortex	Mostly cortex centered May extend to pelvis
Preoperative diagnosis	Ureteroscopic biopsy	CT-guided percutaneous needle core biopsy
Pelvic involvement	Always	Uncommon
Gross appearance	Tan, yellow papillary mass or thickened urothelial mucosa	Mass in renal parenchyma Clear cell RCC bright yellow
Tumor border	Poorly defined border	Well-defined border No capsule
Histology		
Surface component (CIS or papillary UC)	Present	Absent
High-grade component	Often present, mixed with low-grade component	Isolated areas from low-grade component
Glandular differentiation	Occasional	Always
Squamous differentiation	Possible	Rare
Markers		
P63	Positive	Negative
HWMCK	Positive	Negative
GATA3	Positive	Negative
S100P	Positive	Negative
PAX2/PAX8	Negative	Positive
CA9	Negative or focally positive	Strong membranous staining (CRCC)
AMACR	Negative or focally positive	Diffusely positive (PRCC)
Treatment		
Nephrectomy	Yes, radical	Yes, partial or radical
Ureterectomy	Possible	No
Bladder cuff resection	Possible	No

AMACR, α-methylacyl-CoA racemase; CA9, carbonic anhydrase 9; CIS, carcinoma in situ; CRCC, chromophobe renal cell carcinoma; CT, computed tomography; HWMCK, high molecular cytokeratins; PAX2/PAX8, paired box gene 2 or 8; PRCC, papillary renal cell carcinoma; RCC, renal cell carcinoma; UC, urothelial carcinoma.

- When under pressure to make such a difficult distinction on frozen sections, a mistake by confusing an RCC with a urothelial carcinoma can happen. As a result, the entire ureter and bladder cuff were unnecessarily removed along with the kidney
- In an uncertain situation about the nature of renal tumor as possible urothelial carcinoma during surgery, it may be wise to put surgery on hold until a definitive diagnosis is established
- Obviously, it is much more difficult to put back the ureter, bladder, and other structures when resected
- Tumor stages: T1 (lamina propria invasion); T2 (muscularis propria invasion); T3 (peripelvic fat or renal parenchyma); and T4 (adjacent organs or through kidney to perinephric fat)

INVASIVE SQUAMOUS CELL CARCINOMA

Definition

- Primary invasive squamous cell carcinoma involving the renal pelvis or ureter
- No evidence of urothelial carcinoma

Clinical features

- Similar to invasive high-grade urothelial carcinoma
- Hematuria and possible flank mass
- Ureteroscope can be used to detect a mass lesion involving the renal pelvis or ureter

Gross pathology

- Large mass with poorly defined borders
- Necrosis with yellow-white "cheesy" keratin debris can be seen (Fig. 43-14*a*)

Histology

- The tumor involving the renal pelvis or ureter (Fig. 43-14*b*)
- Squamous cell carcinoma is characterized by the presence of keratin pearls, intercellular bridges (Fig. 43-14*c*)
- Malignant squamous cells, keratinized or nonkeratinized, can be seen (Fig. 43-14*c*)
- Invasion of lamina propria or renal parenchyma is generally present
- No evidence of invasive or in situ urothelial carcinoma. In the case with both urothelial and squamous cell carcinoma, the diagnosis should be *urothelial carcinoma with squamous differentiation*
- Squamous metaplasia (keratinized or nonkeratinized) may be present (Fig. 43-15)
- As we discussed before in the bladder chapter, the claim that only keratinized squamous metaplasia is associated with squamous cell carcinoma cannot be substantiated since we have seen the presence of nonkeratinized squamous metaplasia associated with many cases of squamous cell carcinomas of the upper urinary tract

Clinical relevance (prognosis and treatment options)

- It is generally an aggressive disease
- Radical nephrectomy is indicated
- Chemotherapy may be helpful; however, the experience is limited

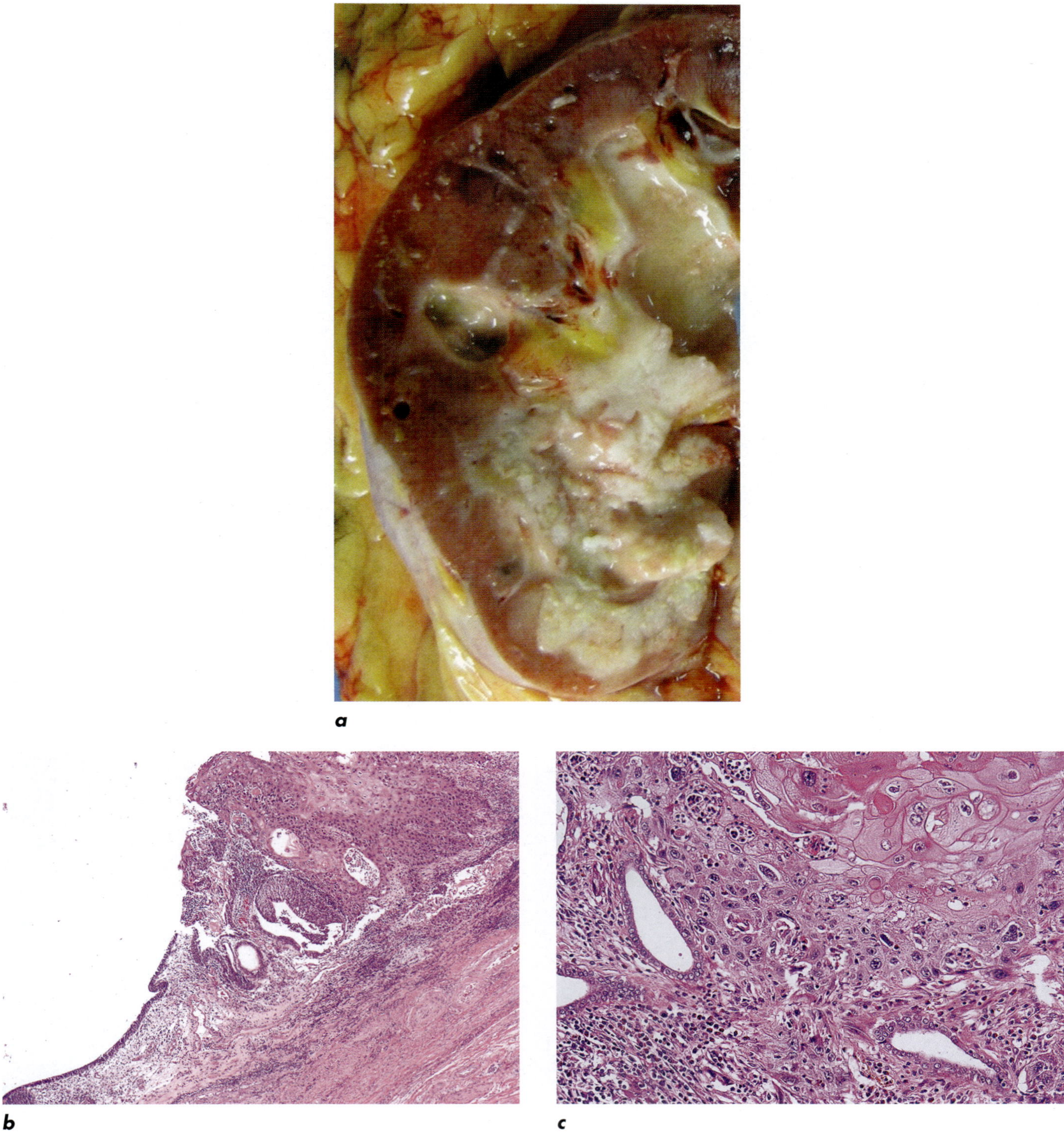

Figure 43-14.

Squamous cell carcinoma of the kidney appears to develop from the renal pelvis (*a*). The tumor has a poorly defined infiltrating border and some areas of cheesy necrosis. Microscopically, invasive tumor cells involving renal pelvis without any urothelial carcinoma components (*b*). High-grade squamous cell carcinoma cells invading renal parenchyma (*c*).

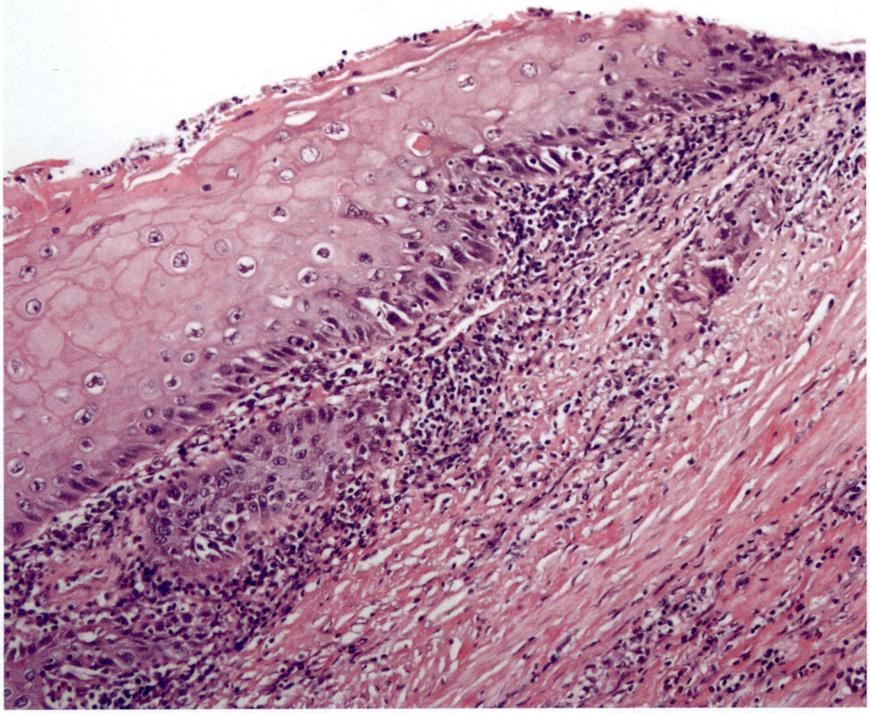

Figure 43-15.
Nonkeratinized squamous metaplasia of the renal pelvic urothelium associated with invasive squamous cell carcinoma.

SECTION 6
The Bladder

CHAPTER 44 Normal Bladder Histology

Anatomy

- Bladder is a bag-like structure
- Connected to both ureters in the upper portion
- Connected to the urethra in the lower portion
- The area between the two openings of the ureters (ureteral orifices) and the one opening of the urethra is called the trigone
- The top portion of the bladder is the dome

Adjacent organs

- In men, the prostate is located in the inferior aspect of the bladder. The urethra is longer and passing through the prostate
- In women, the bladder, located in the anterior aspect of the uterus, connects to the short urethra

Histology

- The bladder wall is composed of multiple layers from the luminal side to outside as the following (Figs. 44-1 and 44-2)
  - Urothelium
  - Lamina propria
  - Muscularis propria
  - Perivesicle adipose tissue
- *Urothelium*, the most inner lining of the bladder (Fig. 44-3), consists of
  - Umbrella cells (Fig. 44-4)
    - Umbrella cells have dense cytoplasm membrane and form a protective surface layer
    - They have abundant cytoplasm with a low nucleus/cytoplasm (N/C) ratio
  - Basal cells
    - The major component of the urothelium
    - Containing four to six layers of well-organized epithelial cells
    - Nuclear grooving can be seen
    - No keratinization or intracellular bridges
- Lamina propria
  - Since the muscularis mucosa (Fig. 44-5) is incomplete and signified by the smaller discontinuous smooth muscle bundles, the true lamina propria and submucosa of the bladder cannot easily be distinguished
  - Therefore, for all practical purposes, the lamina propria of the bladder actually includes the *true lamina propria, muscularis mucosa, and submucosal connective tissue*
  - There may be scattered adipocytes in the lamina propria (Fig. 44-2), which should not be confused with the perivesicle adipose tissue
- Muscularis propria
  - The muscularis propria, generally referred to as *muscle layer*, is composed of larger smooth muscle bundles (Fig. 44-6)
  - By our experience, the muscle bundles of muscularis are generally thicker than 100-200 μm (0.1-0.2 mm) in diameter (Fig. 44-7)
  - Muscularis propria smooth muscle is positive for smoothelin, while the lamina propria wispy smooth muscle is negative for smoothelin. This difference has some diagnostic value in determining the depth of tumor invasion
  - Adipose tissue may also be present in muscularis propria (Fig. 44-2)
- Perivesicle adipose tissue
  - Mostly adipose tissue with larger blood vessels

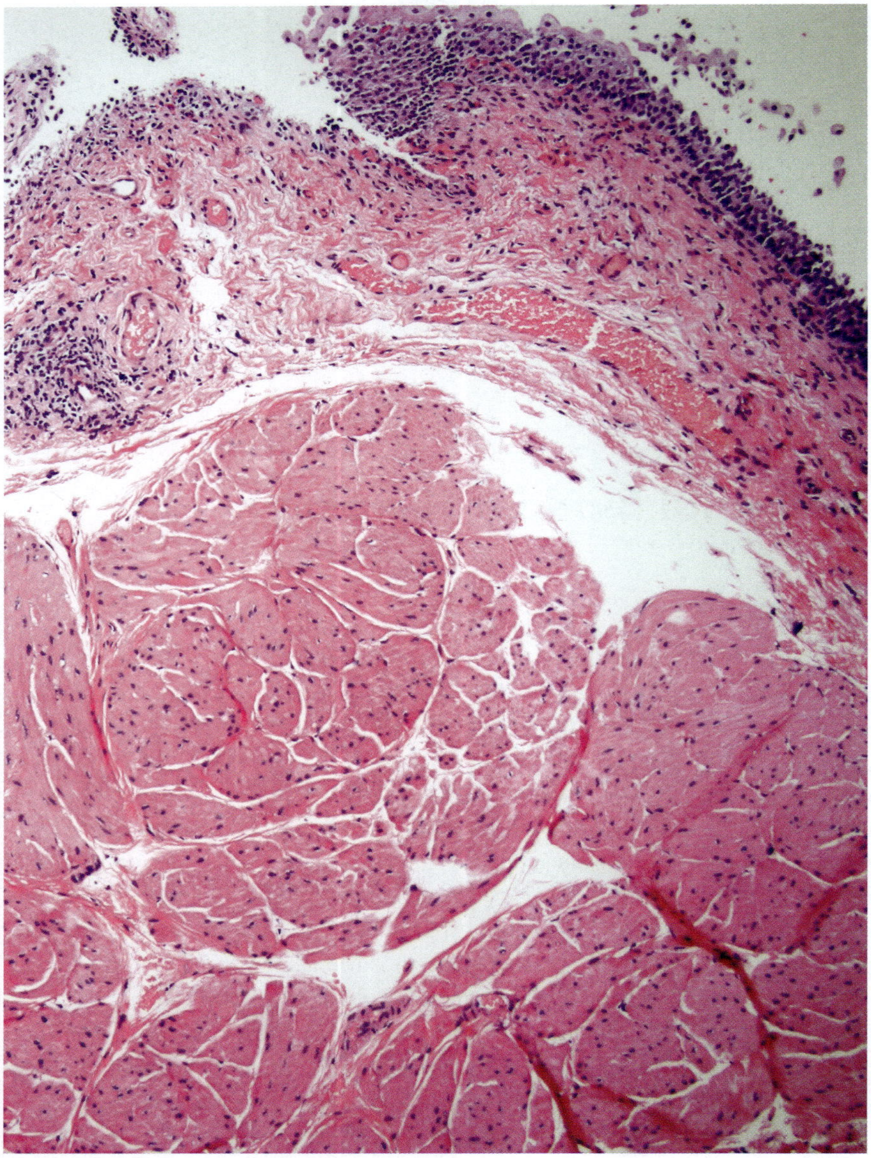

Figure 44-1.
The bladder wall contains large smooth muscle bundle in the muscularis propria.

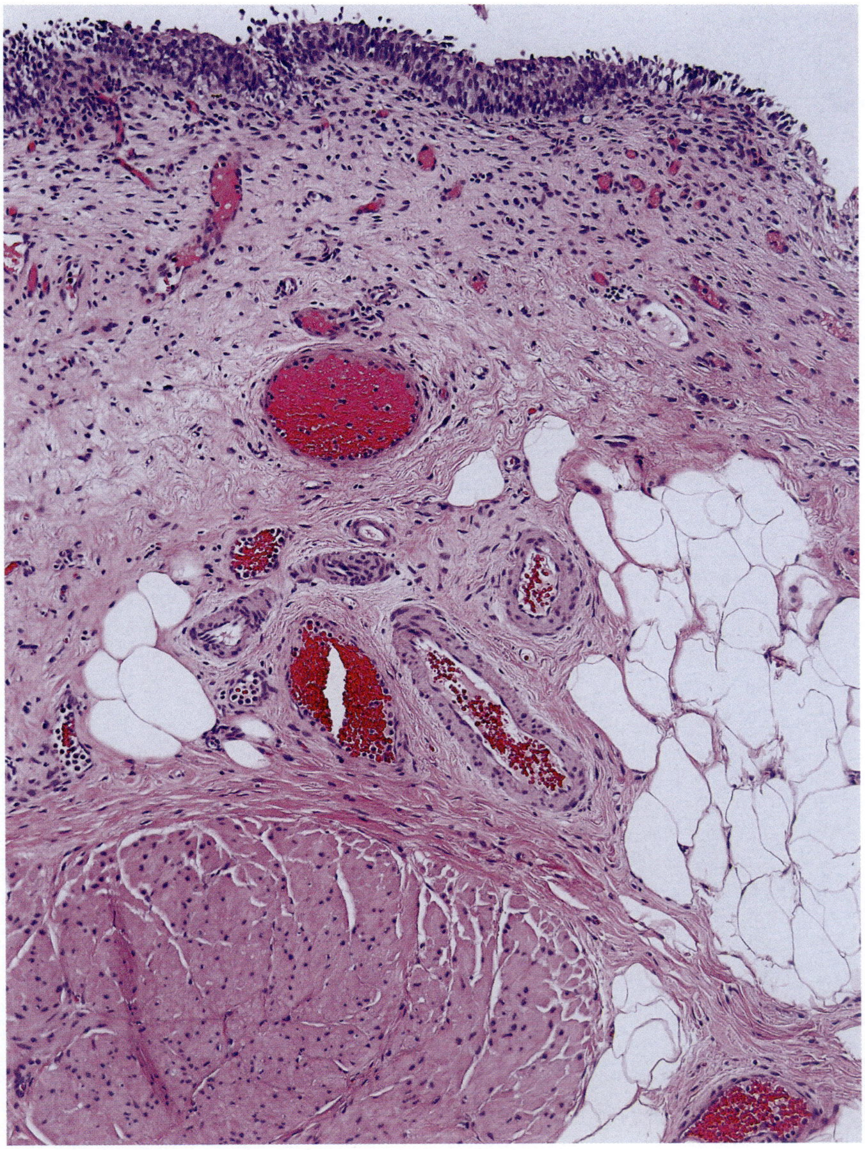

Figure 44-2.
Presence of adipose tissue in the lamina propria and muscularis propria of the bladder wall.

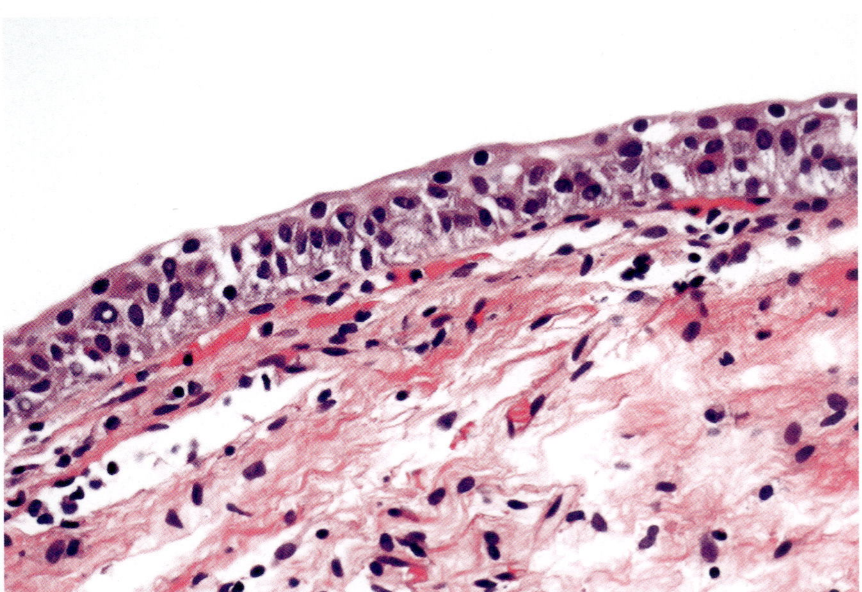

Figure 44-3.
Epithelial lining of the bladder composed of several layers of benign urothelial cells.

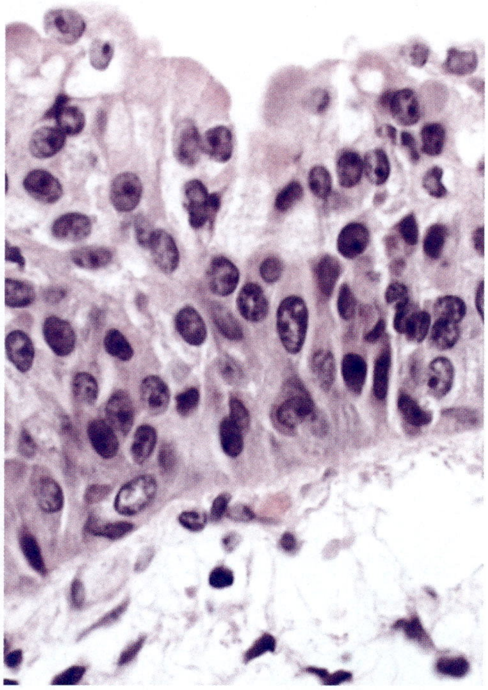

Figure 44-4.
High magnification shows the presence of umbrella cells on the surface with abundant cytoplasm and a dense cell membrane.

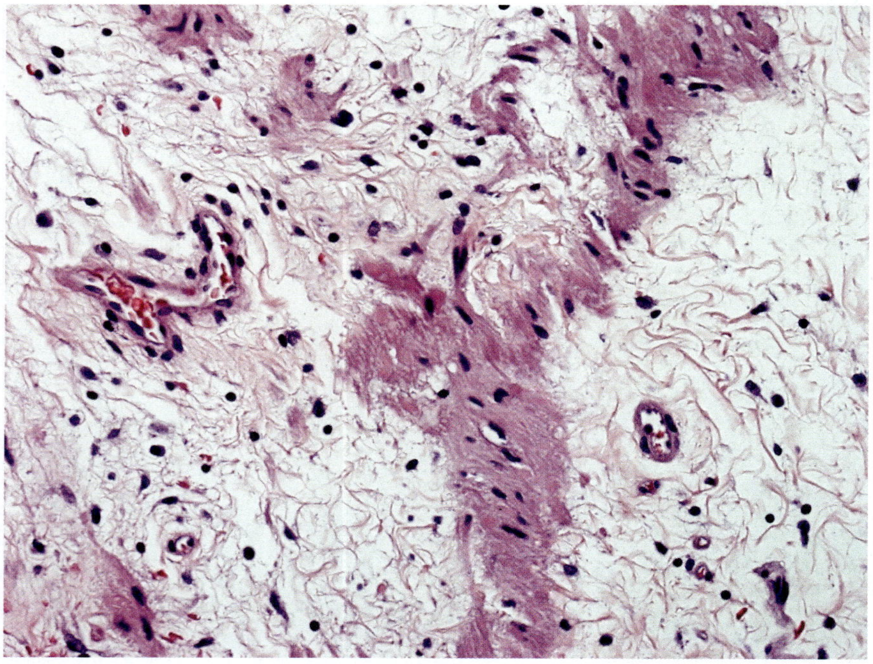

Figure 44-5.
Lamina propria containing thin and wispy smooth muscle bundles.

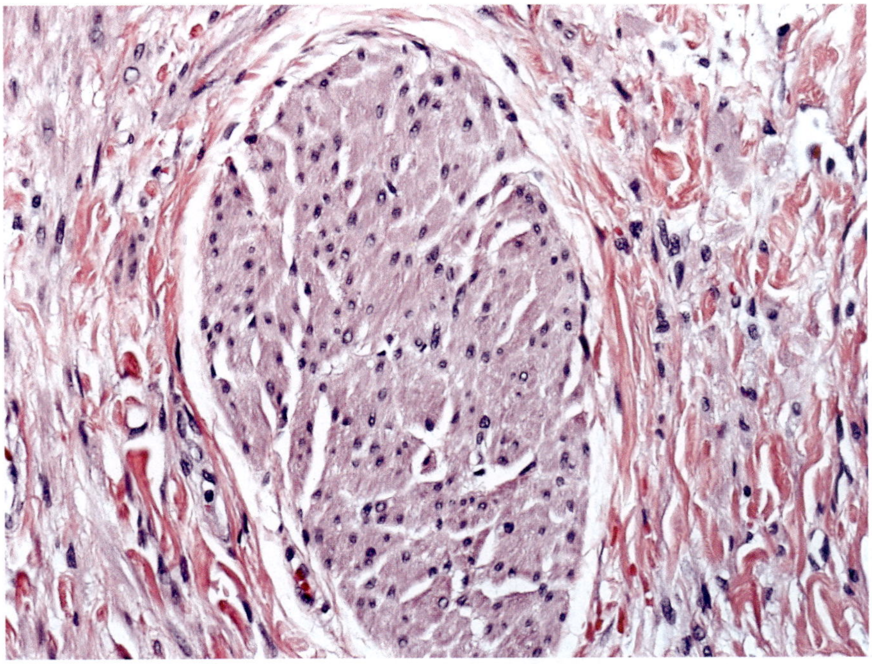

Figure 44-6.
A large smooth muscle bundle of muscularis propria in the bladder wall.

Figure 44-7.
Comparison of smaller muscular bundle (<200 μm) in the lamina propria (*a*) and large muscle bundles (*b*) of muscularis propria in the bladder wall.

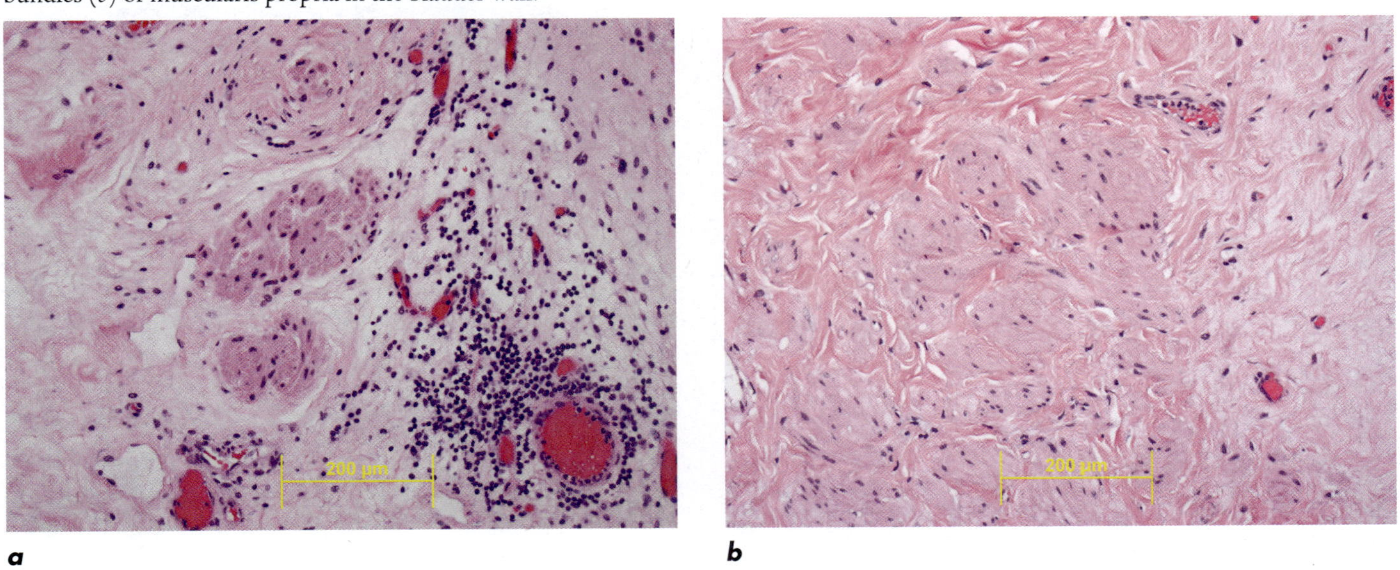

CHAPTER 45

Immunohistochemical Markers Used for Urothelial Lesions

CK20 (cytokeratin 20)

- Positive in umbrella cells only (Fig. 45-1*a*)
- Negative in basal cells in urothelium
- Positive in the majority of cases of urothelial carcinoma (Fig. 45-1*b*)

P53

- Weakly positive (wild-type staining) in the basal layer of urothelium (Fig. 45-1*c*)
- Strongly positive in urothelial carcinoma in situ (CIS) (Fig. 45-1*d*) and high-grade urothelial carcinoma
- Weak or moderate reactivity in the low-grade urothelial carcinoma

Figure 45-1.
CK20 labels umbrella cells on the surface of the normal urothelium (*a*) and tumor cells in urothelial carcinoma in situ (*b*). P53 immunostaining of normal urothelium with only basal cells weakly positive for p53 (*c*), and urothelial carcinoma in situ is strongly positive for p53 (*d*).

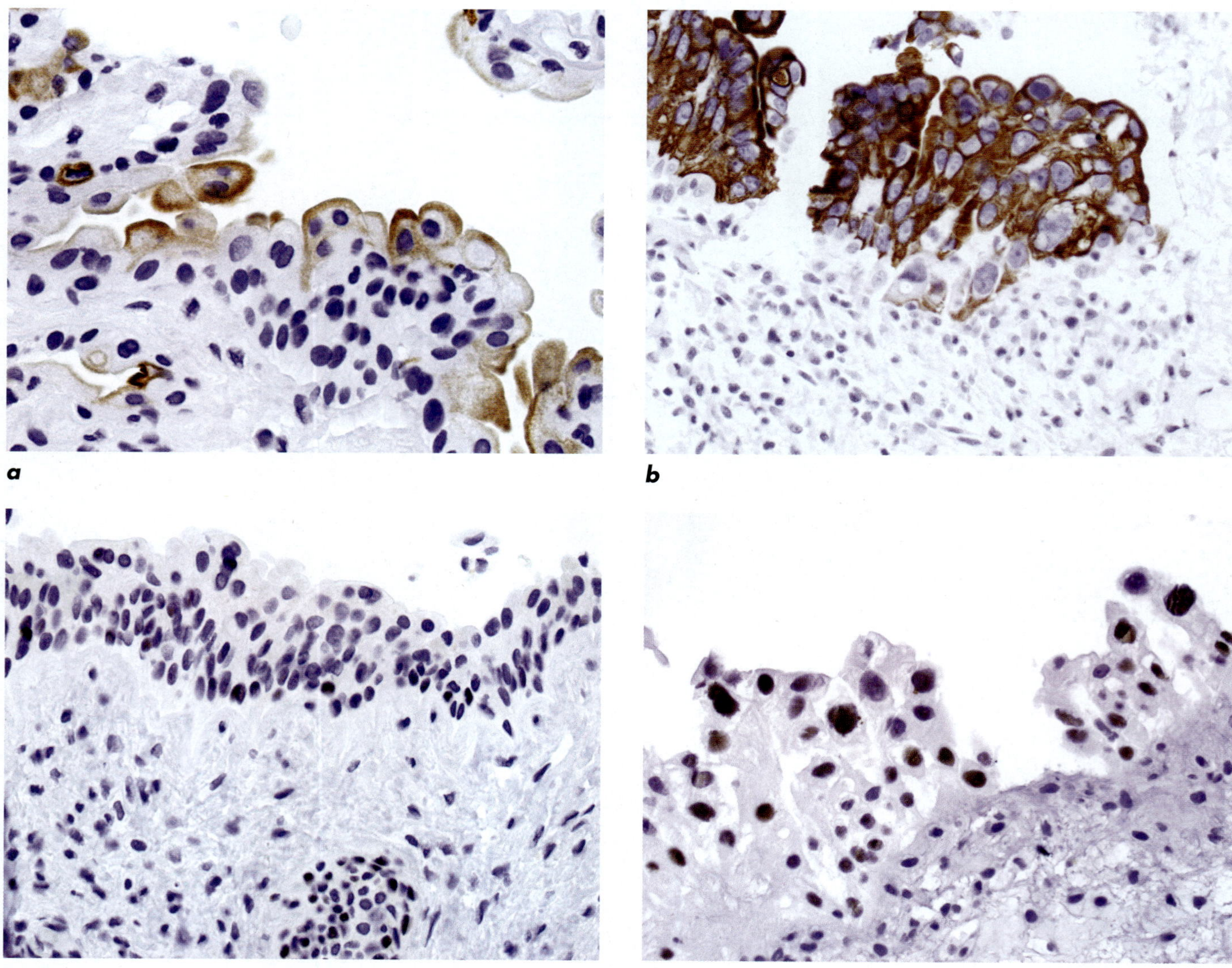

a *b* *c* *d*

P63

- Nuclear staining in urothelial cells
- Positive in benign urothelium both umbrella cells and basal cells
- Positive in urothelial carcinoma (Figs. 45-2 and 45-3)
- Positive in benign prostatic basal cells and squamous cells
- Positive in squamous cell carcinoma
- Negative in prostatic adenocarcinoma, although rare cases of adenocarcinoma positive for p63 have been seen

HMWCK (high molecular weight cytokeratin)

- Distribution is similar to p63, cytoplasmic staining
- Positive in benign urothelium both umbrella cells and basal cells
- Positive in urothelial carcinoma (Fig. 45-2)
- Positive benign prostatic basal cells and squamous cells
- Negative in prostatic adenocarcinoma

AMACR (α-methylacyl-CoA racemase)

- An enzyme for fatty acid metabolism
- Best known as prostate cancer marker: positive in prostatic adenocarcinoma and negative or weakly positive in benign prostatic glands
- Positive in papillary renal cell carcinoma
- Positive in renal tubules and nephrogenic adenoma
- Positive in colonic adenocarcinoma
- Negative in normal urothelium

Figure 45-2.
Urothelial carcinoma (*a*) demonstrates the positivity for both HMWCK (cytoplasm) and p63 (nuclear), but is negative for AMACR (*b*, triple staining). Another case of urothelial carcinoma (*c*) shows the positivity for p63 and HMWCK (brown) as well as weak positivity for AMACR (red) (*d*, triple staining).

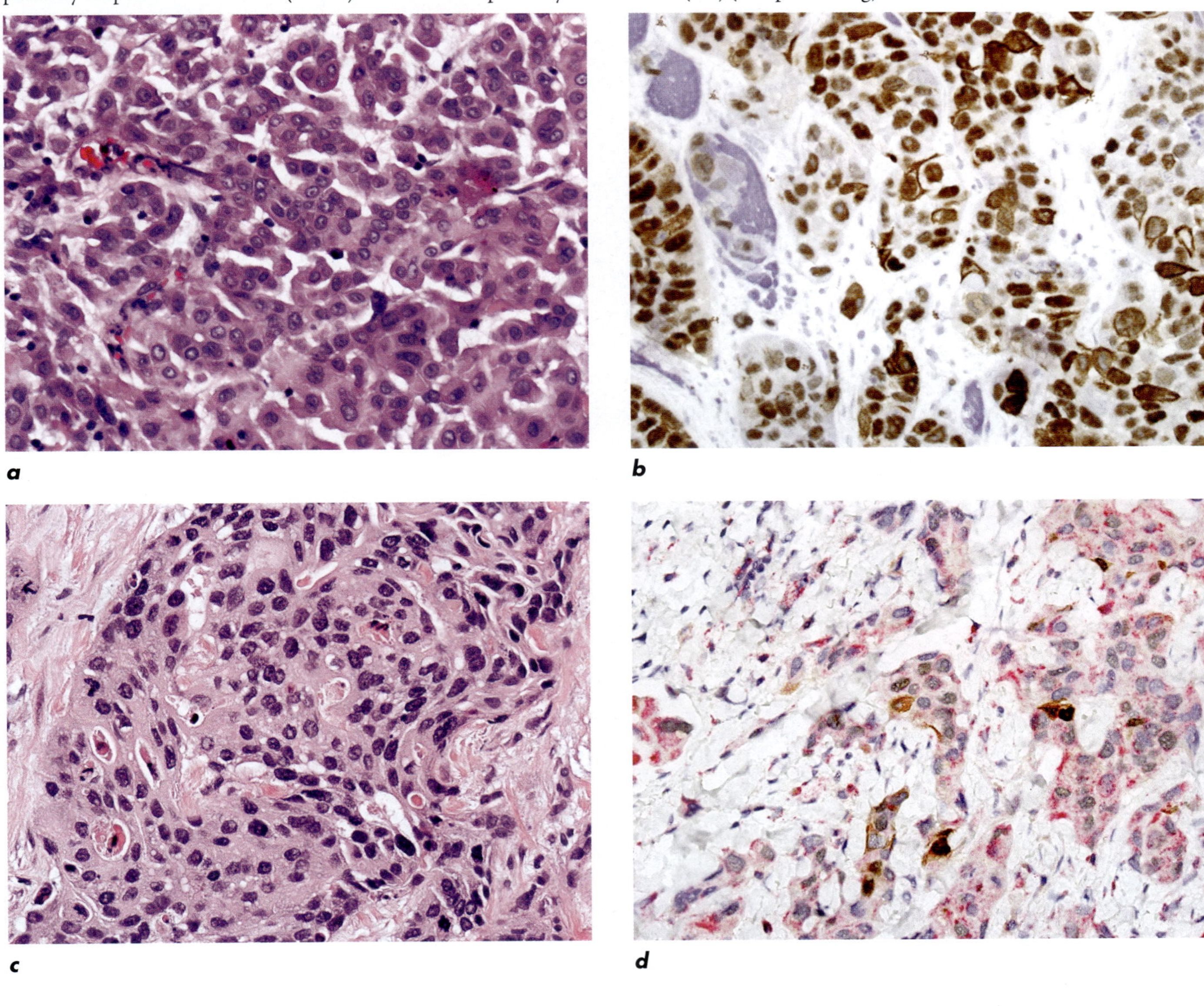

a b c d

- Often used together with p63 and HMWCK as a triple staining
- Negative or weakly positive in urothelial carcinoma (Fig. 45-2*b* and *d*)

S100P

- A variant of S100 originally found to be expressed in placental trophoblasts
- Positive in benign urothelium and benign urothelial lesions
- Positive in the majority of urothelial carcinoma (Fig. 45-3*c*)
- Uncommon activity in other types of carcinomas

GATA3

- Positive in benign urothelium
- Positive in urothelial carcinoma, both low and high grade, invasive and noninvasive tumors (Fig. 45-3*d*)
- Probably the best marker for urothelial carcinoma but it does not distinguish benign from malignant urothelial lesions
- Positive in breast adenocarcinoma
- Negative in the vast majority of other epithelial malignancies

AE1/AE3

- Pan keratin markers
- Positive in both benign and malignant urothelial cells as well as other epithelial cells
- Used to confirm the presence of malignant epithelial cells (Fig. 45-4)

Ki67

- Measuring proliferative activity
- Low proliferative index in benign urothelium

Figure 45-3.
Urothelial carcinoma (*a*) is positive for p63 (*b*, nuclear), S100p (*c*, mostly nuclear staining), and GATA3 (*d*, nuclear).

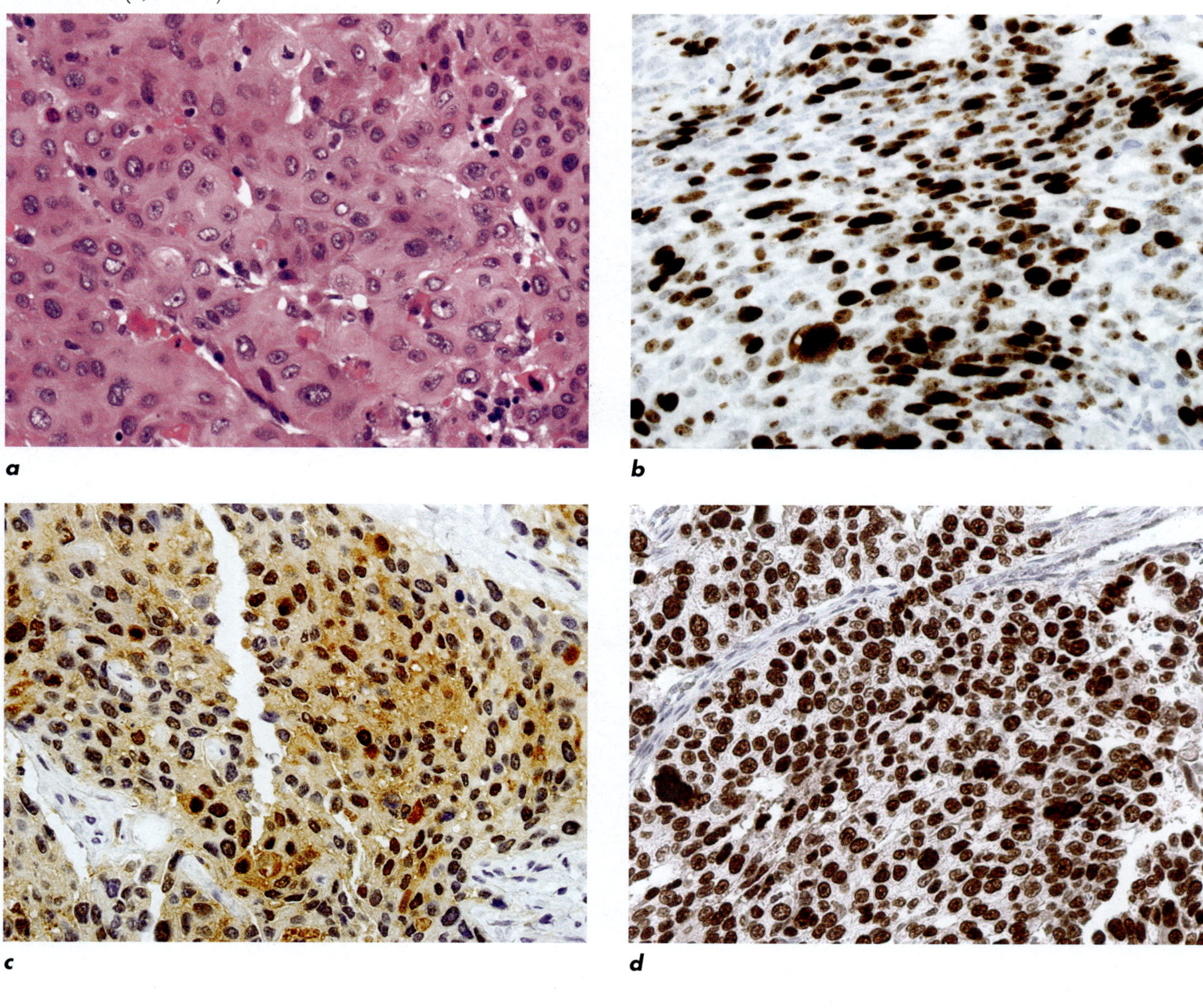

a b c d

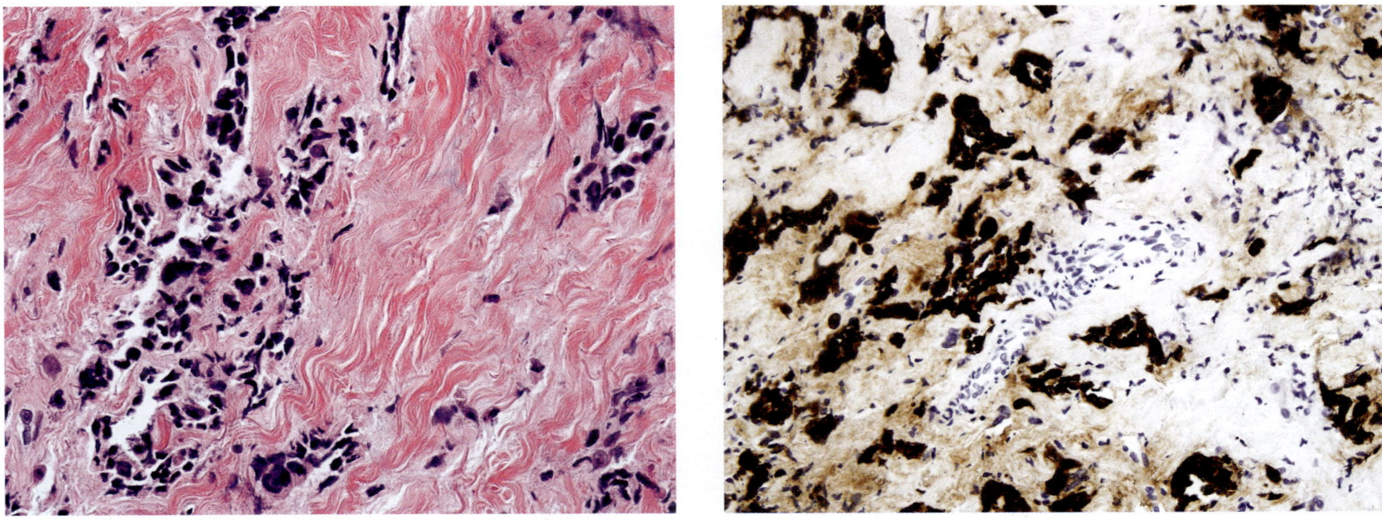

Figure 45-4.
Invasive urothelial carcinoma with crushing artifact (*a*) is confirmed by the positive staining for AE1/AE3 (*b*).

- Increased proliferative index in low-grade urothelial carcinoma
- High proliferative index in CIS and high-grade urothelial carcinoma

Smoothelin

- Positive in muscularis propria muscle
- Negative in lamina propria muscle
- Helpful marker for identifying muscle invasive cancer: positive smoothelin staining associated with urothelial carcinoma cells in a case would favor muscularis invasion (90% cases positive) than lamina propria invasion (20% to 30% cases positive)
- Common markers used for urothelial lesions are listed in Table 45-1

Table 45-1. Comparison of Immunohistochemical Markers Used for Urothelium

Marker	*Benign urothelium (and stroma)*	*Urothelial carcinoma (UCa)*
P53	Basal cell weakly positive	Positive Low grade (UCa) weaker High grade (UCa) strong
CK20	Umbrella cells positive	Diffusely positive
CD44	Positive	Negative
Smoothelin	Positive in muscularis propria Negative in lamina proria	Positive in muscularis propria invaded by (UCa)
S100p	Positive	Positive
GATA3	Positive	Positive
AMACR	Negative	Negative or weakly positive
P63	Positive	Positive
HMWCK	Positive	Positive

CHAPTER 46

Benign Glandular Lesions of the Bladder

CYSTITIS GLANDULARIS AND CYSTITIS CYSTICA

Definition

- Reactive urothelial lesion with glandular or cystic changes
- Cystitis glandularis (CG): a metaplastic lesion with benign glandular structures present in von Brunn nests or replacing the surface urothelium
- Cystitis cystica (CC): a lesion characterized by cystic dilatation of von Brunn nests or benign glandular structures
- However, the terms cystitis glandularis and cystitis cystica are often used interchangeably
- CG and CC can also be divided into two types
  - Non-mucinous type, which will be discussed in this entity
  - Mucinous type (intestinal type), which will be discussed as a separate entity (colonic metaplasia) in this chapter

Other term

- Cystitis cystica et glandularis

Pathogenesis

- A very common reactive lesion of the bladder in reaction to chronic stimuli
- Chronic inflammatory cells may or may not present in CG and CC
- There is a speculation that CG and CC are precursor lesions of adenocarcinoma
- However, the evidence for this causative relationship is weak since CG and CC are commonly seen in the bladder, while adenocarcinoma of the bladder is uncommon. Therefore, this weak association between CG/CC and adenocarcinoma has a very poor predicative value

Clinical features

- No specific associated symptoms

Gross pathology

- CC and CG are microscopic findings; therefore, they are not visible macroscopically

Histology

- CG is characterized by benign glandular differentiation of urothelium in von Brunn nests (Fig. 46-1) or in surface urothelium
- CC shows cystic dilatation of benign glandular structures or von Brunn nests in the bladder (Fig. 46-2)
- There is no cytological atypia or infiltrating patterns in either CG or CC, which often coexist (Figs. 46-1 and 46-2)
- Intestinal metaplasia, characterized by the presence of intestinal-type epithelium, particularly the presence of goblet cells in the urothelium, often develops in the background of CC or CG (see Colonic Metaplasia in this chapter)
- Acute or chronic inflammation may be present but not required for the diagnosis of CG or CC

Immunohistochemistry

- Not applicable

Clinical relevance

- No particular treatment is known, but clinical follow-up may be necessary
- The presence of colonic metaplasia should be specified if present in CG, because of its closer relationship to adenocarcinoma

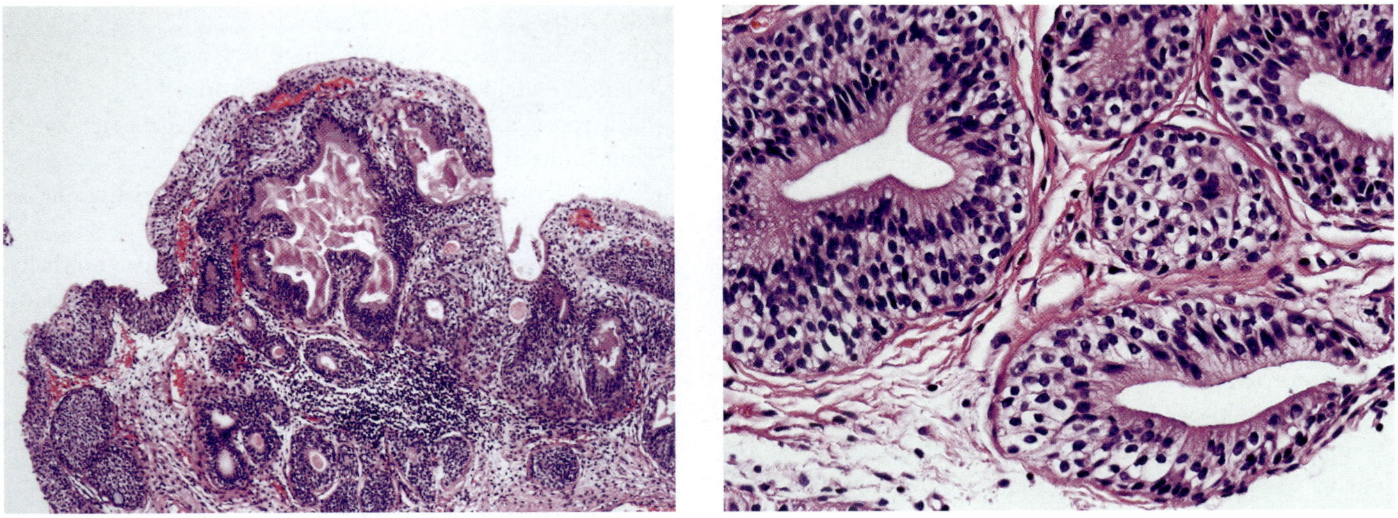

a ***b***

Figure 46-1.
Cystitis glandularis with some solid von Brunn nests, and some von Brunn nests with glandular formation. Chronic inflammation is present (*a*). Several von Brunn nests are replaced by glandular cells. There is no cytological atypia in these glandular cells (*b*).

Figure 46-2.
Cystitis cystica with multiple dilated von Brunn nests (*a*). Higher magnification shows several dilated von Brunn nests lined by tall columnar cells and filled with pink secretions (*b*).

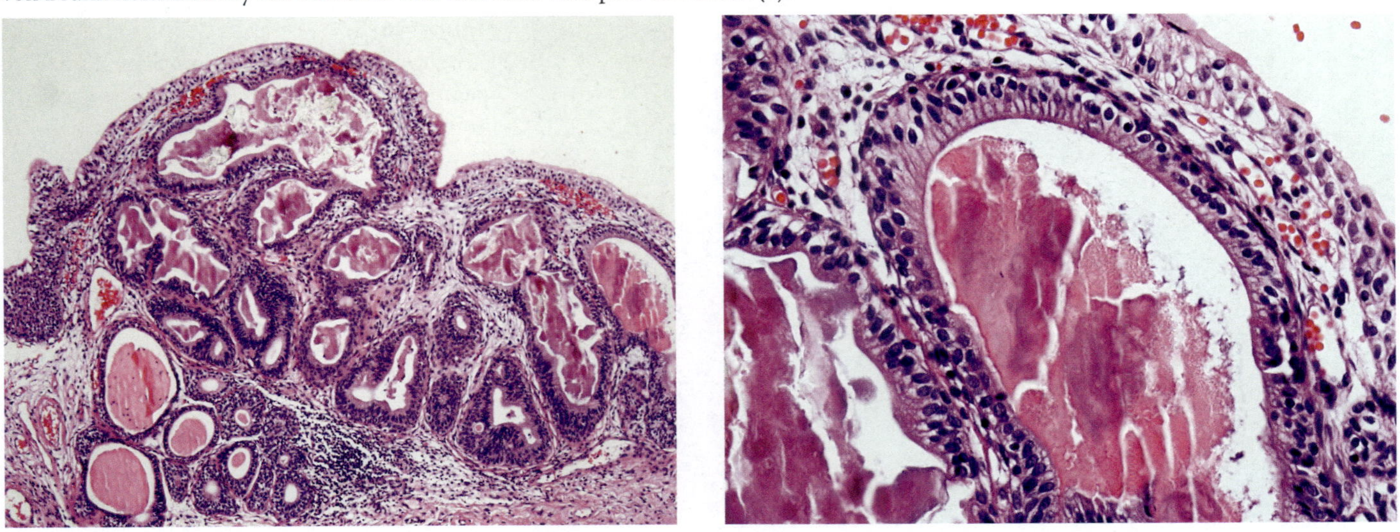

a ***b***

PSEUDOGLANDULAR DIFFERENTIATION

Definition

- Histological findings of small cystic spaces present in reactive urothelium or a urothelial neoplasm

Other terms

- Microcysts, microcyst formation

Pathogenesis

- Because of degenerative changes and cell drop out, the small cystic spaces are created within the urothelium
- This phenomenon can be observed in both reactive urothelium and urothelial carcinoma

Clinical features

- It is a microscopic finding, which can be associated with benign or malignant lesions of the bladder

Gross pathology

- No specific gross findings

Histology

- In the reactive urothelium, there is a single, occasionally multiple small spaces (Figs. 46-3 and 46-4)
- The space is either empty or filled with degenerative cells, mucinous or necrotic debris (Fig. 46-4)
- The cells surrounding the spaces are not palisading or forming a bona fide glandular structure
- The microcystic formation in a papillary urothelial carcinoma is also commonly seen, which may represent a degenerative process of the tumor cells (Figs. 46-5 and 46-6)

Immunohistochemistry

- Not applicable

Clinical relevance (prognosis and treatment options)

- This is a common microscopic finding in the majority of reactive urothelium and a significant subset of urothelial carcinoma, which should not be considered glandular differentiation

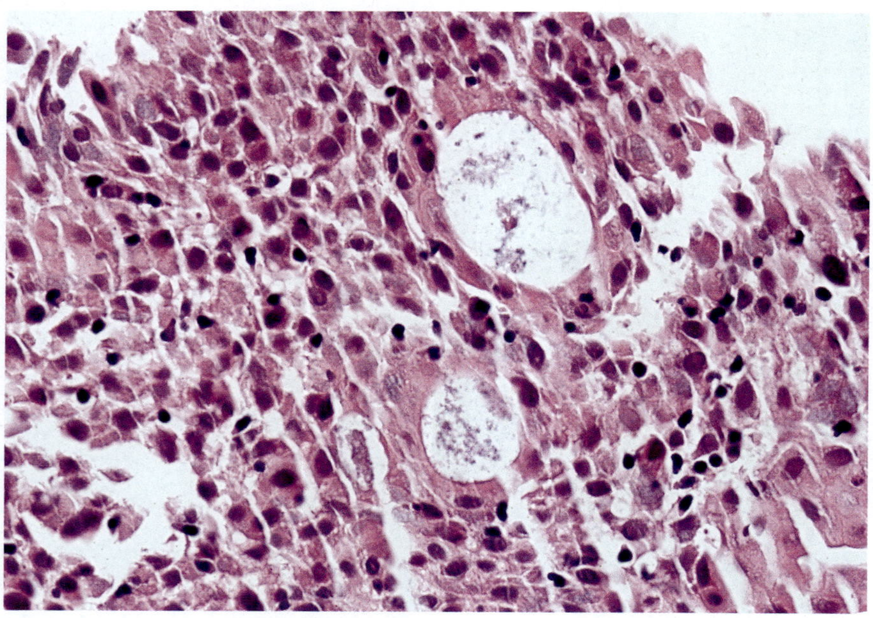

Figure 46-3.
Pseudoglandular differentiation. Several small spaces containing some cell debris in a reactive urothelium with spongiosis.

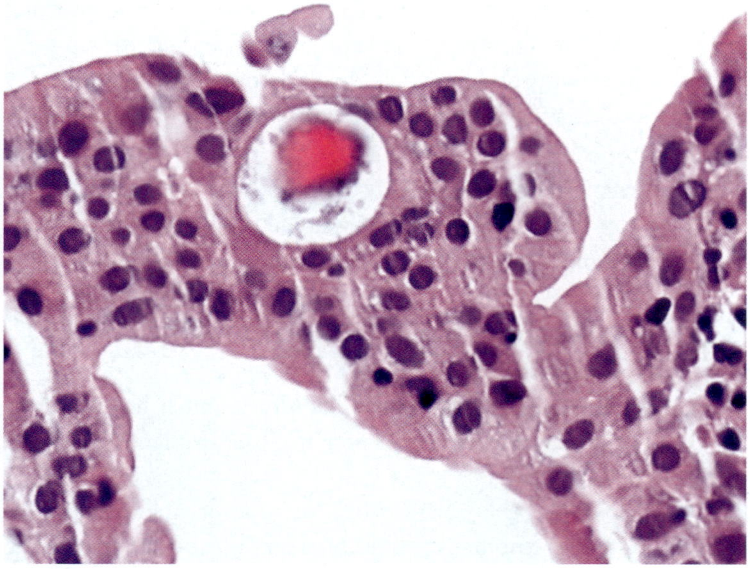

Figure 46-4.
A microcyst (pseudoglandular differentiation) containing cell debris in reactive urothelium.

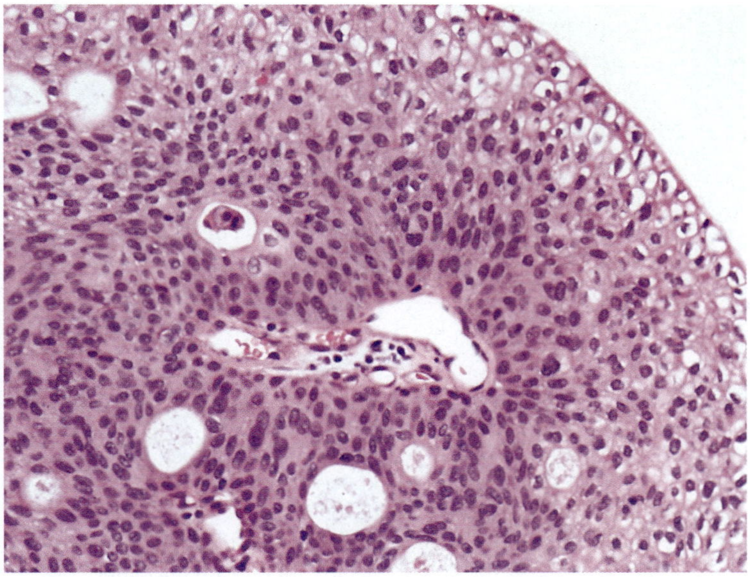

Figure 46-5.
Pseudoglandular differentiation in a low-grade papillary urothelial carcinoma. Multiple small spaces filled with cell debris can be seen without glandular lining cells.

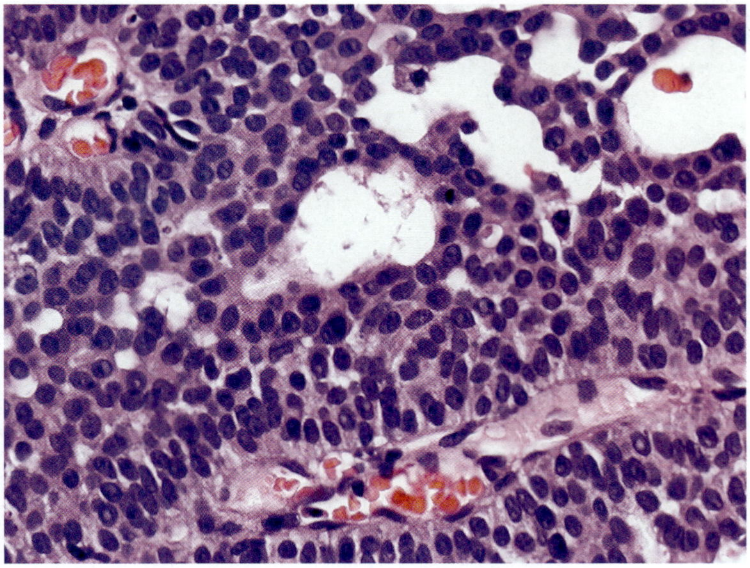

Figure 46-6.
Pseudoglandular differentiation of a papillary urothelial carcinoma contains several spaces without true glandular formation.

COLONIC METAPLASIA

Definition

- A metaplastic process in which urothelium is transformed to colonic epithelium with goblet cells. It may be considered a special form of CG

Other terms

- Intestinal metaplasia, mucinous metaplasia, mucinous cystitis glandularis

Pathogenesis

- Reactive changes to some chronic stimuli
- It may be a precursor of adenocarcinoma
- It can be found in the bladder and other organs of the urinary tract with urothelial lining

Clinical features

- Chronic irritating symptoms similar to CG

Gross pathology

- No lesion grossly identifiable

Histology

- Presence of tall columnar cells with basally located nuclei and a variable number of goblet cells (Fig. 46-7)
- Intestinal metaplasia can involve full thickness of urothelium (Fig. 46-8*a*) or present focally in the background of CG (Fig. 46-8*b*)
- Glandular cells are similar to normal colonic mucosa, without cytological atypia (Figs. 47-7 and 46-8)
- Reactive urothelium (Fig. 46-8*c*) and chronic inflammatory cells may be present in the lamina propria (Fig. 46-8*d*)

Immunohistochemistry

- Not well established. The lesional cells can be positive for colonic markers such as CDX2

Clinical relevance (prognosis and treatment options)

- Colonic metaplasia in the bladder is much less common than CG, which may be one step closer to adenocarcinoma, enteric type
- However, the relationship of colonic metaplasia and adenocarcinoma of the bladder is still controversial, which is less clear than the relationship between Barrett esophagus and adenocarcinoma
- There is a frequent finding of colonic metaplasia in cases of bladder adenocarcinoma, enteric type
- Although there is no agreement on the degree of risk that carcinoma can develop in the background of colonic metaplasia, we believe that the patients with colonic metaplasia in the bladder should be closely followed clinically to monitor the potential development of adenocarcinoma

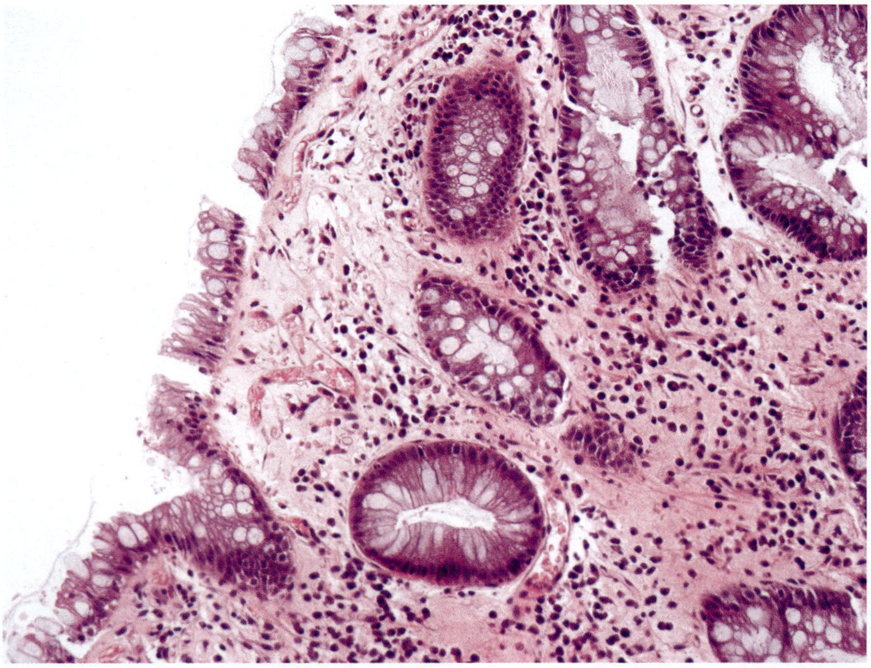

Figure 46-7.
Colonic metaplasia of the bladder, individual metaplastic glands are indistinguishable morphologically from normal colonic glands.

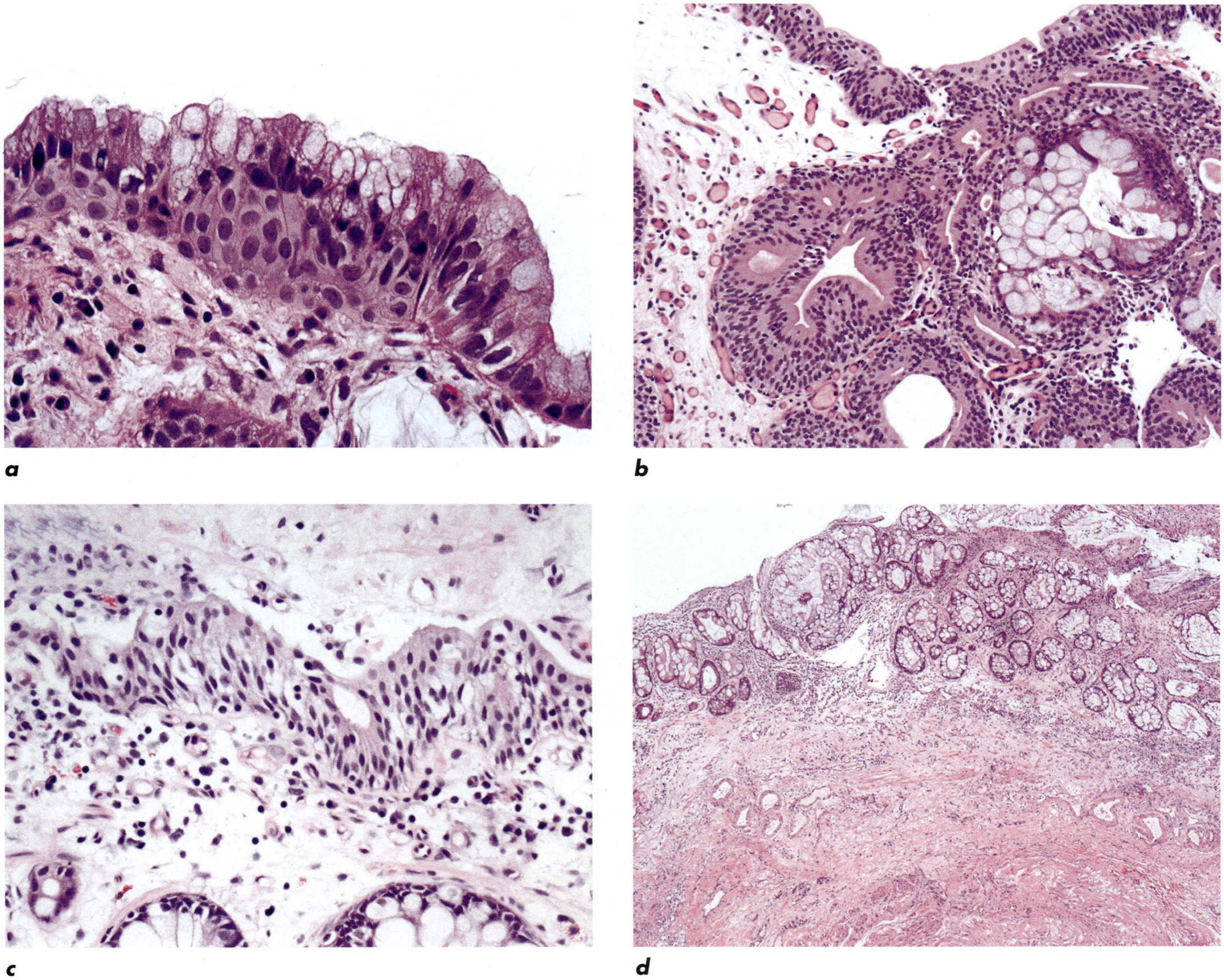

Figure 46-8.
Colonic metaplasia of the urothelium containing columnar cells with a few goblet cells on the top of urothelial basal cells (*a*). The presence of colonic metaplasia in the background of cystitis glandularis (*b*). Reactive urothelium present adjacent to colonic metaplasia (*c*). The entire urothelial lining of the bladder is replaced by colonic epithelium (*d*), which is difficult to distinguish from a colonic mucosa. But the discontinuous muscular mucosae of the bladder is present.

PROSTATIC-TYPE POLYP

Definition

- Benign prostatic glands present in the bladder mucosa as a polypoid lesion
- This lesion can be seen in the bladder or prostatic urethra

Other term

- Ectopic prostatic tissue in the bladder

Clinical features

- Only seen in males
- In young patients, it usually presents as a polypoid lesion, which may be ectopic in nature
- In an older man, benign prostatic hyperplasia can protrude into the bladder neck or prostatic urethra, giving the appearance of a mass lesion

Gross pathology

- Mostly located in the trigone or bladder neck as a polypoid or small mass lesion

Histology

- Benign urothelial lining of the polypoid lesion
- Clusters of prostatic-type glandular structures in a lobular pattern (Fig. 46-9*a*)
- Two types cells: tall columnar (secretory) cells and basal cells are present as seen in a benign prostatic gland (Figs. 46-9*b* and 46-10)
- With or without corpora amylacea

Immunohistochemistry

- PSA positive, P63 and HMWCK positive (in basal cells) (Fig. 46-10)
- AMACR, p53 negative
- Low Ki67 proliferative activities

Differential diagnosis

Cystitis glandularis

- Not convoluted as prostatic glands
- Only one population of cells (no basal cells)
- PSA negative

Prostatic ductal adenocarcinoma

- Tall columnar cells with nuclear atypia
- Arranged in papillary or cribriform patterns
- No basal cells (p63 and HMWCK negative)
- AMACR positive (strong to weak)

Clinical relevance (prognosis and treatment options)

- Benign
- Surgical removal if symptomatic or suspicious for malignancy

Figure 46-9.
Prostatic-type polyp is composed of glandular structures under papillary reactive urothelium (*a*). High magnification shows the presence of prostatic glands with both columnar secretory cells and basal cells without cytological atypia (*b*).

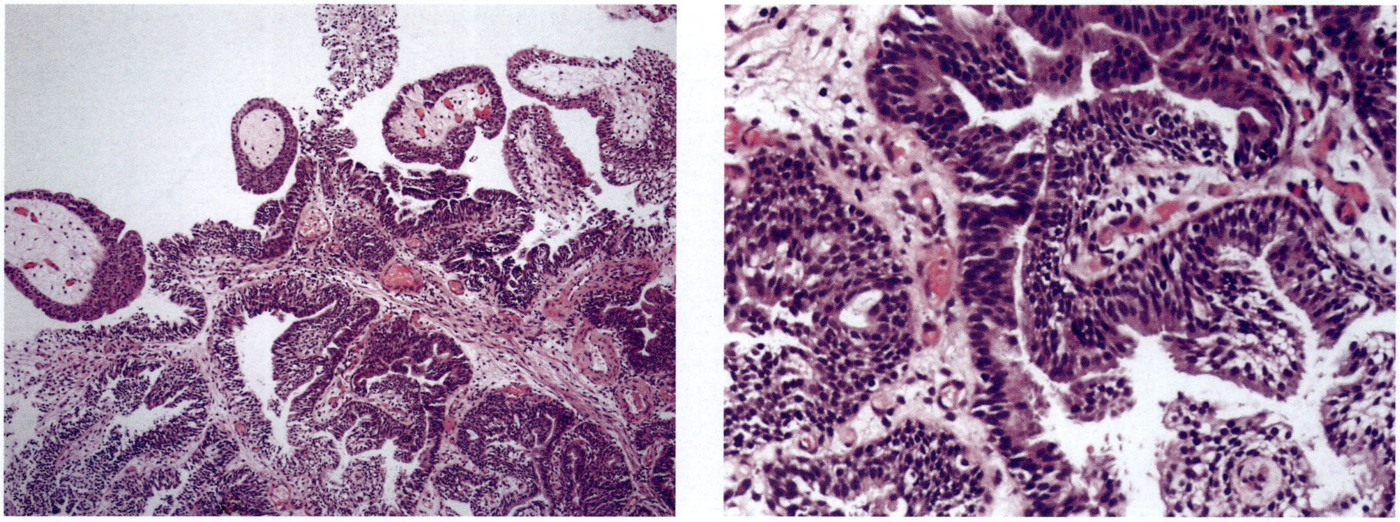

a **b**

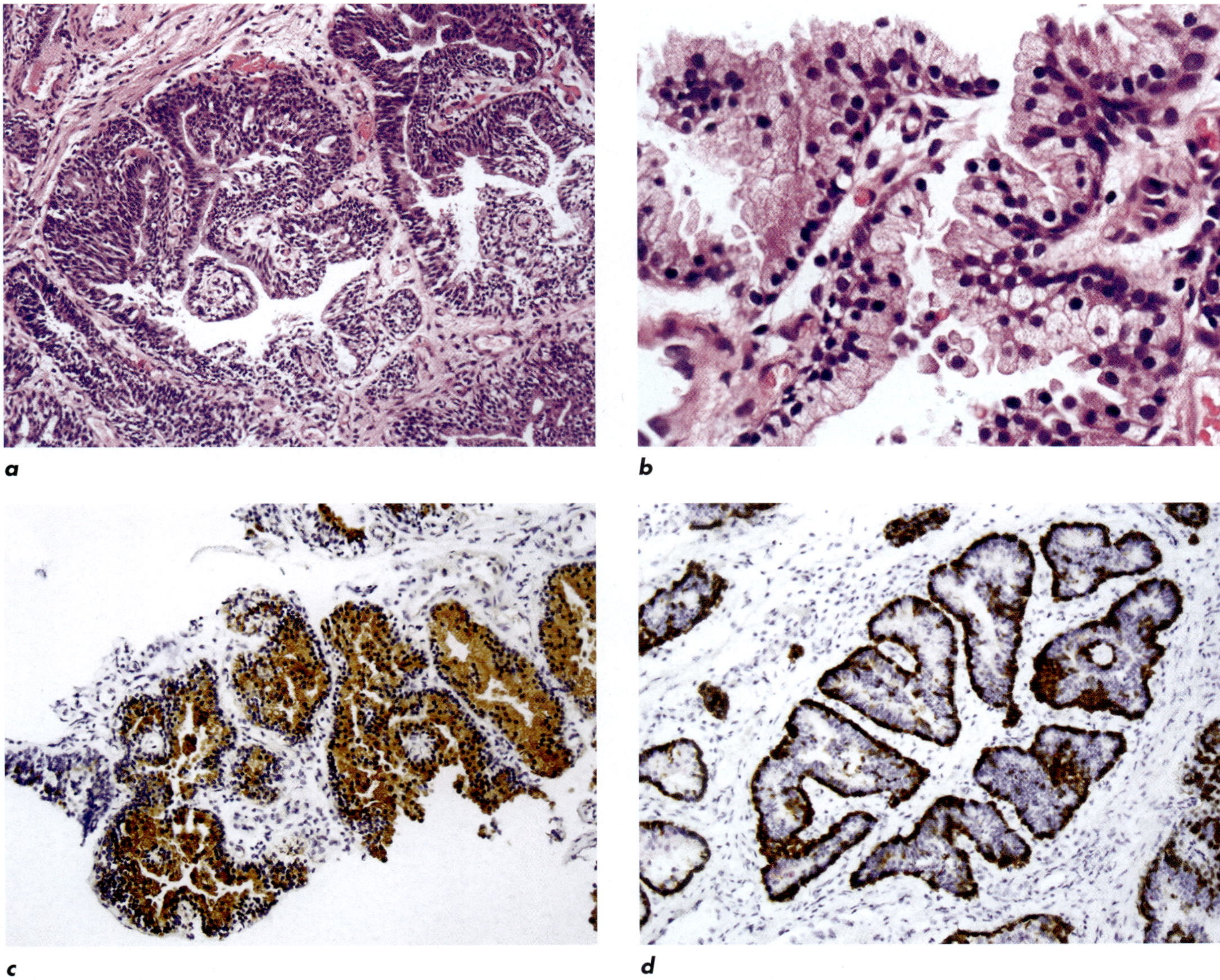

Figure 46-10.
Prostatic-type polyp with glandular structures in the bladder (*a*). High magnification shows the presence of prostatic glands (*b*), which are positive for PSA (*c*), positive for basal cell markers (p63 and HMWCK), and negative for AMACR (*d*, triple stain).

ENDOMETRIOSIS OF THE BLADDER

Definition

- Presence of benign endometrium in the bladder

Clinical features

- Females of reproductive age
- Low abdominal pain intensified with menstrual cycles
- Hematuria if the bladder mucosa is interrupted

Gross pathology

- Hemorrhagic spots or cysts in bladder mucosa
- Mass lesion if involving deep muscularis propria and associated with fibrosis

Histology

- Clusters or individual glands with infiltrating appearance (Fig. 46-11). Glandular cells are tall columnar and mitotically active, which may have secretion or cilia (if tubal metaplasia is present). The glandular cells are surrounded by spindle endometrial stroma (Fig. 46-12)
- The presence of hemorrhage or hemosiderin-laden macrophages is a common finding (Fig. 46-13)

Immunohistochemistry

- ER and PR positive in both epithelial and stromal cells
- CD10 positive in stromal cells

Clinical relevance (prognosis and treatment options)

- Benign condition, which may require treatment such as hormonal therapy for endometriosis

Figure 46-11.
Bladder endometriosis is composed of glands with columnar cells and short spindle stroma cells (*a*). High magnification shows benign tall columnar epithelial cells and spindle stromal cells, associated with hemorrhage (*b*).

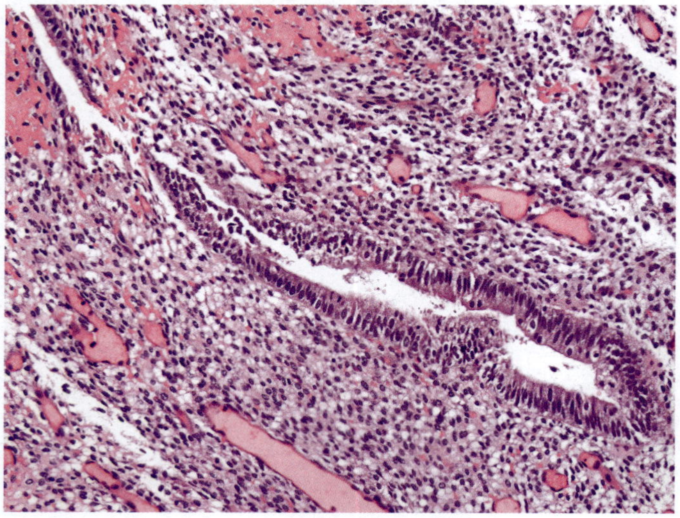

a

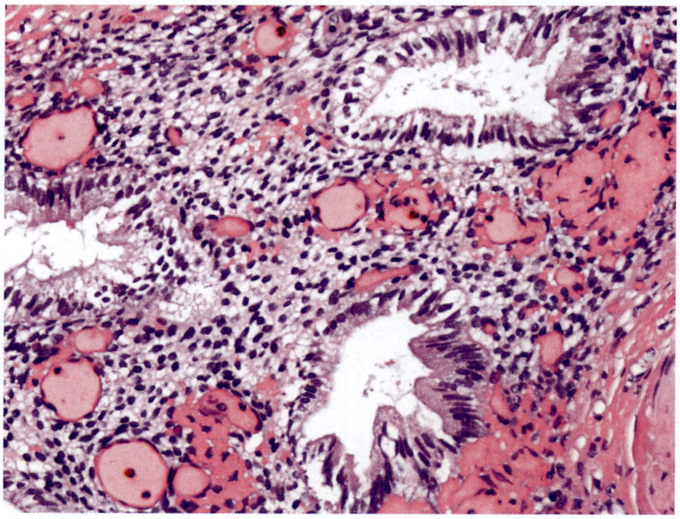

b

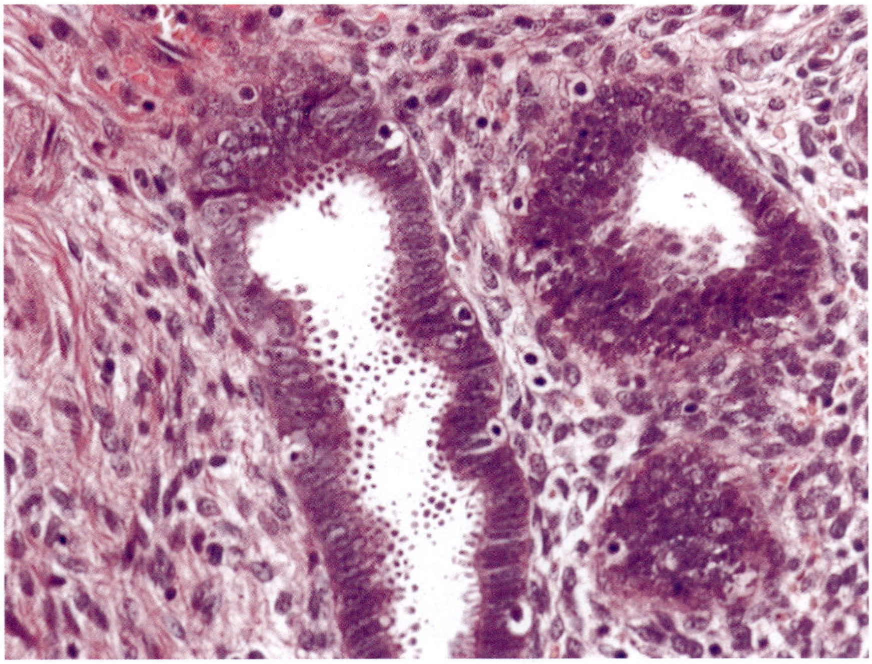

Figure 46-12.
Bladder endometriosis with tubular metaplasia.

Figure 46-13.
Bladder endometriosis with dilated endometrial gland and chronic inflammation (*a*). High magnification shows the presence of hemosiderin-laden macrophages (*b*).

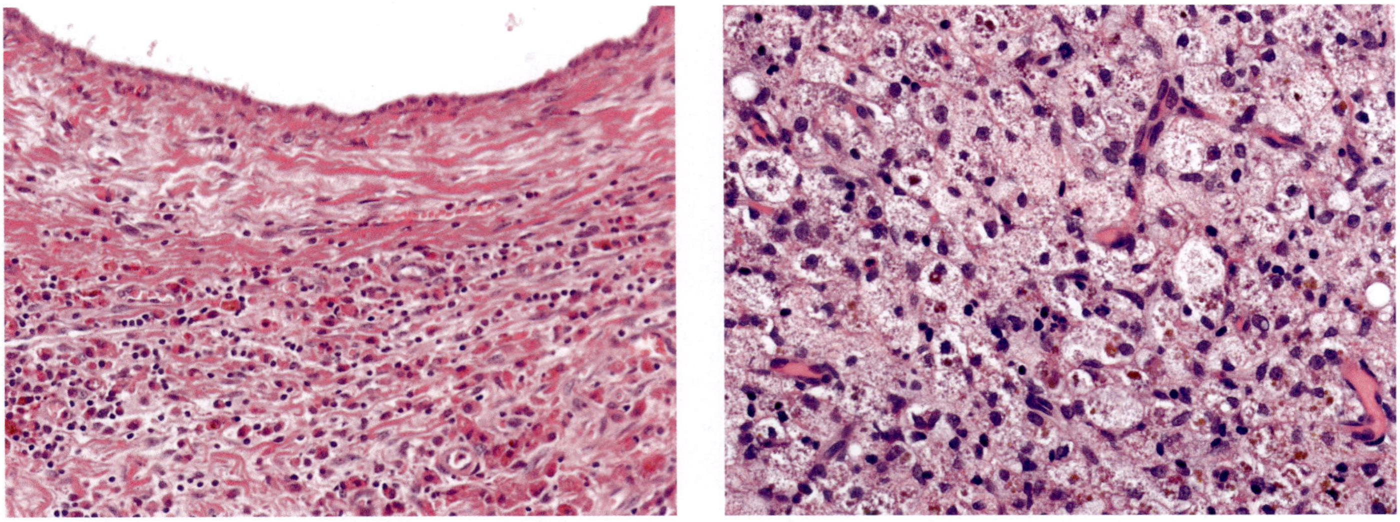

a **b**

NEPHROGENIC ADENOMA

Definition

- Nephrogenic adenoma is a benign lesion developed in the urothelium, characterized by small clusters of glandular structures resembling renal tubules

Other term

- Nephrogenic metaplasia

Pathogenesis

- In most cases, the epithelial components of lesions are derived from implants of shed renal tubules in a damaged urothelial mucosa
- It is a reactive process rather than a neoplastic process
- In some cases, metaplastic changes derived from the urothelial lining are possible

Clinical features

- There is usually a history of urothelial injury, such as instrumentation, calculi, or following a biopsy or transurethral resection (TUR)
- In immunocompromised particularly renal transplant patients, the risk is higher
- The majority of the cases are seen in immune-competent individuals

Gross pathology

- Nephrogenic adenoma is typically a small polypoid or papillary lesion, ranging from 1 to 10 mm

Histology

- Typically two components present: glandular cells similar to renal tubules and granulation tissue background (Fig. 46-14)
- The two common patterns are papillary (Fig. 46-15) and tubular (Fig. 46-16)
- The glandular epithelial cells of this lesion are ranging from flat (capillary type), cuboidal to occasionally columnar (Figs. 46-14 and 46-16)
- There are many different patterns such as capillary, flat, thyroid-like, or signet-ring-cell like patterns (Fig. 46-17). Most often, multiple patterns are mixed in a nephrogenic adenoma
- Hobnail cells, cells with cytological vacuoles (signet-ring like), or isolated cells with prominent nucleoli can be seen (Fig. 46-17*d*)
- Diffuse cytological atypia is generally absent
- Occasionally, nephrogenic adenoma may coexist with urothelial carcinoma or adenocarcinoma (Fig. 46-18)
- Two common features in nephrogenic adenomas are
  - Granulation-tissue-like background with prominent stroma edema and inflammatory cell infiltrates (Fig. 46-17)
  - Thick basement membranes or hyaline sheets around the tubules

Figure 46-14.
Nephrogenic adenoma of the bladder is composed of glandular structures lined by columnar cells in an edematous stromal background (*a*). The lining epithelium is tall columnar with basally located nuclei (*b*).

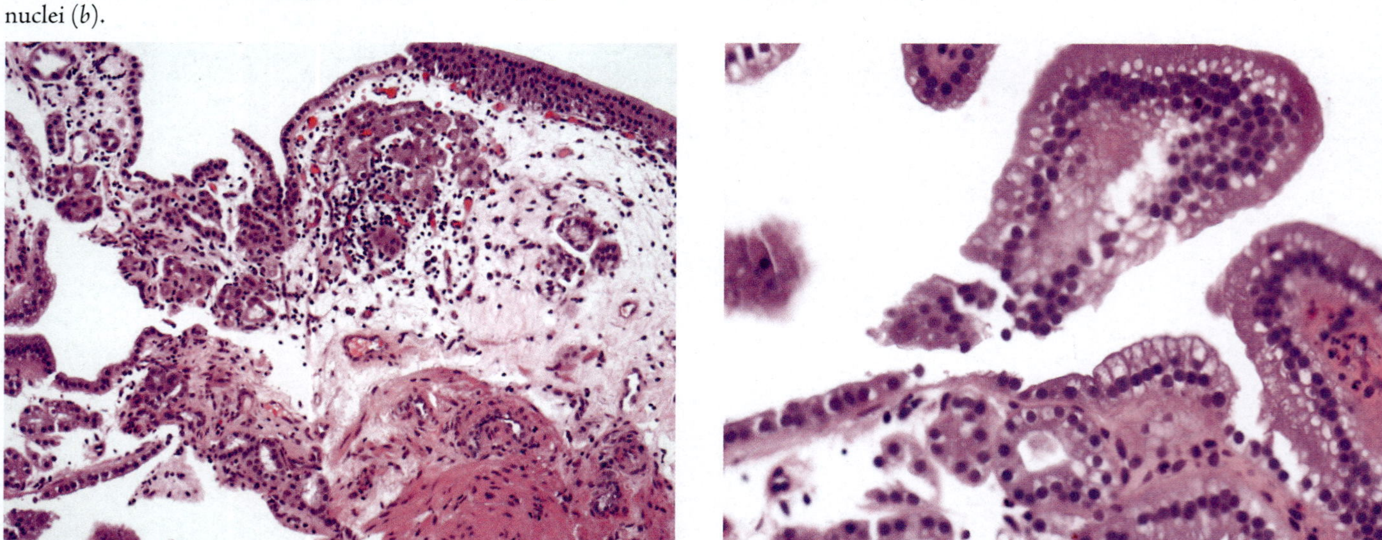

a **b**

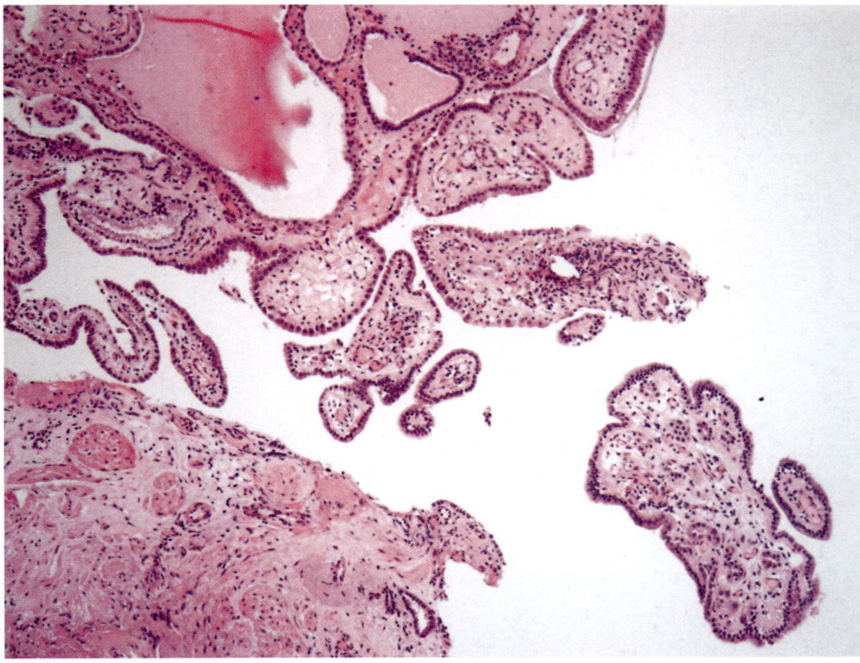

Figure 46-15.
Nephrogenic adenoma showing papillary structures with fibrovascular cores, lined by a single layer of columnar epithelium.

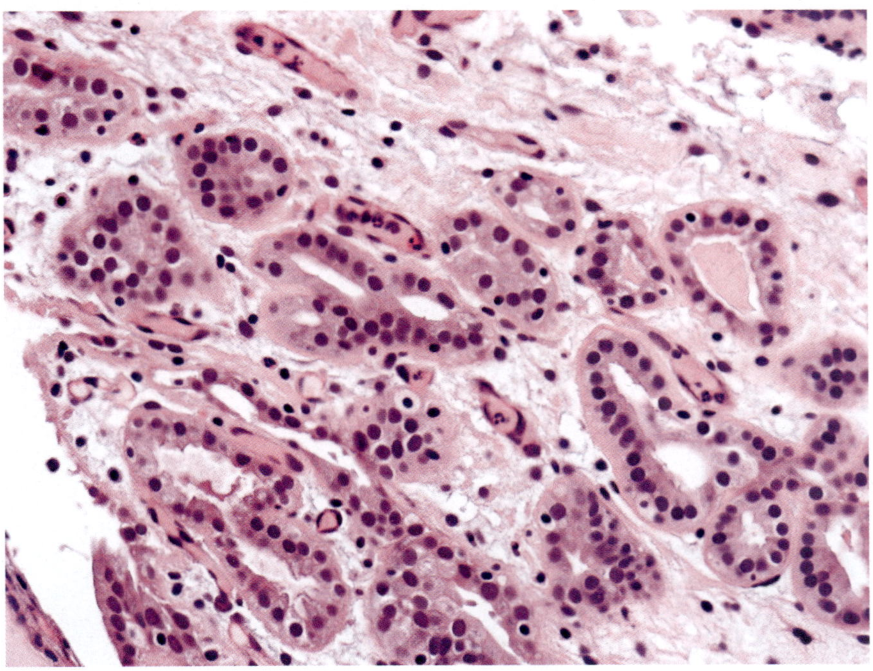

Figure 46-16.
Nephrogenic adenoma, tubular type, is composed of tubules with hyalinized basement membrane surrounded by edematous stroma.

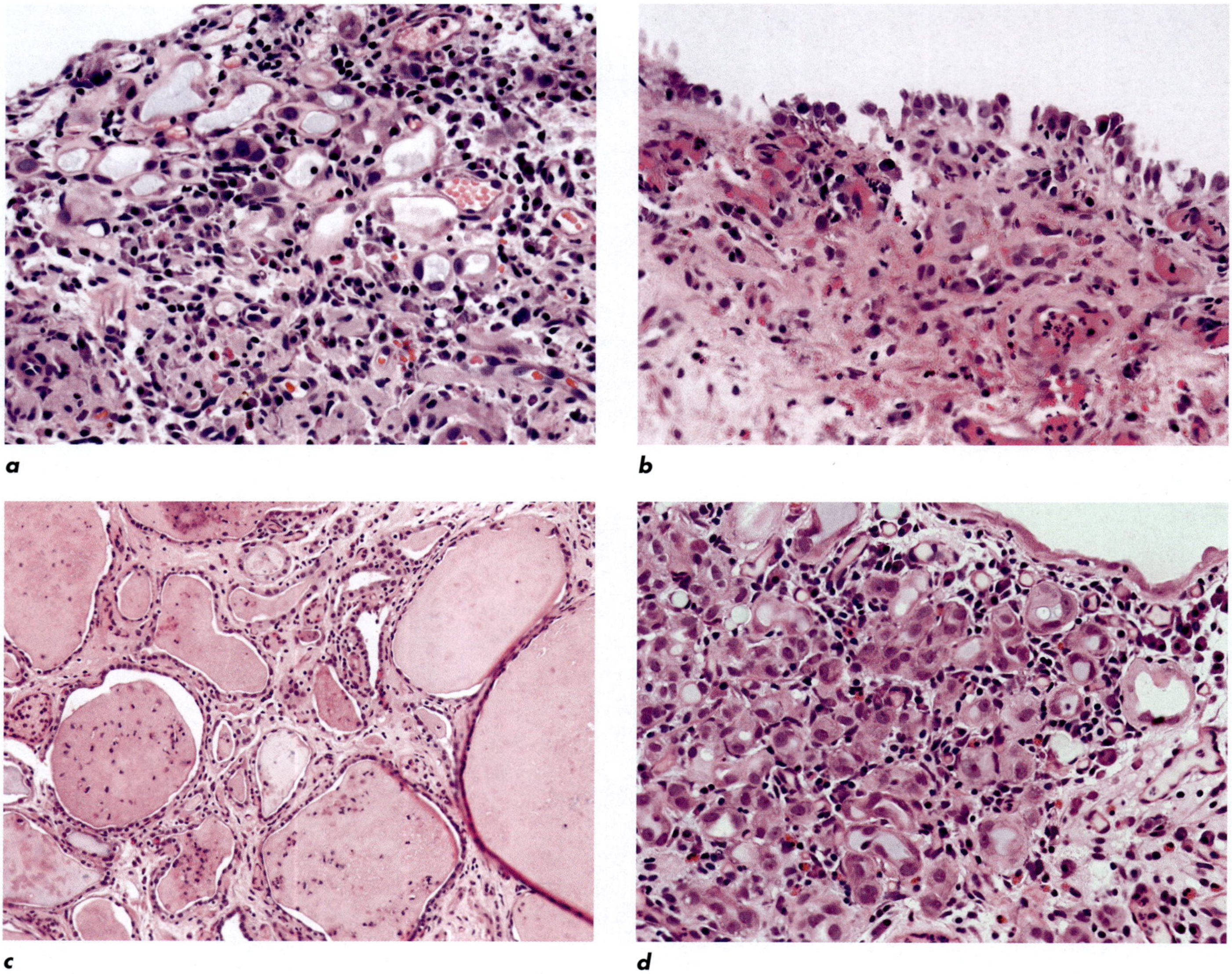

Figure 46-17.

Histological variants of nephrogenic adenoma. Endothelium-like type, composed of cystic dilated glands resembling capillaries (*a*), flat type, a single layer of columnar cells covering the surface (*b*), thyroid-like type, resembling the thyroidization of renal tubules in the end-stage kidney (*c*), and signet-ring type, containing mucinous secretion in the cells or glands (*d*).

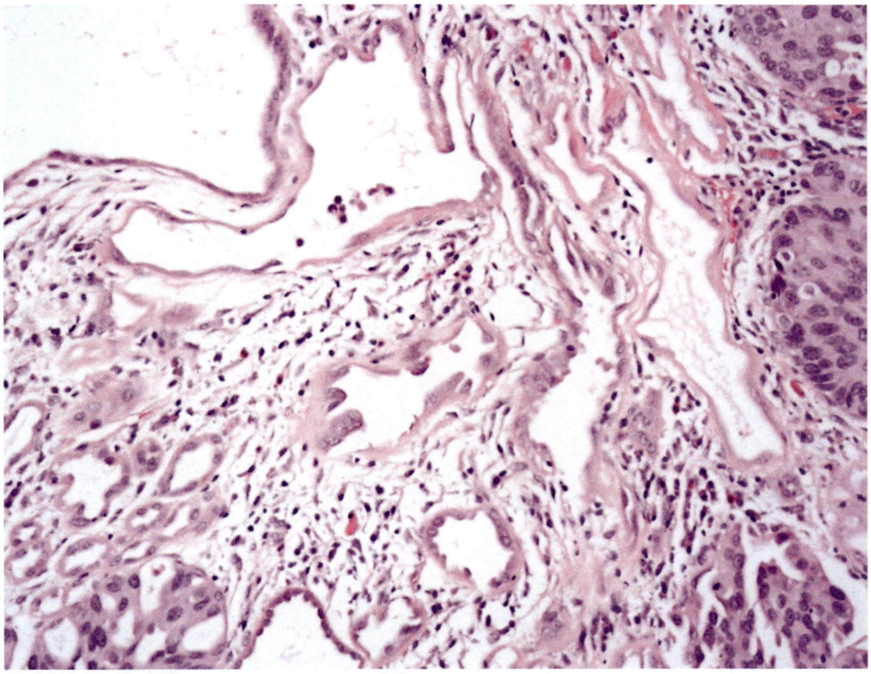

Figure 46-18.
Nephrogenic adenoma coexisting with low-grade urothelial carcinoma (right).

Immunohistochemistry

- Diagnosis of nephrogenic adenoma should be primarily based on H&E, because its immunoprofiles are variable and can be overlapping with adenocarcinoma
- Positive for PAX8, AMACR (50%) (Fig. 46-19), and HMWCK (30% to 50%), positive for CK7
- Negative for PSA (Fig. 46-19*c*) or p53

Differential diagnosis

- Adenocarcinoma of the bladder (see Table 46-1)
- Prostatic-type polyp and prostatic adenocarcinoma (see Table 46-2)

Clinical relevance (prognosis and treatment options)

- This is a benign reactive lesion, not a neoplasm as the name suggests
- No particular treatment necessary
- In most cases, the lesions are removed because they are suspicious for tumors
- Histologically, it can be mistaken for bladder adenocarcinoma or prostatic adenocarcinoma

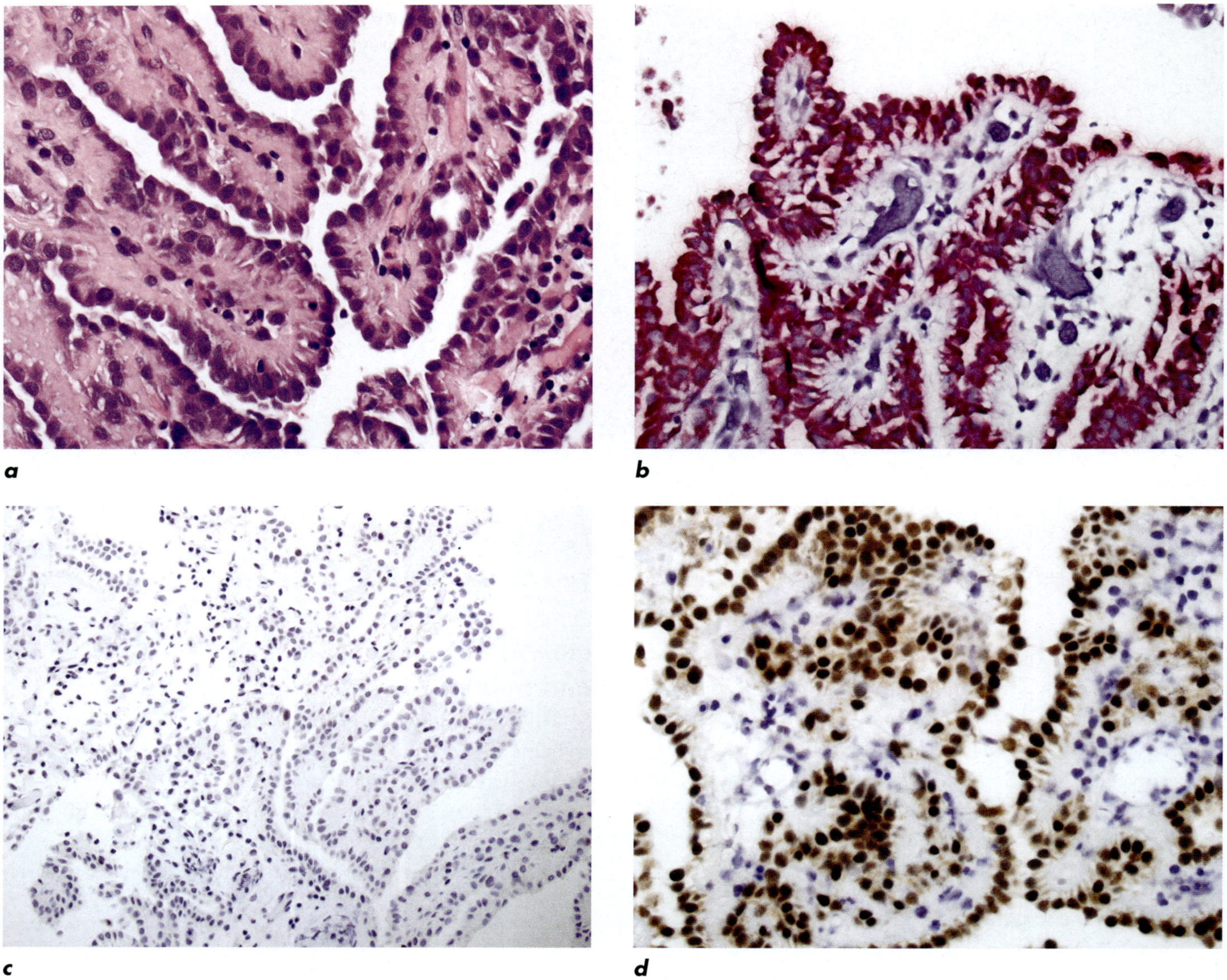

Figure 46-19.
Nephrogenic adenoma (*a*), showing positivity for AMACR, negative for basal cell markers (*b* triple stain), negative for PSA (*c*), and positive for PAX8 (*d*).

Table 46-1. Comparison of Nephrogenic Adenoma and Bladder Adenocarcinoma

Features	*Nephrogenic adenoma*	*Bladder adenocarcinoma*
Size	Small	Large
	Usually <1 cm	
Gross configuration	Papillary or flat	Mass lesion
History	Procedures	Not specific
	Injury of urothelium	
Urine cytology	Negative	Positive
Background of granulation tissue	Yes	No
Hyalinized basement membrane	Yes	No
Patterns	Many, papillary, signet ring, tubular	Uniform glandular
Atypia	Mild	Marked
Immunomarkers		
AMACR	Strongly positive (50% of cases)	Negative or weakly positive
P63	Negative/positive	Positive
HMWCK	Negative/positive	Strongly positive
P53	Negative	Strongly positive
PAX8	Positive	Negative
PSA	Negative	Negative

AMACR, α-methylacyl-CoA racemase; HMWCK, high molecular cytokeratins; PAX8, paired box gene 8; PSA, prostate-specific antigen.

Table 46-2. Differential Diagnosis Using Immunohistochemical Markers

Marker	*Nephrogenic adenoma*	*Prostatic polyp*	*Prostatic adenocarcinoma*
AMACR	Positive (50%)	Negative	Positive
P63	Negative	Positive	Negative
HMWCK	Positive or negative	Positive	Negative
PSA	Negative	Positive	Positive
PAX8	Positive	Negative	Negative

AMACR, α-methylacyl-CoA racemase; HMWCK, high molecular cytokeratins; PAX8, paired box gene 8; PSA, prostate-specific antigen.

URACHAL REMNANTS AND URACHAL CYST

Definition

- The urachal remnants are residual tissues from the urachus or embryonic allantoic stalk (precursor of urachus) connecting the umbilicus and bladder
- Urachal cysts are dilated urachal remnants

Pathogenesis

- After embryonic development, the urachal epithelium still remains
- After birth, most urachal ducts will be closed, but with remnant epithelium in place
- Other urachal anomalies caused by incomplete urachal closure include patent urachus (persistent urachus), urachal diverticulum (outpouching urothelium), and urachal abscess (infected urachal cyst with pus formation)

Clinical features

- Urachal remnants are usually indolent without symptoms
- A midline low abdominal palpable mass lesion located between umbilicus and bladder dome, if the lesion is dilated or infected
- Tenderness and fever may be present when urachal cysts are infected
- Persistent discharge of mucous material from the umbilicus
- Pain during urination
- Symptoms associated with low urinary tract infection if the infected urachal cysts are open to the bladder
- Imaging studies reveal a cystic lesion located between the umbilicus and the dome of the bladder
- Urachal abscess is defined as acute inflammation of urachal cysts with pus formation

Gross pathology

- Urachal remnants cannot be identified grossly unless it is dilated or infected
- Urachal cyst, with smooth inner surface, contains clear or mucous content

Histology

- Urachal remnants are small tubular or glandular structures lined by flat or cuboidal epithelium (Fig. 46-20)
- Urachal remnants can be cystically dilated and become urachal cysts (Fig. 46-21)
- Acute or chronic inflammation may be found in the cystic wall if infected. An abscess can be formed (Fig. 46-22)
- Colonic metaplasia can be occasionally seen in the urachal remnants or cysts
- Dysplastic changes may be present, which is the precursor lesion of adenocarcinoma

Clinical relevance (prognosis and treatment options)

- Urachal remnants do not need treatment if asymptomatic
- The treatment of choice for urachal cysts or infected urachal cysts is surgical removal
- Presence of the urachal remnants is the evidence for the diagnosis of urachal carcinoma

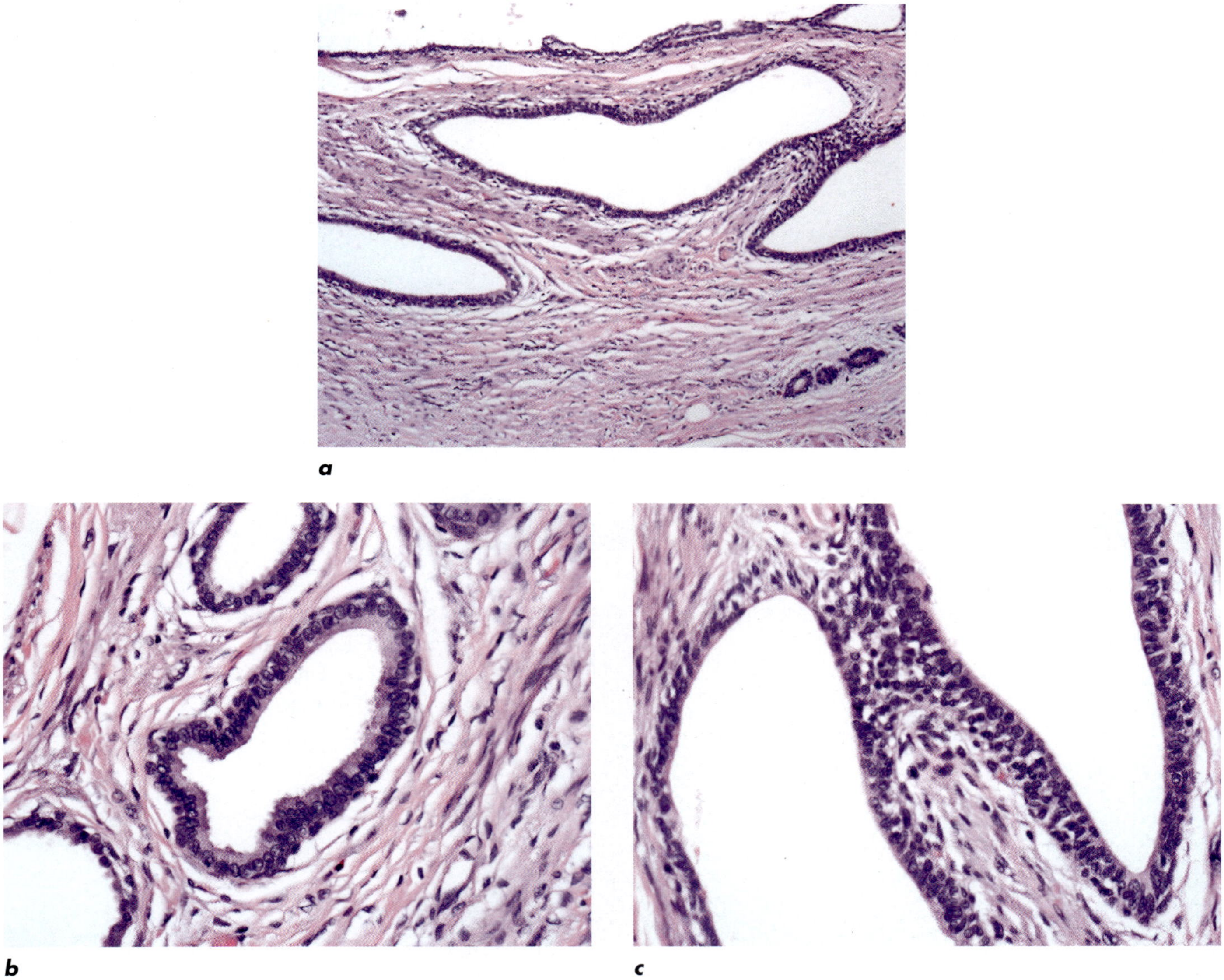

Figure 46-20.

Urachal remnants are glandular structures located in the bladder dome or area between bladder and umbilicus (*a*). Two layers of lining epithelium can be seen: columnar with single layer of basal cells (*b*) or columnar cells with multiple layers of basal cells (*c*).

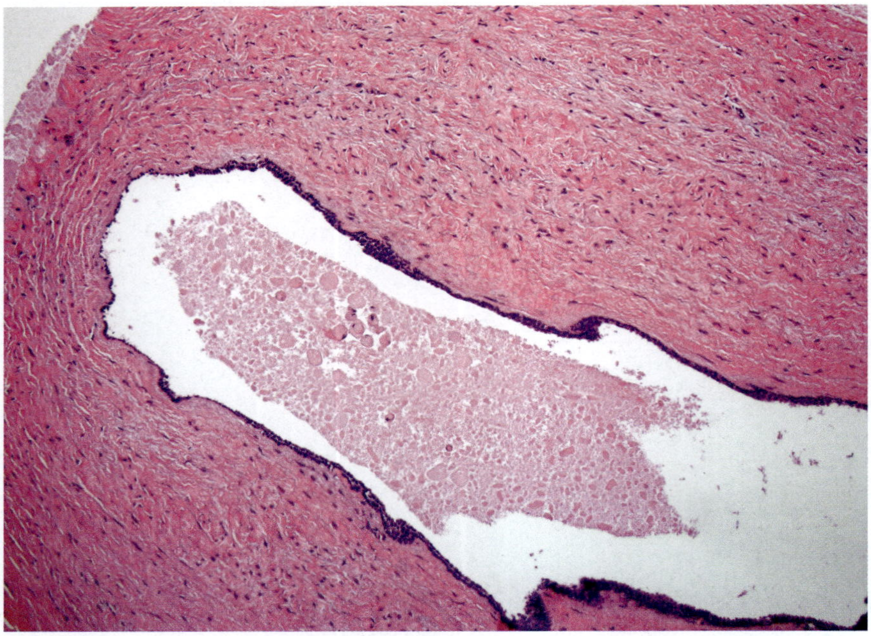

Figure 46-21.
Urachal cyst lined by multiple layers of epithelium.

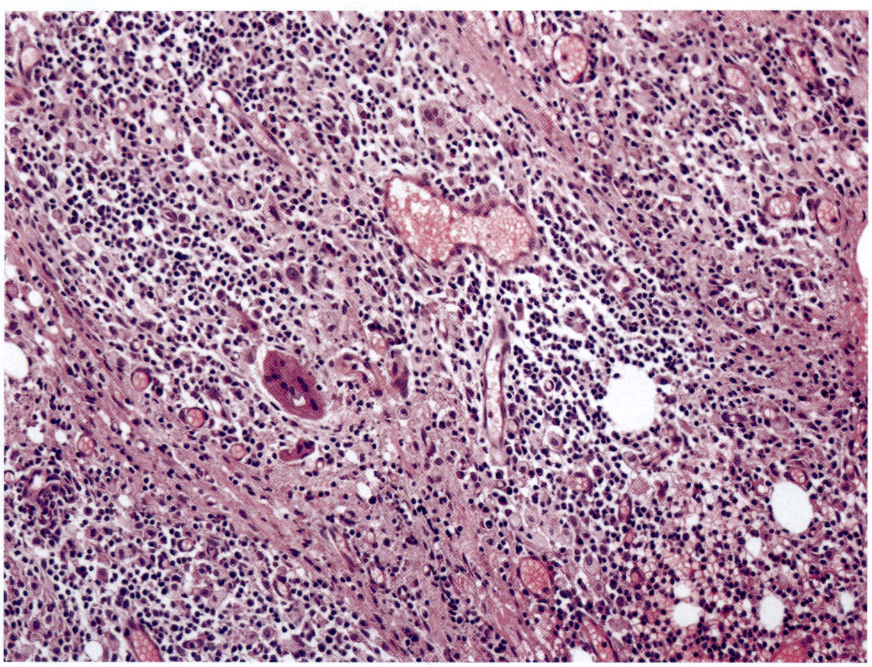

Figure 46-22.
Urachal abscess. Infected urachal cyst with marked acute and chronic inflammation, and abscess formation.

VILLOUS ADENOMA

Definition

- Benign glandular epithelial neoplasm of the bladder, similar to tubular or villous adenoma of the colon in morphology

Other terms

- Tubular adenoma
- Tubovillous adenoma

Pathogenesis

- It is believed to be derived from intestinal metaplasia of urothelium of the bladder
- It is very likely that there is a colonic metaplasia-adenoma-adenocarcinoma transition

Clinical features

- Uncommon condition, most common in elderly men, mean age 65 years
- Hematuria and irritative symptoms
- Mucosuria (mucus in urine) possible if the tumor is mucinous
- Cystoscopy shows a polypoid or papillary lesion

Gross pathology

- Polypoid or exophytic lesion, mostly single
- A fixed base would suggest no invasive component
- Occasionally mucinous appearance

Histology

- Villous, papillary projections covered by tall columnar cells with basally located cigar-shaped nuclei (Fig. 46-23)
- Goblet cells or intracellular mucin can be seen
- Mild or moderate dysplastic changes similar to tubular adenoma of the colon can be seen, but the presence of significant cytological atypia, loss of polarity or cribriform pattern would suggest adenocarcinoma in situ (high-grade dysplasia) (Fig. 46-24)
- The presence of high-grade dysplasia should be reported additionally

Immunohistochemistry

- CK20 positive , CDX2 positive, and CEA positive

Differential diagnosis

- All the benign glandular conditions discussed in this chapter are summarized in Table 46-3

Clinical relevance (prognosis and treatment options)

- Biologically this tumor, similar to tubular adenoma of the colon, is a dysplastic lesion
- In approximately one-third of cases, tubular adenomas may progress to invasive adenocarcinoma. Therefore, tubular adenoma is a precursor to adenocarcinoma of the bladder
- Local resection is the treatment of choice
- The patients with a history of this tumor should be clinically followed
- Cystoscopic examination is necessary in a fashion similar to the one for patients with colon tubular adenomas

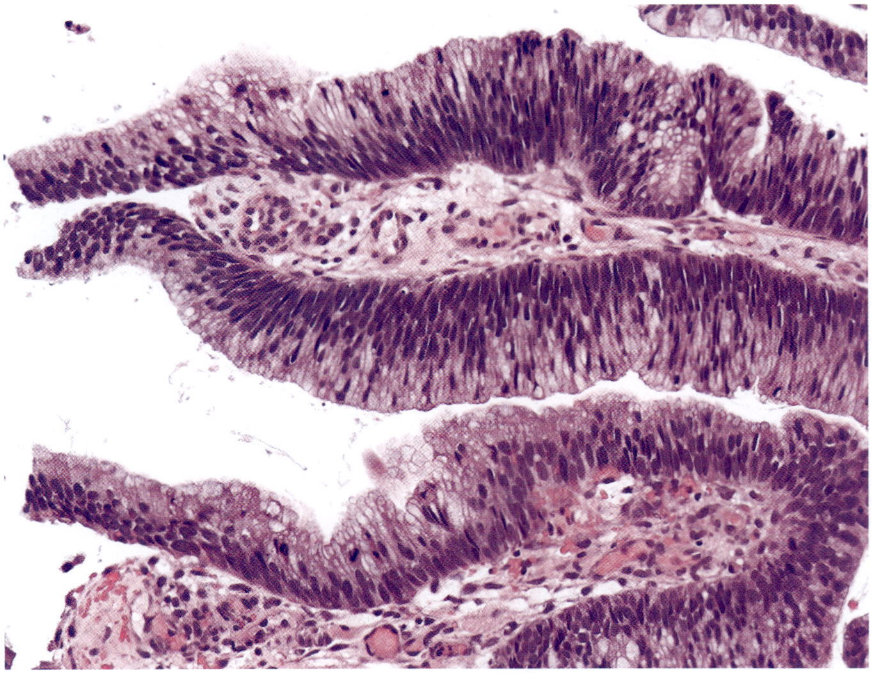

Figure 46-23.
Villous adenoma with elongated villous structures lined by pseudostratified tall columnar cells with cigar-shaped nuclei, identical to the villous adenoma of the colon.

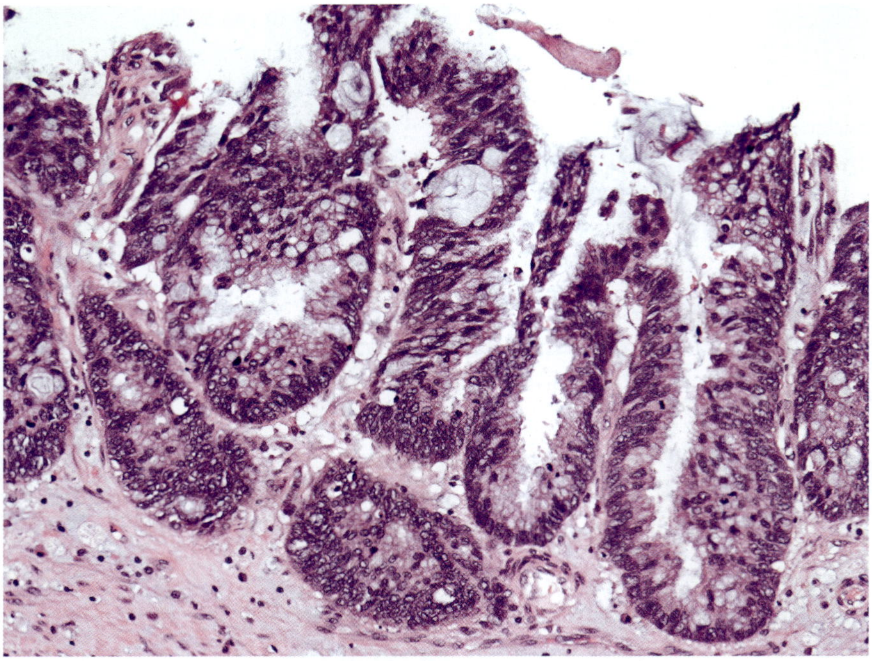

Figure 46-24.
High-grade dysplasia of villous adenoma in the bladder. The tumor cells lose the polarity with cribriform formation.

Table 46-3. Benign Glandular Lesions of the Bladder

Lesion	*Frequency*	*Histology*	*Other key feature*
Cystitis glandularis/cystica	Very common	Gland/cyst formation	
Microcysts	Common	Microcyst formation	Reactive or neoplastic urothelium
Colonic metaplasia	Uncommon	Colonic epithelium	Goblet cells
Prostatic-type polyp	Uncommon	Prostatic epithelium	Male PSA positive
Endometriosis	Uncommon	Endometrial epithelium and stroma	Female, ER/PR CD10 positive
Nephrogenic adenoma	Relatively common	Renal tubule implants	History of injury AMACR positive PSA negative
Urachal remnants	Uncommon	Flat or columnar epithelium	Located in the dome or adjacent soft tissue
Villous adenoma	Uncommon	Enteric-type adenoma	Similar to tubular adenoma of the colon

AMACR, α-methylacyl-CoA racemase; ER, estrogen receptor; PR, progesterone receptor; PSA, prostate-specific antigen.

CHAPTER 47 Inflammatory Lesions of the Bladder

NONSPECIFIC CHRONIC CYSTITIS

Definition

- There are several morphological variants of chronic cystitis with the following definitions:

Chronic cystitis (not otherwise specified)

- Chronic inflammation of the bladder with lymphocytic infiltrates without other specific features

Follicular cystitis

- Chronic inflammation of the bladder with lymphoid follicle formation

Eosinophilic cystitis

- Chronic inflammation of the bladder with prominent eosinophilic infiltrates

Etiology and epidemiology

- Infectious with predominantly gram-negative bacteria
- Induced by stone, catheterization, instrumentation, or other treatments such as BCG
- Very frequent findings in the bladder biopsies, TUR, or cystectomy specimens

Clinical features

- Nonspecific urinary stimulating syndrome
- Urine culture may be positive
- Negative cytology for malignancy

Gross pathology

- Absence of a mass lesion
- Bladder wall may be edematous, erythematous, or thickened

Histology

Chronic cystitis

- Presence of predominantly lymphocytic infiltrate in the lamina propria (Fig. 47-1*a*)
- In addition, plasma cells, neutrophils, or eosinophils can be seen
- Stromal edema and dilated vessels are commonly observed (Fig. 47-1*b*)
- Reactive urothelial changes including spongiosis may be present (Fig. 47-2)

Figure 47-1.
Nonspecific chronic cystitis caused by bacterial infection showing prominent lymphocytic infiltrate and dilated capillaries with neutrophil margination in the lamina propria (*a*). Another area shows urothelial spongiosis, edematous stroma, and chronic inflammatory cell infiltrates (*b*).

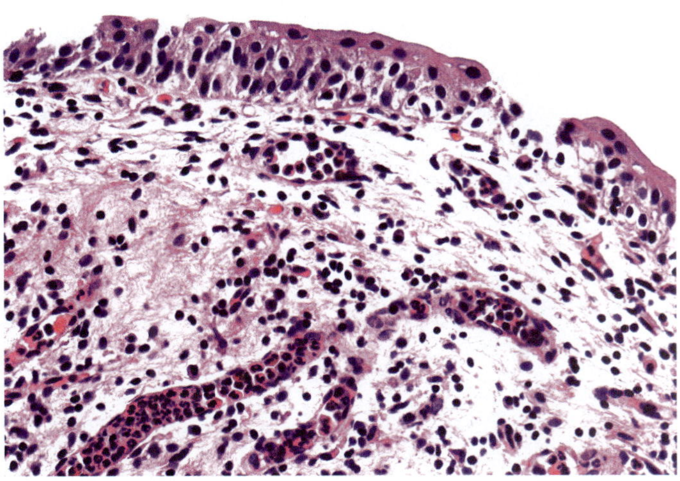

a

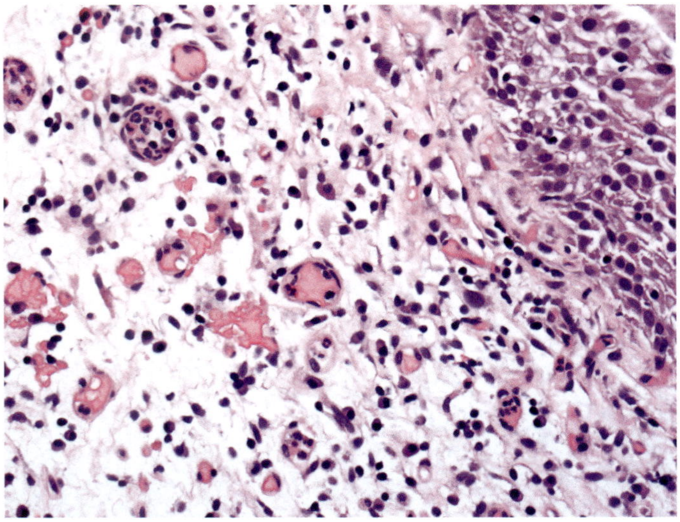

b

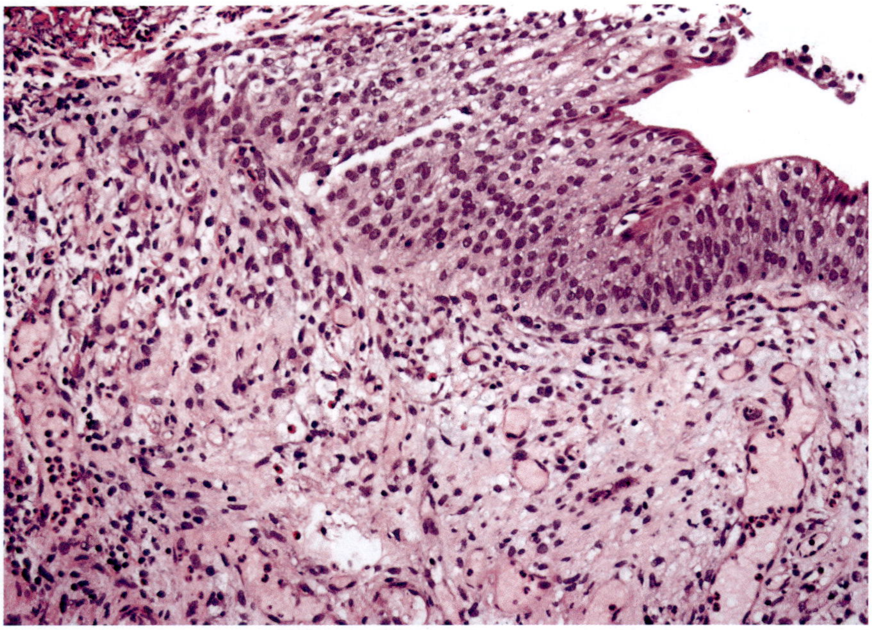

Figure 47-2.
Nonspecific chronic cystitis with infiltrate including lymphocytes and some eosinophils as well as reactive urothelium.

Follicular cystitis

- Similar to the nonspecific chronic cystitis, but with the presence of lymphoid follicles with or without germinal centers in lamina propria (Figs. 47-3 and 47-4)
- Other nonspecific chronic inflammatory cells such as plasma cells, neutrophils, or eosinophils may be present
- Stromal edema or dilated vessels may be seen
- Reactive urothelial changes may be present (Fig. 47-3*b*)
- Most of the reactive lymphocytes are mature B cells (Fig. 47-4*d*)

Eosinophilic cystitis

- Presence of prominent eosinophilic infiltrate (Fig. 47-5)
- The eosinophil count can be up to 50 to 100 per high power field (Fig. 47-5)
- It is not clear how many eosinophils are required for the diagnosis of eosinophilic cystitis (EC). Using the cutoff value of 25 eosinophils per high power field may be reasonable
- Other nonspecific chronic inflammatory cells may be present
- Reactive urothelial changes may be present
- EC is also observed in case of urothelial carcinoma and/or BCG treatment. Both carcinoma and BCG may contribute to the presence of eosinophilic infiltrate (Fig. 47-6)
- EC can be caused by systemic eosinophilia or a localized reaction to parasite infestation or treatment, which cannot be distinguished based on bladder histology alone

Differential diagnosis

- Lymphoma
  - Monotonous populations of lymphocytes
  - Some degree of cytological atypia
  - Lymphoma markers showing kappa or lambda light chain restriction will be helpful
- Small cell carcinoma
  - With high mitotic activity
  - Molding and nuclear atypia
  - Immunostaining positivity for keratins and neuroendocrine markers such as chromogranin, synaptophysin, or neuron-specific enolase can be helpful

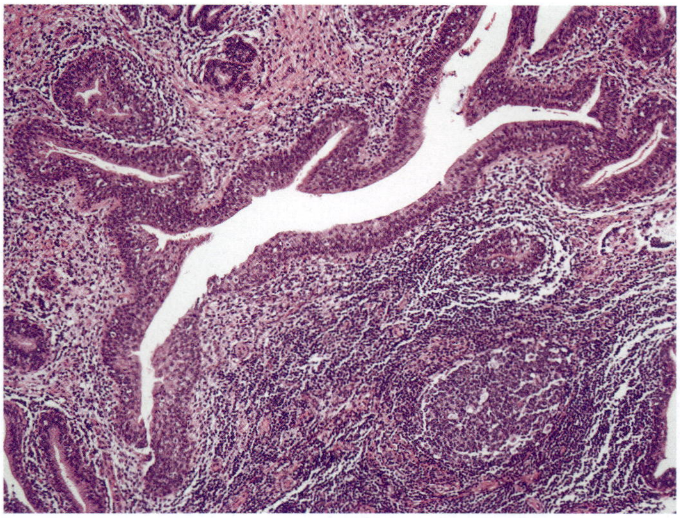

a

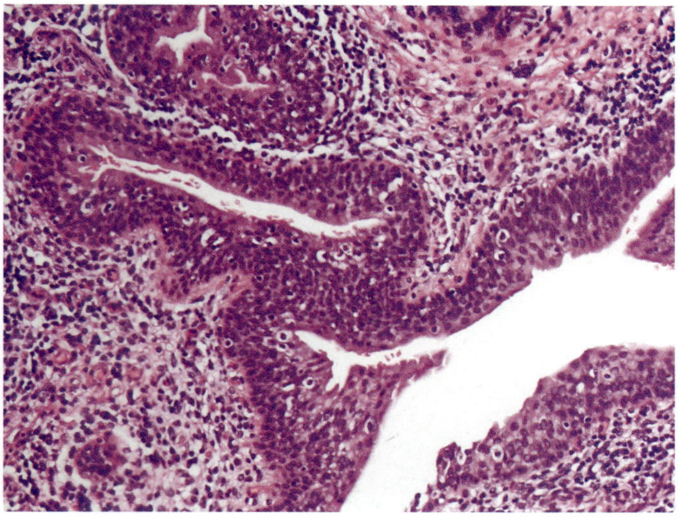

b

Figure 47-3.
Follicular cystitis containing lymphoid aggregates with germinal centers in the lamina propria (*a*). High magnification showing the presence of intraurothelial lymphocytes and urothelial reactive atypia (*b*).

Clinical relevance (prognosis and treatment options)

Chronic cystitis and follicular cystitis

- It is a nonspecific chronic inflammation
- Many infectious or noninfectious causes
- Can be coexisting with CIS or other bladder cancers
- Best treatment would be to remove the cause of disease if it is known

Eosinophilic cystitis (EC)

- EC is not a specific diagnosis for etiology based on the current knowledge
- EC could be a part of systemic eosinophilia such as parasite infection or immunological disorders
- EC could also be an isolated local reaction to a previous biopsy, parasite infestation, or invasive carcinoma
- The presence of EC should suggest a clinical work-up to rule out systemic disorder, parasite infestation, or allergic or autoimmune conditions

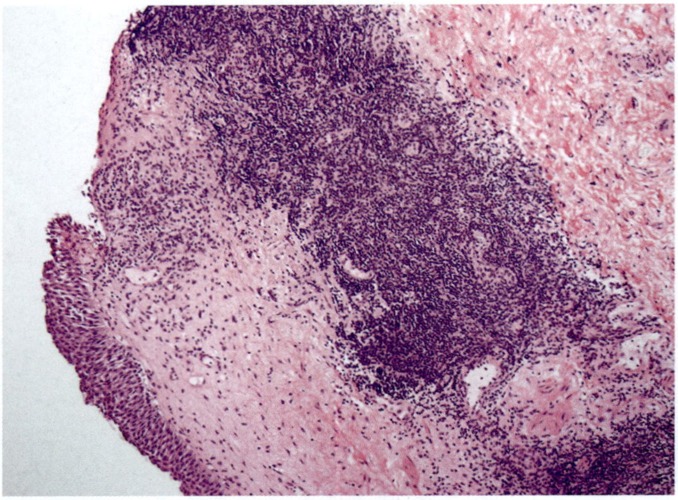

a

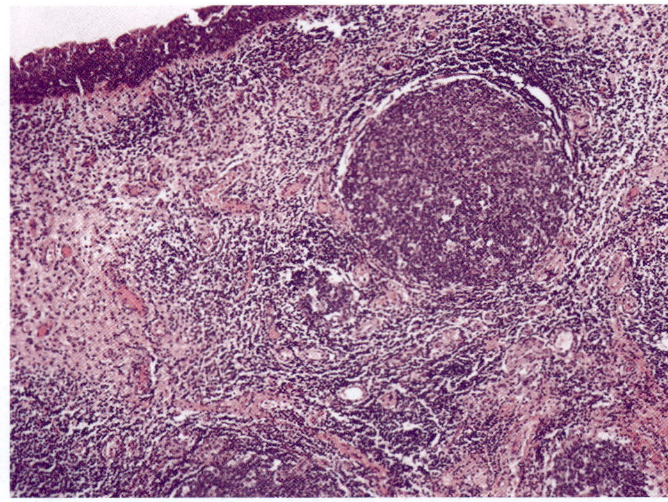

b

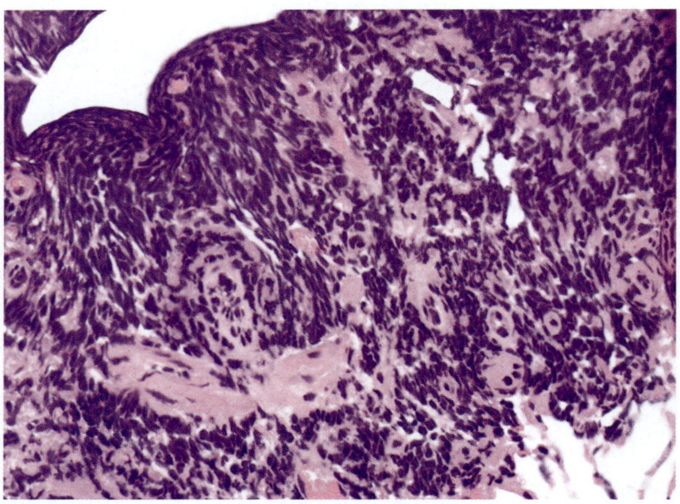

c

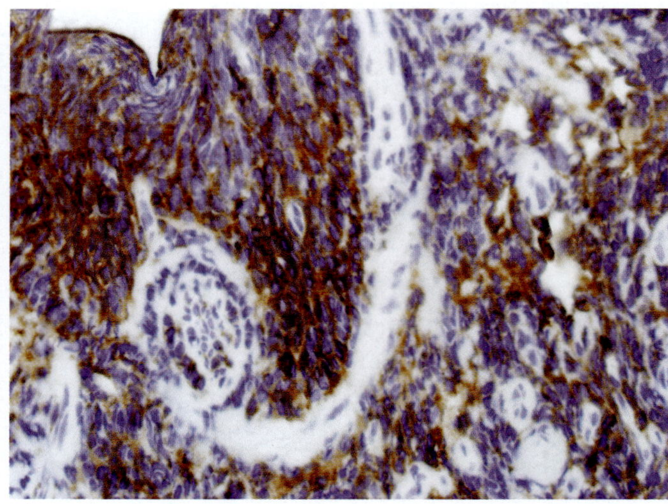

d

Figure 47-4.
Follicular cystitis with lymphoid aggregates (*a*) and lymph follicles with germinal centers (*b*). When severe crushing artifact is present (*c*), CD20 immunostaining was performed to confirm the B-cell nature of this lesion (*d*).

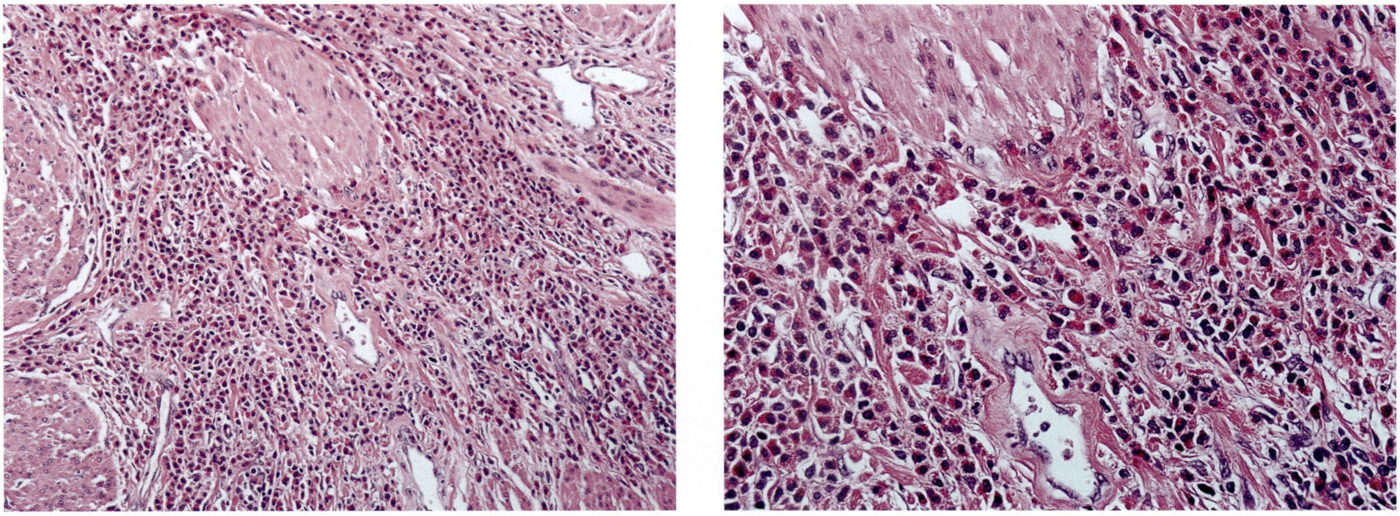

a *b*

Figure 47-5.
Eosinophilic cystitis with heavy eosinophilic infiltrates in the lamina propria (*a*). High magnification confirms more than 100 eosinophils per high power field (*b*).

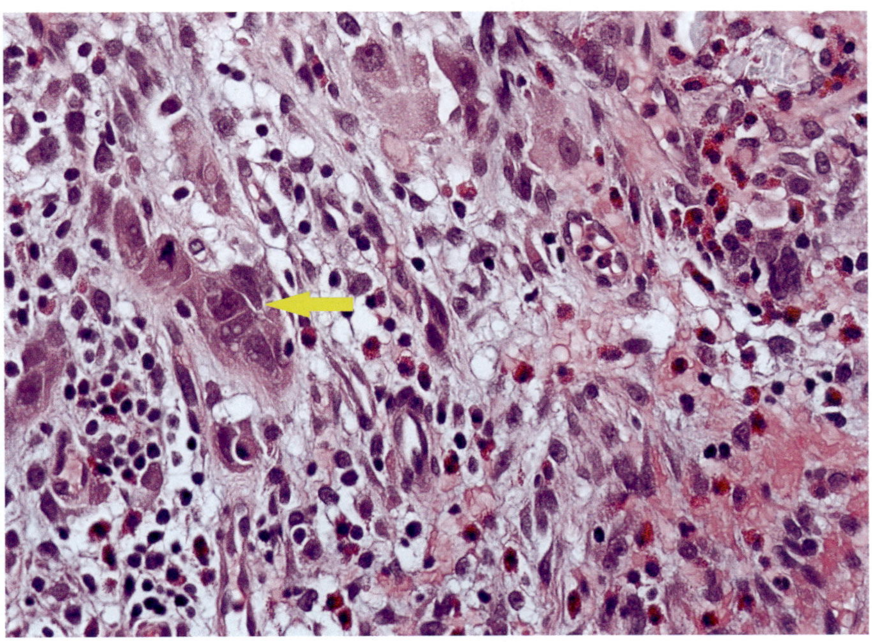

Figure 47-6.
Eosinophilic cystitis associated with high-grade invasive urothelial carcinoma (arrow) after BCG treatment.

INTERSTITIAL CYSTITIS

Definition

- Interstitial cystitis (IC) is an idiopathic inflammatory condition that may lead to ulceration and chronic inflammation of bladder mucosa

Other terms

- Hunner cystitis or Hunner ulcer, painful bladder syndrome

Pathogenesis

- Unknown etiology. It is neither infectious nor related to the presence of malignancy

Clinical features

- Typically affecting middle-aged women
- Chronic pelvic pain, particularly related to bladder filling, may be accompanied by persistent urge to void or increased urinary frequency
- Mostly female patients, more common in Caucasians
- No evidence of infection including negative urine culture
- No evidence of malignancy particularly urothelial carcinoma in situ

Gross pathology

- Classic (Hunner) type shows an ulcer or scar with radiating small vessels. Sometimes, erythematous areas or edematous mucosa can be seen
- Nonulcer type: normal-appearing and erythematous areas

Histology

- Histological features are not specific. It is basically a diagnosis of exclusion
- Infectious or neoplastic etiology needs to be excluded by negative urine culture, negative urine cytology, and confirmative biopsy
- Histologically, interstitial cystitis can be divided into two pathologic types although the clinical significance of such classification is unknown
  - Hunner type with ulceration and nonspecific chronic inflammation, with an increased number of mast cells (Fig. 47-7)
  - Nonulcer type with intact bladder mucosa and nonspecific chronic inflammation, with increased mast cells (Fig. 47-8*a*), although this finding is not specific
- Pathologists are still being asked to count the number of mast cells for diagnosis or for monitoring the disease progression and or treatment effect, although the diagnosis of IC based on the mast cell count alone is no longer accepted in clinical practice

Immunohistochemistry

- CD117 (C-kit) will highlight mast cells (Fig. 47-8*b*)

Clinical relevance (prognosis and treatment options)

- Controlling the pain is important
- Medical therapies include nonspecific anti-inflammatory drugs, antihistamines, or tricyclic agents. Can be a long-standing chronic disease
- Surgical intervention such as urinary diversion occasionally necessary

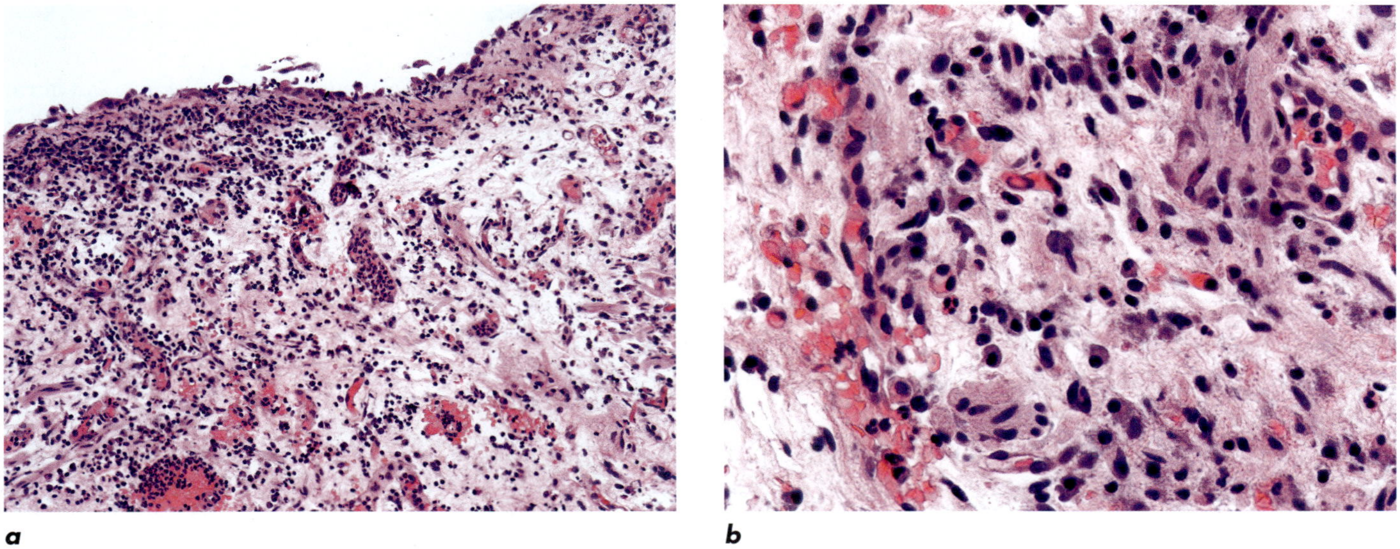

Figure 47-7.
Interstitial cystitis with partially ulcerated bladder mucosa (*a*). High magnification shows chronic inflammatory infiltrate (*b*).

Figure 47-8.
Interstitial cystitis showing mast cells in the lamina propria (*a*, arrow). Immunostaining for C-kit confirms the presence of increased mast cells in the lamina propria (*b*).

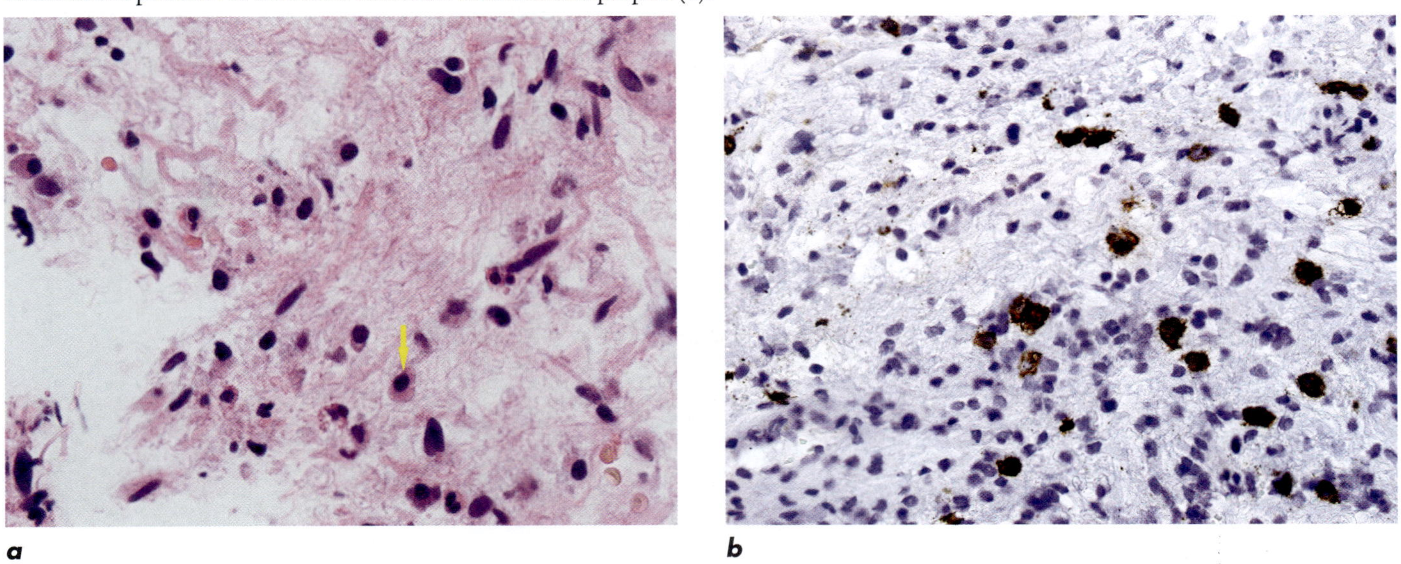

RADIATION CYSTITIS

Definition
- Inflammation of the bladder associated with radiation

Other term
- Hemorrhagic cystitis associated with radiation, postradiation cystitis

Pathogenesis
- Cystitis caused by the radiation-induced injury of the bladder mucosa

Clinical features
- History of radiation, mostly external beam for prostate cancer, cervical cancer, or low abdominal radiation
- Latent period from a few weeks to several years. Acute inflammation develops in a few days while chronic inflammation occurs a few weeks to several years after radiation
- Typical radiation cystitis encountered in clinical practice is a chronic process a few years after radiation treatment
- Symptoms include irritation symptoms such as pain, increased frequency, and urgency
- Gross or microscopic hematuria may occur

Gross pathology
- Cystoscopy shows prominent dilated blood vessels with spots of hemorrhage
- Edema and ulceration may be present

Histology
- Stromal changes (Fig. 47-9)
  - In acute phase, edema, neutrophilic infiltrates, and fibrin deposit can be seen
  - In chronic phase, there are mixed inflammatory infiltrates
  - Hemorrhage is prominent either fresh or old one which is characterized by the presence of hemosiderin-laden macrophages
  - Large multinuclear stromal cells (atypical fibroblasts) with degenerative features are often present
- Vascular changes (Fig. 47-10)
  - Endothelial swelling or hyperplasia
  - Vascular ectasia may be present
  - Thickened wall of blood vessels with intimal proliferation, fibrosis, and hyalinization of the wall
  - Similar stromal and epithelial changes can been seen in cystitis caused by other agents such as chemotherapy drugs, but vascular changes are typically not present in other conditions
- Epithelial changes (Fig. 47-11)
  - Reactive changes such as nuclear enlargement or disorganization
  - Nest of squamoid cells, known as pseudocarcinomatous epithelial hyperplasia, can be seen
  - The presence of significant cytological atypia should be distinguished from carcinoma in situ

Figure 47-9.
Radiation cystitis shows the prominent hemorrhage (*a*) and chronic inflammation in the lamina propria (*b*).

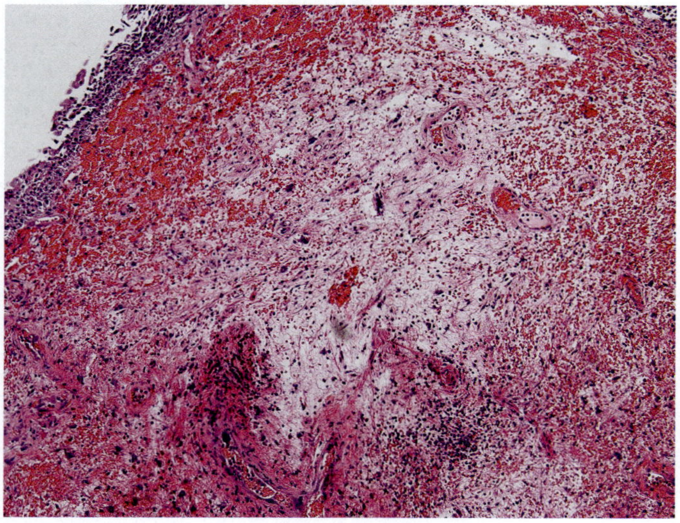

a

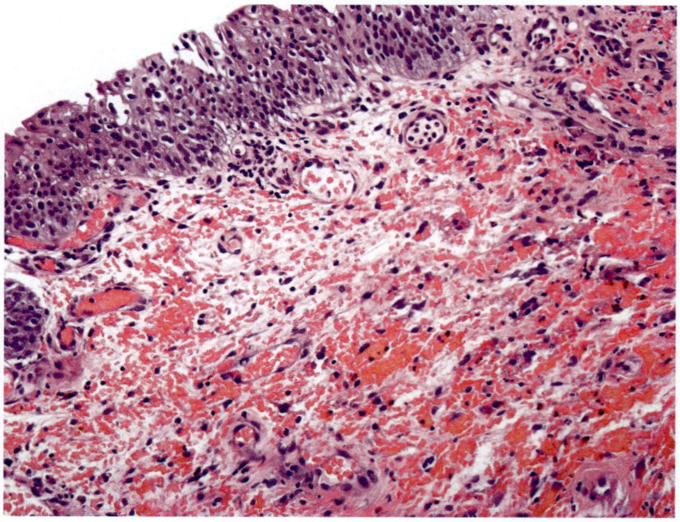

b

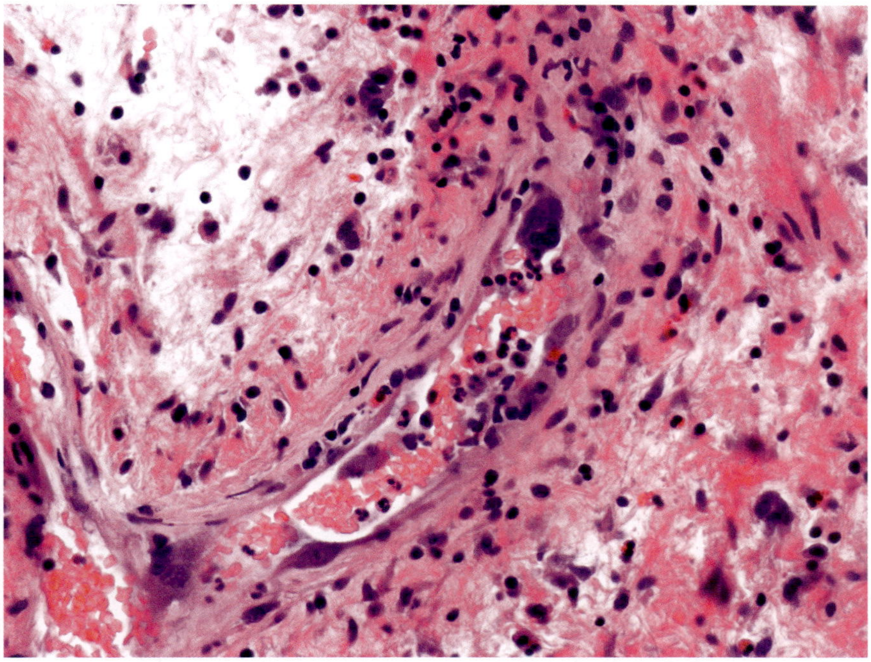

Figure 47-10.
Radiation cystitis with thickened vessels and prominent endothelial atypia.

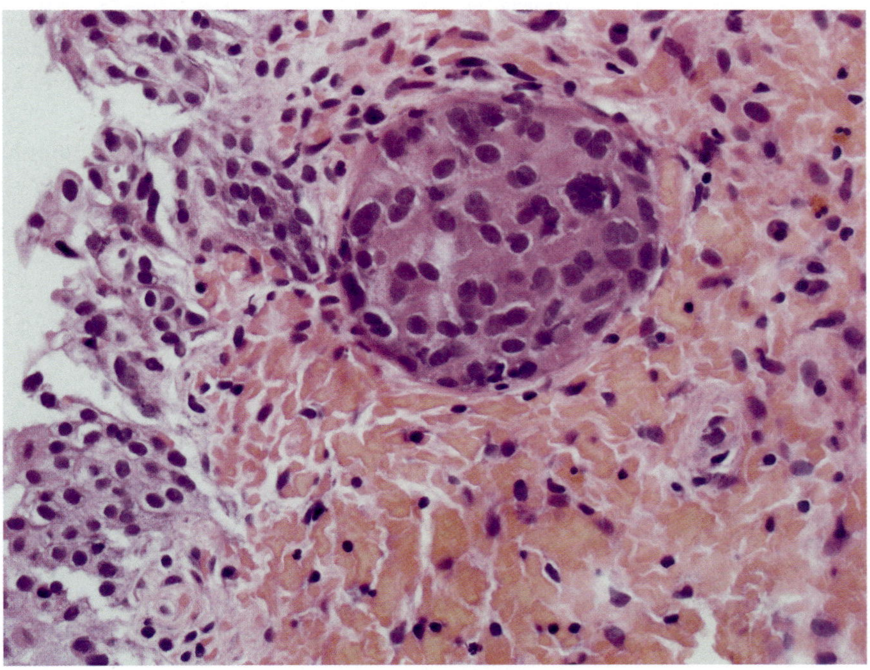

Figure 47-11.
Radiation cystitis with urothelial cells in a von Brunn nest showing cytological atypia.

Immunohistochemistry and molecular analysis

- P53 negative
- CK20 negative or weakly positive

Differential diagnosis

- Urothelial carcinoma in situ (CIS)
  - Generally no history of radiation (only a small subset of urothelial CIS cases may have a history of radiation)
  - No prominent hemorrhage, usually microscopic hematuria rather than gross hematuria
  - Endothelial atypia not present
  - More severe and diffuse cytological atypia rather than isolated cytological atypia
  - P53 positive, CK20 positive (full thickness)
  - In the postradiation cases exhibiting significant cytological atypia of urothelium, the diagnosis of urothelial atypia with unknown significance should be used and clinical follow-up is necessary

Clinical relevance (prognosis and treatment options)

- There is an increased risk of bladder cancer in the patients that received radiation
- Because postradiation urothelial atypia can be prominent, the diagnosis of urothelial carcinoma should be made with great caution
- If the cytological atypia of urothelium is prominent in a patient with radiation cystitis, but it is short of diagnosis of carcinoma in situ, close clinical follow-up and rebiopsy are necessary
- Recently, some new therapies such as recombinant activated factor VII show some promising treatment results

POLYPOID CYSTITIS

Definition

- Inflammation of the bladder with prominent polypoid appearance of the bladder mucosa
- Similar lesions may occur in other parts of the urinary tract, particularly urethra

Pathogenesis

- Chronic cystitis associated with prominent lamina propria edema

Clinical features

- More often multiple polypoid lesions
- Edematous appearance

Gross pathology

- Polypoid projections of bladder mucosa
- Single or multiple
- Mobile with nonfixed base

Histology

- Polypoid bladder mucosa (Fig. 47-12)
- Edematous stroma (lamina propria) is typically acellular or paucicellular with occasional small vessels (Figs. 47-12 and 47-13)
- Urothelial hyperplasia can be seen, with increased thickness but without cytological atypia (Fig. 47-12*b*). Chronic inflammation can be minimal within polypoid lesions, mostly found in the base of the lesion
- Von Brunn nests and cystitis cystica are commonly associated

Immunohistochemistry and molecular analysis

- Not indicated

Differential diagnosis

- Papillary urothelial carcinoma
  - Thickened urothelium with thin fibrovascular cores
  - Significant cytological atypia

Clinical relevance (prognosis and treatment options)

- Benign reactive lesion
- Anti-inflammatory medication may be needed as a conservative measure
- No recurrence if resected

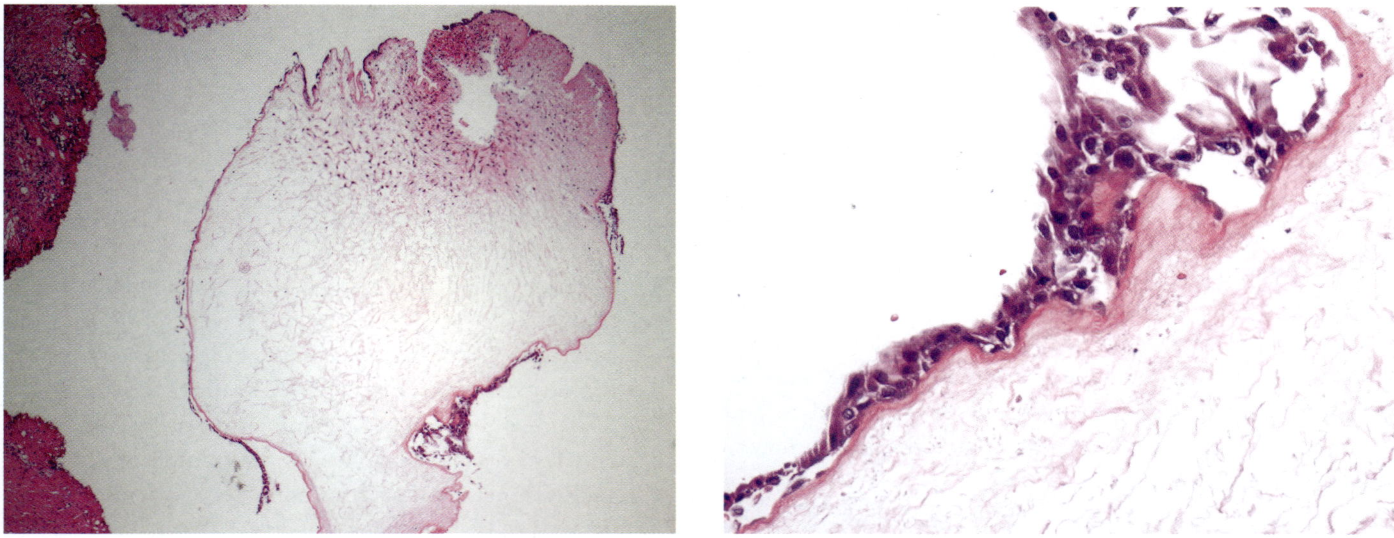

a b

Figure 47-12.
Polypoid cystitis is characterized by a large polypoid lesion with extremely edematous stroma and almost no vessel (*a*). High magnification shows lining urothelium with mild reactive changes (*b*).

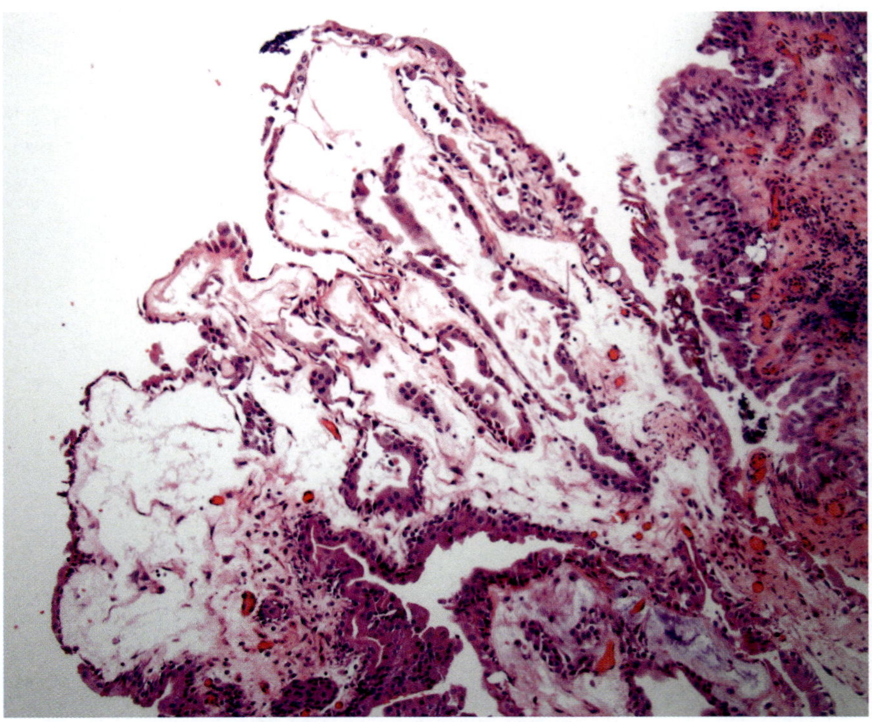

Figure 47-13.
Polypoid cystitis with multiple papillary projections mimicking papillary neoplasm. The stroma is edematous with dilated small vessels.

CYSTITIS RELATED TO SCHISTOSOMIASIS

Definition

- Bladder inflammation caused by the deposition of Schistosoma eggs in the bladder wall

Pathogenesis

- Infected fresh water snails release Schistosoma larvae into water, which attach and penetrate human skin, the larvae will mature in the lungs or liver of the host and travel to pelvic vein to lay eggs, which will be circulated to and deposited in the bladder wall, where the inflammatory reaction will be induced

Clinical features

- All the patients had a history of *Schistosoma haematobium* infestation, which is common in Africa and the Middle East, particularly in Egypt
- Symptoms are nonspecific, including suprapubic pain, dysuria, increased urine frequency, and hematuria
- In advanced stages, the severe fibrosis of bladder wall may lead to urinary obstruction, secondary bacterial urinary tract infection, hydronephrosis, and renal failure
- Increased risk for developing squamous cell carcinoma

Gross pathology

- Thickened mucosa because the eggs are mostly located in the lamina propria

Histology

- Early phase of infection, the eggs induce eosinophilic inflammation, necrosis, and ulceration
- Late phase of infection, chronic inflammation and fibrosis are present
- Identification of *S. haematobium* eggs is necessary for the pathologic diagnosis. Eggs are oval shaped, measuring 110 to 170 μm embedded in the lamina propria (Fig. 47-14)
- Eventually, eggs may be calcified and surrounded by fibrosis
- Squamous metaplasia is commonly seen. The presence of squamous cell carcinoma is possible

Clinical relevance (prognosis and treatment options)

- Antihelminths for early disease
- Surgical treatment may be necessary in the advanced stage associated with urinary obstruction
- Because of the long-standing chronic inflammation, squamous metaplasia associated with Schistosoma eggs is a risk factor for development of squamous cell carcinoma

Figure 47-14.
A bladder mucosa with multiple Schistosoma eggs surrounded by fibrosis (*a*). Higher magnification shows the two oval-shaped eggs with calcifications (*b*).

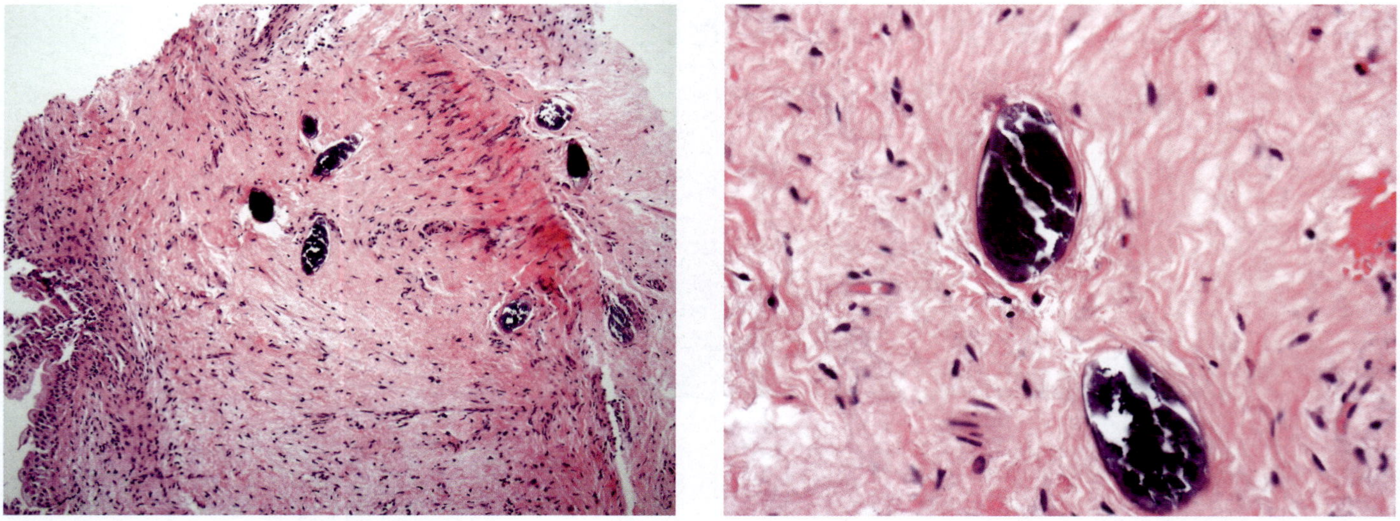

a *b*

MALAKOPLAKIA

Definition

- An inflammatory lesion is predominantly composed of abnormal macrophages containing special structures (Michaelis-Gutmann bodies)
- The most common site is the bladder, other GU organs such as testis and kidney or non-GU organs such as gastrointestinal tract, central nervous system, or female genital tract can be affected

Pathogenesis

- The formation of Michaelis-Gutmann bodies is the result of bacteria ingested but not digested by macrophages
- The bacteria in macrophage are subjected to calcium or iron deposits

Clinical features

- Signs of infection, such as fever and urinary irritation symptoms
- Typically presents as a mass lesion

Gross pathology

- White to yellow plaques or elevated spots in the bladder mucosa

Histology

- Background of chronic inflammatory cell infiltrate with numerous macrophages (Fig. 47-15)
- The presence of Michaelis-Gutmann (MG) bodies is a pathognomonic feature of malakoplakia (Fig. 47-16, arrows)
- MG bodies is characterized by bluish targetoid structures, ranging from 2 to 5 μm in diameter in the cytoplasm of macrophages (Fig. 47-17)

Histochemistry and microbiology studies

- Iron stain shows the presence of iron deposit in the MG bodies
- Bacteria culture may be necessary for identification of the infectious organisms

Clinical relevance

- Benign condition
- Sometimes surgically removed as a mass lesion

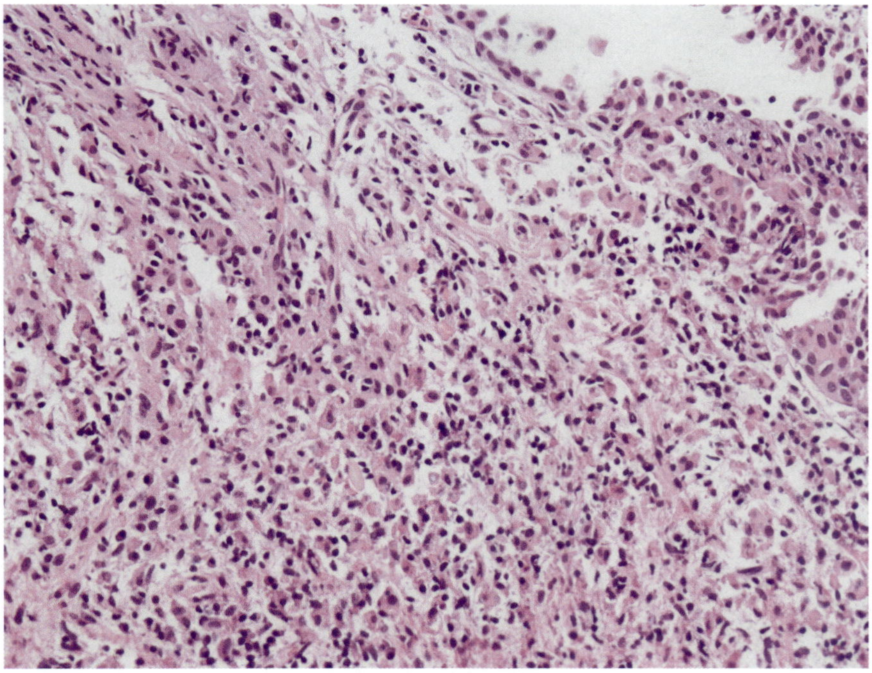

Figure 47-15.
Malakoplakia of the bladder is composed of mostly macrophages and chronic inflammatory cells.

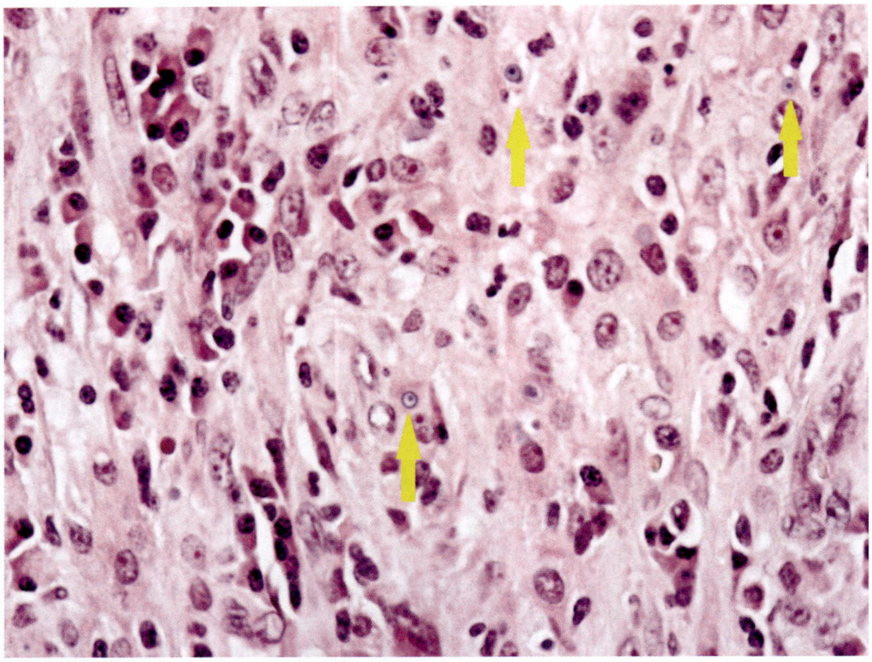

Figure 47-16.
Malakoplakia showing macrophages containing blue targetoid Michaelis-Gutmann bodies inside the macrophages (arrows).

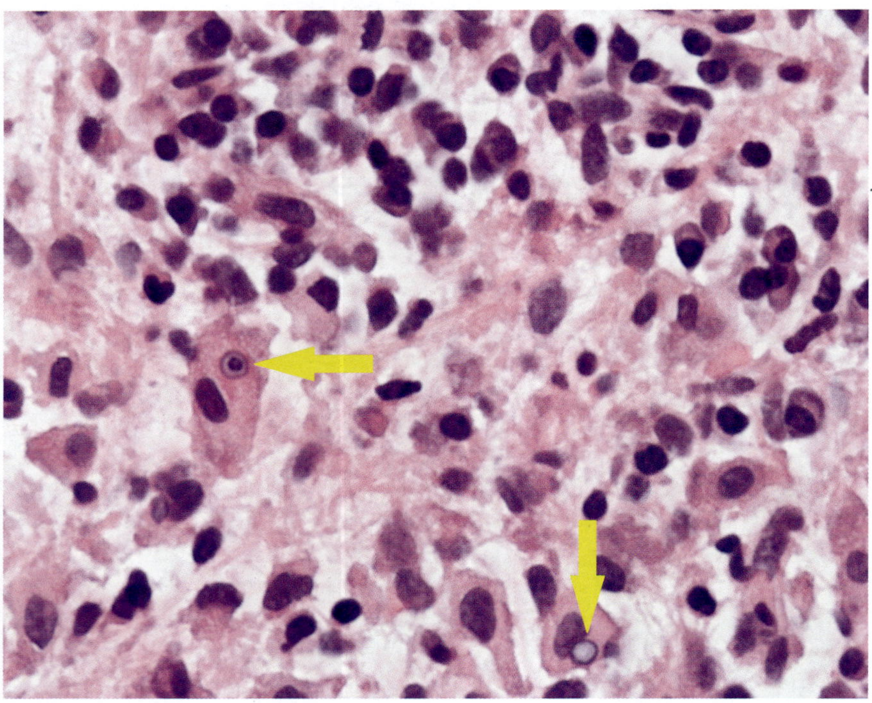

Figure 47-17.
Malakoplakia with several Michaelis-Gutmann bodies inside the macrophages. Lymphocytes and plasma cells are also present in the background.

BCG GRANULOMATOUS CYSTITIS

Definition

- Bladder granulomatous inflammation caused by bacillus Calmette-Guerin (BCG) therapy

Pathogenesis

- BCG is a weaker strain of mycobacteria, which has been used by many countries as a vaccine to prevent TB infection
- A liquid drug containing live BCG bacteria is injected intravesically through a catheter into a patient with superficial bladder cancer such as urothelial carcinoma in situ or after resection of papillary urothelial carcinoma
- BCG as expected will induce granulomatous inflammation

Clinical features

- All the patients had a history of intravesical BCG installation
- No specific symptoms
- Cystoscopy shows erythematous bladder mucosa

Histology

- Typically seen in the posttreatment biopsy to evaluate the presence or absence of residual tumor
- Caseating or noncaseating granulomas seen in the bladder mucosa
- The granuloma is composed of epithelioid histiocytes and multinucleated Langerhans giant cells (Fig. 47-18), morphologically identical to a TB granuloma (Fig. 47-19)
- Urothelium may show inflammation and reactive changes

Immunohistochemistry and histochemistry

- AFB stain may confirm the presence of mycobacteria, but it is rarely necessary for diagnosis with a history of BCG treatment

Clinical relevance (prognosis and treatment options)

- No treatment necessary
- Unless systemic granulomatous inflammation develops in an immunocompromised individual
- Therefore, the diagnosis of BCG granulomas should be made with caution when history is unknown, since some patients without BCG treatment will contain granulomas in the bladder caused by biopsy or TURs

Figure 47-18.
A BCG granuloma of the bladder is located in the lamina propria (*a*). High magnification shows the granuloma is composed of epithelioid histiocytes without necrosis (*b*).

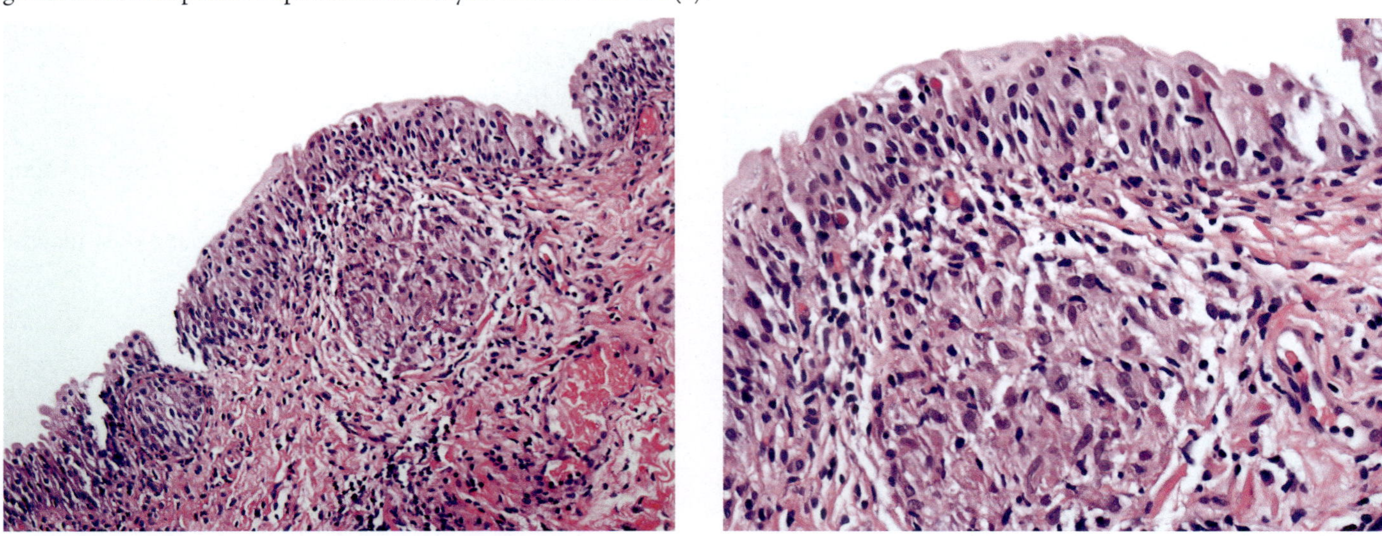

a *b*

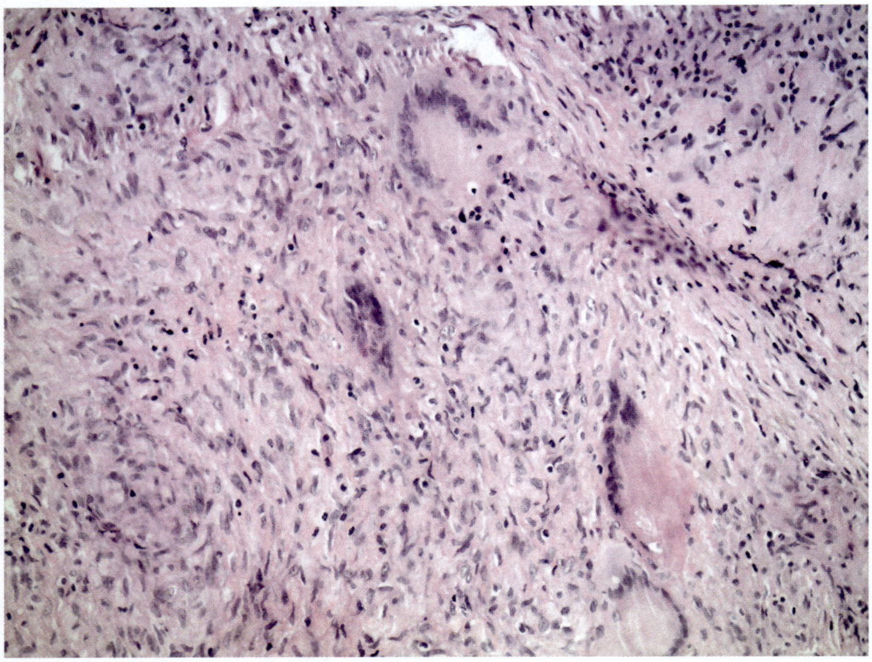

Figure 47-19.
A tuberculosis granuloma in the bladder with Langerhans giant cells and epithelioid histiocytes, which is almost identical to the BCG granulomas histologically.

POSTBIOPSY GRANULOMA

Definition

- Granulomatous inflammation of the bladder mucosa in response to a prior biopsy or transurethral resection

Other term

- Post-TUR granuloma

Pathogenesis

- Reparative changes after the tissue damage caused by invasive procedures such as biopsy or transurethral resection of the bladder
- Granuloma reaction surrounding the damaged tissue

Clinical features

- May have nonspecific irritation syndrome

Gross pathology

- Ulcer may be present
- No mass lesion seen

Histology

- One or multiple granulomas composed of central necrosis and histiocytes
- Central fibrinoid necrosis showing irregular "geographic" shapes, which is not the same as caseating necrosis (Fig. 47-20)
- Within the necrotic areas, ghost cells and vessel may be seen
- Necrotic areas are immediately surrounded by palisading histiocytes
- Foamy macrophages or foreign body giant cells may be present

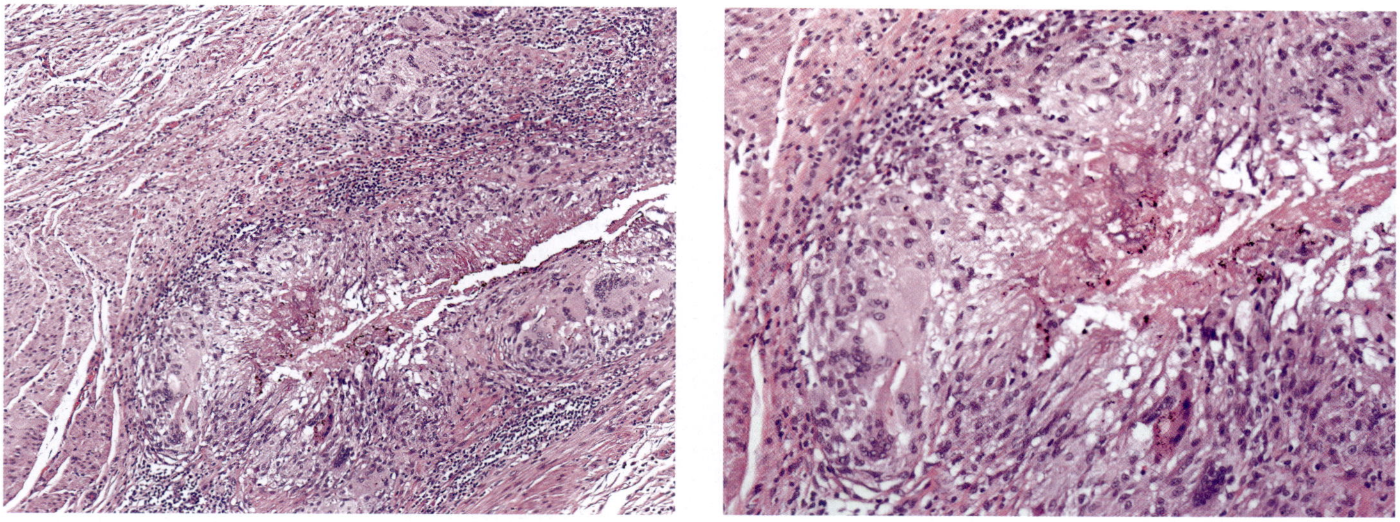

a b

Figure 47-20.
A postbiopsy granuloma is composed of fibrinoid necrosis, rimmed by epithelioid histiocytes and occasional multinuclear giant cells (*a*). High magnification shows the epithelioid histiocytes and multinuclear giant cells (*b*).

Immunohistochemistry

- CD68 positive for histiocytes/macrophages
- GMS, AFB are negative for microorganisms, but rarely necessary

Clinical relevance (prognosis and treatment options)

- No treatment necessary, it will heal over time
- Sometimes, postbiopsy granulomas may resemble BCG granulomas
- Therefore, the diagnosis of BCG granulomas should be made with great caution since some patients without BCG treatment will contain granulomas caused by biopsy or TURs

CHAPTER 48

Other Reactive Lesions of the Bladder

UROTHELIAL HYPERPLASIA

Definition

- Increased thickness of urothelial cells as a reactive change

Pathogenesis

- Reactive changes to the stimuli

Clinical features

- Inflammation-related symptoms but specific features

Gross pathology

- No specific features

Histology

- Increased layers of urothelium (Fig. 48-1) without papillary structures seen
- There is no evidence of loss of polarity or presence of cytological atypia (Fig. 48-2)
- May be associated with chronic inflammation (Fig. 48-2)

Immunohistochemistry

- Usually not necessary
- P53 negative and Ki67 index low

Clinical relevance (prognosis and treatment options)

- Benign reactive change, no specific treatment

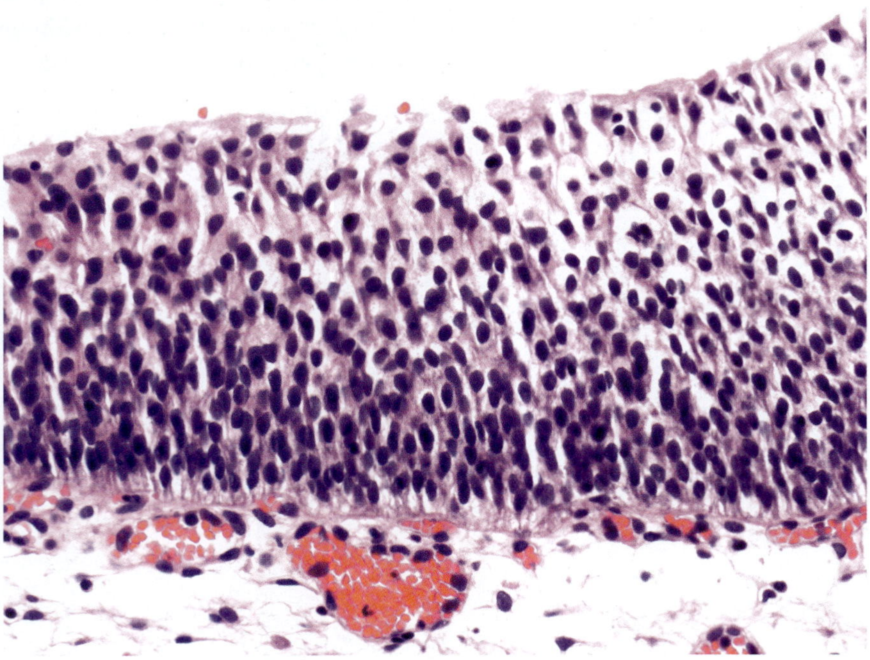

Figure 48-1.
Urothelial hyperplasia is characterized by the increased layers of urothelial cells, with no cytological atypia.

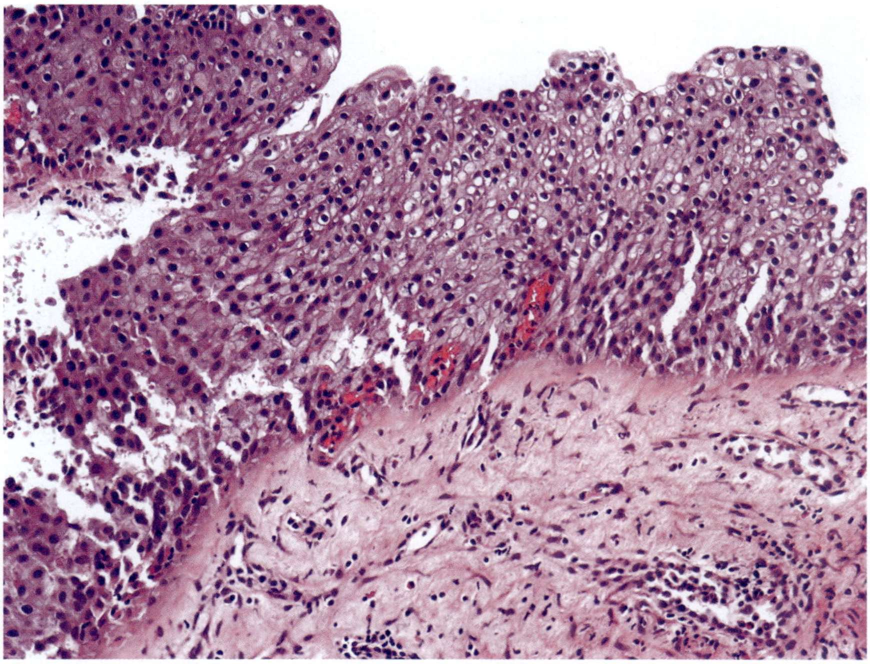

Figure 48-2.
Urothelial hyperplasia showing thickened urothelium without cytological atypia, associated with mild chronic inflammation.

VON BRUNN NESTS AND FLORID VON BRUNN NESTS

Definition

- Von Brunn nests are benign solid urothelial cell nests budding underneath overlying urothelium or present in the lamina propria
- Florid von Brunn nests are numerous von Brunn nests, probably a proliferative process of urothelium responding to the local inflammation or as reactive changes
- Typical and florid von Brunn nests may present anywhere throughout the urinary tract

Clinical features

- Asymptomatic
- Symptoms may present when von Brunn nests are associated with neoplasm, inflammation, or other injuries

Gross pathology

- Usually a von Brunn nest is not grossly identifiable, while florid von Brunn nests may appear as opaque plaques (Fig. 48-3)

Histology

- Small solid nests of normal urothelium with defined contours in the lamina propria (Figs. 48-4 and 48-5)
- With or without connection to overlying benign urothelium (Fig. 48-6)
- When glandular structures develop within von Brunn nests, it is considered to be cystitis glandularis (Fig. 48-5). In reality, von Brunn nests often coexist with cystitis glandularis or cystitis cystica
- In florid von Brunn nests, there are many solid nests evenly spaced with some edematous stroma between them (Figs. 48-7 and 48-8)
- Inflammatory cells may be present in the surrounding lamina propria
- Cytological atypia is absent
- Urothelial dysplasia and carcinoma in situ may involve von Brunn nests

Immunohistochemistry and molecular analysis

- Positive for urothelial markers such as HMWCK, p63 (Fig. 48-6*c*), S100P, or GATA3
- P53 negative, Ki67 proliferative index is low

Clinical relevance (prognosis and treatment options)

- No significant clinical relevance, no treatment is necessary
- Should be distinguished from invasive or urothelial carcinoma in situ

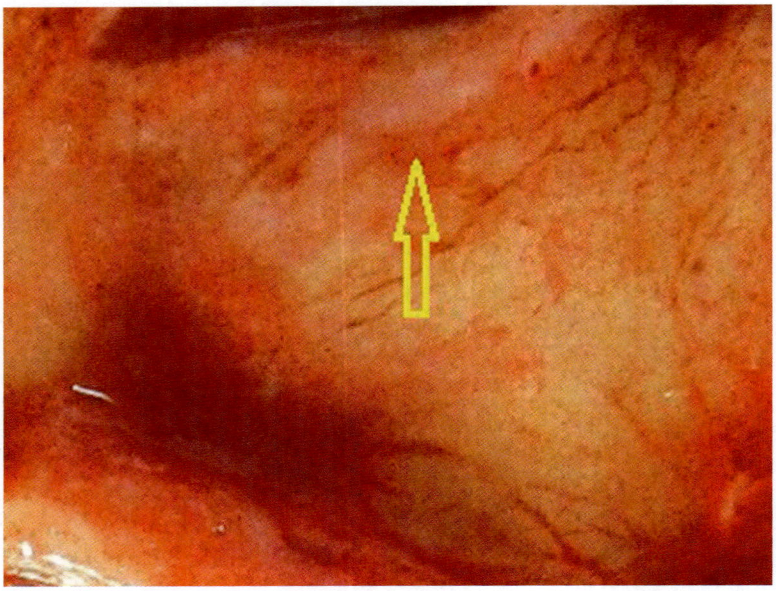

Figure 48-3.
Gross appearance of florid von Brunn nests as white opaque plaques.

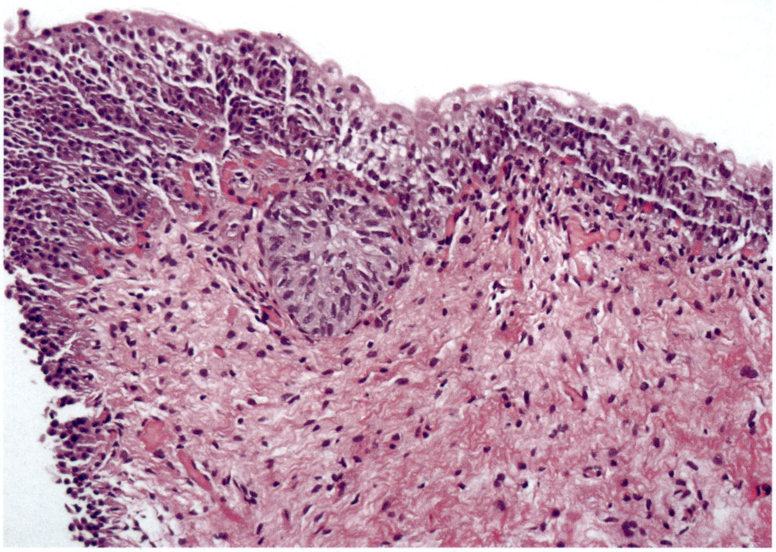

Figure 48-4.
Von Brunn nest is a solid cluster of urothelial cells located underneath the urothelium.

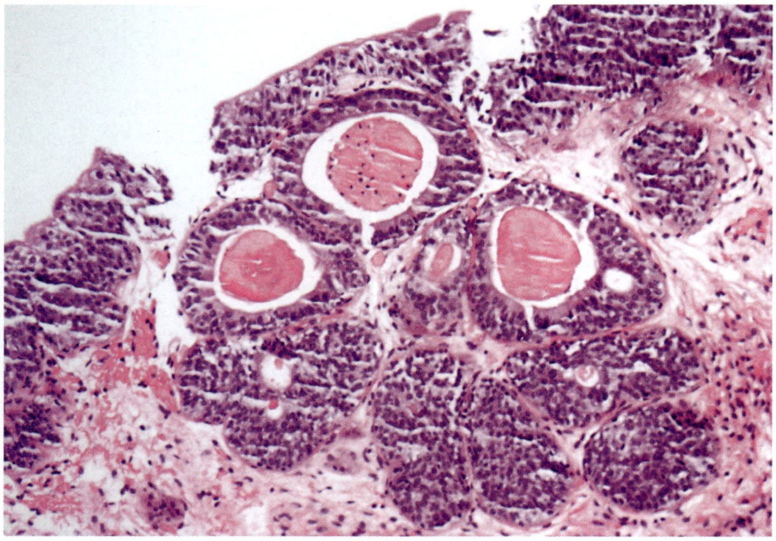

Figure 48-5.
Multiple von Brunn nests containing solid urothelial nests confined within the basement membrane as well as nests with glandular differentiation (cystitis glandularis, upper portion).

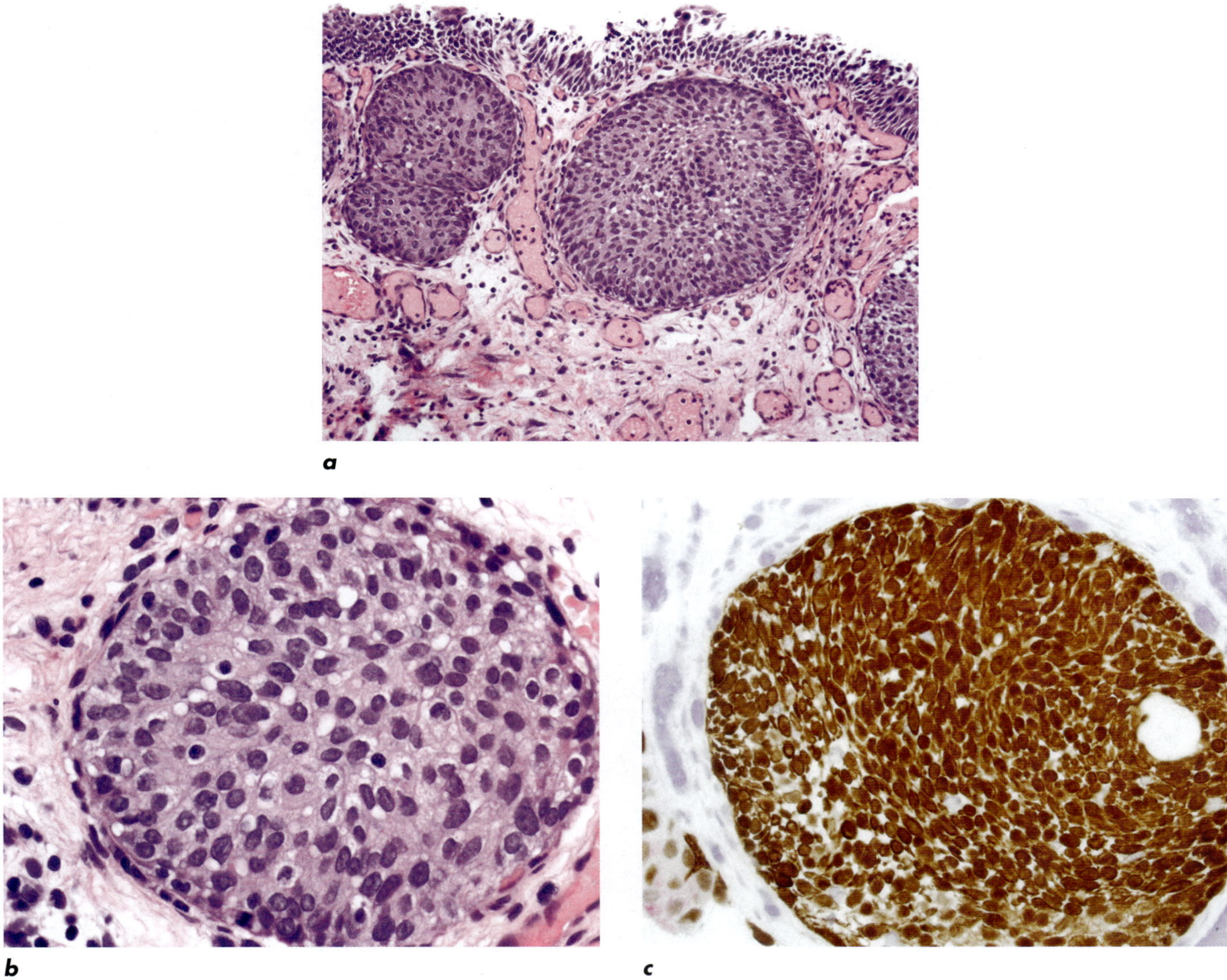

Figure 48-6.
Von Brunn nests in the lamina propria (*a*). High magnification of a von Brunn nest shows many of the urothelial cells with nuclear grooves, but no significant cytological atypia (*b*). HMWCK and p63 immunostains are positive in the urothelial cells in the nest (*c*, triple stain).

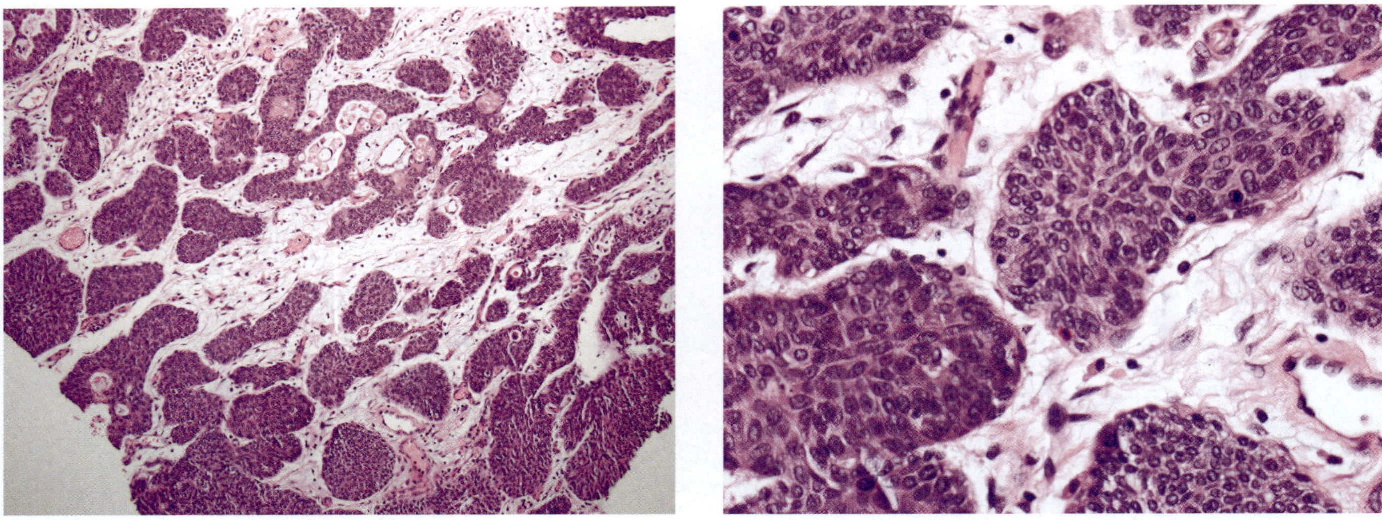

a b

Figure 48-7.
Florid von Brunn nests in the lamina propria with edema (*a*). High magnification shows the regularly shaped nests consisting of benign urothelial cells without atypia (*b*).

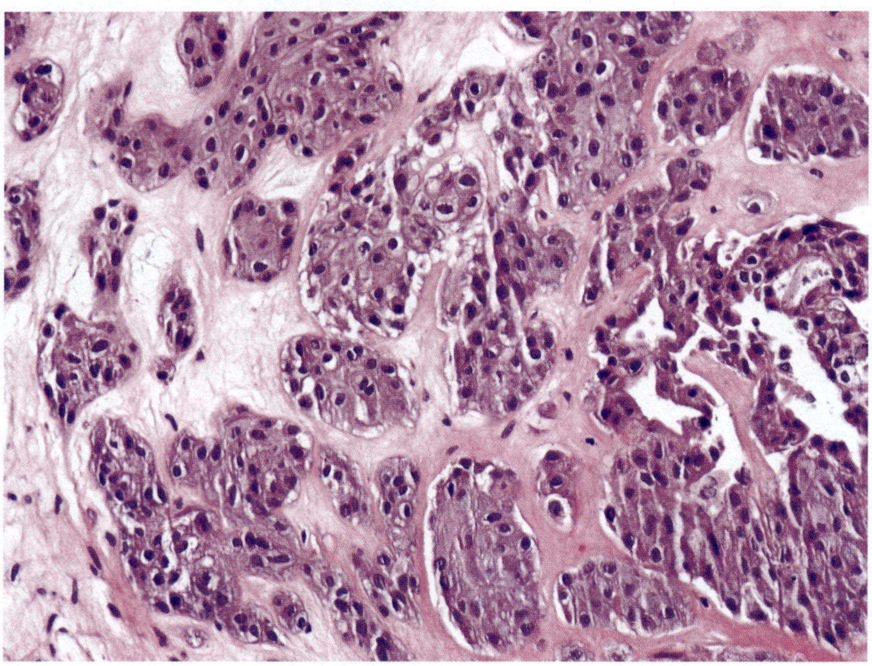

Figure 48-8.
Florid von Brunn nests of the bladder exhibits regularly shaped islands of urothelial cells with low N/C ratio, separated by the edematous and hyalinized stroma.

SQUAMOUS METAPLASIA

Definition

- Benign metaplastic process replacing urothelium with squamous epithelium

Pathogenesis

- Squamous metaplasia is a reactive change of urothelium in response to chronic stimuli, such as indwelling catheters, calculi, or neurogenic bladder
- In the highly infested areas, Schistosoma is the major cause of squamous metaplasia of the bladder
- It is more common in women than men (5:1)

Clinical features

- Typically urinary symptoms such as hematuria and urinary frequency or urgency
- Associated conditions such as calculi or indwelling catheters are present

Gross pathology

- Very smooth surface or thickened mucosa (Fig. 48-9*a*). Sometimes, the keratin layer can be very thick and results in the appearance of "wrinkled skin" (Fig. 48-10*a*)

Figure 48-9.
Bladder squamous metaplasia. Gross photo shows the mucosal surface is thickened and with white plaque appearance. A white pearly elevated lesion is indicated by an arrow (*a*). Microscopically, hyperplastic squamous epithelium is seen (*b*, right) in a background squamous metaplasia. Higher magnification demonstrates the significantly thickened metaplastic squamous epithelium of the pearly lesion (*c*, right) adjacent to the normal thickness of metaplastic squamous epithelium (*b*, left). High magnification also shows koilocytic changes in this lesion (*d*).

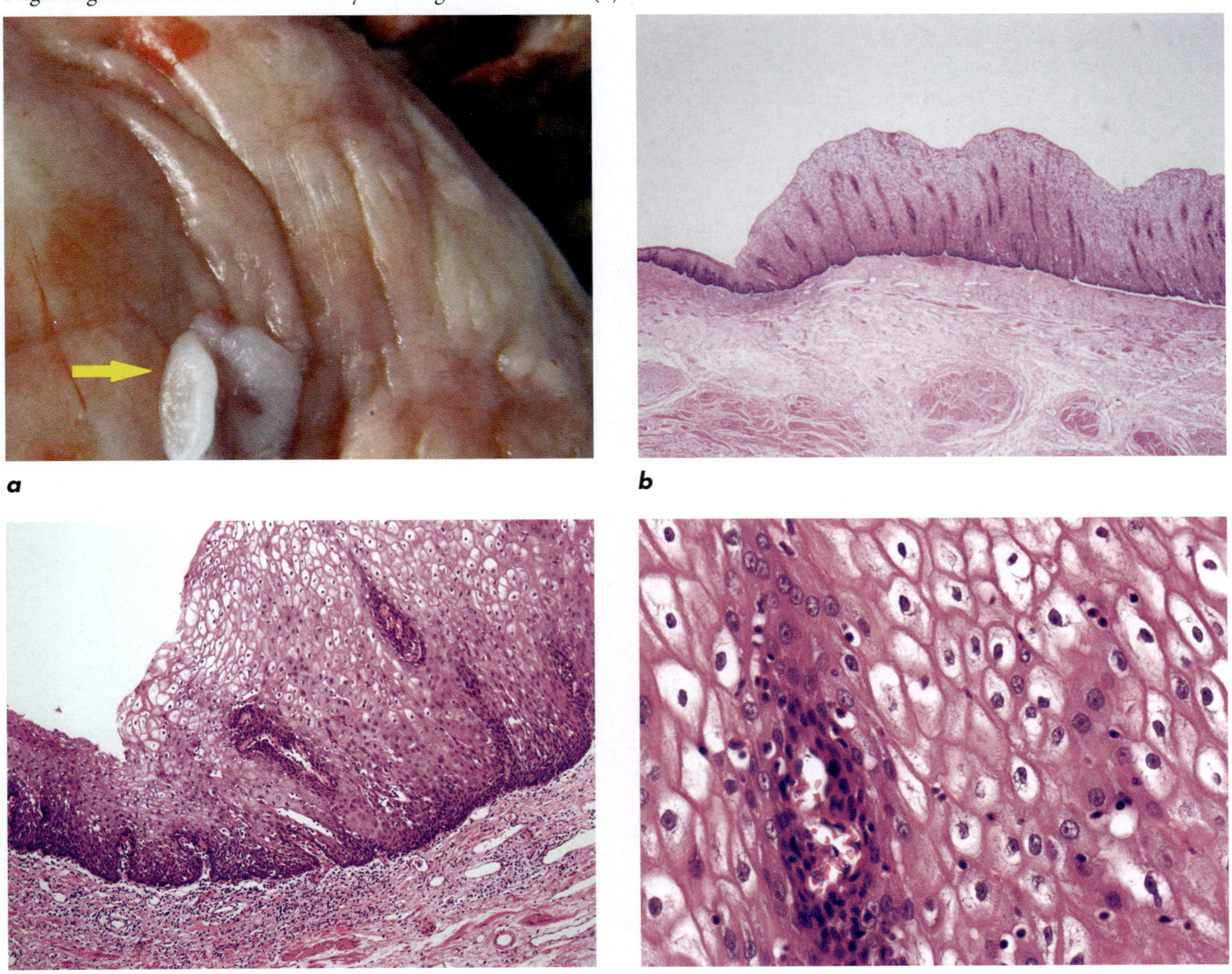

a b c d

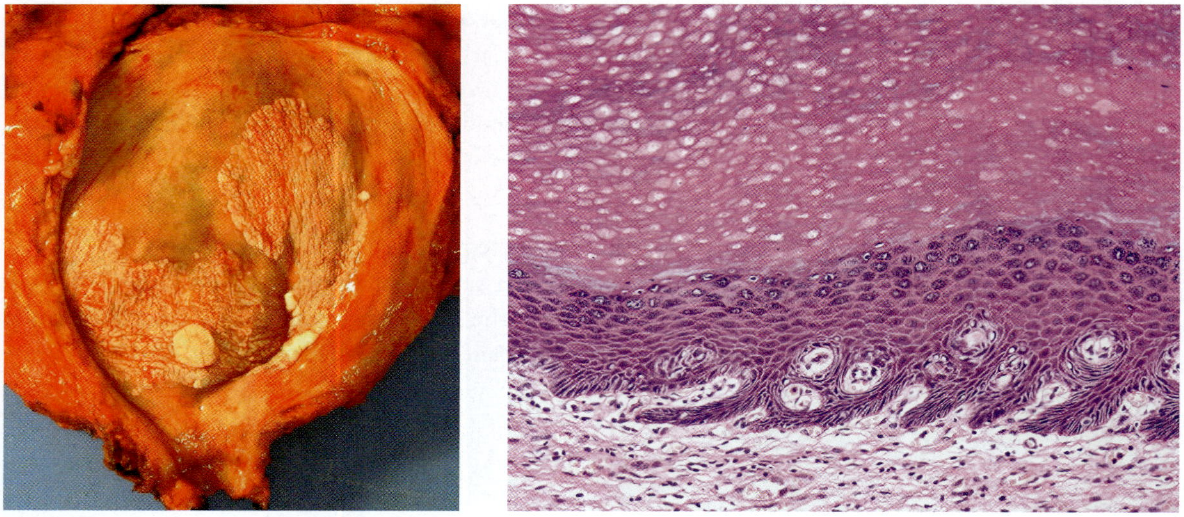

a *b*

Figure 48-10.
Gross photo of keratinizing squamous metaplasia of the bladder exhibits extensive keratin layer on the mucosal surface with the appearance of "wrinkled skin" (*a*). Microscopically, thick keratin layer and granular layer can be seen (*b*).

Histology

- The lesion can be focal or involving the entire bladder mucosa
- The presence of squamous epithelium, either normal or increased thickness (Fig. 48-11)
- Squamous metaplasia can be keratinizing (Fig. 48-10*b*) or nonkeratinizing (Fig. 48-11)
- Squamous metaplasia may involve von Brunn nests (Fig. 48-12*a*) or be associated with cystitis glandularis (Fig. 48-12*b*) or lymphocytic infiltrate
- In keratinized squamous metaplasia, there is a prominent granular layer underneath the keratin material on the surface resembling the epidermis (Fig. 48-12*c*)
- The squamous cells can be glycogenated or nonglycogenated, which does not have clinical relevance
- Squamous metaplasia, both keratinizing and nonkeratinizing forms, can be seen associated with squamous cell carcinoma (Fig. 48-12*d*)

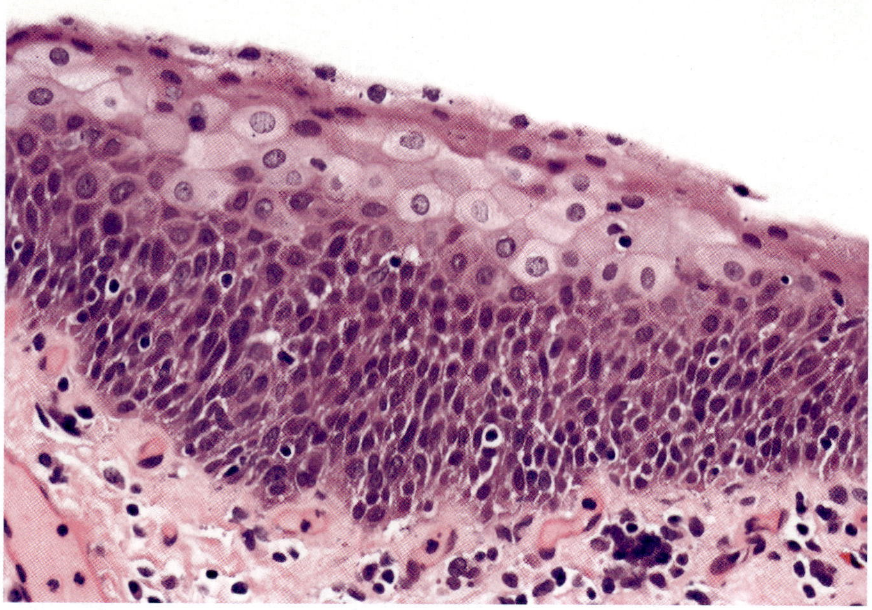

Figure 48-11.
Nonkeratinized squamous metaplasia of the bladder.

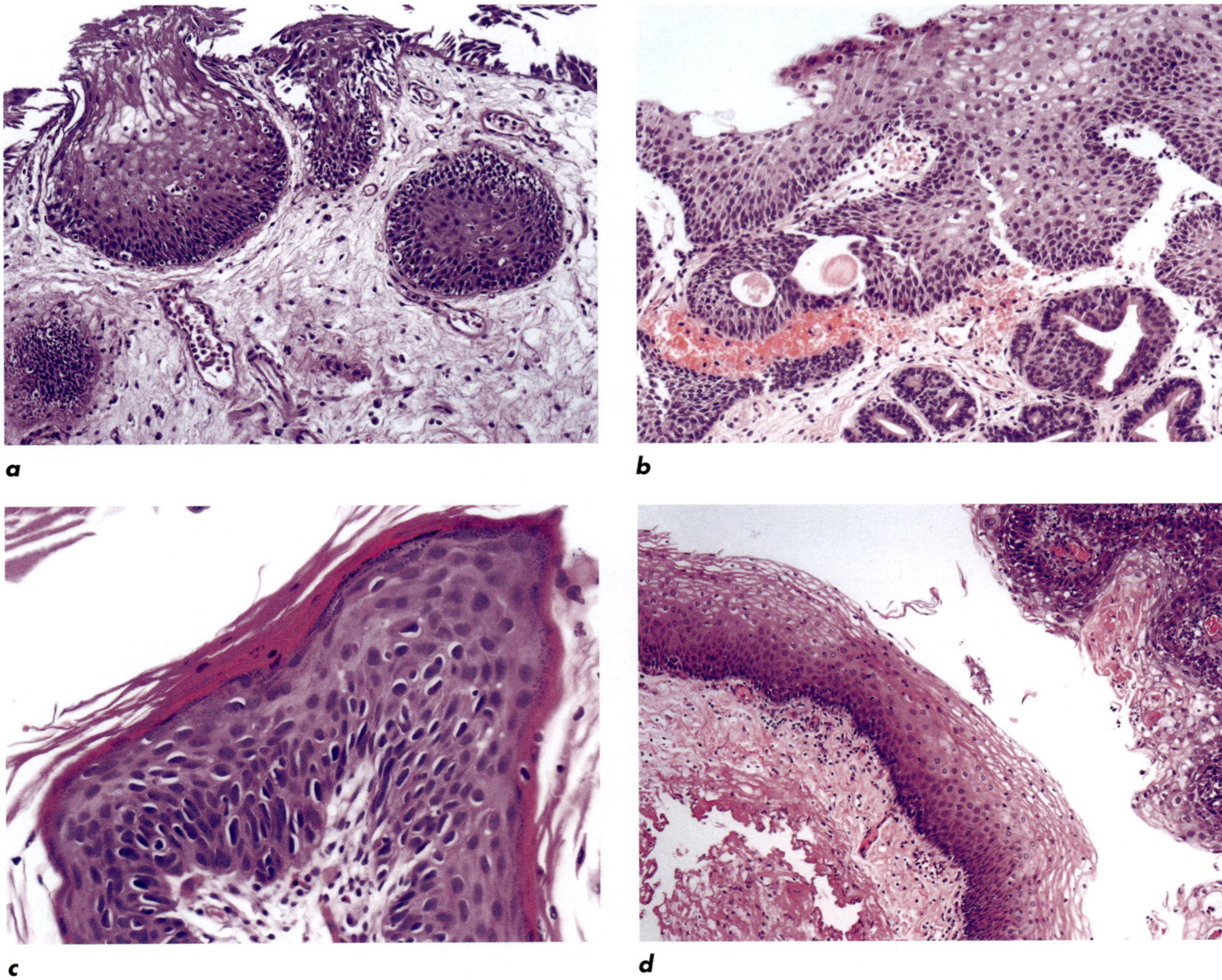

Figure 48-12.
Squamous metaplasia of the bladder involving von Brunn nests (*a*) and cystitis glandularis (*b*). Keratinizing squamous metaplasia with a prominent granular layer similar to the epidermis (*c*). Nonkeratinizing squamous metaplasia (left) of the bladder is associated with invasive squamous cell carcinoma (right) in the same case (*d*).

Immunohistochemistry

- Usually not necessary. p63 positive, p53 negative

Differential diagnosis

Squamous cell carcinoma

- Showing significant cytological atypia
- Loss of polarity and disorganization
- Stroma invasion is also present in invasive squamous cell carcinoma

Clinical relevance (prognosis and treatment options)

- Squamous metaplasia is considered to be the precursor lesion of squamous cell carcinoma
- It may also be at a high risk for condylomas, particularly in a patient with a history of condyloma of external genital areas
- The notion that nonkeratinizing squamous metaplasia is not associated with the risk of squamous cell carcinoma may be originated from some old data, but it cannot be substantiated in our experience
- Significant numbers of cases of squamous cell carcinoma of the bladder are associated with nonkeratinizing squamous metaplasia
- Therefore, all patients, both male and female, with nonkeratinizing or keratinizing squamous metaplasia should be followed and monitored clinically

PSEUDOCARCINOMATOUS HYPERPLASIA OF THE UROTHELIUM

Definition

- Benign urothelial proliferative lesions of the bladder, demonstrating a growth pattern mimicking invasive carcinoma
- With or without association of radiation or chemotherapy

Other terms

- Pseudoeptheliomatous proliferation of urothelium
- Pseudocarcinomatous epithelial hyperplasia
- Pseudocarcinomatous urothelial hyperplasia

Pathogenesis

- The patient may or may not have a history of radiation or chemotherapy
- Radiation and chemotherapy are known to damage urothelium, and subsequently cause a urothelial proliferation
- Sometimes, when the history of radiation or chemotherapy is uncertain, an unknown insulting agent may be responsible for this lesion

Clinical features

- Symptoms of chronic inflammation
- With or without a known history of radiation or chemotherapy
- A history of other injury may be identified
- Typically polypoid edematous lesion by endoscopy

Gross pathology

- Flat or polypoid bladder mucosal surface
- Soft and edematous appearance
- Without a solid firm mass in cut surface

Histology

- Small nests of epithelial cells deep in the lamina propria, appearing to be infiltrative (pseudoinfiltrating) (Fig. 48-13)

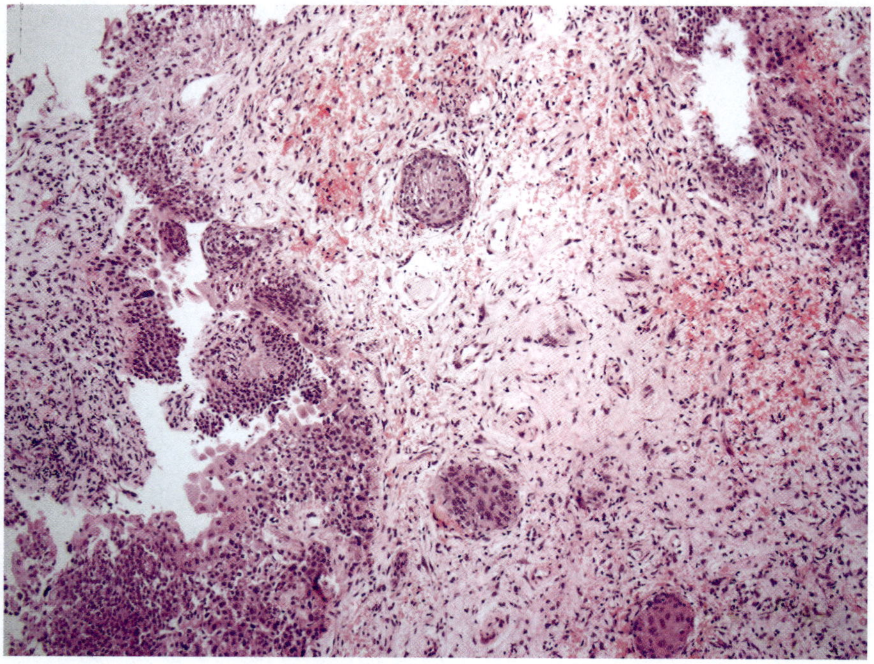

Figure 48-13. Pseudocarcinomatous hyperplasia with marked chronic inflammation and nests of squamoid cells in the lamina propria.

- The nests are round or slightly irregular with epithelial cells showing squamoid differentiation (Fig. 48-14)
- No significant cytological atypia
- Intact surface urothelium without atypia
- Edematous stroma with chronic inflammatory infiltrate
- Hemorrhage, fibrin deposition, vascular congestion are common features, which suggest previous injury to bladder mucosa
- No evidence of urothelial carcinoma in situ or squamous cell carcinoma in situ

Immunohistochemistry

- P53 negative and Ki67 proliferative index low

Figure 48-14.
Pseudocarcinomatous hyperplasia showing disorganized urothelium and small epithelial clusters of the lamina propria with prominent stromal reaction (*a*). The nest of cells showing squamoid features, but minimal cytological atypia although they appear to be infiltrating (*b*).

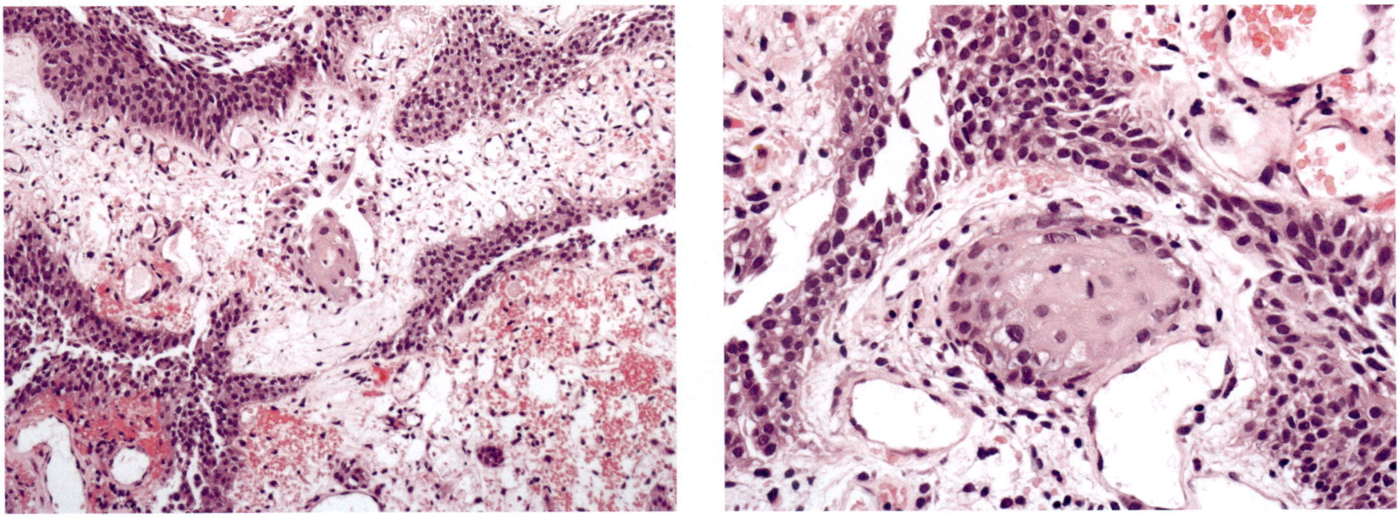

a **b**

Differential diagnosis

- Urothelial carcinoma
  - Cytological atypia and pleomorphism are more prominent in urothelial carcinoma (differential diagnosis is summarized in Table 48-1)
- Squamous cell carcinoma
  - Presence of carcinoma in situ
  - Presence of keratin pearls
  - P53 positivity and high proliferative activity
  - Coexisting squamous metaplasia

Clinical relevance (prognosis and treatment options)

- Clinical history of urothelial injury is important
- Benign conditions
- Immunostains such as p53, Ki67, or CK20 may be helpful
- In cases with significant suspicion, close clinical follow-up is necessary
- A benign condition mimicking invasive carcinoma
- Clinical follow-up necessary

Table 48-1. Distinction Between Pseudocarcinomatous Hyperplasia and Urothelial Carcinoma

	Pseudocarcinomatous Hyperplasia	*Invasive Urothelial Carcinoma*
History	Injury or no known injury	Prior dysplasia or carcinoma
Inflammation	Yes	No
Urothelial carcinoma in situ	No	Yes
Surface urothelium	Reactive	Dysplastic or carcinoma in situ
Squamous changes	Yes	Yes or no
Stromal edema	Yes	No
Stromal desmoplastic reaction	No	Yes
P53	Negative	Positive
Vascular invasion by CD31	No	Possible

DIVERTICULUM

Definition

- Benign urothelial outpouching into the bladder wall

Clinical features

- Mostly asymptomatic, diverticulum is found incidentally
- If associated with inflammation or calculus, there will be nonspecific urinary symptoms

Gross pathology

- Outpouching may be detectable grossly or cystoscopic examination

Histology

- Diverticulum is covered by benign urothelium (Figs. 48-15 and 48-16)
- Urothelium may be seen adjacent to thick muscle bundles in muscularis propria or perivesicle adipose tissue microscopically
- In diverticulum, urothelial-lined mucosa may be close to the perivesicle fat with just a thin layer of fibrous band between urothelium and perivesicle fat
- Reactive urothelium, chronic inflammation, or ulceration may be present
- Urothelial carcinoma may develop within diverticulum. In such a case, the tumor can invade perivesicle adipose tissue more easily (Fig. 48-17)
- Other conditions such as calculus, squamous metaplasia, or nephrogenic adenoma can also develop within a diverticulum

Immunohistochemistry

- Not indicated

Clinical relevance (prognosis and treatment options)

- Surgical resection for symptomatic cases
- The rupture of diverticulum is associated with acute and chronic inflammation of the bladder and serositis
- Invasive urothelial carcinoma developing within a diverticulum should be treated more aggressively as muscle invasive disease, because the defects in the bladder wall provide minimal protection against cancer invasion to perivesicle fat

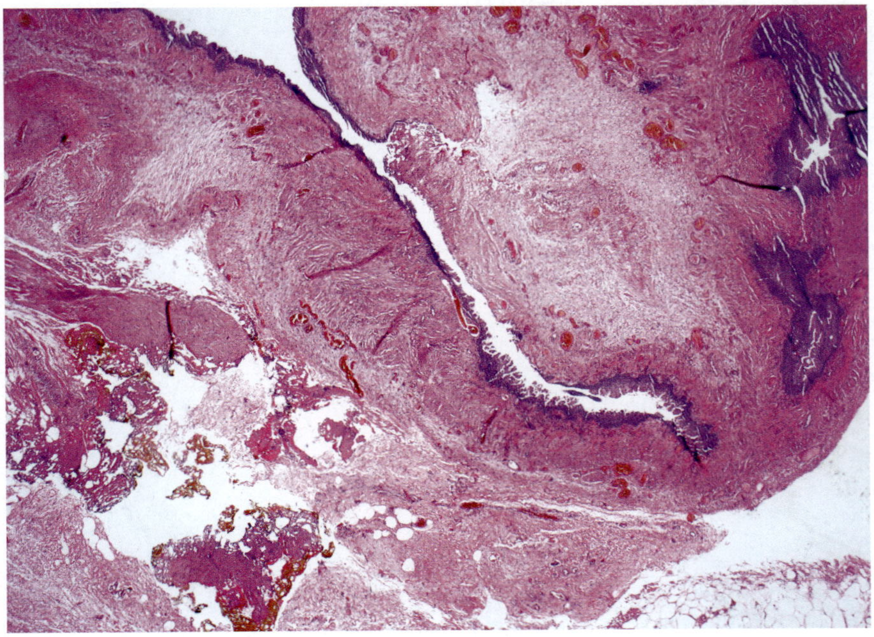

Figure 48-15.
A bladder diverticulum with outpouching urothelium almost through the bladder wall to the perivesicle tissue.

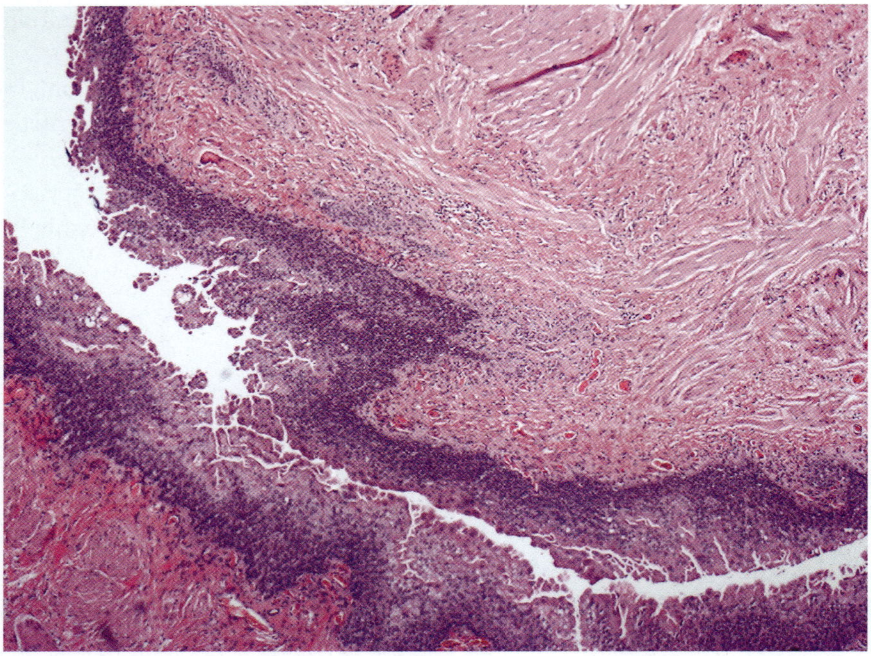

Figure 48-16.
Bladder diverticulum is associated with chronic inflammation and urothelial hyperplasia.

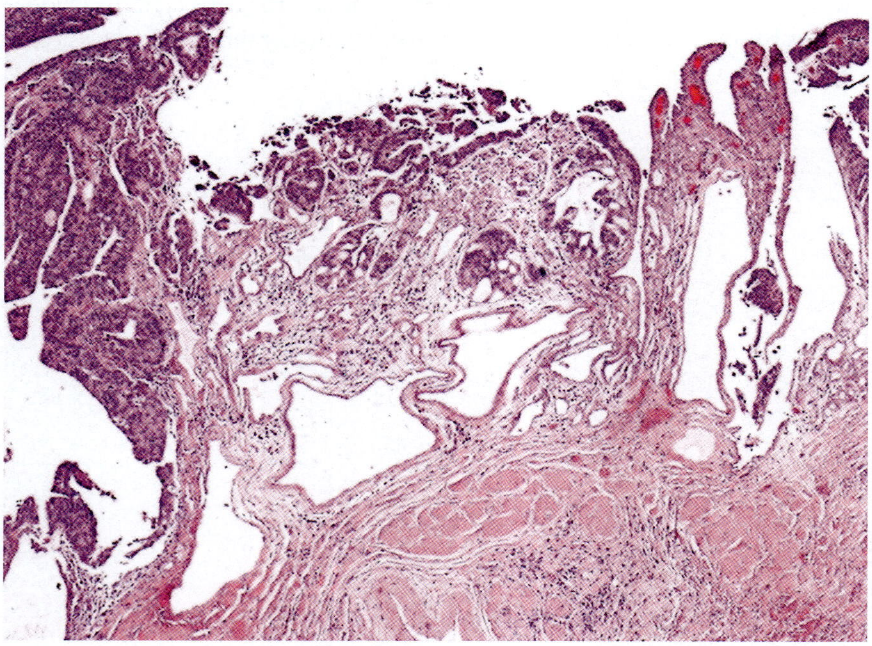

Figure 48-17.
A low-grade papillary urothelial carcinoma develops within a diverticulum (left). The dilated cystic structures represent a nephrogenic adenoma (right).

AMYLOIDOSIS

Definition

- Amyloid deposits in the bladder
- The presence of amyloid deposits, in the seminal vesicles, which increase with age, is a normal finding. However, amyloid deposits in other GU organs are considered abnormal
- Amyloidosis can be systemic or localized

Pathogenesis

- Systemic amyloidosis is associated with multiple myeloma or autoimmune diseases
- There are different types of amyloid material (see Table 48-2)
- Localized amyloidosis without other organ involvement has unknown etiology

Clinical features

- Painless hematuria mimicking the symptoms of bladder cancer
- Occurs mostly in older patients (>50 years)
- Imaging and cystoscopy reveal poorly defined mass lesions or thickened bladder wall
- The lesions preferentially affect the posterior bladder wall

Gross pathology

- Areas of diffuse erythema, petechiae in the mucosa, or nodular surface
- Rigid or hard mucosa with poorly defined mass lesions in the wall, resembling an infiltrating tumor

Histology

- Areas of amorphous eosinophilic material replacing connective tissue in lamina propria (Fig. 48-18)
- Amyloid deposits may be seen in or around vessels (Fig. 48-19), in such a case, the histological recognition may be difficult without clinical information
- No obvious inflammatory cells but foreign body giant cell reaction may be present
- Urothelium shows reactive changes
- Perivascular amyloid deposits typically seen in systemic amyloidosis

Table 48-2. Types of Amyloidosis

Type		*Association*	*Amyloid type*
Systemic	Primary	Multiple myeloma	AL
	Secondary	Autoimmune diseases	AA
	Familial	Mutations of *transthyretin* gene	ATTR
Localized	Primary	Unknown	AL

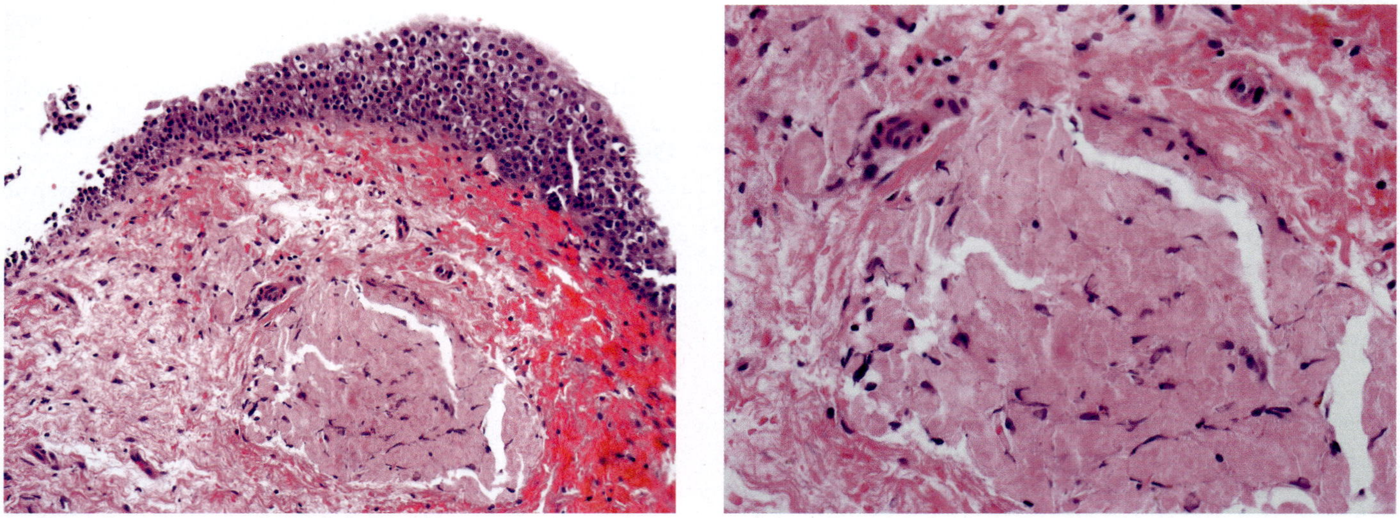

a *b*

Figure 48-18.
Amyloid deposit in the bladder lamina propria associated with hemorrhage (*a*). High magnification shows homogenous pink amyloid deposit (*b*).

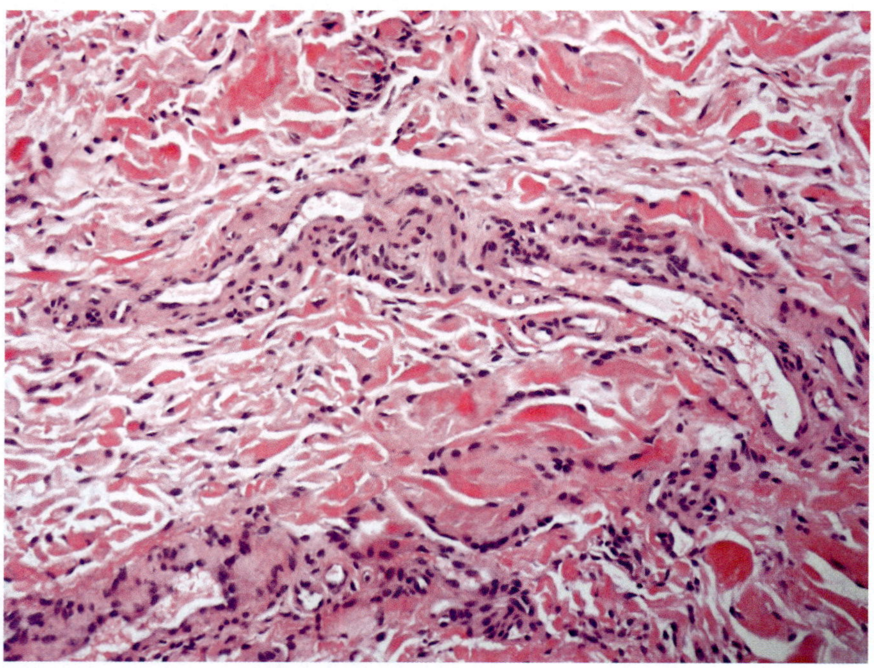

Figure 48-19.
Bladder amyloidosis with perivascular amyloid deposit seen as in thickened walls (*a*).

Immunohistochemistry and histochemistry

- Congo red stain demonstrates apple-green birefringence under polarized light (Fig. 48-20)
- Immunostains for kappa and lambda light chains may be used
- Multiple myeloma work-up can be helpful

Differential diagnosis

Bladder urothelial carcinoma (clinical)

- In bladder amyloidosis, sometimes the clinical suspicion is high; however, pathology report may be negative (amyloid material might be mistaken for fibrosis when a specimen is very small)
- Presence of malignant cells are relatively easy to be distinguished from amyloidosis
- Request Congo red if there is a clinical suspicion for amyloidosis

Fibrosis

- Hyalinized fibrous tissue sometimes can be confused with amyloid deposit
- Trichrome stain is positive
- Congo red is negative

Clinical relevance (prognosis and treatment options)

- Transurethral resection and fulguration for localized amyloid areas
- Partial cystectomy for large massive deposits comprising bladder function
- Systemic amyloid may recur after resection
- Systemic treatment of the underlining disease such as multiple myeloma is necessary

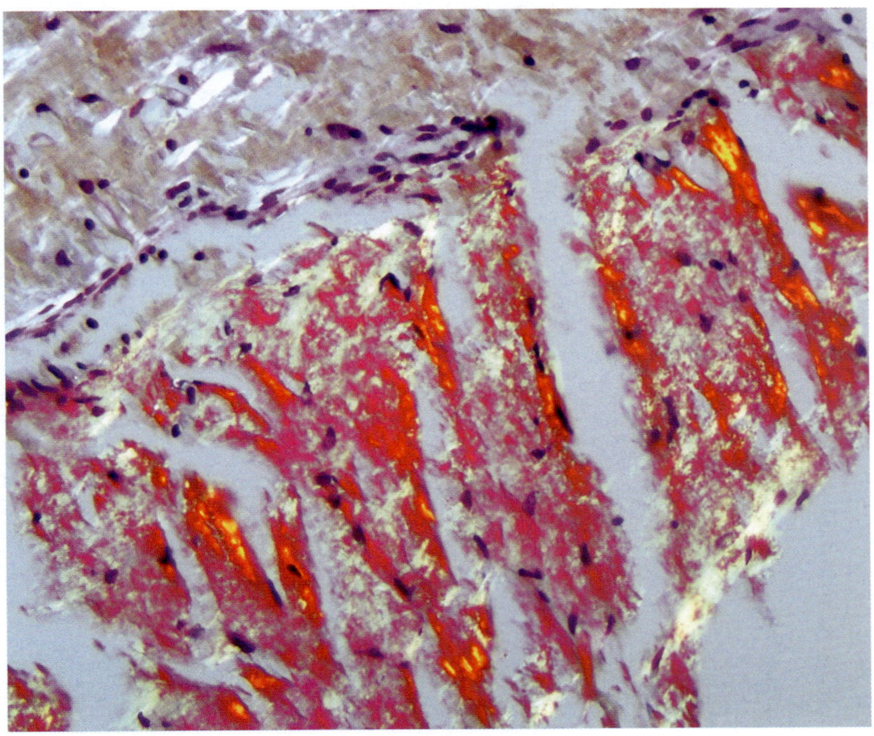

Figure 48-20.
By Congo red stain the "apple-green" amyloid deposit can be demonstrated under polarized light.

REACTIVE STROMAL CHANGE

Definition

- A benign condition of stromal cells of the bladder showing degenerative atypia

Other term

- Stromal atypia

Pathogenesis

- Stromal reaction to chronic stimulus, which can be seen in chronic inflammation, postbiopsy, or presence of malignancy

Clinical features

- No specific clinical findings

Gross pathology

- Not grossly detectable

Histology

- Isolated large stromal cells, fibroblasts, or myofibroblasts
- Scattered stromal cells showing nuclear enlargement with smudged chromatic patterns (Fig. 48-21) in a background stroma with low cellularity
- Hemorrhage or chronic inflammation may be present in the stroma (Fig. 48-22*a*)
- May or may not be associated with reactive epithelial changes

Immunohistochemistry

- Usually not indicated. In a case suspicious for carcinoma, the stromal cells are negative for keratins (Fig. 48-22*b*)

Differential diagnosis

- High-grade urothelial (or sarcomatoid) carcinoma
  - Occasionally, it can be confused with high-grade invasive urothelial carcinoma or metastatic carcinoma
  - Carcinoma will be more diffuse with prominent cytological atypia
  - Immunostaining for keratins can be confirmative

Clinical relevance (prognosis and treatment options)

- The reactive stromal change is a very common finding in bladder biopsy or TUR, which should not be confused with malignance
- No specific clinical significance

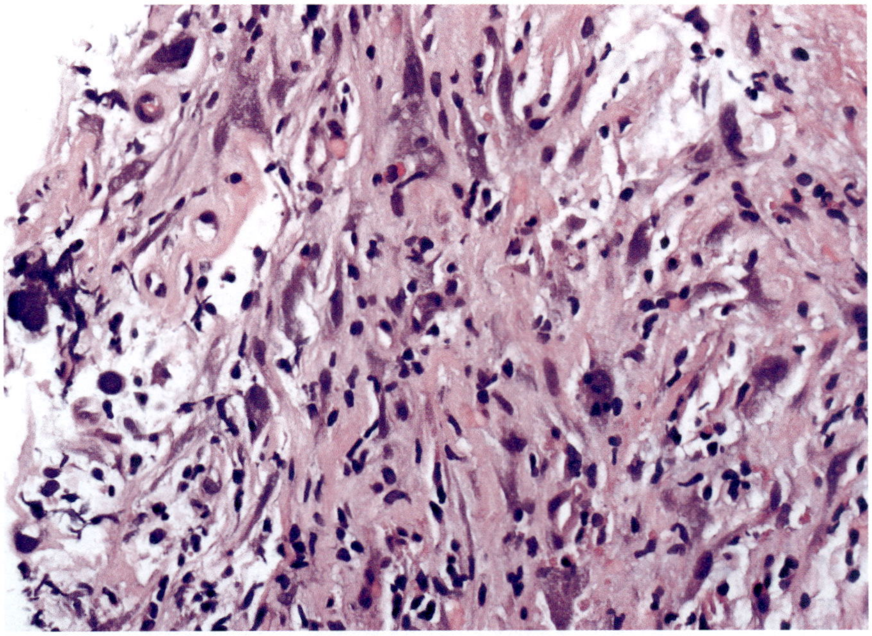

Figure 48-21.
Reactive bladder stroma with chronic inflammation and occasional enlarged spindle stromal cells.

Figure 48-22.
Atypical stromal cells seen in the lamina propria with hemorrhage (*a*). Immunostaining negativity for AE1/AE3 in the atypical stromal cells confirms nature of the nonepithelial cells (*b*).

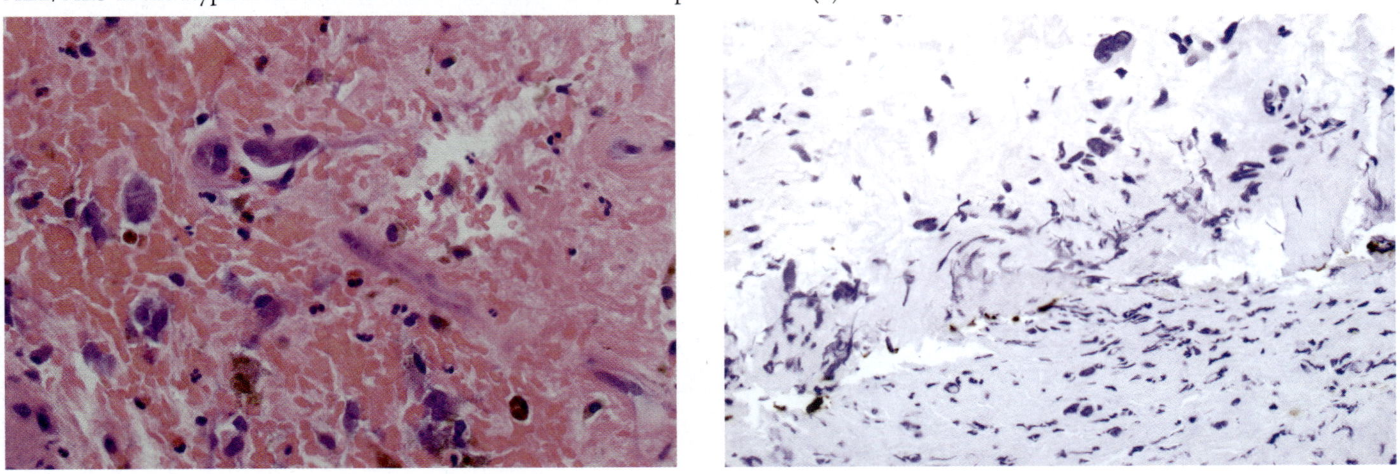

a **b**

POSTBIOPSY SPINDLE CELL PROLIFERATION

Definition

- Reactive stromal proliferative lesion after bladder biopsy or transurethral resections

Other terms

- (Postoperative) spindle cell nodules
- Pseudosarcomatous myofibroblastic proliferation

Pathogenesis

- Reactive process by the bladder stromal cells in response to the tissue damages caused by the invasive procedure such as biopsy or TUR

Clinical features

- History of biopsy, transurethral resection, or other invasive procedures
- May present with hematuria or obstructive voiding symptoms
- Most cases without specific symptoms
- As an incidental finding in a follow-up biopsy

Gross pathology

- The lesion may not be visible grossly if deeply located
- If present in mucosa, it is a friable small lesion, typically less than 1 to 2 cm in size
- The lesion may be ulcerated

Histology

- Cellular stroma with plump or elongated spindle cells, which may show high mitotic rates, but without significant cytological atypia (Fig. 48-23)
- The spindle cells may be deep in the muscularis propria
- Delicate network of small blood vessels and edematous or myxoid stroma
- Acute and chronic inflammatory cell infiltrates, particularly eosinophils, are present (Fig. 48-23*b*)
- Focal hemorrhage (Fig. 48-24) or fibrinoid necrosis (Fig. 48-23*a*) caused by the previous injury may be present adjacent to the lesion
- This lesion morphologically resembles inflammatory myofibroblastic tumor, but this lesion is typically much smaller
- Often coexisting with postbiopsy granulomas and reactive urothelial changes

Immunohistochemistry

- Keratin markers may be focally positive

Differential diagnosis

Inflammatory myofibroblastic tumor

- Microscopically, both inflammatory myofibroblastic tumor (IMFT) and reactive stromal proliferation are similar
- But IMFT is a larger mass lesion with infiltrating borders
- In most cases of inflammatory myofibroblastic tumor, no obvious history of surgical procedures or injury
- Focal hemorrhage and fibrinoid necrosis associated with the previous injury are not evident

Clinical relevance (prognosis and treatment options)

- Benign, with excellent prognosis
- No recurrence if resected

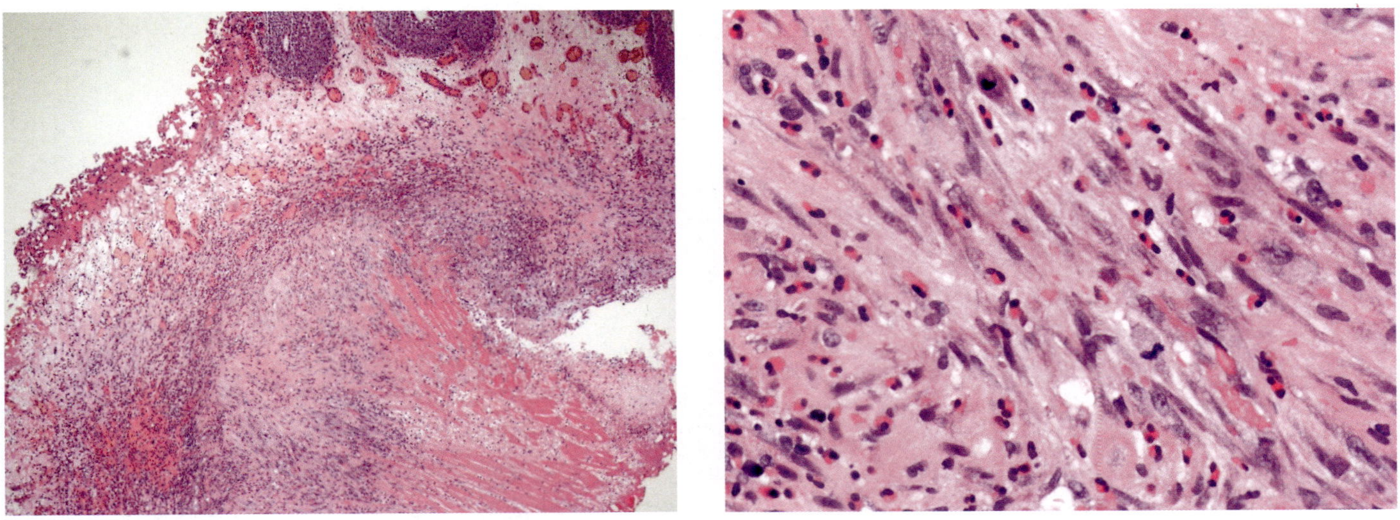

a *b*

Figure 48-23.
Postbiopsy changes in the bladder mucosa consist of spindle cell proliferation and inflammatory infiltrates (*a*). High magnification shows spindle cells (mostly myofibroblasts) associated with inflammatory infiltrate with numerous eosinophils (*b*).

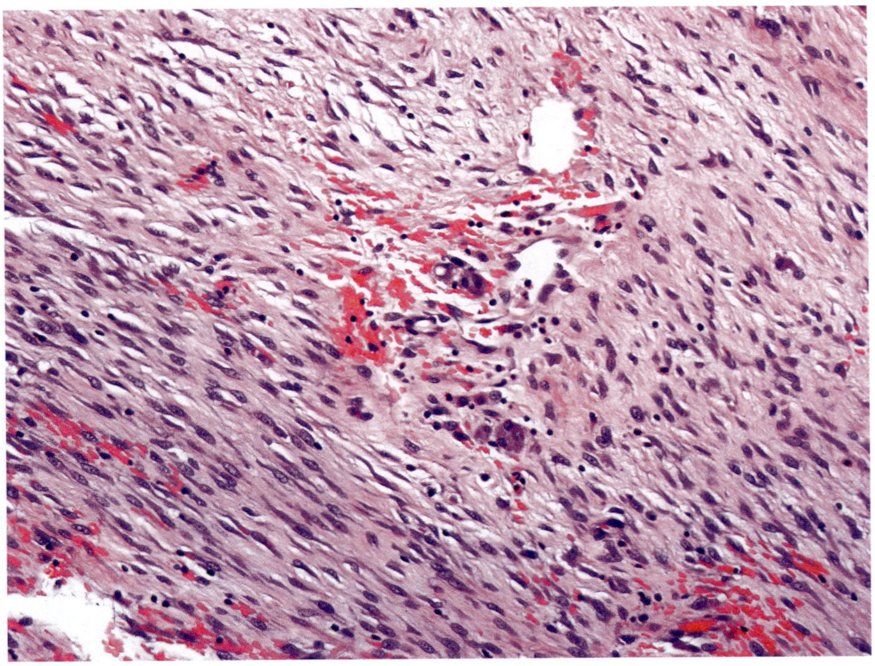

Figure 48-24.
Spindle cell proliferation in the bladder biopsy site associated with hemorrhage and foreign body giant cell reaction.

CONDYLOMA ACUMINATA

Definition

- HPV-induced lesion in the bladder, histologically similar to condyloma acuminata in other locations
- Subtypes 6 and 11 are responsible

Clinical features

- Condyloma is rare in the bladder, mostly occurs as direct extension from genital condylomas
- Presence of squamous metaplasia, related to stones, indwelling catheters, or fistulas, is often seen in the patients with condyloma. It is more commonly seen in females because of the shorter urethra
- Immunocompromised patients are at a higher risk
- Multiple lesions and recurrences after resections are typical
- Association with carcinoma is rare with only a few cases reported

Gross pathology

- Cauliflower-like lesions in the bladder

Histology

- The lesional cells form papillary fronts with hyperkeratosis and acanthosis (thickened epithelium) (Fig. 48-25*a*)
- Koilocytic cells, characterized by wrinkled nuclei and perinuclear halos, are present (Fig. 48-25*b*)
- Squamous metaplasia in the adjacent bladder mucosa
- Failure to recognize the severely cauterized condyloma may lead to a misdiagnosis as a papillary urothelial carcinoma (Fig. 48-26)
- Squamous dysplasia should be reported if present (Fig. 48-27)

Immunohistochemistry and molecular analysis

- HPV staining positive
- P53 weakly positive
- P16 positive

Differential diagnosis

- Low-grade papillary urothelial carcinoma
  - When condyloma is cauterized severely, it may be mistaken for a papillary urothelial carcinoma. Especially, condyloma is much less common than papillary urothelial carcinoma in the bladder
  - Careful examination looking for noncauterized areas is necessary
  - The absence of koilocytic changes and presence of cytological atypia is the key for diagnosis
- Squamous cell carcinoma
  - Significant cytological atypia involving full thickness of epithelium (CIS)
  - Presence of stromal invasion by malignant squamous cells is diagnostic of invasive squamous cell carcinoma

Clinical relevance (prognosis and treatment options)

- Excision is the treatment of choice
- The recurrence chance is high, while the chance to progress to squamous cell carcinoma is present, but probably relatively low
- Follow-up is necessary because of its potential to be associated with dysplasia and squamous cell carcinoma

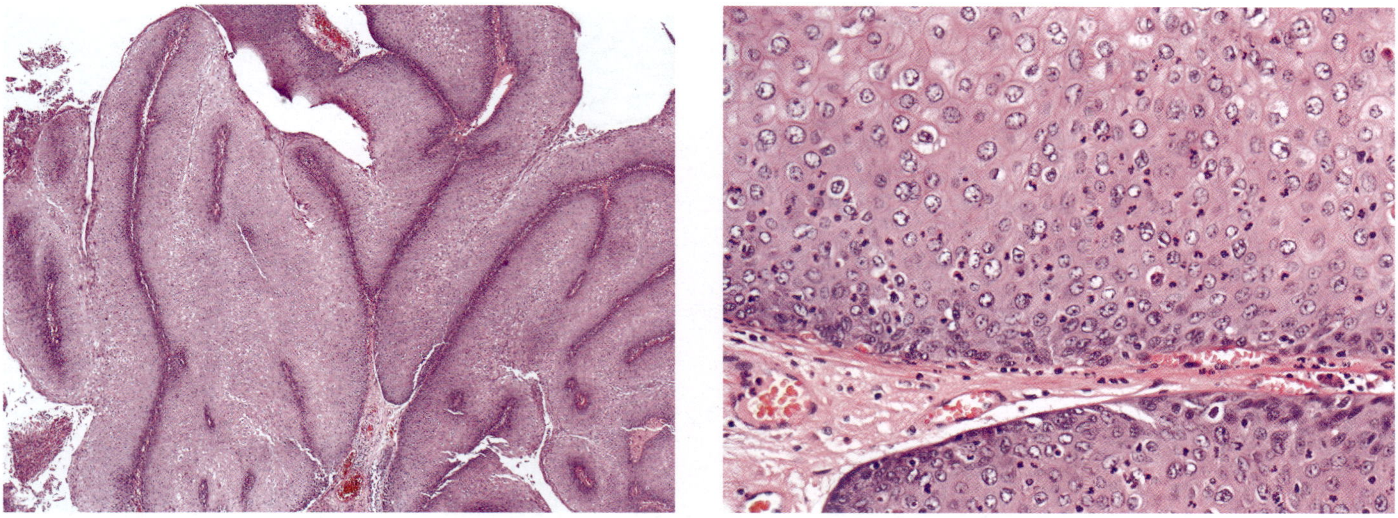

Figure 48-25.
A large condyloma in the bladder displays a papillary configuration (*a*). High magnification shows prominent koilocytic changes with raisinoid nuclei and perinuclear halos (*b*).

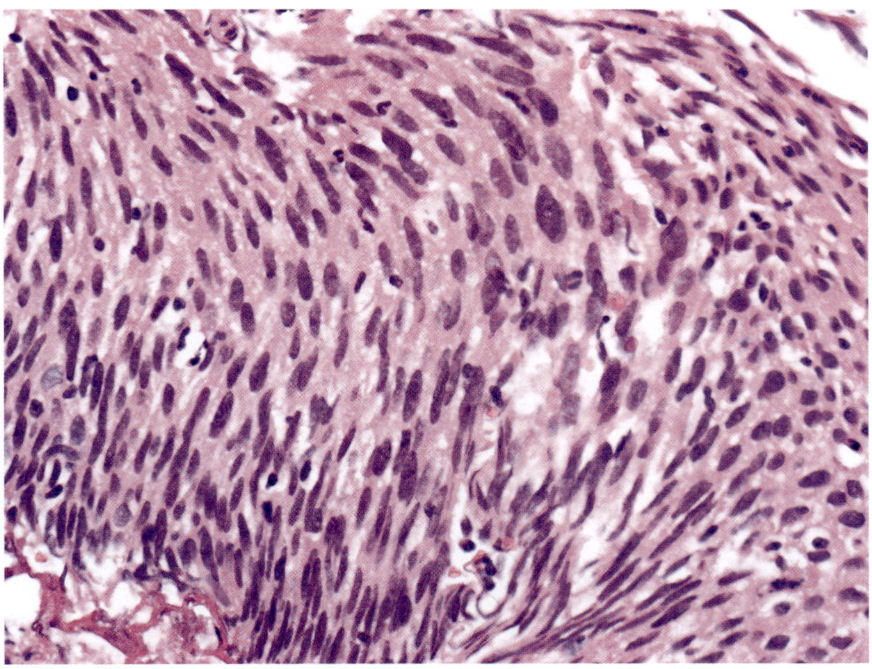

Figure 48-26.
Bladder condyloma resected by TUR with severe thermal effects, which mimics a papillary urothelial carcinoma because koilocytic changes are masked by the thermal damage.

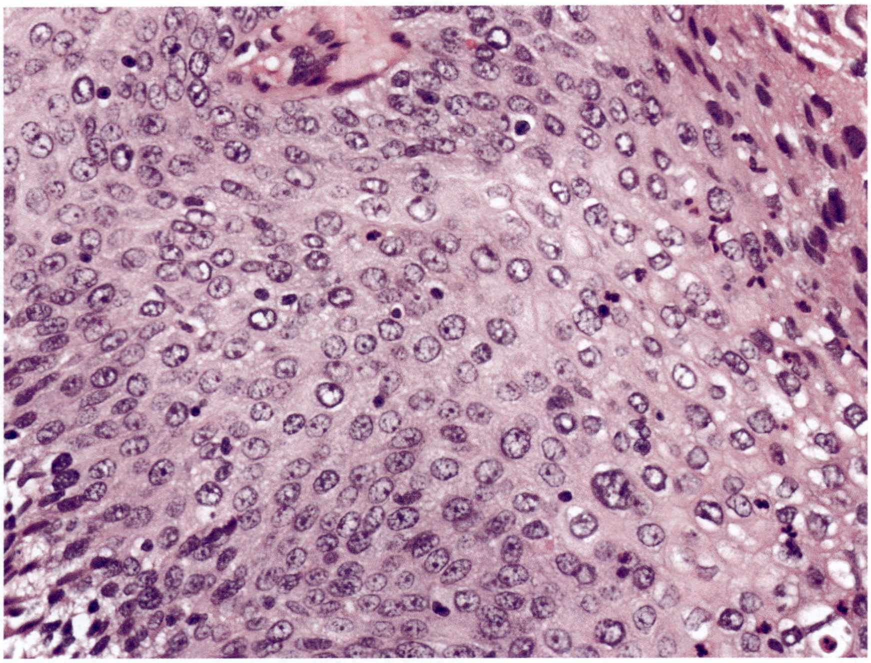

Figure 48-27.
A bladder condyloma displays mild squamous dysplasia.

CHAPTER 49 Flat Atypical Urothelial Lesions of the Bladder

UROTHELIAL ATYPIA

Definition

- Abnormal flat urothelial lesions with cytological atypia, but with uncertainty about its neoplastic nature

Other terms

- Reactive urothelial atypia, flat urothelial atypia

Pathogenesis

- These lesions are common in the bladder. In the majority of cases, they are representing reactive changes to stimuli
- They are, along with dysplasia, probably the most difficult lesions for pathologists to diagnose in bladder biopsy

Clinical features

- No specific symptoms, hematuria or inflammatory symptoms may be present
- Negative or atypical cytology and no evidence of papillary lesions
- Erythematous areas may be seen on cystoscopic examination

Gross pathology

- Not gross lesions seen

Histology

- Two lesions fall into this category with the difference being the presence or absence of associated inflammation
- Urothelial atypia with unknown significance
  - A flat lesion with cytological atypia but does not readily fit into either reactive or dysplastic category
  - Morphologically, it shows nuclear enlargement and disorganization, without obvious inflammation (Figs. 49-1 and 49-2), but difficult to be distinguished from dysplasia
  - It requires clinical follow-up. Most of these lesions will not progress to carcinoma
- Reactive urothelial atypia
  - Associated with previous procedures, infection, catheter, or stone
  - Chronic inflammatory cells may be present (Fig. 49-3)
  - Urothelial cells slightly enlarged and nuclei with fine chromatin and prominent nucleoli (Fig. 49-3)

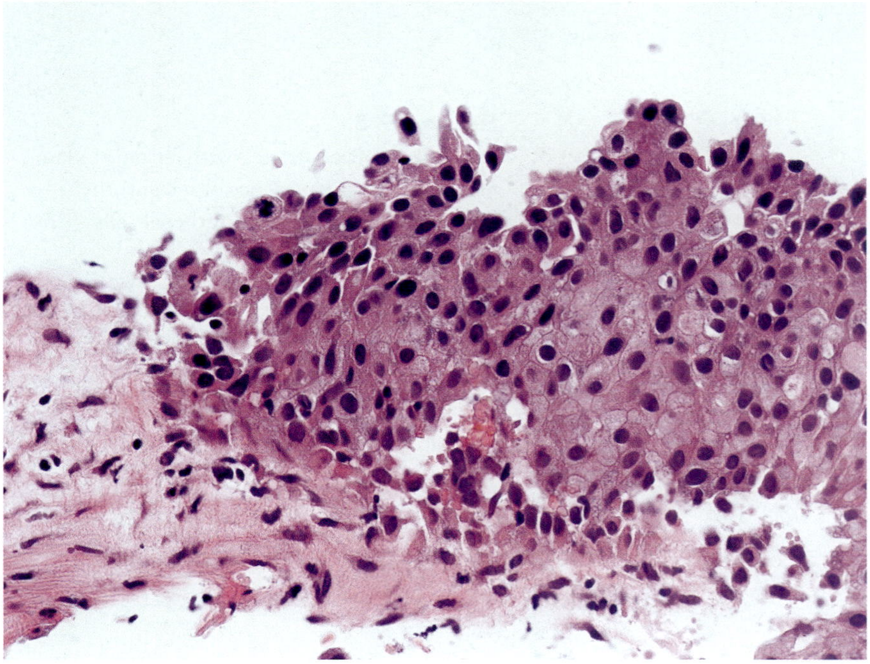

Figure 49-1.
Urothelial atypia of unknown significance. There is disorganization and mild cytological atypia in this flat lesion. It is uncertain that this presents reactive or dysplastic lesions.

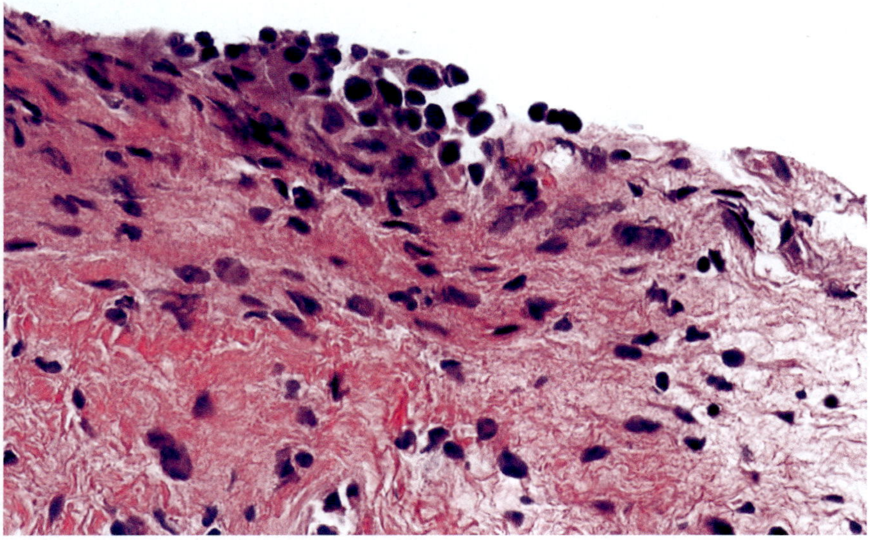

Figure 49-2.
Urothelial atypia of unknown significance. In a patient with a history of radiation, there are atypical urothelial cells with hyperchromatic nuclei present. However, the nuclear sizes of these cells are not sufficient for diagnosis of carcinoma in situ.

- One of the known agents causing reactive atypia is BK virus. BK virus infected urothelial cells show nuclear enlargement, hyperchromasia, and smudged chromatin (Fig. 49-4*a* and *b*), mimicking carcinoma in situ (CIS)
- The clinical management for urothelial atypia of unknown significance or for BK virus associated atypia is similar
- The lesion may resolve after the offending agent is removed
- The chance for reactive atypia to progress to neoplastic lesions is minimal
- It is well known that radiation may induce cytological atypia in benign urothelial cells. It is also well documented that radiation may induce bladder cancer
- In a postradiation biopsy case, when it is difficult to determine whether it is reactive or dysplastic, we also use the term urothelial atypia with unknown significance
- Similar situations when the atypia is present in cases with stones or catheters are mostly reactive (Fig. 49-4*c* and *d*), but it may be difficult to determine its nature in some cases

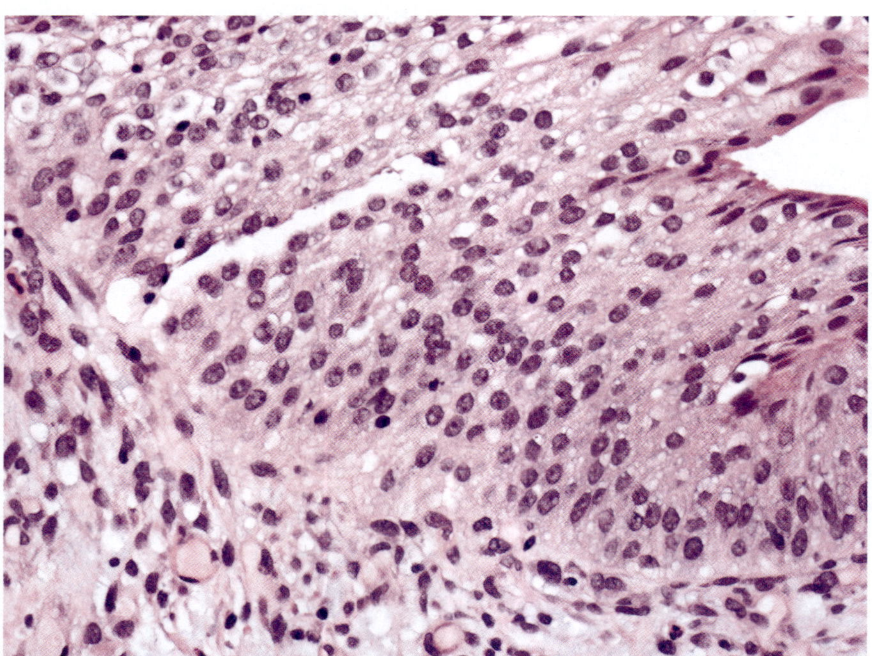

Figure 49-3.
Reactive atypia associated with chronic inflammation shows the presence of intraurothelial lymphocytes and reactive urothelial cells with distinct nucleoli.

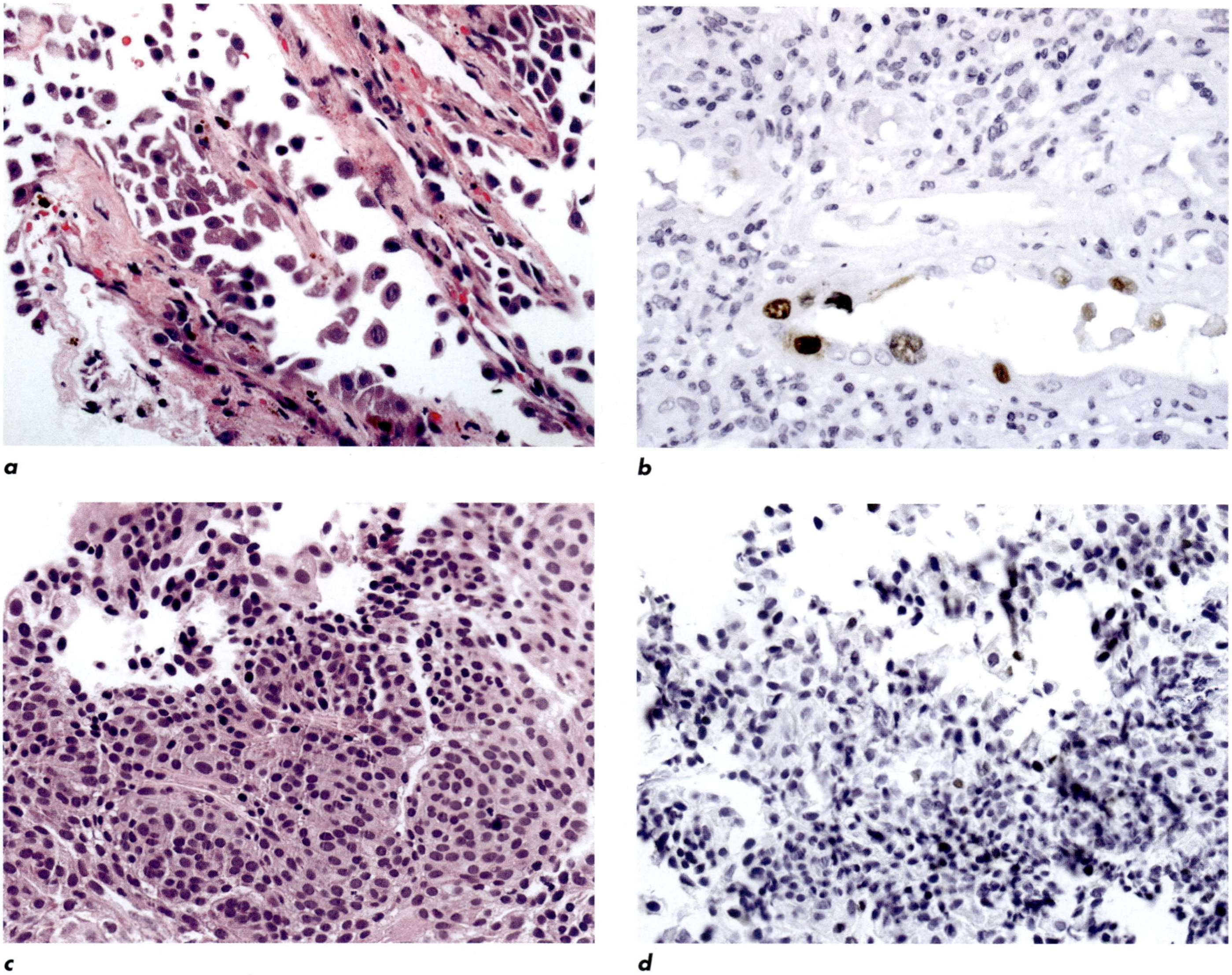

Figure 49-4.

Reactive urothelial atypia induced by BK virus infection is signified by discohesive urothelial cells with prominent nucleoli and high N/C ratio (*a*), mimicking carcinoma in situ. However, these reactive cells are positive for the BK-specific immunostaining (*b*). Urothelial atypia associated with a calculus. There are prominent urothelial hyperplasia and mild cytological atypia (*c*), and the p53 immunostaining is negative (*d*). It is most likely a reactive process related to the stimulus by the calculus.

Immunohistochemistry

- P53 negative, CK20 negative or focally positive, and Ki67 activity is low

Clinical relevance (prognosis and treatment options)

- This is a group of flat lesions that are very difficult to distinguish from each other by histology. Previous studies have shown a poor interobserver and intraobserver reproducibility even among the urological experts
- Most flat atypical lesions will be followed clinically and most of these cases will not progress to urothelial carcinoma with follow-up
- It is important to distinguish this group of lesions from urothelial CIS because of the significance in clinical management (Table 49-1)
- Clinical follow-up with or without repeat biopsies are recommended

Table 49-1. Comparison of Flat Urothelial Lesions

Flat urothelial lesions	*Definition*	*Nature*	*Clinical significance*
Hyperplasia	Increased urothelial cells (thickened layers)	Reactive	Benign
Mild dysplasia	A term to avoid	Reactive	Benign
Reactive atypia	Reactive change with inflammation	Reactive	Benign
Atypia of unknown significance	Not sure benign or premalignant	Reactive or precancerous	Follow-up required
Dysplasia (primary)	Significant atypia but short of carcinoma in situ	Precancerous	Follow-up and rebiopsy required
Carcinoma in situ	High-grade carcinoma cells confined within urothelium	Cancer	Treatment required
Flat lesions adjacent to papillary urothelial carcinoma (secondary dysplasia)	Atypical cells similar to adjacent low-grade urothelial carcinoma	Precancerous or early low-grade carcinoma	Follow-up and rebiopsy required

UROTHELIAL DYSPLASIA

Definition

- A flat neoplastic lesion of the urothelium with appreciable cytological and architectural changes, but short of carcinoma in situ (CIS)
- Dysplasia is believed to be the precursor lesion of urothelial carcinoma
- Dysplasia can be divided into two types
  - Primary (de novo) dysplasia: present alone without urothelial carcinoma. In this chapter, dysplasia refers to primary dysplasia unless it is specified otherwise
  - Secondary dysplasia: present adjacent to a low-grade papillary urothelial carcinoma. The dysplastic cells have the same degree of cytological atypia as low-grade papillary urothelial carcinoma but they do not form papilla

Other terms

- Moderate urothelial dysplasia, low-grade intraurothelial neoplasia, low-grade intraepithelial neoplasia of the bladder
- Mild dysplasia should be diagnosed as benign

Pathogenesis

- Urothelial dysplasia is considered to be preneoplastic in nature
- Therefore, its etiology is supposed to be similar to that of bladder cancer
- However, many of these lesions may not progress to carcinoma

Clinical features

- Nonspecific irritative bladder symptoms and microscopic hematuria may be present for primary dysplasia
- Secondary dysplasia, which is associated with carcinoma, will have the symptoms and signs of urothelial carcinoma

Gross pathology

- Flat lesion, not easy to identify grossly
- The dysplastic lesion may be present alone as erythematous lesions and erosion, with or without an adjacent papillary urothelial carcinoma

Histology

- Dysplastic cells show nuclear hyperchromasia and nuclear enlargement, but only 2-3 (<4) times the diameter of a lymphocyte (Figs. 49-5 and 49-6)
- Dysplastic cells are disorganized with nuclear crowding and loss of polarity and mitosis may be seen occasionally (Fig. 49-7)
- The nuclear atypia is moderate in degree but insufficient for diagnosis of CIS (Figs. 49-7 and 49-8)
- Urothelial dysplasia typically lacks intraurothelial inflammatory cells
- In reality, it is important to distinguish dysplasia from CIS. However, the distinction between dysplasia and atypia sometimes can be very difficult
- Both urothelial dysplasia and atypia require clinical follow-up, while CIS needs treatment

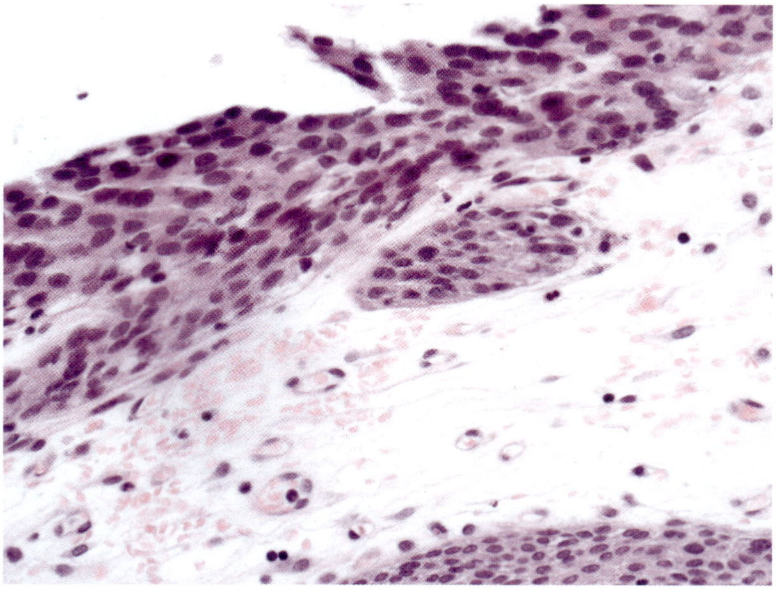

Figure 49-5.
Urothelial dysplasia. The dysplastic urothelial cells (upper portion) are disorganized, with nuclear enlargement and hyperchromasia, clearly different from the benign urothelial cells (lower portion).

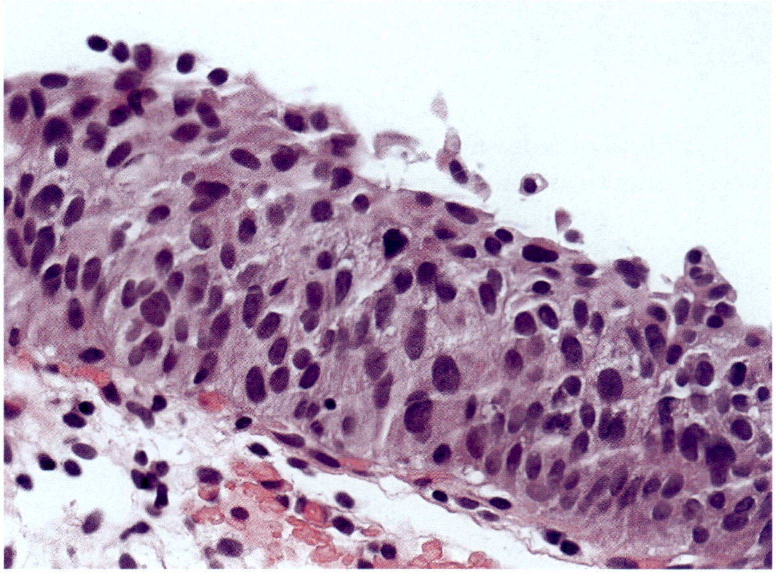

Figure 49-6.
Urothelial dysplasia with disorganized atypical cells. The degree of nuclear atypia is suspicious but not sufficient for the diagnosis of carcinoma in situ.

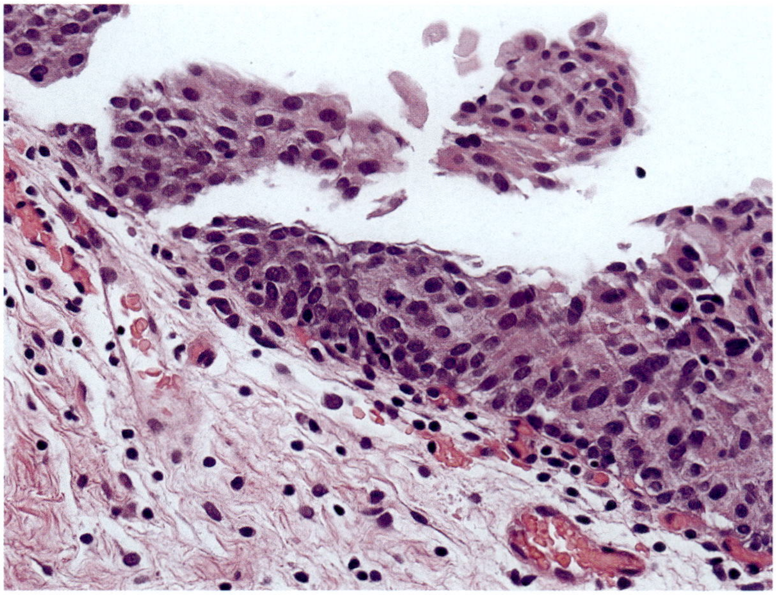

Figure 49-7.
Urothelial dysplasia with loss of polarity, cytological atypia, and occasional mitosis.

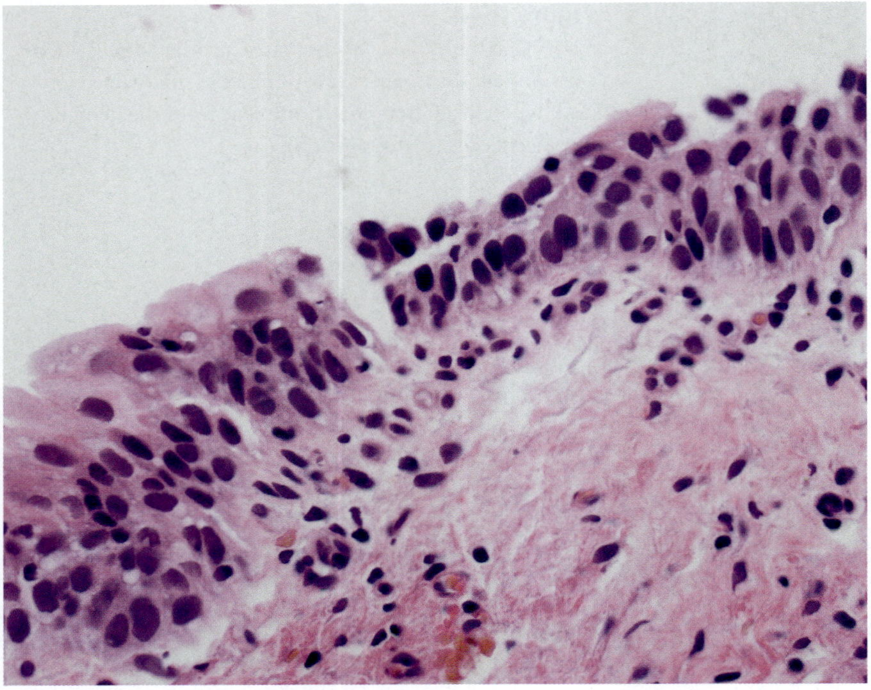

Figure 49-8.
Urothelial dysplasia with cytological atypia and hyperchromasia, but insufficient for diagnosis of carcinoma in situ.

Immunohistochemistry

- No reliable IHC markers have been established, essentially, CIS needs to be ruled out
- P53 negative
- CK20 staining and Ki67 proliferative activity are variable (Fig. 49-9)

Differential diagnosis

- Other flat urothelial lesions are summarized in Table 49-1

Molecular analysis

- No consistent findings

Clinical relevance (prognosis and treatment options)

- There is a risk for developing noninvasive bladder cancer such as CIS or low-grade papillary urothelial carcinoma
- Risk ranging from 5% to 20% based on reports in literature. The rate is probably depending on the distinction between reactive atypia and dysplasia
- Based on our experience, the risk is on the lower end of this range even without treatment
- Clinical follow-up is necessary

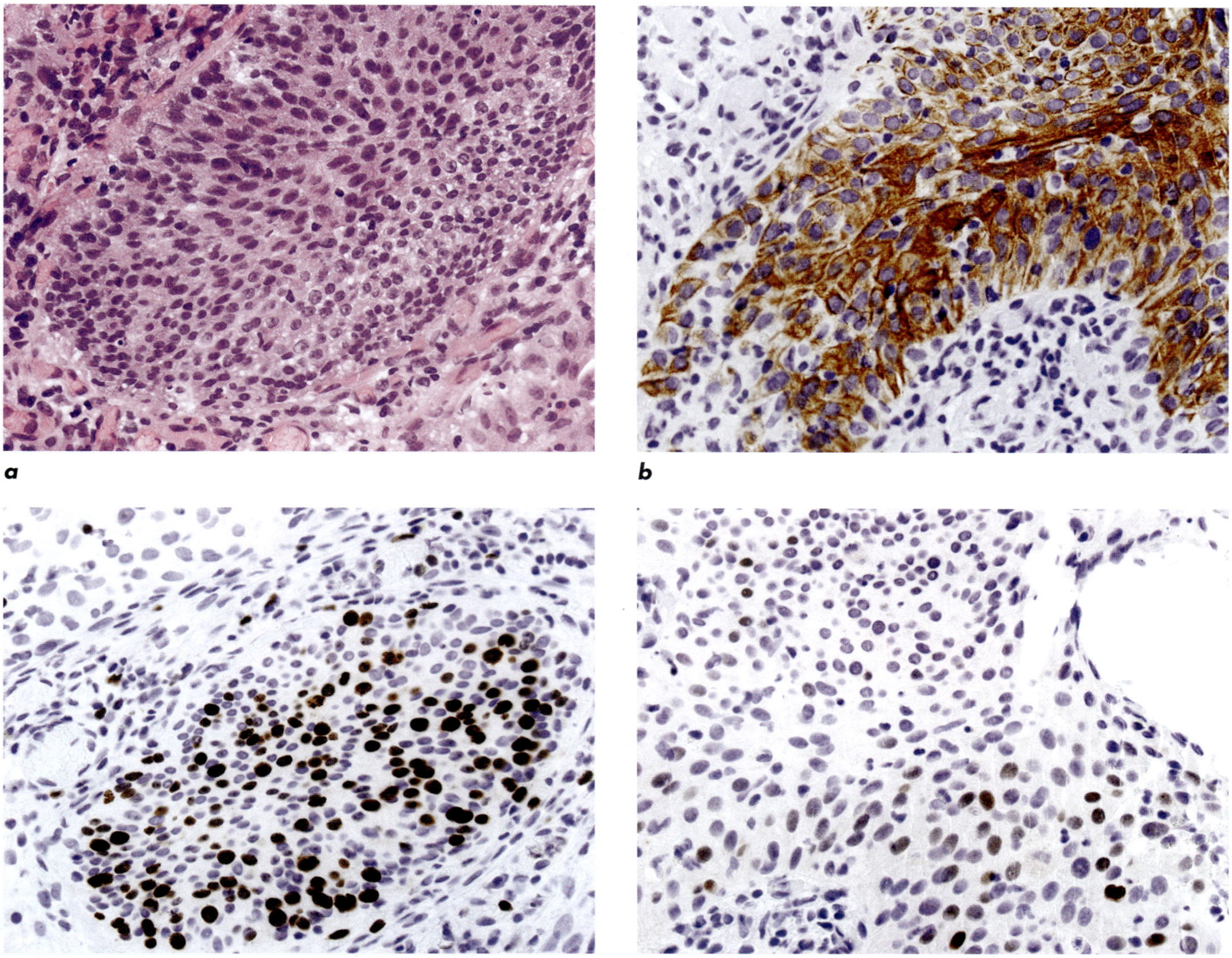

a b c d

Figure 49-9.
Urothelial dysplasia with crowded and disorganized urothelial cells showing cytological atypia (*a*), positive for CK20 (*b*), high Ki67 proliferative activity (*c*), but negative for p53 (*d*). This is a flat lesion adjacent to a low-grade papillary urothelial carcinoma (secondary dysplasia)

CHAPTER 50

Papillary Urothelial Lesions of the Bladder

PAPILLARY UROTHELIAL HYPERPLASIA

Definition

- Benign papillary urothelial proliferation is signified by the presence of nonbranching papillary structures and thickened urothelium

Pathogenesis

- It is a reactive change in response to inflammation, calculi, catheter, instrumentation, or other therapies
- It is a controversial entity. In some cases, it may also represent a very early papillary neoplastic lesion, which is difficult to be distinguished from a reactive process

Clinical features

- Nonspecific inflammatory symptoms
- Microscopic hematuria occasionally

Gross pathology

- Irregularity or granularity of bladder mucosal surface

Histology

- Nonbranching papilla with thickened but normal appearance urothelial lining (similar to urothelial hyperplasia) (Figs. 50-1 and 50-2)
- May be associated with chronic inflammation (Fig. 50-3)
- Generally there is no or minimal cytological atypia

Figure 50-1.
Papillary hyperplasia with nonbranching papilla in a patient with calculus (*a*). High magnification shows the presence of thickened urothelium but without cytological atypia (*b*).

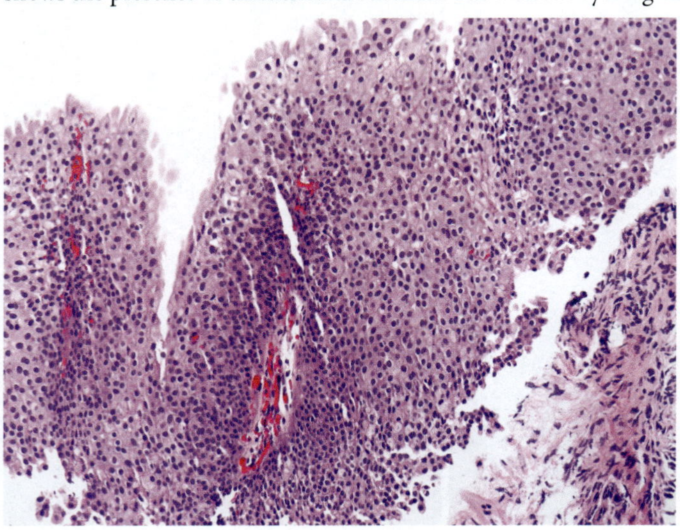

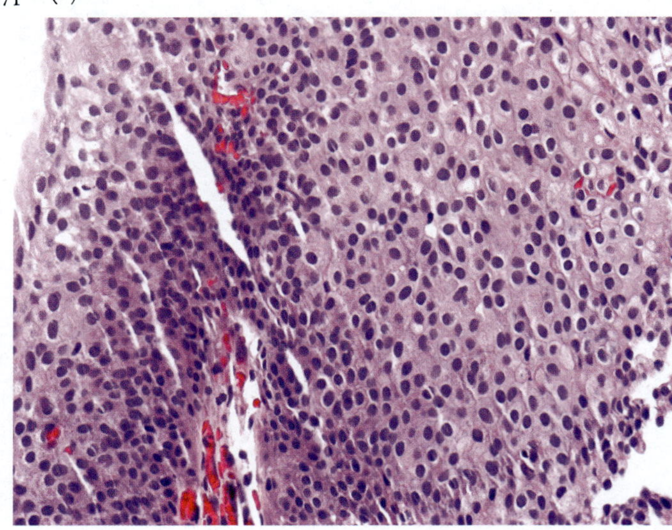

a *b*

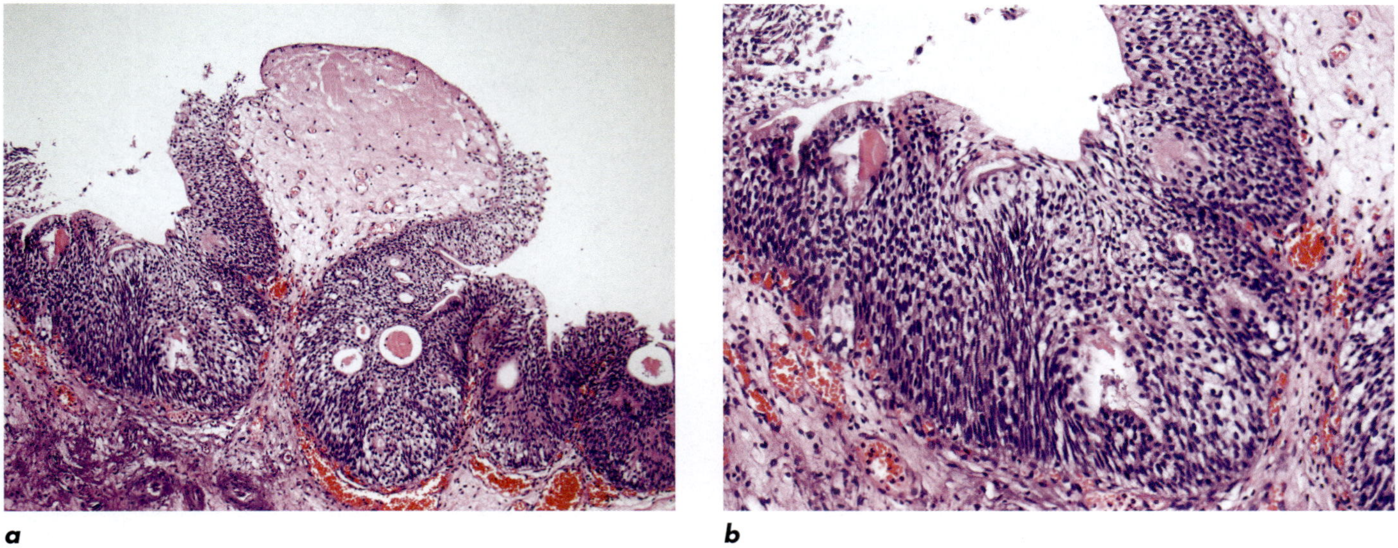

Figure 50-2.
Papillary urothelial hyperplasia is composed of a polypoid lesion with cystitis glandularis and fibrotic stroma (*a*). High magnification shows the reactive urothelium with cystitis glandularis (*b*). This may be the late phase of polypoid cystitis with urothelial proliferation.

- When atypia present in papillary urothelial hyperplasia, it is considered atypical papillary urothelial hyperplasia (Fig. 50-4)

Immunohistochemistry

- Generally not indicated
- To distinguish from papillary urothelial carcinoma (UC)
  - P53 negative (wild type)
  - Ki67 low proliferative index (Fig. 50-4*d*)
  - CK20 negative or focally positive

Clinical relevance (prognosis and treatment options)

- Benign, similar to urothelial hyperplasia
- Treatment for chronic inflammation
- A small subset of the atypical cases may have a risk to develop low-grade papillary neoplasm or difficult to be distinguished from low-grade papillary neoplasms. So that in the cases of atypical papillary hyperplasia, a close clinical follow-up with rebiopsy is necessary

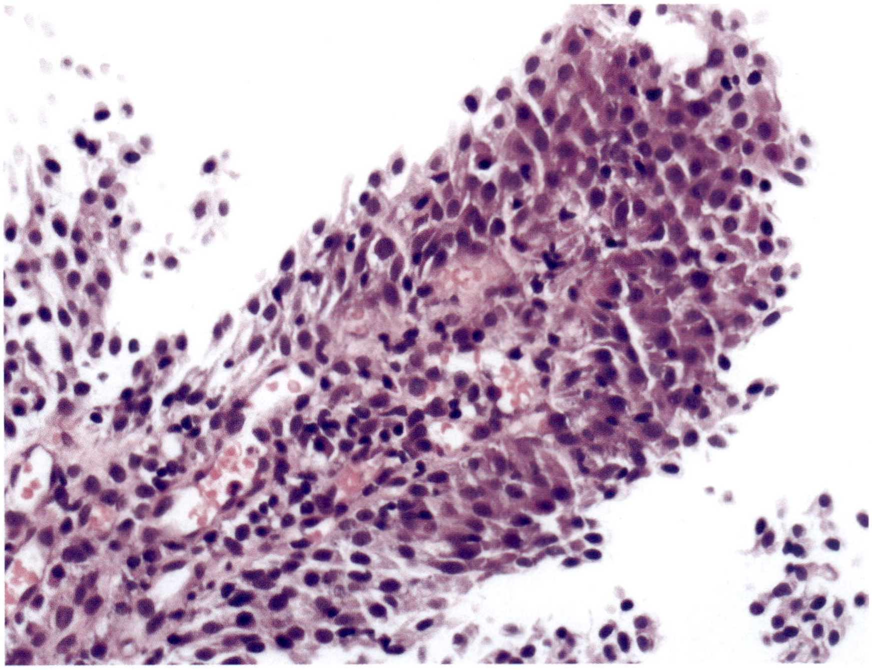

Figure 50-3.
Papillary hyperplasia with prominent chronic inflammation and reactive urothelium.

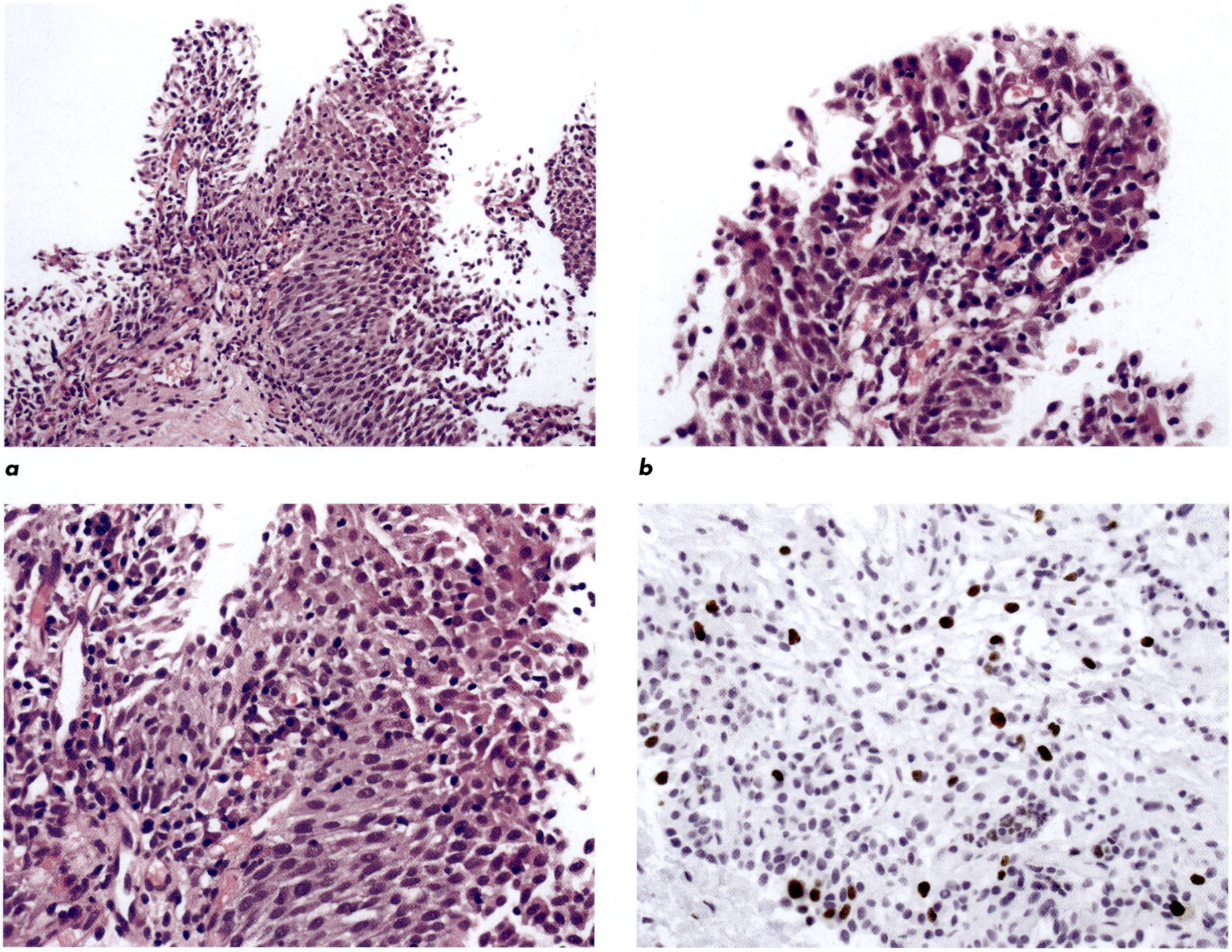

a b c d

Figure 50-4.
Atypical papillary urothelial hyperplasia with nonbranching papillae (*a*). High magnification shows prominent chronic inflammation and reactive urothelium (*b*), while other area shows the urothelial hyperplasia and atypia (*c*). The Ki67 proliferative activity is moderately increased (*d*).

UROTHELIAL PAPILLOMA

Definition

- Benign exophytic urothelial lesion composed of normal-appearing urothelium in a papillary configuration

Pathogenesis

- The low end of the spectrum for papillary tumors

Clinical features

- Nonspecific
- May be present in the younger patients
- Microscopic or gross hematuria

Gross pathology

- Relatively small lesions
- Elongated or pedunculated lesions, with delicate fibrovascular cores
- Simple rather than complex papilla
- Rare condition

Histology

- Simple branching papillary structures with slender fibrovascular cores (Fig. 50-5)
- Covered by the normal appearing urothelium with no cytological atypia (Fig. 50-6)

Immunohistochemistry

- CK20 positive only in umbrella cells similar to that of normal urothelium
- P53 negative or weakly positive in basal layers

Clinical relevance (prognosis and treatment options)

- Benign, but it may recur
- Small chance to develop into carcinoma

Figure 50-5.
Urothelial papilloma as a small lesion with papilla with a fibrovascular core (*a*). The lining urothelium of this lesion is almost normal without cytological atypia (*b*). The lamina propria blood vessels are dilated in the papilla.

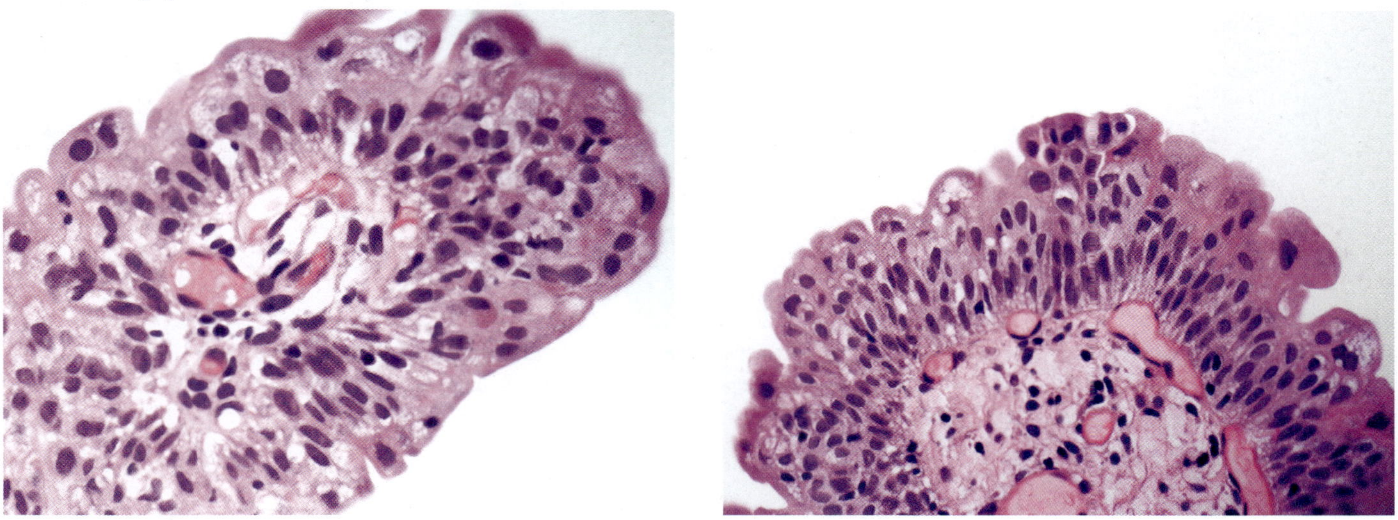

a *b*

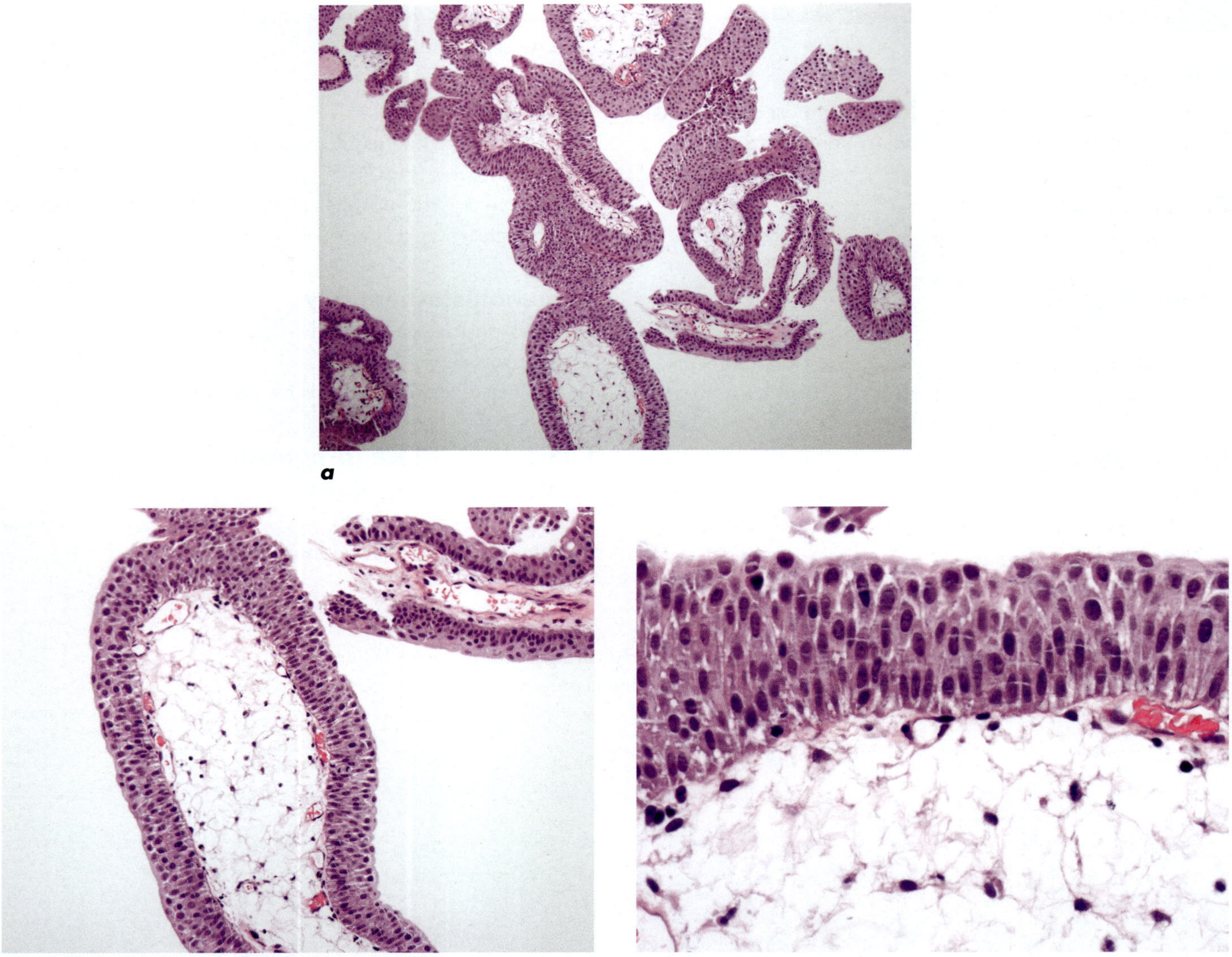

a

b

c

Figure 50-6.

Urothelial papilloma with delicate fibrovascular cores (*a*). The core is covered by benign-looking urothelium without significant increase of thickness (*b*). High magnification shows urothelial cells without significant atypia or increased thickness (*c*).

INVERTED PAPILLOMA

Definition

- Benign urothelial neoplasm with predominantly endophytic growth patterns

Pathogenesis

- Unknown
- It may include benign urothelial neoplasms, very low grade urothelial neoplasms and reactive urothelial lesions

Clinical features

- Uncommon, less than 1% of bladder urothelial tumors
- Wide age range

Gross pathology

- Hematuria
- Dome-shaped or slightly elevated lesion
- Mostly located in the trigone and bladder neck
- Typically less than 3 cm in size

Histology

- Endophytic growth patterns (Fig. 50-7)
- Islands of urothelial or anastomosing nests separated by fibroconnective tissue (Fig. 50-8)
- Peripheral palisading in the nests (Fig. 50-9)
- Smooth border, not desmoplastic reaction
- Minimal cytological atypia with rare mitosis
- May be associated with cystitis glandularis or squamous metaplasia

Immunohistochemistry

- CK20 negative
- Ki67 proliferative index low (Fig. 50-9c)
- P53 negative or weakly negative in basal layer

Clinical relevance (prognosis and treatment options)

- Complete resection (TUR) needed
- Recurrence very common if resected incompletely

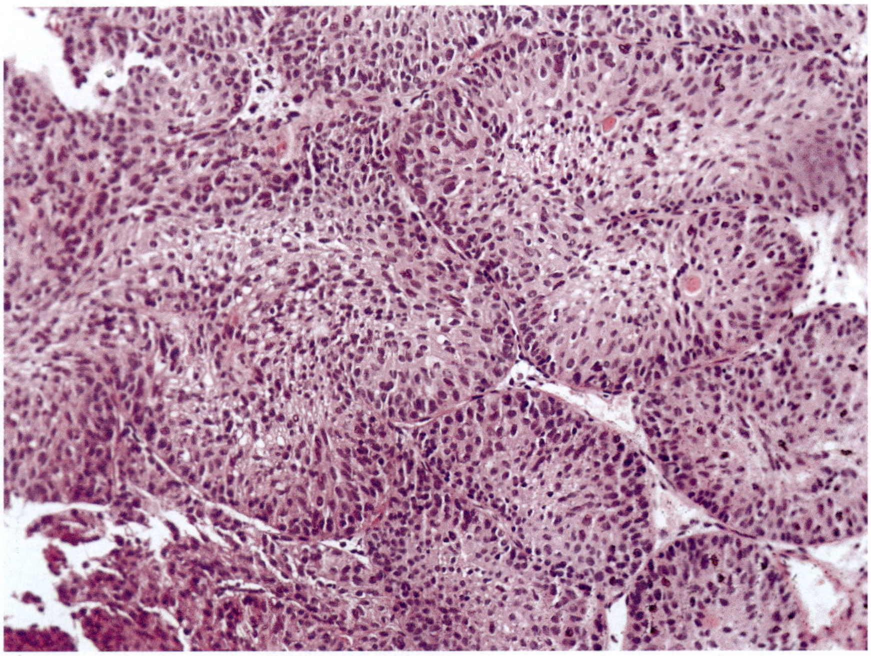

Figure 50-7.
Inverted papilloma of the bladder is characterized by the large islands of proliferative urothelial cells with minimal cytological atypia, separated by the thin fibrovascular cores.

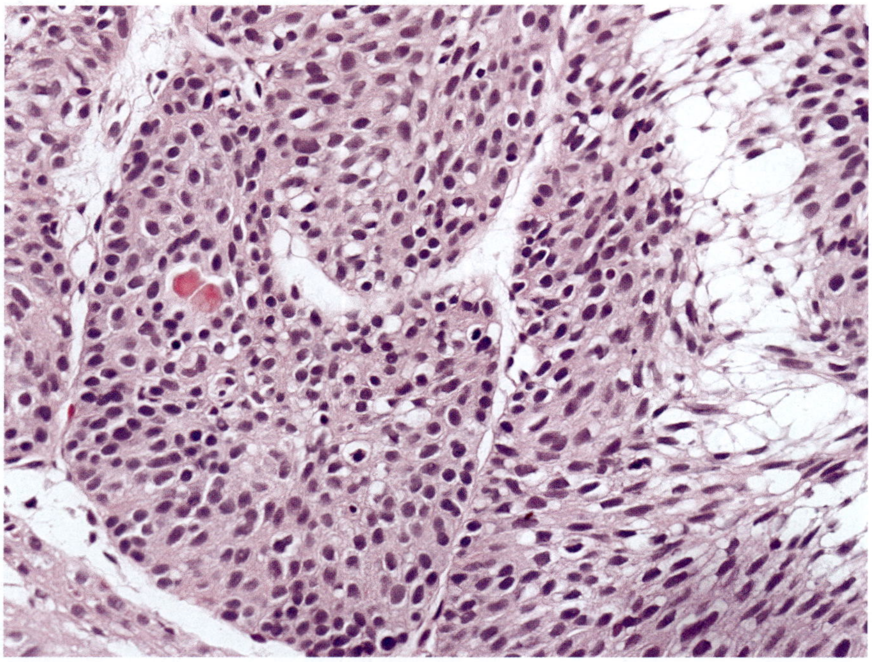

Figure 50-8.
Inverted papilloma of the bladder with the "jigsaw-puzzle" pattern formed by the tumor cells islands.

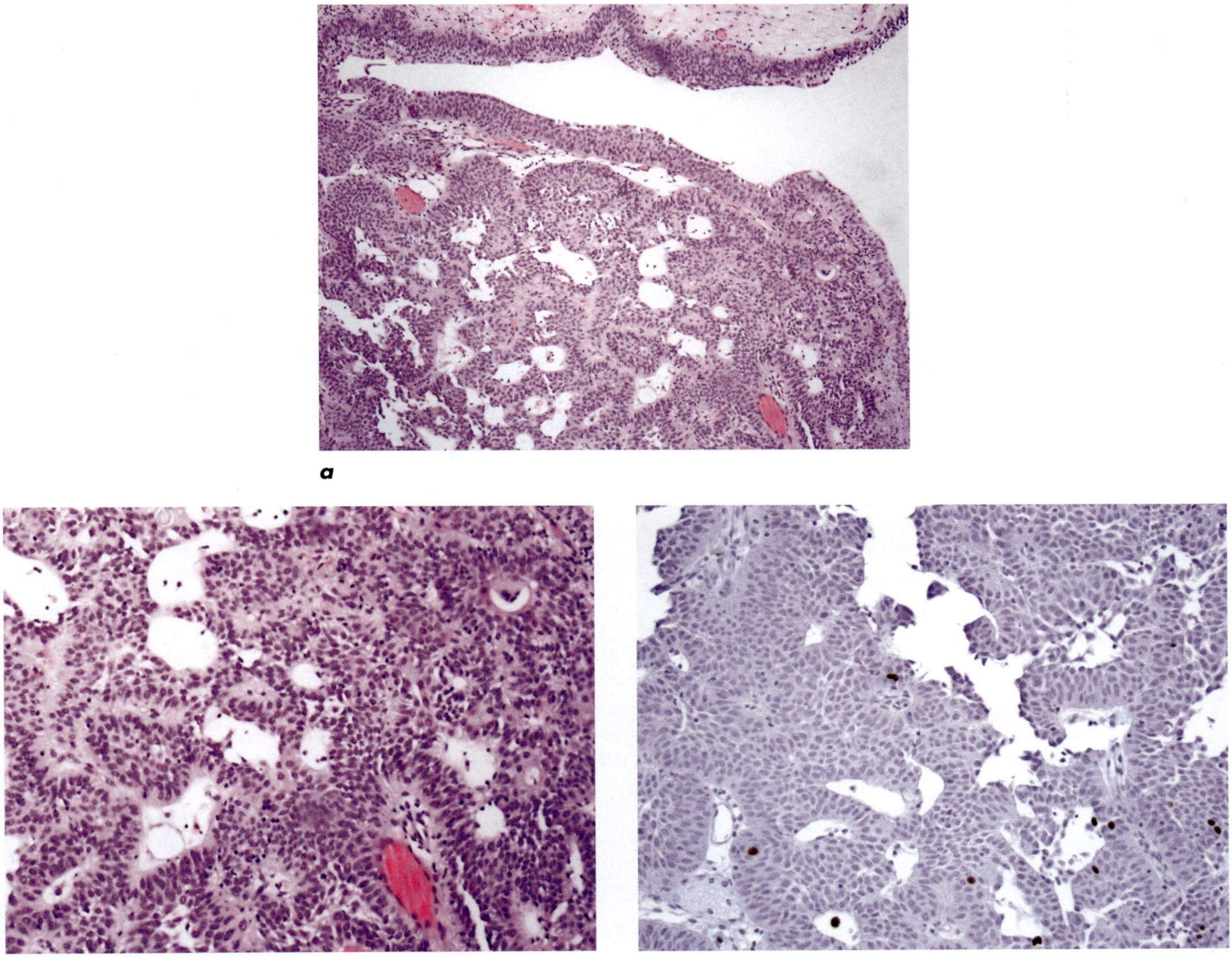

a b c

Figure 50-9.

Inverted papilloma is a dome-shaped lesion composed of nests of proliferating urothelial cells in inverted growth patterns (*a*). High magnification shows the palisading periphery of the urothelial cell islands or nests, without significant cytological atypia (*b*). The Ki67 proliferative activity is low (*c*).

PAPILLARY UROTHELIAL NEOPLASM OF LOW MALIGNANT POTENTIAL

Definition

- Papillary urothelial neoplasm of low malignant potential (PUNLMP) is a urothelial neoplasm with papillary configuration, and thickened abnormal urothelium lacking significant cytological atypia

Other terms

- Papillary UC, grade 1 (old term, only a subset)
- However, other cases of grade 1 carcinomas will be classified as low-grade UC
- The comparison of old and new classification systems is listed in Table 50-1

Pathogenesis and epidemiology

- Uncertain, probably similar to low-grade UC
- Less common than low-grade UC in daily practice
- Male:female = 5:1
- This is a controversial entity. There is no molecular or biochemical evidence so far to support the notion that PUNLMP is a true entity different from low-grade UC
- Many investigators feel that this may represent a very low-grade UC with a good prognosis

Clinical features

- Hematuria or asymptomatic
- Negative urine cytology
- Positive cystoscopic finding of papillary lesion(s), predominantly in the lateral and posterior walls of the bladder

Gross pathology

- Smaller papillary lesion(s), typically less than 2 cm

Histology

- Monotonous urothelial cells are in papillary configuration (Fig. 50-10)
- Cell proliferation leads to increased cell density and thickened urothelium (Fig. 50-11)

Table 50-1. Comparison of the Current with the Old WHO Classification System for Bladder Cancer

Old WHO classification	*New WHO classification*
Papilloma	Papilloma
Papillary transitional cell carcinoma grade 1	Papillary urothelial neoplasm with low malignant potential Low-grade papillary urothelial carcinoma
Papillary transitional cell carcinoma grade 2	Low-grade papillary urothelial carcinoma High-grade papillary urothelial carcinoma
Papillary transitional cell carcinoma grade 3	High-grade papillary urothelial carcinoma

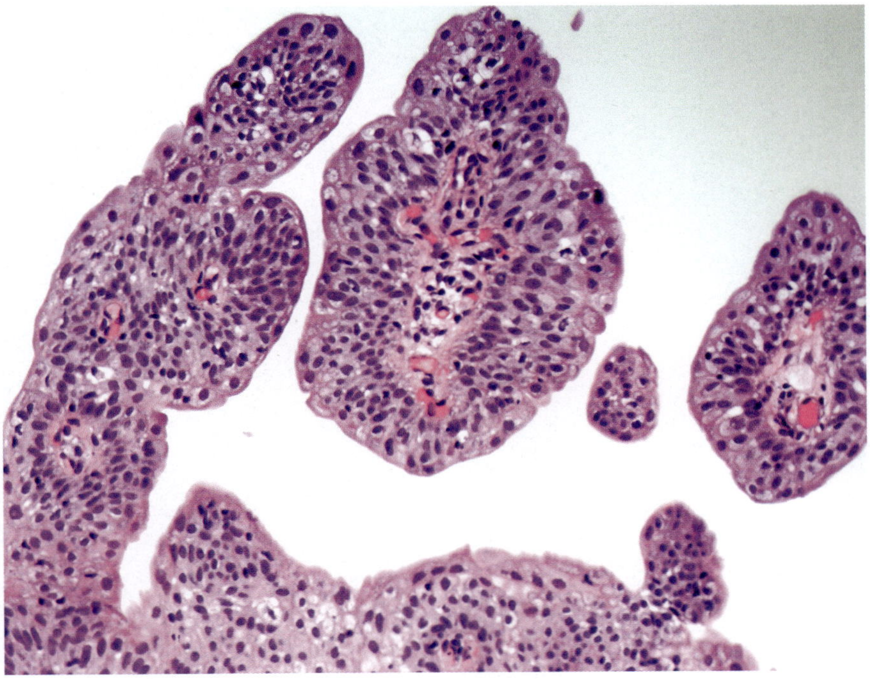

Figure 50-10.
Papillary urothelial neoplasm of low malignant potential (PUNLMP). A small lesion composed of several papillary fonts covered by thickened urothelium with mild cytological atypia.

- Only mild cytological atypia is preserved, but the polarity of urothelial cells is retained (Fig. 50-12)
- Mitosis is uncommon, and it is confined in the basal layer if present
- The histological distinction between PUNLMP and low-grade papillary UC is difficult, even among urological pathology experts. So that the interobserver or intraobserver reproducibility is poor

Immunohistochemistry

- Not contributory

Molecular analysis

- Similar to low-grade papillary UC

Differential diagnosis

- Low-grade UC: lost polarity and increased cytological atypia
- Urothelial papilloma: less complex configuration, no increase of thickness, nor cytological atypia (see Table 50-2)

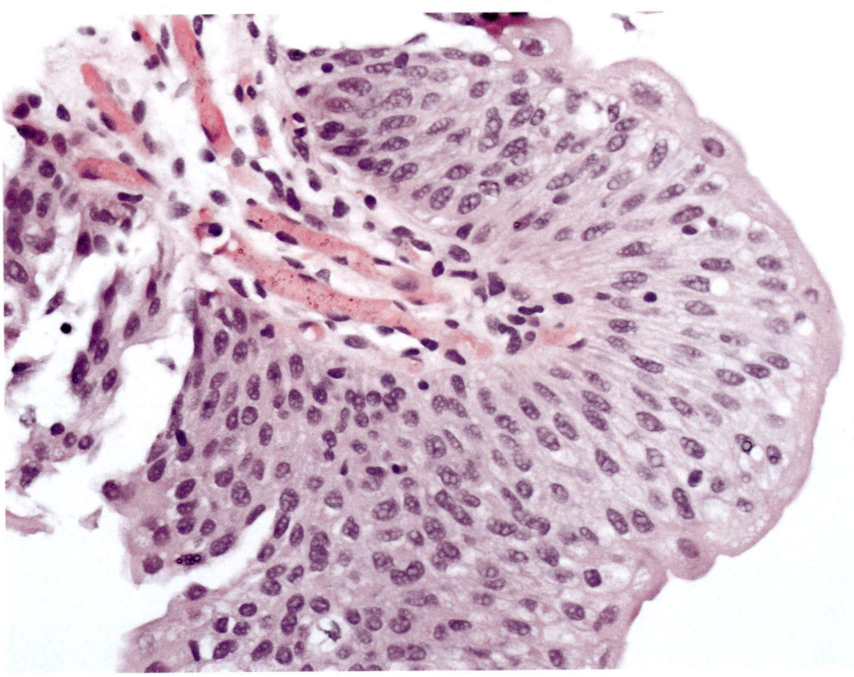

Figure 50-11.
PUNLMP with abnormally thickened urothelial cells covering the fibrovascular core. The neoplastic urothelial cells retain the polarity.

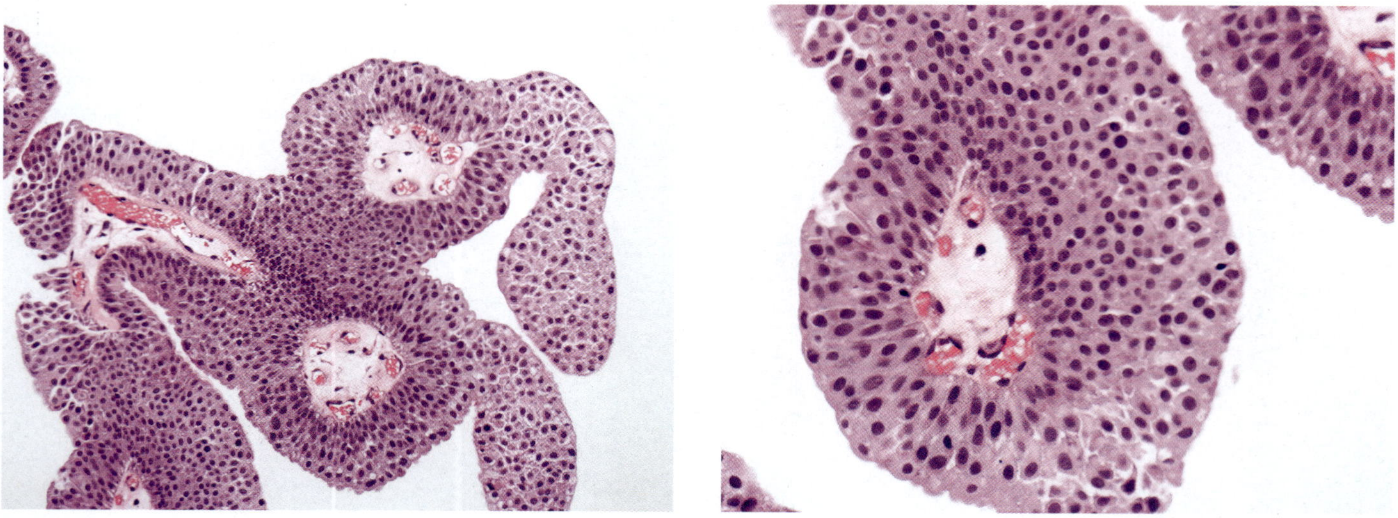

a b

Figure 50-12.
PUNLMP is composed of papillary structures covered by abnormal urothelial cells (*a*). High magnification of PUNLMP shows the presence abnormally thickened urothelium with mild cytological atypia (*b*).

Table 50-2. Urothelial Neoplasms of the Bladder

Lesions	*Gross appearance*	*Histology*
Papilloma	Papillary, slender, and delicate	Lining urothelial cells almost normal
Inverted papilloma	Dome shaped	Inverted growth patterns Bland cytology Palisading periphery
Papillary urothelial neoplasm with low malignant potential	Small papillary	Bland or mild cytological atypia, retained polarity
Low-grade papillary urothelial carcinoma	Papillary, small or large	Mild cytological atypia + loss of polarity
High-grade papillary urothelial carcinoma	Papillary, mostly large	Marked cytological atypia Papillary with fibrovascular cores
Urothelial carcinoma in situ	Flat, erythematous	Marked cytological atypia Flat
Invasive urothelial carcinoma	Masses with flat, ulcerated, or papillary surface	Marked cytological atypia with invasion, mostly cases high grade occasionally low grade

Clinical relevance (prognosis and treatment options)

- The histological distinction between PUNLMP and low-grade papillary UC is difficult because of the overlapping features
- TUR is the treatment of choice
- These patients need to be followed after the initial resection, since there is a high recurrent rate (20% to 50%)
- Because of the difficulty in distinguishing PUNLMP and low-grade papillary UC, a patient may have diagnoses of both low-grade papillary UC and PUNLMP in multiple repeat biopsies, which does not necessarily indicate progression or regression
- Progression to invasive and/or high-grade UC is lower than low-grade papillary UC; therefore, there is a good prognosis after treatment

LOW-GRADE PAPILLARY UROTHELIAL CARCINOMA

Definition

- A malignant papillary neoplasm derived from urothelium
- The tumor is characterized by an orderly appearance of tumor cells lining the papillary structure still resemble urothelium, but with recognizable architectural and cytological atypia
- Low-grade cytologically and biologically

Other terms

- Grade 1 or grade 2 papillary UC (some grade 2 papillary UCs in the old classification system may be classified as high grade based on the current classification system)
- Low-grade papillary transitional cell carcinoma

Pathogenesis and epidemiology

- Most common form of bladder cancer
- Smoking is a high risk factor for bladder cancer

Clinical features

- Painless hematuria
- Cystoscopy shows one or multiple exophytic lesions. May be coexisting with dysplasia or CIS
- May be coexisting with upper GU tract tumors

Gross pathology

- Papillary or cauliflower-like lesion(s), usually it is small (Figs. 50-13 and 50-14), but can be large
- The tumor has a flexible base (no invasion) or fixed base (invasive)

Histology

- Slender papillary fronts with branching fibrovascular cores (Figs. 50-14 and 50-15)
- Tumor cells are orderly in architecture and slightly disorganized, but still resemble urothelium
- The neoplastic urothelium can be thickened or normal in thickness (counting more than seven layers of cells is not necessary)

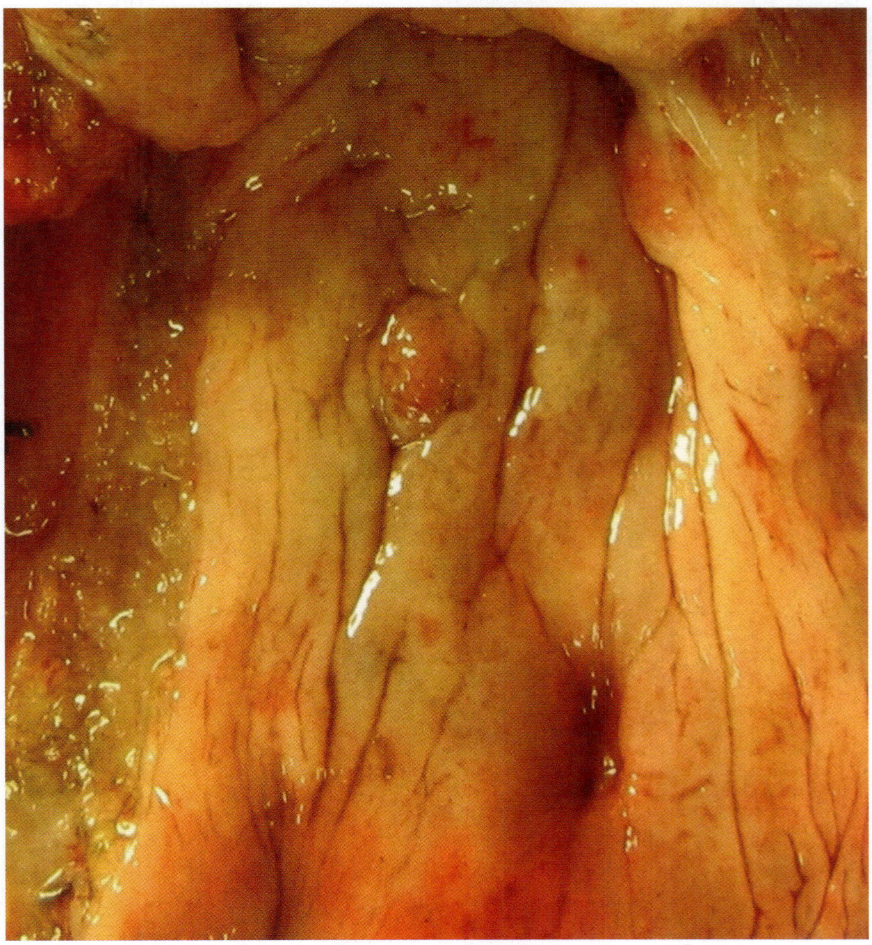

Figure 50-13.
This low-grade papillary urothelial carcinoma of the bladder is a small polypoid lesion.

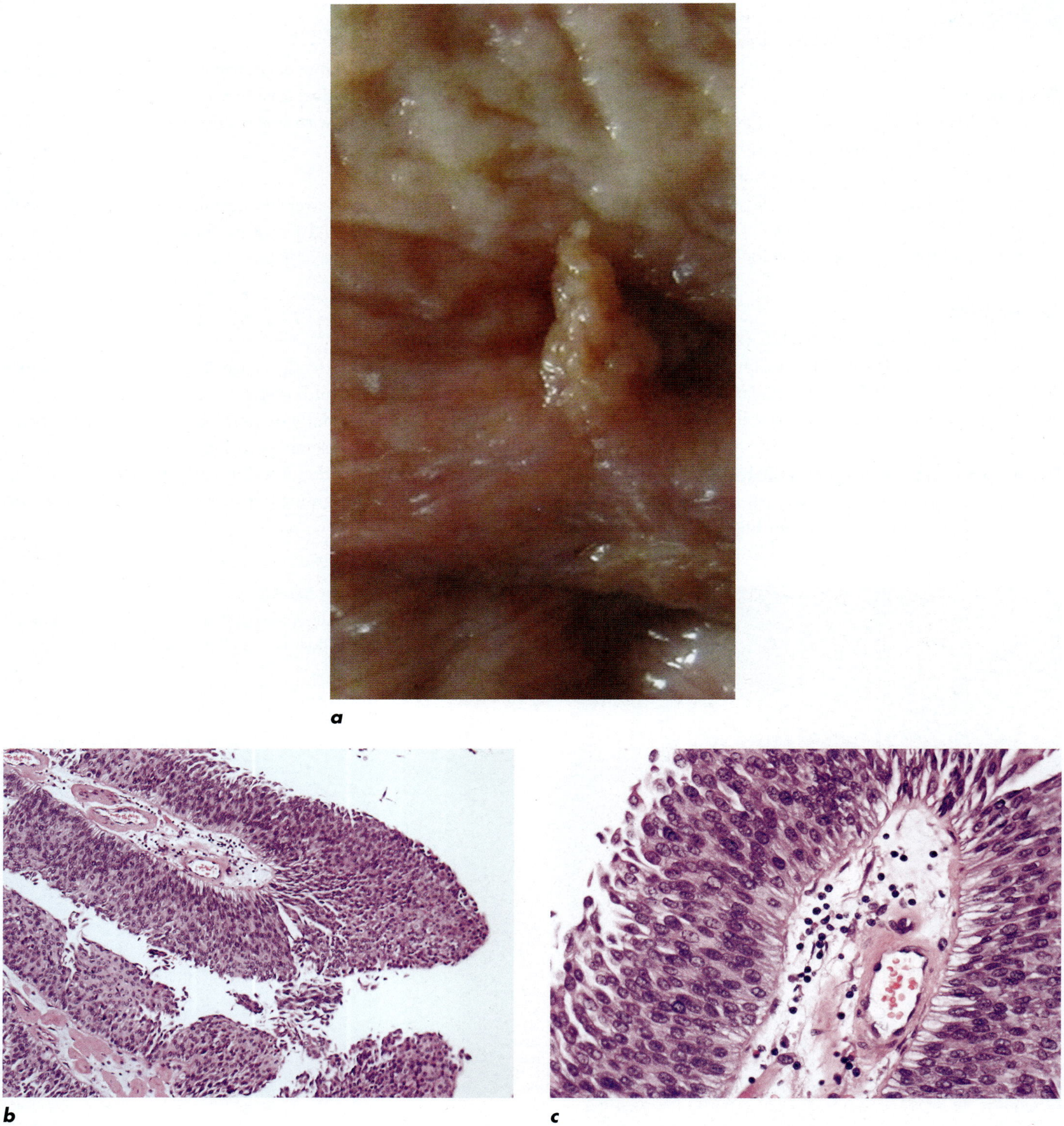

Figure 50-14.
Low-grade papillary urothelial carcinoma of the bladder as a small papillary lesion with a stalk (*a*). The tumor is composed of papillary fronds with edematous fibrovascular cores (*b*), covered by malignant urothelial cells with moderate cytological atypia (*c*).

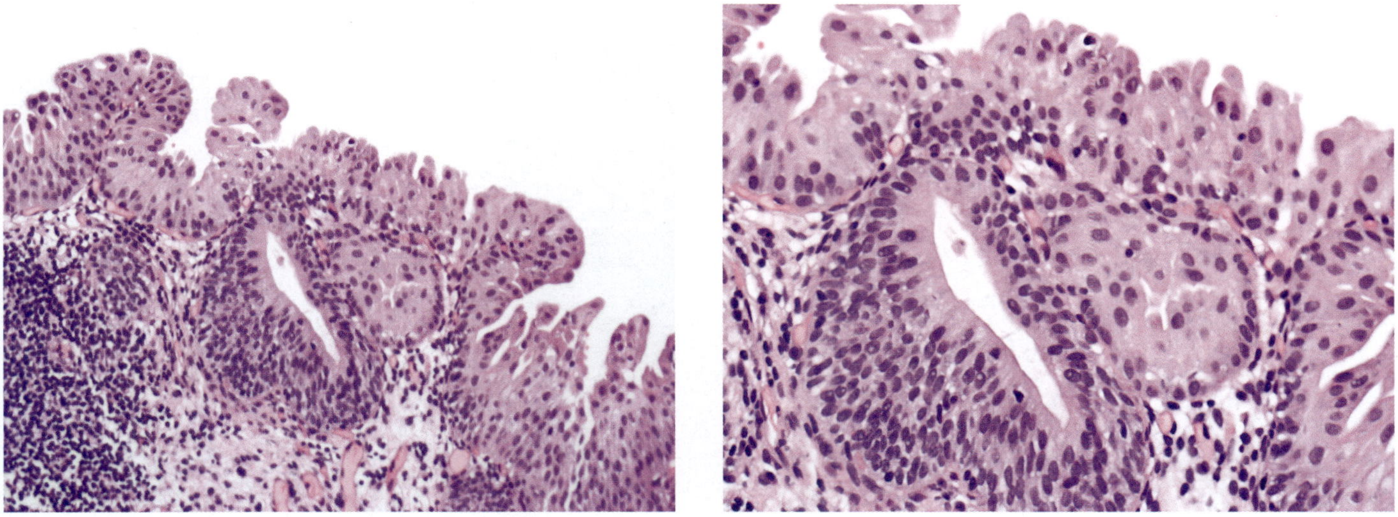

a b

Figure 50-15.
Low-grade papillary urothelial carcinoma consists of multiple small papillae covered by abnormal urothelial cells (*a*). High magnification shows the malignant neoplastic urothelial cells on the surface with mild cytological atypia and loss of polarity (*b*), which are different from benign urothelial cells in the von Brunn nest below.

- Cytological atypia is moderate in degree but it is easily recognizable, such as nuclear enlargement, variation of shape, contour, and chromatin distribution in tumor cells (Fig. 50-16)
- Small nucleoli and nuclear grooving can be seen, and mitoses can be found in all layers
- Sometimes, the tumor cells are denuded from the papillary structures, and give the appearance of "naked papillae" (Fig. 50-17*a* and *b*)
- Microcalculi may be seen associated with papillary tumor (Fig. 50-17*c* and *d*)

Figure 50-16.
Low-grade papillary urothelial carcinoma demonstrates the branching papillae covered by malignant urothelial cells (*a*). In another area of the tumor, there are complex papillary structures covered by the same type of malignant urothelial cells (*b*).

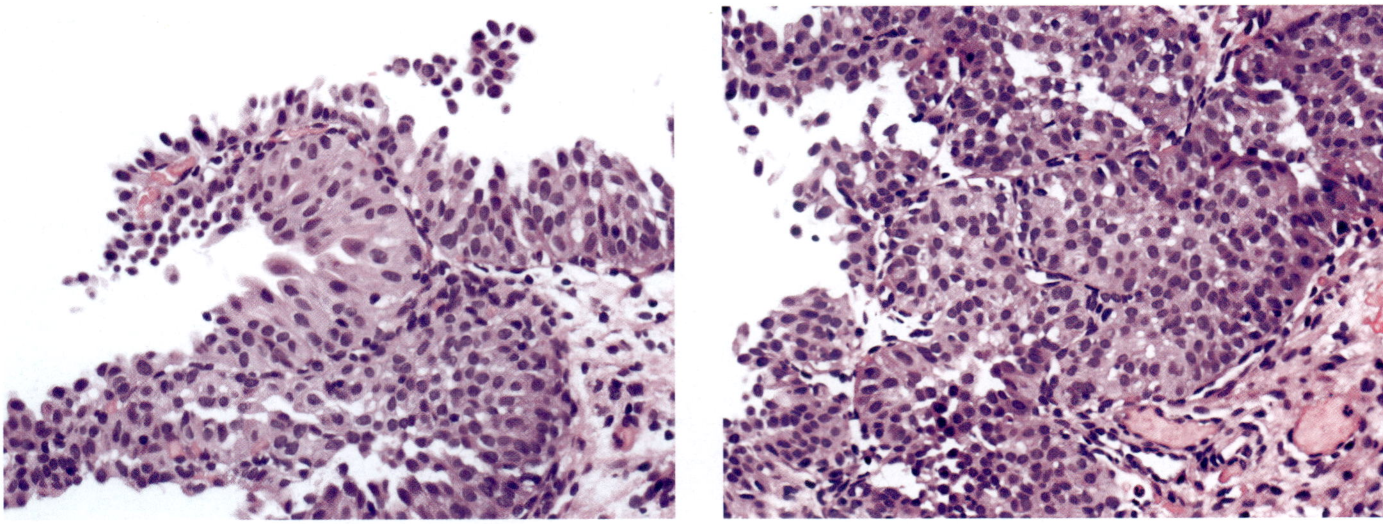

a b

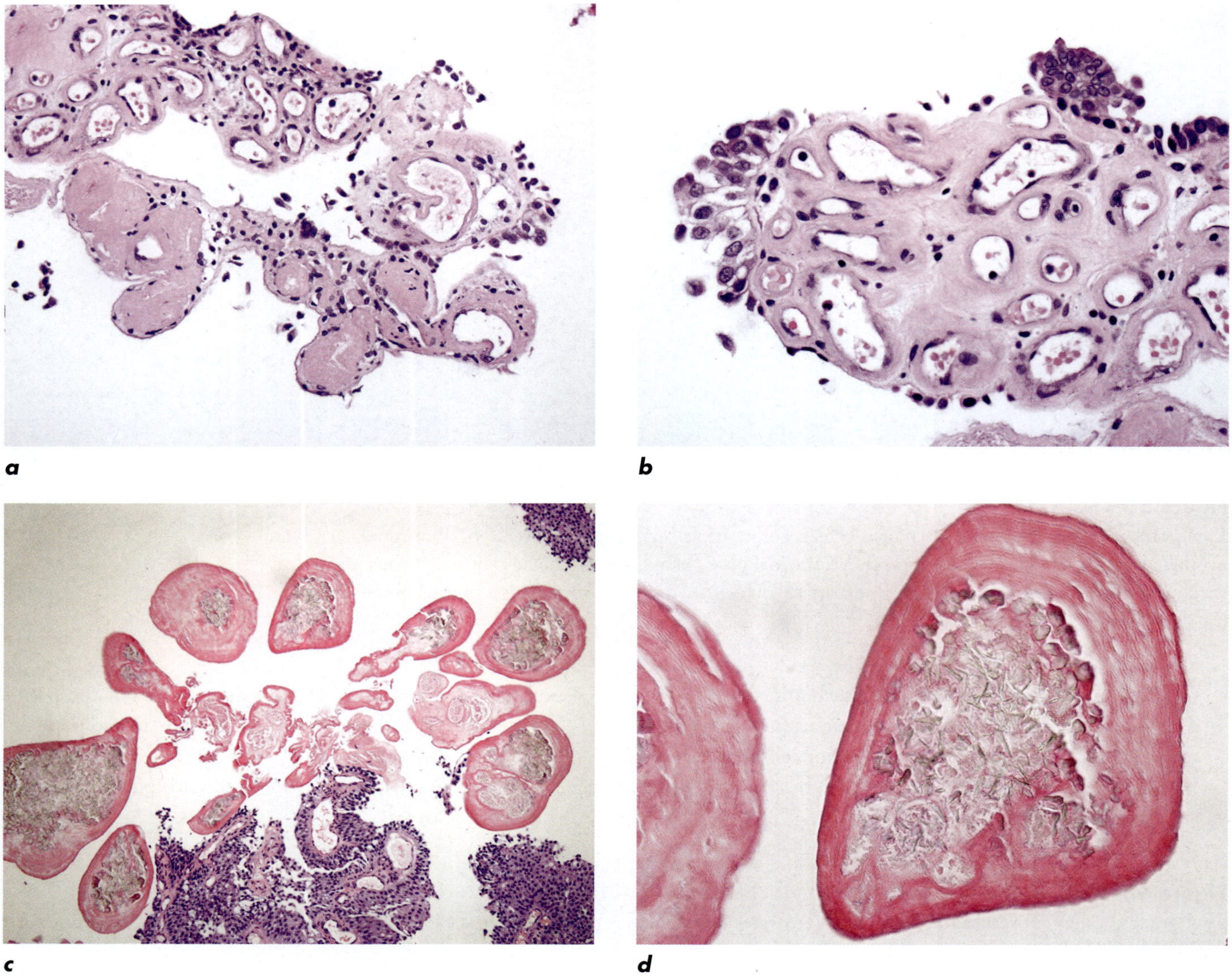

Figure 50-17.
Low-grade papillary urothelial carcinoma contains a naked papilla with mostly denuded urothelial lining (*a*). High magnification shows occasional tumor cells on the surface, sufficient for diagnosis (*b*). Calcified papillae in a low-grade papillary urothelial carcinoma (*c*). These structures may fall off from the tumor forming the core of calculi (*d*).

- If a tumor contains 1% high-grade component, it should be classified as a high-grade carcinoma
- If a tumor contains a few high-grade cells but less than 1%, there is a disagreement among the experts how to classify this tumor
- In our experience, a tumor with a few high-grade cells (<1%), if not completely resected, will propagate to a tumor with dominant high-grade component when it recurs
- Therefore, we prefer the diagnosis of low-grade papillary UC with a comment that a few high-grade tumor cells (<1%) are seen, which suggests a close clinical follow-up and resection if indicated
- If there are more than a couple of high-grade cells, within in the range of 1% to 5% , we call it high-grade UC
- Low-grade papillary UC may develop invasive component, although is uncommon, in our experience it accounts for 5% to 10% cases (Figs. 50-18 and 50-19) of low-grade papillary UC
- Therefore, a large papillary UC with predominantly low-grade component requires a careful search for (a) high-grade component and (b) invasive component to lamina propria
- Glandular and squamous differentiation can be seen in low-grade UC (Fig. 50-20)

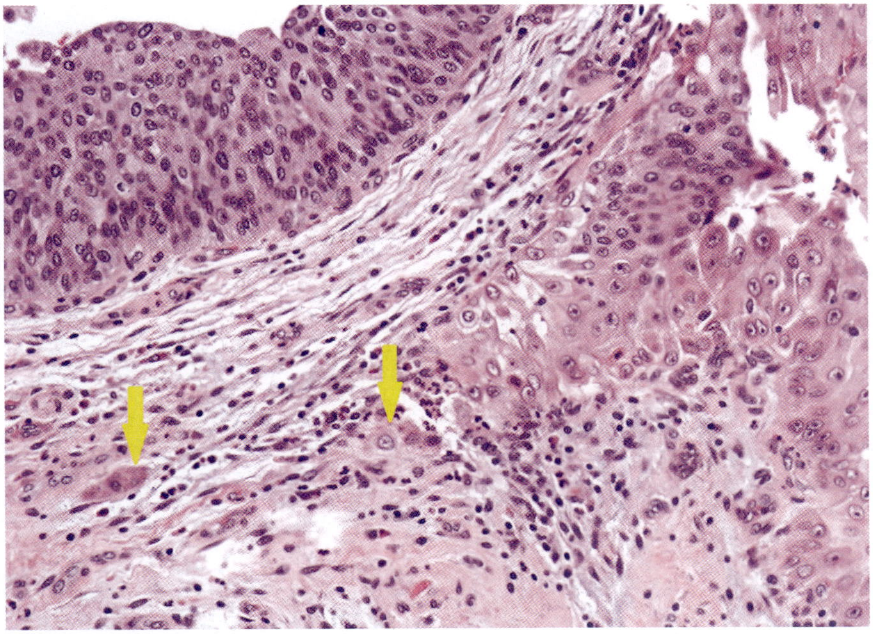

Figure 50-18.
Low-grade papillary urothelial carcinoma showing early invasion of the lamina propria. The invasive tumor cells appear to have more eosinophilic and abundant cytoplasm (arrows).

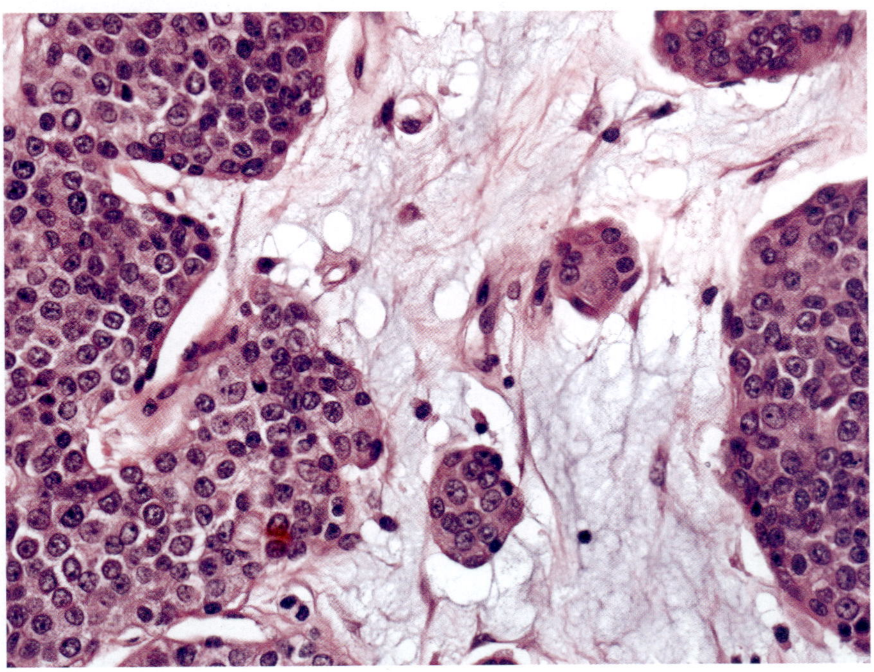

Figure 50-19.
Early lamina invasion by low-grade urothelial carcinoma.

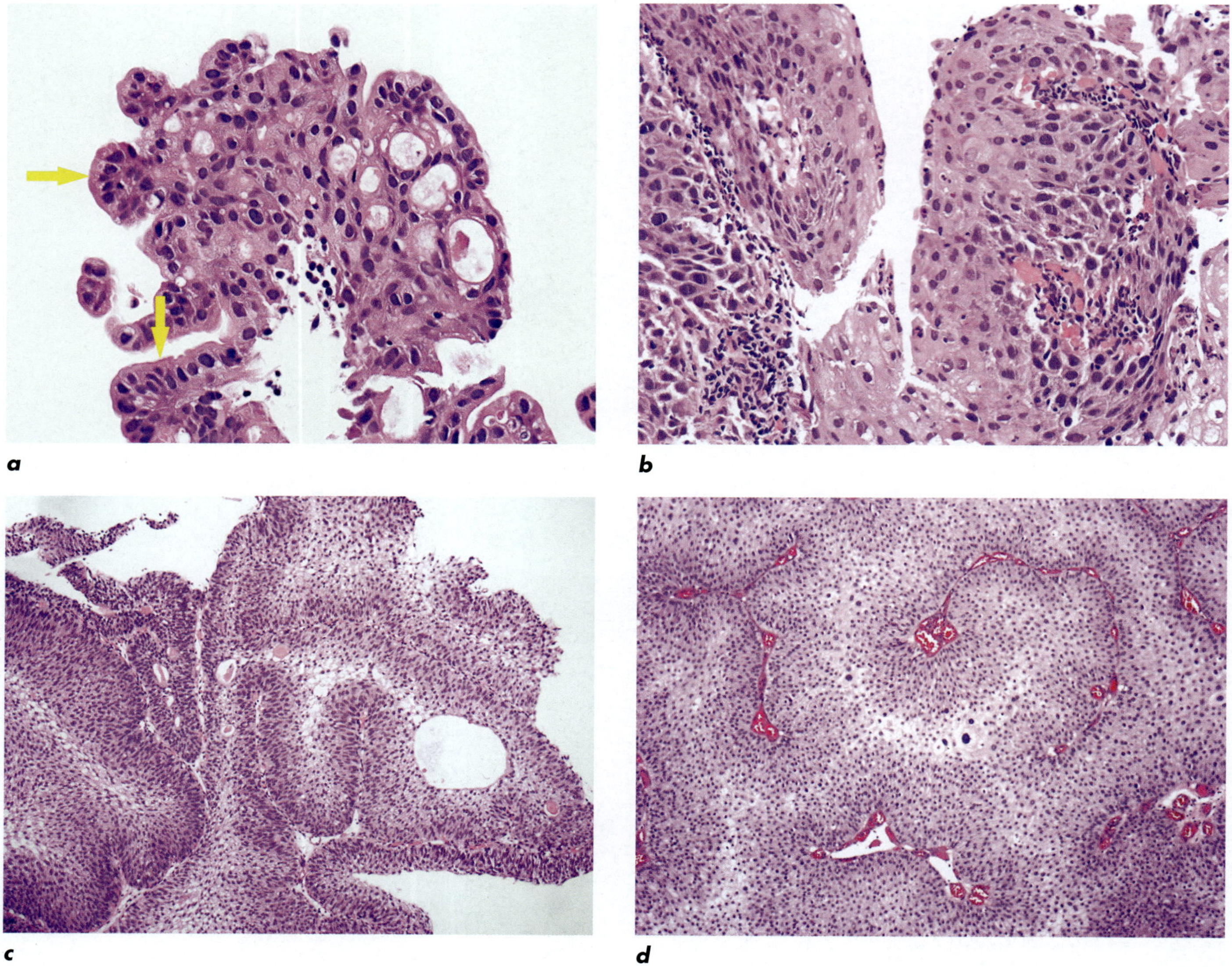

Figure 50-20.
Low-grade papillary urothelial carcinomas display glandular differentiation on the surface (*a*, arrows), squamous differentiation (*b*), exophytic and endophytic patterns (*c*), and solid pattern (*d*).

- Inverted growth or solid patterns can be seen in low-grade papillary UC (Fig. 50-21), which should be distinguished from inverted papilloma
- Although not diagnostic, these structures are highly suspicious for papillary UC because of their complex fibrovascular core

Immunohistochemistry

- P53 positive, but less intensely, CK20 positive (Fig. 50-22)
- Ki67 proliferative index is moderate to low

Molecular analysis

- Chromosomal abnormalities less frequent than CIS or high-grade UC

Clinical relevance (prognosis and treatment options)

- Treatment of choice is transurethral resection to visual completion
- The recurrent rate ranging from 50% to 70%, which is higher than PUNLMP
- Progression to high-grade and/or invasive diseases is greater than 10%, also higher than PUNLMP
- The presence of flat neoplastic lesions (secondary dysplasia) adjacent to the main papillary tumor is the basis for recurrence, although these lesions are difficult to detect grossly
- Cytology is not sensitive for detecting low-grade papillary UC
- Urovision (FISH) test is also less sensitive for low-grade tumors than high-grade tumors
- BCG post-TUR should be considered to eradicate flat dysplastic lesions
- Intravesical chemotherapy or immunotherapy may provide other options in some selected cases

Figure 50-21.
Low-grade papillary urothelial carcinoma with both exothytic (left) and endothytic (inverted) growth patterns (*a*). High magnification shows tumor cells with moderate cytological atypia attached to the fibrovascular core (*b*).

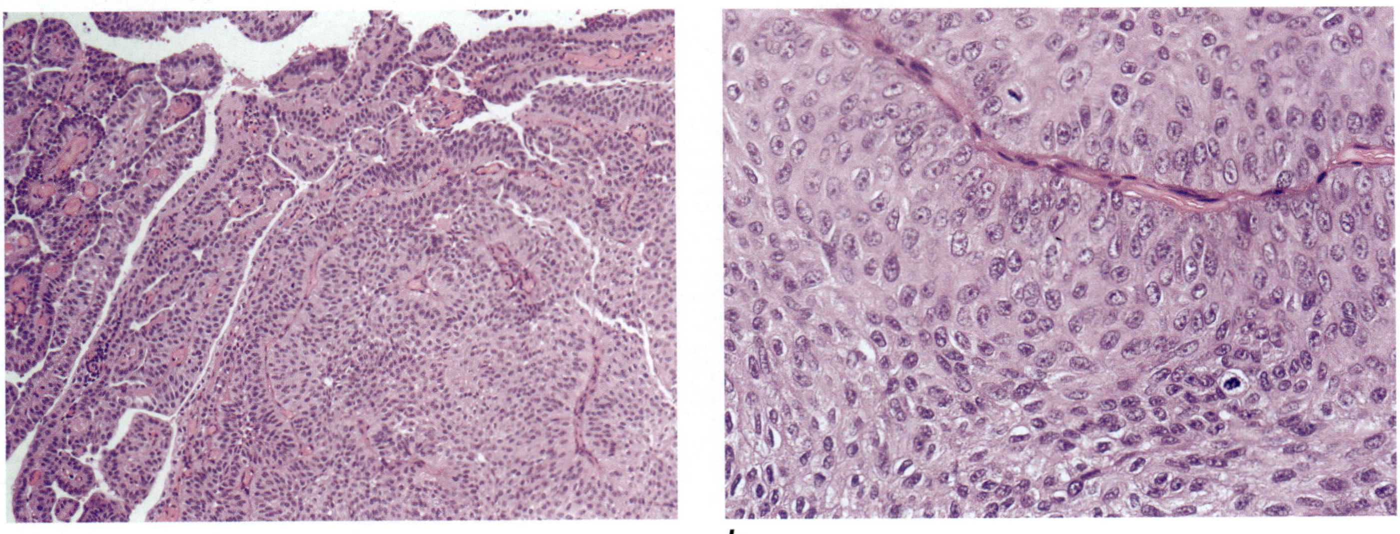

a b

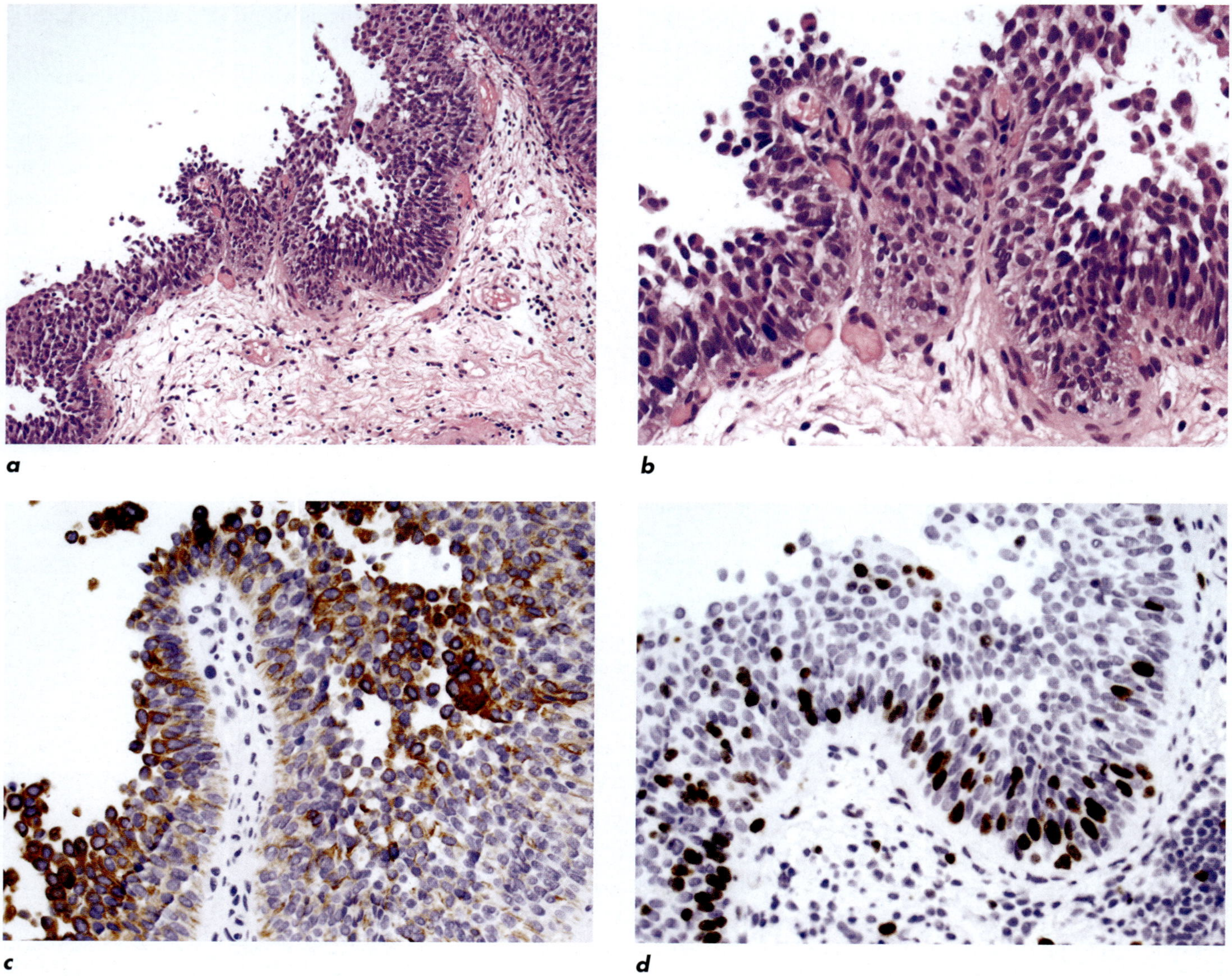

Figure 50-22.
Low-grade papillary urothelial carcinoma with typical branching papillary structures (*a*) and significant cytological atypia (*b*). The tumor cells are positive for CK20 (*c*) and exhibit relatively high K67 proliferative activity (*d*).

HIGH-GRADE PAPILLARY UROTHELIAL CARCINOMA

Definition

- High-grade papillary UC (noninvasive) is a malignant urothelial neoplasm
- It is characterized by a disorderly appearance of urothelium lining papillary fronds
- There is moderate to severe degree of cytological atypia

Other term

- High-grade transitional carcinoma

Pathogenesis

- Unclear, smoking is the major risk factor

Clinical features

- Hematuria, gross or microscopic
- Cystoscopic findings of papillary, sessile lesions
- Single or multiple lesions
- Flexible base (no invasion) rather than fixed base (with invasion) seen on cystoscopy
- Tumors located close to the ureteral orifice or bulky tumors may cause urinary obstruction, and lead to hydroureterosis and hydronephrosis
- Urine cytology positive for malignancy

Gross pathology

- High-grade tumors tend to be larger than low-grade tumors (Fig. 50-23)
- Papillary tumor, solitary or multiple (Fig. 50-24*a*)
- In a large tumor, sufficient sampling and careful microscopic examination is necessary for detecting microscopic invasion

Histology

- The presence of papillary architecture and marked cytological atypia are characteristic of high-grade papillary UC, which can be easily recognized at low magnification (Fig. 50-24*b* and *c*)

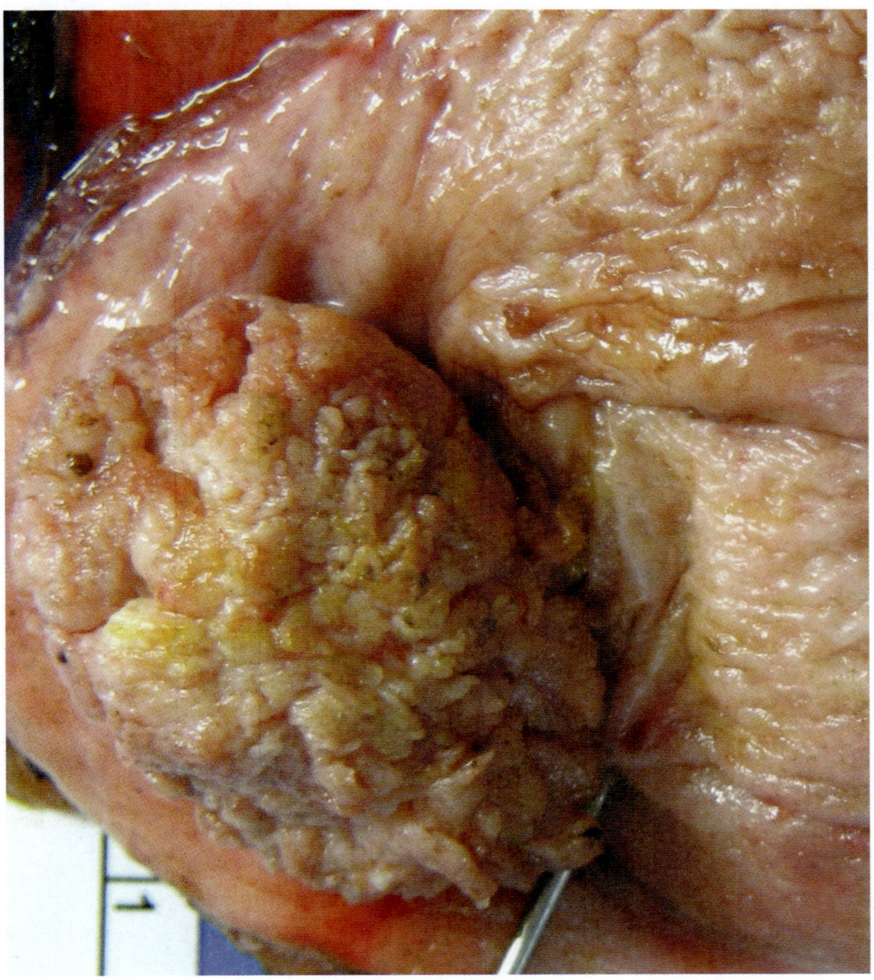

Figure 50-23. Gross photos of high-grade papillary urothelial carcinoma reveal a large papillary mass.

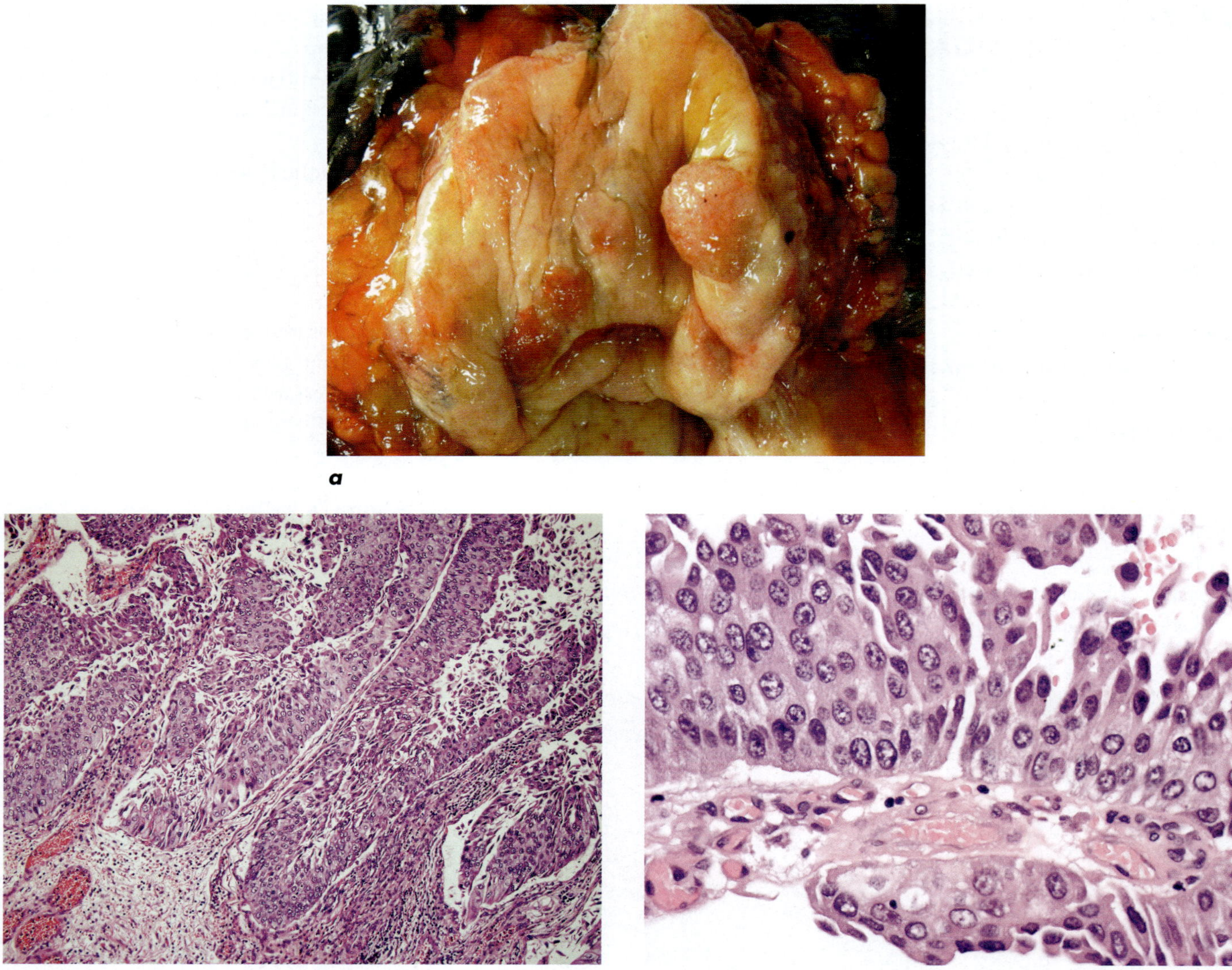

a

b

c

Figure 50-24.
High-grade papillary urothelial carcinoma is present as multiple broad-based masses (*a*). Microscopically, the tumor is composed of complex papillary structures (*b*) covered by neoplastic urothelial cells with marked cytological atypia (*c*).

- The papillae are irregular, and may be fused with variable thickness of the tumor cell covering the papillae
- Tumor cells demonstrated marked nuclear pleomorphism with variable size and shapes of the cells, prominent nucleoli and mitoses are commonly seen (Fig. 50-25*a*)
- Flat urothelial CIS adjacent to the papillary tumor is often present (Fig. 50-25*b*)
- The presence of a minor component of high-grade tumor cells should be diagnosed as a high-grade UC (Fig. 50-26)
- Hemorrhage or necrosis may be present
- The presence of invasion should be carefully searched in case of high-grade papillary UC (Fig. 50-27), since invasive high-grade UC is much more common than that in a low-grade UC or a high-grade noninvasive UC

Immunohistochemistry

- P53 positive, diffuse
- CK20 positive, full thickness
- CD44 negative (loss of staining) in majority of cases

Molecular analysis

- Trisomy
- Urovision (FISH) is available for detecting the majority of cases

Clinical relevance (prognosis and treatment options)

- This tumor has a high risk for progression to invasive disease
- Although the reported progression rate of invasion is 20% to 40%, without treatment or resection, the majority of cases will develop into invasive high-grade tumor
- TUR with visual completion
- Intravesical BCG postoperatively is recommended
- Clinical follow-up with urine cytology (sensitive) and regular cystoscopy

Figure 50-25.
High-grade papillary urothelial carcinoma with fibrovascular core surrounded by malignant urothelial cells (*a*) associated with adjacent urothelial carcinoma in situ (*b*).

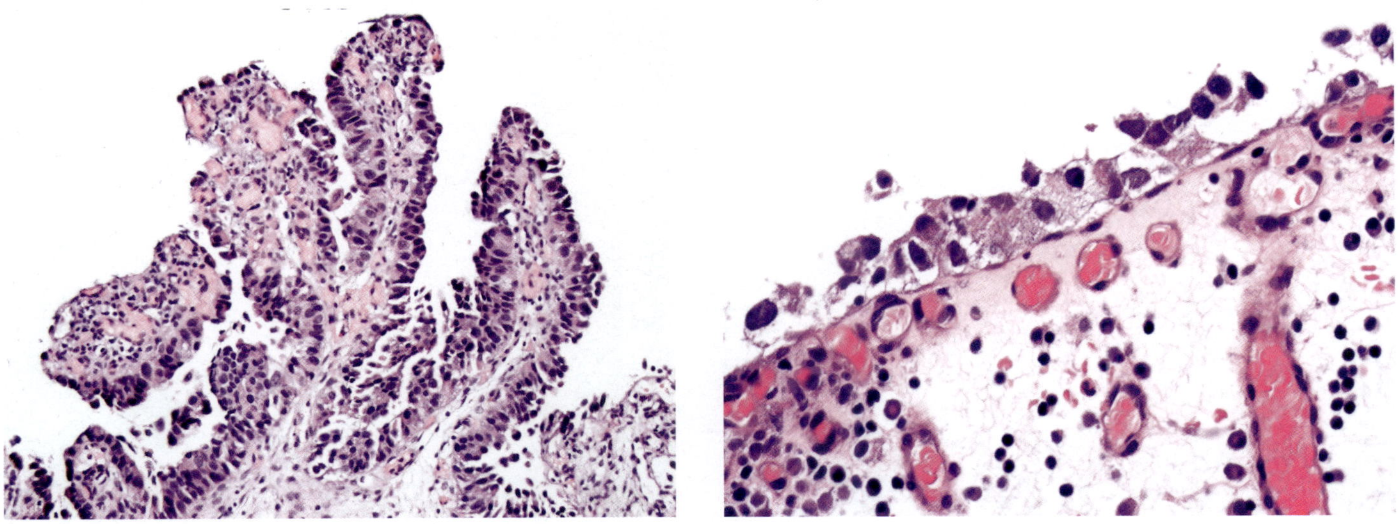

a *b*

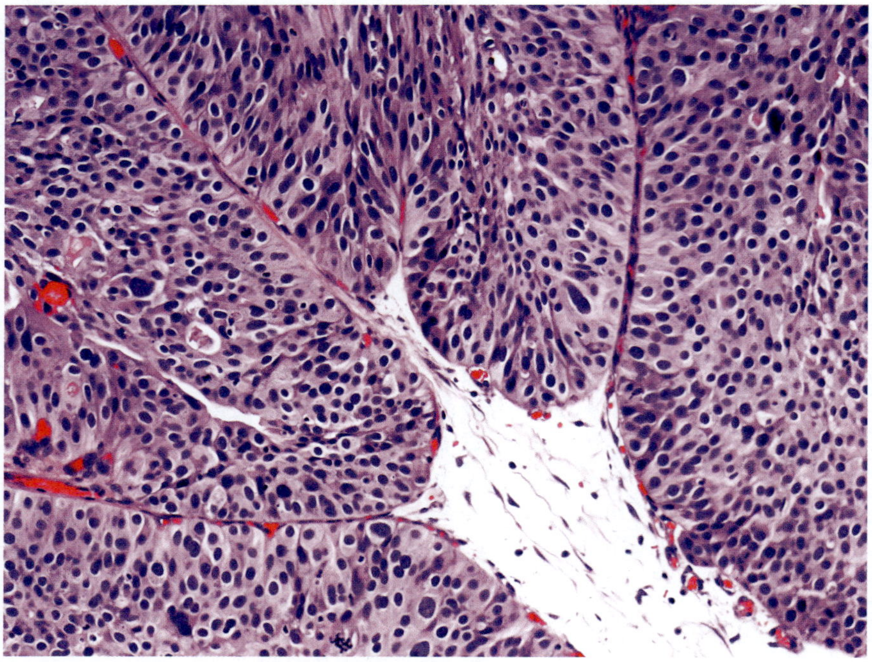

Figure 50-26.
High-grade papillary urothelial carcinoma is composed of predominantly low-grade components with a number of tumor cells with high-grade large nuclei.

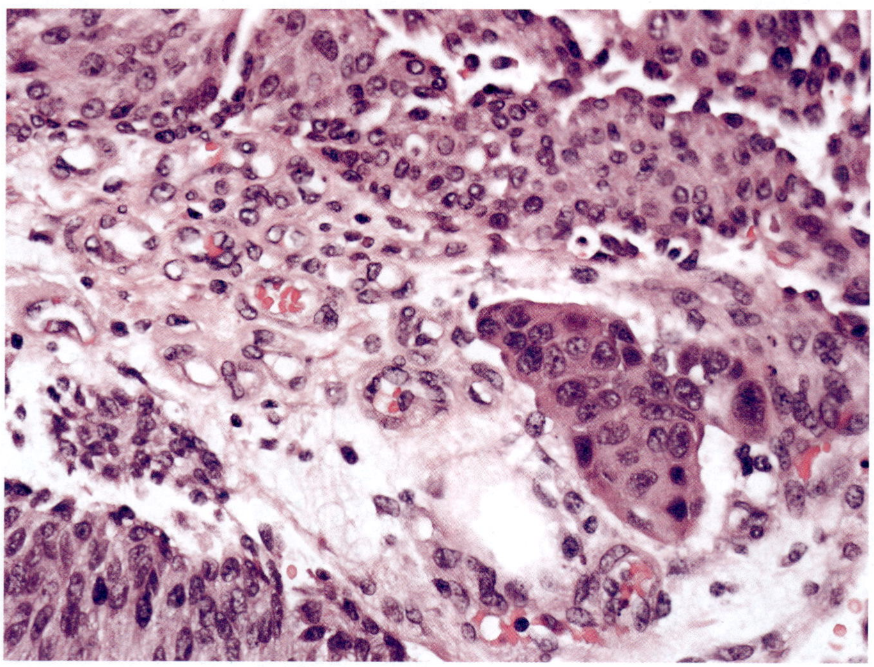

Figure 50-27.
High-grade papillary urothelial carcinoma with early lamina propria invasion. The invasive component appears to have more pink cytoplasm and more pleomorphism than the noninvasive component.

CHAPTER 51 Carcinoma In Situ of the Bladder

UROTHELIAL CARCINOMA IN SITU

Definition

- Flat high-grade urothelial carcinoma confined within the urothelium without invasion
- There are at least three types of carcinoma in situ (CIS), which can develop within the urothelium: urothelial CIS, squamous cell CIS, and adenocarcinoma in situ (which will be discussed in Chapter 53)

Other terms

- High-grade urothelial dysplasia or severe urothelial dysplasia (not recommended)

Clinical features

- Nonspecific urinary symptoms such as hematuria, urinary urgency or frequency
- Cystoscopy showing erythematous changes
- Positive cytology

Gross pathology

- No mass lesion, but there may be areas of rough or erythematous appearance
- The diagnosis is not possible from the gross appearance alone

Histology

- The urothelium is replaced completely or partially by highly atypical neoplastic cells (Fig. 51-1) but confined within the basement membrane
- The tumor cells are disorganized and show a loss of polarity (Fig. 51-2)
- The tumor nuclei are enlarged (greater than four times the diameter of a lymphocyte), with irregular nuclear membrane and hyperchromasia, which could mask the nuclear details
- Tumor cells associated with increased mitosis and apoptosis
- Involvement of urothelial infolds (Fig. 51-3) and von Brunn nests (Fig. 51-4) or cystitis glandularis (Figs. 51-5 and 51-6) by CIS cells are commonly observed, which can mimic invasive tumors with or without glandular differentiation. Denuded urothelium or discohesiveness is often seen in CIS due to the loss of cell adhesion of malignant cells (Fig. 51-7)

Figure 51-1.
Multifocal urothelial carcinoma in situ (CIS) in a cystectomy specimen is signified by the erythematous and hemorrhagic spots indicated by arrows (*a*). Microscopically, CIS is characterized by large tumor cells with high N/C ratio, hyperchromasia, and irregular nuclei within the basement membrane (*b*).

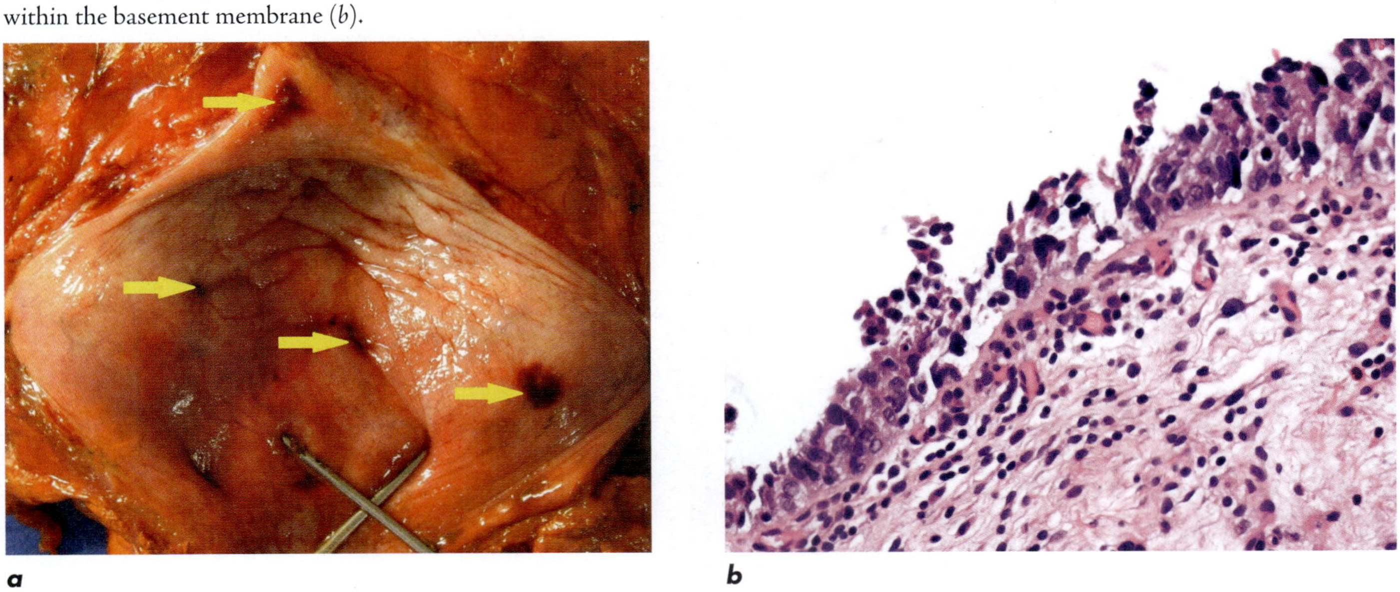

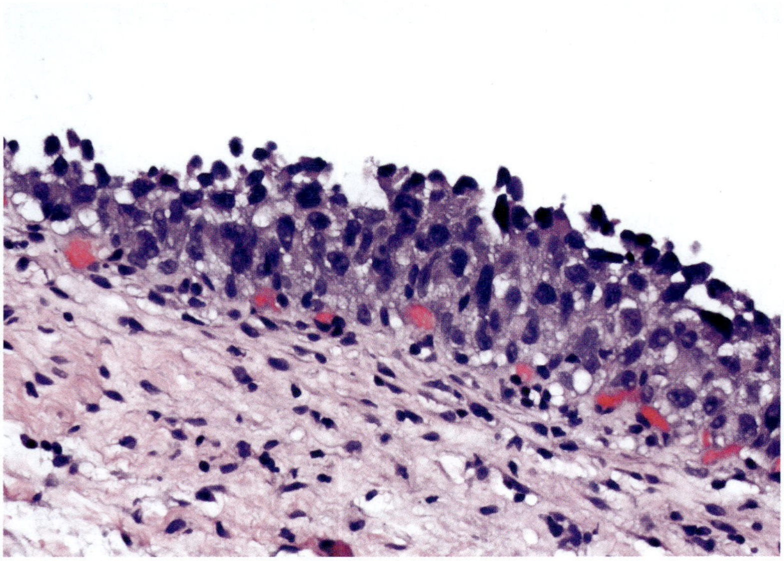

Figure 51-2.
Urothelial CIS. The urothelium is entirely replaced by disorganized tumor cells with prominent nuclear enlargement and hyperchromasia.

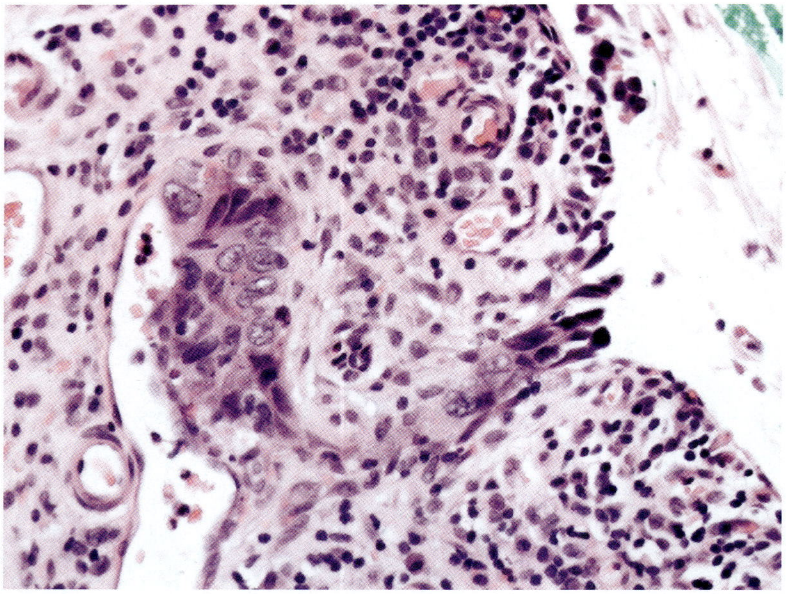

Figure 51-3.
Urothelial CIS with only a few discohesive atypical cells on the surface, but tumor cells involving an infolding of the urothelium (not invasive).

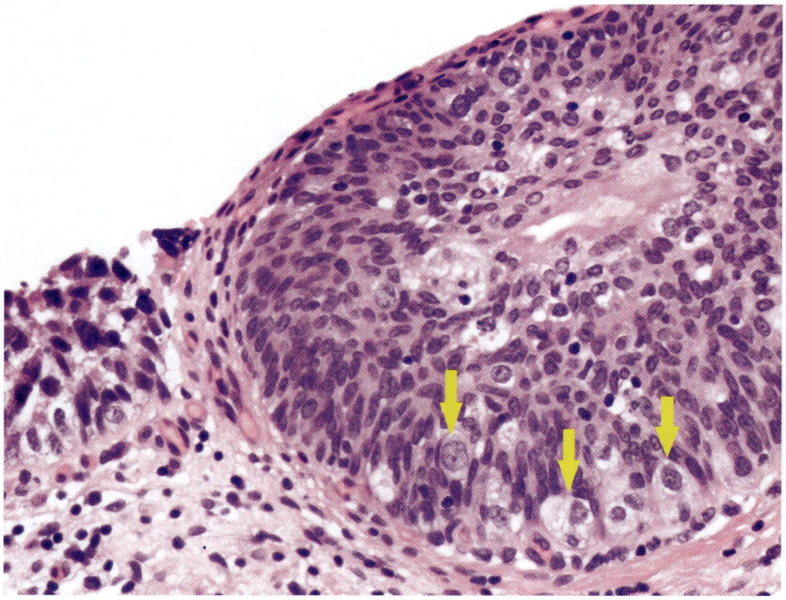

Figure 51-4.
Urothelial CIS cells involving the surface urothelium (left) and a von Brunn nest as pagetoid cells (indicated by arrows).

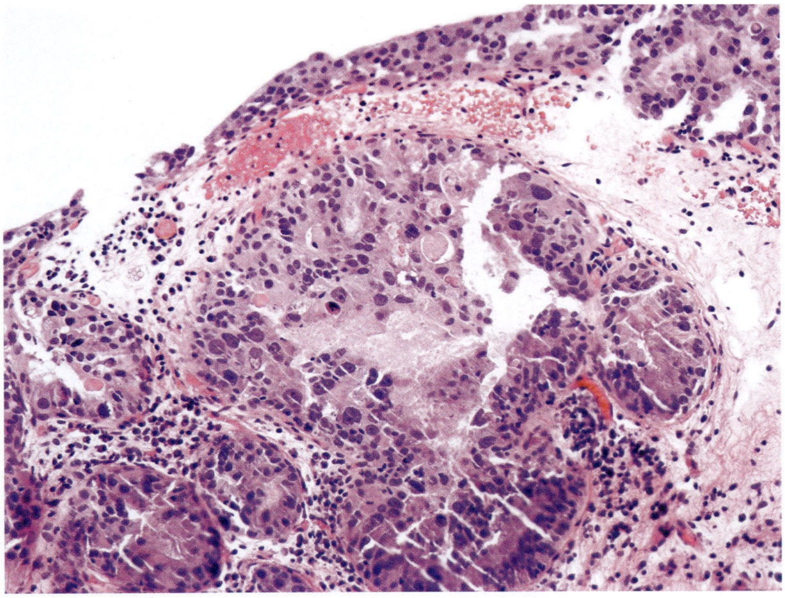

Figure 51-5.
Urothelial CIS cells involving von Brunn nests with glandular differentiation.

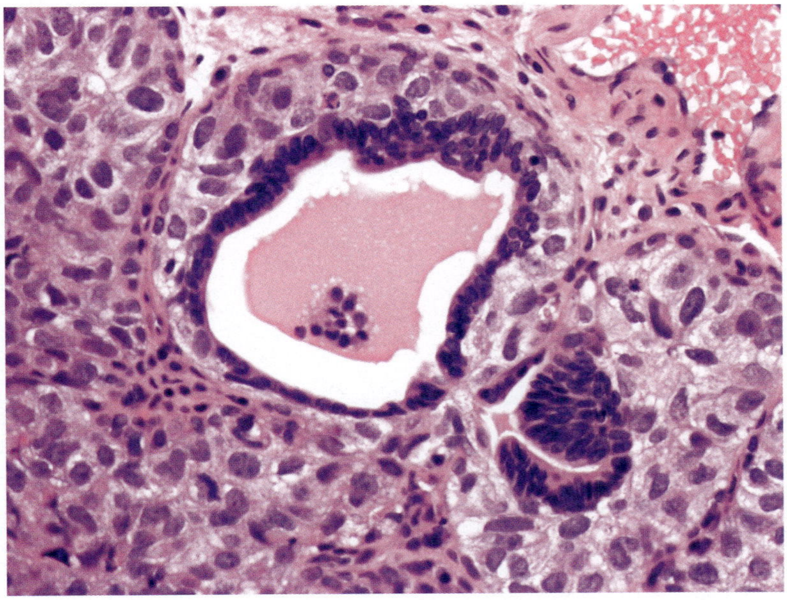

Figure 51-6.
Urothelial CIS involving the glandular structures in cystitis glandularis, mimicking urothelial neoplasm with glandular differentiation.

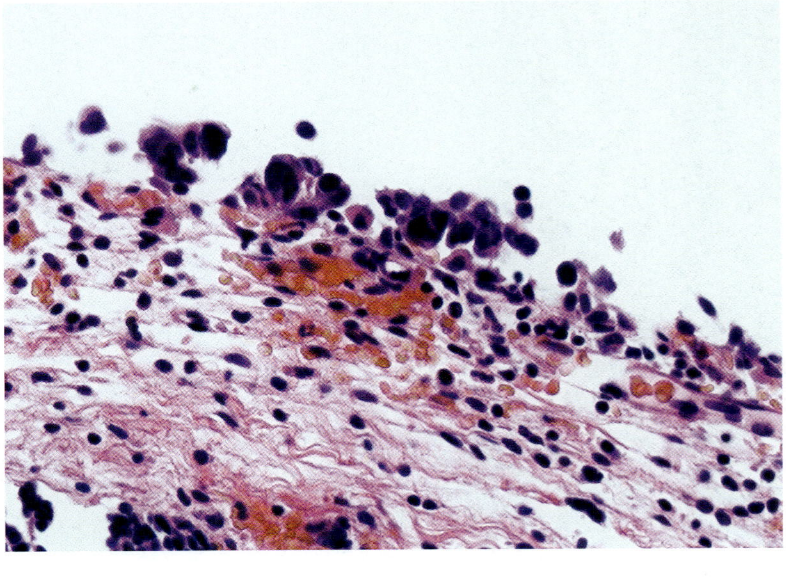

Figure 51-7.
Urothelial CIS with mostly denuded urothelium. The tumor cells are hyperchromatic with high N/C ratio and detached from the basement membrane. The nuclei of these tumor cells are more than four times of a lymphocyte.

- CIS is oftentimes associated with dilated capillaries or hemorrhage in the superficial lamina propria, which contributes to erythematous appearance macroscopically (Figs. 51-1 and 51-2)
- The presence of intact umbrella cells does not exclude the diagnosis of CIS, because the tumor cells can grow undermining the umbrella cells (Fig. 51-8). Pagetoid spread of CIS is characterized by the presence of individual large malignant cells scattered in the background of smaller cells in benign urothelium (Fig. 51-9)
- Unusual patterns of urothelial CIS have been reported, such as micropapillary CIS, small cell CIS, or plasmacytoid CIS (Fig. 51-10)
- Urothelial CIS contributes to one of the most common mistakes made by pathologists, typically underdiagnosis (false negative)
- The consequence of underdiagnosis is the development of extensive and invasive disease

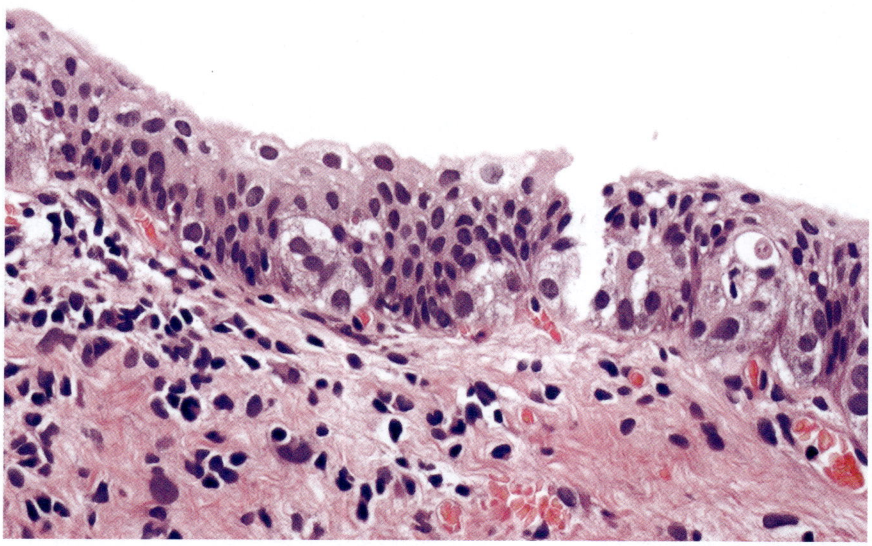

Figure 51-8.
Urothelial CIS present in clusters or individual pagetoid cells underneath the intact umbrella cells.

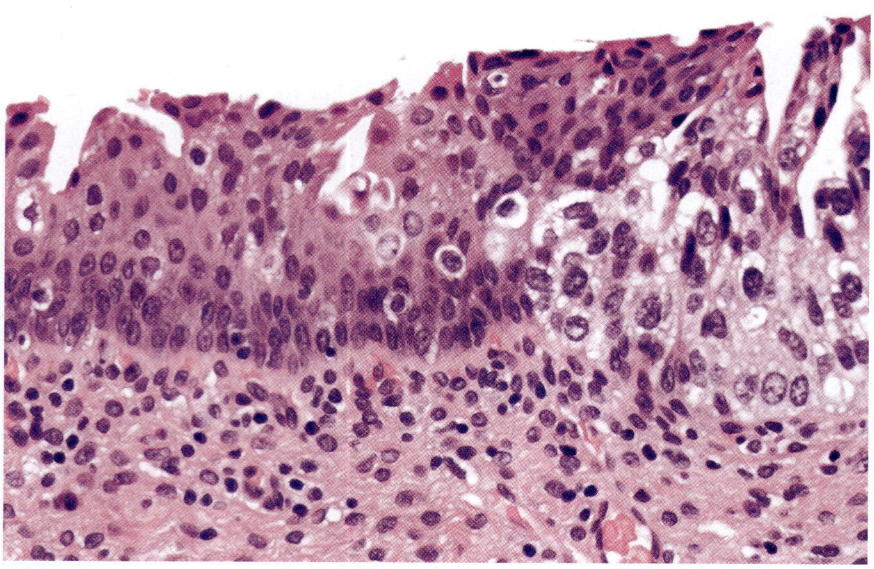

Figure 51-9.
Interface between benign urothelium (left) and pagetoid CIS (right).

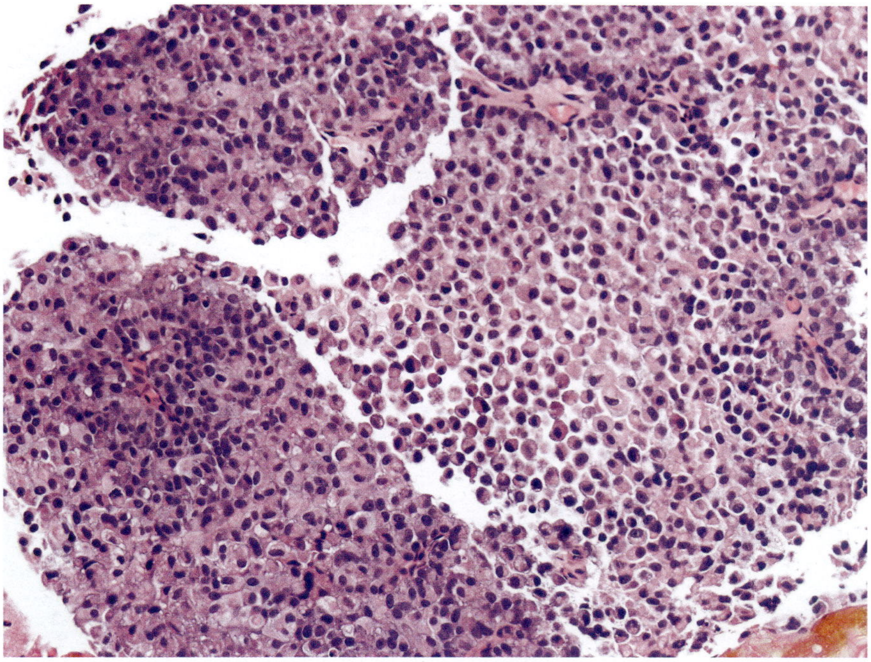

Figure 51-10.
Plasmacytoid urothelial CIS. The urothelium is significantly thickened and replaced by plasmacytoid tumor cells confined within the basement membrane.

Immunohistochemistry

- P53 positive and CK20 positive (Fig. 51-11). CD40 negative

Differential diagnosis

Reactive urothelial atypia (see Table 51-1)

- BCG treatment is not known for inducing cytological atypia of urothelium
- However, chemotherapy, radiation, and viral infection such as BK virus may induce significant cytological atypia, which can be very difficult to distinguish from CIS
- In those difficult cases, a clinical history of previous treatment is important
- Radiation is associated with reactive vascular changes (described in Chapter 47), which is not present in CIS
- Immunostaining for BK virus protein will be helpful if available

Molecular analysis

- In most cases, urothelial CIS shows trisomy

Clinical relevance (prognosis and treatment options)

- CIS in most organs other than the urinary tract is considered an early or indolent lesion. However, urothelial CIS is an aggressive cancer without treatment
- Some important issues regarding biological behavior of urothelial CIS
  - It is always high grade histologically
  - It may progress to high-grade invasive carcinoma in weeks or months without treatment
  - It may quickly spread into the entire bladder mucosa from a localized lesion without appropriate treatment
  - CIS may also spread upstream (by reflux) to the ureter and renal pelvis, or more frequently downstream to the prostate and urethra
- A low-grade papillary urothelial carcinoma should not be diagnosed as CIS even though it is noninvasive
- The mainstream treatment for urothelial CIS is instillation of live BCG in the bladder, which will induce extensive granulomatous inflammation and subsequently eradicate the urothelium along with urothelial CIS
- In BCG refractile cases, intravesical chemotherapy or even cystectomy may be considered
- Close follow-up with urine cytology and biopsy after treatment is essential to monitor recurrence or progression to invasive urothelial carcinoma

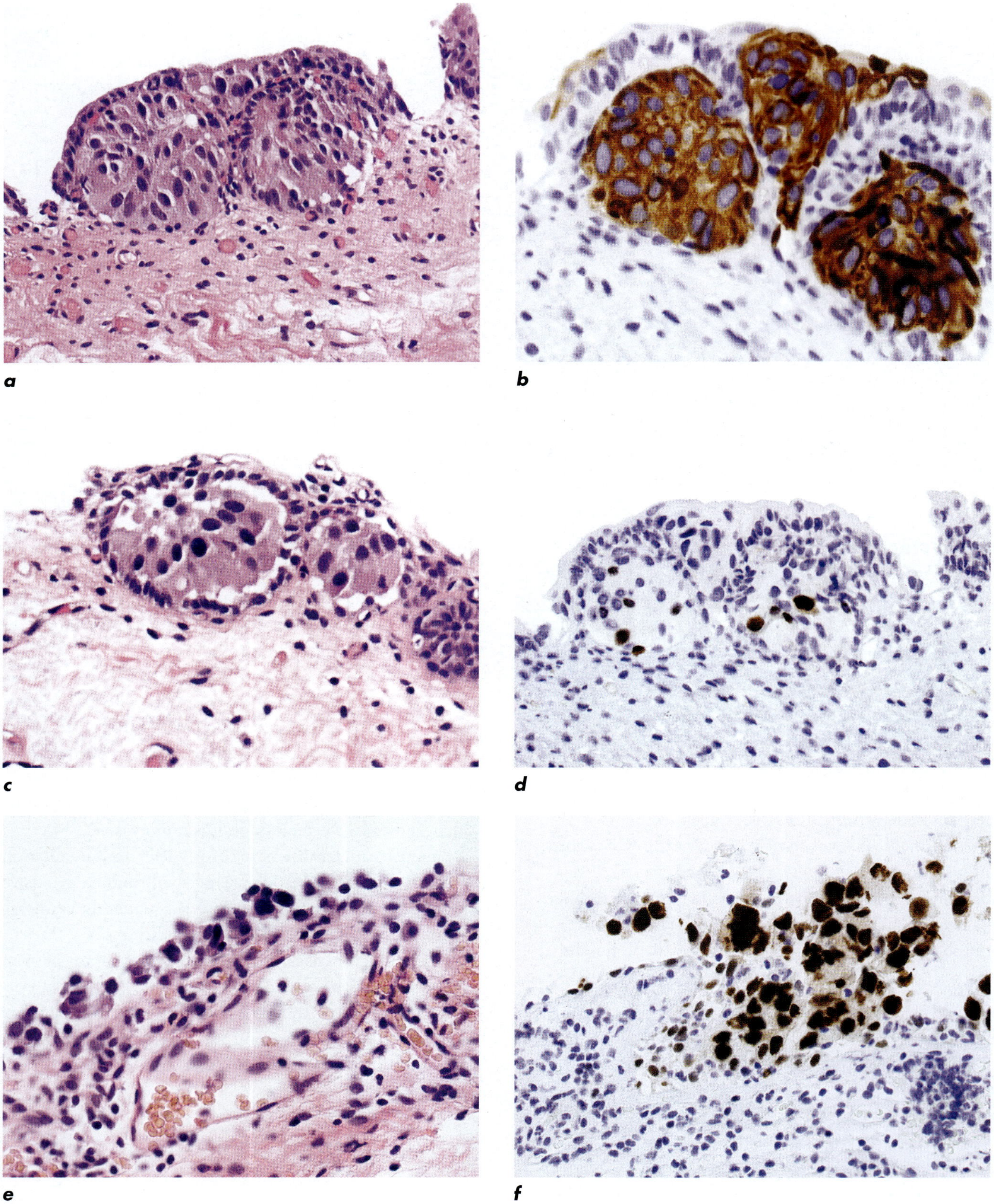

Figure 51-11.
Urothelial CIS with involvement of surface and von Brunn nests (*a*) is confirmed by diffuse CK20 staining (*b*); CIS with von Brunn nest involvement (*c*) is confirmed by positive p53 staining (*d*); CIS with typical denuded appearance (*e*) is confirmed by strong p53 positivity (*f*).

Table 51-1. Comparison of Urothelial CIS and Reactive Atypia

Features	*Urothelial carcinoma in situ*	*Urothelial reactive atypia*
Low power	Single layer, partially denuded or thickened	Thickened
Inflammation	Absent	Present
Nuclear chromatin	Hyperchromatic	Vesicular
Nuclear size	Four to six times of lymphocyte	<3 times of lymphocytes
Nucleoli	Enlarged, but not easy to see	Small but easily seen
Mitosis	Frequent	Possible
Polarity	Lost	Retained
P53	Strongly positive	Negative or weakly positive
CK20	Positive, full thickness	Positive in umbrella cells
CD44	Negative	Diffusely positive

SQUAMOUS CELL CARCINOMA IN SITU

Definition

- Squamous cell carcinoma of the bladder without invasion

Other terms

- High-grade squamous intraepithelial neoplasia, high-grade squamous dysplasia (not recommended)

Pathogenesis

- Long-standing chronic inflammation leading to squamous metaplasia, which undergoes dysplastic changes and subsequent malignant transformation

Clinical features

- A history of chronic inflammation by infectious etiology
- Or other causes of long-standing catheterization in a patient with spina bifida or paralyzed with spinal cord injury (paraplegia or quadriplegia)
- Cystoscopy shows the sign of inflammation, such as erythematous changes and mucosal thickening
- History of atypical cytology

Gross pathology

- White or opaque patches in the bladder mucosa with no evidence of papillary or exophytic lesions
- Ulceration may be present sometimes

Histology

- Presence of dysplastic squamous cells in the full thickness (Fig. 51-12)
- Significant cytological atypia is evident and intracellular bridges are present (Fig. 51-13)
- No evidence of invasion or in situ urothelial carcinoma. In the case with urothelial CIS, it will be diagnosed as urothelial CIS with squamous metaplasia
- Coexisting chronic inflammation, keratinized or nonkeratinized squamous metaplasia are often present
- Transition from squamous metaplasia to squamous dysplasia can be seen

Immunohistochemistry

- P53 positive

Clinical relevance (prognosis and treatment options)

- Squamous cell CIS may be associated with subsequent or concurrent invasive tumor
- Squamous cell CIS is difficult to control medically. BCG has not been shown to be effective in the eradication of squamous cell CIS
- Coexisting invasive squamous cell carcinoma can be found in some patients undergoing cystectomy although the invasive components are not present in biopsy
- The treatment option includes cystectomy, considering the risk of invasive tumor

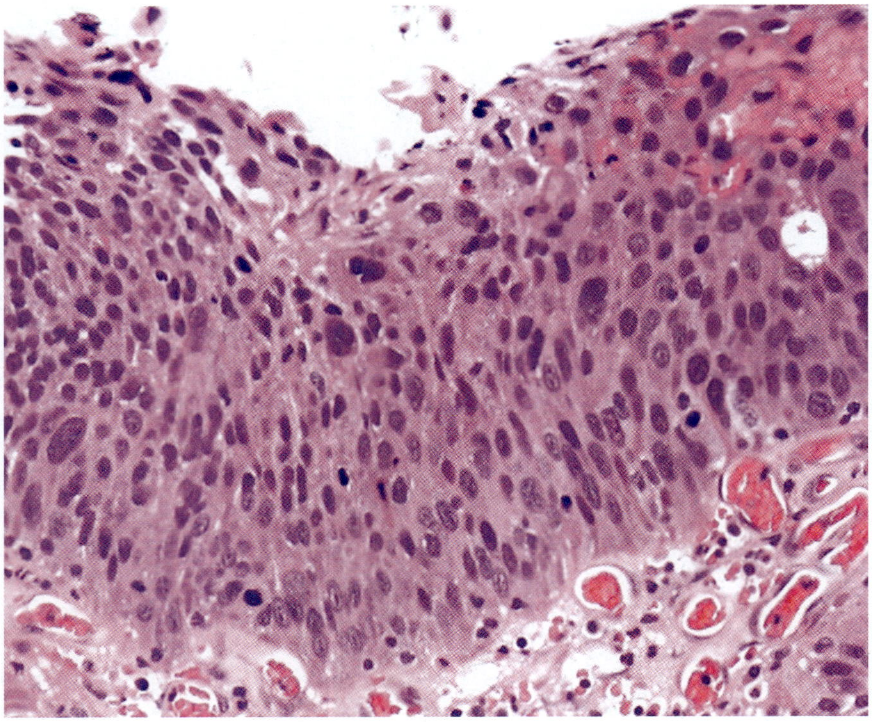

Figure 51-12. Squamous cell carcinoma in situ (CIS) consists of full thickness involvement by atypical squamous cells with brisk mitoses. Dilated capillaries are present in the lamina propria.

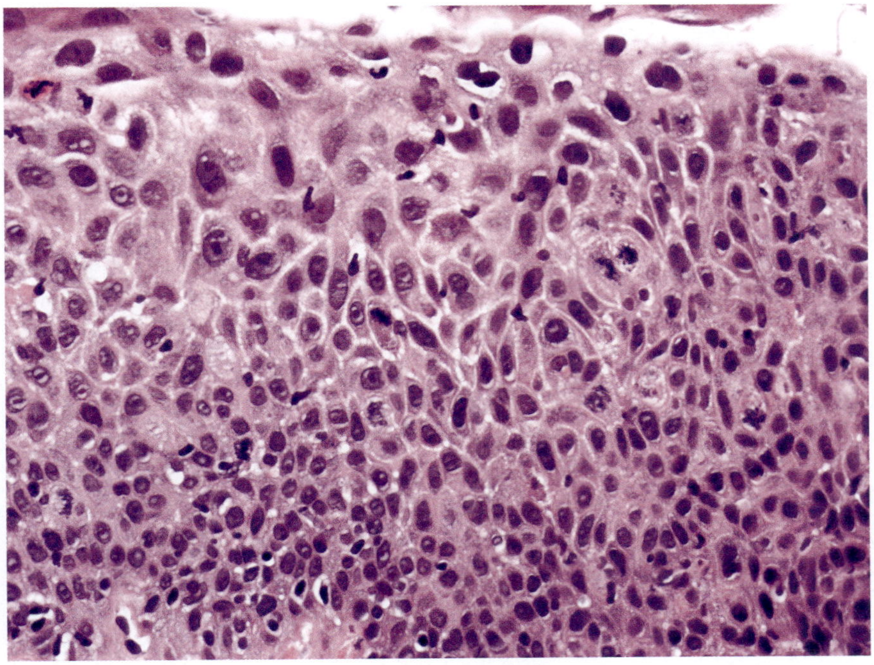

Figure 51-13.
Squamous cell CIS with prominent cytological atypia in full thickness. The tumor cells display the intracellular bridges.

CHAPTER 52 Invasive Urothelial Carcinoma and Its Variants of the Bladder

INVASIVE UROTHELIAL CARCINOMA

Definition

- Urothelial carcinoma invading beyond the basement membrane to the underlying tissues of the bladder

Other terms

- Infiltrating urothelial carcinoma, invasive (infiltrating) transitional cell carcinoma

Pathogenesis

- Invasive urothelial carcinoma can be derived from either urothelial carcinoma in situ (CIS) or papillary carcinoma (low grade and high grade) when they develop an invasive component

Clinical features

- Hematuria, either gross or microscopic
- Cystoscopic findings of one or multiple papillary or sessile lesions
- Fixed base of the tumor suggestive of invasion
- Tumors located close to the ureteral orifice or bulky tumors may cause urinary obstruction, and lead to hydroureterosis and hydronephrosis
- Tumor cells may detach from the bladder mucosa to implant downstream in the prostatic urethra or distal urethra

Gross pathology

- Large or small papillary lesions, single or multiple, usually with a fixed or broad base (Fig. 52-1). The cut surface of the tumor is pale and granular and irregular interface between epithelium and stroma (Fig. 52-1*b*)
- Ulceration may be present either as treatment effect or caused by tumor necrosis

Histology

- There are three types of invasive tumors
  - High-grade invasive urothelial carcinoma associated or derived from CIS
  - High-grade invasive urothelial carcinoma derived from noninvasive high-grade papillary urothelial carcinoma
  - Low-grade invasive urothelial carcinoma derived from noninvasive low-grade papillary urothelial carcinoma, which is the least common type
- Three levels of invasion are

Lamina propria invasion (T1)

- Characterized by small nests of tumor cells (Figs. 52-1 and 52-2) breaking the smooth contours of the basement membrane into the connective tissue of the lamina propria (LP) (Fig. 52-3)
- The LP contains small wispy smooth muscles, which should not be confused with muscularis propria (MP)
- Histological changes associated with early LP invasion
  - Increased cytological atypia
  - Eosinophilic change and increased volume in cytoplasm of the tumor cells (Figs. 52-2 and 52-4)
  - Broken smooth contours of urothelial basement membrane. Inverted growth patterns of large tumor cell islands, with smooth contours of endophytic growth (Fig. 52-5), should not be confused with LP invasion
  - Desmoplastic reaction and chronic inflammation may be present at the site of invasion (Figs. 52-3, 52-6, and 52-7)
- Necrosis can be seen in invasive urothelial carcinoma (Fig. 52-8)

Muscularis propria invasion (T2)

- Tumor cells invading big smooth muscle bundles (Fig. 52-9)
- Typically, the smooth muscle bundles of the MP are greater than 0.1 mm in diameter (Figs. 52-10 and 52-11)
- Distinguishing LP (wispy muscle bundles) from MP (thick muscle bundles) is important for clinical management
- The presence of bladder urothelial carcinoma with MP invasion, often referred to as "muscle invasive" disease, is an indication for cystectomy in most practices
- The presence of MP with or without tumor invasion should be reported, because a specially deep bite to sample MP is a common clinical practice during biopsy

Perivesical tissue invasion (T3)

- Tumor cells invading through MP the perivesical adipose tissue (Fig. 52-12)
- However, the presence of tumor cells in the fat does not necessarily mean perivesical invasion. As we discussed earlier, adipose tissue may also be seen in LP or MP of the bladder
- Therefore, it is rarely possible to diagnose perivesical invasion in the biopsy or TUR specimens
  - In a large or high-grade papillary urothelial carcinoma, the chance of invasion is high, so ample sampling and careful microscopic examination are warranted

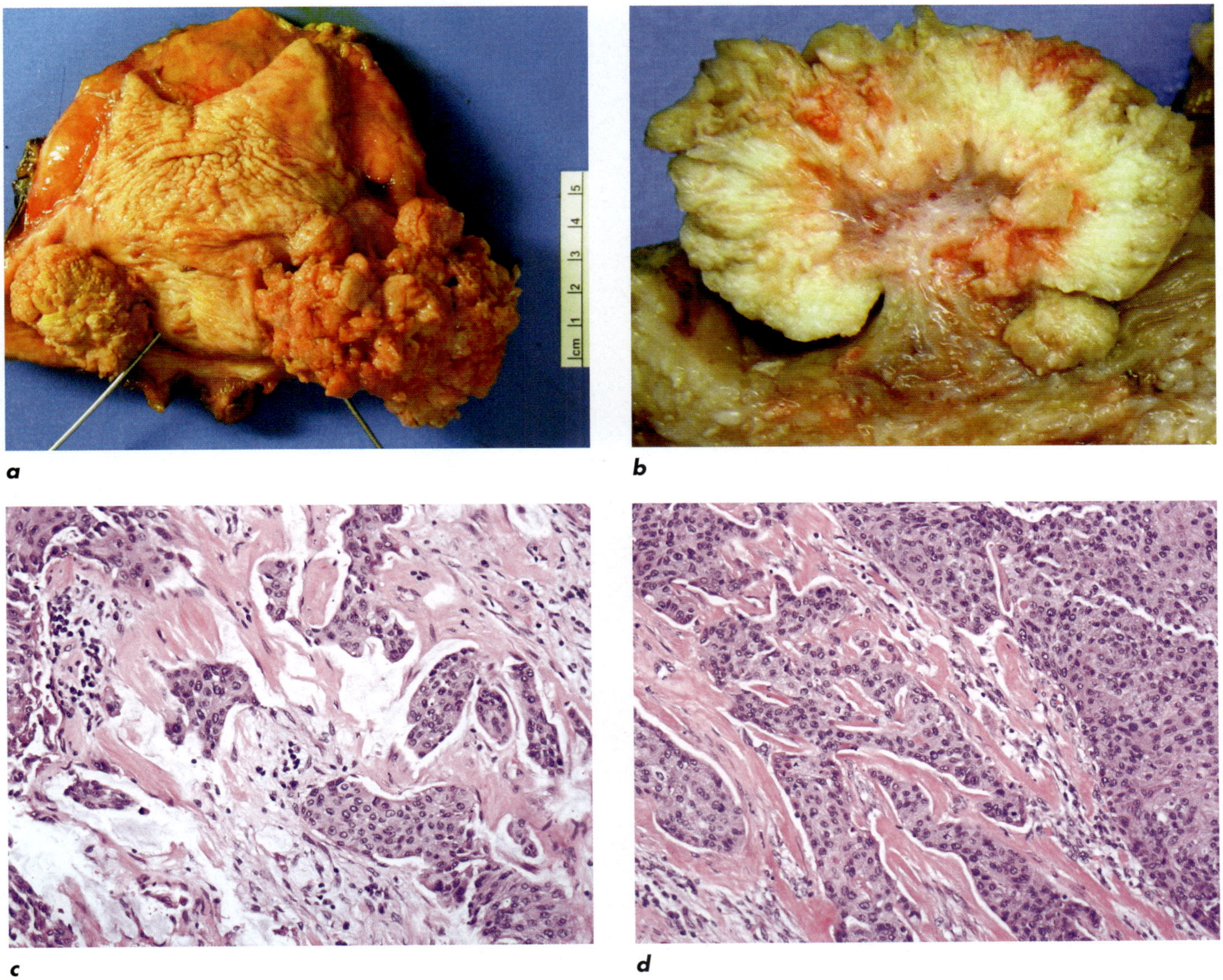

Figure 52-1.
Invasive papillary urothelial carcinoma includes two masses with broad bases (*a*) and the cut surface of one of the cauliflower-shaped tumors showing irregular base (*b*). Microscopically, lamina propria invasion by tumor nests and desmoplastic reaction is evident (*c*). Stromal reaction and irregular invasive tumor cell nests are present (*d*).

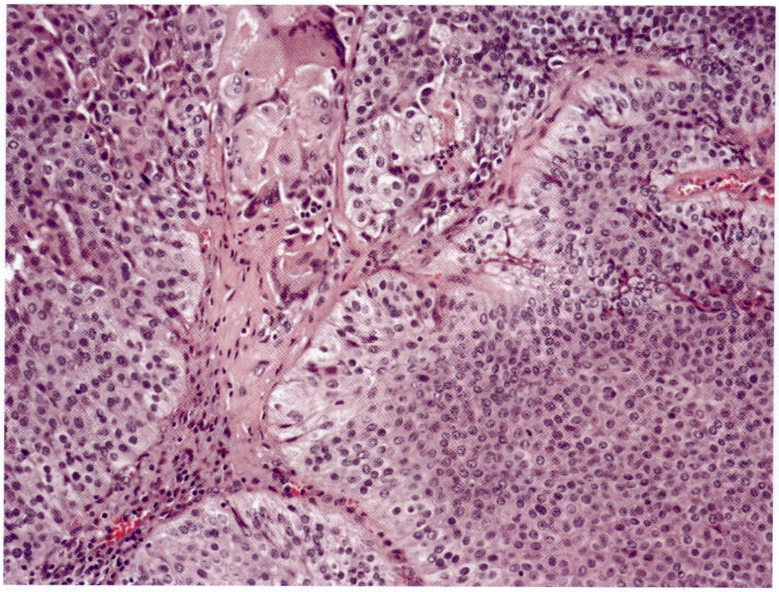

Figure 52-2.
High-grade urothelial carcinoma with early lamina propria invasion exhibiting eosinophilic cytoplasmic changes of the invasive cells.

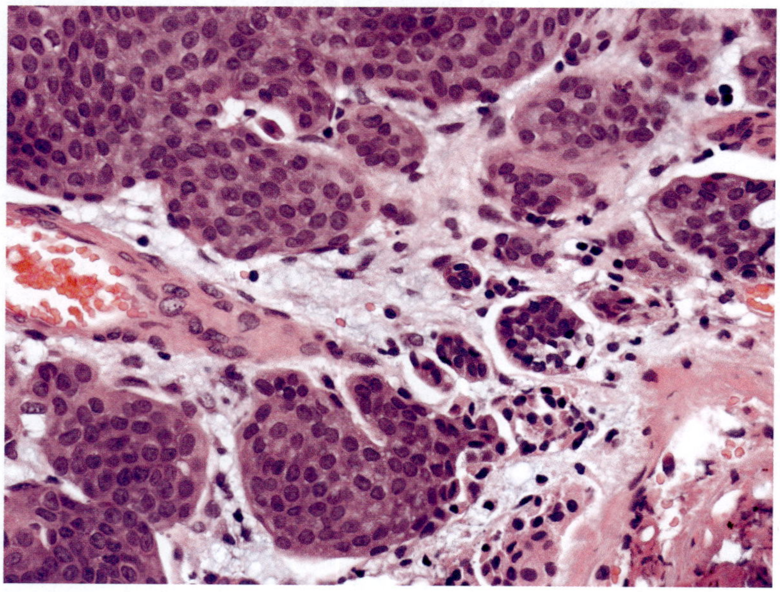

Figure 52-3.
Low-grade urothelial carcinoma with lamina propria invasion, although uncommon, shows stromal reaction.

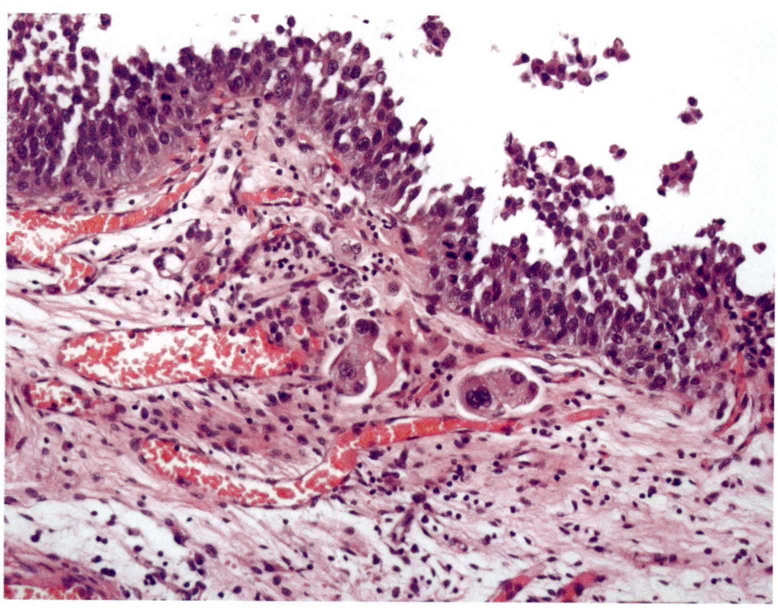

Figure 52-4.
High-grade urothelial carcinoma cells invading lamina propria show abundant eosinophilic cytoplasm and more prominent nuclear atypia.

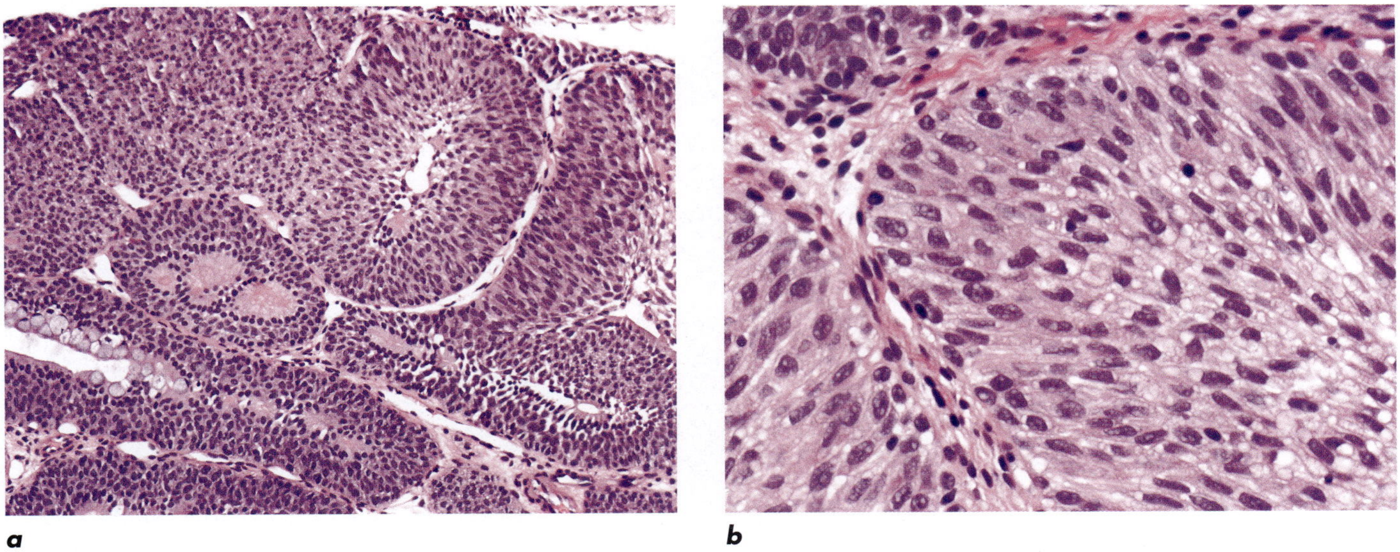

Figure 52-5.
Inverted growth pattern of noninvasive tumor cells forming nests with smooth borders (*a*). High magnification showing smooth borders of the tumor nests (*b*).

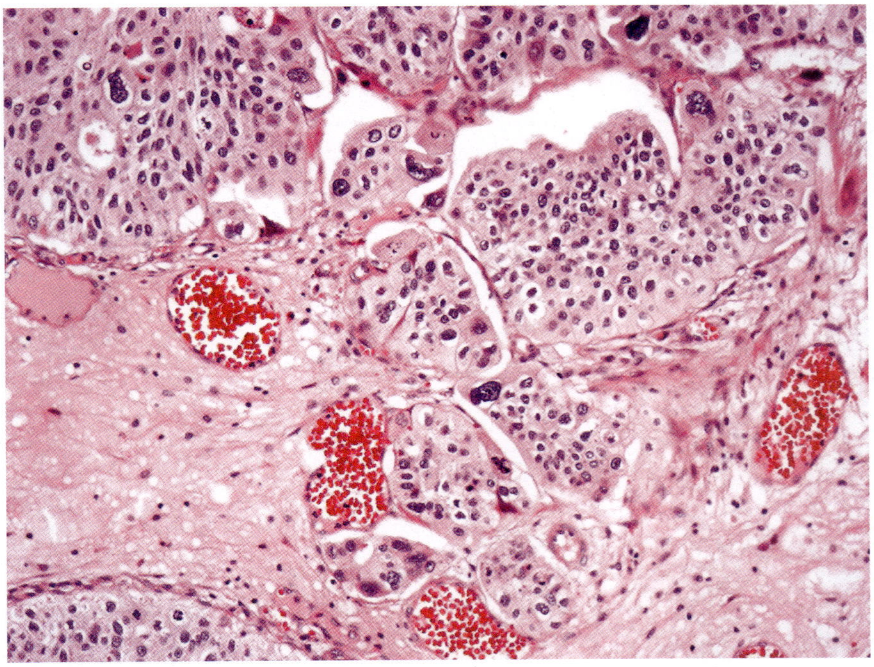

Figure 52-6.
High-grade urothelial carcinoma with lamina propria invasion, next to dilated vessels.

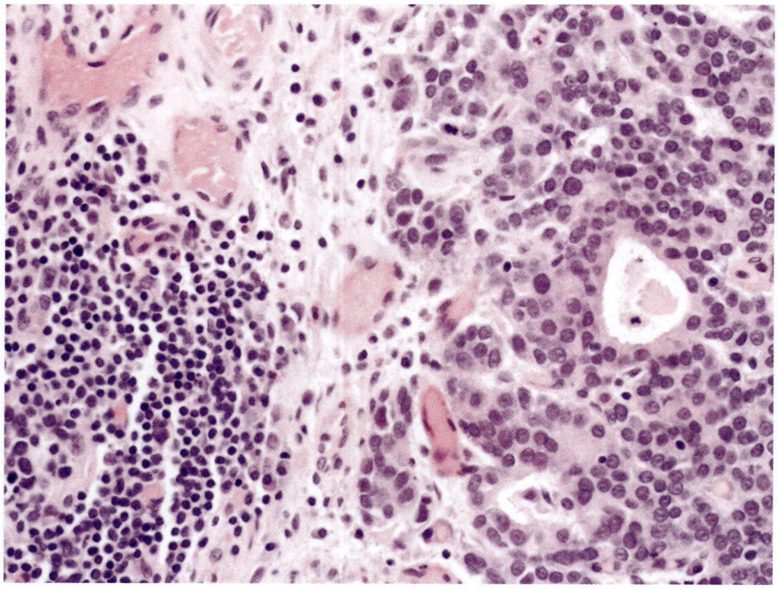

Figure 52-7.
Invasive urothelial carcinoma with lamina propria invasion, associated with chronic inflammatory infiltrate.

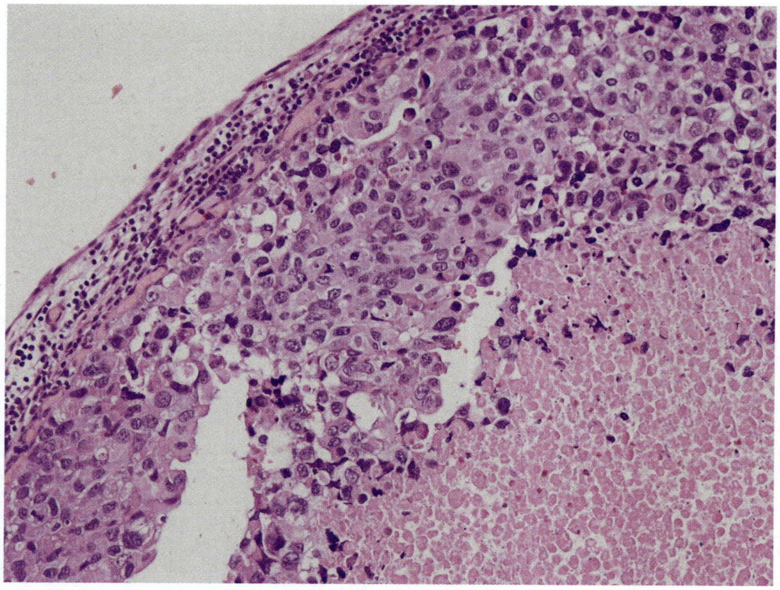

Figure 52-8.
Invasive high-grade urothelial carcinoma with necrosis.

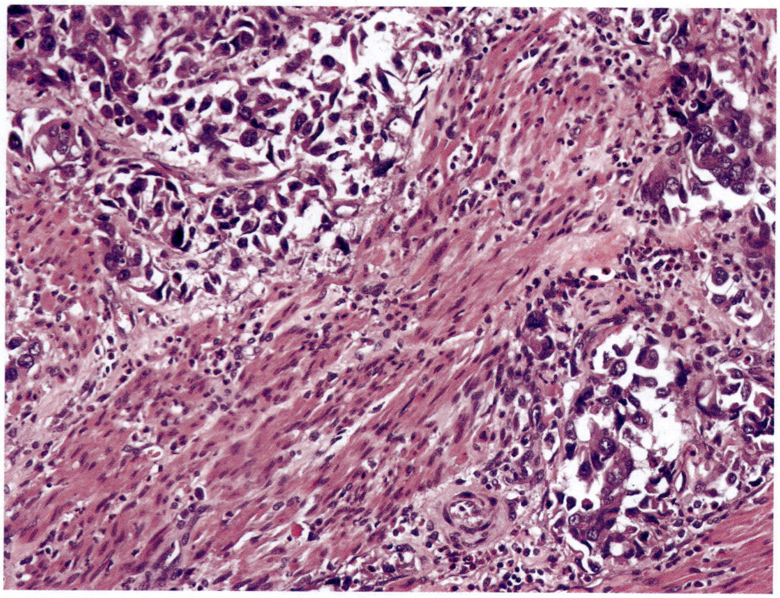

Figure 52-9.
High-grade urothelial carcinoma with muscularis propria invasion. The tumor cells are present within the large smooth muscle bundles.

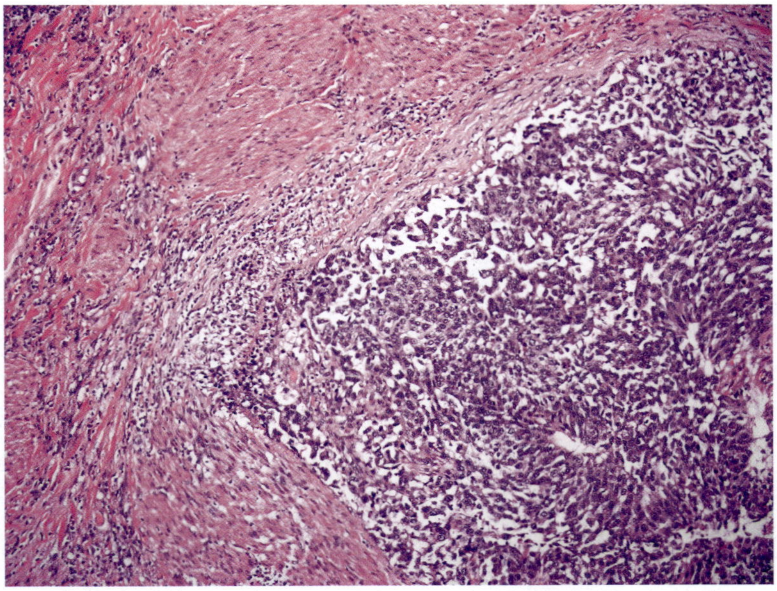

Figure 52-10.
High-grade urothelial carcinoma, with a nesting pattern, with smooth border but invading muscularis propria.

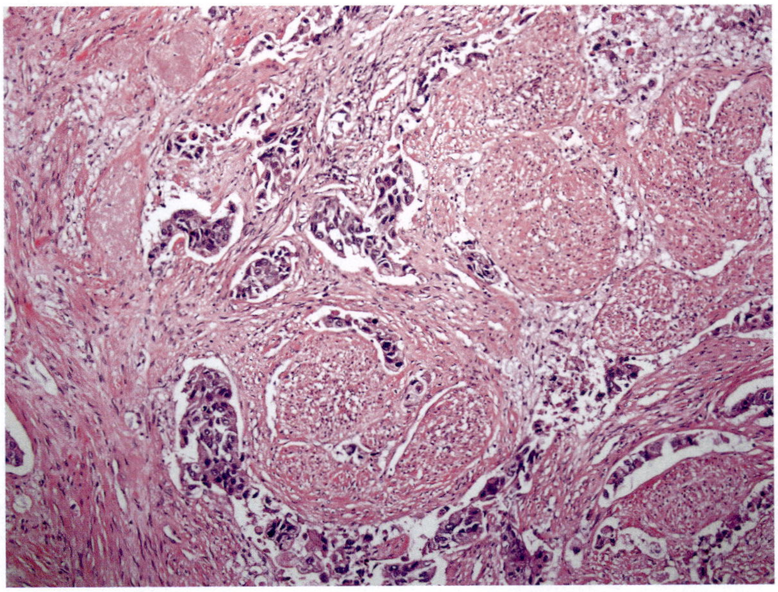

Figure 52-11.
High-grade urothelial carcinoma with muscularis propria invasion and lymphovascular invasion.

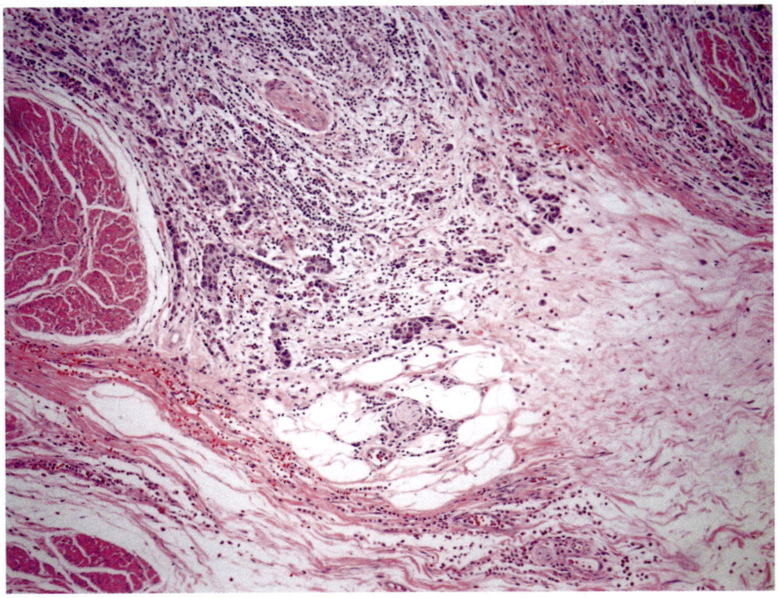

Figure 52-12.
High-grade urothelial carcinoma with invasion into perivesical adipose tissue.

- The diagnosis of lymphovascular invasion (Fig. 52-13) should be made with caution because retraction artifacts are more common in invasive urothelial carcinoma
- In the advanced stage (Stage IV) of urothelial carcinoma, the invasion of prostatic stroma (Fig. 52-14), seminal vesicles, vagina, or other adjacent tissues may be present
- Sometimes, tumor cells extensively invade the LP, and destroy the MP. In this case, we will report "tumor extensively invading LP, although no definitive MP invasion is identified" (Fig. 52-15)
- We also report the presence of urothelial CIS if present based on the belief that invasive urothelial carcinoma associated with CIS may have a worse prognosis
- The important information and pathologic findings should be included in a bladder biopsy/TUR report as listed in Table 52-1

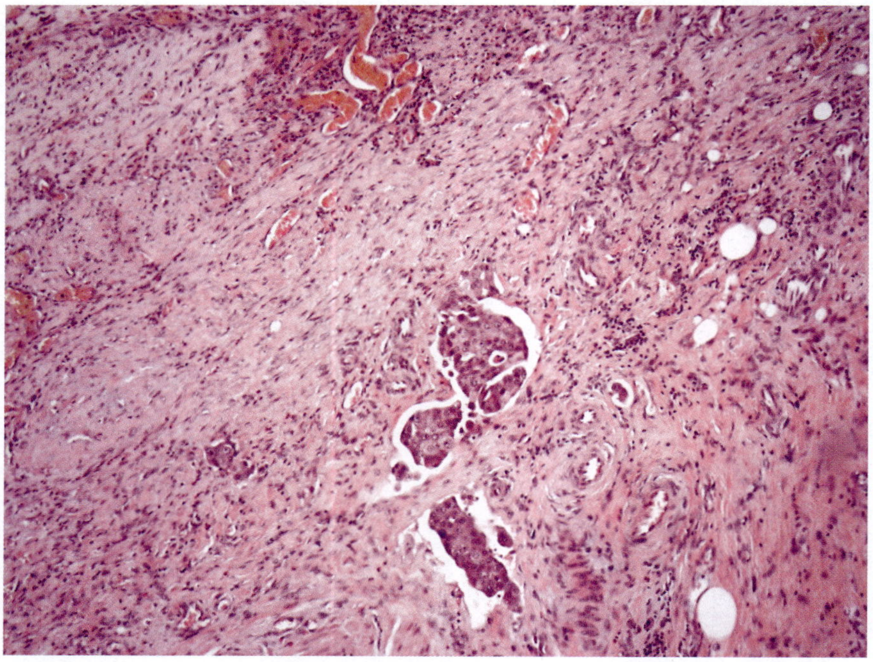

Figure 52-13.
High-grade urothelial carcinoma with lymphovascular invasion.

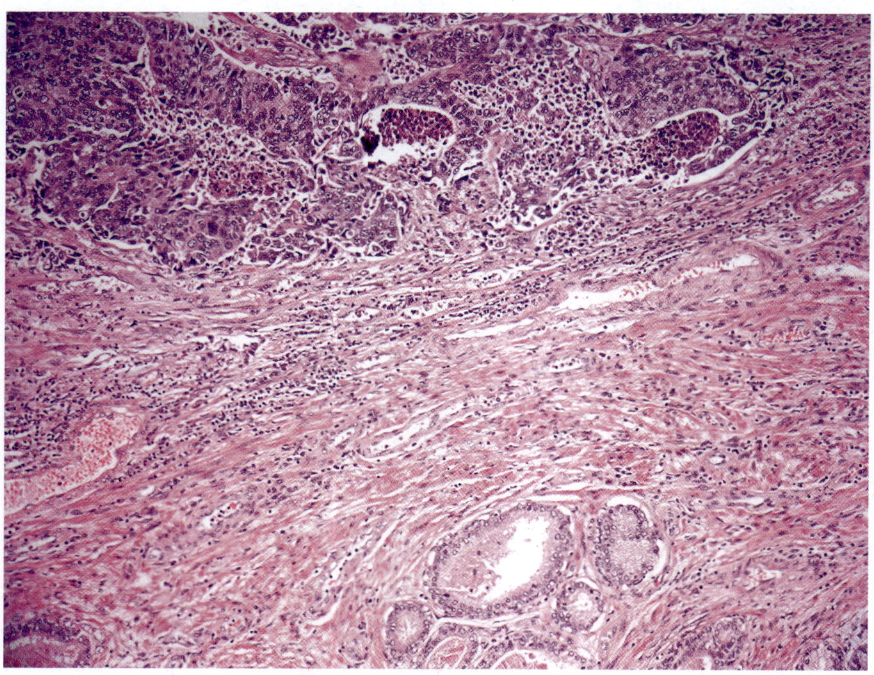

Figure 52-14.
High-grade urothelial carcinoma with invasion of the prostatic stroma.

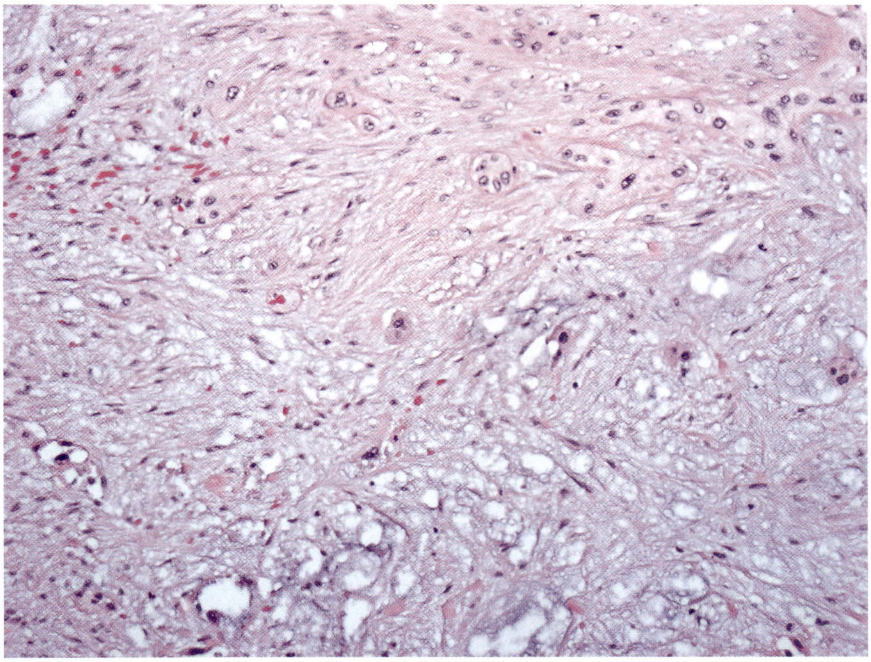

Figure 52-15.
Invasive urothelial carcinoma with myxoid stroma, but is still considered to be lamina propria invasion.

Table 52-1. Diagnostic Information in a Bladder Biopsy/TUR Pathology Report

In the case of carcinoma present	*These pathological findings should be included in the report*
	Urothelial carcinoma or other types
	Papillary configuration and size of the tumor
	Grade of tumor (high or low)
	Depth of invasion (lamina propria or muscularis propria)
	Presence or absence of muscularis propria
	Presence (or absence) and degree of divergent differentiation, such as squamous, glandular, micropapillary, and small cell carcinoma (focal or extensive)
	Presence (or absence) of necrosis
	Presence (or absence) of carcinoma in situ
	Presence (or absence) of lymphovascular invasion

Immunohistochemistry

- P53 diffusely positive, CK20 and CK7 positive in the majority of cases
- P63 and high molecular weight cytokeratins positive
- CD44 negative (loss of staining) in majority of cases
- GATA3 and S100P are new urothelial markers useful to determine the urothelial origin, but they cannot be used to distinguish benign from malignant urothelial lesions
- No reliable markers can be used for detecting tumor invasion
- Smoothelin, present in MP not LP, is useful for determining muscular propria invasion
- The cases with MP invasion are most likely positive for smoothelin (80% to 90%) than those with LP invasion only (20% to 30%), although a significant overlapping is present in difficult cases
- HER2/neu immunostaining may show positive membranous staining in a small subset of invasive UC cases

Molecular genetics

- Complex molecular alterations including numerous chromosomal losses and gains and oncogene mutations, but mostly found in the minority of cases
- FISH analysis is helpful for diagnosis
- HER2/neu can be amplified in a small subset of cases
- H-ras mutations have been detected in approximately 50% of urothelial carcinoma cases

Clinical relevance (prognosis and treatment options)

- Low-grade (LP) invasive urothelial carcinoma may be cured by TUR with intravesical BCG. But if it is not completely removed, it may recur
- High-grade invasive urothelial carcinoma will have a higher rate of recurrence rate after TUR with or without local therapies such as intravesical chemotherapy or BCG.
- A significant number (approximately 20% to 30%) of cases are understaged in biopsy or TUR specimens because of sampling issues
- Therefore, high-grade invasive urothelial carcinoma, particularly the ones with extensive LP invasion, should be treated more aggressively by surgical resections
- Neoadjuvant (before cystectomy) and adjuvant (after cystectomy) therapies are effective in some cases and should be considered
- Stages for bladder cancer
  - For noninvasive tumors: Ta—noninvasive papillary urothelial carcinoma; Tcis—urothelial CIS
  - For invasive tumors: T1—LP invasion; T2—MP invasion; T3—perivesical invasion; T4—invasion of other organs outside the bladder including prostate (stroma)

INVASIVE SQUAMOUS CELL CARCINOMA AND UROTHELIAL CARCINOMA WITH SQUAMOUS DIFFERENTIATION

Definition

Squamous cell carcinoma

- Malignant epithelial neoplasm composed of pure squamous component

Urothelial carcinoma with squamous differentiation

- The squamous metaplasia develop in a urothelial carcinoma
- The presence of both urothelial carcinoma and squamous cell carcinoma components

Other term

- Transitional cell carcinoma with squamous metaplasia

Pathogenesis

- Pure squamous cell carcinoma usually develops in the background of chronic inflammation and squamous metaplasia
- Squamous cell carcinoma (SqCC) accounts for the vast majority of bladder cancer associated with schistosomiasis, which results in chronic inflammation and squamous metaplasia of the urothelium
- Urothelial carcinoma may undergo squamous differentiation without specific causes

Clinical features

- Hematuria
- Other symptoms similar to urothelial carcinoma

Gross pathology

- Large mass with necrosis and hemorrhage
- Cheesy (keratin debris) material can be seen (Fig. 52-16)
- Uninvolved bladder mucosa may show thickness and fibrosis

Histology

Squamous cell carcinoma

- Pure squamous cell carcinoma without urothelial component (Fig. 52-16)
- Keratinized or nonkeratinized malignant squamous cells can be present (there is no difference in their biological behaviors) (Fig. 52-17). Squamous metaplasia and chronic inflammation usually present (Fig. 52-17) although squamous metaplasia can also be seen in urothelial carcinoma with squamous metaplasia

Figure 52-16.
Squamous cell carcinoma of the bladder as a large mass with necrosis on the surface and cheesy material in the center (*a*). Microscopically, this tumor is composed entirely of keratinized malignant squamous cells with lamina propria invasion (*b*).

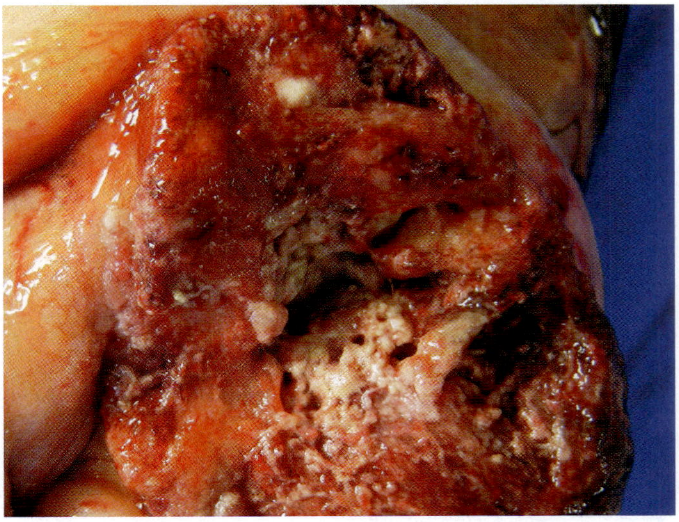

a

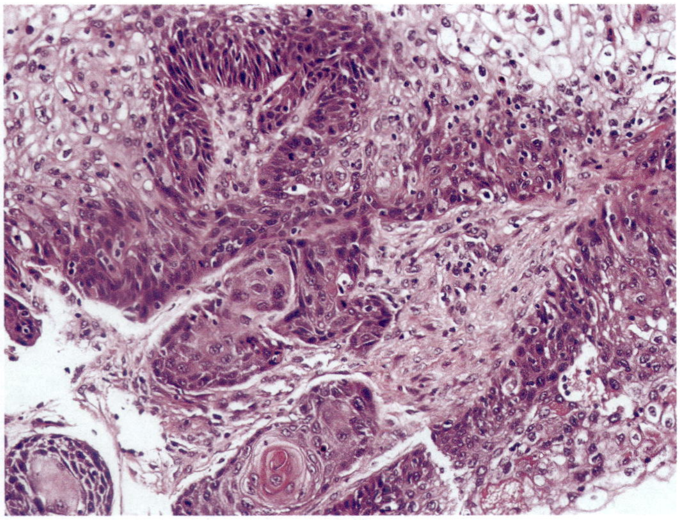

b

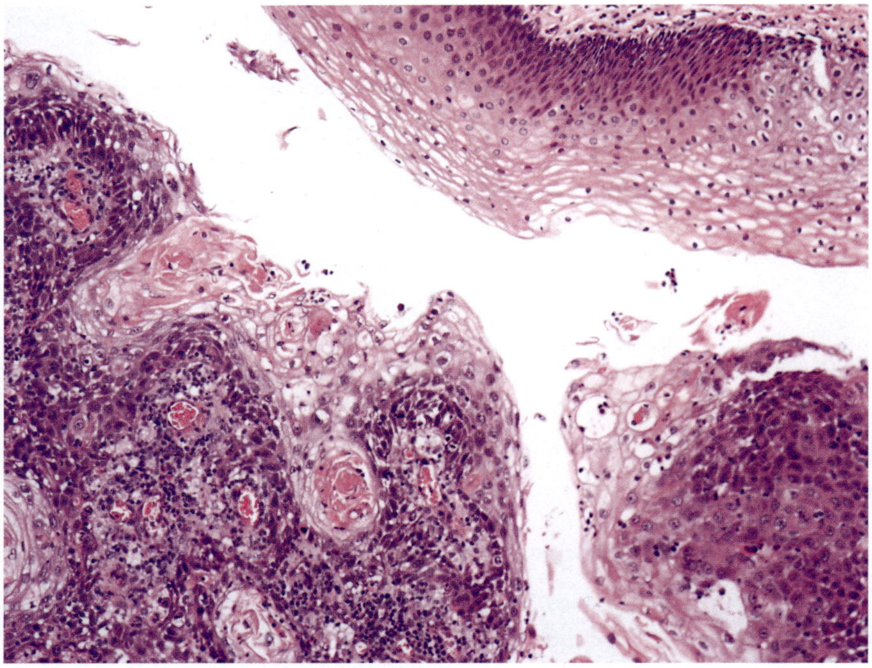

Figure 52-17.
Invasive keratinized squamous cell carcinoma of the bladder (lower portion) coexisting with nonkeratinized squamous metaplasia (upper portion).

- Squamous cell CIS (Fig. 52-18) with or without early invasion can be seen (Fig. 52-19)
- Keratin pearls (keratinization of tumor cells), characterized by the central keratinization surrounded by concentric layer of malignant epithelial cells, are often seen in invasive SqCC (Fig. 52-20)
- Intracellular bridges (tight junctions) are prominent between tumor cells (Fig. 52-21) and desmoplastic stromal reaction present

Urothelial carcinoma with squamous differentiation

- All the above features of squamous cell carcinoma can be seen, except presence of a urothelial component (Figs. 52-22 and 52-23)
- Squamous differentiation can be seen in both low-grade or high-grade urothelial carcinoma, but more commonly in high-grade ones

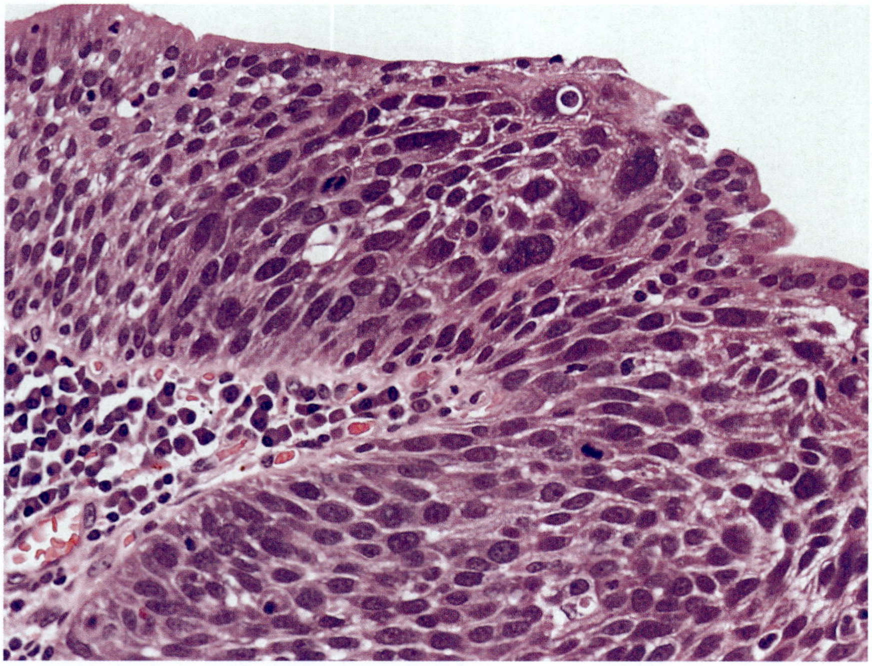

Figure 52-18.
Squamous cell carcinoma in situ found in a case with invasive squamous cell carcinoma of the bladder.

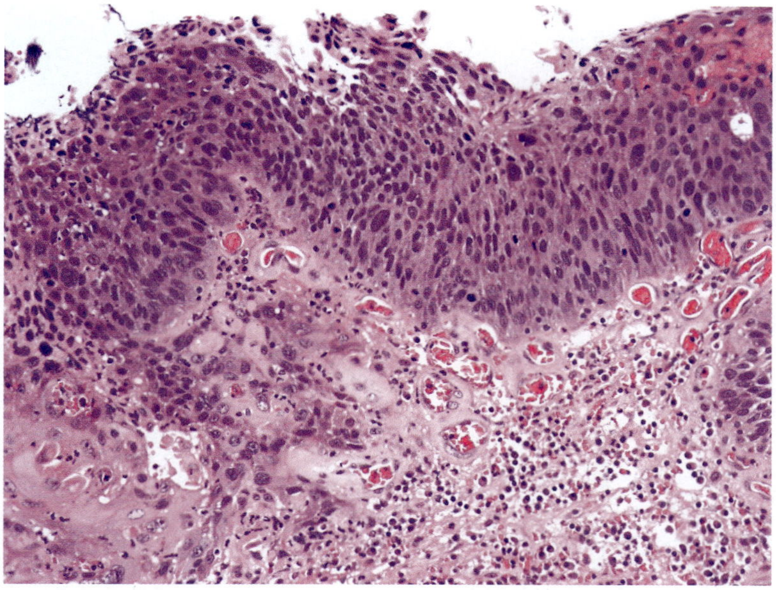

Figure 52-19.
Squamous cell carcinoma in situ with early lamina propria invasion.

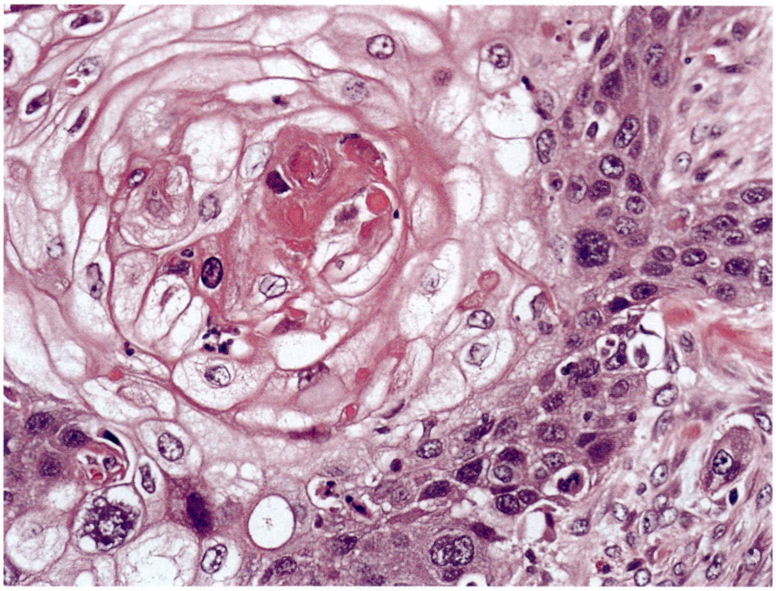

Figure 52-20.
Invasive squamous cell carcinoma of the bladder with a keratin pearl.

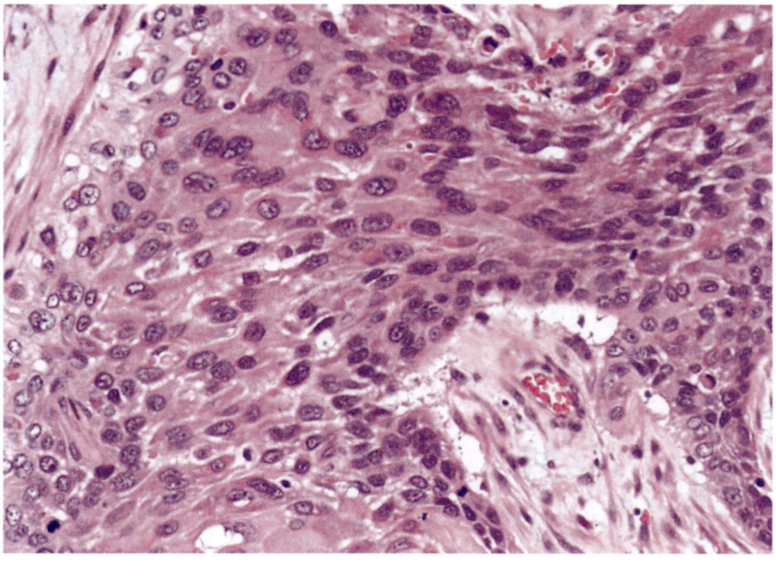

Figure 52-21.
Invasive squamous cell carcinoma of the bladder with intercellular bridges and desmoplastic reaction.

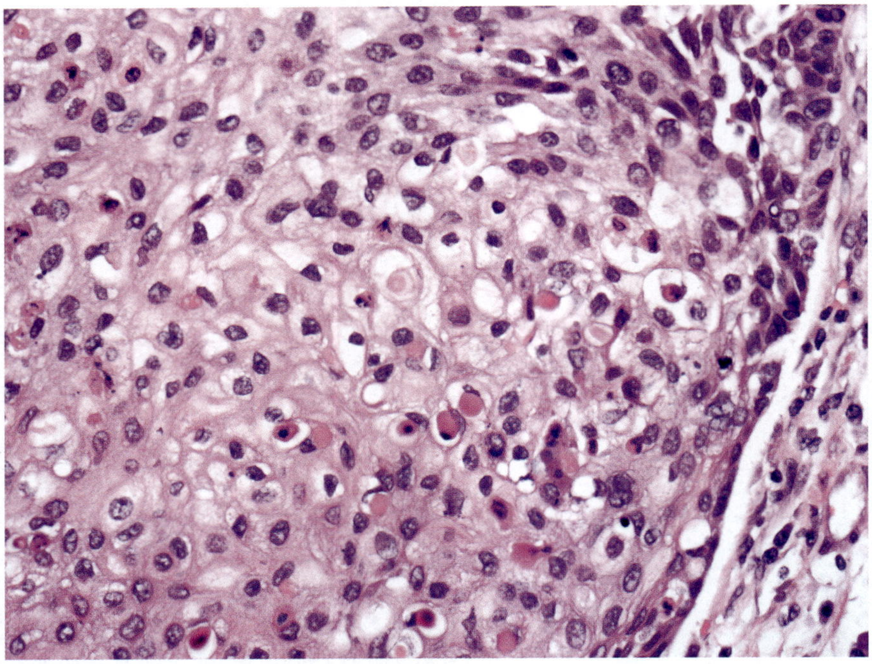

Figure 52-22.
Urothelial carcinoma with squamous differentiation.

- Several features would be favoring urothelial carcinoma with squamous differentiation
  - Presence of urothelial CIS
  - Presence of glandular differentiation (Fig. 52-23)
  - Presence of urothelial CIS or adenocarcinoma in situ
  - Lack of benign squamous metaplasia
  - If both urothelial and squamous carcinomatous components are observed (Fig. 52-24), the diagnosis of urothelial carcinoma with squamous differentiation can be established
- There are some differences between these two entities (summarized in Table 52-2). It is difficult to distinguish pure squamous cell carcinoma and urothelial carcinoma with squamous differentiation on a limited biopsy specimen
- In an invasive carcinoma with extensive squamous differentiation of the bladder, the differential diagnosis includes squamous cell carcinoma and urothelial carcinoma with squamous differentiation

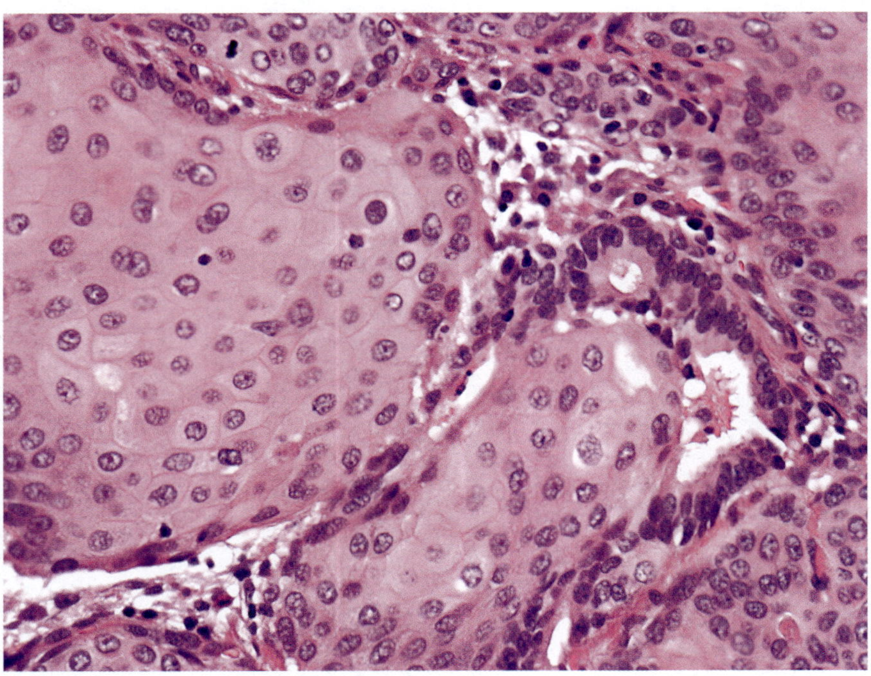

Figure 52-23.
Urothelial carcinoma with squamous differentiation and glandular differentiation.

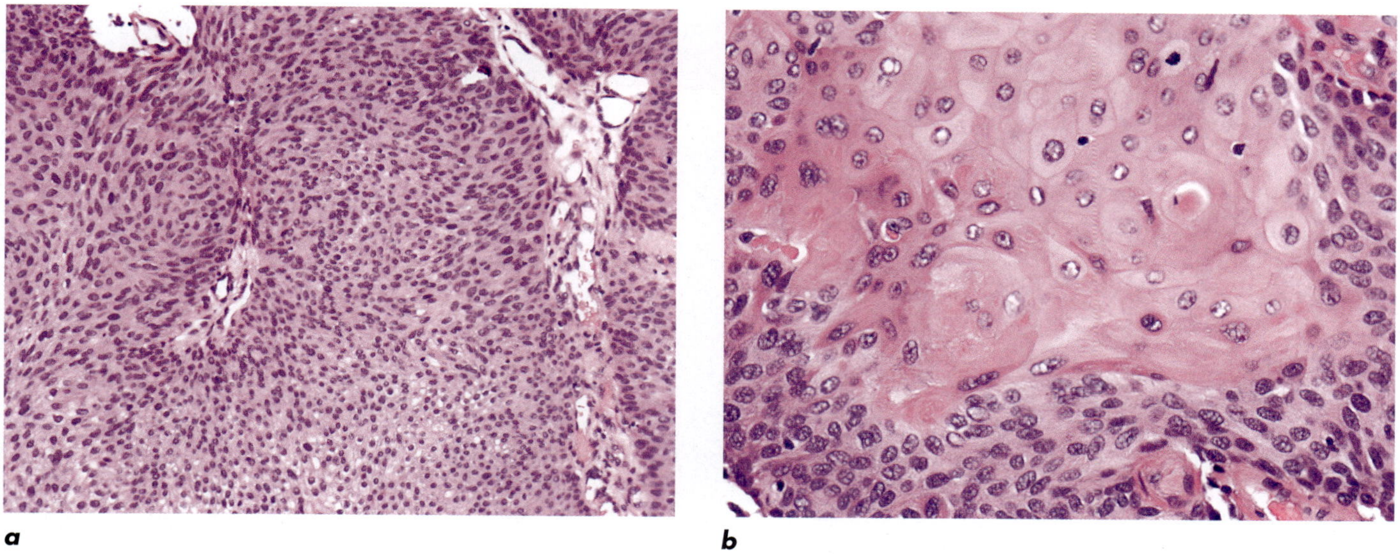

Figure 52-24.
Urothelial carcinoma with squamous differentiation, both low-grade tumor cells (*a*) and tumor cells with squamous differentiation (*b*) can be seen.

Immunohistochemistry

- It is not well documented whether there are specific markers to distinguish squamous cell carcinoma from urothelial carcinoma with squamous differentiation
- Typically, both will be positive for p63 and p53

Differential diagnosis

Secondary squamous cell carcinoma

- SqCC of anal, cervical, vaginal, or vulvar primary can involve bladder by direct extension or metastasis
- The morphological features of primary and secondary squamous cell carcinomas are essentially the same
- Primary bladder squamous cell carcinoma is often associated with the preexisting benign squamous metaplasia, while the secondary tumor is not
- Secondary squamous cell carcinoma may not inovolve the surface urothelium
- Clinical correlation is essential for making a distinction

Clinical relevance (prognosis and treatment options)

- Pure squamous cell carcinoma is associated with a poor prognosis and requires cystectomy
- It is controversial that urothelial carcinoma with squamous differentiation has a worse or the same prognosis than conventional urothelial carcinoma of the same grade
- In our observation of the limited number of cases, urothelial carcinoma with extensive squamous differentiation did not respond well to neoadjuvant chemotherapy. They probably behave more like a squamous cell carcinoma than a urothelial carcinoma
- Therefore, the degree of squamous component should be reported (at least reporting focal or extensive squamous differentiation)
- In a biopsy specimen, because of this difficulty, we use "poorly differentiated carcinoma with extensive squamous differentiation; the differential diagnosis includes invasive squamous cell carcinoma and urothelial carcinoma with squamous differentiation"

Table 52-2. Comparison of Squamous Cell Carcinoma of the Bladder and Urothelial Carcinoma with Squamous Differentiation

	Squamous cell carcinoma	*Urothelial carcinoma with squamous differentiation*
Pathogenesis	Chronic cystitis	Unknown
	Indwelling catheters or calculi, schistosomiasis	Smoking
	HPV infection	
Gross	Bulky mass	Papillary or bulky mass
	Cheesy keratin debris	Necrosis may be present
Histology		
Squamous component	Pure (100%)	With urothelial component
Invasive	Yes	Yes
Keratin pearls	Yes	Yes (focal)
Intercellular bridges	Yes	Yes (focal)
Invasive urothelial carcinoma	Absent	Present
Urothelial carcinoma in situ	Absent	Present
Glandular differentiation	Rare	Common
Other urothelial variants		
such as small cell or micropapillary components	Absent	May be present
Squamous metaplasia	Always	Mostly not
Prognosis	Poor, may be worse than urothelial carcinoma	Poor
Cystectomy	Indicated	May be indicated
Chemotherapy for urothelial carcinoma	May not be effective	Depending on the degree of squamous differentiation

HPV, human papillomavirus.

PLASMACYTOID UROTHELIAL CARCINOMA

Definition

- A variant of urothelial carcinoma composed of tumor cells resembling plasma cells

Pathogenesis

- Unknown
- Small-sized urothelial carcinoma cells similar to plasma cells although they do not have any biomedical features of plasma cells

Clinical features

- Same as invasive high-grade urothelial carcinoma

Gross pathology

- Same as invasive high-grade urothelial carcinoma

Histology

- Plasmacytoid urothelial carcinoma is composed of discohesive tumor cells of smaller size and shape. The tumor can be invasive or in situ
- They have scant and eccentric cytoplasm, morphologically similar to plasma cells (Figs. 52-25 and 52-26)
- This tumor (Fig. 52-27) can be difficult to distinguish from other lesions such as chronic cystitis or lymphoma, or plasmacytoma especially on a small biopsy
- Sometimes, tumor cells will form single-file cords as Indian filing
- Typical high-grade invasive urothelial carcinomas are often present

Immunohistochemistry

- Keratins positive (Figs. 52-26*b*, 52-27*c*, *d*)
- P63, HMWCK positive
- Plasma cell markers negative and neuroendocrine markers negative

Figure 52-25.
Plasmacytoid urothelial carcinoma of the bladder exhibits diffuse patterns and tumor cells with relatively uniform sizes and shapes (*a*). High magnification shows the tumor cells with scant cytoplasm and slight variability in size and shape (*b*).

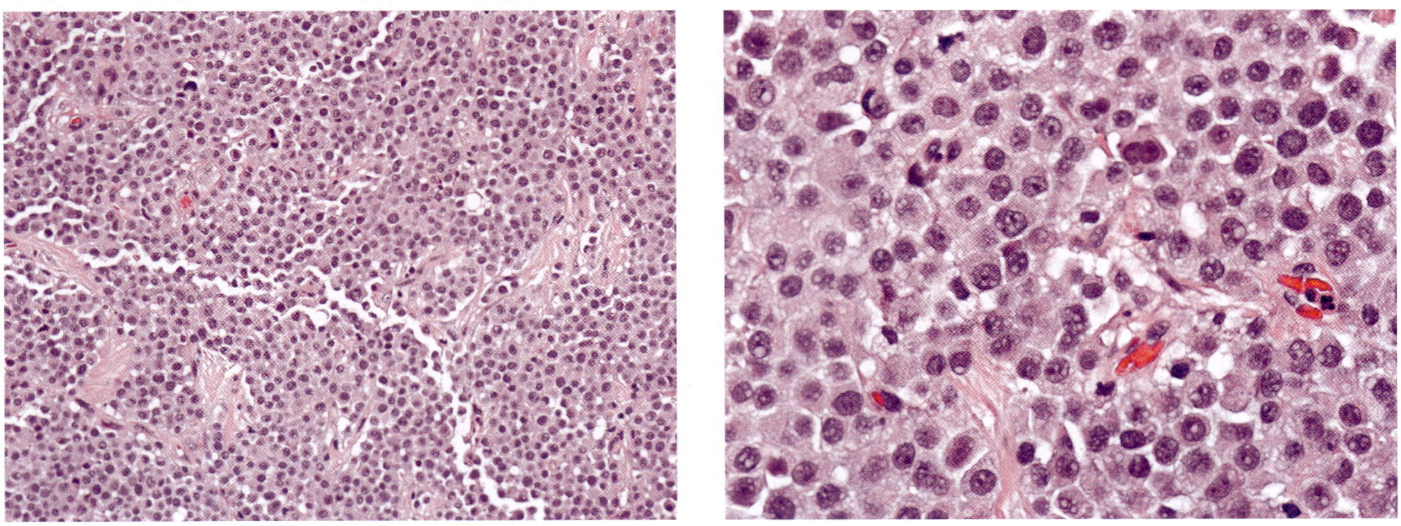

a b

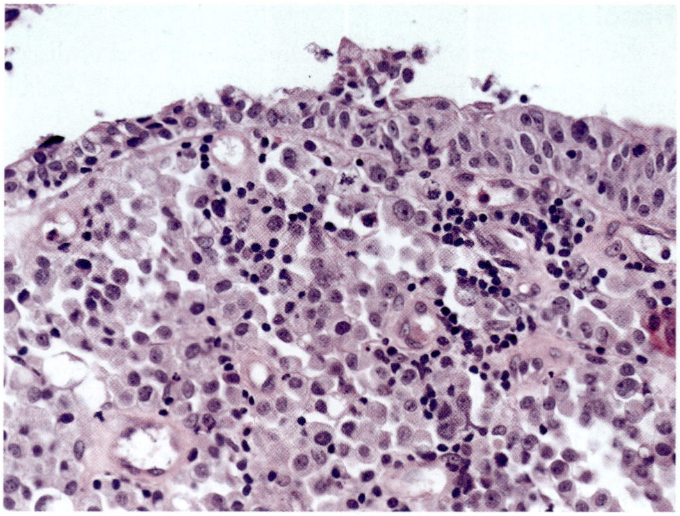

a

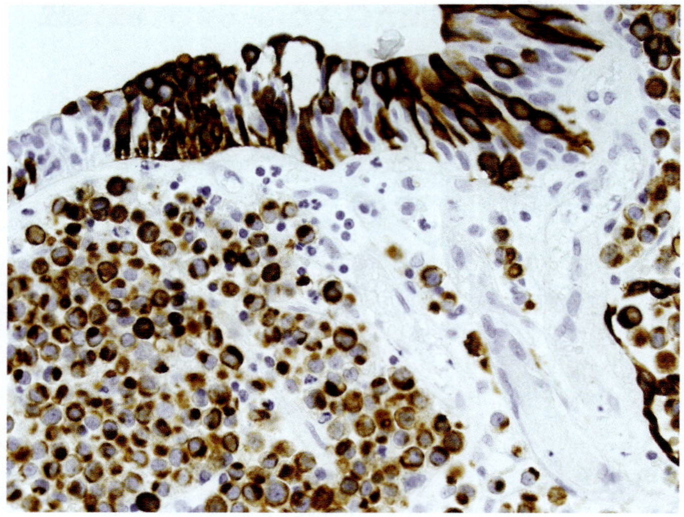

b

Figure 52-26.
Invasive plasmacytoid urothelial carcinoma involving the urothelium and lamina propria (*a*). The diagnosis of carcinoma is confirmed by positive CK20 immunoreactivity in the tumor cells (*b*).

Differential diagnosis

Lymphoma

- Negative for keratins and positive for lymphoma without typical UC components

Plasmacytoma

- Plasmacytoma or multiple myeloma is composed of uniform neoplastic with perinuclear halos
- This tumor is keratin negative but positive for plasma cell markers CD138 and kappa or lambda light chain positive
- Plasmacytoid carcinoma often contains a typical urothelial carcinoma component
- In addition, plasmacytoid carcinoma shows more variation in size and shape of the tumor cells than malignant plasma cells

Clinical relevance (prognosis and treatment options)

- Aggressive behavior as a high-grade urothelial carcinoma

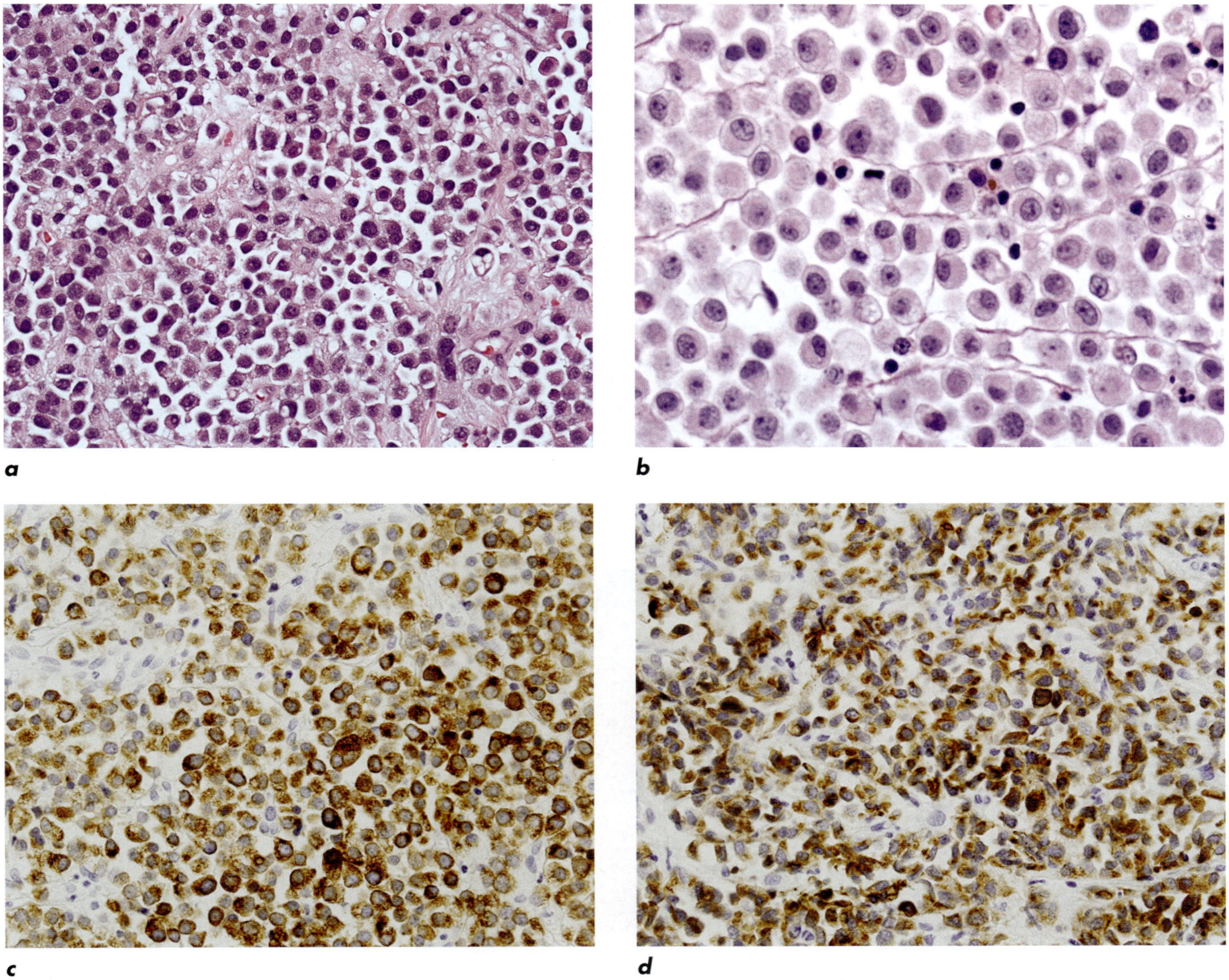

Figure 52-27.

Plasmacytoid urothelial carcinoma is composed of dissociated smaller tumor cells resembling plasma cells (*a*). High magnification shows the individual tumor cells with eccentric cytoplasm mimicking plasma cells (*b*), but they are three to four times larger than lymphocytes. Tumor cells are positive for both CK20 (*c*) and CK7 (*d*).

SMALL CELL CARCINOMA

Definition

- Highly malignant carcinoma primarily composed of small neuroendocrine cells
- Morphologically similar to the pulmonary small cell carcinoma

Pathogenesis

- In at least 50% of the cases, small cell carcinoma is derived from a high-grade urothelial carcinoma, representing dedifferentiation

Clinical features

- Similar to high-grade urothelial carcinoma
- Serum neuroendocrine markers may be elevated
- Paraneoplastic syndrome may be present

Gross pathology

- Poorly defined infiltrating mass with white, yellow, or brown cut surface (Fig. 52-28)

Histology

- Composed of small neuroendocrine cells with scant cytoplasm and a high N/C ratio (Fig. 52-29)
- Salt-and-pepper chromatin patterns as well as high mitotic counts and high apoptosis rate are evident (Fig. 52-30)
- Invasive to bladder wall and adjacent organs
- Typically, invasive or urothelial carcinoma in situ can be detected in approximately one-half of the cases of small cell carcinomas of the bladder

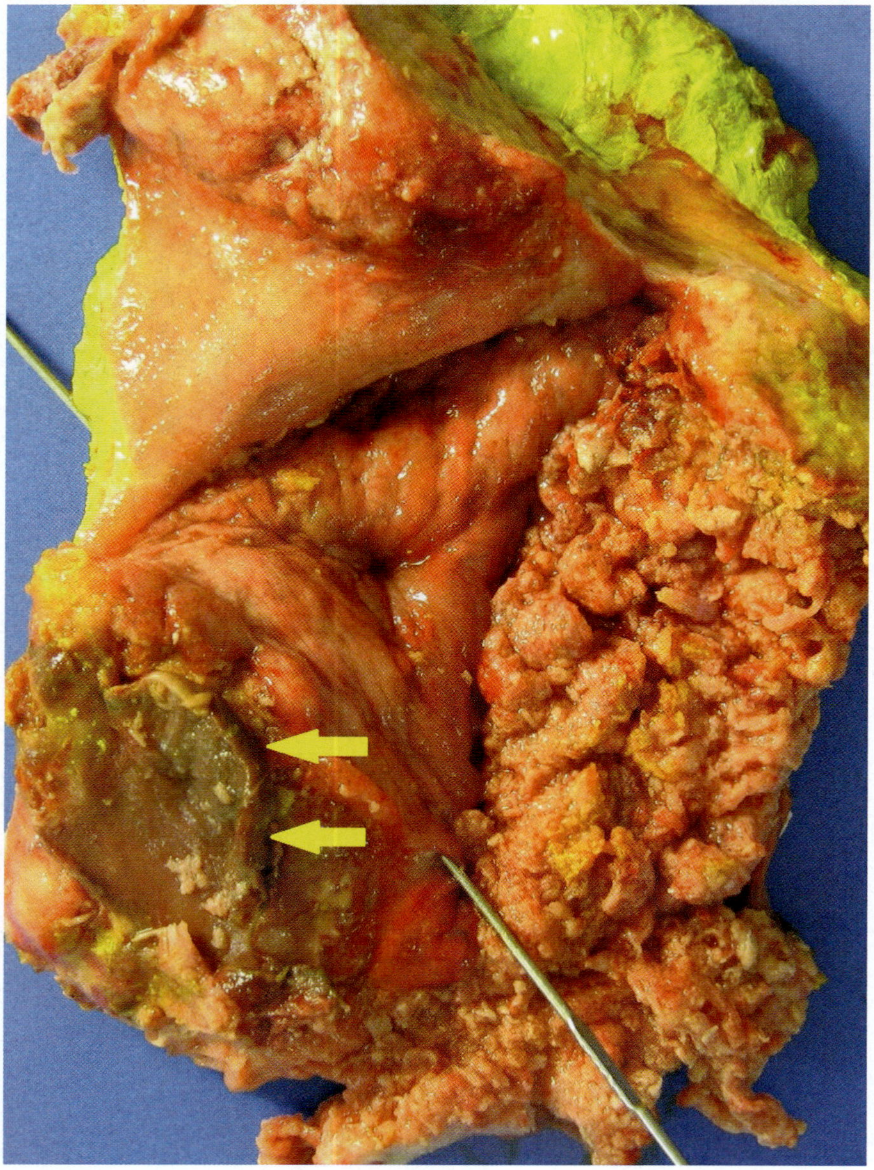

Figure 52-28.
Small cell carcinoma of the bladder as a mass with a chocolate-color cut surface is indicated by arrows. The typical papillary urothelial carcinoma is on the right side.

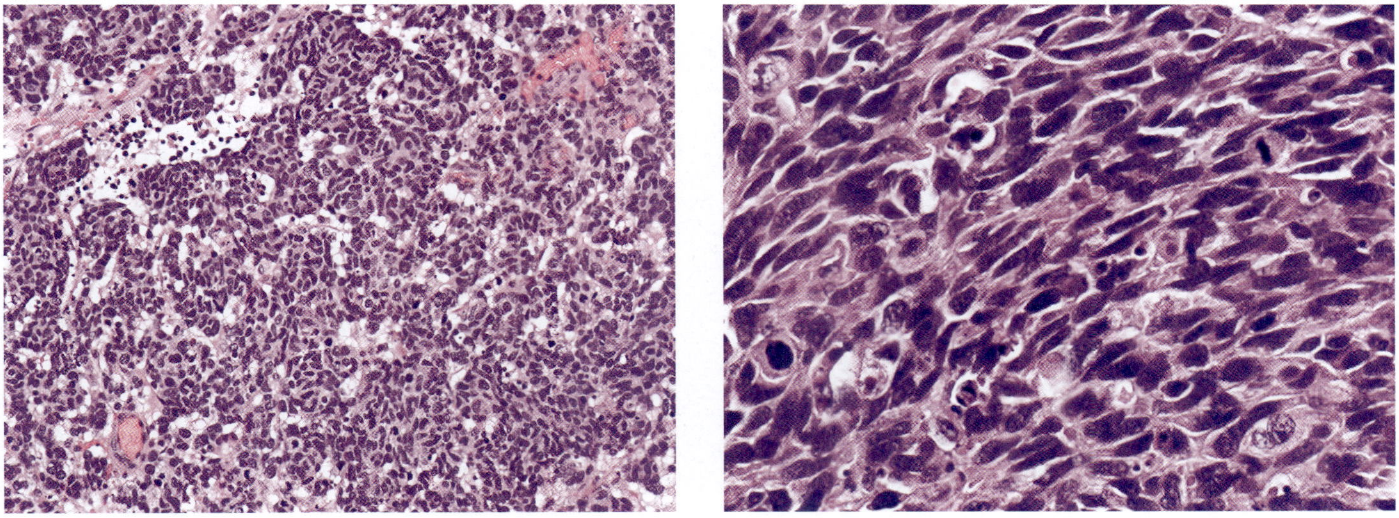

a b

Figure 52-29.
Small cell carcinoma demonstrates diffuse nests of small blue cells with fine chromatin (*a*). High magnification shows fine "salt-pepper" chromatin and frequent mitoses; some cells have the appearance of spindle cells (*b*).

Immunohistochemistry

- Neuroendocrine markers positive, at least one or two (Fig. 52-30), such as NSE, chromogranin, synaptophysin, and CD56
- Only 50% of cases are positive for TTF1
- Keratin positive
- Urothelial carcinoma markers positive for the component of urothelial cell carcinoma but not for small cell carcinoma component

Clinical relevance (prognosis and treatment options)

- Aggressive systemic disease
- Half of the cases are associated with typical high-grade invasive urothelial carcinoma
- Serum neuroendocrine markers, such as chromogranin, may be positive
- Need systemic chemotherapy with or without surgery

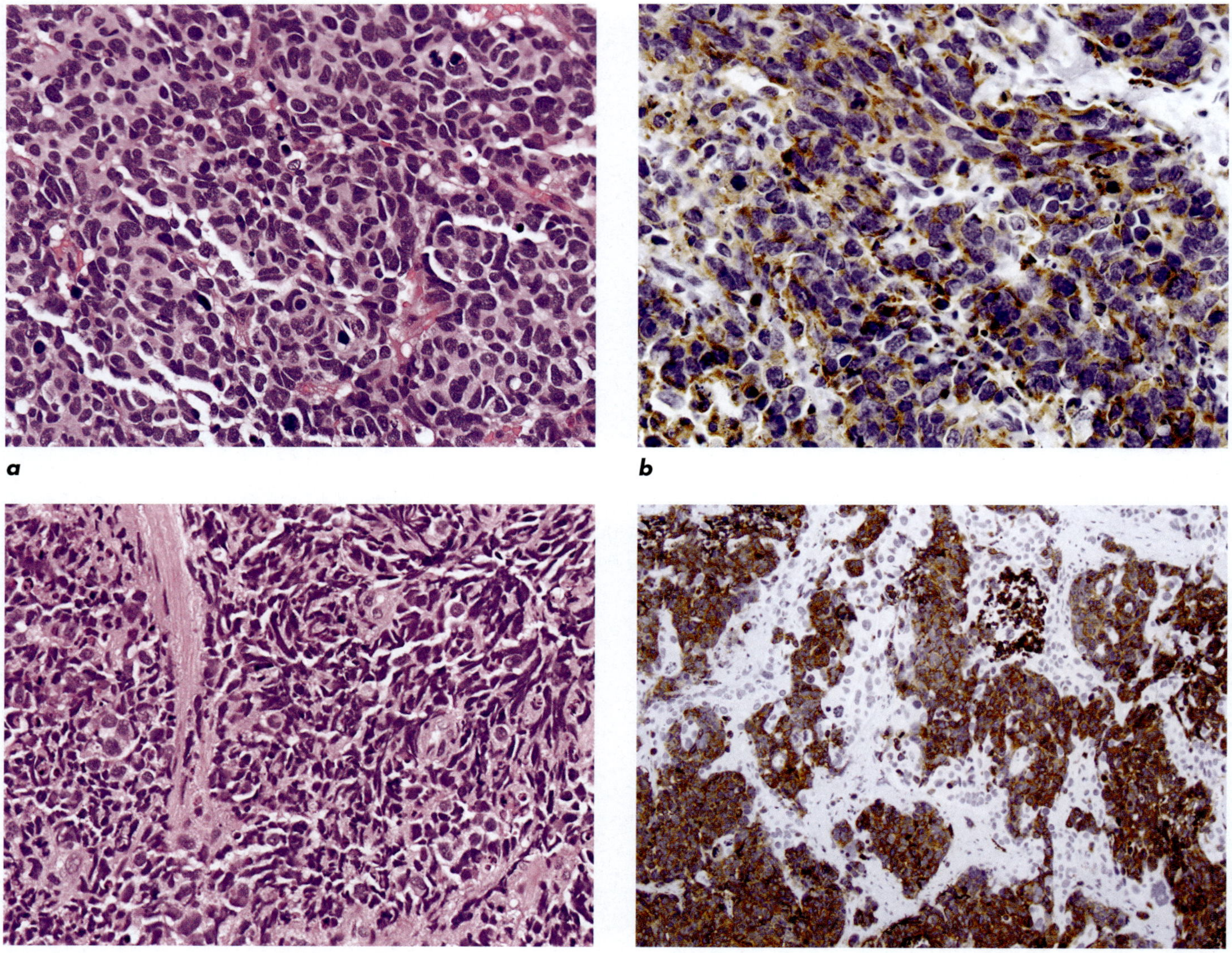

a b c d

Figure 52-30.

Small cell carcinoma is composed of small tumor cells with "salt-pepper" chromatin, scant cytoplasm, and frequent mitoses (*a*). Immunostaining for chromogranin is strongly positive in tumor cells (*b*). Cauterization of small cell carcinoma masking the nuclear details (*c*), but the diagnosis is confirmed by the strong synaptophysin immunoreactivity (*d*).

CARCINOSARCOMA

Definition

- A malignant neoplasm of the bladder contains both carcinomatous and sarcomatous components

Other terms

- Sarcomatoid urothelial carcinoma
- Urothelial carcinoma with sarcomatoid differentiation

Pathogenesis

- Urothelial carcinoma undergoing dedifferentiation to transform to a high-grade malignancy
- The association with radiation or chemotherapy is reported but the relationship is not fully established

Clinical features

- Hematuria
- History of low-grade or high-grade urothelial carcinoma
- If detected initially without history of bladder tumor, typically present as an advanced stage of malignancy
- Imaging or cystoscopic studies show bulky mass lesion(s) with or without metastasis

Gross pathology

- Large bulky mass (Fig. 52-31) with a fixed nonmobile base indicating the invasive component
- Areas of papillary appearance, ulceration, hemorrhage, and necrosis are common
- Cut surface may show myxoid or fleshy areas representing malignant stromal components in addition to typical white hard areas of carcinoma

Histology

- The presence of both carcinomatous and sarcomatous components in the same tumor is required for diagnosis (Fig. 52-32)
- Carcinomatous components are typically high-grade invasive urothelial carcinoma

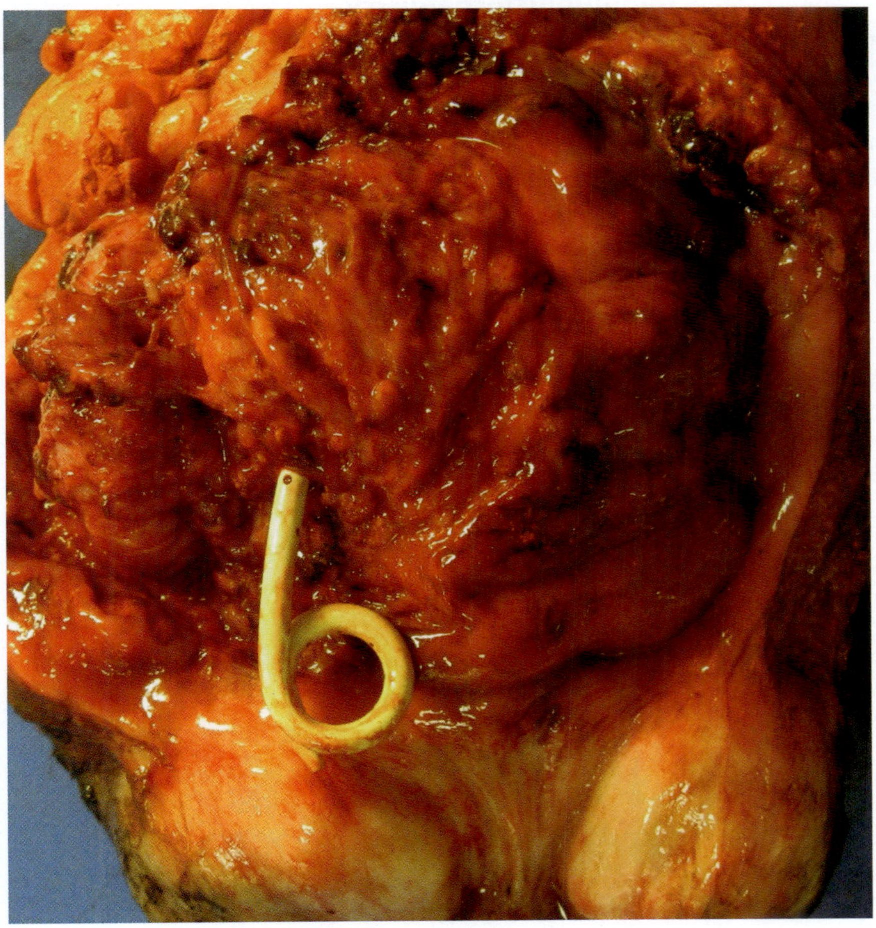

Figure 52-31.
Carcinosarcoma of the bladder is a bulky mass occupying most of the bladder mucosal surface.

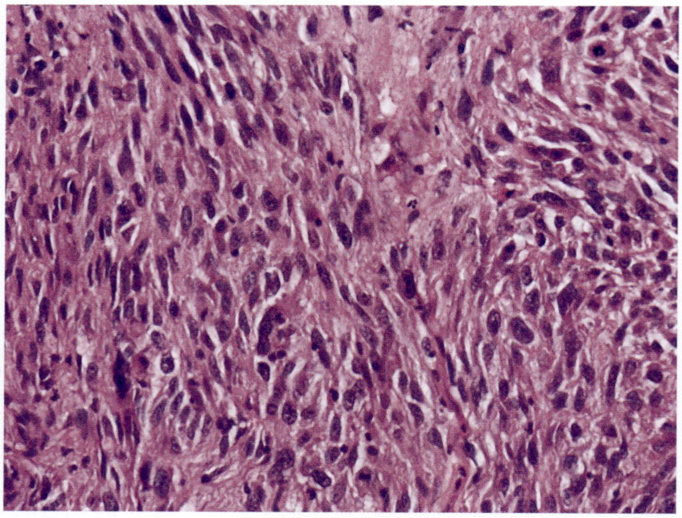

a

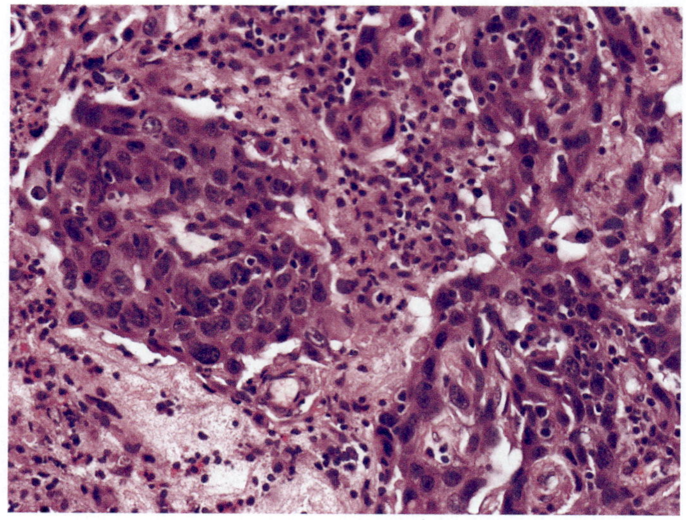

b

Figure 52-32.
Carcinosarcoma of the bladder is characterized by the presence of malignant spindle cells (*a*) mimicking a sarcoma. However, the presence of carcinomatous component is required for the diagnosis (*b*).

- Occasionally, only CIS tumor (Fig. 52-33) or low-grade urothelial carcinoma, squamous or glandular differentiation may be identified
- Sarcomatoid components are typically high-grade malignant spindle cells in high cellularity and high mitotic counts without specific differentiation (Figs. 52-34 and 52-35)
- Sometimes, heterologous elements such as malignant cartilage (chondrosarcoma), bone (osteosarcoma), or skeletal muscle differentiation (rhabdomyosarcoma)

Immunohistochemistry

- Carcinomatous components will be similar to urothelial carcinoma: p63 positive, p53 positive, HMWCK positive
- Sarcomatous components can be positive for keratins (Fig. 52-35*b* and *d*)
- Sarcomatous components may be positive for muscle markers such as desmin, smooth muscle actin
- ALK-1 negative

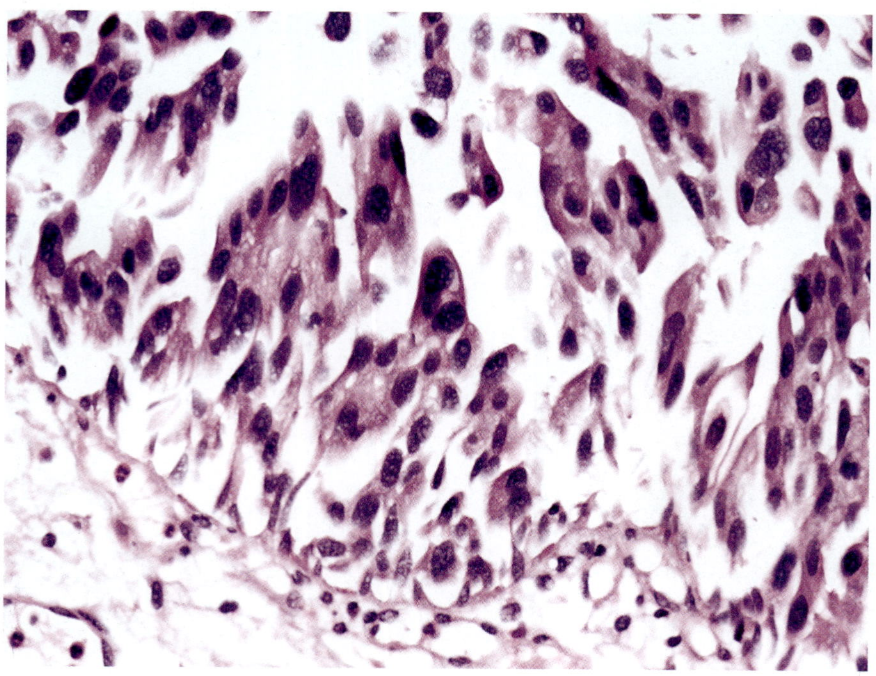

Figure 52-33.
Urothelial CIS present in a carcinosarcoma.

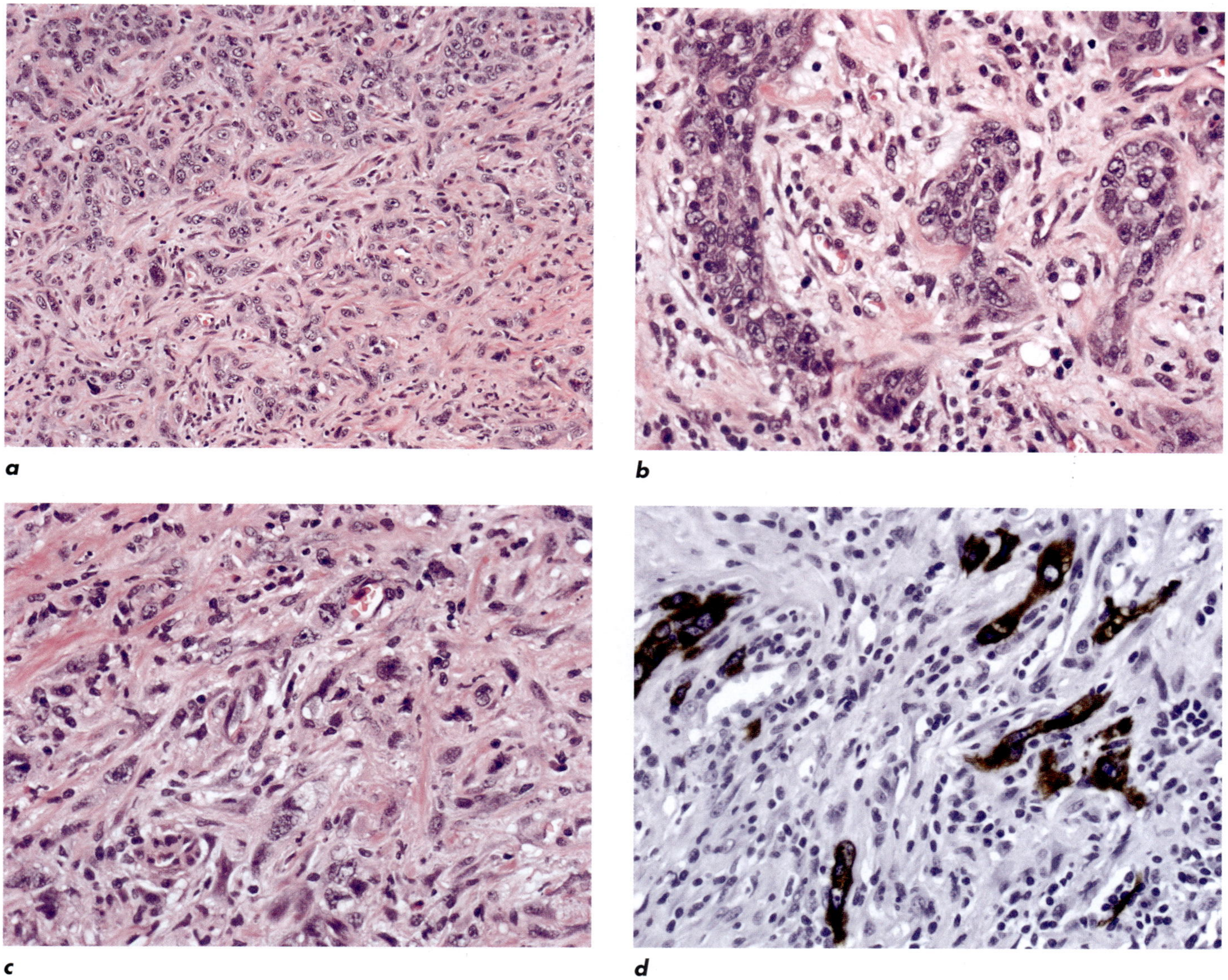

Figure 52-34.
Carcinosarcoma of the bladder (*a*) exhibits both carcinomatous (*b*) and sarcomatoid components (*c*). The sarcomatoid cells are positive for AE1/AE3 (*d*).

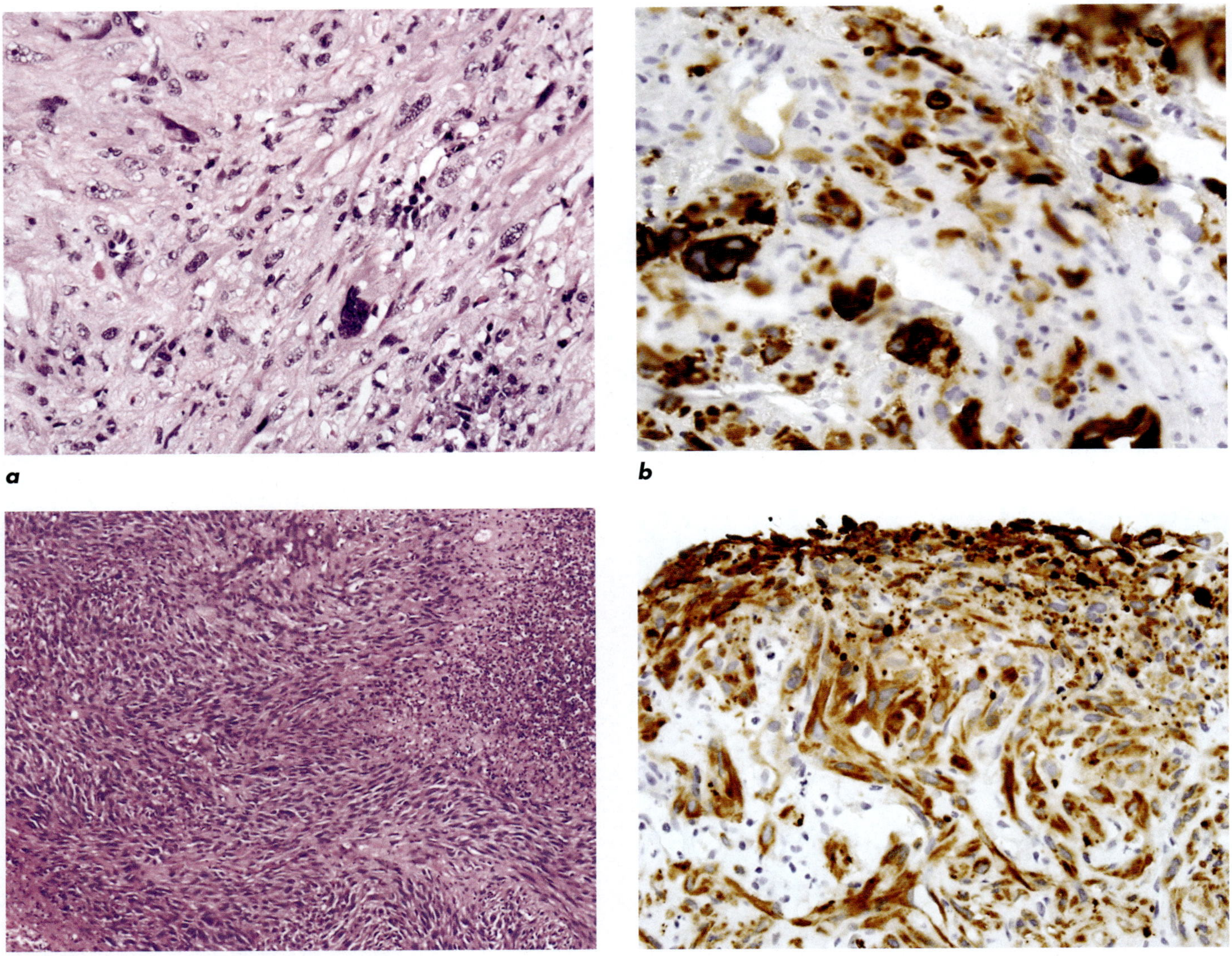

Figure 52-35.
Carcinosarcoma of the bladder is signified by the pleomorphic sarcomatoid component (*a*), which is positive for CK20 (*b*), or a spindle cell sarcomatoid component (*c*), which is confirmed by the positive AE1/AE3 immunoreactivity (*d*).

Molecular analysis

- Molecular analysis has shown that both carcinomatous and sarcomatous components are derived from the same cell origin, suggesting the dedifferentiation

Clinical relevance (prognosis and treatment options)

- Worse prognosis than typical high-grade urothelial carcinoma
- Cystectomy with or without adjuvant therapy should be considered

METASTATIC UROTHELIAL CARCINOMA FROM THE BLADDER

Definition

- Urothelial carcinoma metastasizes from the bladder (or another site of the urinary tract) to other organs
- A clinical history of bladder urothelial carcinoma is preferred for such a diagnosis

Histology

- Urothelial carcinoma may display a wide range of morphologic variants, which makes the diagnosis and identification of a urothelial primary very difficult with a history
- The most common sites include pelvic lymph nodes (Fig. 52-36)
- The metastatic tumor can be bulky or a minute focus as individual cells, similar to breast lobular carcinoma, which can easily escape recognition
- The size of the metastatic foci and presence of extranodal extension should be documented
- Urothelial carcinoma with lymph node metastasis carries a very poor prognosis with only less than 10% survival for more than 5 years without effective treatment
- The second most common site is the lung. Many other organs are possible sites for metastatic urothelial carcinoma
- The primary tumors are always high grade. Without a clinical history, the urothelial carcinoma can be difficult to recognize in a metastatic site (Figs. 52-37 and 52-38)
    - Sometimes, there is resemblance of urothelium (Fig. 52-39). But oftentimes, the tumor cells are highly pleomorphic with relatively abundant cytoplasm (Fig. 52-40)
- Squamous and glandular differentiation in metastatic urothelial carcinoma is possible but uncommon

Immunohistochemistry

- Several urothelial markers may be helpful such as p63, CK20, GATA3, and S100P (Figs. 52-39 and 52-40)

Figure 52-36.
Metastatic urothelial carcinoma in a pelvic lymph node, which is entirely replaced by the tumor (*a*). High magnification shows the presence of a high-grade carcinoma that can be different to determine the origin (*b*).

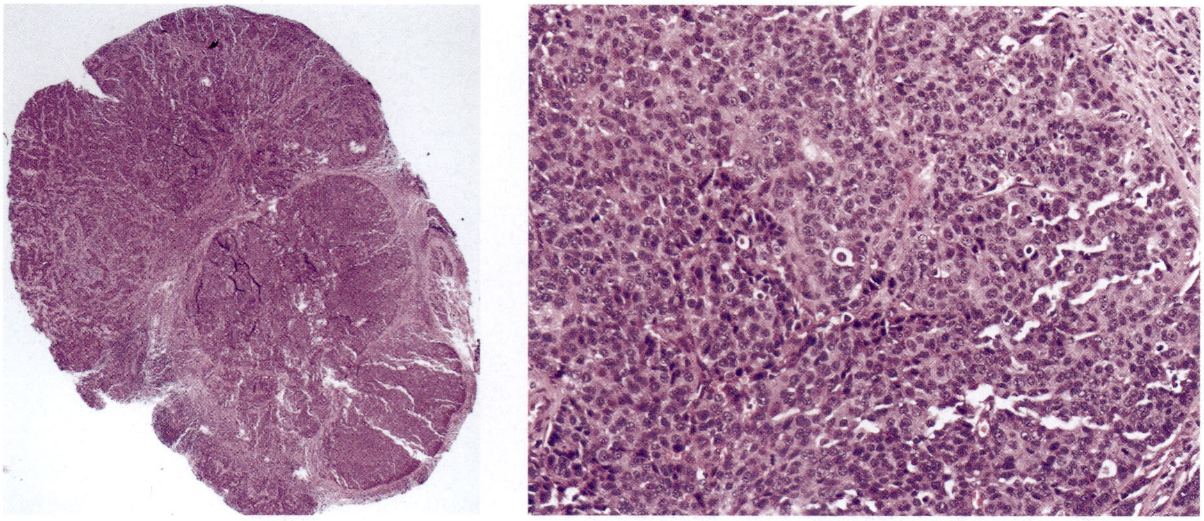

a **b**

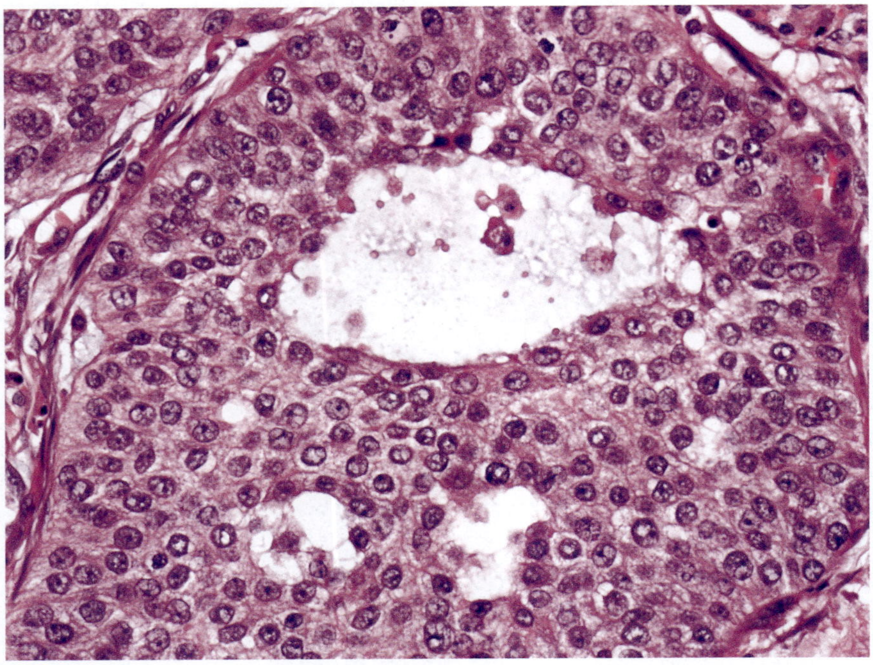

Figure 52-37.
Metastatic urothelial carcinoma can mimic adenocarcinoma or squamous cell carcinoma.

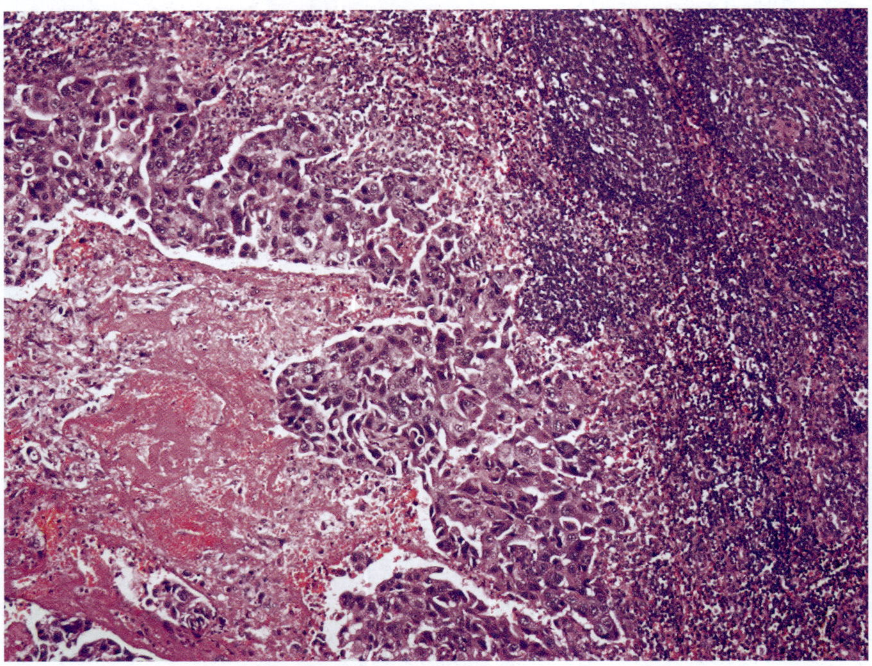

Figure 52-38.
Metastatic urothelial carcinoma in a pelvic lymph node with necrosis.

Clinicopathological features

- High-grade invasive urothelial carcinomas are responsible for the vast majority of metastasis from the bladder
- Metastasis in regional lymph nodes should be recognized and reported specifically (specifying a metastatic urothelial carcinoma, not metastatic prostatic adenocarcinoma). Generally, metastatic urothelial carcinoma carries a very poor prognosis. The survival may be improved with contemporary chemotherapy

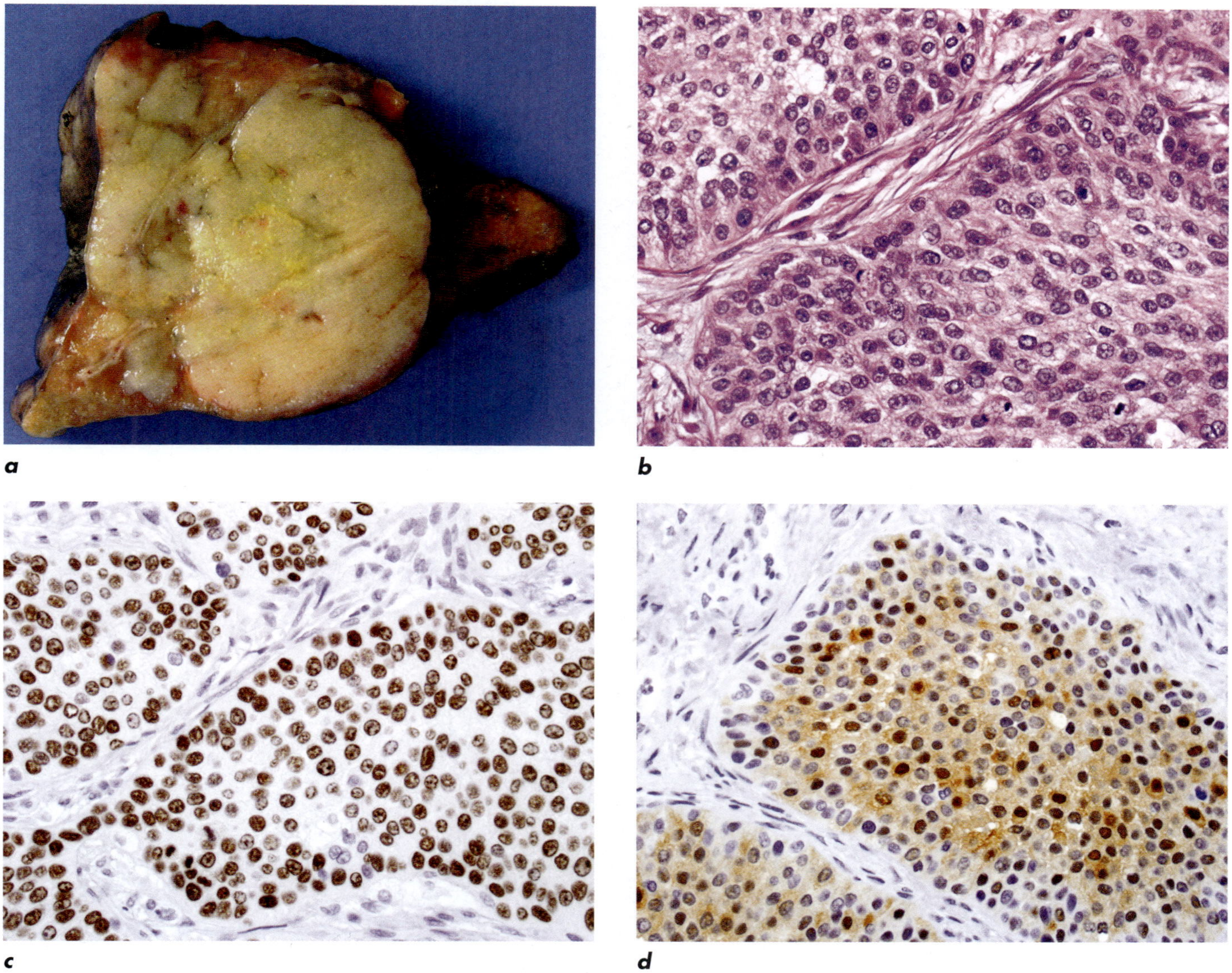

Figure 52-39.
Gross photo of metastatic urothelial carcinoma in the lung demonstrates a large solid well-defined mass in the lung (*a*). Microscopically, the tumor shows the features of urothelial carcinoma with large islands of cells (*b*). Immunostains highlight the tumor cells positive for p63 (*c*) and S100P (*d*).

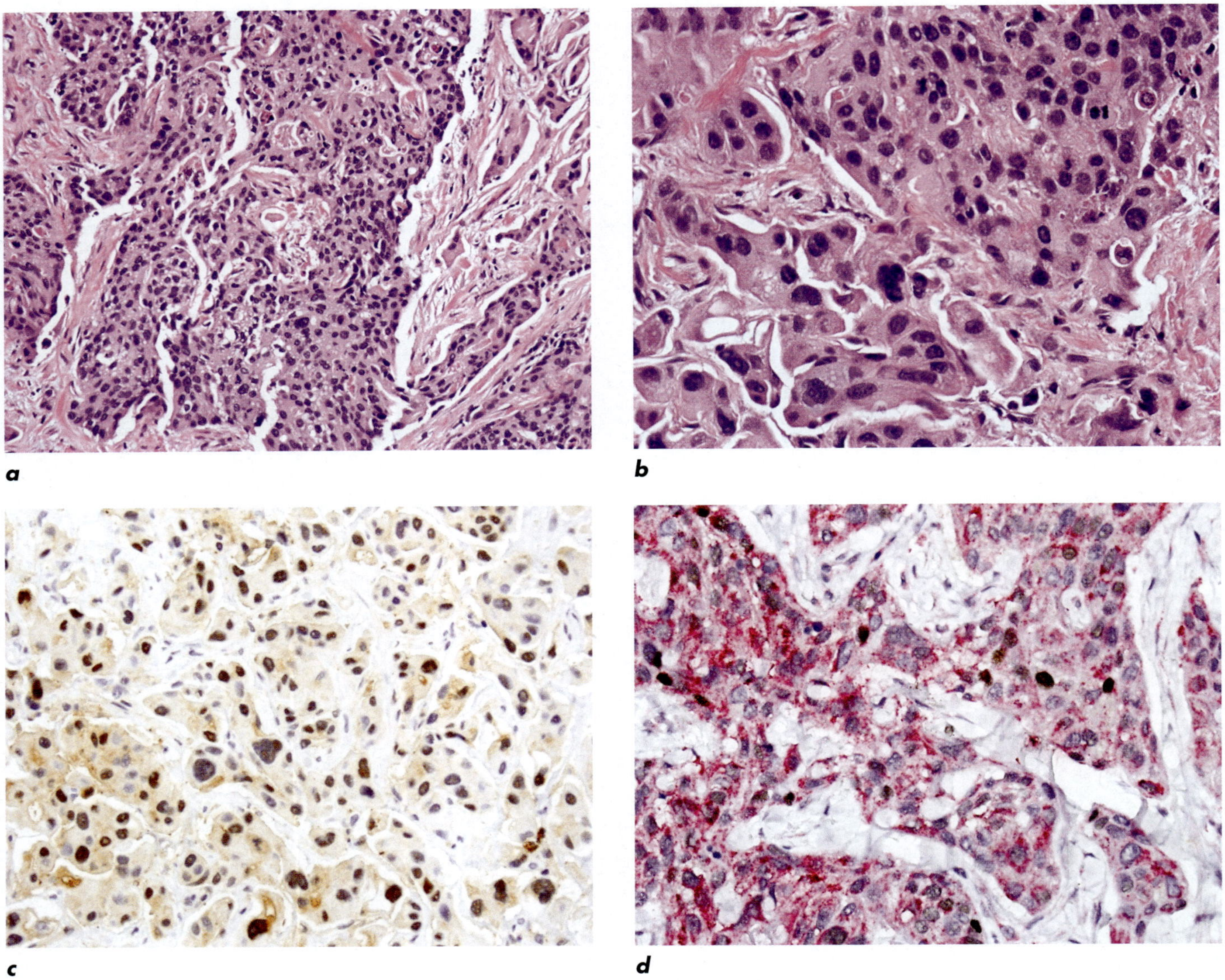

Figure 52-40.
Metastatic urothelial carcinoma in the retroperitoneal area. The tumor cells form large nests (*a*). High magnification shows the large pleomorphic tumor cells with abundant cytoplasm (*b*). Immunostains confirm the diagnosis of urothelial carcinoma with S100P nuclear positivity (*c*) and immunoreactivity for both p63 and HMWCK and mild AMACR staining (*d*, triple staining).

CHAPTER 53

Malignant Glandular Lesions of the Bladder

UROTHELIAL CARCINOMA WITH GLANDULAR DIFFERENTIATION

Definition

- Glandular differentiation of urothelial carcinoma is defined as the presence of true glandular spaces lined by tumor cells within urothelial carcinoma
- Both urothelial and glandular carcinomatous components are present

Pathogenesis

- Urothelial carcinoma has a great capacity for morphological plasticity. Particularly, high-grade invasive urothelial carcinoma often shows divergent differentiation, such as glandular, squamous, or neuroendocrine differentiation
- Glandular differentiation, less common than squamous differentiation, is the second most common form of divergent differentiation of urothelial carcinoma

Clinical features

- Same as typical urothelial carcinoma

Gross pathology

- Same as typical invasive urothelial carcinoma, typically one or multiple large papillary masses

Histology

- Different from adenocarcinoma, which is composed of entirely malignant glandular structures (a pure adenocarcinoma) without typical urothelial carcinoma component, urothelial carcinoma with glandular differentiation is classified as urothelial carcinoma with glandular differentiation regardless of the extent of the glandular differentiation (Figs. 53-1 and 53-2)
- Some findings may help distinguish urothelial carcinoma with glandular differentiation from adenocarcinoma of the bladder (in additional to malignant glandular component)
  - Presence of invasive urothelial carcinoma (Fig. 53-3)
  - Presence of squamous components (Fig. 53-3)
  - Presence of urothelial carcinoma in situ
- The glandular structures are lined by cuboidal or columnar tumor cells
- Urothelial carcinoma with goblet cell differentiation is considered a special form of glandular differentiation, although its significance is less known (Fig. 53-4)

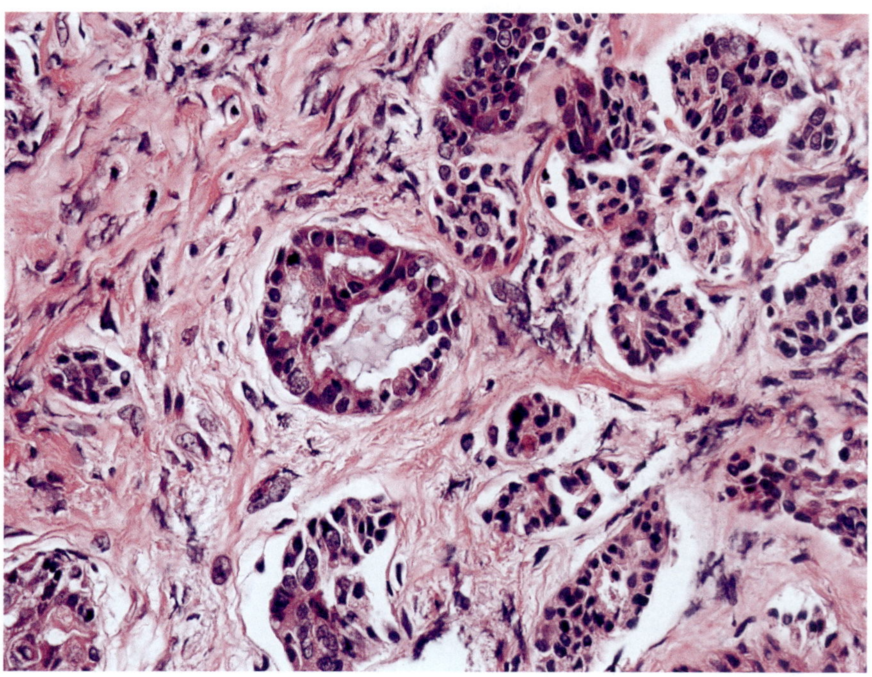

Figure 53-1.
High-grade urothelial carcinoma with glandular differentiation. Several clusters of invasive urothelial carcinoma cells exhibit glandular differentiation and a small amount of mucinous secretion in the lumen.

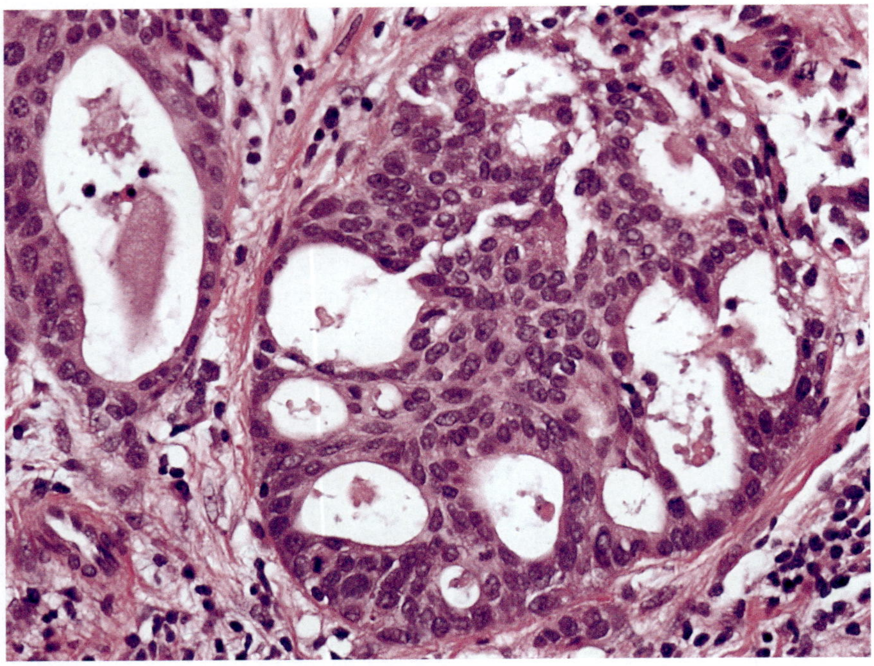

Figure 53-2.
Urothelial carcinoma with glandular differentiation as cribriform pattern.

- However, it can be difficult to differentiate urothelial carcinoma with glandular differentiation from adenocarcinoma on bladder biopsies because of the limited sampling

Immunohistochemistry

- Not well studied

Differential diagnosis

Pseudoglandular differentiation in benign urothelium

- Benign urothelium can occasionally show glandular differentiation
- It is a reactive change to inflammation or other stimulus
- This lesion is generally very small within reactive urothelium, without cytological atypia

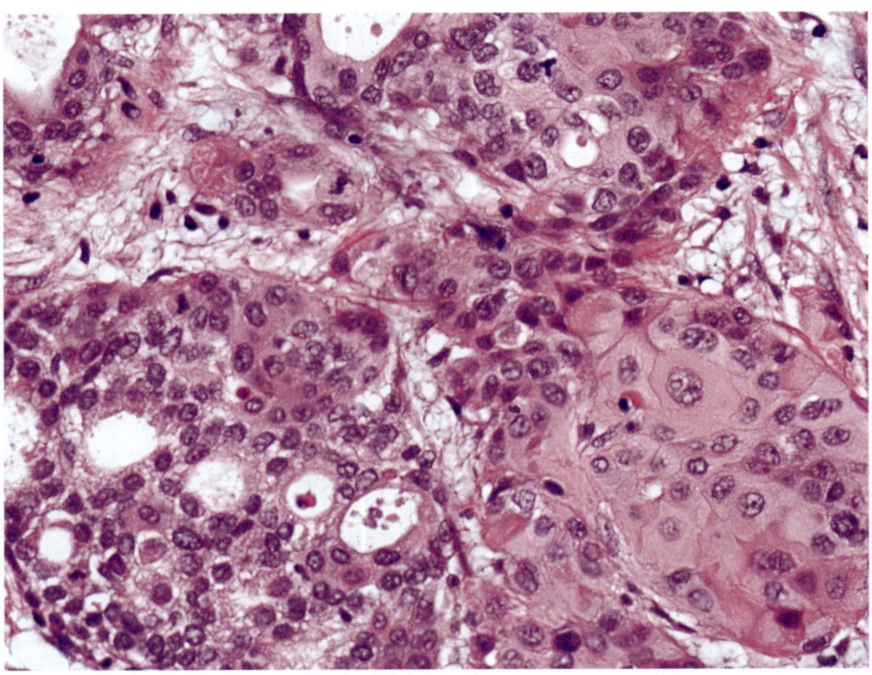

Figure 53-3.
Urothelial carcinoma with both glandular (left) and squamous differentiations (right).

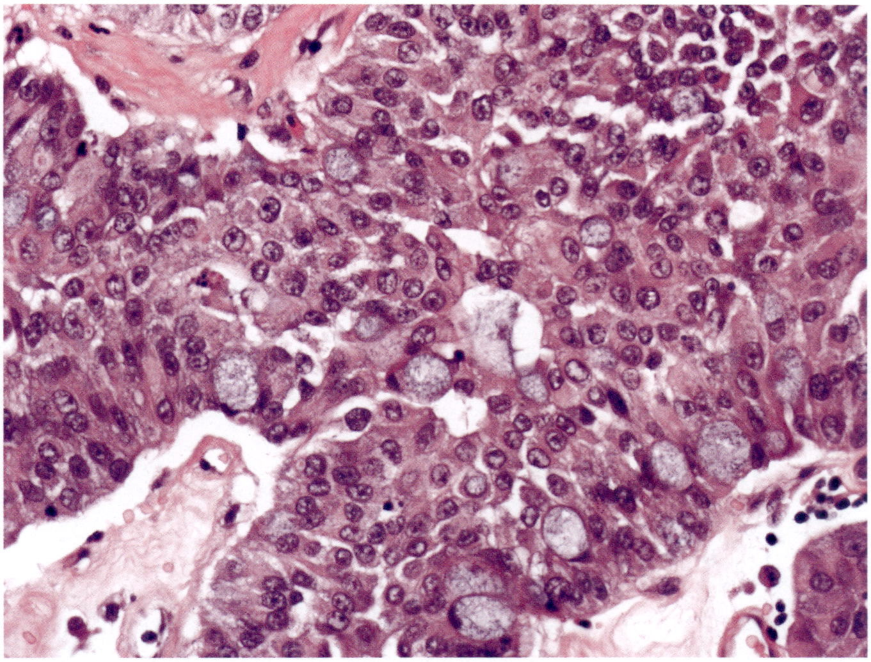

Figure 53-4.
Urothelial carcinoma with goblet cell differentiation.

Urothelial CIS involving von Brunn nests (Fig. 53-5)

- Urothelial CIS involving von Brunn nests with glandular differentiation (cystitis glandularis). The presence of benign urothelium in the nest is the key

Pseudoglandular differentiation in urothelial carcinoma (Figs. 53-6 and 53-7)

- Urothelial carcinoma, both low grade and high grade, may show small intracytoplasmic spaces (microcysts), which are very common in urothelial carcinoma
- The microcysts are often filled with cell debris, but lacking cuboidal or columnar epithelial lining
- Because its high frequency in the majority of urothelial carcinoma, these structures should not be classified glandular differentiation

Adenocarcinoma

- Pure malignant glandular patterns, no urothelial carcinoma component

Clinical relevance (prognosis and treatment options)

- Similar to typical urothelial carcinoma. Radical cystectomy is indicated if muscle invasive tumor is identified
- The clinical significance of glandular differentiation remains unclear. It may be depending on the extent of glandular differentiation, which may affect the choice of therapy
- Some studies suggested that focal glandular differentiation of urothelial carcinoma did not correlate with a poor prognosis in patients with radical cystectomy
- However, more recent studies suggested that the presence of glandular differentiation in urothelial carcinoma may be associated with a poorer response to systemic neoadjuvant chemotherapy than typical urothelial carcinoma.
- More studies are necessary to substantiate these observations

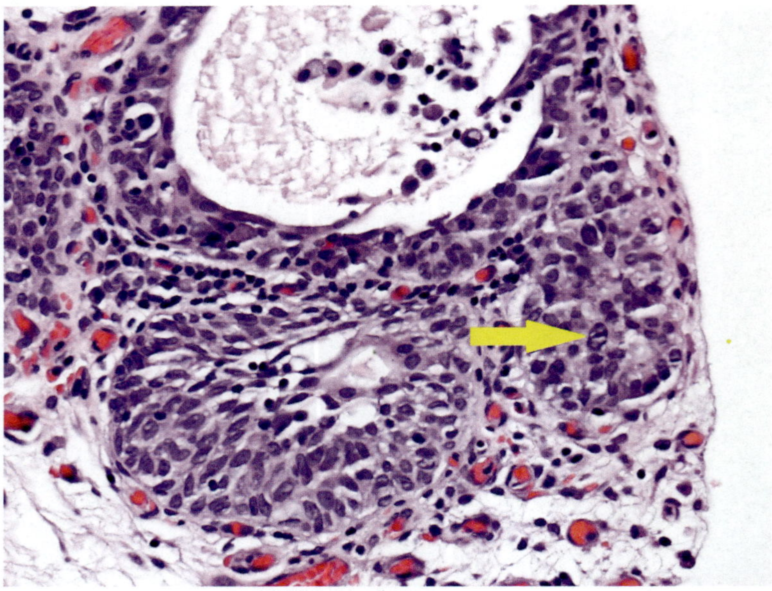

Figure 53-5.
Urothelial carcinoma in situ (arrow) involving cystitis glandularis mimicking glandular differentiation.

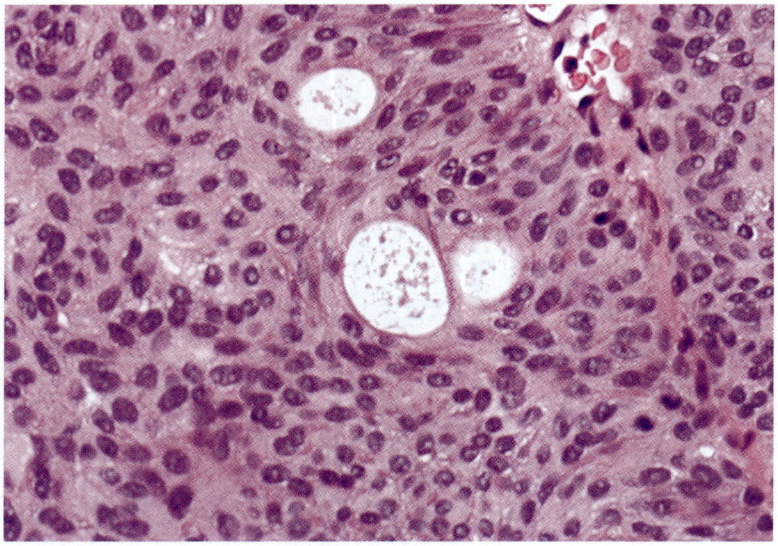

Figure 53-6.
Microcyst formation (pseudoglandular differentiation) in a low-grade noninvasive urothelial carcinoma mimicking glandular differentiation.

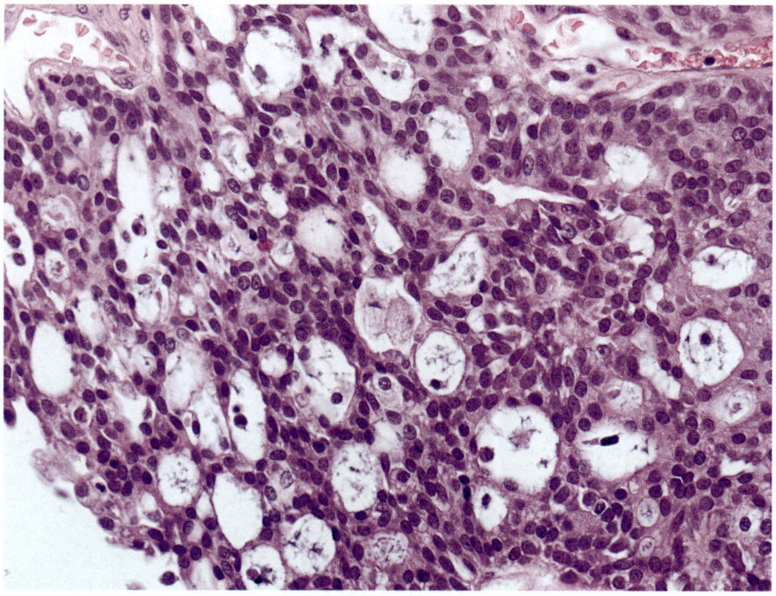

Figure 53-7.
Urothelial carcinoma with extensive microcyst formation (pseudoglandular differentiation). Cell debris can be seen in most of the spaces.

ADENOCARCINOMA IN SITU OF THE BLADDER

Definition

- Adenocarcinoma in situ is a noninvasive glandular lesion derived from urothelium, characterized by malignant columnar epithelium with apical cytoplasm

Other term

- Noninvasive urothelial carcinoma with glandular differentiation

Clinical features

- Adenocarcinoma in situ, an uncommon entity, is usually associated with invasive urothelial carcinoma of the bladder. Therefore, the term *noninvasive urothelial carcinoma with glandular differentiation* may be more appropriate
- The clinical outcome is most determined by the invasive carcinoma component
- We have observed adenocarcinoma in situ coexisting with invasive urothelial carcinoma and small cell carcinoma in the same case

Gross pathology

- Often a small lesion with papillary, cribriform, and flat architectural patterns
- It may also depend on the appearance of associated invasive component

Histology

- Adenocarcinoma in situ of the bladder is characterized by the malignant cuboidal or columnar epithelial cells (Figs. 53-8 and 53-9) confined within the basement membrane
- The tumor cells are single layer or pseudostratified, resembling adenocarcinoma in situ of the colon (Figs. 53-9 and 53-10)
- In most cases, adenocarcinoma in situ cells are high nuclear grade, arranged in flat or papillary patterns (Fig. 53-11)
- Other types of carcinoma components are often coexisting, such as typical invasive urothelial carcinoma (Fig. 53-12), small cell carcinoma (Fig. 53-13), or micropapillary carcinoma
- Urothelial carcinomas with microcystic changes or urothelial carcinoma involving von Brunn nests, neither of which is lined by columnar epithelium and, therefore, they should not be confused with adenocarcinoma in situ

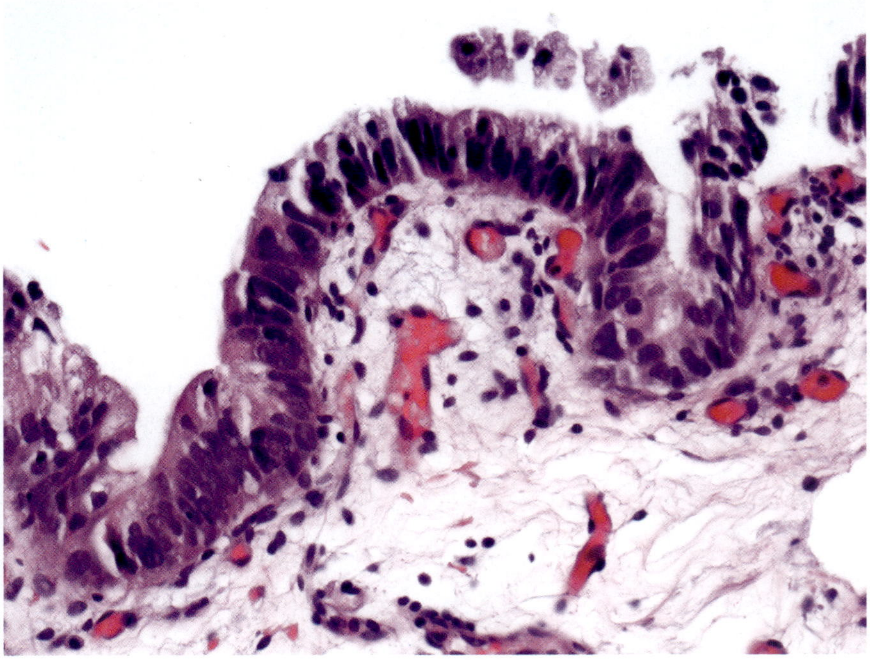

Figure 53-8.
Adenocarcinoma in situ of the bladder is characterized by the presence of malignant columnar cells confined within the basement membrane. The tumor cells have elongated nuclei with hyperchromasia and cytological atypia.

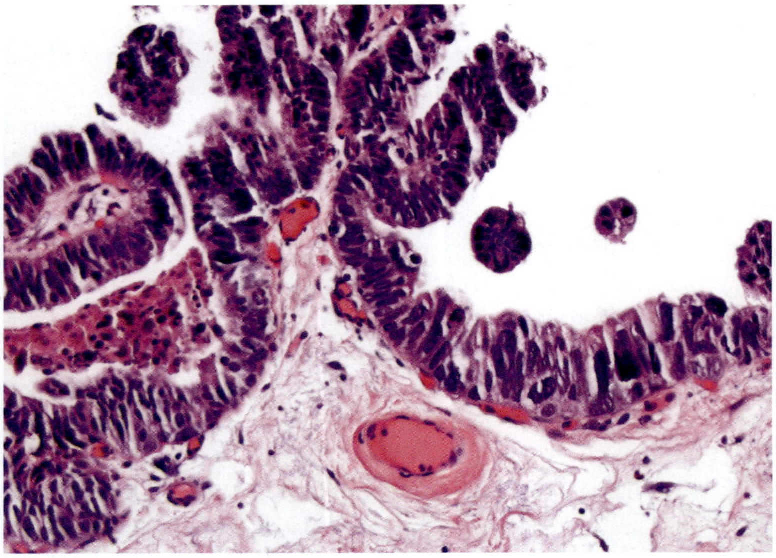

Figure 53-9.
Adenocarcinoma in situ with malignant columnar cells in a papillary configuration confined within the basement membrane.

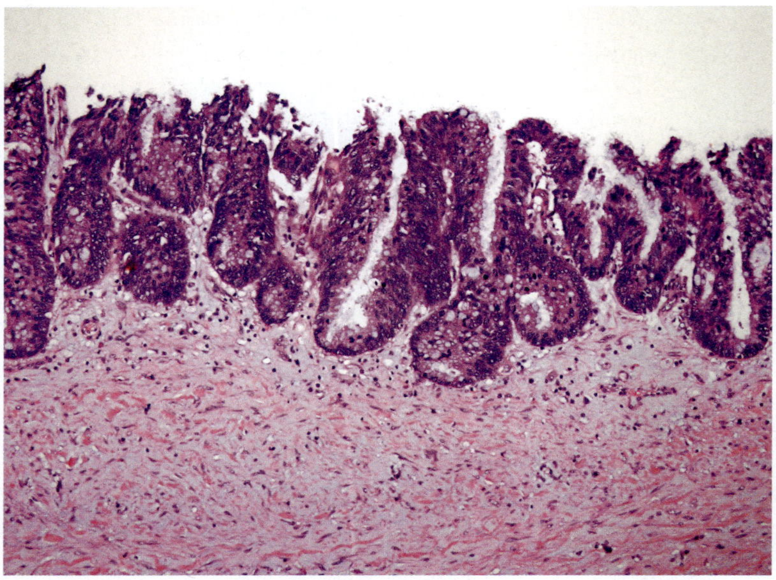

Figure 53-10.
Adenocarcinoma in situ composed of a single layer of cuboidal malignant cells covering fibrovascular cores of the papillary structures.

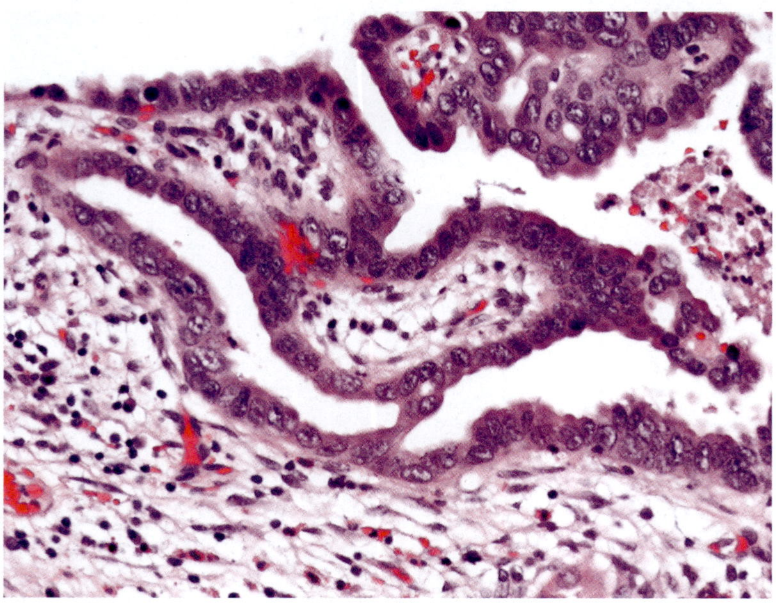

Figure 53-11.
Adenocarcinoma in situ composed of pseudostratified columnar malignant cells, with focal mucinous differentiation without invasion.

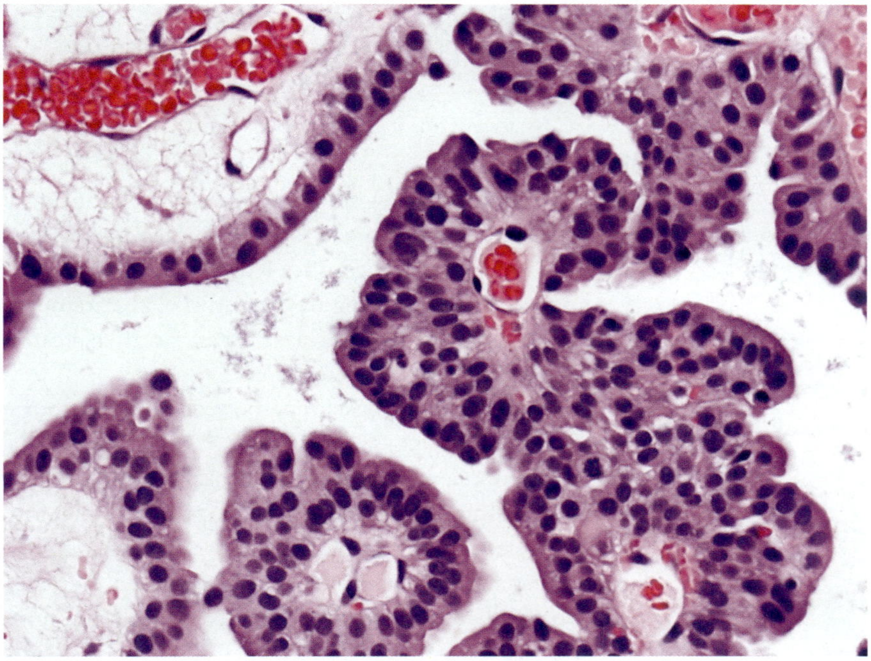

Figure 53-12.
Adenocarcinoma in situ (left) associated with noninvasive papillary urothelial carcinoma (right).

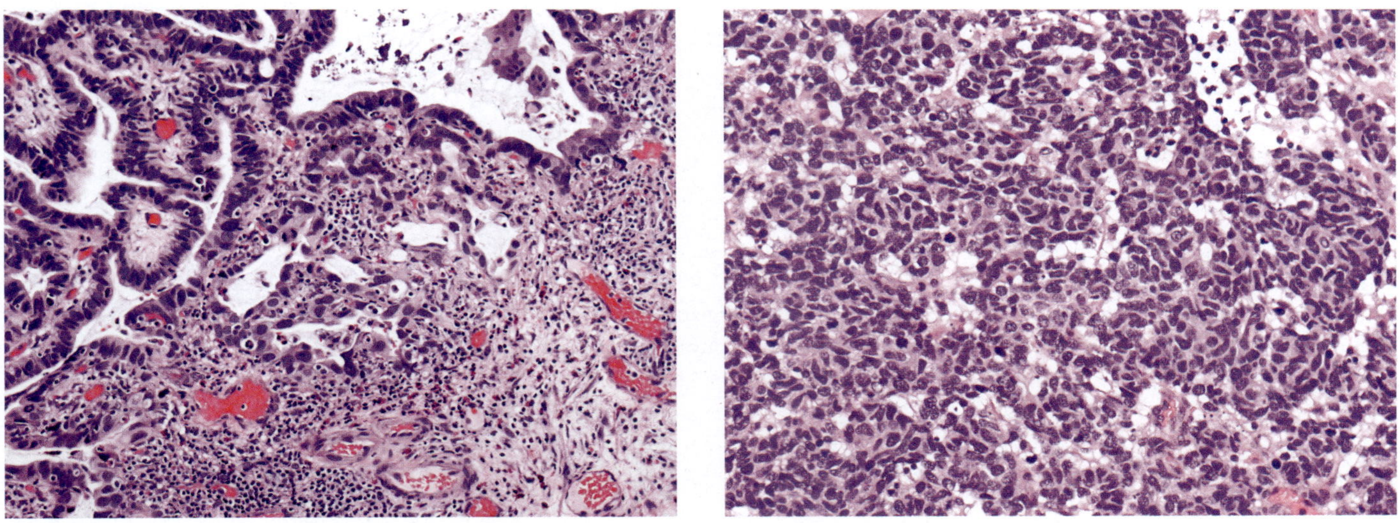

a **b**

Figure 53-13.
Adenocarcinoma in situ (*a*, left) coexisting with invasive urothelial carcinoma (*a*, middle) and small cell carcinoma component (*b*) in one case.

Immunohistochemistry

- Not known, probably similar to invasive urothelial carcinoma

Clinical relevance (prognosis and treatment options)

- If adenocarcinoma in situ is detected on a biopsy without invasive tumor, rebiopsy should be considered because of its frequent association with high-grade invasive carcinoma
- The patient with adenocarcinoma in situ of the bladder usually has a poor prognosis because of its association high-grade invasive tumors with an aggressive behavior
- Treatment is dependent on the invasive urothelial carcinoma, in most cases radical cystectomy is indicated when muscle invasive tumor is present
- The systemic chemotherapy may be necessary if small cell carcinoma component is present

PRIMARY ADENOCARCINOMA

Definition

- Malignant epithelial neoplasm is entirely composed of glandular component (100% or pure adenocarcinoma) in the bladder
- No typical urothelial carcinoma component present. Otherwise, it should be named as urothelial carcinoma with glandular differentiation

Pathogenesis and epidemiology

- The pathogenesis of primary adenocarcinoma of the urinary bladder is still unknown
- Intestinal metaplasia has been speculated as a precursor lesion, because its high concurrence rate with primary adenocarcinoma of the urinary bladder
- Primary adenocarcinoma of the urinary bladder is a rare malignancy
- This tumor is more common in males than females with a mean age 60 years

Clinical features

- Hematuria, dysuria, and lower abdominal mass
- Occasionally mucosuria if the tumor is predominantly mucinous

Gross pathology

- Large mass with necrosis and ulceration with mucinous cut surface

Histology

- Diagnosis of a primary adenocarcinoma of the urinary bladder should only be made for a carcinoma with a pure glandular component (Figs. 53-14 and 53-15)
- A tumor contains a recognizable urothelial carcinoma component, which should be classified as urothelial carcinoma with glandular differentiation
- Benign intestinal metaplasia may be seen adjacent to the tumor
- Tubular adenoma may be seen in the background
- Adenocarcinoma cells form glands, papillary, cribriform, or tubular structures, sometimes signet rings (Fig. 53-16)
- Several histological variants have been observed. But they can be basically divided into two groups (enteric and non-enteric types) based on histology

Enteric type

- Typical intestinal type
  - Composed of tall columnar tumor cells with abundant eosinophilic cytoplasm
  - With or without central necrosis

Figure 53-14.
Primary bladder adenocarcinoma, enteric type, is composed of malignant glands (*a*). High magnification shows the tall columnar tumor cells with goblet cells invading lamina propria (*b*).

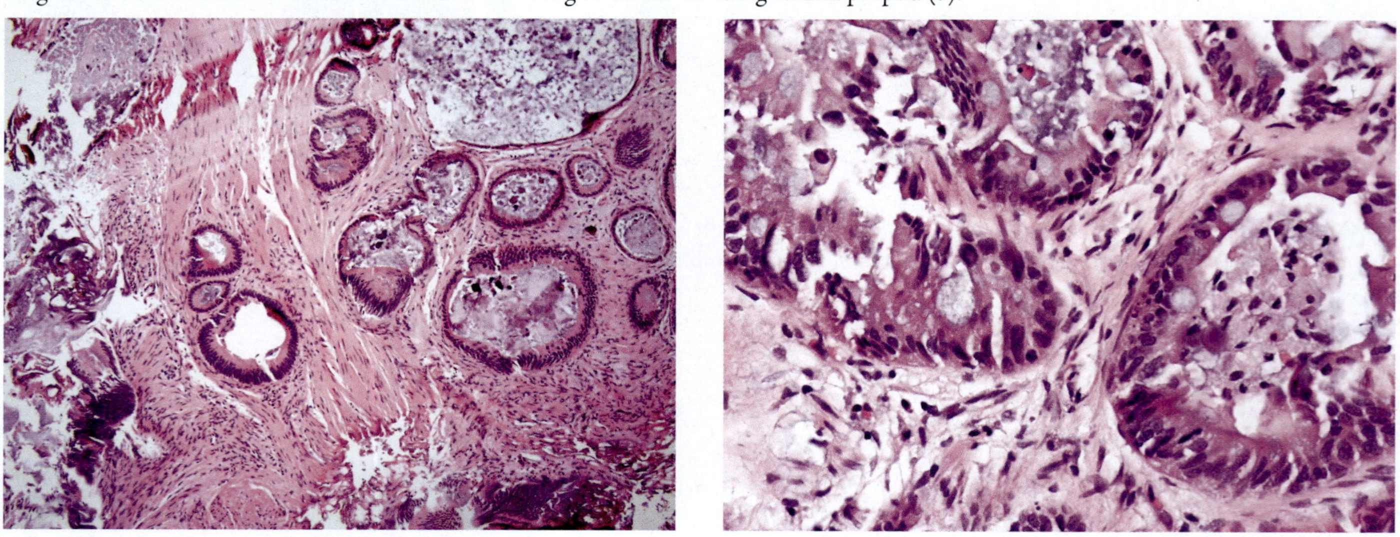

a **b**

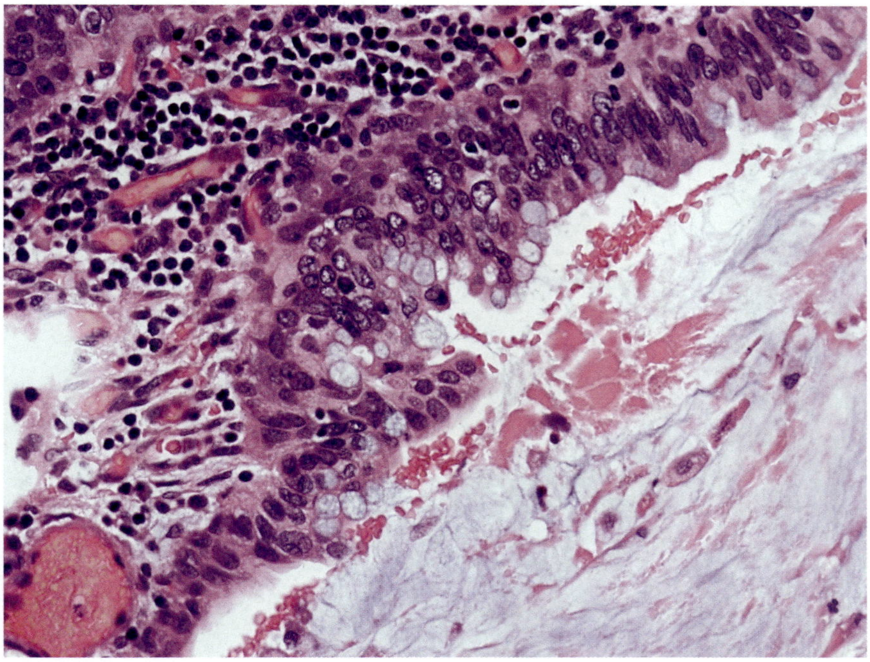

Figure 53-15.
Primary bladder adenocarcinoma, enteric type, with goblet cell differentiation and mucinous pool.

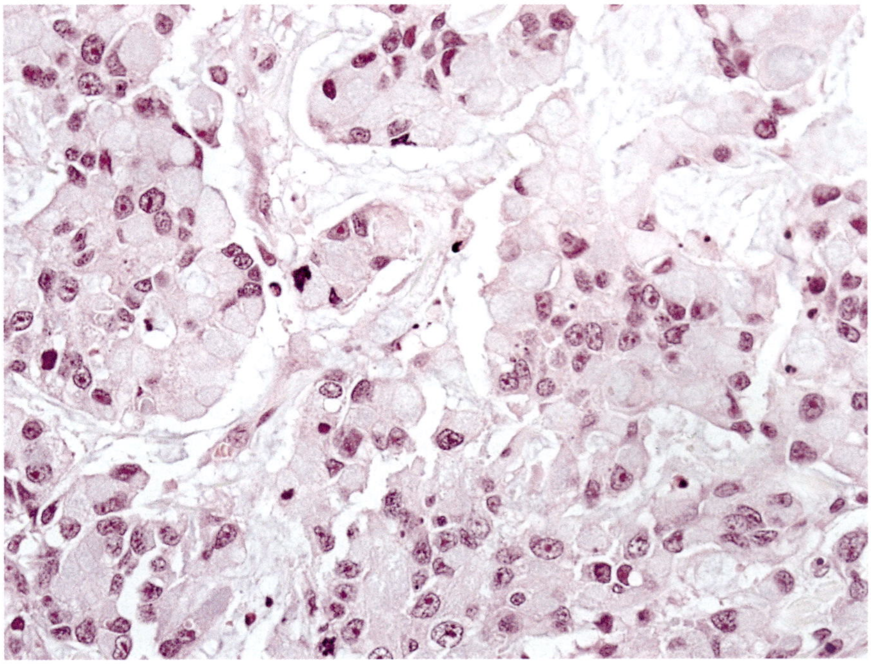

Figure 53-16.
Primary signet ring cell adenocarcinoma of the bladder with mucin-containing signet ring cells.

- With focal goblet cell differentiation
- Morphologically identical to colon adenocarcinoma (Fig. 53-14)

- Mucinous type

Predominant mucinous component

- Large pools of extracellular mucin mixed with collections of tumor cells (Figs. 53-15 and 53-17*a*)
- The mucinous components should constitute at least half of the tumor mass

- Signet ring type
    - Presence of mucin-containing signet ring tumor cells (Fig. 53-16)
    - The signet ring cells may demonstrate a plasmacytoid or monocytoid appearance with a large cytoplasmic vacuole
    - Diffuse patterns
    - Often associated with mucinous-type or enteric-type adenocarcinoma

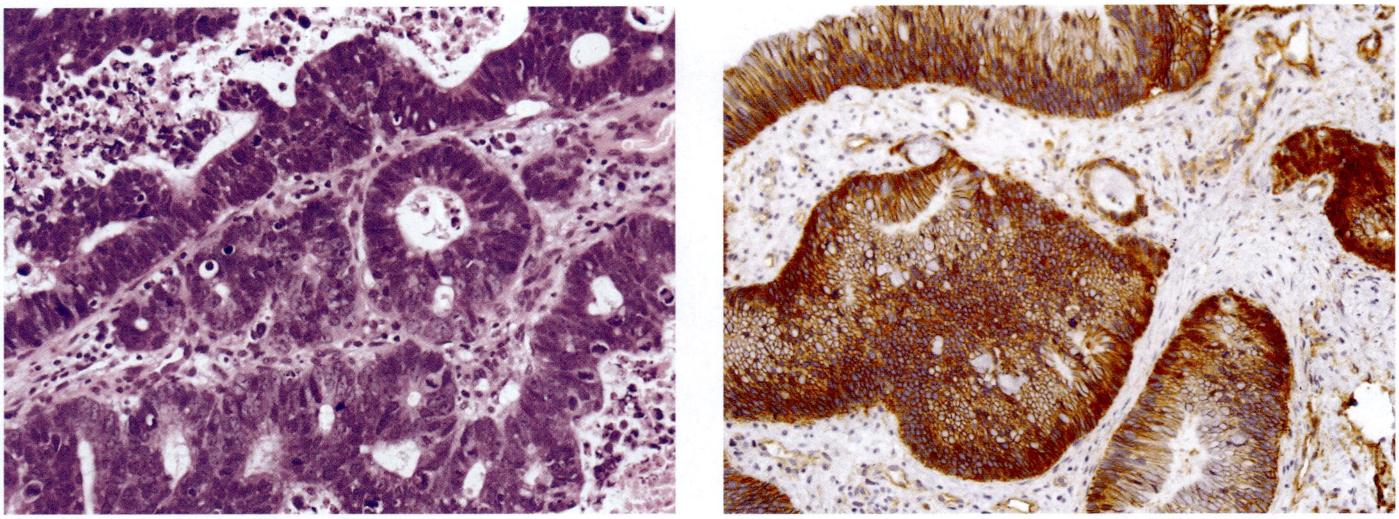

a b

Figure 53-17.
Primary adenocarcinoma of the bladder, enteric type, composed of colonic-type tall columnar cells (*a*). β-Catenin stain shows negative nuclear staining (*b*).

Nonenteric type

- Not otherwise specified
  - Composed of malignant cuboidal or columnar cells (Fig. 53-18)
- Clear cell adenocarcinoma (will be discussed later in this chapter)
  - Composed of clear cells
  - Similar to be in female genital organs

Immunohistochemistry

- Enteric type similar to colonic adenocarcinoma, nonenteric type displays variable immunostaining
- Generally tumor cells are
  - Positive for CK20, CDX2, variable positivity for CK7
  - Positive for p63, HMWCK, CK5/6
  - Positive for AMACR. β-Catenin negative (no nuclear staining) (Fig. 53-17*b*)

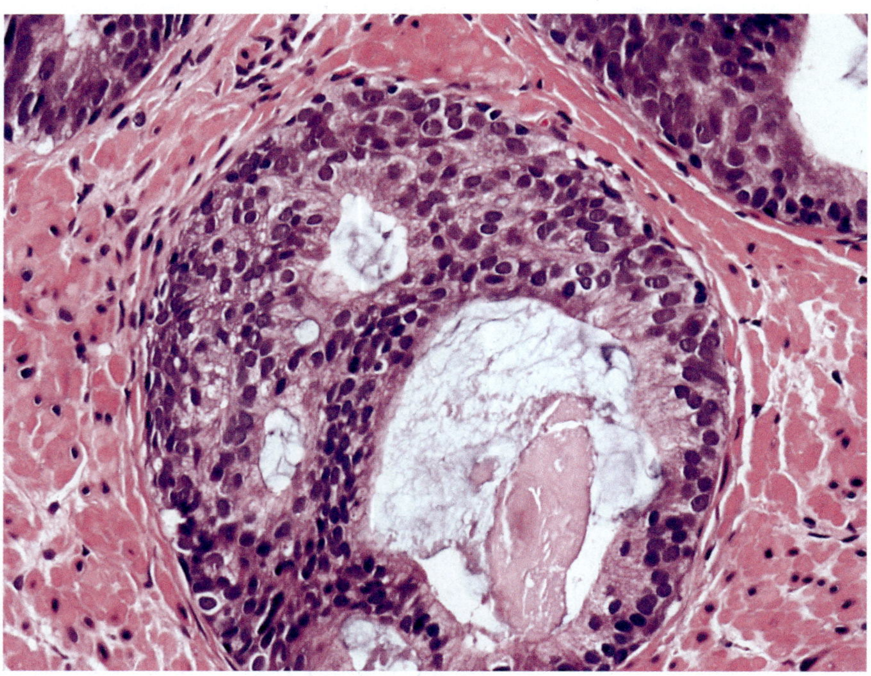

Figure 53-18.
Adenocarcinoma of the bladder, not otherwise specified.

Differential diagnosis (see Table 53-1)

Secondary adenocarcinoma

- The most common secondary adenocarcinomas involving the bladder are prostatic adenocarcinoma and colonic adenocarcinoma
- Other common secondary adenocarcinomas in the bladder are carcinoma of the breast, lung, and endometrium

Clinical relevance (prognosis and treatment options)

- When a diagnosis of adenocarcinoma of the bladder is made, one cannot assume that it is a primary tumor
- Typically a GI work up with image studies are required to exclude adenocarcinoma from other organs secondarily involve the bladder
- As pathologists, we should try our best to apply immunohistochemical markers to obtain some important information of the origin of the tumor
- Adenocarcinoma of the bladder is generally an aggressive tumor, with metastatic rate of up to 40%
- They are usually present at an advanced stage at diagnosis, therefore, with a poor prognosis
- However, in large studies, stage- and grade-adjusted cancer-specific mortality is the same between patients with primary adenocarcinomas or advanced urothelial carcinomas
- With limited cases, we also noticed that adenocarcinoma of the bladder did not respond well to the neoadjuvant therapy designed for urothelial carcinoma
- Radical cystectomy is treatment of choice if it is localized disease

Table 53-1. Comparison of Urachal Adenocarcinoma with Primary Bladder Adenocarcinoma and Colonic Adenocarcinoma

	Urachal adenocarcinoma	*Primary adenocarcinoma*	*Secondary colonic adenocarcinoma*
Urachal remnants	May be present	Absent	Absent
Location at dome	Yes	Anywhere	Anywhere
Umbilicus involved	Possible	No	No
Urothelial CIS	No	Possible	No
Extensive cystitis glandularis	No	Yes	No
Glandular dysplasia	Possible in urachal remnant	Yes	No
Colonic metaplasia	Uncommon	Common	No
CK7	Positive	Positive/negative	Negative
CK20	Positive	Positive/negative	Positive
CDX2	Positive/negative	Positive	Positive
β-Catenin	Negative	Negative	Positive

CK7, cytokeratin 7; CK20, cytokeratin 20.

URACHAL ADENOCARCINOMA

Definition

- A special type of primary adenocarcinoma derived from urachal remnants
- The strict diagnostic criteria should be the adenocarcinoma arises in the background of urachal remnants
- However, for many cases without urachal remnants, the following criteria for urachal adenocarcinoma are used:
  - Location in the bladder dome
  - Sharp demarcation between tumor and surface benign urothelium
  - Exclusion of other primary adenocarcinoma
- Some features favoring urachal carcinoma including
  - The tumor centered in the muscularis propria with or without involving urothelium
  - Absence of extensive cystitis glandularis
  - Absence of urothelial carcinoma in situ
  - Presence of transition from dysplasia to carcinoma

Pathogenesis

- Urachal carcinoma is a carcinoma derived from urachal remnants
- However, urachal urothelial carcinoma is rarely diagnosed because it has no morphological difference or clinical significance from typical urothelial carcinoma
- Presence of urothelial carcinoma does not exclude the diagnosis of urachal adenocarcinoma

Clinical features

- Usually in the fifth and sixth decades of life, approximately 10 years younger than patients with primary adenocarcinoma of the bladder. More common in men than in women
- Typical symptoms and signs of bladder urothelial carcinoma, such hematuria, urgency, and frequency, can be present in patients with urachal adenocarcinoma
- One specific symptom is leaking mucinous material from the umbilicus or mucosuria (mucinous urine)
- Another sign highly suggestive of urachal adenocarcinoma is the presence of a mass located between the umbilicus and bladder dome

Gross pathology

- Tumor located in the dome of the bladder, often deep in the muscularis propria or superior portion of the bladder (Figs. 53-19 and 53-20)
- In the case with urothelial involvement, an ulcerative mass is present
- Mucinous or myxoid cut surface is common (Fig. 53-20*b*)

Histology

- Practically, urachal adenocarcinoma is primary adenocarcinoma located in the dome, after the exclusion of other types of malignant glandular lesions of the bladder
- Presence of invasive adenocarcinoma, enteric type with or without mucinous differentiation (Figs. 53-19 and 53-20)
- Mostly high-grade enteric-type adenocarcinoma including mucinous and signet ring types with extensive extravasated mucin may be seen (Fig. 53-20*e*)
- Urachal remnants with or without dysplasia are observed only in a subset of cases (Fig. 53-21)

Immunohistochemistry

- CK20/CK7: positive (similar to urothelial carcinoma)
- CDX2: positive (similar to colon carcinoma)
- β-Catenin: negative nuclear staining (different from colon carcinoma)

Clinical relevance (prognosis and treatment options)

- Overall and disease-specific mortality is slightly better in patients with urachal adenocarcinoma compared to patients with nonurachal adenocarcinoma
- The prognosis is worse if the tumor is signet ring type
- Treatment of choice is partial cystectomy (for localized disease) or radical cystectomy (for extensive disease) with or without resection of umbilicus
- Adjuvant chemotherapy may have some value

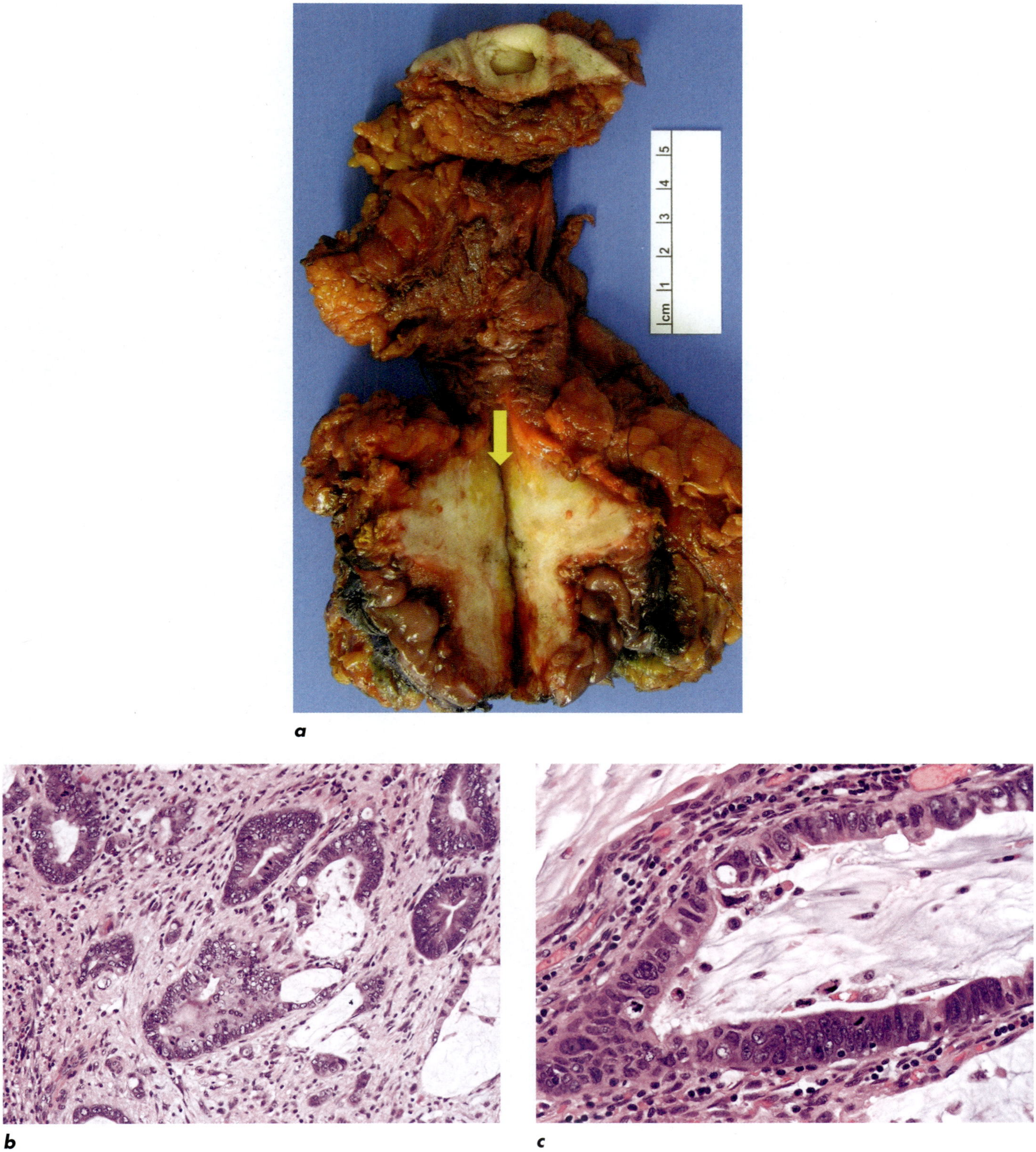

Figure 53-19.
Urachal adenocarcinoma of the bladder dome from a partial cystectomy. The tumor (*a*, arrow) is deeply seeded with intact mucosa; the umbilicus is at the top. Microscopically, this is an invasive enteric-type adenocarcinoma (*b*) with mucinous differentiation (*c*).

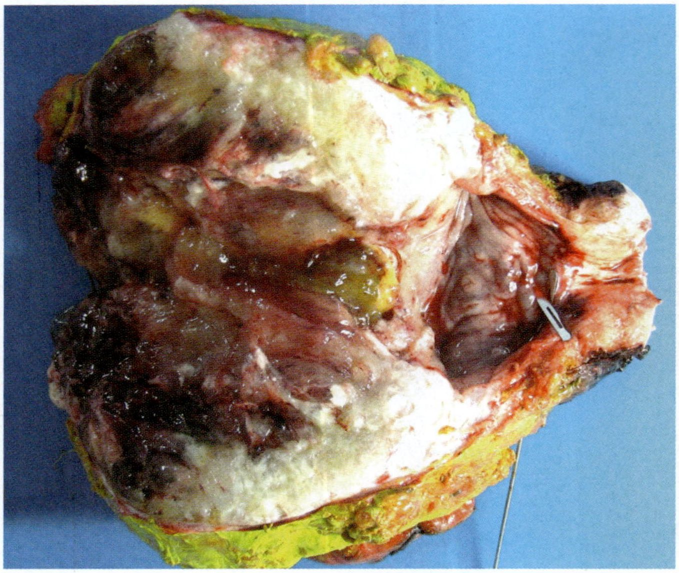

a

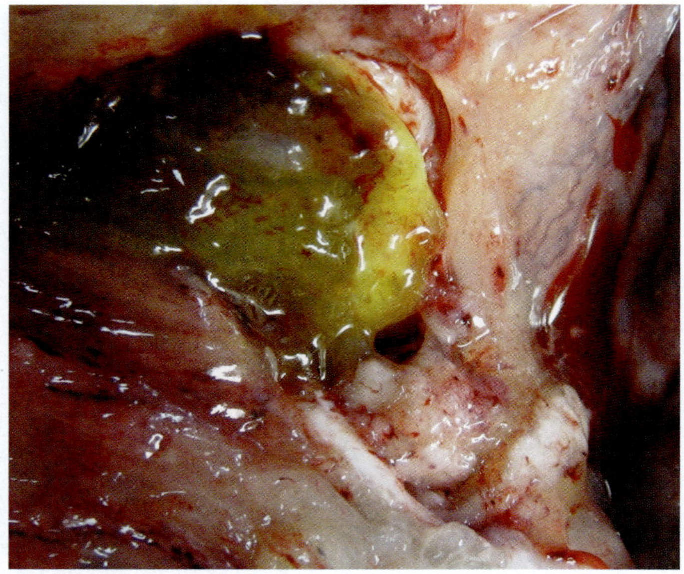

b

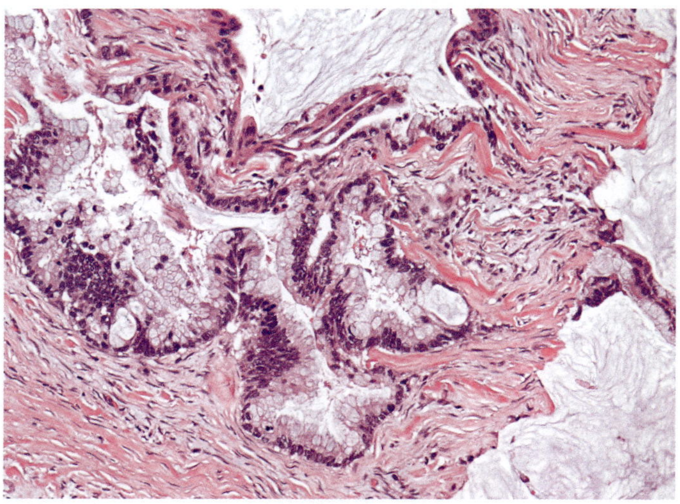

c

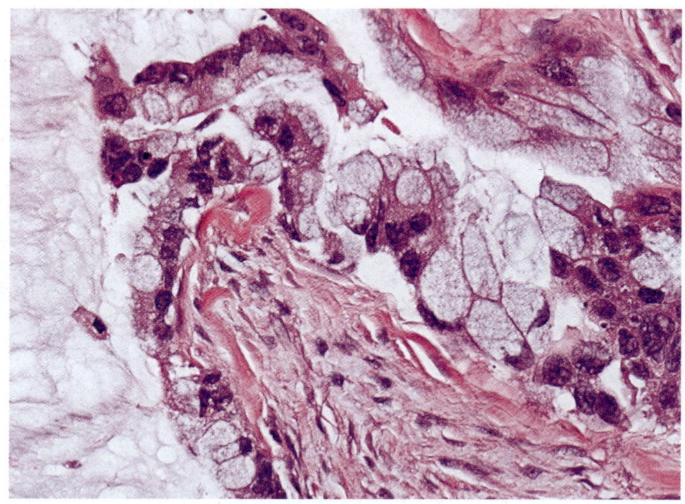

d

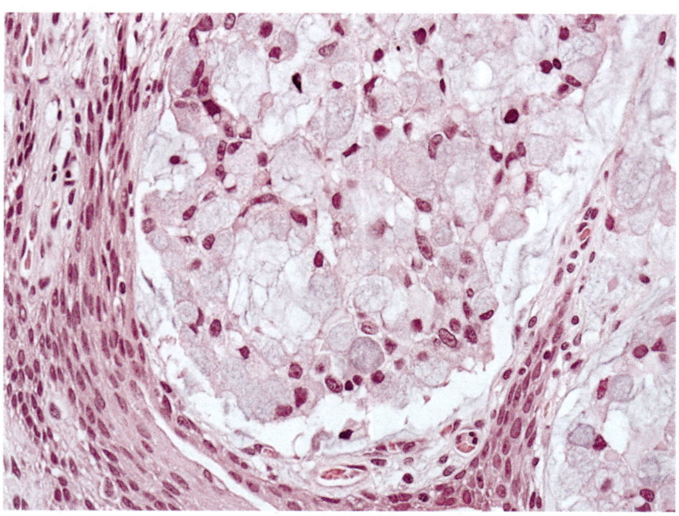

e

Figure 53-20.
Urachal adenocarcinoma showing a mass located in the muscularis propria of the bladder dome (*a*). A close-up photo (*b*) demonstrates yellow mucinous material on the surface. Microscopically, invasive adenocarcinoma, enteric type (*c*) with focal goblet cells (*d*) and signet ring cells (*e*).

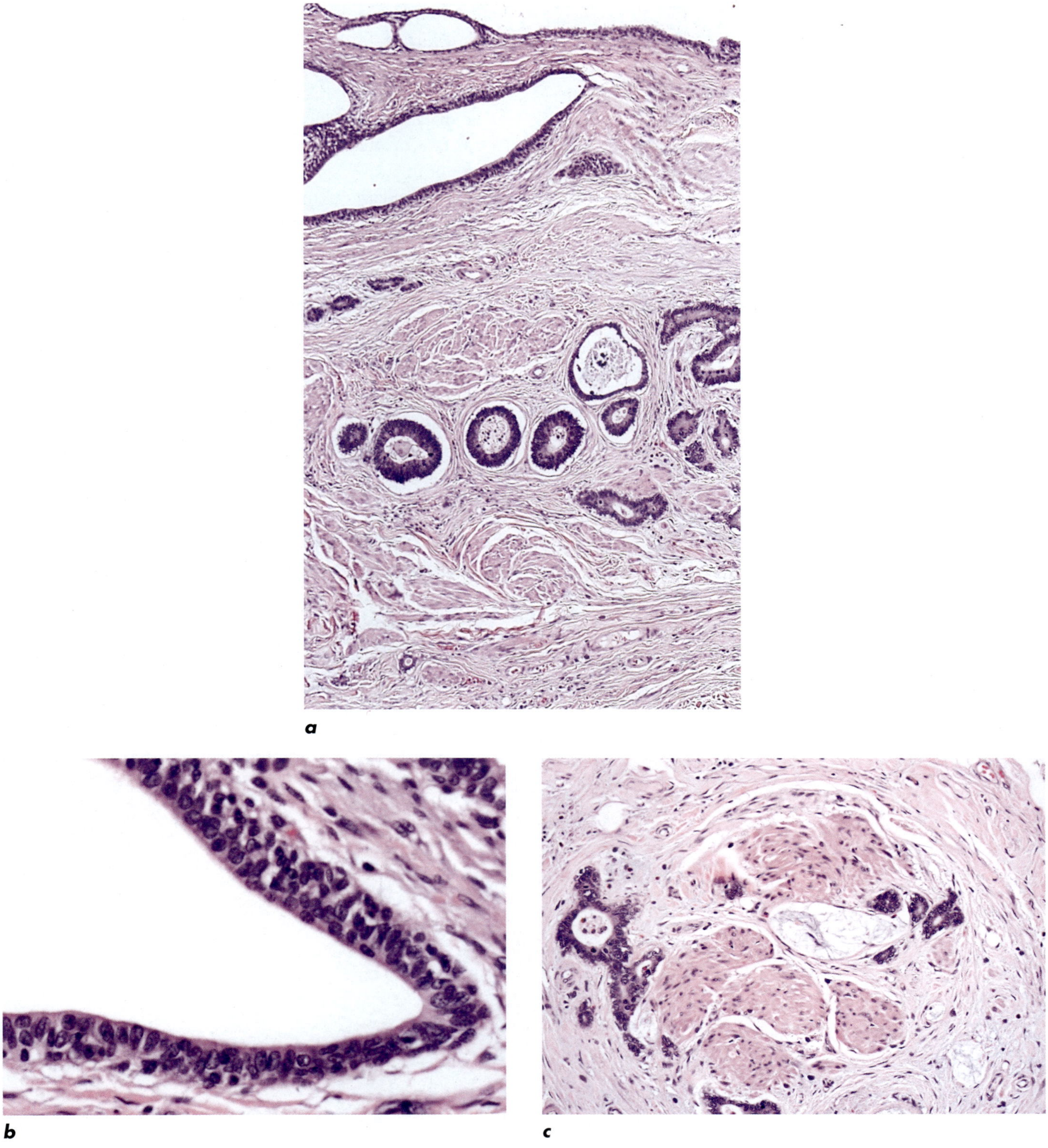

Figure 53-21.
Urachal adenocarcinoma shows the presence of both urachal remnants (*a*, upper) and invasive adenocarcinoma (*a*, lower). High magnification confirms the benign urachal remnant (*b*) and adenocarcinoma invading the muscularis propria (*c*).

MICROPAPILLARY CARCINOMA

Definition

- A variant of urothelial carcinoma with micropapillary features
- Pure form of micropapillary carcinoma is very rare, most cases are associated with typical high-grade urothelial carcinoma

Pathogenesis

- Unknown
- Micropapillary carcinoma cells are prone to invade vessels, which is related to early lymph node metastasis and deep invasion

Clinical features

- Symptoms such as hematuria, mass, and urinary irritations similar to typical urothelial carcinoma
- May present early metastasis

Gross pathology

- The exophytic lesion may be small, but deeply invasive components are prominent
- Grossly, it is not possible to make diagnosis of micropapillary carcinoma

Histology

- Small clusters of tumor cells with or without central fibrovascular cores (Fig. 53-22)
- Clusters of tumor cells with moderate degree of cytological atypia are located in a lacuna space (Fig. 53-23)
- Surface urothelium may or may not be involved by the tumor in biopsy
- Micropapillary carcinoma in situ can be occasionally seen
- Very frequent lymphovascular invasion
- Often associated with CIS and/or other high-grade invasive urothelial carcinoma

Immunohistochemistry

- P53 positive
- P63 negative (which is different from conventional high-grade urothelial carcinoma)
- CD31 can be used to highlight the lymphovascular invasion

Clinical relevance (prognosis and treatment options)

- Aggressive variant of bladder cancer
- Early and extensive lymphovascular invasion present

Figure 53-22.
Micropapillary carcinoma of the bladder with intact urothelium (*a*). Higher magnification shows clusters of tumor cells in lymphatics (*b*).

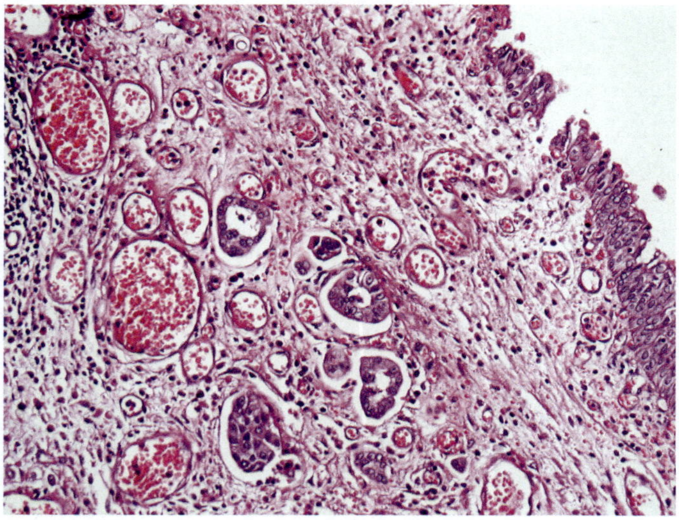

a

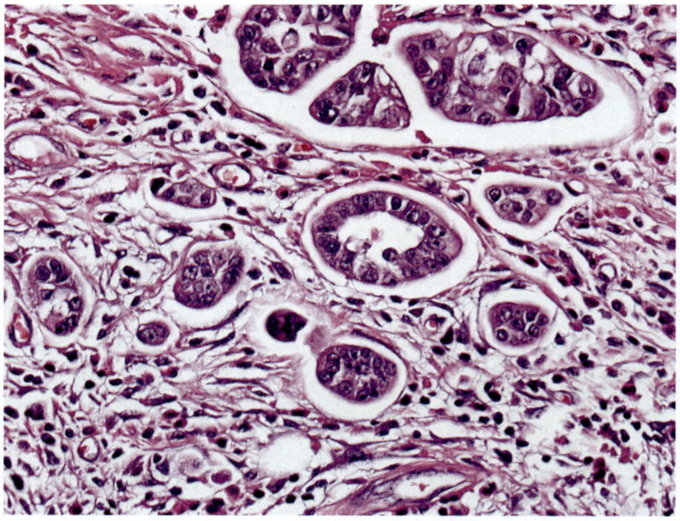

b

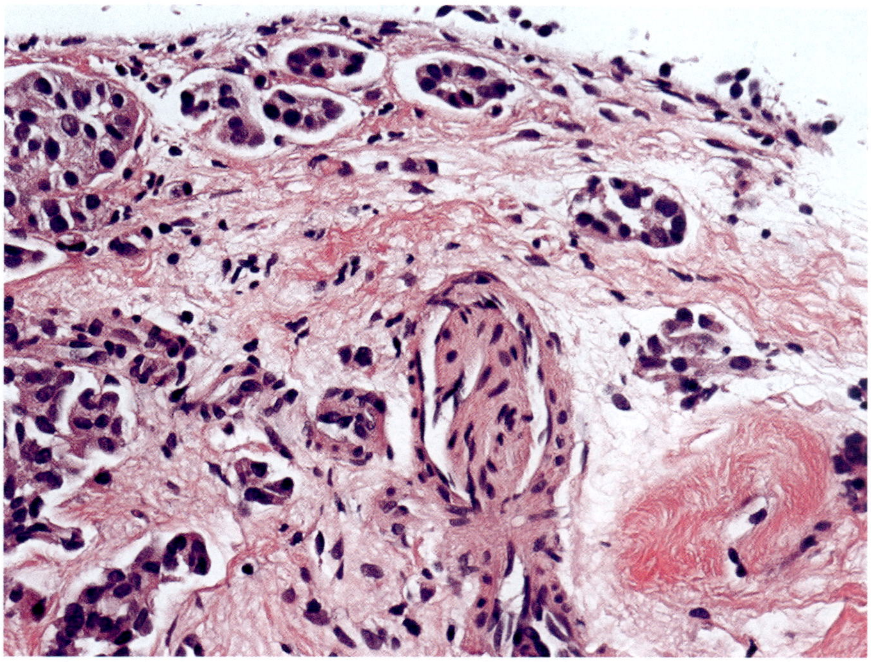

Figure 53-23.
Micropapillary carcinoma is composed of small clusters of tumor cells, some with fibrovascular cores present in lacuna spaces.

CLEAR CELL ADENOCARCINOMA

Definition

- A special type of adenocarcinoma composed of clear cells resembling its Mullerian counterpart of the female genital tract

Other terms

- Mesonephric carcinoma
- Primary adenocarcinoma composed of clear cells

Pathogenesis and epidemiology

- Most are female patients (mean age 57 years)
- It is suggested that this tumor is derived from mesonephric origin although convincing evidence is lacking
- The tumor may be derived from the preexisting endometriosis or Mullerian remnants

Clinical features

- Hematuria or dysuria

Gross pathology

- No specific features

Histology

- This tumor is almost morphologically identical to the clear cell carcinoma of the female genital tract
- Three common patterns are tubulocystic, papillary, and diffuse
- Tumor cells with clear cytoplasm (Figs. 53-24 and 53-25)
- Hobnail appearance may be present
- Moderate to severe cytological atypia
- Brisk mitotic activity

Immunohistochemistry

- CK7, CK20, CEA, CA125 positive
- LeuM1 negative
- ER/PR negative
- P53 positive

Clinical relevance (prognosis and treatment options)

- Early staged tumors can be treated effectively by surgery, if detected
- Late stage tumors have a poor prognosis

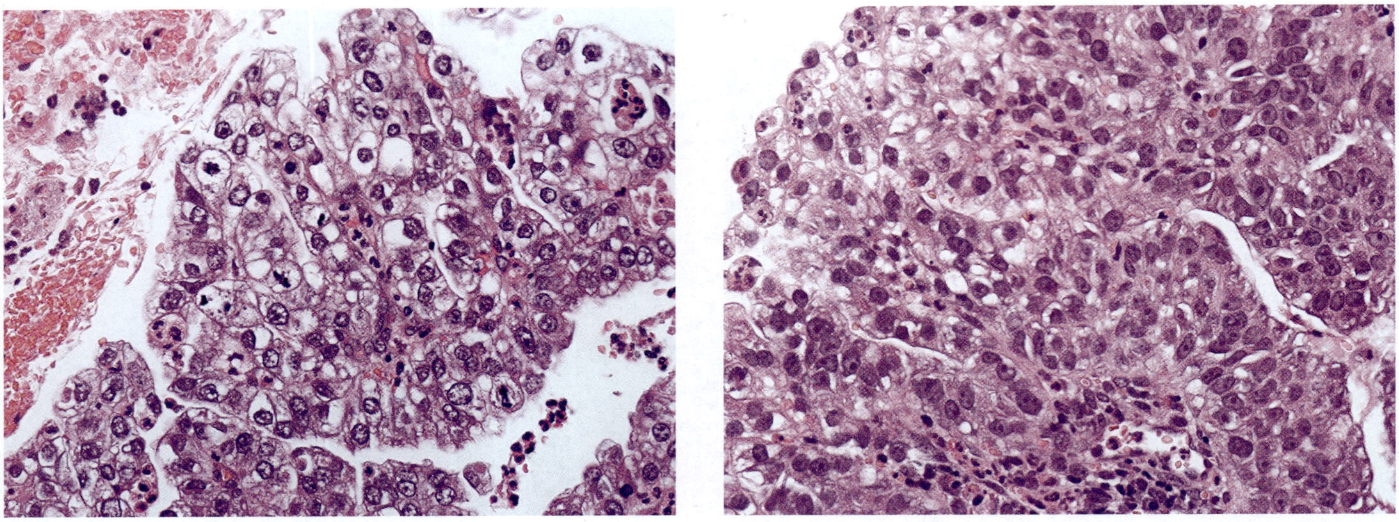

a **b**

Figure 53-24.
Clear cell adenocarcinoma of the bladder is composed of tumor cells with clear cytoplasm and prominent cytological atypia in a diffuse pattern (*a*). In another area, the tumor cells form a vague papillary pattern (*b*).

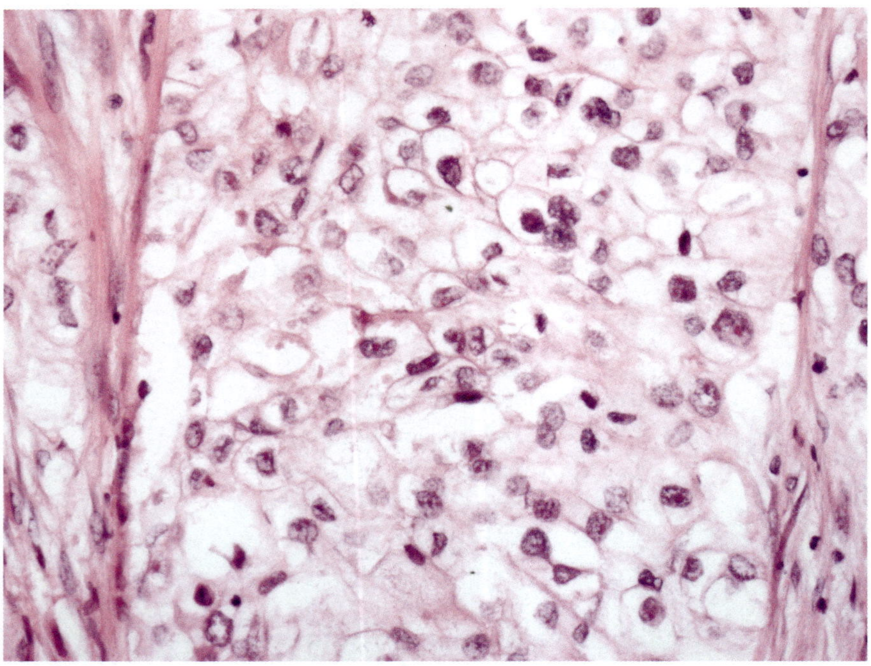

Figure 53-25.
Clear cell carcinoma consists of high-grade tumor cells with clear cytoplasm, resembling clear cell RCC although they do not have the typical "chicken-wire" vasculature.

PROSTATIC ADENOCARCINOMA INVOLVING THE BLADDER

Definition

- Prostatic adenocarcinoma involving the bladder by direct extension or metastasis

Other terms

- Secondary adenocarcinoma of the bladder, metastatic prostatic adenocarcinoma in the bladder

Pathogenesis

- Prostatic adenocarcinoma in the bladder can come from several origins: direct extension (most common cause), metastasis, or malignant transformation of ectopic prostate tissue or prostate-type polyp
- But in the vast majority of cases, a primary prostatic adenocarcinoma is also present, indicating the bladder tumor is secondary
- Since prostatic adenocarcinoma is the most common malignancy in the United States, it is by far the most common form of secondary adenocarcinomas of the bladder in our practice

Clinical features

- Male patients only with history of prostatic adenocarcinoma, typically high grade
- Previously treated or without treatment
- Elevation of serum PSA
- Hematuria
- Bladder mass lesions identified by imaging or cystoscopy
- Presence or absence of metastatic lesions in other organs such as bone or lung

Gross pathology

- Mass lesions in the bladder mucosa, flat, ulcerated or papillary, sometimes indistinguishable from urothelial carcinoma
- Lesions may range from a few millimeters to centimeters

Histology

- Pathologists should always keep in mind the possibility of prostatic adenocarcinoma, in the case of a high-grade carcinoma present in the bladder of a male of 50 to 90 years old
- The following features may suggest a prostatic primary:
  - The presence of relatively uniform size and shape of tumor cells
  - Prominent cribriform or glandular patterns with prominent "cherry-red" nucleoli (Fig. 53-26)
  - Nonenteric-type adenocarcinoma (Fig. 53-27)
  - The absence of urothelial carcinoma in situ although the tumor cells may undermine the lining epithelium
  - Intact urothelium (Fig. 53-26*a*)
  - Ductal adenocarcinoma features tall columnar "endometrioid" tumor cells (Figs. 53-28 and 53-29)
- In addition to the histological features, elevated serum PSA and prior diagnosis of high-grade prostatic adenocarcinoma should provide enough suspicion for prostatic primary to start a work up for the differential diagnosis

Figure 53-26.
Secondary (prostatic) adenocarcinoma in the bladder is characterized by the presence of tumor nodules in lamina propria with an intact urothelium (*a*). High magnification shows the cribriform pattern of the tumor cells (*b*).

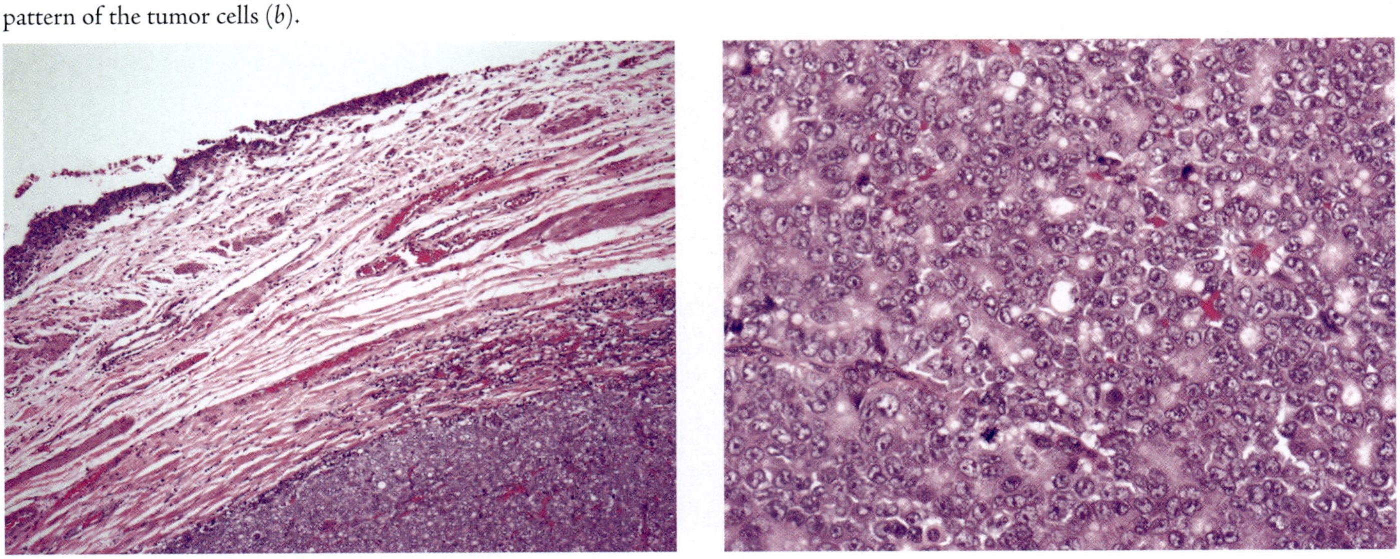

a **b**

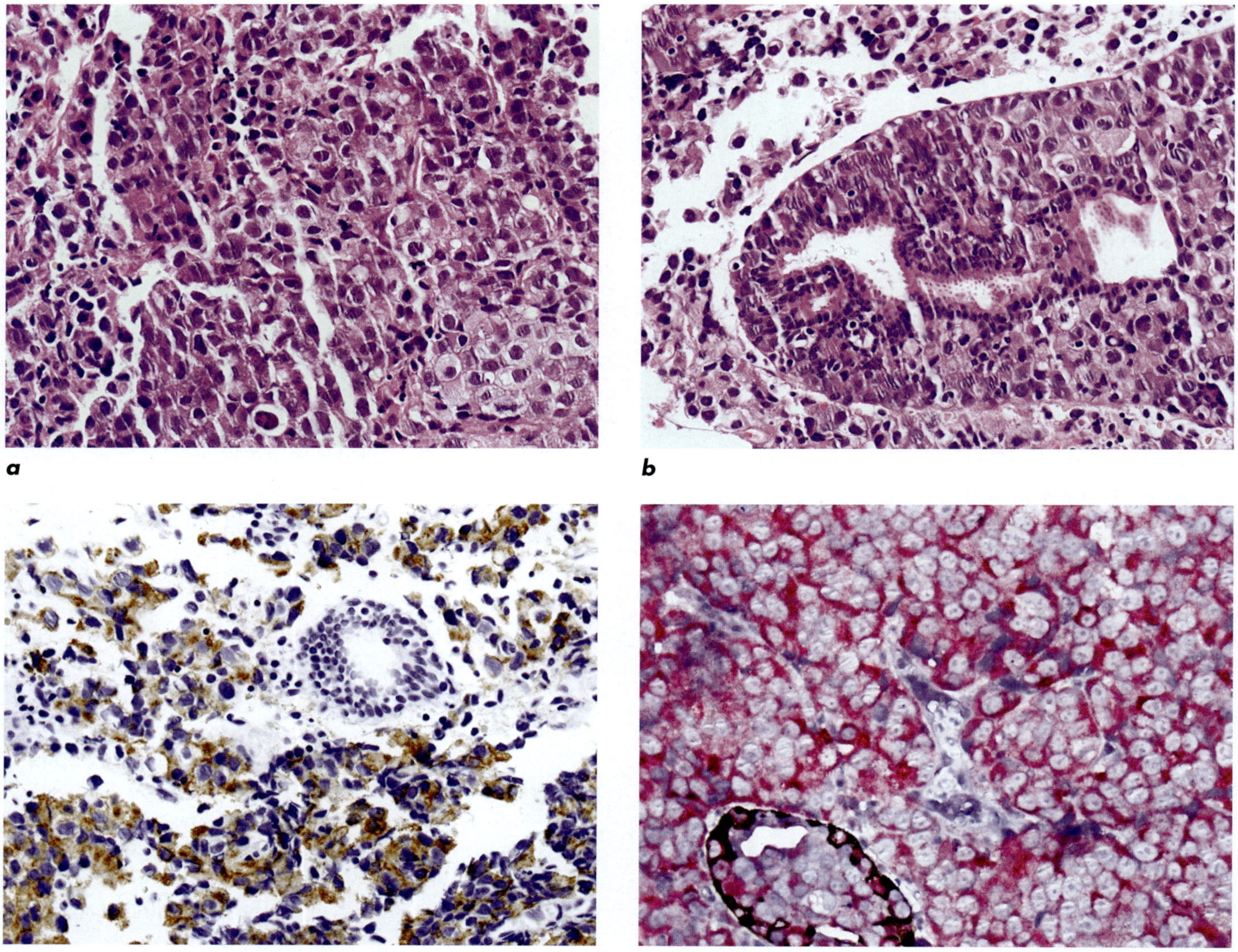

a b c d

Figure 53-27.

Prostatic adenocarcinoma in the bladder exhibits a diffuse pattern (*a*), and tumor cells growing undermining the benign glandular cells of cystitis glandularis, mimicking urothelial carcinoma in situ (*b*). By immunohistochemistry, the tumor cells are positive for PSA (*c*) and AMACR, negative for p63 and HMWCK (*d*) confirming the diagnosis.

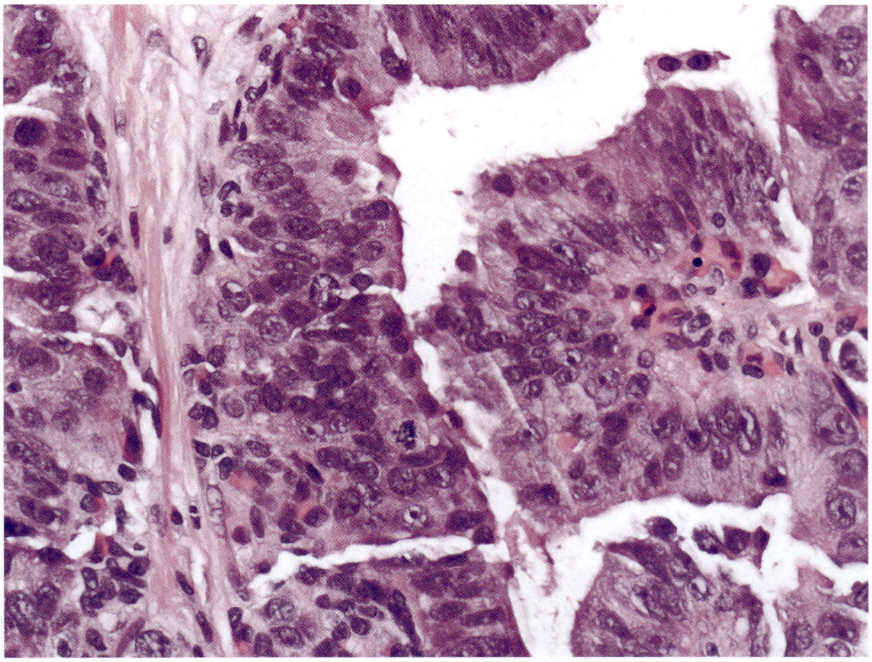

Figure 53-28.
Prostatic ductal adenocarcinoma secondarily involving the bladder is signified by the tall columnar cells in a papillary pattern.

- The following features are not favoring a prostatic primary:
  - The presence of squamous differentiation in the tumor (unless prostate cancer treated with estrogen)
  - Highly pleomorphic tumor cells (unless prostate cancer treated with hormonal therapy)
  - History of bladder carcinoma
  - Presence of urothelial dysplasia or CIS
- The application with IHC markers is important for establishing the definitive diagnosis because of importance for treatment

Immunohistochemistry

- PSA positivity is highly specific. But the positivity tends to be focal, particularly in high-grade and treated prostatic adenocarcinoma (Figs. 53-27*c* and 53-29*c*)
- AMACR positivity is highly sensitive (Fig. 53-27*d*), even in most high-grade prostatic adenocarcinoma cases. But it is less specific because other carcinomas such as colon adenocarcinoma, papillary RCC can be positive
- P63 and HMWCK negative
- However, rare cases of p63 positive and HMWCK positive prostatic adenocarcinomas have been reported

Differential diagnosis

- Differential diagnosis of prostatic adenocarcinoma and urothelial carcinoma is summarized in Table 53-2

Clinical relevance (prognosis and treatment options)

- Urologists and oncologists are obligated to provide the history of prostate cancer if it is known, even though they may not think the bladder lesion is related to the history of prostate cancer
- Hematuria and bladder mass can be the initial presentation of prostate cancer patients
- Distinction of prostate cancer from bladder cancer has a major impact on treatment selection
- Prostatic adenocarcinoma in the bladder may be responsible for hormonal therapy, while bladder cancer will not
- Radiation may be another choice for prostatic adenocarcinoma, but unlikely for urothelial carcinoma

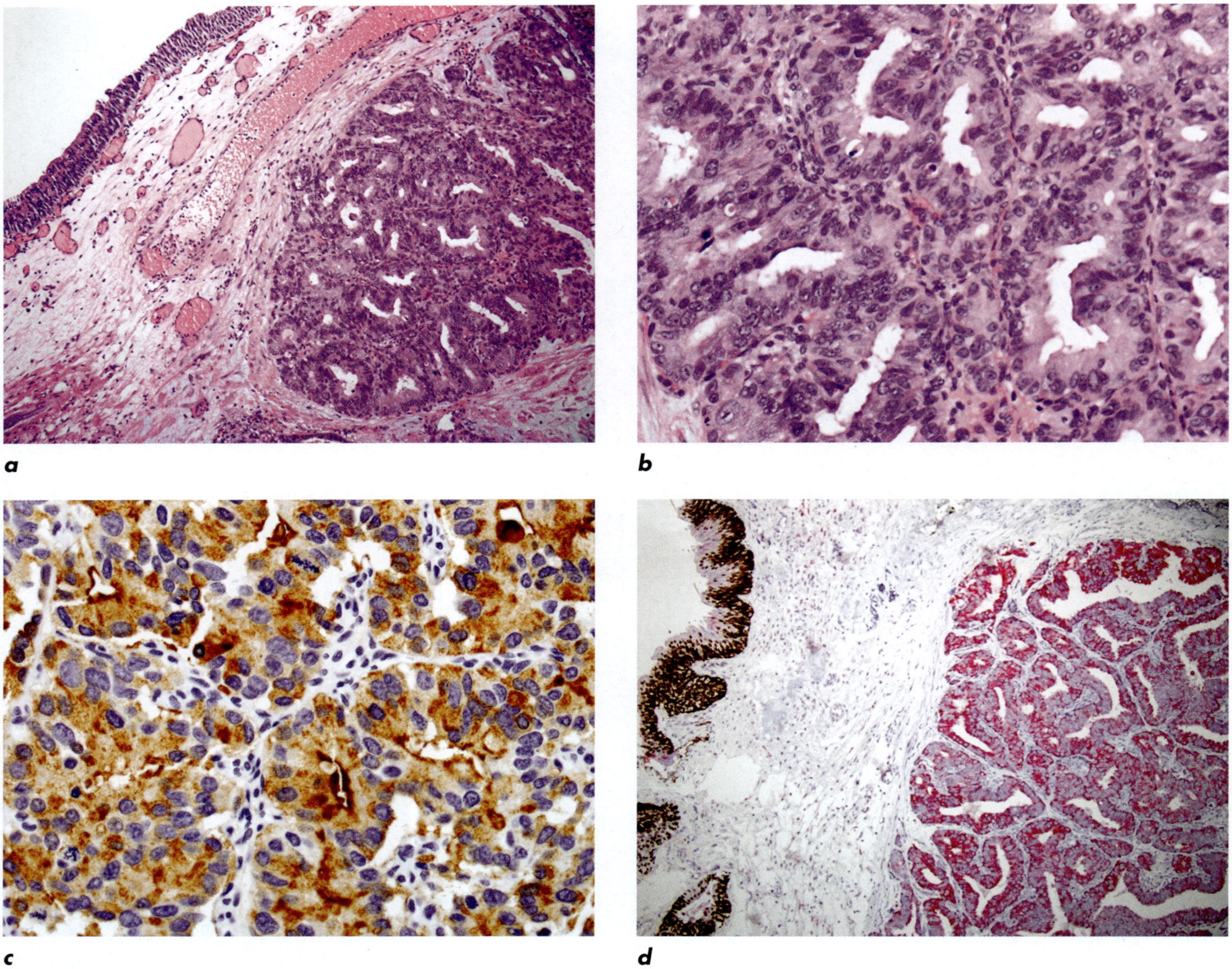

Figure 53-29.
Metastatic prostatic (ductal) adenocarcinoma in the bladder, characterized by a large nest of tumor cells is present in the lamina propria with an intact urothelium (*a*). High magnification shows that the tall columnar cells with cytological atypia with prominent nucleoli arranged in a cribriform pattern (*b*). The tumor cells are positive for PSA (*c*) and AMACR (*d*), negative for p63 and HMWCK (triple staining).

Table 53-2. Differential Diagnosis of Prostatic Adenocarcinoma and Urothelial Carcinoma in the Bladder

	Prostatic adenocarcinoma	*Urothelial carcinoma*
Serum PSA	Elevated	Not elevated
Prior history	Prostate cancer possible	Bladder cancer possible
Sex	Male	Male or female
Patterns	Cribriform or glandular	Solid sheets
Cell pleomorphism	Less prominent	Greater
Nucleoli	Cherry red	Any size and shape
Squamous differentiation	Uncommon	Common
Urothelial carcinoma	Absent	May be present
AMACR	Strongly positive	Negative or weakly positive
PSA	Positive, could be focal	Negative
PSMA	Positive	Negative
P63	Negative (rare case positive)	Positive
HMWCK	Negative (rare case positive)	Positive
P53	Negative	Positive
S100P	Negative	Positive
GATA3	Negative	Positive
Hormonal treatment	Could be effective	Not indicated

AMACR, α-methylacyl-CoA racemase; HMWCK, high molecular weight cytokeratins; PSA, prostate-specific antigen; PSMA, prostate-specific membrane antigen.

OTHER SECONDARY CARCINOMAS INVOLVING THE BLADDER

Definition

- In addition to prostatic adenocarcinoma, many other carcinomas from different organs can involve the bladder either by metastasis (such lung, breast) or by direct extension (colon, endometrial, or ovarian carcinomas)

Clinical features

- The diagnosis of a secondary carcinoma of the bladder is very difficult without clinical information
- The reason is the great capacity of divergent differentiation of bladder cancer, which can mimic adenocarcinoma, squamous cell carcinoma, small cell carcinoma, poorly differentiated carcinoma, or even sarcoma from other organs
- Therefore, clinical information is essential for differential diagnosis between a primary versus secondary carcinoma in the bladder

Gross pathology

- Not specific for distinguishing a secondary carcinoma from a high-grade urothelial carcinoma

Histology

- Depending on the type of the original carcinoma
- However, some features may suggest secondary carcinoma
  - Intact bladder mucosa or urothelium
  - Absence of urothelial carcinoma in situ or dysplasia
  - A prior history of malignancy
  - Presence of prominent intravascular tumor thrombi
- Colonic adenocarcinoma (Fig. 53-30)
  - The second most common secondary carcinoma involving the bladder
  - Composed of tall columnar cells with a variable number of goblet cells (Fig. 53-31)
  - Central "dirty" necrosis is common
  - It can infiltrate benign urothelium, mimicking urothelial carcinoma (Fig. 53-32)
- Breast adenocarcinoma
  - Can be either ductal or lobular
  - Glandular formation often not obvious (Figs. 53-33 and 53-34)
  - Intracellular lumens can be seen in some cases (Fig. 53-33*b*)
  - ER/PR and other breast markers are positive (Fig. 53-33*c*)
  - GATA3 positive (similar to urothelial carcinoma)
- Endometrial adenocarcinoma (Fig. 53-35)
  - Can be confused with urothelial carcinoma, primary or other secondary adenocarcinomas (such as prostatic duct adenocarcinoma) of the bladder
  - ER and PR are positive in most of endometrioid adenocarcinoma (Fig. 53-36)
- Mucinous adenocarcinoma and signet ring cell carcinoma
  - Mostly from gastrointestinal tract (Fig. 53-37)
  - Mucin-containing signet ring cells can be seen
  - Ideally, the original material including H&E-stained slides along with immunostains should be reviewed before making the decision of a primary or secondary carcinoma

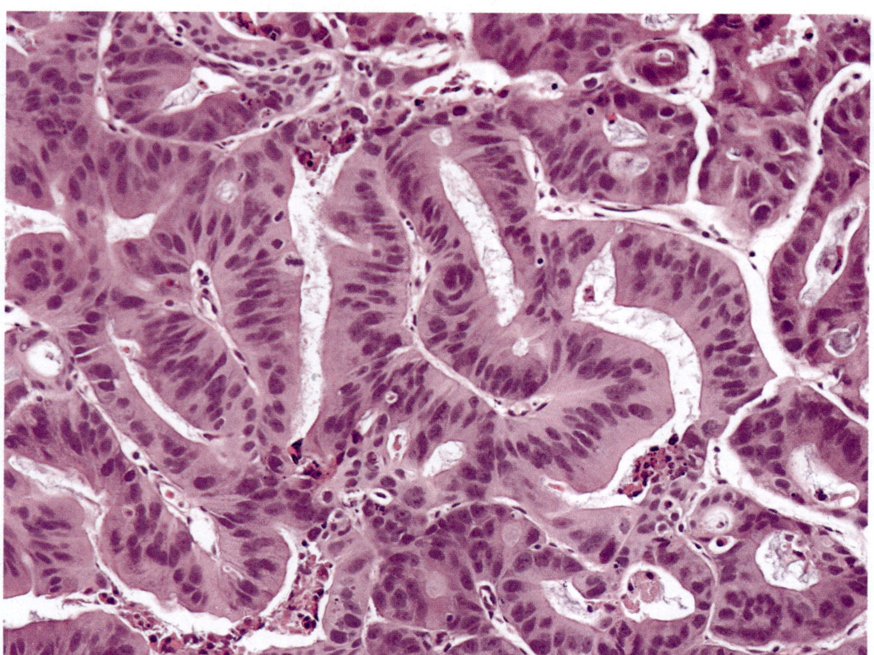

Figure 53-30.
Secondary colonic adenocarcinoma in the bladder demonstrates typical tall columnar cells with cribriform patterns.

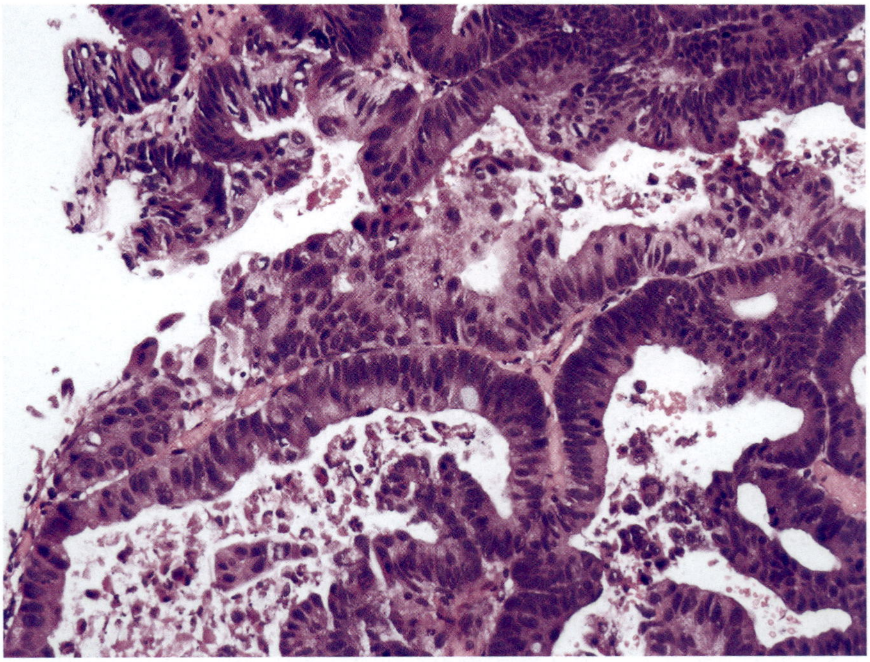

Figure 53-31.
Metastatic colonic adenocarcinoma in the bladder containing goblet cells with cribriform patterns and "dirty" necrosis in the lumen.

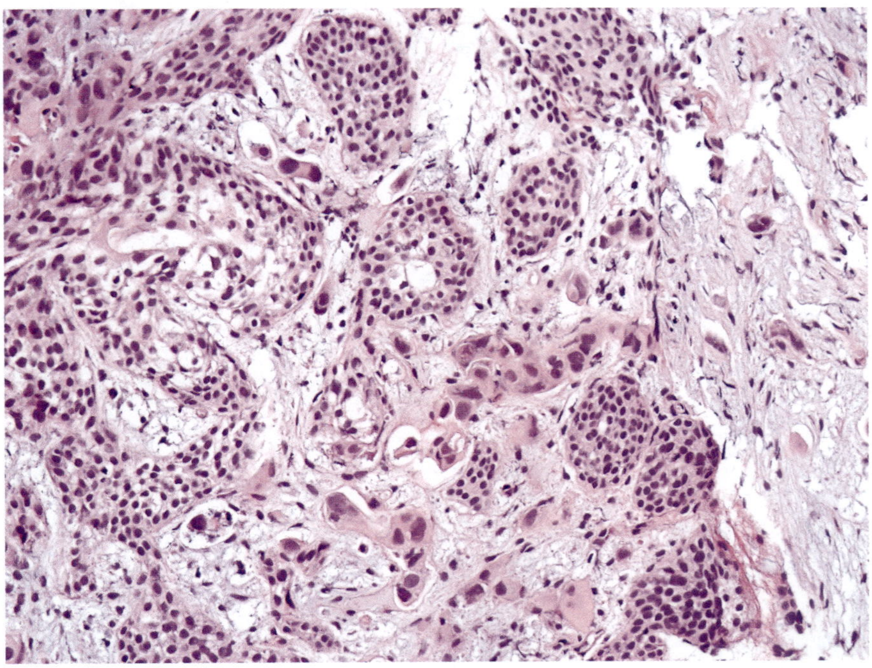

Figure 53-32.
Metastatic colonic adenocarcinoma with lymphatic thrombi in the bladder mucosa, mimicking infiltrating urothelial carcinoma.

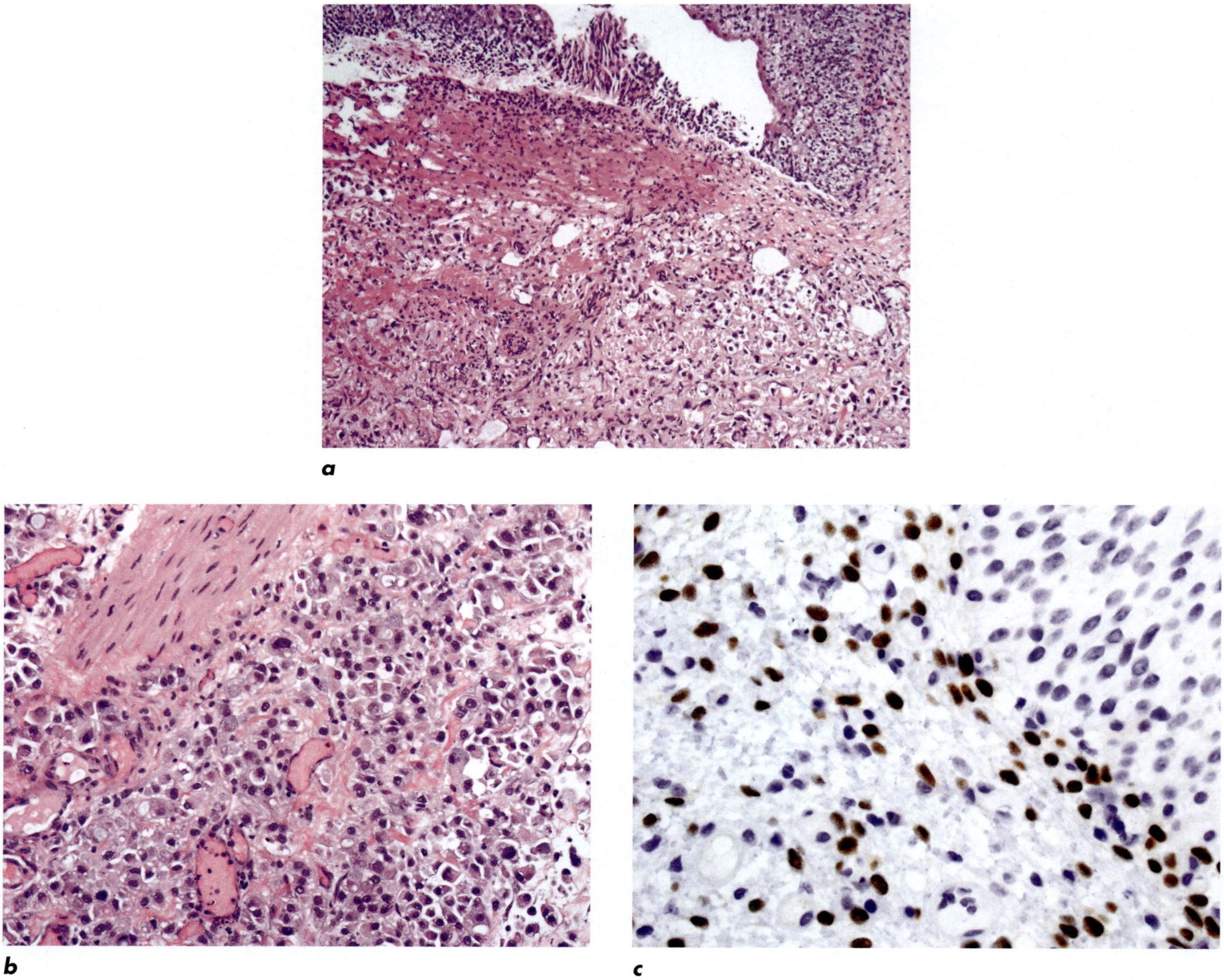

Figure 53-33.
Metastatic breast adenocarcinoma of the bladder involving the lamina propria (*a*). High magnification shows tumor cells with intracellular lumens (*b*). Immunostaining confirms the tumor cells positive for ER (*c*).

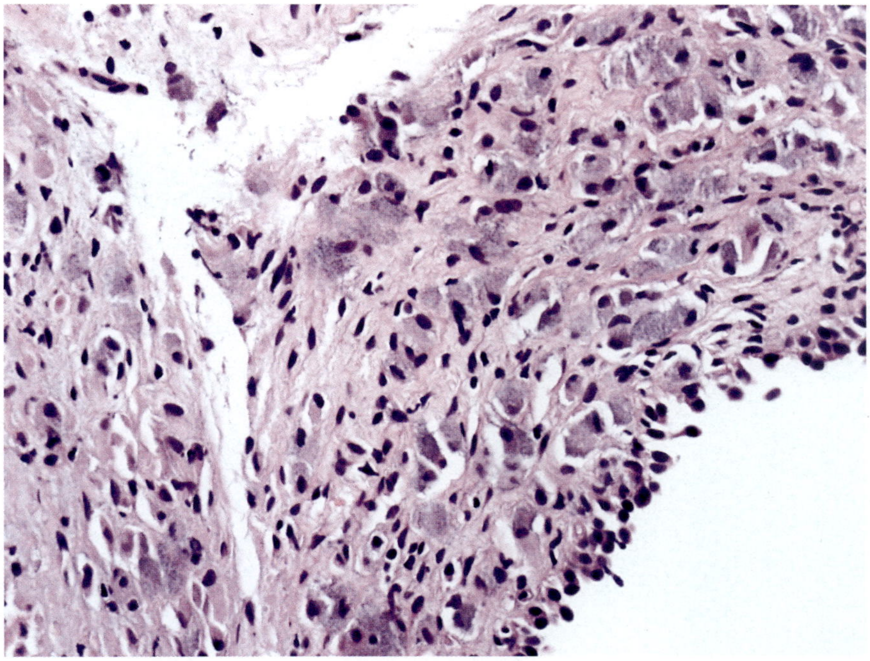

Figure 53-34.
Metastatic breast adenocarcinoma with glandular patterns in the lamina propria of the bladder.

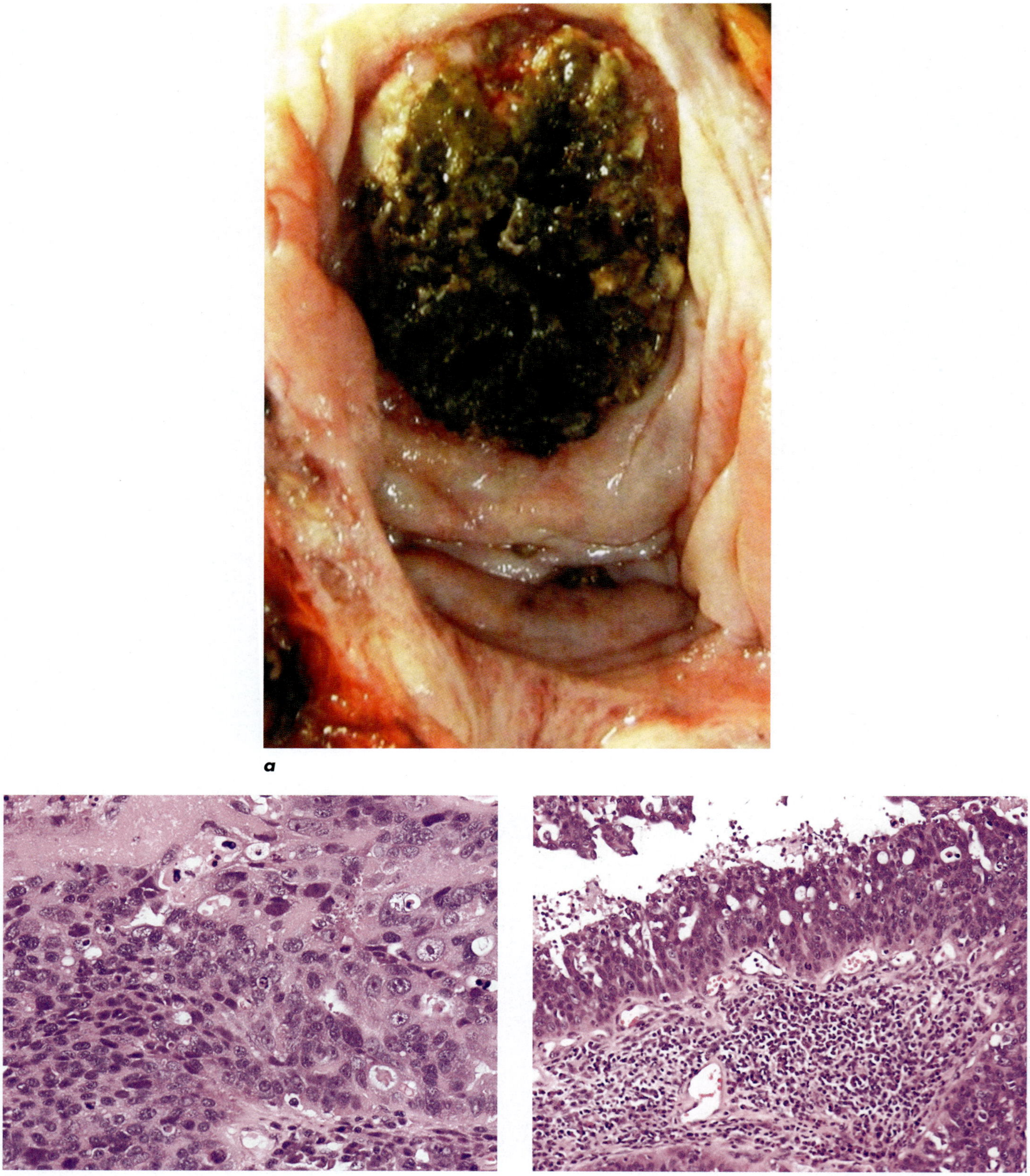

Figure 53-35.
Secondary endometrial adenocarcinoma in the bladder appears to be a large ulcerated mass mimicking urothelial carcinoma (*a*). Microscopically, it is a high-grade carcinoma with subtle glandular differentiation (*b*). Metastatic endometrial carcinoma in the pelvic lymph node displays more obvious glandular patterns (*c*).

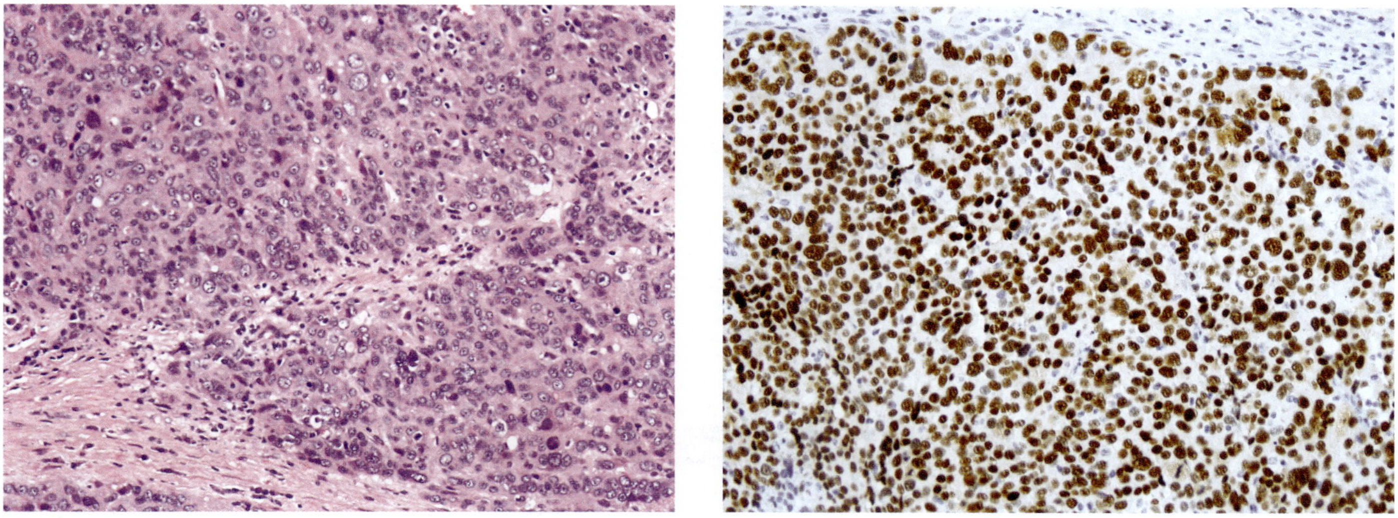

a ***b***

Figure 53-36.
Metastatic endometrial adenocarcinoma in the bladder (*a*) is highlighted by the ER immunostaining (*b*).

Figure 53-37.
Metastatic carcinoma from the stomach in the bladder with intact urothelium (*a*). High magnification shows the presence of occasional intracellular mucin and signet ring cells (*b*).

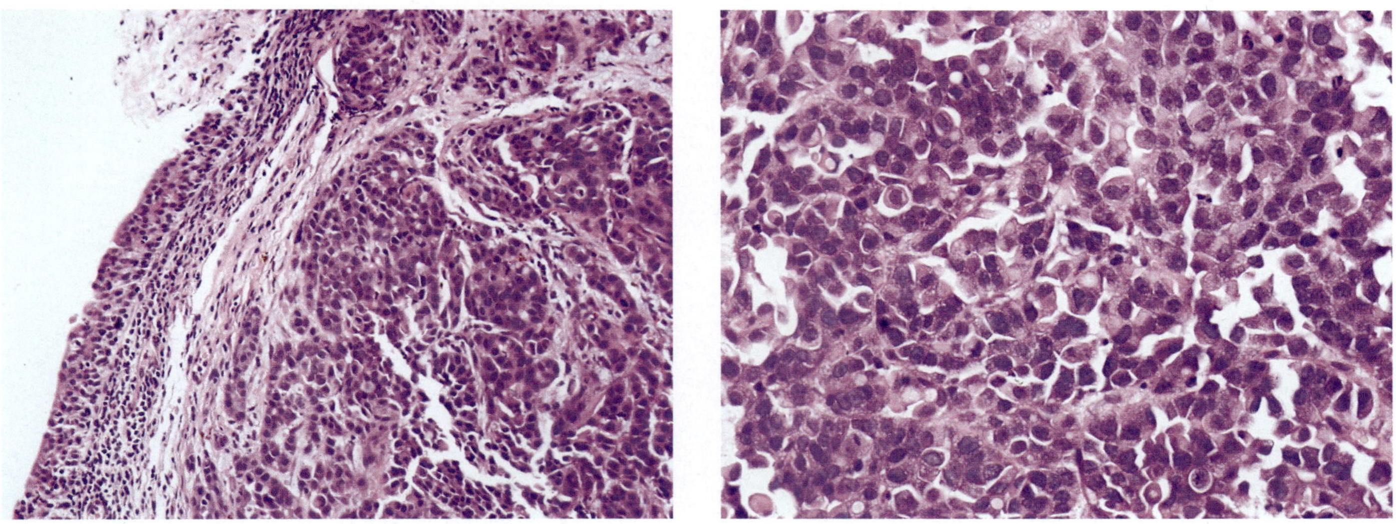

a ***b***

Differential diagnosis and immunohistochemistry

- Including primary benign and malignant glandular lesions (see Table 53-3)
- The special features of common secondary carcinomas of the bladder is summarized in Table 53-4

Clinical relevance

- The diagnosis of secondary adenocarcinoma of the bladder is often difficult without a clinical history
- So the detailed clinical history and review of the original primary tumor histology are essential if the determination of primary versus secondary adenocarcinoma is clinically important
- Surgery or radiation may not be effective for a metastatic cancer in the bladder, but it may be used as a palliative measure to control symptoms such as bleeding

Table 53-3. Summary of Benign and Malignant Glandular Lesions of the Bladder

	Glandular lesions of the bladder	*Key features*
Benign	Cystitis glandularis and cystitis cystica	Benign glandular epithelium on surface or in von Brunn nests
	Colonic metaplasia	Benign glandular epithelium with goblet cells
	Prostatic-type polyp	Benign prostatic glands in the bladder (PSA positive)
	Endometriosis	Benign endometrial glands and stroma (ER/PR, CD10 positive)
	Nephrogenic adenoma	Benign renal-tubule-like epithelium in granulation background (PAX8 positive)
	Urachal remnants and urachal cysts	Deeply seeded benign glandular cells in the wall of the bladder dome
	Mesonephric remnants	Clusters of benign glands with secretion
	Tubular or villous adenoma	Dysplastic glandular neoplasm similar to colon tubular adenoma
Malignant	Urothelial carcinoma with glandular differentiation	Presence of both urothelial carcinoma and malignant glandular components
	Adenocarcinoma in situ	Noninvasive malignant glandular epithelium, but often associated with high-grade urothelial carcinoma
	Primary adenocarcinoma	Enteric and nonenteric adenocarcinoma originated in the bladder, β-catenin negative
	Urachal adenocarcinoma	Special form of primary dome-located or deeply seeded adenocarcinoma
	Clear cell carcinoma	Adenocarcinoma with clear glycogenated cells similar to endometrial/ovary clear cell carcinoma
	Micropapillary carcinoma	High-grade urothelial carcinoma with micropapillary pattern
	Prostatic adenocarcinoma	Adenocarcinoma with prostatic features (PSA and AMACR positive)
	Secondary adenocarcinoma	Adenocarcinoma from other organs by direct extension or metastasis

AMACR, α-methylacyl-CoA racemase; ER/PR, estrogen receptor/progesterone receptor; PAX8, paired box gene 8; PSA, prostate-specific antigen.

Table 53-4. Differential Diagnosis of Common Secondary Carcinoma

Primary	*Rout*	*Clue*	*Positive marker*
Colonic adenocarcinoma	Direct extension or metastasis	Dirty necrosis	CDX2 β-Catenin
Breast adenocarcinoma	Metastasis	Intracellular lumens	ER/PR
Lung adenocarcinoma	Metastasis		TTF1, napsin
Endometrial carcinoma	Direct extension or metastasis	Tall columnar cells	ER/PR, vimentin

ER/PR, estrogen receptor/progesterone receptor; TTF1, thyroid transcription factor 1.

CHAPTER 54 Other Neoplasms of the Bladder

INFLAMMATORY MYOFIBROBLASTIC TUMOR

Definition

- A neoplasm in the bladder with predominant spindle myofibroblasts as well as inflammatory cells including lymphocytes, eosinophils, and plasma cells. It can be seen in other organs such as lung or soft tissue
- Uncertain malignant potential

Pathogenesis

- It may include a group of lesions that may include reactive lesion, benign and malignant neoplasms

Other terms

- Inflammatory pseudotumor, pseudosarcoma, plasma cell granuloma

Clinical features

- Gross hematuria
- Wide range of age groups, mostly occurs in young adults
- A history of recent bladder injury absent in the majority of cases

Gross pathology

- Polypoid or nodular lesion, typically less than 4 to 5 cm in size (Fig. 54-1*a*)
- White or tan in cut surface, sometimes edematous or myxoid appearance
- The lesion is not well circumscribed, occasional ulceration present

Histology

- Predominantly spindle cell proliferation (Figs. 54-1 and 54-2)
- The lesion is located deep in the bladder wall. Urothelium is mostly intact (Fig. 54-3)
- Haphazard arrangement of tumor cells in the loose edematous background, giving the appearance of "fibroblast cell culture" (Figs. 54-1*b* and 54-3*b*)
- Minimal cytological atypia of the spindle cells, often degenerative in nature, but a higher cellularity, mitoses, and atypia can be seen occasionally (Fig. 54-2)
- Background of mixed inflammatory cells or fibrosis (Figs. 54-1*b* and 54-3*b*)
- Urothelial cells often display reactive atypia (Fig. 54-2*d*)

Figure 54-1.
Inflammatory myofibroblastic tumor from partial cystectomy specimen as an ulcerated mass (*a*). Microscopically, spindle tumor cells mixed with inflammatory cells are arranged in a loose background, giving a typical "cell-culture" appearance (*b*).

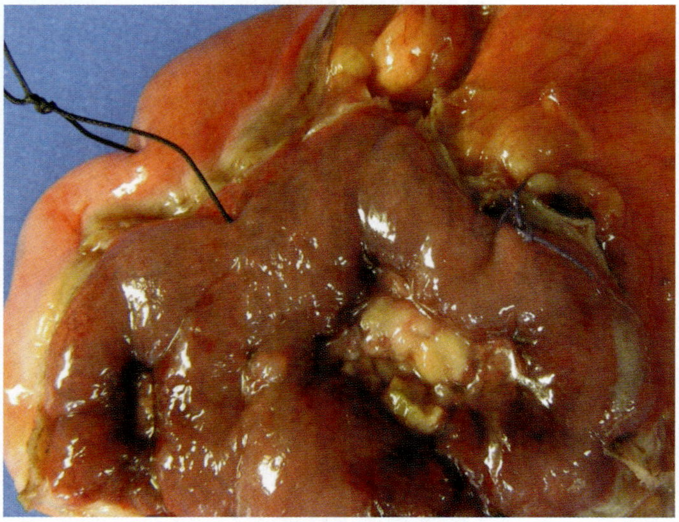

a

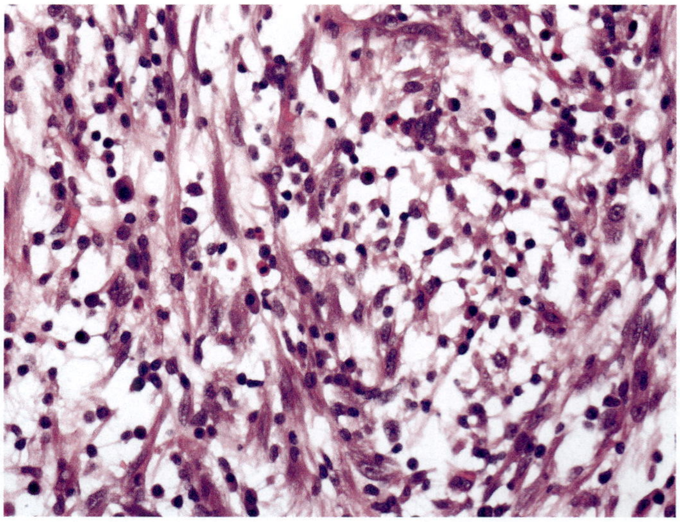

b

Immunohistochemistry

- Variable keratin positivity (Fig. 54-3*c*)
- ALK (anaplastic lymphoma kinase) positive in the majority of cases (Fig. 54-3*d*)
- Smooth muscle actin positive
- P53 negative

Differential diagnosis

- Sarcoma: more cellular and atypical, not cell culture background, inflammatory cells are usually not present
- High-grade urothelial carcinoma: nested malignant epithelial cells, rare to see bland spindle cells

Molecular analysis

- ALK rearrangement can be detected in the most cases

Clinical relevance (prognosis and treatment options)

- It is considered a tumor with an uncertain malignant potential, especially the ones with histological atypia
- Most cases take a benign course
- Recurrence can happen although uncommon
- Resection of the tumor is necessary
- However, therapies such as radical cystectomy, radiation, or chemotherapy are not indicated without extensive disease

Figure 54-2.
Inflammatory myofibroblastic tumor is composed of spindle cells and inflammatory cells in a relatively high cellularity (*a*). High magnification shows the proliferating spindle cells with frequent mitoses mixed with inflammatory cells (*b*) and occasional spindle cells with degenerative nuclear atypia (*c*). The urothelium overlying the lesion shows hyperplasia and atypia (*d*).

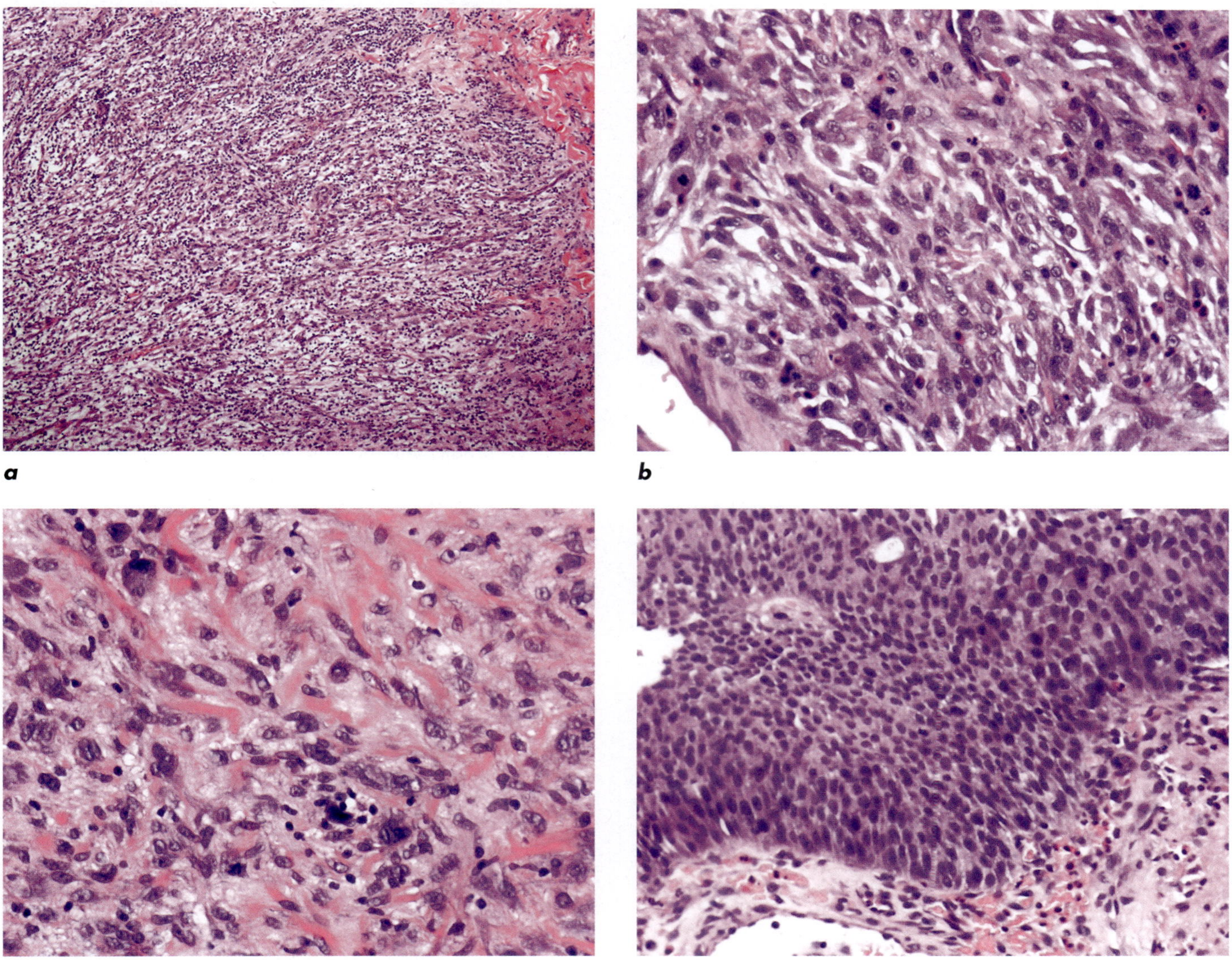

a b c d

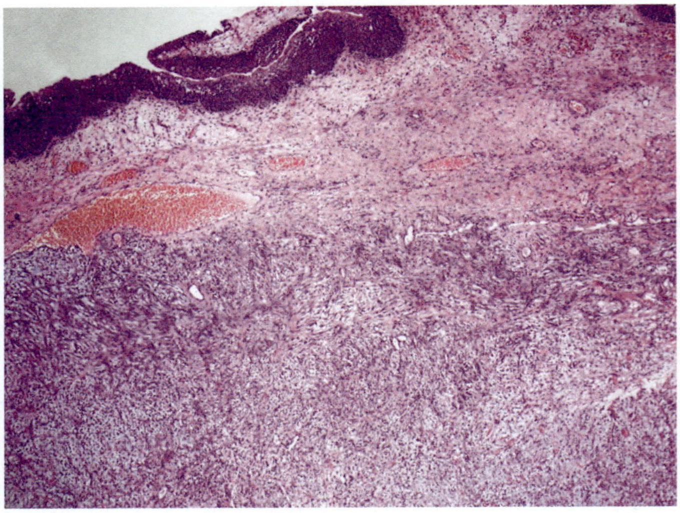

a

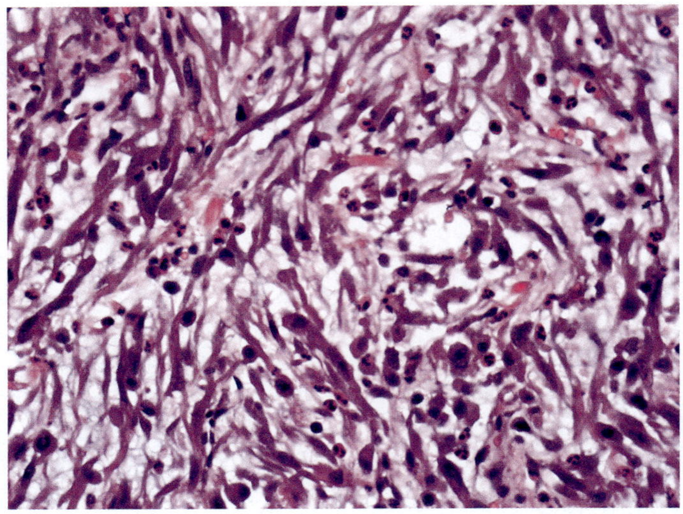

b

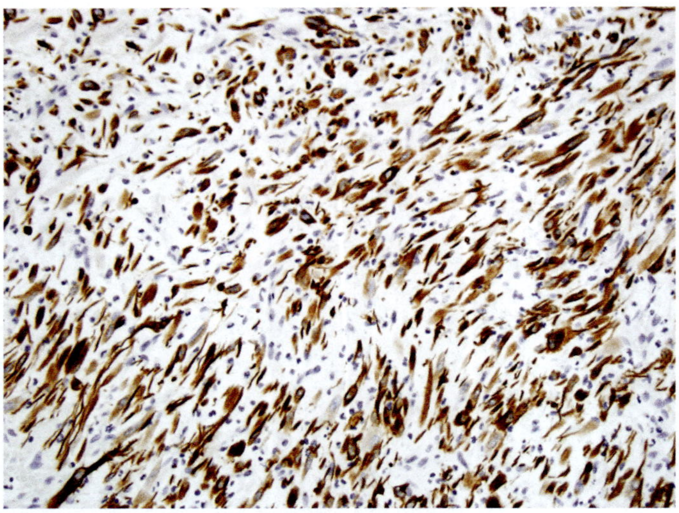

c

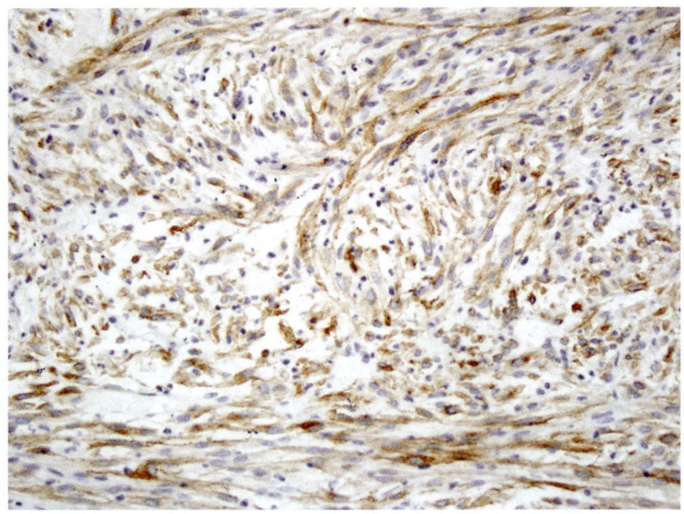

d

Figure 54-3.
Inflammatory myofibroblastic tumor infiltrates deeply the bladder wall with intact urothelium (*a*). High magnification shows the spindle cells with loose edematous background and inflammatory cells including eosinophils (*b*). Tumor cells are positive for AE1/AE3 (*c*) and ALK-1 (*d*).

PARAGANGLIOMA

Definition

- Neoplasm derived from paraganglion cells in the bladder
- Paraganglioma can be seen in other GU organs, such as the kidney or prostate but most commonly seen in the bladder

Other term

- Extra-adrenal pheochromocytoma

Clinical features

- Other locations including the prostate and kidney
- A wide range of ages of the patients
- Hypertension in the majority of cases, which would be a particular suspicious sign for paraganglioma in a young patient with a bladder mass
- Hypertensive symptoms such as blurred vision, lightheadedness, especially associated with urination
- Typical symptom is micturition attack, in which the patient experiences bursting headache, sweating, or even syncope
- Hematuria in a patient if the tumor breaks the urothelium
- Some familial cases are associated with genetic syndromes

Gross pathology

- Early lesion centered in the lamina propria or muscularis propria
- Well-demarcated mass with white to yellow fleshy cut surface (Fig. 54-4*a*)
- Hemorrhage, necrosis, and ulceration may be present (Fig. 54-5*a*)

Histology

- The tumor grows underneath the urothelium (Fig. 54-5*b*)
- Typically nests of large polygonal tumor cells separated by thin wall blood vessels (Figs. 54-4*b* and 54-5*c*) as "Zellballen" (cell ball) pattern is characteristic (Fig. 54-6)
- Tumor cells with abundant granular to clear cytoplasm (Figs. 54-4*b* and 54-6*b*)
- Isolated nuclear atypia is common (Fig. 54-6*b*)
- May invade smooth muscle, perivesical fat, or vessels
- Hyaline globules can be seen
- Metastasis to lymph nodes (Fig. 54-7) or other organs only occur in the minority of cases, which is the definitive evidence of malignancy
- Unlike adrenal cortical tumor, the malignant potential of paraganglioma cannot be predicated based on histology. We do not report benign or malignant paraganglioma unless metastasis is present

Figure 54-4.
Paraganglioma of the bladder of a partial cystectomy is a well-circumscribed mass with fleshy cut surface (*a*). The urothelium surface on the top is most intact. Tumor cells with granular cytoplasm are organized in cell balls (Zellballen) separated by fine capillaries (*b*).

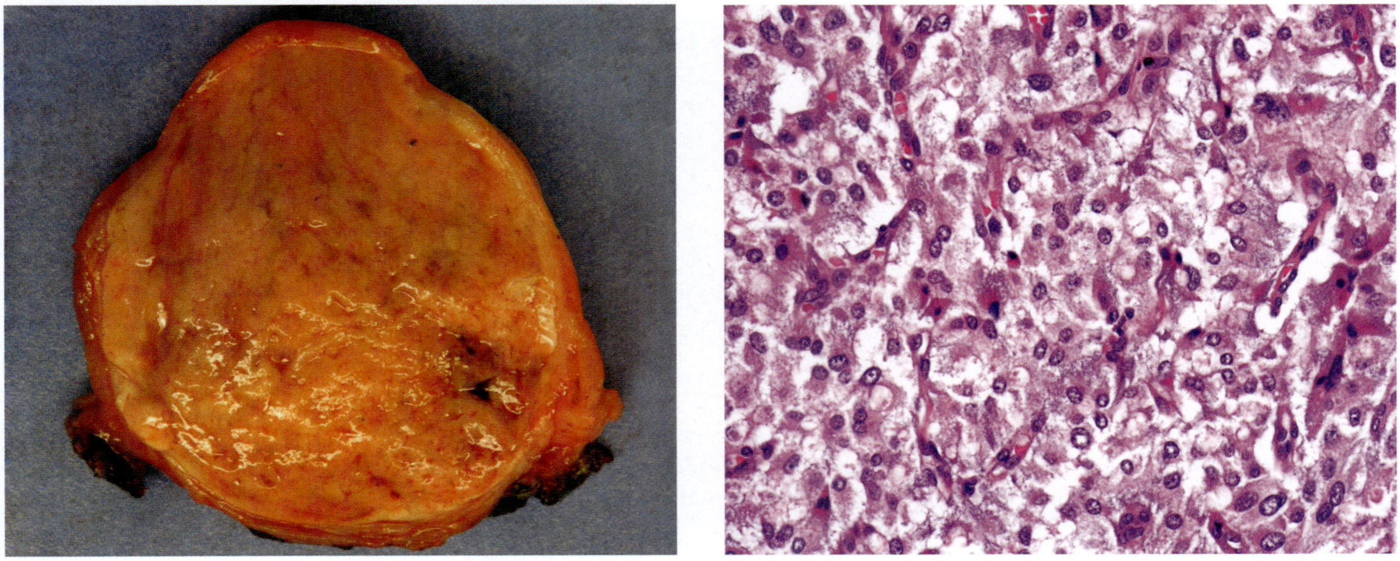

a *b*

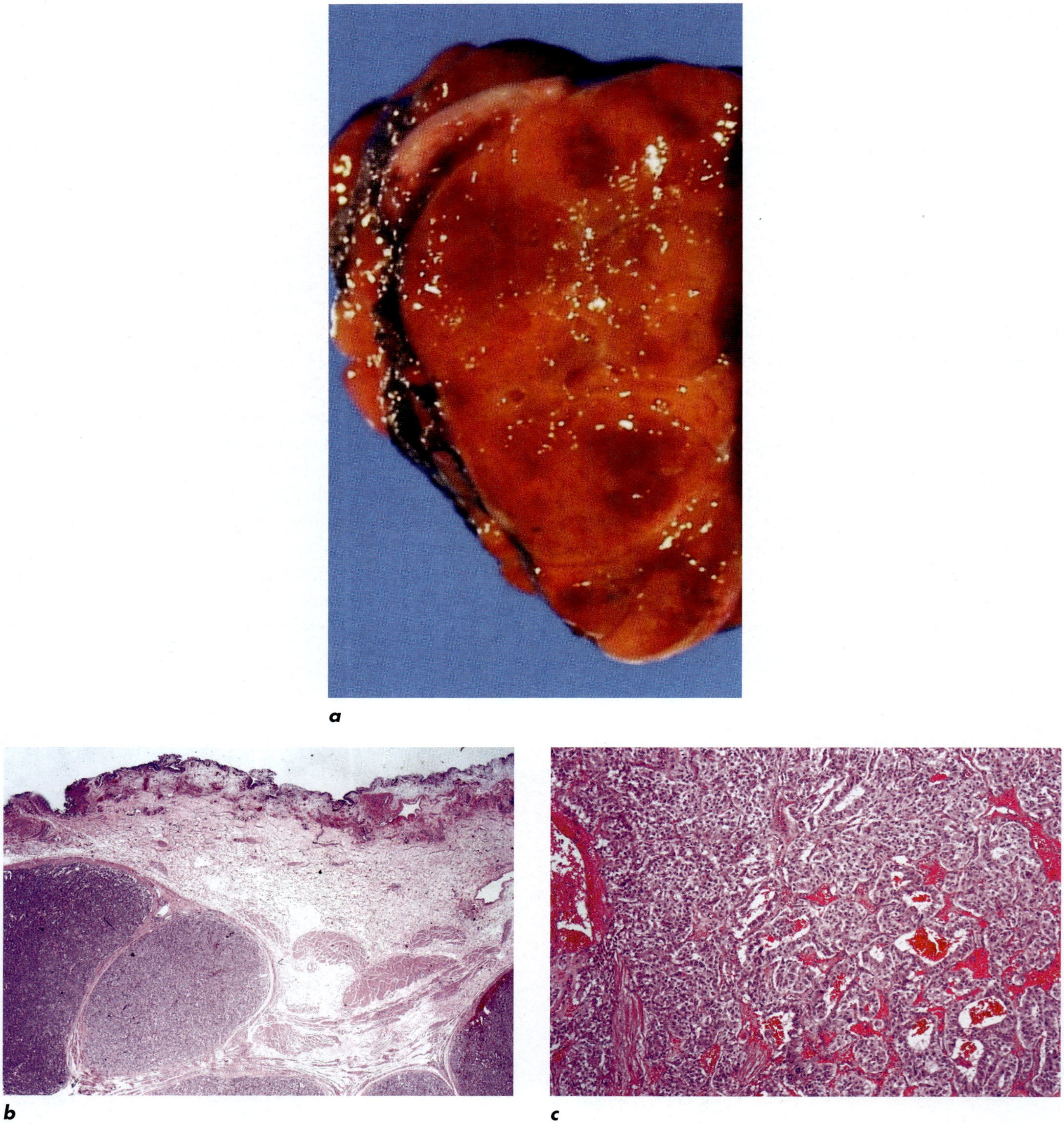

Figure 54-5.
Paraganglioma as a large fleshy mass with focal hemorrhage in the bladder wall (*a*). Microscopically, large islands of cells are located in the bladder wall with the intact urothelium (*b*). High magnification shows the nests of tumor cells with rich vasculature (*c*).

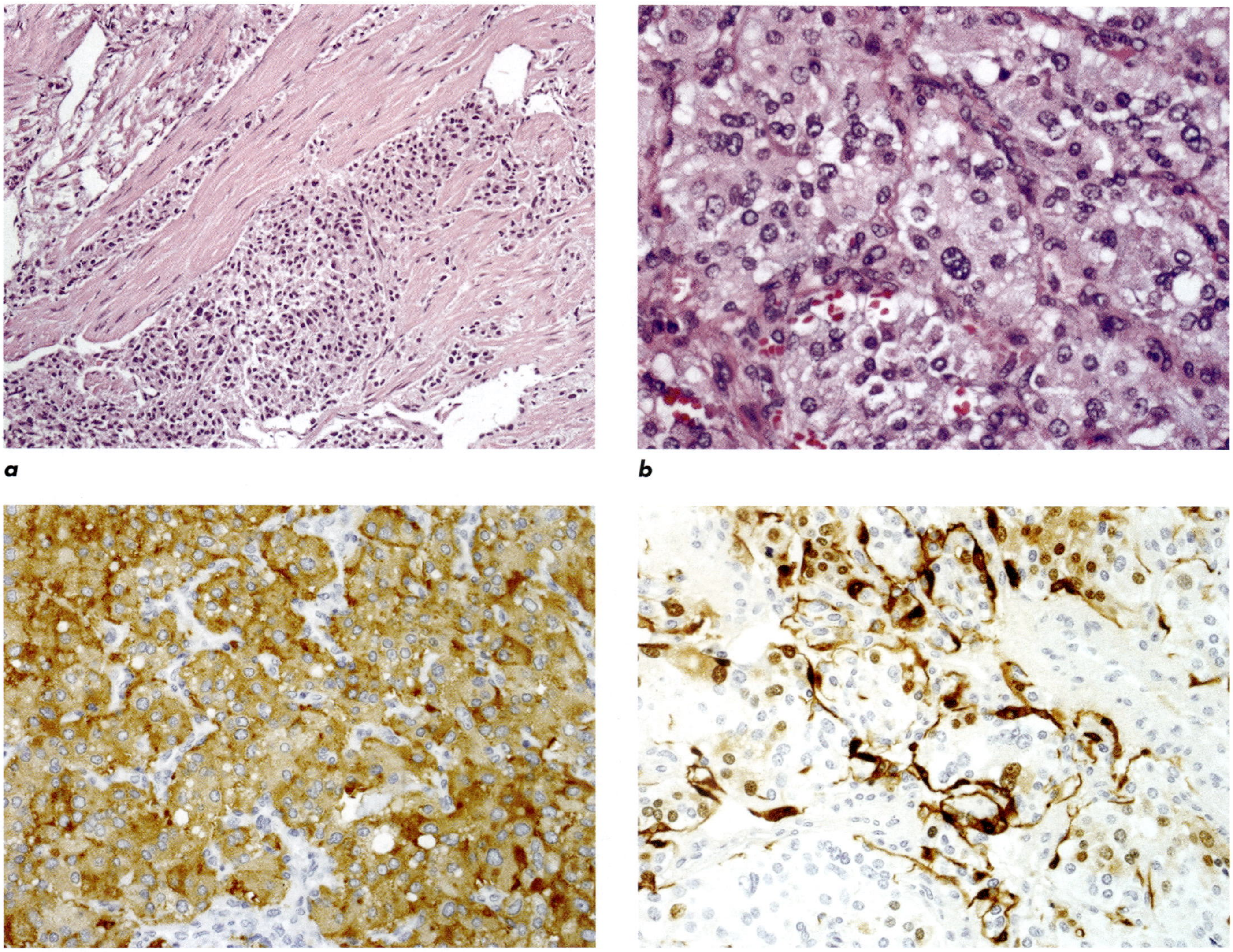

a b c d

Figure 54-6.

Paraganglioma cells are infiltrating muscularis propria (*a*). Tumor cells with granular cytoplasm and occasional nuclear atypia form typical Zellballen separated by thin septa (*b*). Tumor cells are positive for synaptophysin (*c*), and sustentacular cells are positive for S100 (*d*).

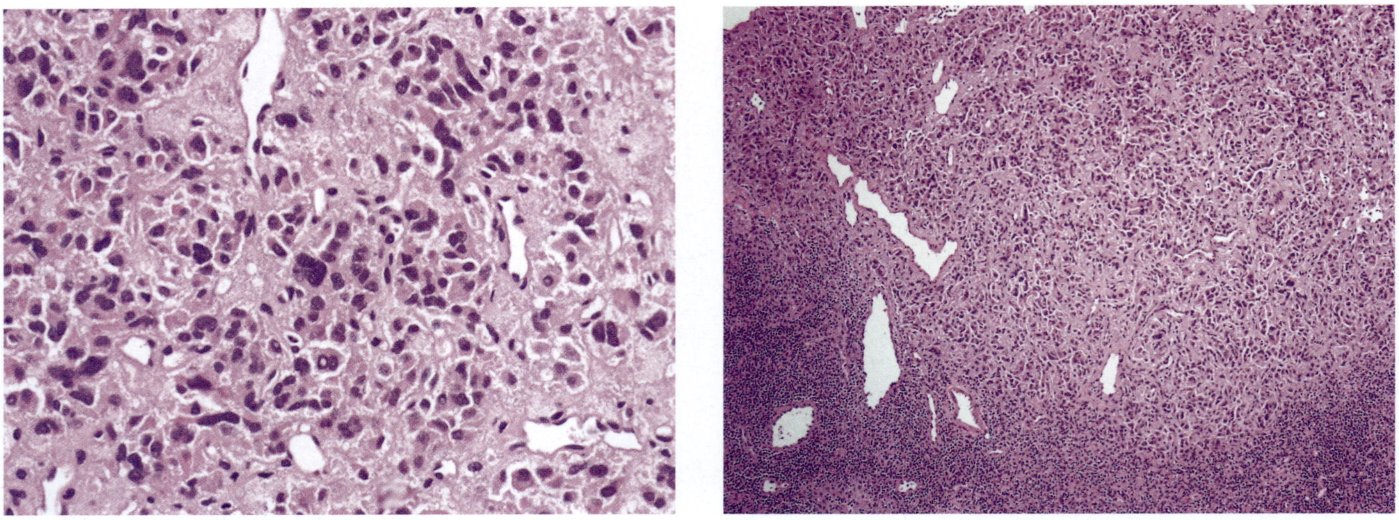

a *b*

Figure 54-7.
Paraganglioma shows prominent cytological atypia (*a*). However, the diagnosis of malignant paraganglioma can be made only when lymph node metastasis is identified in this case (*b*).

Immunohistochemistry

- Neuroendocrine markers such as chromogranin, synaptophysin, or NSE (Fig. 54-6*b*)
- Patchy sustentacular (supporting) cells positive for S100 (Fig. 54-6*d*)
- Epithelial markers such as AE1/AE3, Cam5.2, CK20, HMWCK negative
- Other urothelial markers such as S100p, GATA3, and p63 negative

Clinical relevance (prognosis and treatment options)

- Paragangliomas in the GU organs, morphologically indistinguishable from pheochromocytoma, have a slightly higher rate of malignancy (15% to 30%) than the adrenal counterpart (10%)
- Malignant paraganglioma can be diagnosed only when metastasis develops
- Surgical resection, partial or radical cystectomy is indicated
- Radiation may be used for cases with multiple recurrences
- Chemotherapy designed for bladder cancer has not been shown to be effective for paraganglioma, if paraganglioma is misdiagnosed as urothelial carcinoma

PRIMARY SARCOMAS

Definition

- Sarcoma is a malignant mesenchymal tumor developing in the bladder

Pathogenesis and epidemiology

- Primary bladder sarcoma is rare, accounting for less than 1% of bladder malignancies
- Rhabdomyosarcoma (sarcoma of skeletal muscle) and leiomyosarcoma (sarcoma of smooth muscle) are the most common sarcomas in the bladder
- Rhabdomyosarcoma is more common in children, while leiomyosarcoma is more common in adults
- Other sarcoma types such as angiosarcoma and malignant fibrous histiocytoma have been seen in the bladder

Clinical features

- Hematuria, irritative symptoms, or obstructive symptoms
- Large mass by cystoscopic or imaging studies
- Bladder mucosa biopsy may be negative if deeply seeded

Gross pathology

- If a tumor is deeply located in the bladder wall, bladder mucosa surface will be intact
- Late stage tumors will show large bulky mass (average size 7 cm) with hemorrhage, necrosis, and ulceration (Fig. 54-8*a*)
- Some cases of rhabdomyosarcoma in children may appear grape-like (sarcoma botryoid) lesions
- No typical papillary appearance of urothelial tumors

Histology

Rhabdomyosarcoma

- It may consist of
  - Small round or spindle cells (embryonal type, Fig. 54-8*b*) with hyperchromatic nuclei and diffuse arrangement (Fig. 54-9)
  - Large tumor cells with cross striations

Leiomyosarcoma

- Composed of infiltrative interlacing fascicles of long spindle cells (Fig. 54-10)
- High cellularity, pleomorphism, and increased mitoses (Fig. 54-11)
  - Low grade: <5 mitoses/10 HPF, moderate cytological atypia
  - High grade: >5 mitoses/10 HPF, marked cytological atypia
- Tumor necrosis may be present
- Invading adjacent tissue such as perivesical adipose tissue or eroding mucosal surface may be present

Figure 54-8.
Rhabdomyosarcoma of the bladder from an 18-year-old boy is a polypoid mass (*a*, arrow). Microscopically, the tumor cells are small spindle shaped with hyperchromatic nuclei in a loose background (*b*).

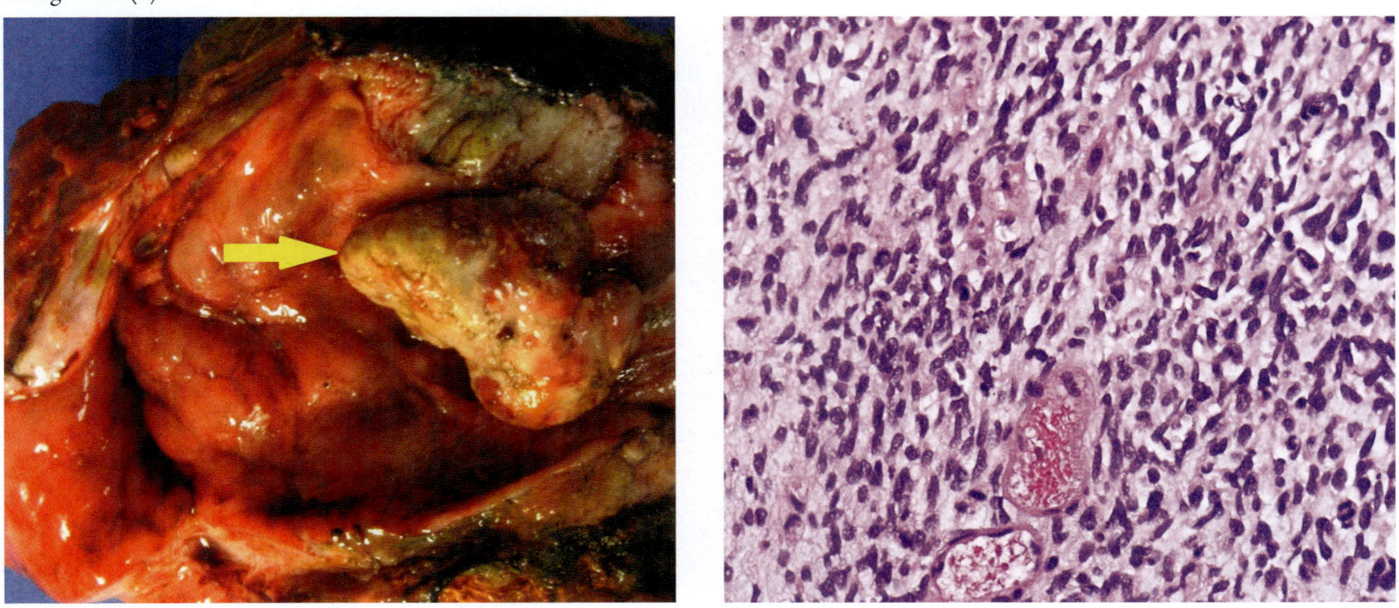

a *b*

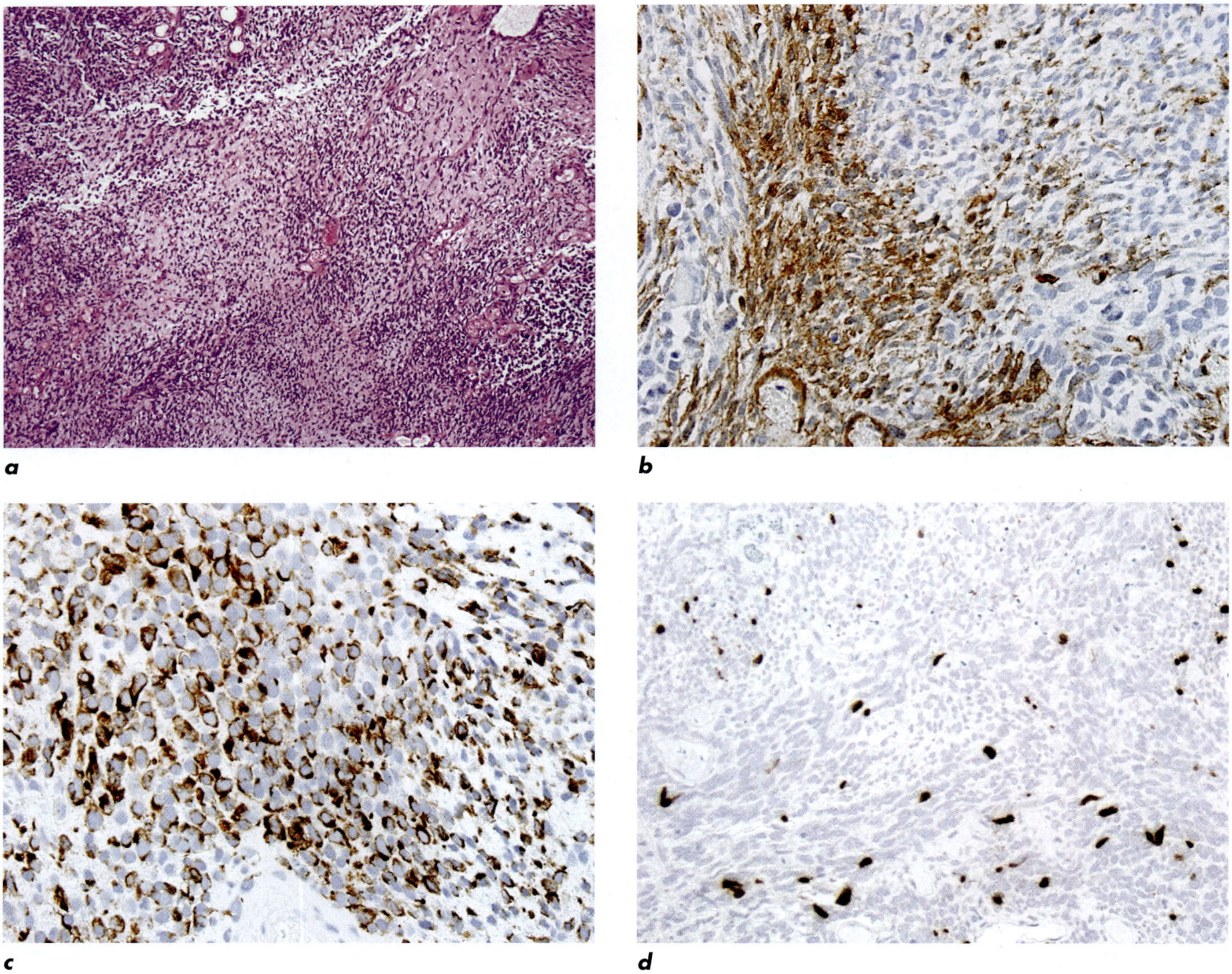

Figure 54-9.
Rhabdomyosarcoma of the bladder with small spindle tumor cells in diffuse patterns (*a*). The tumor cells are positive for desmin (*b*) and muscle-specific actin (*c*) and focally positive for myogenin (*d*).

Immunohistochemistry

- Smooth muscle actin, desmin (Fig. 54-9), vimentin positive
- Keratin markers negative

Clinical relevance (prognosis and treatment options)

- Prognosis remains to be poor with 5-year survival rate 50% to 70% after treatment
- Treatment of choice is surgical resection
- Chemotherapy and radiation may have benefits

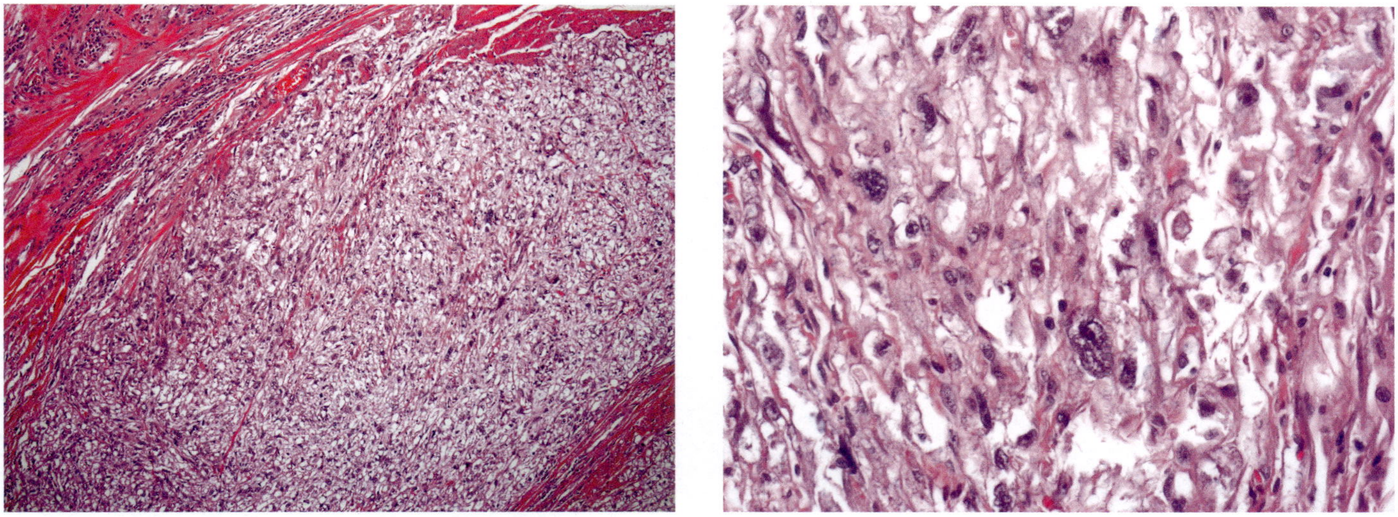

a **b**

Figure 54-10.
Leiomyosarcoma of the bladder is composed of malignant spindle cells infiltrating the bladder wall (*a*). Nuclear atypia of the leiomyosarcoma cells is prominent (*b*).

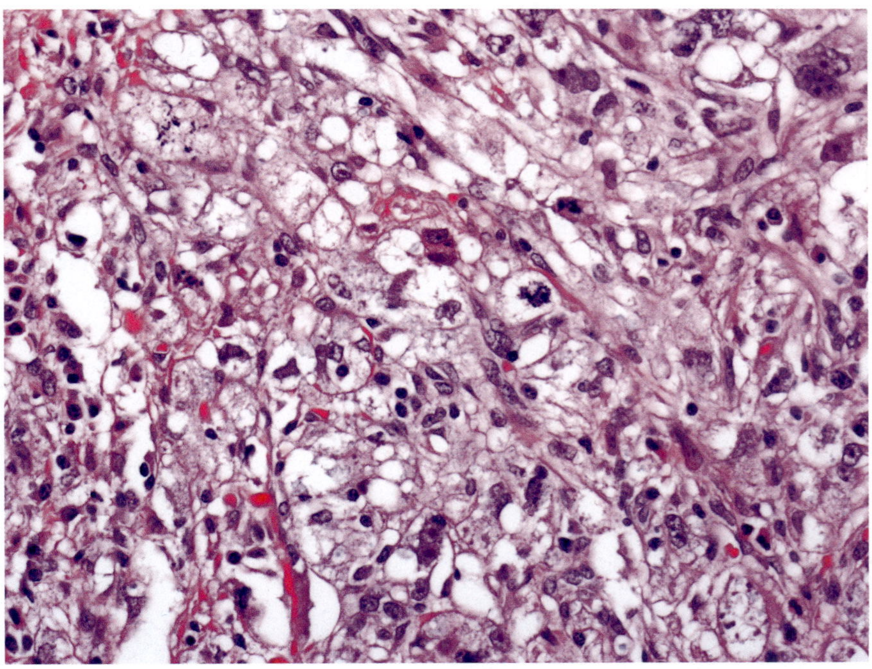

Figure 54-11.
Leiomyosarcoma of the bladder demonstrates frequent mitotic figures and cytological atypia.

MELANOMA

Definition

- Malignant melanocytic neoplasm develops in the bladder

Pathogenesis

- The primary melanoma is a very rare and many of the reported cases are metastatic melanomas

Clinical features

- Hematuria
- Bladder mass detected by imaging studies or cystoscopy
- The features of primary melanoma of the bladder
  - Lack of history of cutaneous melanoma
  - No evidence of regressed melanoma of the skin (by Woods lamp examination)
  - No evidence of a visceral melanoma in other organs
  - Patterns of the spread consistent with a bladder primary

Gross pathology

- Darkly pigmented lesion of variable size from 1 to 8 cm
- May involve urothelium or deeply seeded in the bladder wall

Histology

- Melanoma is composed of large pleomorphic cells with prominent nucleoli and dusty cytoplasm. Melanin pigment may be present in tumor cells (Fig. 54-12)
- Pagetoid melanoma in situ can be seen in urothelium (Fig. 54-13), either with or without invasive components, which does not necessarily define a primary melanoma
- Melanoma can display many unusual patterns, mimicking plasmacytoid urothelial carcinoma, small cell carcinoma, lymphoma, spindle cell tumor, or other malignant tumors (Fig. 54-14).
- Because of the diverse histological appearance, pathology diagnosis of a bladder melanoma can be difficult without a clinical history (Fig. 54-15). When a malignant tumor in the bladder is unusual and does not fit any typical types of bladder carcinoma, the possibility of a melanoma involving bladder should be excluded by obtaining a clinical history and using immunostains

Immunohistochemistry

- S100 positive (Figs. 54-13*b* and 54-15*b*), melan A positive, and HMB45 positive (Fig. 54-13*d*)
- Keratins negative

Clinical relevance (prognosis and treatment options)

- Clinical history of a known melanoma is very important
- Without clinical history or immunohistochemistry, melanoma can be easily mistaken for high-grade urothelial carcinoma or other malignancies
- The definition of a melanoma in the bladder is based on clinical information, histological features, and immunohistochemistry
- Very poor prognosis, the majority of patients with bladder melanoma die within a few years after diagnosis

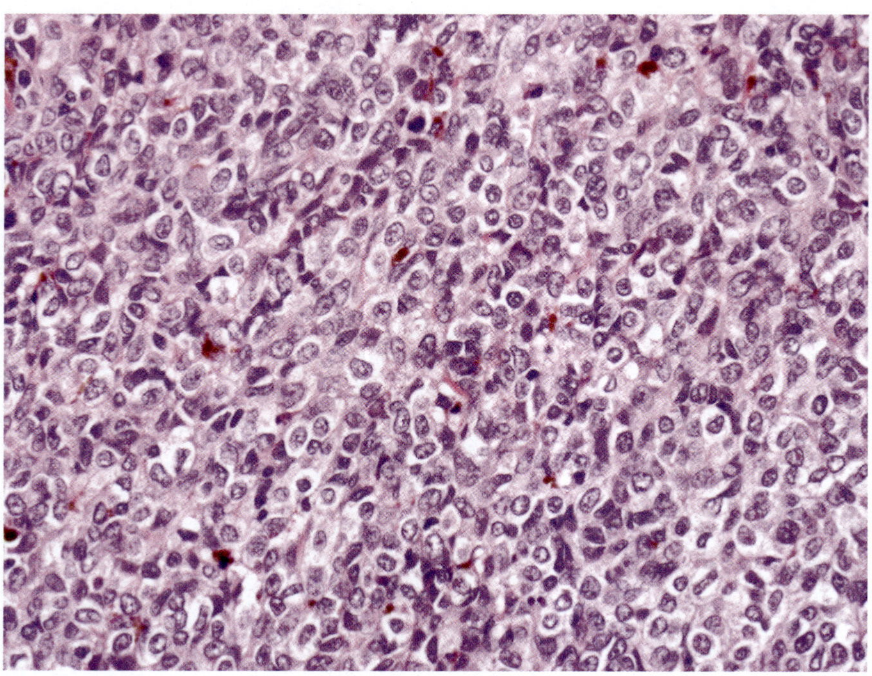

Figure 54-12.
A bladder melanoma is composed of epithelioid tumor cells displaying diffuse patterns. Occasionally, pigmented tumor cells can be seen.

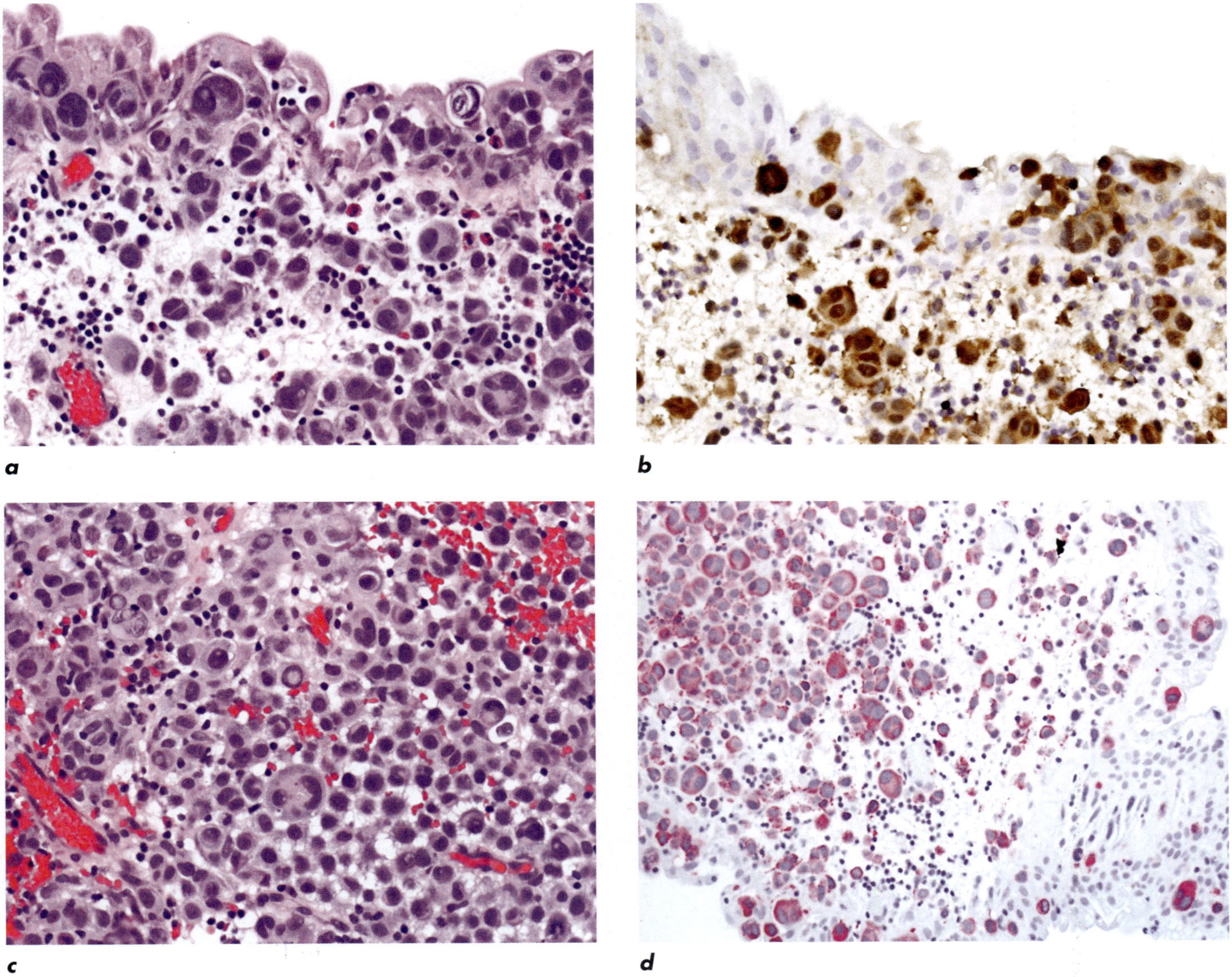

Figure 54-13.
Bladder melanoma involving urothelium as pagetoid spread (*a*); the tumor cells in the urothelium and lamina propria are positive for S100 (*b*). Another area of this melanoma is composed of plasmacytoid tumor cells (*c*), which are positive for HMB45 (*d*).

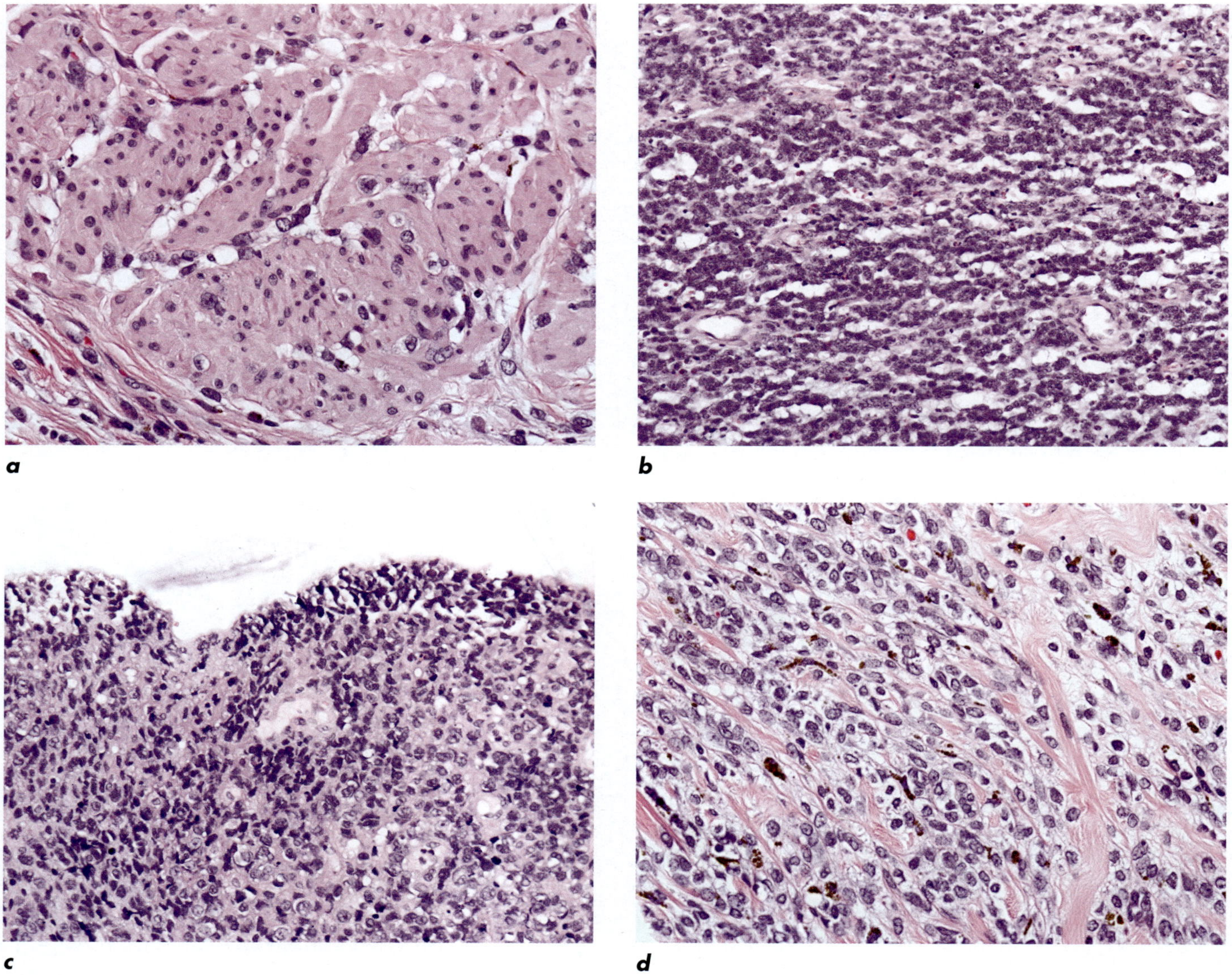

Figure 54-14.
Histological variations of bladder melanomas. A melanoma infiltrates muscularis propria, mimicking urothelial carcinoma (*a*). A melanoma consists of small tumor cells, mimicking small cell carcinoma (*b*). A melanoma underneath the intact urothelium with diffuse growth patterns, resembling lymphoma (*c*). Typical melanoma with pigmented tumor cells may also be present (*d*).

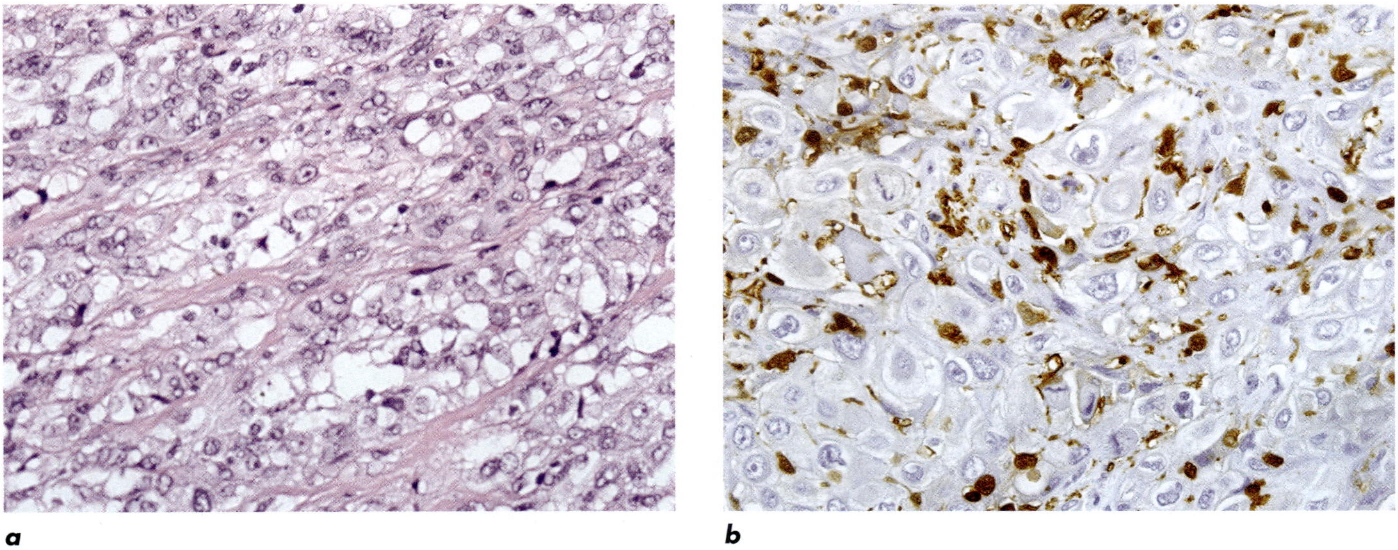

Figure 54-15.
Bladder melanoma, composed of large epithelial tumor cells (*a*). The diagnosis is confirmed by positive S100 immunostaining (*b*).

SECTION 7
The Urethra

CHAPTER 55 Pathology of the Urethra

Ximing J. Yang, Sanjiv V. Prabhu

THE NORMAL STRUCTURE OF THE URETHRA

Anatomy

- The urethra is a tubular organ (Fig. 55-1) connecting the bladder to outside of the body
- In males, the urethra is long and passing through the penis; it can be divided into
  - Prostatic urethra (where semen-containing ejaculatory ducts and prostatic ducts open)
  - Bulbar urethra
  - Penile urethra
    - The male urethra has a dual function, because it carries urine as well as semen
    - The meatus, which is the opening of the urethra, is situated on the glans penis
- In females, the urethra is shorter
  - It only carries urine
  - The meatus is situated in the vulva

Histology

- The proximal portion of the urethra is lined by urothelium (Fig. 55-2) and the distal portion by squamous epithelium
- Lamina propria is situated underneath the urothelium and squamous epithelium
- Periurethral glands are small glands, which secrete mucinous material and open in the urethra (Fig. 55-3)
- Most bladder or penile lesions can also be seen in the urethra. Cowper's glands are a pair of glands located in the bulb urethra. The lesions of the Cowper's glands may also cause urethral obstruction
- Penile urethra is surrounded by corpus spongiosum (Fig. 55-3)

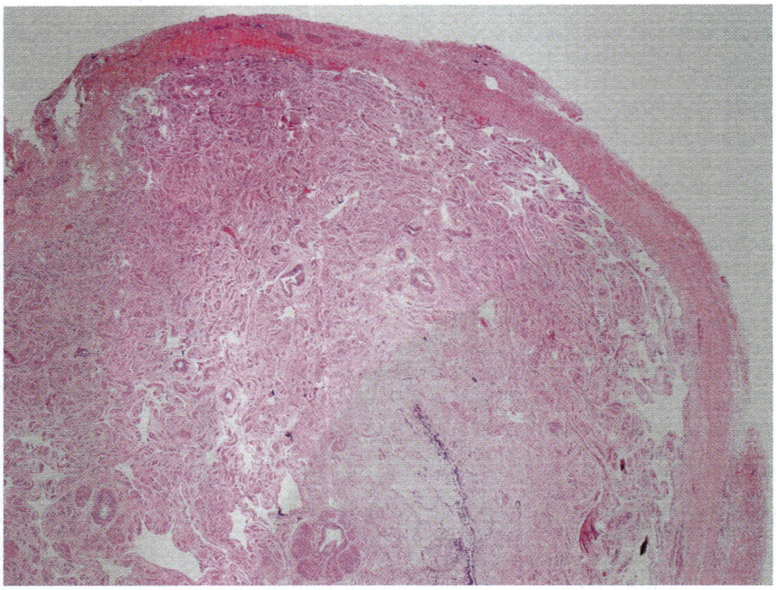

Figure 55-1.
Cross section of penile urethra, which is surrounded by corpus spongiosum.

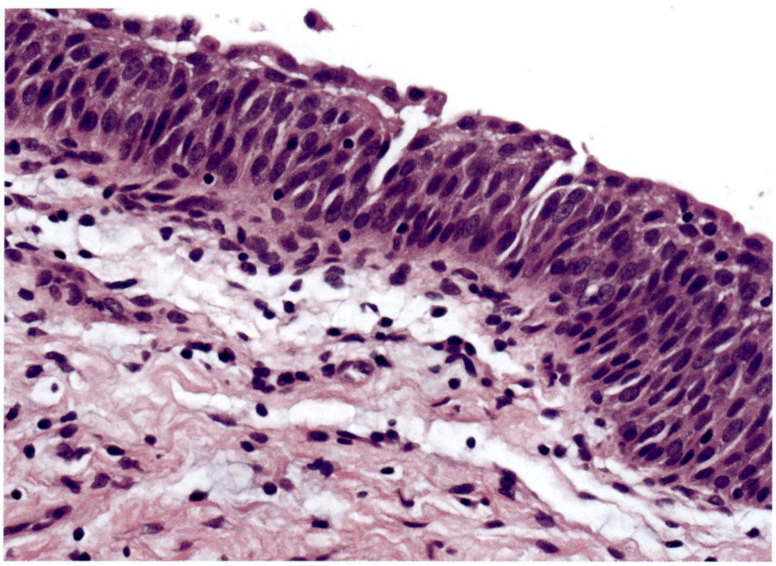

Figure 55-2.
The urethra is lined by urothelium, which is essentially the same as the one in the bladder and upper urinary tract.

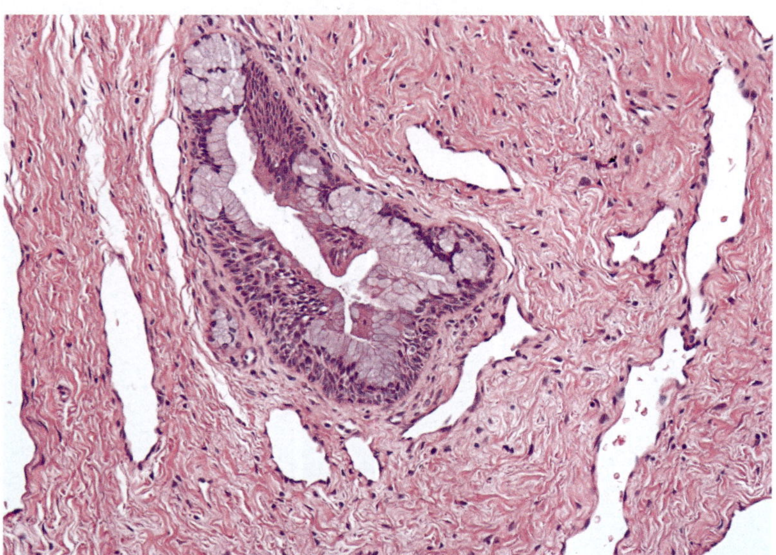

Figure 55-3.
Periurethral gland with a mucinous acinus embedded in erectile tissue of the corpus spongiosum.

CARUNCLE

Definition

- A benign polypoid lesion involving the distal urethra, characterized by the presence of large vessels with thrombosis and chronic inflammation

Pathogenesis and epidemiology

- Benign reactive condition
- Mostly seen in postmenopausal women, rare cases reported in men
- Probably caused by focal mucosal prolapse, with consequent vascular, epithelial, and stromal changes

Clinical features

- Most patients with urethral caruncle are asymptomatic
- Occasionally, patients may present with symptoms such as frequency, urgency, dysuria, and dyspareunia, particularly when the lesion is inflamed
- Hemorrhage, typically bloody spotting, is only seen when there is trauma or damage to the lining epithelium

Gross pathology

- A reddish or fleshy polypoid lesion in the urethra, protruding from the posterior lip of the urethral orifice
- Usually small in size, less than 1 to 2 cm in diameter

Histology

- Caruncle is characterized by a polypoid mucosal lesion representing prolapse (Fig. 55-4)
- Three components
  - Reactive surface epithelium (Fig. 55-5), either urothelial or squamous. The epithelial cells can be hyperplastic, but dysplasia is and viral cytopathic change are not seen
  - Prominent vessels in the lamina propria stroma. Thrombosis or hemorrhage can be seen (Fig. 55-6)
  - Acute or chronic inflammation
- Some investigators have described three histological groups: papillomatous (epithelium as predominant component), angiomatous (blood vessel as predominant component), and granulomatous (inflammation as predominant component). The classification and grouping are not clinically relevant
- Most often, all three histological components are present in a single lesion

Differential diagnosis

Urothelial or squamous cell carcinoma

- Because of the polypoid appearance, a papillary urothelial carcinoma or squamous cell carcinoma needs to be excluded
- Carcinoma or dysplastic lesions differ from caruncle in the presence of cytologically atypical epithelial cells
- Invasive component may be present in carcinoma

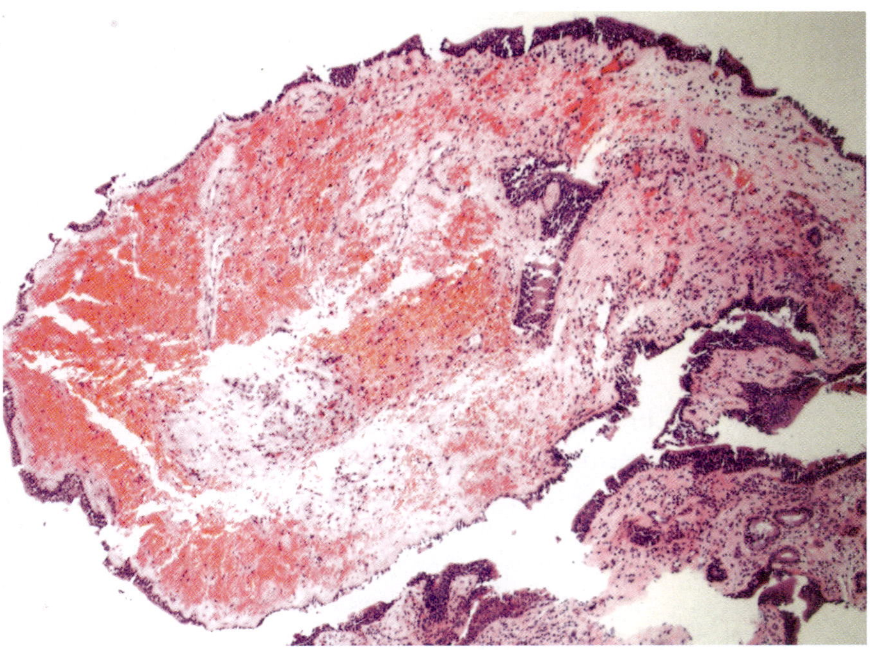

Figure 55-4.
Urethral caruncle with polypoid appearance. Reactive surface urothelium and stromal hemorrhage can be seen.

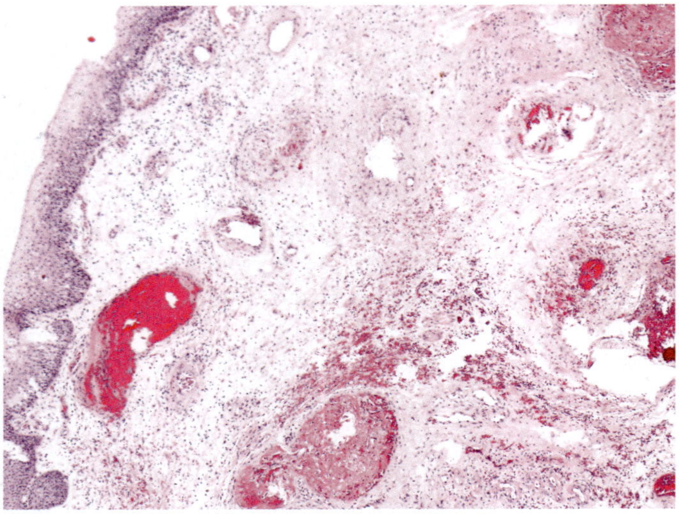

a

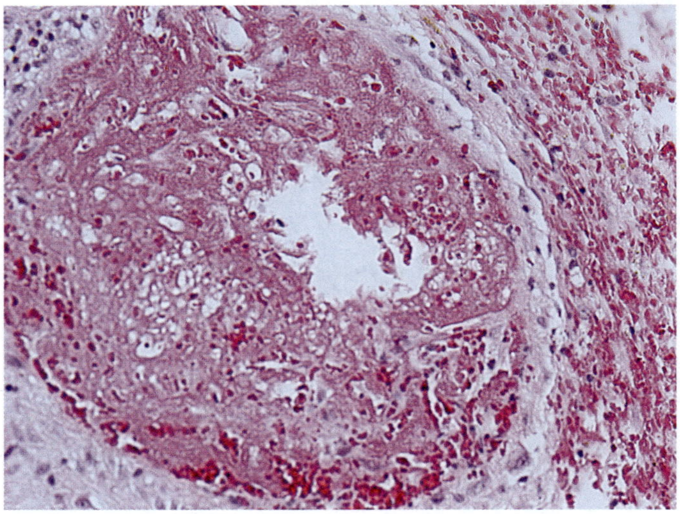

b

Figure 55-5.
Urethral caruncle with reactive urothelium, vascular thrombosis, and chronic inflammation (*a*). High magnification shows organization of a thrombus (*b*).

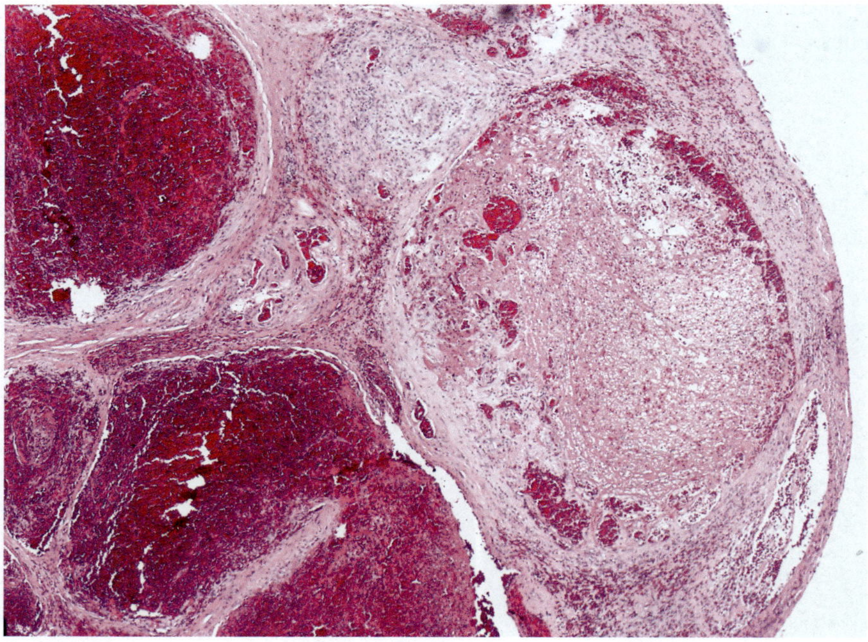

Figure 55-6.
Urethral caruncle showing blood vessel with thrombosis and hemorrhage in the stroma.

Inflammatory myofibroblastic tumor (inflammatory pseudotumor)

- Inflammatory myofibroblastic tumor composed mostly of proliferating spindle myoepithelial cells in a myxoid background
- Background of lymphocytic infiltrates
- In the cases with uncertainty, a biopsy with a panel of immunohistochemical markers including ALK, calponin, and smooth muscle actin may be helpful to establish a diagnosis
- Most cases can be diagnosed based on H&E slides

Clinical relevance (treatment options and prognosis)

- Urethral caruncle is a benign condition with no treatment necessary if asymptomatic
- Conservative treatment such as topical medication or warm sitz bath may relieve the symptoms
- Surgical treatment is performed for symptomatic cases resistant to conservative therapies or cases with suspicion for neoplastic lesions

URETHRAL DIVERTICULUM

Definition

- Characterized by the outpouching or invagination of urothelial mucosa into the urethral wall
- Diverticulitis: inflammation associated with a diverticulum

Pathogenesis

- Mostly affecting women
- Defect or weakness of urethral wall is a risk factor
- Relatively common condition, similar to bladder diverticulum
- May be acquired after injuries including trauma, infection, or obstruction

Clinical features

- May be asymptomatic
- Some patients develop a bulging mass, which may be palpated in the anterior vaginal wall
- Signs of inflammation or obstruction if it is associated with infection or calculi

Histology

- Diverticulum is characterized by the invagination of urothelial mucosa (Fig. 55-7*a*)
- The outpouched mucosa is lined by benign urothelium
- Urothelium may undergo squamous metaplasia
- Often associated with chronic inflammation, which is called diverticulitis (Fig. 55-7*b*)
- Ulceration or fistula may develop
- In the late stage, there might be extensive fibrosis in the wall, resulting in urethral stricture
- Occasionally, other conditions may be harbored in a diverticulum, such as colonic metaplasia, nephrogenic adenoma, condyloma, or even urothelial carcinoma

Clinical relevance (prognosis and treatment options)

- Benign
- Surgical resection if symptomatic or suspicious for other lesions in the diverticulum

Figure 55-7.
Urethral diverticulum with invagination of urothelium (*a*). High magnification shows the diverticulum with reactive urothelial lining and chronic inflammation (*b*).

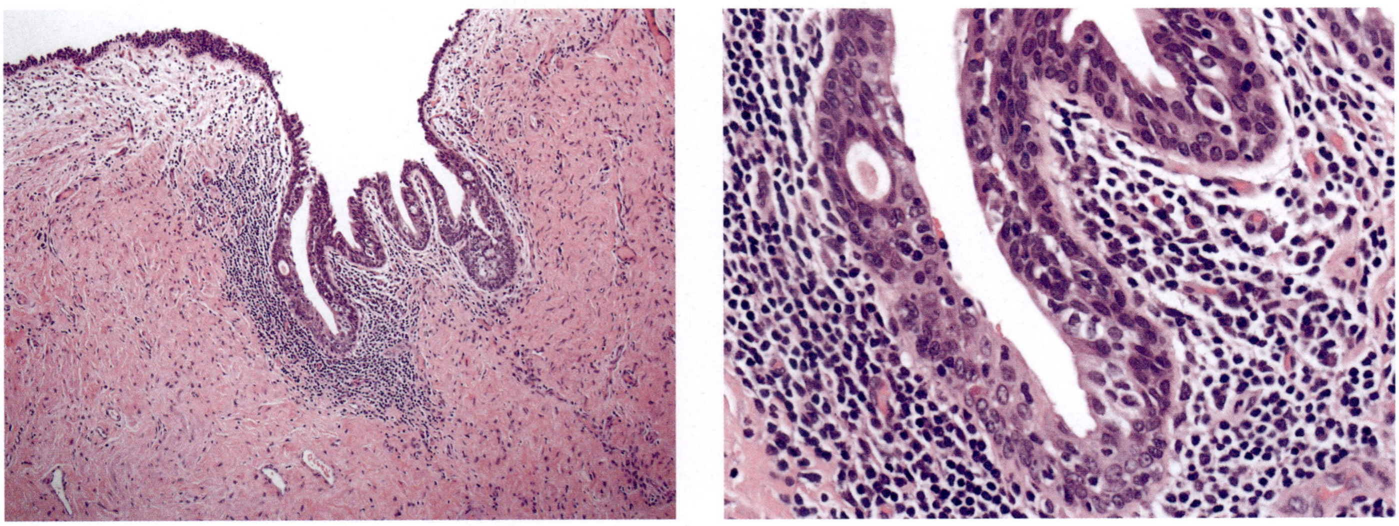

a **b**

INFLAMMATION AND REACTIVE CHANGES OF COWPER'S GLANDS

Definition

- Inflammation associated with Cowper's glands, a pair of mucinous glands located in bulbar urethra
- Cowper's gland metaplasia is characterized by mucin depletion, and hyperplasia is characterized by increased glandular cell number caused by reactive proliferation

Pathogenesis

- Infection or noninfectious etiologies lead to chronic or acute inflammation and reactive cell proliferation of the Cowper's glands

Clinical features

- Urinary obstruction if the lesion is large
- May be associated with an abscess or present as a mass lesion

Histology

- Chronic inflammation of the Cowper's glands is characterized by the lymphocytic infiltrates (Fig. 55-8)
- Normal Cowper's glands are typically arranged in lobular patterns, surrounded by skeletal muscle. There are two histological components: mucinous acini and ducts (Fig. 55-9*a*)
- Glandular metaplasia and hyperplasia of Cowper's glands may be present with or without inflammation (Fig. 55-9*b*)

Figure 55-8.
Cowper's gland is associated with chronic inflammation (*a*). High magnification shows the loss of mucinous features in most acini and dilated ducts become more prominent (*b*).

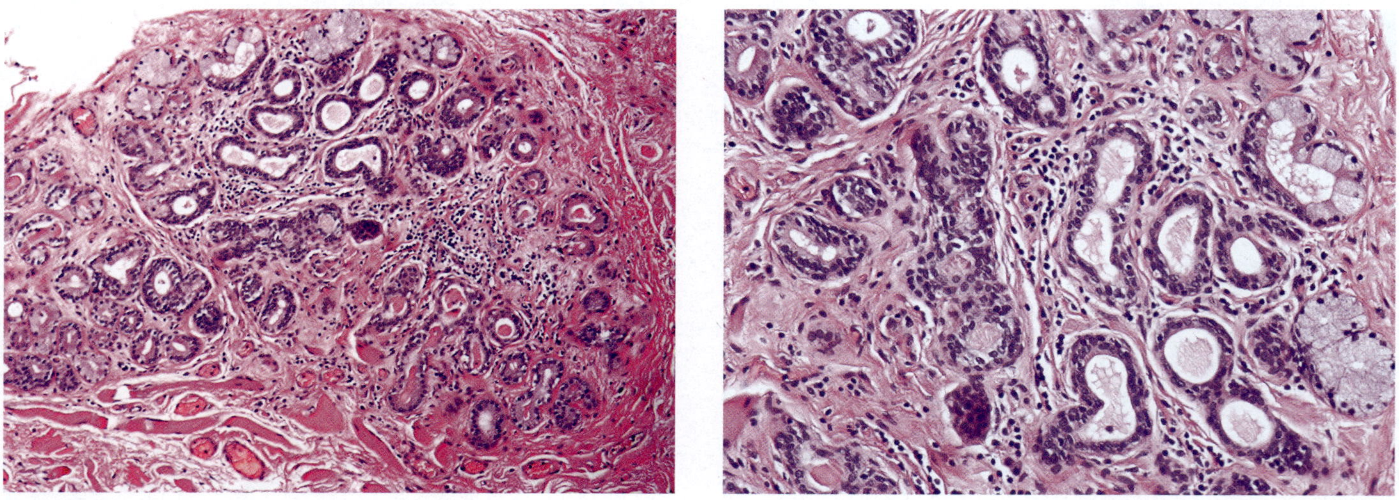

a **b**

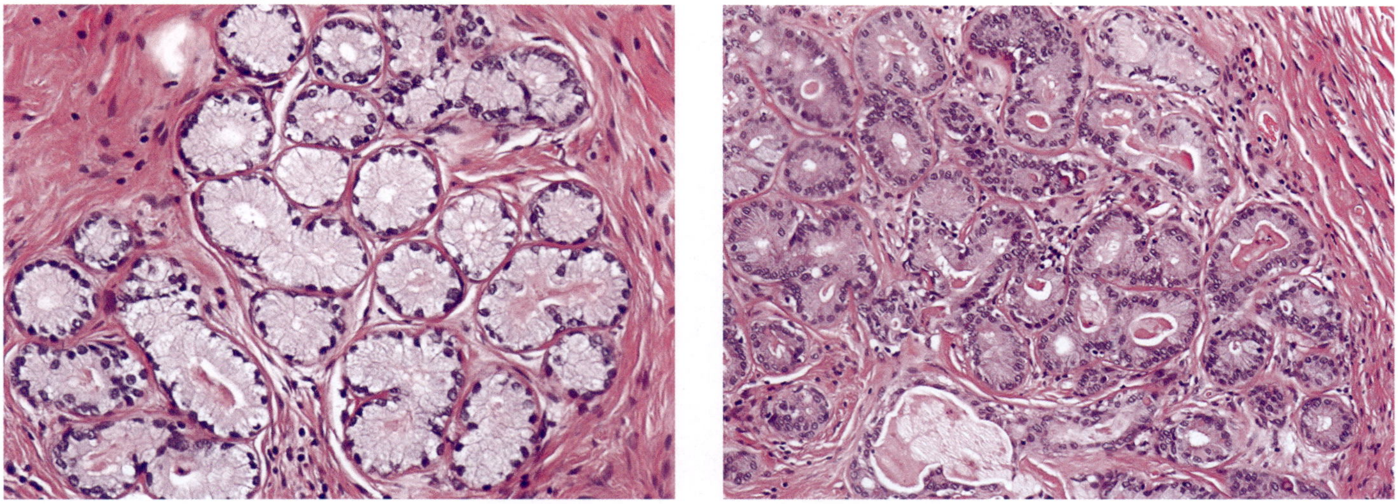

Figure 55-9.
Comparison of uninvolved normal mucinous acini (*a*) and reactive Cowper's gland with mucin depletion and glandular cell proliferation (*b*), which can be confused with adenocarcinoma.

URETHRAL STRICTURE

Definition

- A common clinical condition related to fibrotic narrowing of the urethra caused by various etiologies and pathologic changes

Pathogenesis

- Various injuries to the urethral tissue leading to the fibrosis in which the tissue elasticity is lost
- Risk factors including infection, instrumentation, trauma, and radiation
- Several pathological conditions responsible or associated with urethral stricture are listed in Table 55-1
- One of the most common etiologies is lichen sclerosus
- In rare cases, strictures may be caused by fibrosis related to a malignancy or nephrogenic adenoma

Clinical features

- More common in men
- Urinary obstruction
- Other signs related to the specific etiology

Histology

- Nonspecific chronic inflammation is often present (Fig. 55-10)
- Variable degree of dense fibrosis (Fig. 55-11)
- Hyperplastic squamous or urothelium with squamous metaplasia
- The histological features of lichen sclerosus should be sought, which include loss of basal cells, atrophic epithelium, stromal edema, and fibrosis with hyalinization
- Sometimes, no specific etiology can be detected. Only descriptive diagnosis will be rendered

Lichen sclerosus (lichen sclerosus et atrophicus)

- Lichen sclerosus is also called *balanitis xerotica obliterans* when found in the glans penis. The details of this condition are provided in Chapter 25. However, this condition is not limited to the glans penis; it can be found in other locations such as foreskin or distal urethra. This disease is under-recognized in pathology reports for patients with urethral strictures
- There are two phases (forms)
  - Inflammatory phase, often nonspecific, including loss of basal cells and lichenoid chronic inflammation (Fig. 55-12)
  - Sclerosing phase, characteristic of lichen sclerosus, including atrophic squamous/urothelial mucosa, loss of basal layer, and hyalinized stroma (Fig. 55-13)

Clinical relevance (prognosis and treatment options)

- The diagnosis of lichen sclerosus may lead to specific treatment, such as topical steroids, tacrolimus, and laser treatment
- Early diagnosis and treatment may result in better prognosis
- Late stage may require surgical resection and urethroplasty
- There is a possibility that urethral stricture may be associated with cancer. But the degree of the risk is uncertain

Table 55-1. List of Common Pathology Diagnoses in Cases with Clinical Diagnosis of Urethral Stricture

Pathology diagnosis	*Clinical diagnosis*
Nonspecific chronic inflammation and/or fibrosis	Urethral strictures
Urethral epithelium and stromal fibrosis	Urethral strictures
Lichen sclerosus	Urethral strictures
Other conditions including nephrogenic adenoma associated with inflammation	Urethral strictures
Urothelial carcinoma (rare)	Urethral strictures

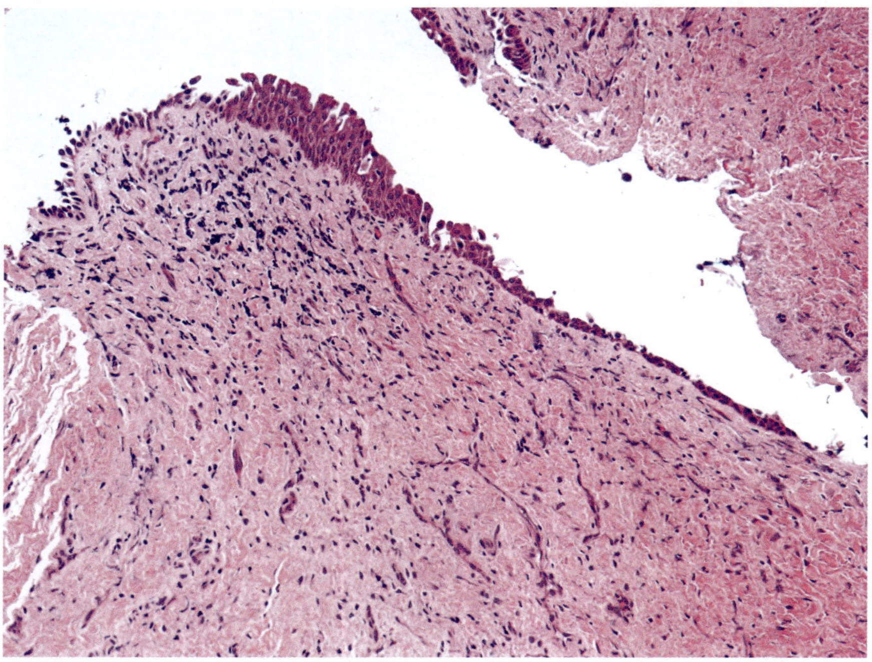

Figure 55-10.
Urethral stricture with nonspecific chronic inflammation and fibrosis.

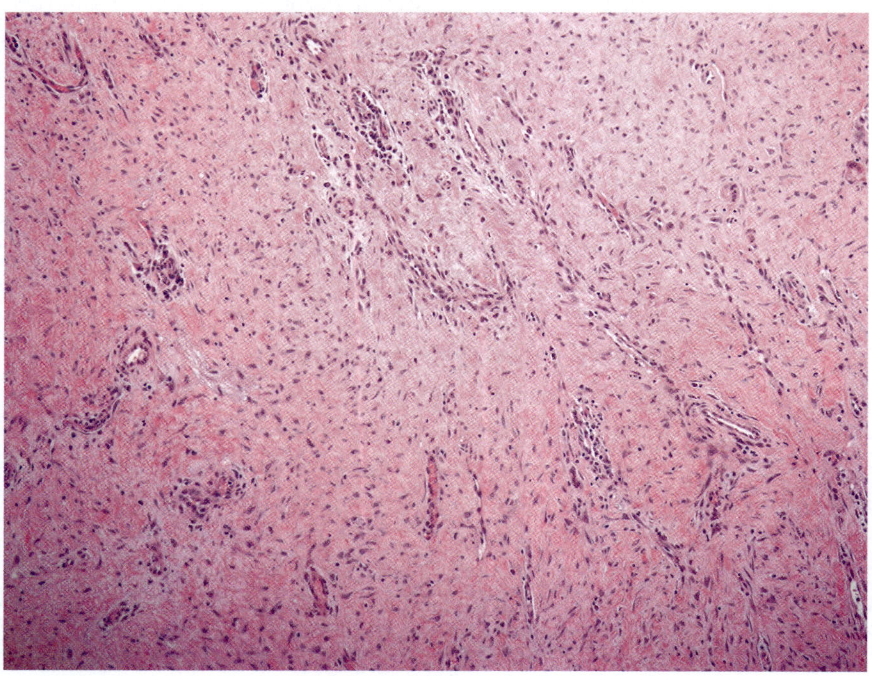

Figure 55-11.
Urethral stricture with prominent submucosal fibrosis without obvious active inflammation.

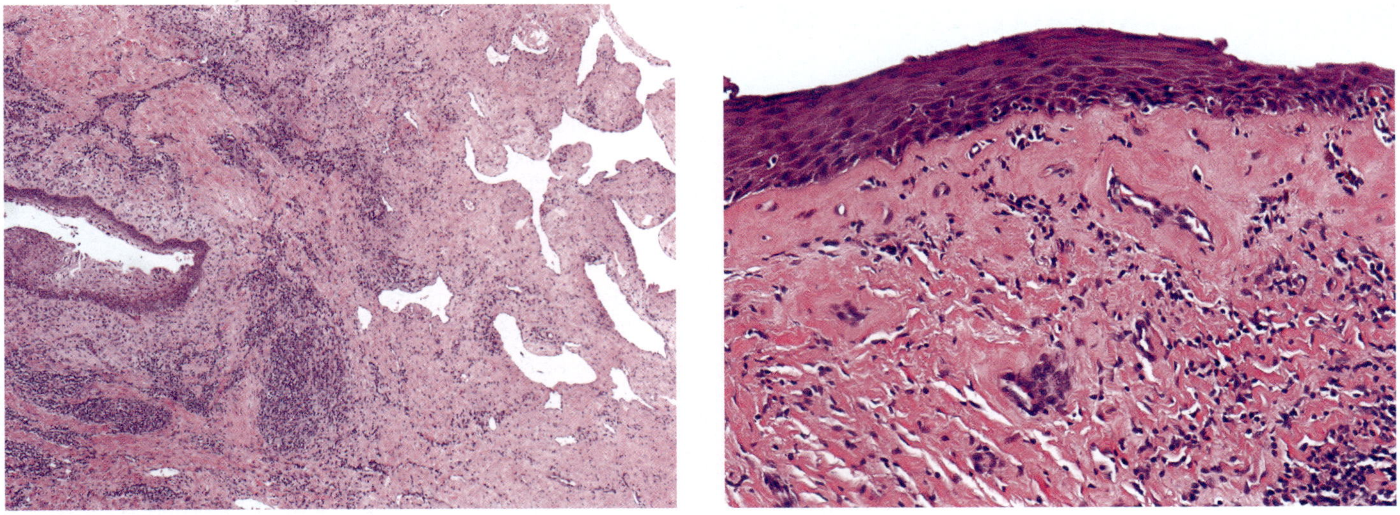

a ***b***

Figure 55-12.
Lichen sclerosus resulting in urethral stricture. The urethral tissue with lichenoid chronic inflammation and reactive squamous changes (*a*). High magnification demonstrates the loss of basal cells, chronic inflammation, and early lamina propria fibrosis (*b*).

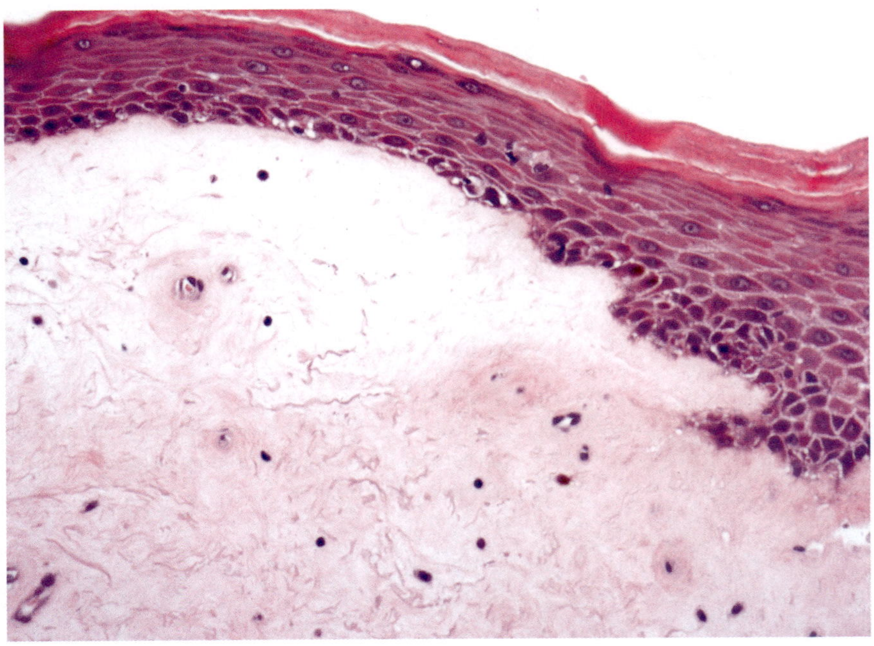

Figure 55-13.
Lichen sclerosus in late stage of urethral stricture showing prominent acellular stromal fibrosis.

OTHER REACTIVE CHANGES IN URETHRA

Definition

- Many inflammatory or reactive changes, which typically occur in the bladder, can also develop in the urethra
- Most of these lesions are discussed in Chapters 46 to 48
- Other lesions occurring in the penis can also involve the urethra such as condyloma acuminata and lichen sclerosus

Pathogenesis

- Developmental: diverticulum, prostatic-type polyp
- Infectious and inflammatory: chronic urethritis, urethritis glandularis, polypoid urethritis, condyloma acuminata
- Other reactive changes: nephrogenic adenoma, lichen sclerosus, squamous metaplasia

Clinical features

- Nonspecific clinical symptoms such as irritation and hematuria
- Polypoid, small nodular, or larger mass lesions

Histology

- Urethritis glandularis (Fig. 55-14)
  - Presence of glandular structures involving surface urothelium, the lamina propria with or without Von Brunn nests
  - Typically associated with chronic inflammatory infiltrates
  - May be associated with colonic metaplasia (Fig. 55-15), which is believed to be the precursor lesion of adenocarcinoma
- Polypoid urethritis (Fig. 55-16)
  - Polypoid lesion in the urethra
  - Histologically, there is prominent edematous or fibrotic stroma
  - Large "feeder" vessels can be seen
  - Associated chronic inflammatory infiltrates
  - Lining urothelium is benign
- Prostatic-type polyp (Fig. 55-17)
  - Polypoid lesion present in the urethral mucosa
  - Clusters of benign prostatic glands
  - Can be confirmed with positive PSA immunostaining
- Nephrogenic adenoma (Figs. 55-18 and 55-19)
  - Usually associated with a history of urethral injury
  - Morphologically similar to the one in the bladder
  - Small lesion composed of benign glandular cells
  - Associated with granulation tissue background and chronic inflammation
  - Can be deep in the stroma
  - Immunohistochemistry: PAX8 positive, AMACR positive, PSA negative

Clinical relevance (prognosis and treatment options)

- Most of the benign conditions are diagnosed in a biopsy specimen
- Treated with conservative medical therapies, local resection surgery, or transurethral resection
- Important to distinguish these benign conditions from malignant neoplasms

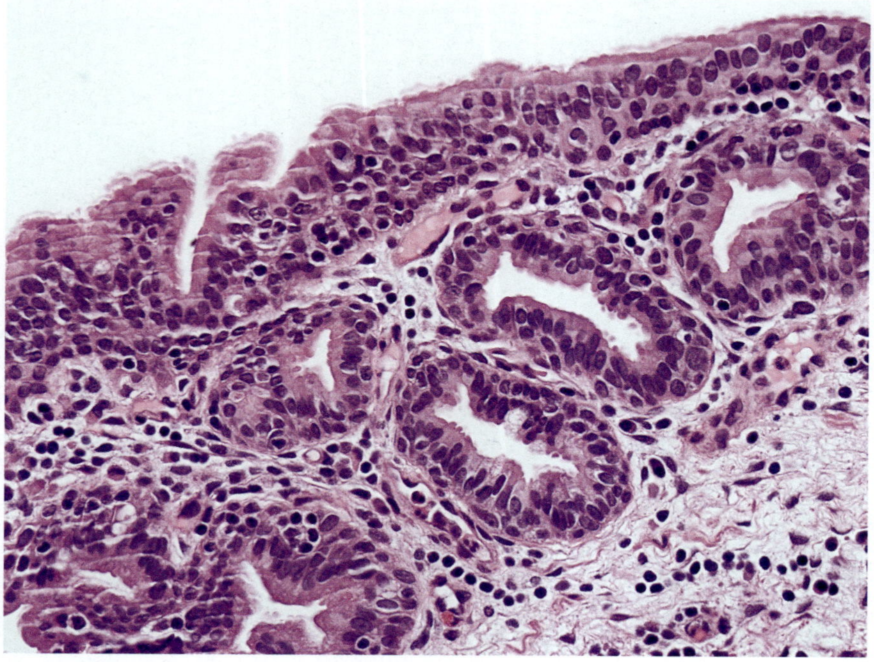

Figure 55-14. Urethritis glandularis characterized by glandular structures involving urothelium, associated with chronic inflammation.

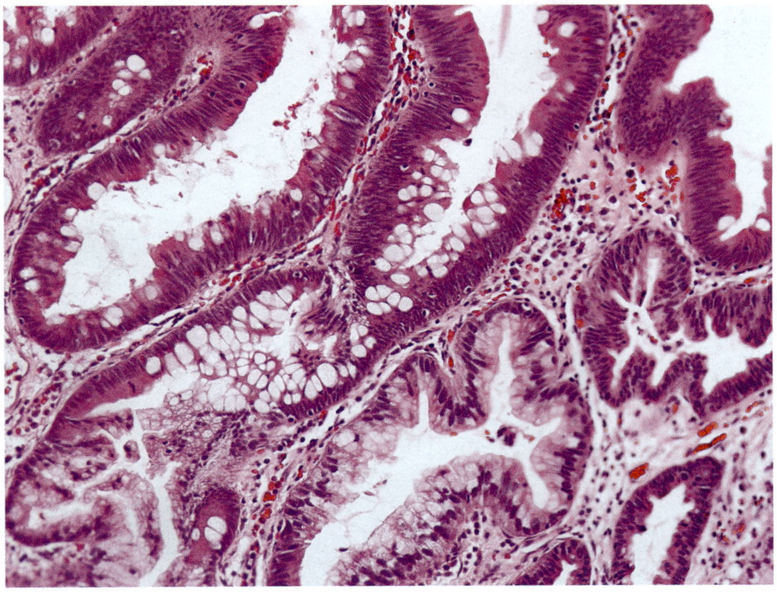

Figure 55-15.
Colonic metaplasia of the urethra is characterized by the presence of intestinal epithelium and goblet cells.

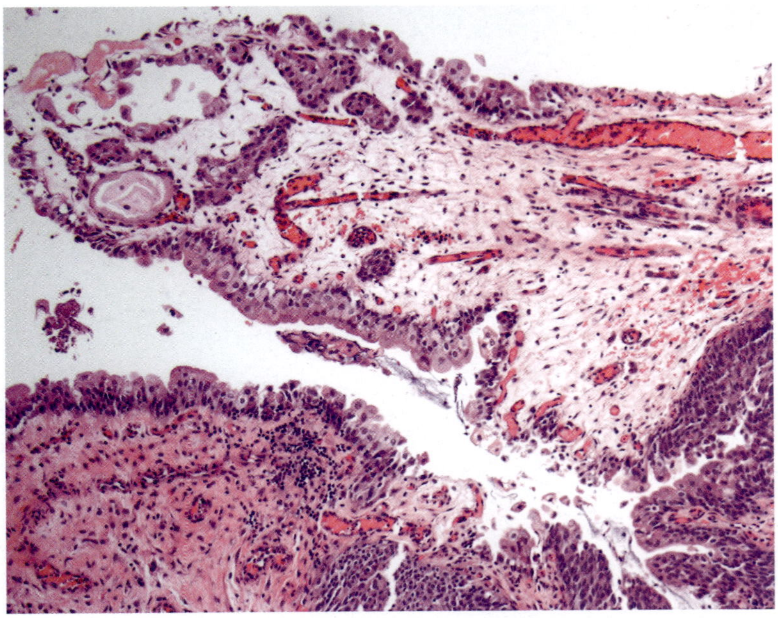

Figure 55-16.
Polypoid urethritis signified by prominent edematous stroma and dilated vessels, reactive urothelium, and occasional chronic inflammatory cells.

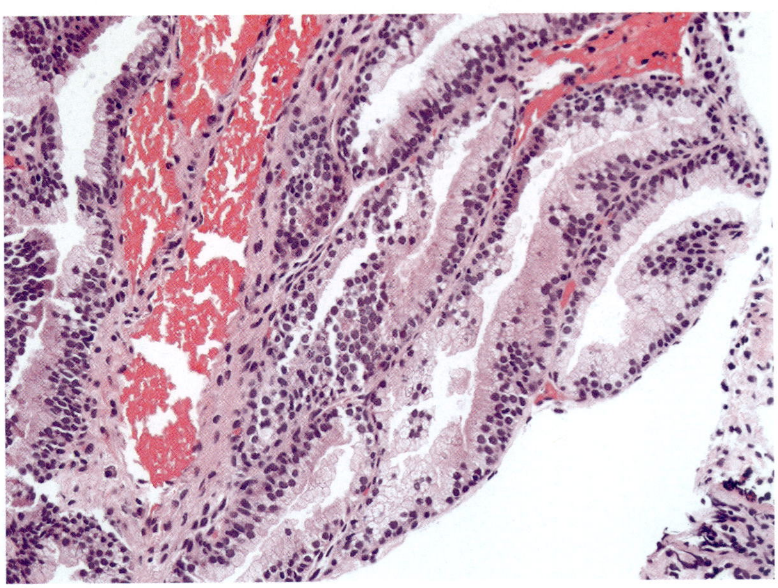

Figure 55-17.
Prostatic-type polyp is characterized by polypoid benign prostatic glands containing prostatic basal cells and secretory cells.

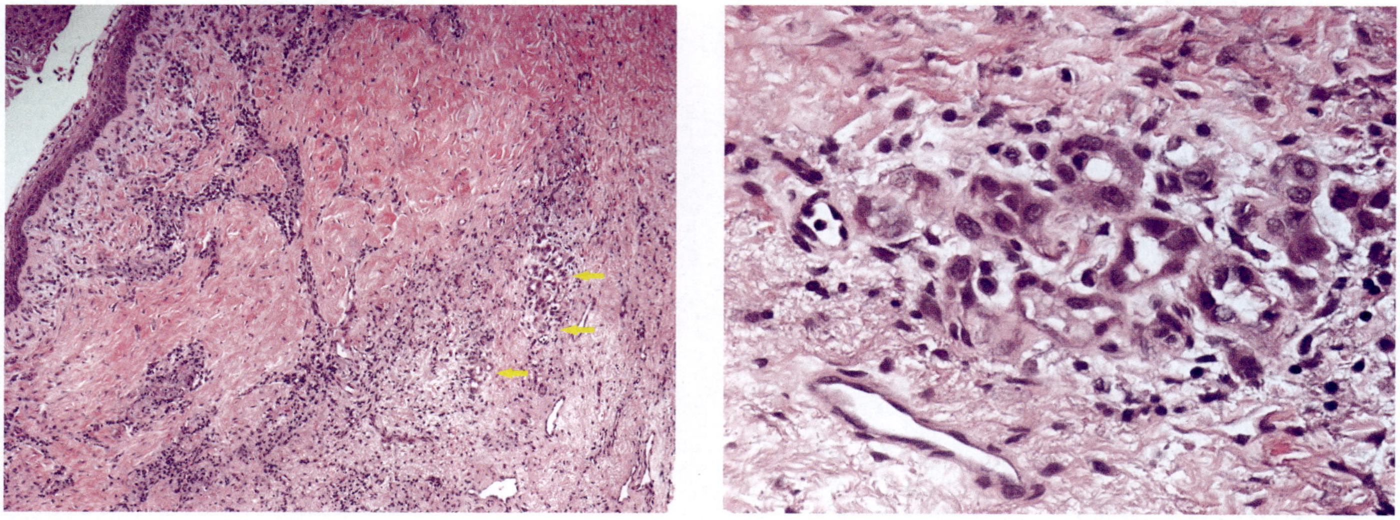

a b

Figure 55-18.
Nephrogenic adenoma of the urethra deep in the stroma indicated by arrows (*a*). High magnification demonstrates the typical bland cytology of the glandular components and granulation tissue-like stroma (*b*).

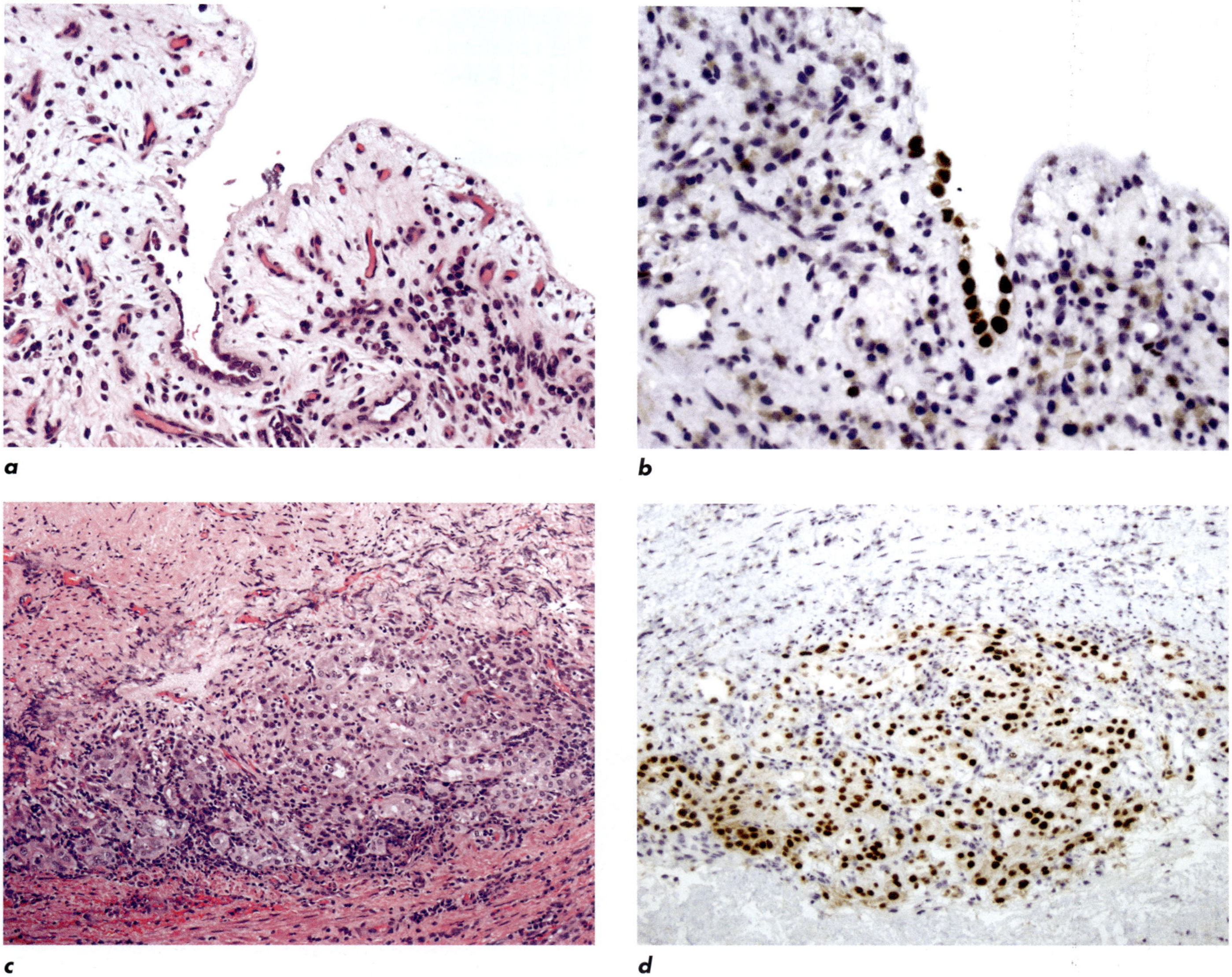

Figure 55-19.
Nephrogenic adenomas of the urethra composed of glandular cells involving surface urothelium (*a*, *b*) or deep in the stroma (*c*, *d*). The lesional cells show strong PAX8 immunoreactivity in surface glandular cells (*b*) and cluster in the stroma (*d*). Prominent chronic inflammation is present in both lesions.

INVERTED PAPILLOMA OF THE URETHRA

Definition

- Benign urothelial neoplasm with predominantly endophytic growth patterns

Clinical features

- May be asymptomatic as an incidental finding
- Hematuria
- Dome-shaped masses in the urethra by cystoscopic examination

Gross pathology

- Small lesions less than 2 to 3 cm in size

Histology

- Similar to the bladder-inverted papilloma
- Large islands or nests of urothelial cells (Fig. 55-20*a*) separated by thin fibrovascular cores or septa
- Tumor cells show nuclear grooving and bland cytological features, and mitosis is rare
- Peripheral palisading is prominent (Fig. 55-20*b*)

Differential diagnosis

Low-grade urothelial carcinoma

- It may show inverted growth patterns, but it has typically more cytologic atypia
- Higher proliferative Ki67 activity and positive for p53 and CK20

Clinical relevance (prognosis and treatment options)

- Benign, but with a low recurrence rate
- Resected if symptomatic or suspicious for malignancy

Figure 55-20.
Inverted papilloma in the prostatic urethra (*a*). The tumor is composed of large nests of neoplastic urothelial cells with peripheral palisading; no significant cytological atypia is seen (*b*).

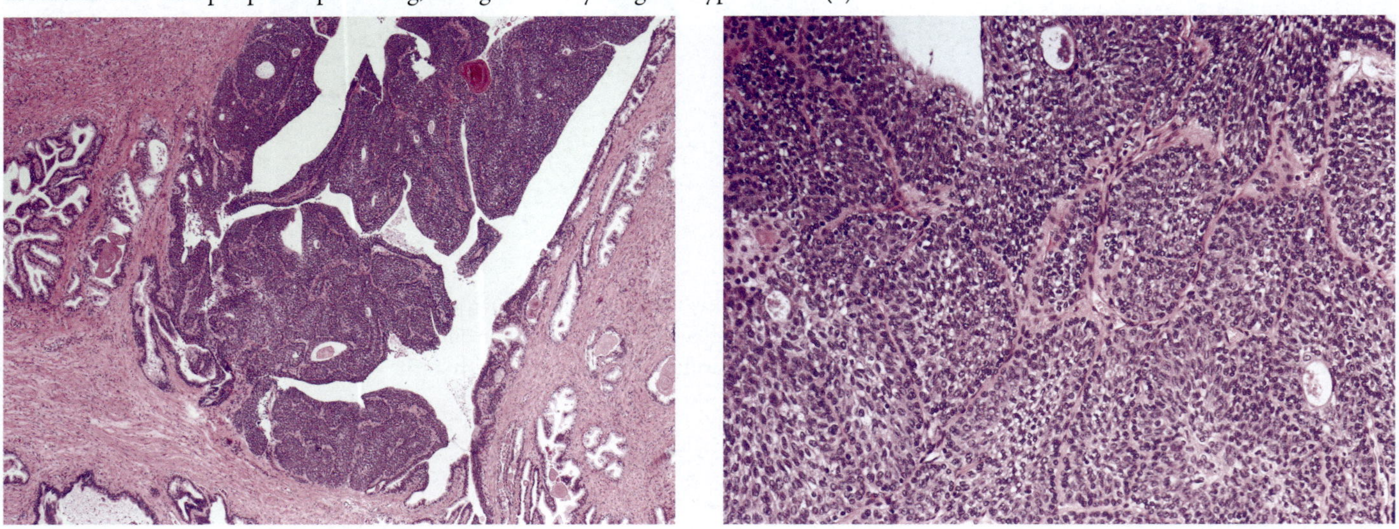

a   *b*

SQUAMOUS CELL CARCINOMA OF THE URETHRA

Definition

- Squamous cell carcinoma arising in the urethra

Other term

- Urethral cancer

Pathogenesis and epidemiology

- It is an uncommon disease, but it is the most common histologic type of urethral cancer
- Most cases arise from the distal urethra
- More common in females, probably because many cases of distal urethral squamous cell carcinoma in men are classified as penile cancer

Clinical features

- Obstructive symptoms may be an early presentation
- Hematuria or irritation symptoms may be present
- Large mass lesions detected by gross examination, endoscopic or imaging studies
- A history of infection, diverticulum, fistula, or stricture is common

Gross pathology

- Large cauliflower-like and ulcerated exophytic mass with keratin debris as cheesy material present (Fig. 55-21)
- Distortion or destruction of the urethra
- Often invasive into adjacent tissues

Histology

- Squamous cell carcinoma (Figs. 55-22 and 55-23), either keratinizing or nonkeratinizing type
- Tumor cells show characteristic intercellular bridges
- The characteristic feature of keratinized squamous cell carcinoma is the keratin pearl (Fig. 55-22*b*), which consists of
  - A center of concentric layers of keratin
  - Surrounding malignant squamous cells
- Squamous CIS may be seen. Invasive to surrounding erectile corpus tissue or fibroadipose tissue
- Squamous metaplasia, chronic inflammation are commonly seen

Immunohistochemistry

Positive for p53 and p63

Differential diagnosis

Urothelial carcinoma with squamous differentiation

- Presence of invasive or in situ urothelial carcinoma component
- Finding of both squamous and glandular differentiation would favor urothelial carcinoma

Clinical relevance (prognosis and treatment options)

- May be difficult to distinguish from squamous cell carcinoma of the penis
- Prognosis is poor. Surgical resection is the treatment of choice, with or without radiation and chemotherapy

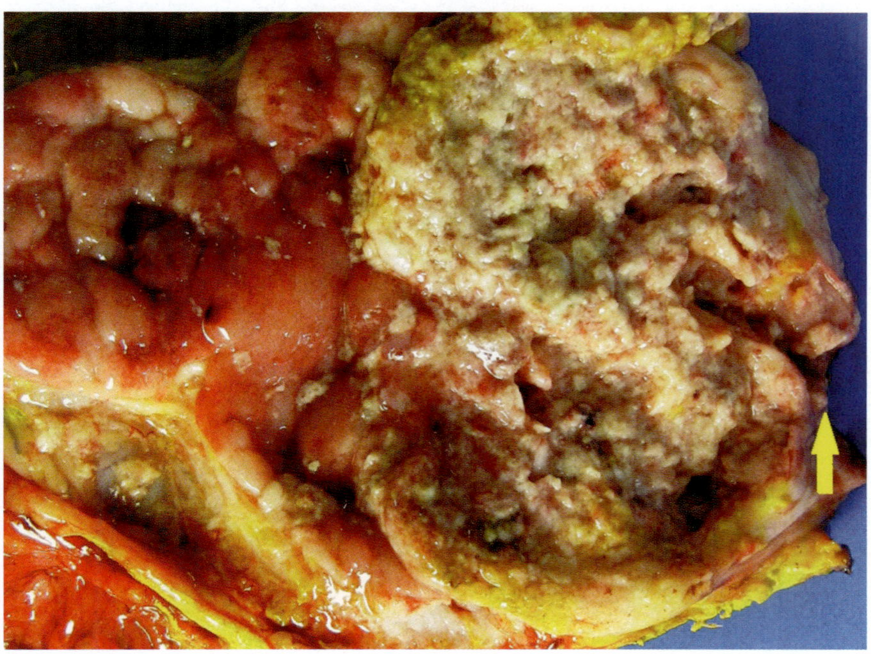

Figure 55-21.
Squamous cell carcinoma of the urethra in a 67-year female. The tumor involves the meatus (arrow) and entire urethra, as well as the distal portion of the bladder (left). The surface of the tumor is covered by cheesy keratin debris.

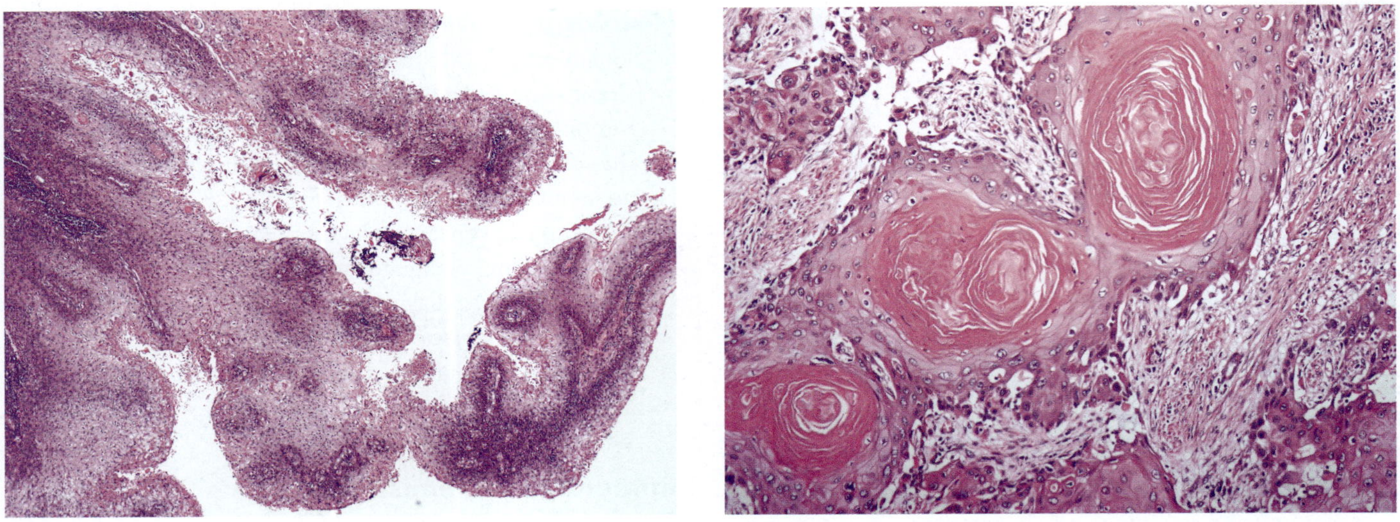

a b

Figure 55-22.
Invasive squamous cell carcinoma demonstrates papillary configurations on the surface (*a*). The characteristic keratin pearls formed by invasive tumor cells are seen (*b*).

Figure 55-23.
Squamous cell carcinoma of the distal urethra in a male. The tumor displays prominent invasion and desmoplastic reaction by the stroma (*a*). High magnification shows the keratinized individual tumor cells invading stroma (*b*).

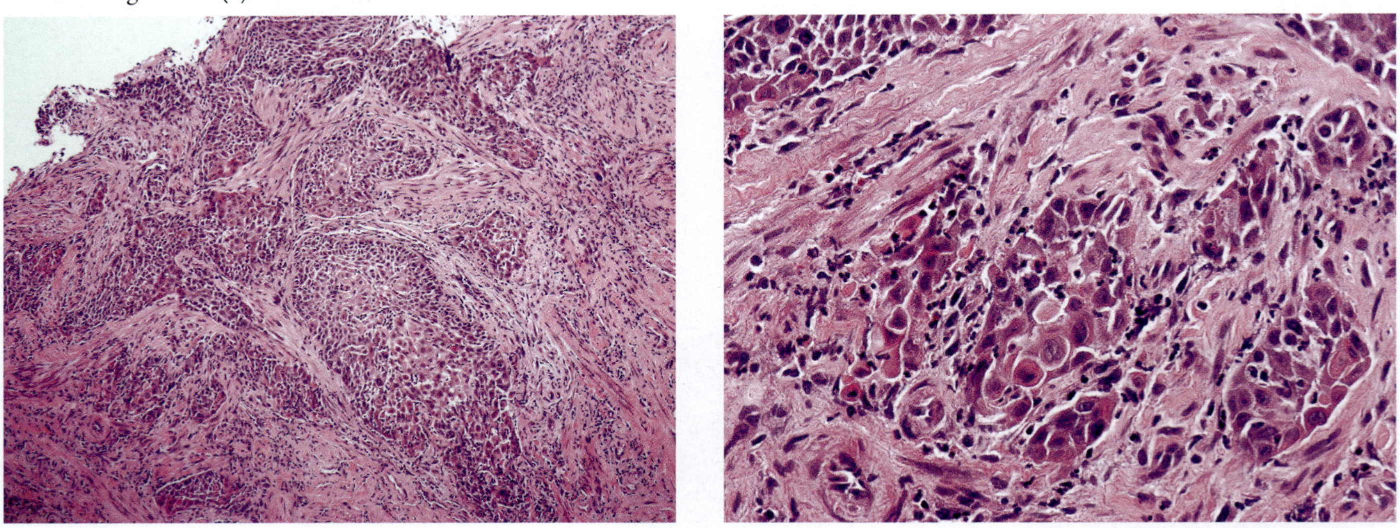

a b

UROTHELIAL CARCINOMA OF THE URETHRA

Definition

- Primary urothelial carcinoma arising from the urethra outside the prostate
- Urothelial carcinoma developing in the prostatic urethra is considered primary prostatic urothelial carcinoma
- Urothelial carcinoma involving the urethra associated with urothelial carcinoma of the bladder and other upper tract is generally considered secondary, by direct extension, seeding, or metastasis, although multifocality is possible

Pathogenesis and epidemiology

- Tumors arising in the proximal urethra are likely to be urothelial carcinoma, while tumors arising in the distal urethra are likely to be squamous cell carcinoma
- More common in women than men and typically occurs in old patients with mean age of 65
- Urothelial carcinoma is the second most common type of urethral cancer after squamous cell carcinoma

Clinical features

- The symptoms may include dysuria, hematuria, and signs of urinary obstruction
- Mass lesions can be seen by gross examination, cystoscopy, or image studies

Gross pathology

- Large polypoid or papillary mass lesion. Ulceration or necrosis is common
- It may invade the adjacent organs

Histology

- Similar to bladder cancer, several types of urothelial carcinoma may be present
  - Carcinoma in situ (Fig. 55-24)
  - Low-grade papillary urothelial carcinoma (Fig. 55-25)
  - High-grade papillary urothelial carcinoma
  - Invasive urothelial carcinoma (Figs. 55-26 and 55-27)
- Most cases are high-grade invasive urothelial carcinoma
- Tumor may have focal glandular or squamous differentiation

Immunohistochemistry

- Same as urothelial carcinoma of the bladder

Differential diagnosis

Squamous cell carcinoma

- Preexisting conditions such as chronic inflammation
- Squamous metaplasia often present
- Keratin pearls or intracellular bridges are present

Adenocarcinoma

- Pure adenocarcinoma without urothelial components

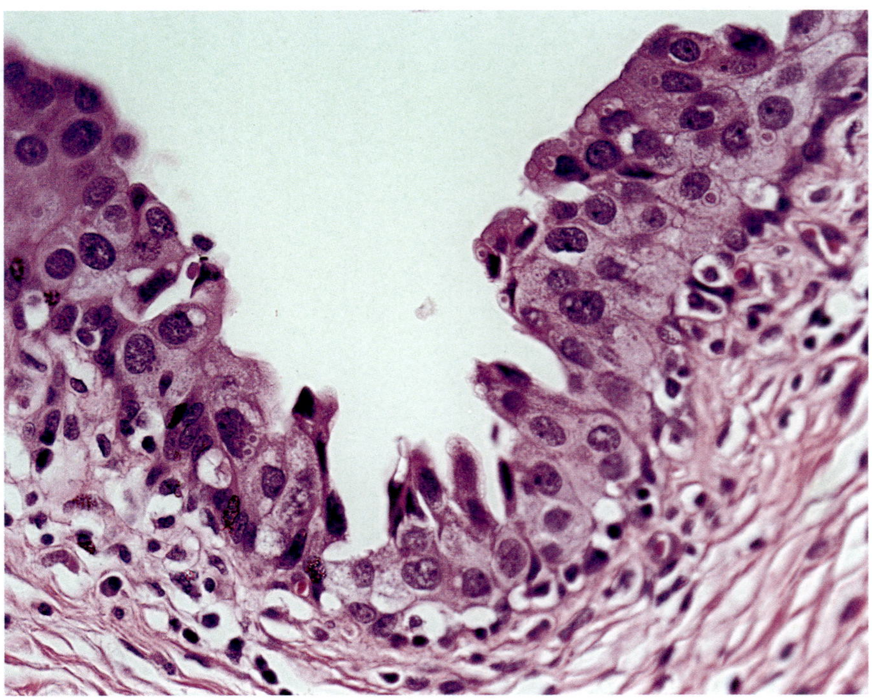

Figure 55-24.
Urothelial carcinoma in situ of the urethra.

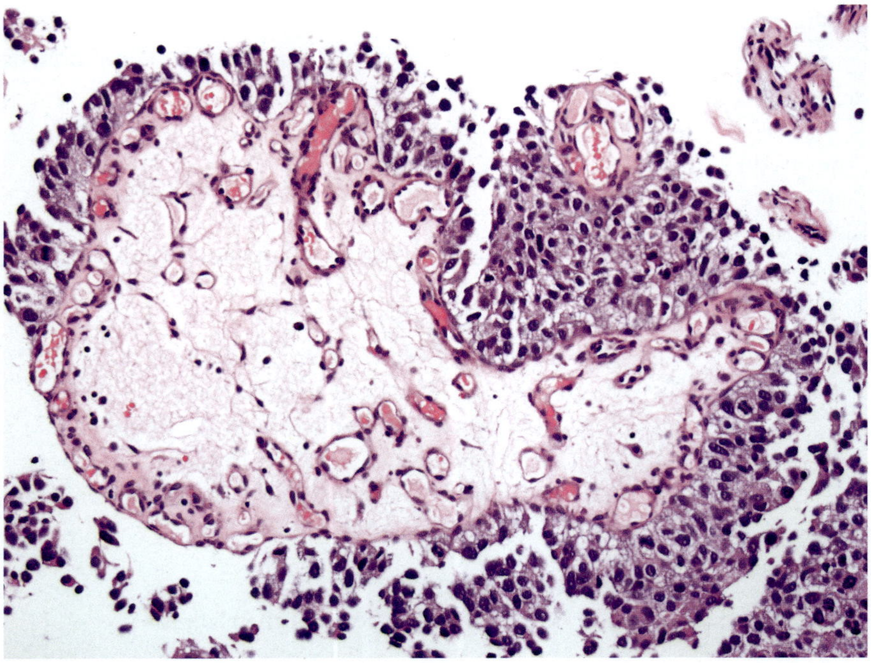

Figure 55-25.
Low-grade papillary urothelial carcinoma of the urethra, no invasion identified.

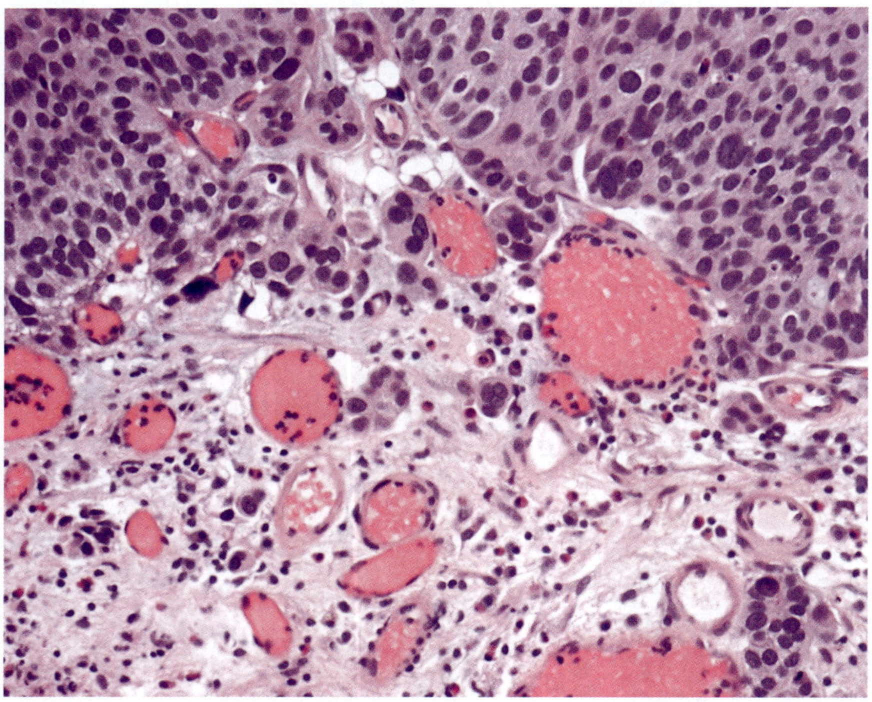

Figure 55-26.
High-grade urothelial carcinoma with focal lamina propria invasion.

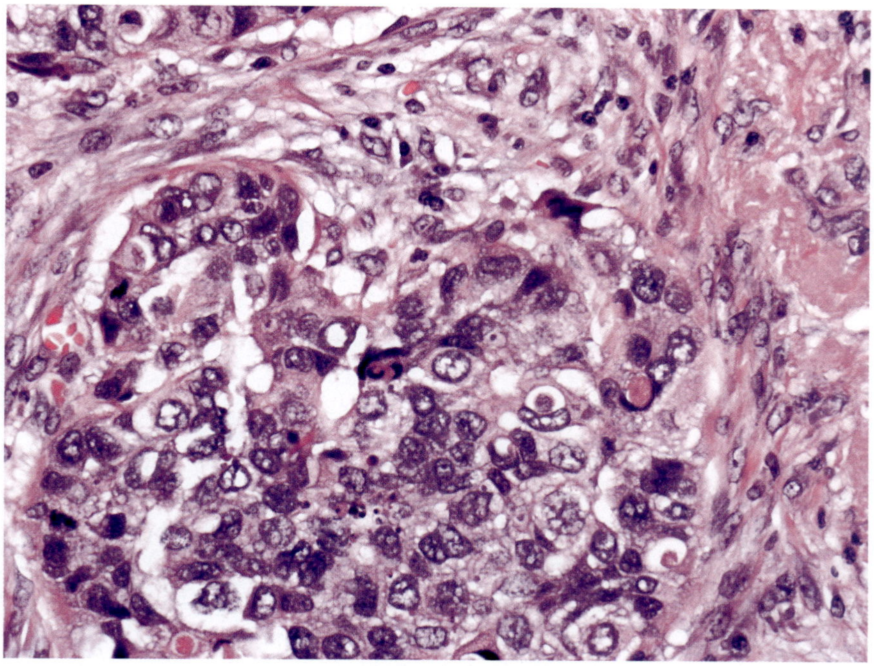

Figure 55-27.
High-grade invasive urothelial carcinoma of the urethra with marked cytological atypia.

Clinical relevance (prognosis and treatment options)

- A diagnosis of urothelial carcinoma in a urethral biopsy should prompt a work up to rule out bladder and upper tract tumors, which may cause implants in the urethra
- The primary invasive urothelial carcinoma, if it is high grade, carries a poor prognosis, worse than bladder cancer
- Death typically occurs in a few years caused by local recurrence and metastasis to inguinal and pelvic lymph nodes, lungs, or other organs
- Proximal urethral carcinoma is usually higher stage because of late detection
- Initial treatment is surgical resection
- Radiation and chemotherapy may play a role

ADENOCARCINOMA OF THE URETHRA

Definition

- Malignant epithelial neoplasm with pure glandular component
- Primary adenocarcinoma: arising from the urethra
- Secondary adenocarcinoma: adenocarcinoma from other organs involving the urethra either by direct extension or by metastasis

Pathogenesis

- Primary adenocarcinoma is rare and accounts for less than 10% of urethral cancer
- Secondary adenocarcinoma is more common than primary
- The most common secondary type in the United States is prostatic adenocarcinoma extending distally or metastatic to the urethra. Particularly, prostatic ductal adenocarcinoma has a greater propensity to involve the urethra

Clinical features

- Urinary irritation symptoms such as dysuria, urinary frequency and urgency
- Obstructive voiding symptoms and hematuria
- Mass lesions by imaging studies. Mucosuria may occur if it is mucinous adenocarcinoma

Gross pathology

- Typical a large mass, with compression of or protrusion into the urethra
- Hemorrhage and necrosis
- May be invasive through the urethral wall and into adjacent tissues
- Distant metastasis may develop in some cases

Histology

Primary adenocarcinoma

- Similar to its bladder counterpart, primary urethral adenocarcinoma can be divided into two types
  - Enteric type, similar to colonic adenocarcinoma
    - Conventional type with goblet cells (Fig. 55-28)
    - Mucinous type and signet ring type
  - Nonenteric type
    - Clear cell adenocarcinoma (Fig. 55-29)
    - Adenocarcinoma not otherwise specific, and poorly differentiated (Fig. 55-30)
- In the majority of cases, invasion can be identified
- Associated colonic metaplasia, villous adenoma, or dysplastic glandular epithelium may be present adjacent to the invasive carcinoma, which suggests that they are precursor lesions

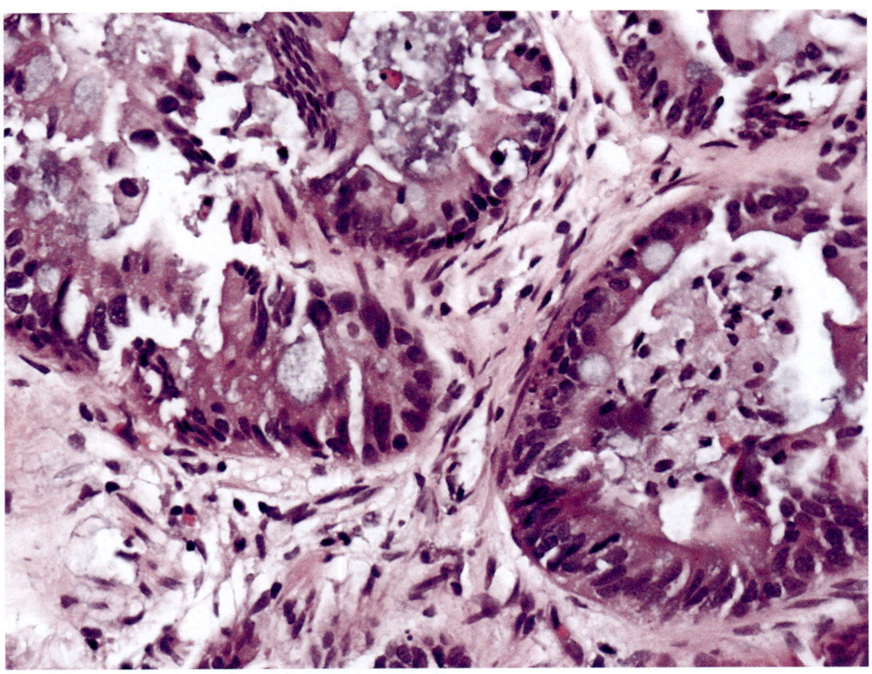

Figure 55-28.
Primary adenocarcinoma of the urethra, enteric type with mild cytologic atypia and occasional goblet cell differentiation.

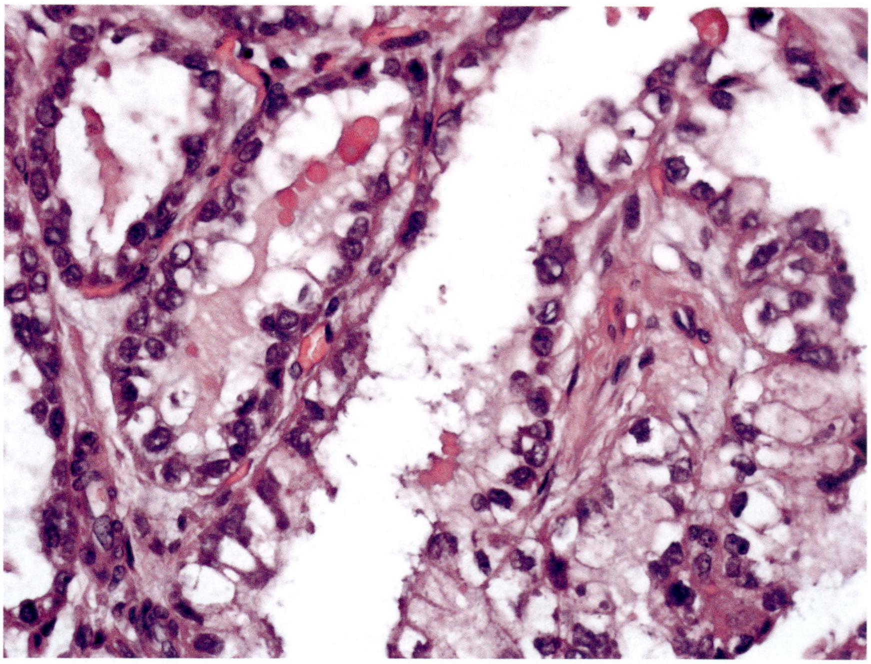

Figure 55-29.
Primary adenocarcinoma of the urethra, clear cell type with glandular and papillary patterns.

Figure 55-30.
Primary adenocarcinoma of the urethra, poorly differentiated, mostly underneath the urethra squamous epithelium (*a*). High magnification shows vague glandular differentiation and cytological atypia (*b*).

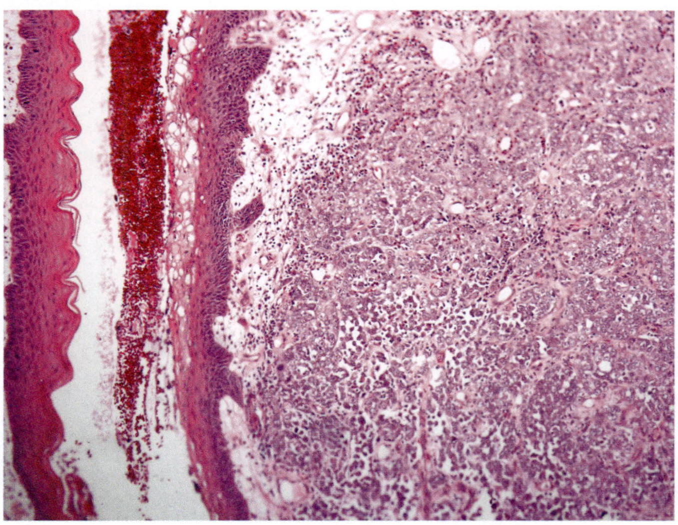

a

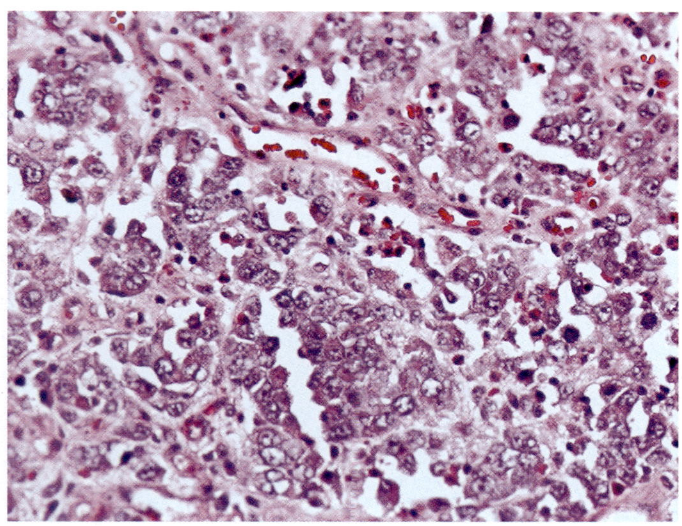

b

Prostatic adenocarcinoma

- Prostatic adenocarcinoma (Fig. 55-31), ductal type or acinar type, involving distal urethra is much more common than primary adenocarcinoma
- They are often polypoid mass lesions or prominent papillary configurations
- Ductal adenocarcinoma with tall columnar cells with prominent nucleoli has a higher propensity involving the urethra
- Relatively uniform in size and shape of the cells without marked cytologic atypia
- Sometimes, they can be deceivingly bland in cytology and confused with a benign lesion
- Adenocarcinoma derived from Skene glands in females is morphologically and immunohistochemically very similar to prostatic adenocarcinoma in males, but it is not appropriate to call these tumors *prostatic* adenocarcinoma

Immunohistochemistry

Primary

- CK20, CK7, and p53 positive
- PSA negative

Differential diagnosis

Primary versus prostatic adenocarcinoma

- It is most important to distinguish prostatic adenocarcinoma from urethral primary adenocarcinoma
- Details have been discussed in Chapters 46 to 48
- Briefly, prostatic adenocarcinoma has a tendency to form cribriform patterns. The tumor cells are less pleomorphic and they have prominent nucleoli
- Immunostains are very helpful to make such a distinction: PSA positive, AMACR positive, p63, and HMWCK negative (Fig. 55-31)

Benign glandular lesions

- Lesions such as urethritis glandularis, nephrogenic adenoma, and prostatic-type polyp should be excluded before making the diagnosis of adenocarcinoma

Clinical relevance (prognosis and treatment options)

- Initial treatment for primary adenocarcinoma includes surgical resection
- The presence or absence of a bladder counterpart should be determined preoperatively
- Radical urethrectomy and cystectomy, if the tumor involves both urethra and bladder
- Adjacent chemotherapy may be necessary for a subset of high-risk patients after surgery
- Distinction of prostatic adenocarcinoma involving urethra from primary adenocarcinoma is very important clinically, because prostate cancer can respond to hormonal therapy

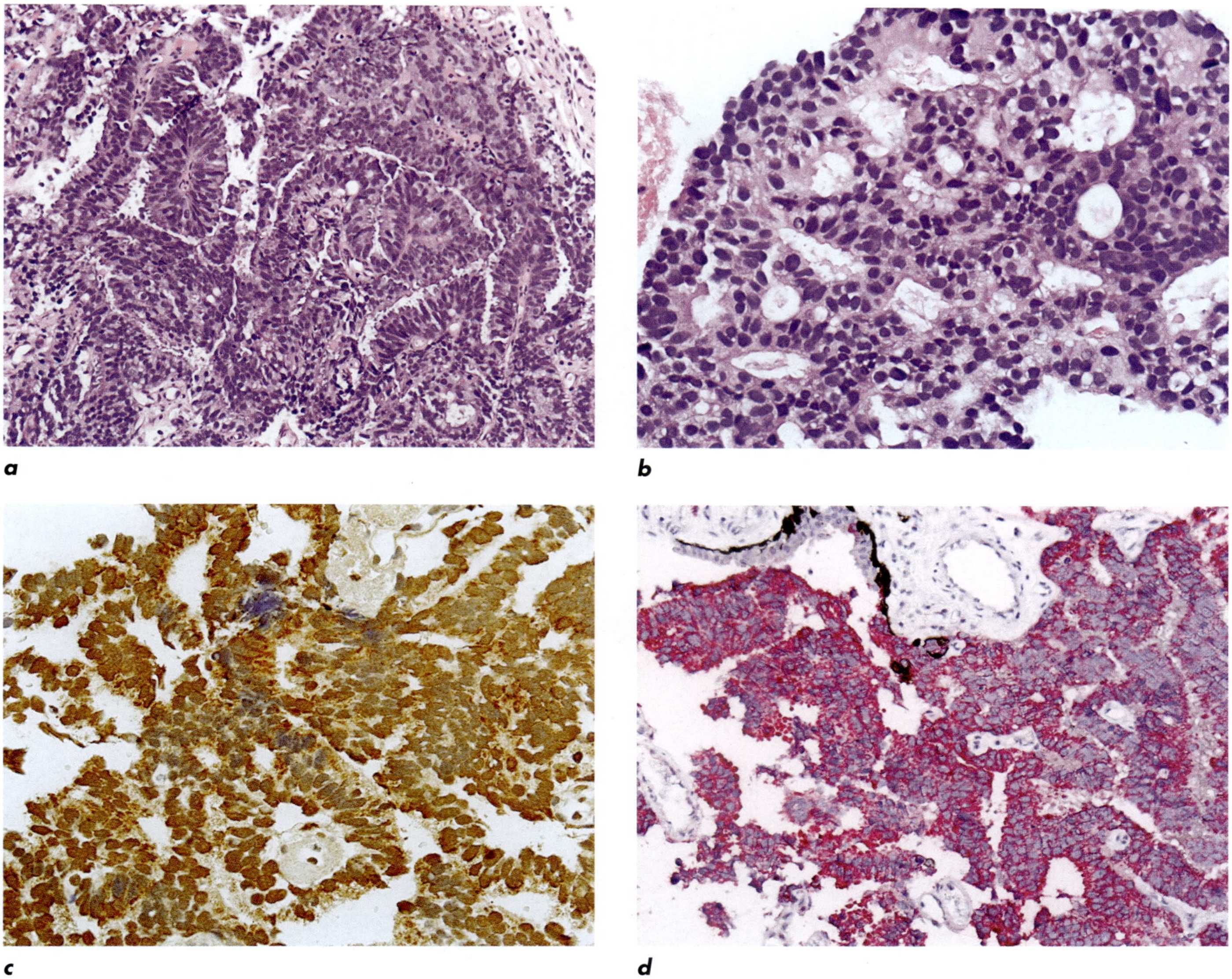

Figure 55-31.
Prostatic adenocarcinoma secondarily involving the urethra, with ductal differentiation (*a*, tall columnar cells) and acinar differentiation (*b*, cribriform pattern). Tumor cells are positive for PSA (*c*) and AMACR (*d*, triple stain), negative for HMWCK and p63 (*d*).

SECTION 8
The Adrenal

CHAPTER 56 Normal Adrenal Histology

Celina Villa, Anjana Yeldandi, Ximing J. Yang

ANATOMY

- Paired endocrine glands located in the retroperitoneum, superior and medial to each kidney
- Each adrenal gland weighs 8 to 9 g
- The adrenal is composed of outer cortex and inner medulla and produces steroid hormones and catecholamines (Table 56-1)
- Strictly speaking, they are not a part of the GU system. However, because of their location, they are often involved by kidney disease and removed as a part of radical nephrectomy

Table 56-1. Adrenal Layers and Hormone Production

Component	*Zone*	*Pattern*	*Hormone*	*Cells*	*% of cortex*
Cortex	Zona glomerulosa	Ovoid	Mineralocorticoids (aldosterone)	Lipid-containing cells	10%
	Zona fasciculata	Columns	Glucocorticoids (cortisol)	Lipid-containing cells	80%
	Zona reticularis	Network	Androgens (DHEA)	Lipid-containing cells	10%
Medulla			Catecholamines	Cells with amphophilic cytoplasm	

CORTEX

- Derived from mesoderm
- Grossly bright yellow due to high lipid content (Fig. 56-1)
- Cortical thickness: 0.7 to 1.3 mm, histologically composed of three zones (Fig. 56-2)
- Cortical cells can be distinguished from medullary cells by the presence of lipid droplets displaying foamy cytoplasm or small vacuoles in the cytoplasm (Fig. 56-3)
- Cells in zona glomerulosa and zona reticularis may have lower lipid contents and more eosinophilic cytoplasm than those in zona fasciculata
- One cannot reliably predict the type of steroid hormones produced at the light microscopic examination of H&E slides alone, on either normal cortical cells or neoplastic cortical cells
- By IHC, cortical cells are immunoreactive to inhibin, melan A and negative for chromogranin

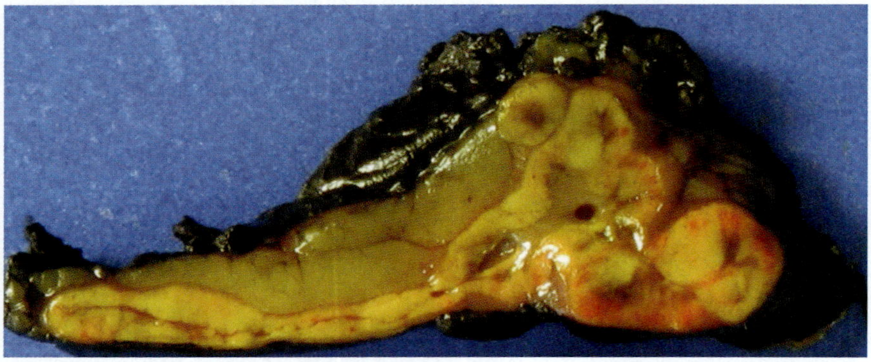

Figure 56-1.
Gross photo of a normal appearing adrenal. The medulla in the middle is surrounded by the bright yellow cortex.

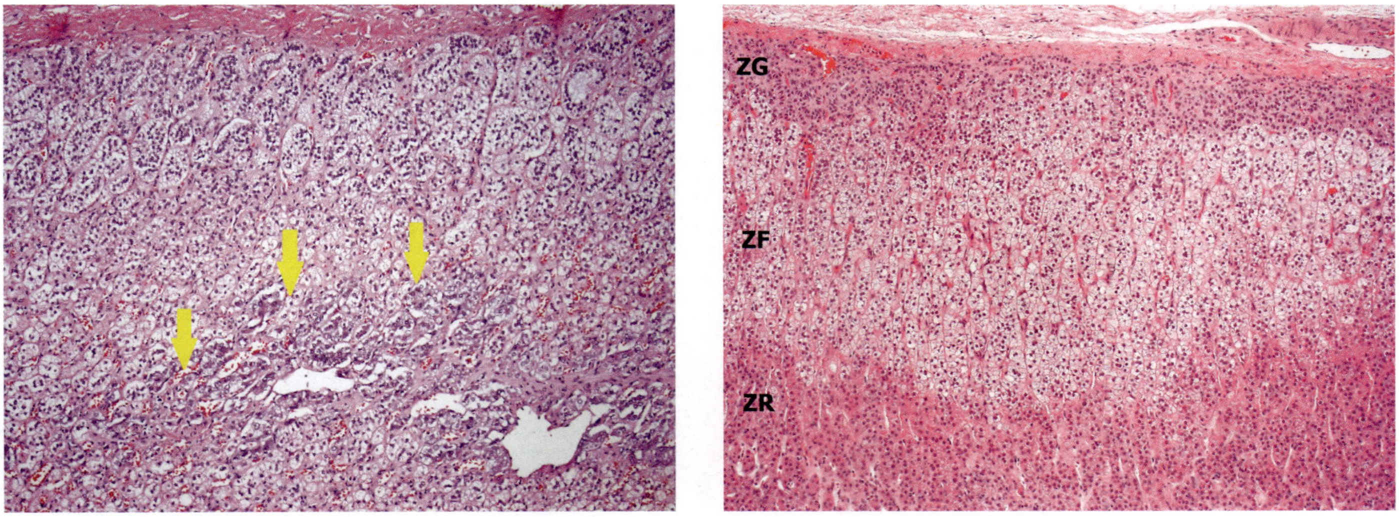

a *b*

Figure 56-2.
Adrenal cortex and medulla (*a*, arrows). The cortex contains zona glomerulosa (ZG, adjacent to the capsule), zona fasciculata (ZF, the major component of the cortex in the middle), and zona reticularis (ZR) with more eosinophilic cytoplasm (*b*).

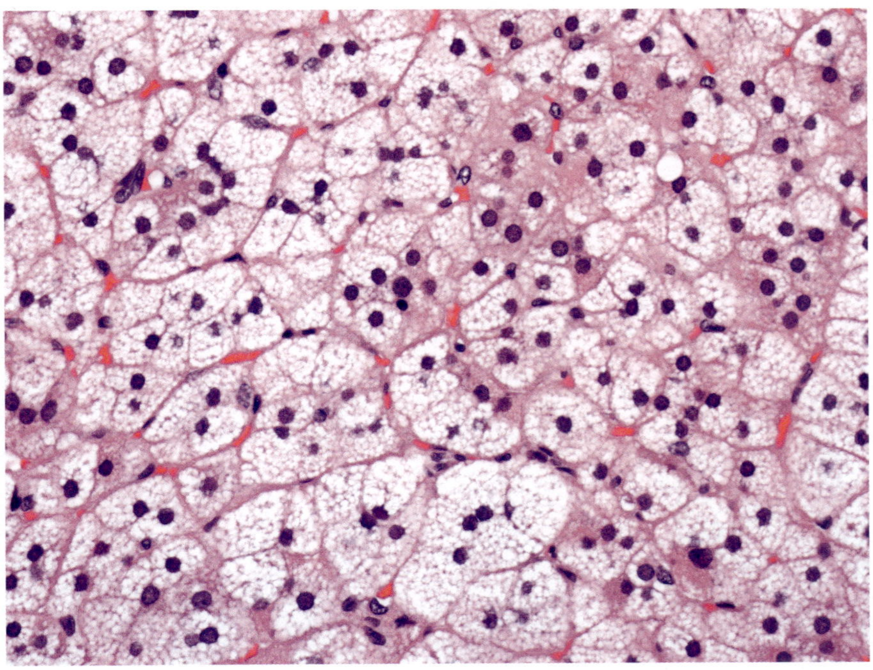

Figure 56-3.
Cortical cells from zona fasciculata have small round nuclei with foamy or vesicular cytoplasm.

MEDULLA

- Neuroectodermal origin
- Grossly gray to tan in color
- Produces catecholamines: norepinephrine and epinephrine, synthesized from amino acids phenylalanine, or tyrosine
- Medullary cells (Figs. 56-4 and 56-5) are mainly chromaffin cells, which are large polygonal cells with abundant amphophilic or basophilic cytoplasm
- Medullary cells may contain hyaline globules that are PAS positive
- Ganglion cells can occasionally be seen in normal medulla
- By IHC, chromaffin cells are positive for chromogranin, synaptophysin, neurofilament, and negative for keratin, vimentin
- Sustentacular cells are second cell population and are S100 positive

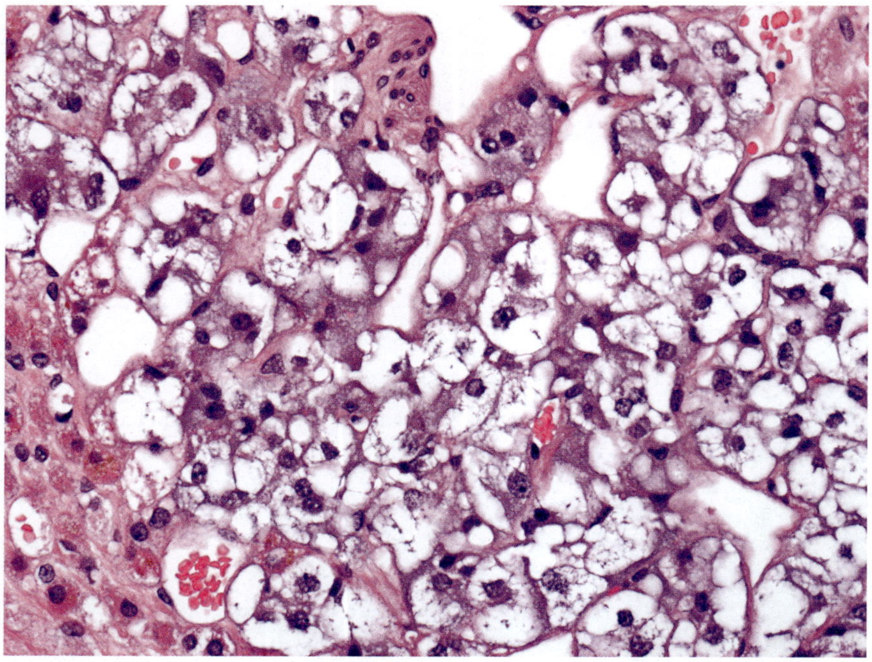

Figure 56-4.
Medullary cells have larger and slightly irregular nuclei with clear to amphophilic cytoplasm.

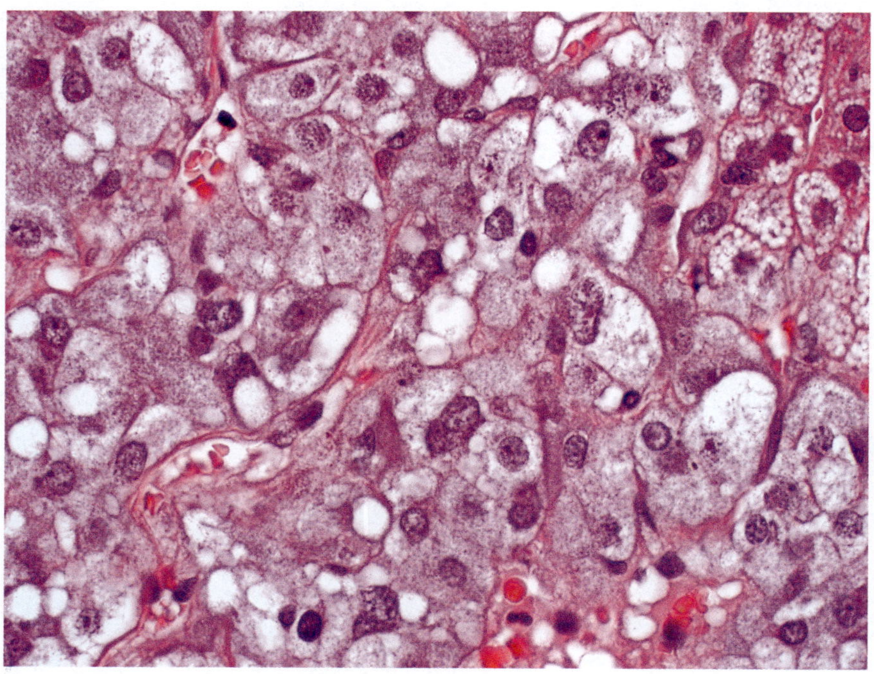

Figure 56-5.
Comparison of medullary cells with larger nuclei and granular cytoplasm and cortical cells (upper right) with vesicular cytoplasm.

CHAPTER 57

Reactive Lesions of the Adrenal

Celina Villa, Anjana Yeldandi, Ximing J. Yang

ADRENAL HEMORRHAGIC NECROSIS

Definition

- Severe hemorrhagic necrosis of the adrenal caused by a variety of infectious and noninfectious processes

Other term

- Adrenal involvement by Waterhouse-Friderichsen syndrome

Pathogenesis

- The anatomy of the adrenal gland vascularity predisposes it to hemorrhage and necrosis
- In situations of increased stress, increased adrenal blood flow, hypotension, and/or coagulopathy, it is believed that central adrenal vein thrombosis occurs and predisposes the adrenal gland to hemorrhagic necrosis
- *Neisseria meningitidis* is the most common infectious cause
- May also be caused by other bacterial infections such as *Haemophilus influenzae, Streptococcus pneumoniae, Staphylococcus aureus*, group A *Streptococcus*, *Neisseria gonorrhoeae*, *Pseudomonas aeruginosa*, and *Klebsiella oxytoca*
- Noninfectious causes include hypercoagulable states, bleeding disorders, burns, trauma, tumor metastasis, pregnancy, and cardiovascular shock

Clinical features

- Septic shock in patients with infectious adrenal hemorrhage
- Signs and symptoms of acute adrenal insufficiency

Gross pathology

- Enlarged adrenal with hemorrhagic necrosis (Fig. 57-1*a*)

Histology

- In the acute phase, there is extensive hemorrhage (Fig. 57-1*b*) with foci of ischemic necrosis
- In the late phase, organization of hemorrhage may be seen
- Rarely foci of inflammation, congestion, or edema may be present

Special stains/other techniques for diagnosis

- GMS may highlight fungal organisms
- PCR may identify infectious agents
- However, in many instances, the infectious agents may not be demonstrated in the necrotic adrenal tissue

Clinical relevance

- May cause adrenal failure, hypotension, and disseminated intravascular coagulation

Figure 57-1.
Gross photo of hemorrhagic necrosis of the adrenal (*a*). Microscopically, the adrenal tissue is replaced by red blood cells and necrotic debris (*b*).

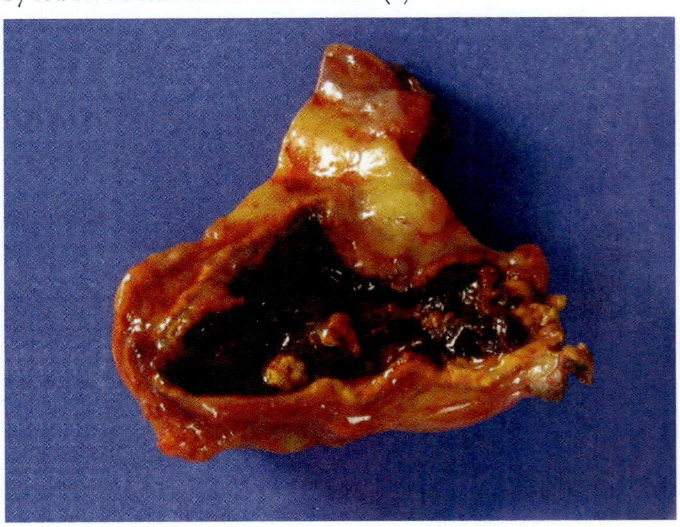

a

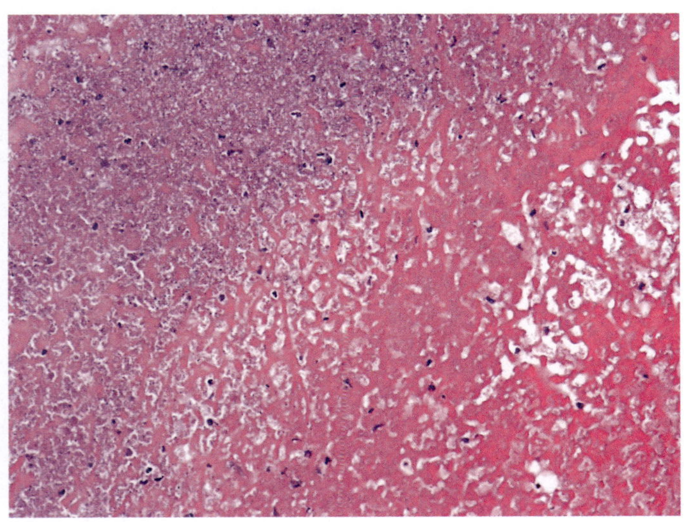

b

GRANULOMATOUS INFLAMMATION OF THE ADRENAL

Definition

- Granulomatous inflammation involving the adrenal
- Granulomas may be infectious, noninfectious, isolated, or systemic

Pathogenesis

Infectious

- Mycobacterial: tuberculosis
- Fungal: histoplasmosis, blastomycosis, mucormycosis, and malassezia furfur
- Parasitic: leishmaniasis (rare)

Noninfectious

- Sarcoidosis, malakoplakia (rare)

Clinical features

- May present as acute adrenal insufficiency
- Symptoms and signs associated with infection if it is infectious etiology
- Granulomas may mimic a neoplasm as a mass lesion

Gross pathology

- Variable, including cystic and hemorrhagic or replacement of the normal adrenal gland by solid, firm white nodular tissue
- Caseating granulomatous lesions will have cheesy necrotic material

Histology

Caseating granuloma

- Three cellular components in a caseating granuloma (Fig. 57-2)
  - Large, elongated, epithelioid histiocytes
  - Langerhans multinucleated giant cells with "horseshoe" like nuclear pattern
  - Peripheral lymphocytic infiltrate, occasionally with neutrophils
- Central necrosis
- Tuberculosis granulomas: contain AFB positive bacilli
- Fungal granuloma: yeast or hyphal structures can be seen and confirmed with fungal stains such as Gomori methenamine silver (GMS)

Noncaseating granuloma

- Similar to caseating granuloma but with no necrosis (Fig. 57-3)
- Sarcoidosis
  - Multiple predominantly noncaseating conglomerate granulomas
  - Sometimes with minimal peripheral lymphocytic infiltrate ("naked" granulomas)
- Malakoplakia
  - Diffuse histiocytic infiltrates
  - Histiocytes containing Michaelis-Gutmann bodies, which are partially digested bacteria with iron and calcium deposits

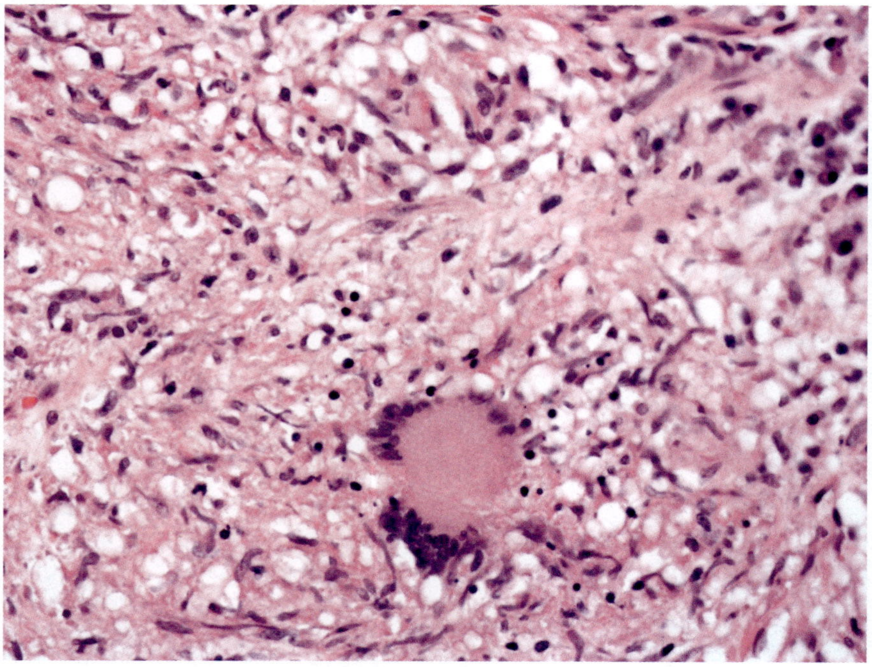

Figure 57-2.
A tuberculosis granuloma is characterized by the presence of caseating necrosis, epithelioid histiocytes, and Langerhans giant cell with "horseshoe"-like nuclei.

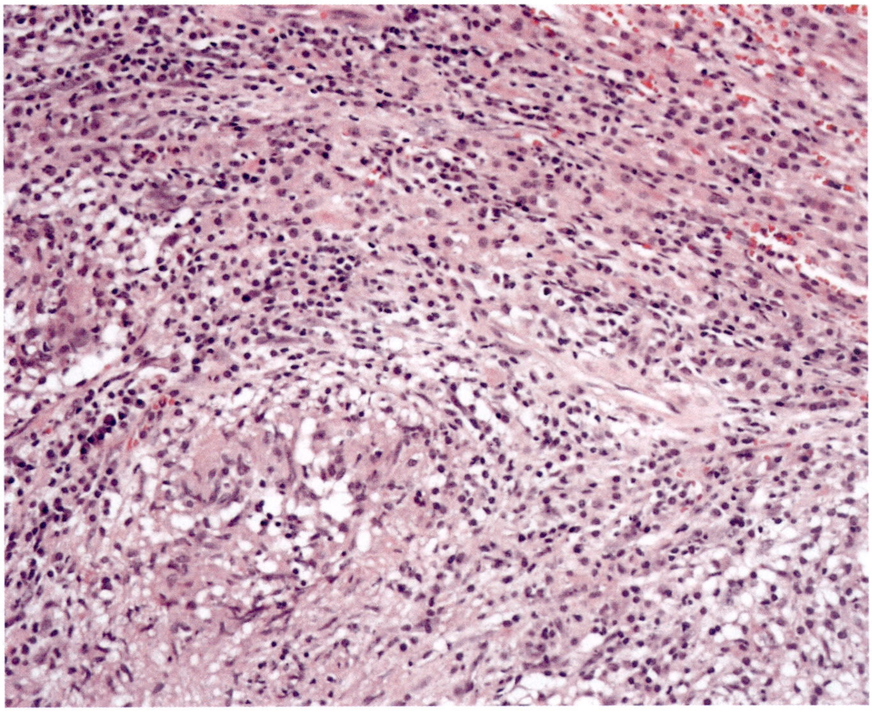

Figure 57-3.
Noncaseating granulomatous inflammation of the adrenal with epithelioid histiocytes and lymphocytes without necrosis.

Diagnostic tests

- Special stains for organisms (GMS, PAS, AFB)
- Other microbiological studies including culture or PCR-based tests may be needed to identify infectious agent

Clinical relevance

- Granulomatous inflammation may solely involve the adrenal or present as multiorgan systemic involvement
- Granulomatous inflammation may mimic a solid or cystic lesion on imaging studies, therefore, biopsy and histologic examination are essential for definitive diagnosis
- Identification of infectious agent is critical to establish the infectious etiology of the granuloma
- Sarcoidosis is a diagnosis of exclusion with all negative microbiological studies and negative stains for microorganisms

ADRENAL CYSTIC LESIONS

Definition

- Four major types
  - Endothelial cysts (45%): considered variants of lymphatic and vascular cysts and can be subtyped into angiomatous, lymphangiomatous, and hamartomatous. Commonly multilocular
  - Pseudocysts (40%): cysts without any epithelial lining, are usually unilocular, and encapsulated
  - Epithelial cysts (<10%): cystic tumors such as cystic adenomas, primary or secondary cystic carcinoma, which are discussed in other chapters
  - Parasitic (hydatid) cysts (<5%): caused by tapeworm (echinococcal) infestation, they are most commonly seen in the liver, but can occasionally involve the adrenal

Pathogenesis

- Adrenal endothelial cysts originate from preexisting vascular or lymphatic malformations
- Adrenal pseudocysts are derived from hemorrhage within an adrenal neoplasm or a normal adrenal gland due to trauma, infection, or toxic injury
- Epithelial cysts are derived from cystic degeneration of an epithelial neoplasm
- Parasitic cysts are caused by infection or parasite infestation

Clinical features

- Typically asymptomatic, cystic mass lesions are detected by imaging studies

Gross pathology

- A cystic lesion, unilocular or multilocular, is located in the adrenal parenchyma
- The inner surface of endothelial and epithelial cysts is smooth (Fig. 57-4), while a pseudocyst has an irregular inner surface
- Hydatid cyst is filled with larva-containing fluid

Histology

- An endothelial cyst is lined by endothelium (Fig. 57-5), which can be either lymphatic or vascular. Calcifications within the multilocular septa are often seen
- Pseudocysts demonstrate a fibrous capsule, hemorrhage, calcifications, thin-walled vessels, and lymphoid aggregates. Calcifications typically seen in the fibrous capsule
- Epithelial cysts are lined by benign or neoplastic epithelial cells. Ample sampling and careful histological examination looking for viable cells are necessary for establishing the diagnosis
- Parasitic cyst is characterized by the presence of echinococcal larva or ova

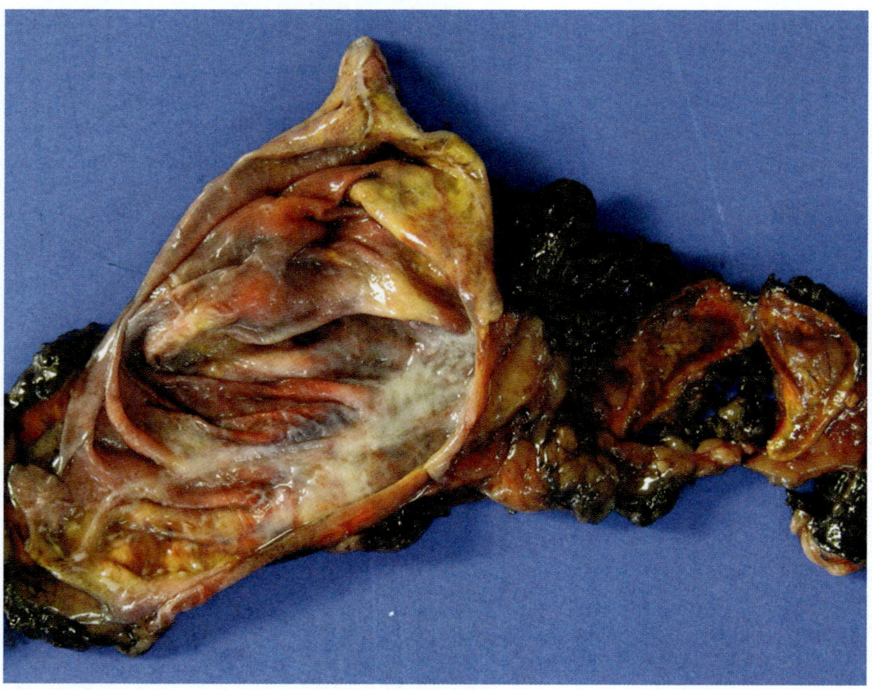

Figure 57-4.
Endothelial cyst of the adrenal with a smooth inner surface.

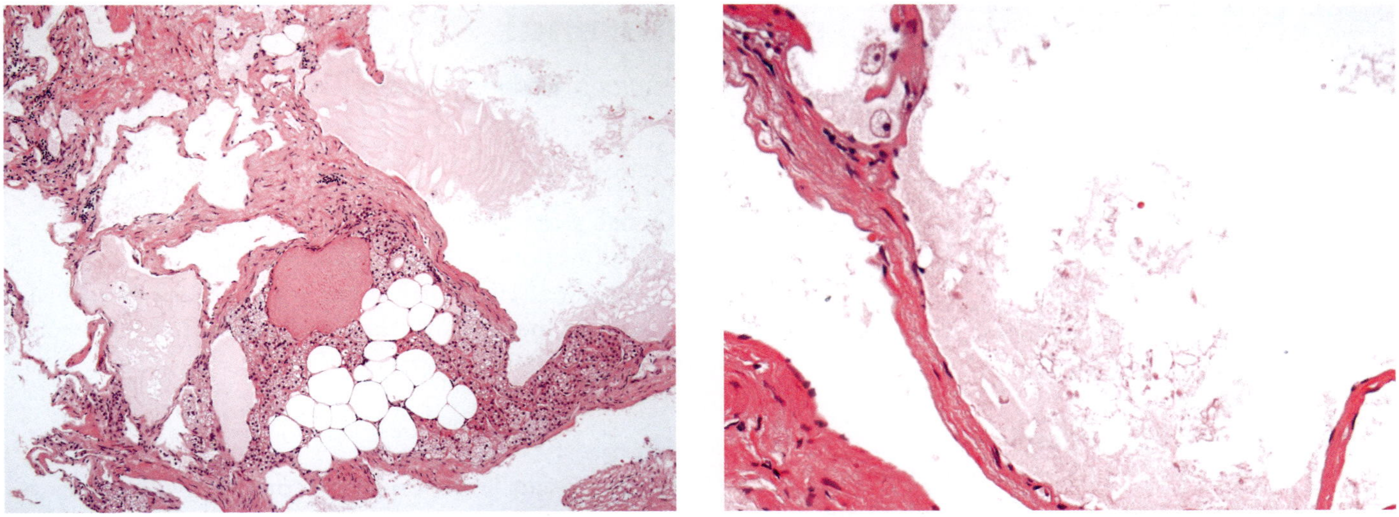

a b

Figure 57-5.
Endothelial cyst of the adrenal (lymphangioma) as a multilocular cyst mingled with normal-appearing cortical tissue (*a*). The flat endothelial lining can be seen (*b*).

Special stains/other techniques for diagnosis

- Immunoreactivity depends on the underlying nature of the cyst
- CD31 or D2-40 immunoreactivity in angiomatous or lymphangiomatous cysts

Clinical relevance

- Observation and follow-up for a small adrenal cyst if asymptomatic
- Surgical removal for cases with symptoms or suspicion for malignancy
- Hydatid cyst requires surgical removal of the cystic contents and sterilization of the cyst cavity by injection of a scolicidal agent. Systemic treatment may also be necessary

CHAPTER 58

Benign Neoplastic Lesions of the Adrenal

Celina Villa, Anjana Yeldandi, Ximing J. Yang

MYELOLIPOMA

Definition

- A benign adrenal tumor composed of hematopoietic elements and mature adipose tissue

Pathogenesis and epidemiology

- The pathogenesis of myelolipoma is not known
- Recent studies suggest that the hematopoietic and lipomatous components are monoclonal. These findings support the neoplastic nature of this tumor
- Other hypothesis suggests that this lesion is most likely a form of extramedullary hematopoiesis
- The tumor is rare with an incidence of less than 0.4%

Clinical features

- Most cases are asymptomatic and detected by imaging studies for other causes
- Large tumors can compress the adjacent tissue and lead to symptoms such as hematuria, flank mass, and pain
- Occasionally, a large tumor may develop necrosis and hemorrhage, leading to peritoneal hemorrhage
- Imaging studies can identify this lesion based on the fat content

Gross pathology

- The majority of these tumors are small
- Mostly, a yellow fatty lesion in the adrenal parenchyma. Within the fatty area, there are reddish areas representing bone marrow elements (Fig. 58-1)

Histology

- No capsule; lesional tissue intermingled with benign adrenal tissue
- Two components of the lesion (Fig. 58-2)
  - Mature adipose tissue can be a dominant (Fig. 58-3) or minor component
  - Trilineage marrow elements (Fig. 58-2*b*) including
    - Myeloid (WBC formation) line
    - Erythroid (RBC formation) line
    - Megakaryocytic (platelet formation) line
- Small microscopic foci of marrow components can be seen in the adrenal with minimal adipose tissue (Fig. 58-4)

Differential diagnosis

Lipoma and liposarcoma

- No bone marrow elements. Liposarcoma often displays cytologic atypia and the presence of lipoblasts

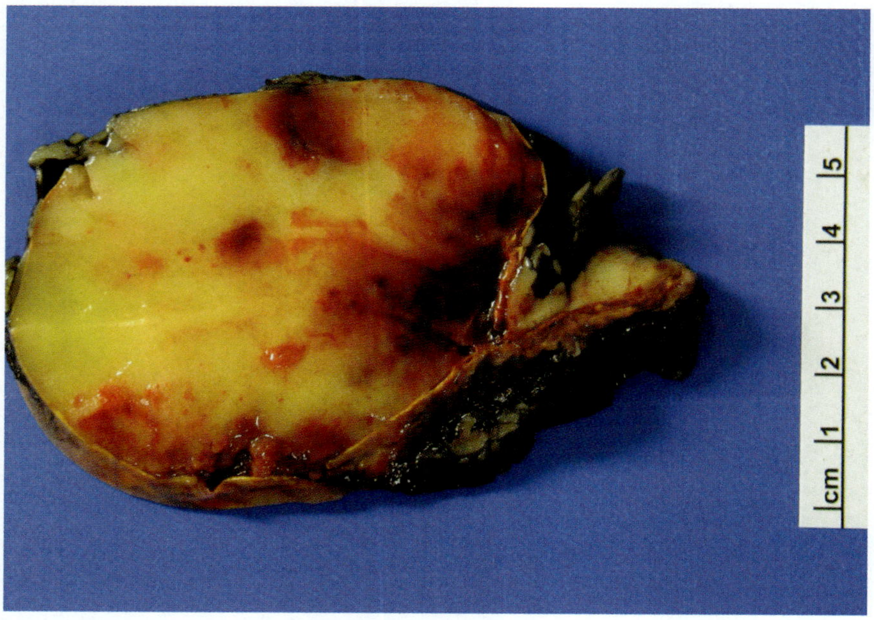

Figure 58-1.
Gross photo of adrenal myelolipoma. The cut surface shows red areas (marrow elements) in a yellow background surrounded by a thin rim of cortical tissue.

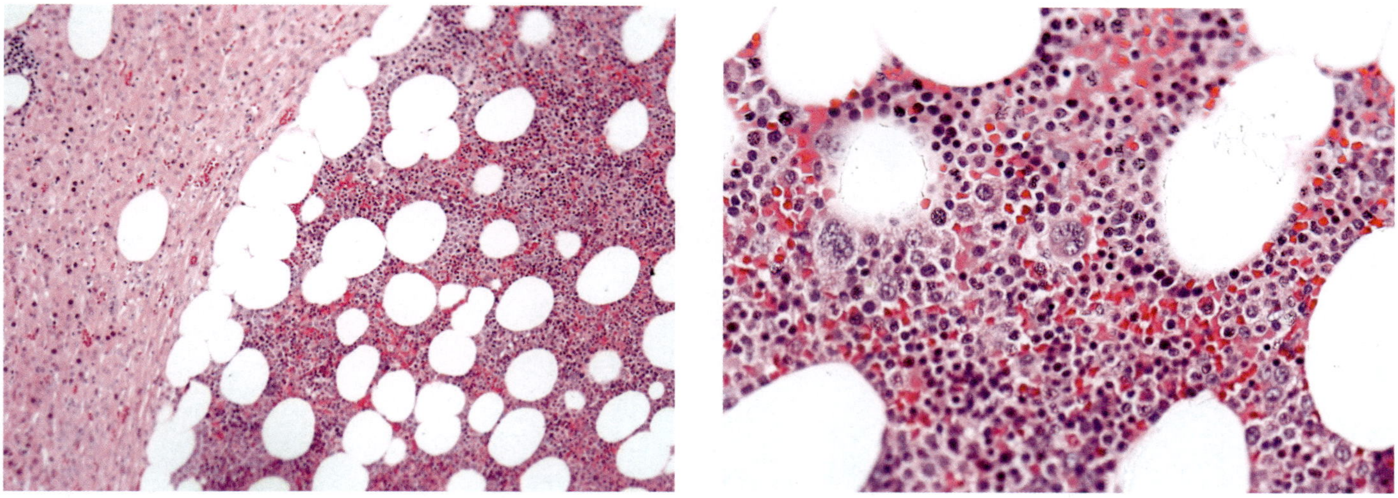

a b

Figure 58-2.
Myelolipoma of the adrenal is characterized by the presence of maturing bone marrow elements and adipose tissue (*a*). High magnification shows all three components including myeloid cells, erythroid cells, and megakaryocytes (multinucleated cells) (*b*).

Angiomyolipoma (AML)

- A renal parenchymal tumor, not found in the adrenal. The tumor consists of spindle cell proliferation and abnormal vessels. No bone marrow elements

Clinical relevance (prognosis and treatment options)

- Benign; no need for surgery if the patient with a small tumor is asymptomatic
- Surgical excision is recommended for large myelolipomas because of the risk of bleeding

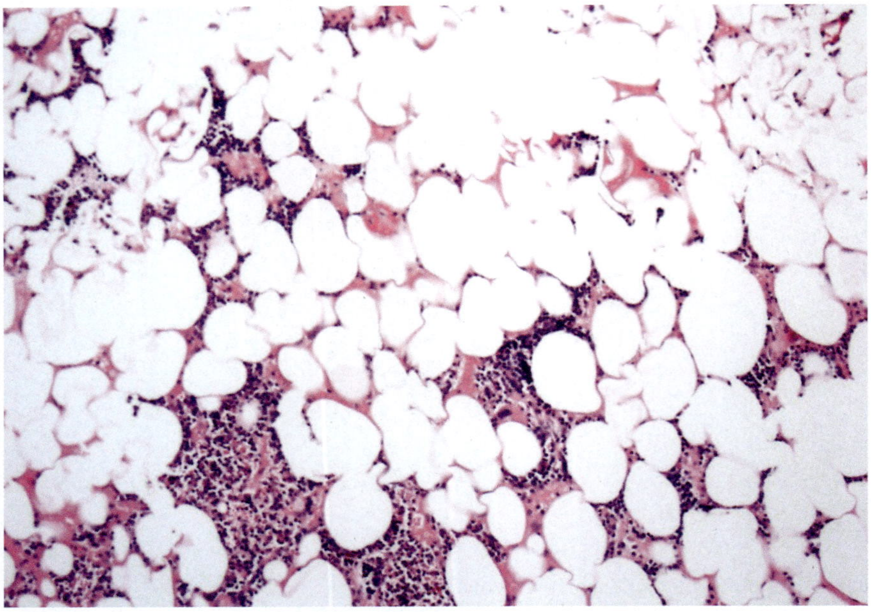

Figure 58-3.
Myelolipoma composed predominantly of adipose tissue with small cluster of hematopoietic cells.

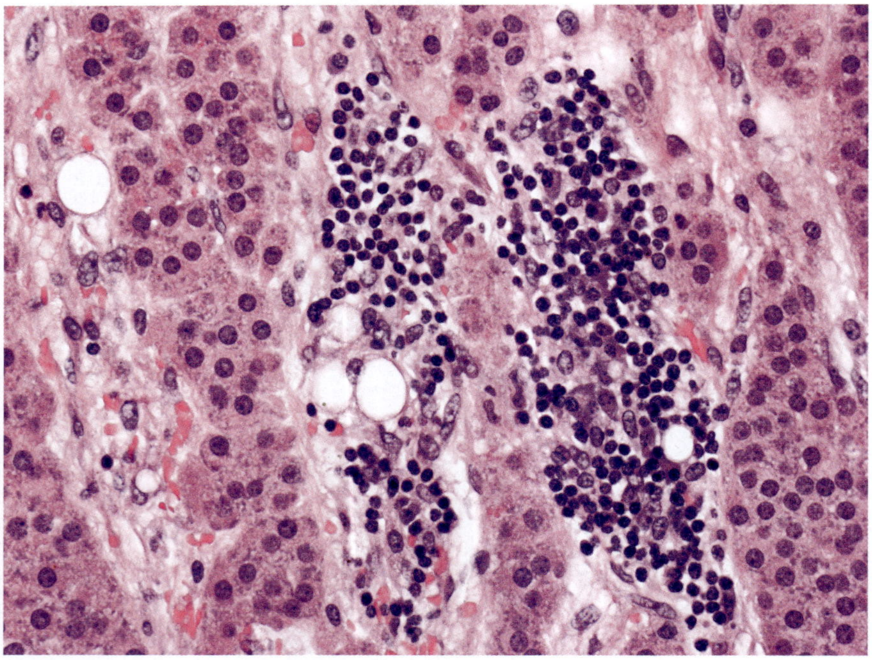

Figure 58-4.
Myelolipomatous focus containing only a cluster of hematopoietic cells and a couple of adipocytes within adrenal cortex.

CORTICAL ADENOMA

Definition

- Benign neoplasm arising from the adrenal cortex
- Usually defined as greater than 1 cm in size

Other terms

- Benign adrenocortical neoplasm, adrenal "incidentaloma" if asymptomatic

Pathogenesis

- Tumor is composed of neoplastic cells that morphologically resemble the normal adrenal cortical cells
- Similar to the normal counterpart, the neoplastic cells are capable of producing steroid hormones, which may result in clinical symptoms related to excess hormone production
- It is unclear whether adenomas progress to adrenocortical carcinomas
- Adrenocortical carcinomas can be distinguished from adenomas based on the Weiss criteria (see Chapter 59)

Clinical features

- Occurs most commonly in adults, rarely in children
- May be found at autopsy, or incidental imaging studies performed for other reasons
- May be functional or nonfunctional
- Majority of cases are detected due to signs or symptoms of hormone dysfunction or mass effect
- Functional adenomas may be associated with adrenogenital syndrome, Cushing syndrome, and hyperaldosteronism (Conn syndrome)

Gross findings

- Usually solitary, less than 5 cm and less than 50 g in weight
- Encapsulated or well circumscribed (Fig. 58-5)
- Cut surface shows solid, homogenous, yellow or gray appearance (Fig. 58-6)
- Hemorrhage may be present (Fig. 58-7)

Histology

- Microscopically, adenoma cells recapitulate the appearance of the adrenal cortical tissue
- The tumor cells resemble normal cortical cells of zona fasciculata, zona glomerulosa, or zona reticularis (Figs. 58-5 and 58-7)
- More commonly, however, the tumor cells constitute a mixture of all three patterns
- The function (the type of steroid hormone produced) cannot be predicated from the histology of the tumor
- Hemorrhage often can be seen (Fig. 58-7), but necrosis is rare in an adenoma
- As in other endocrine tumors, bizarre nuclear atypia may be seen in cortical adenomas without any clinical significance (Fig. 58-8)
- Mitoses are rare or absent

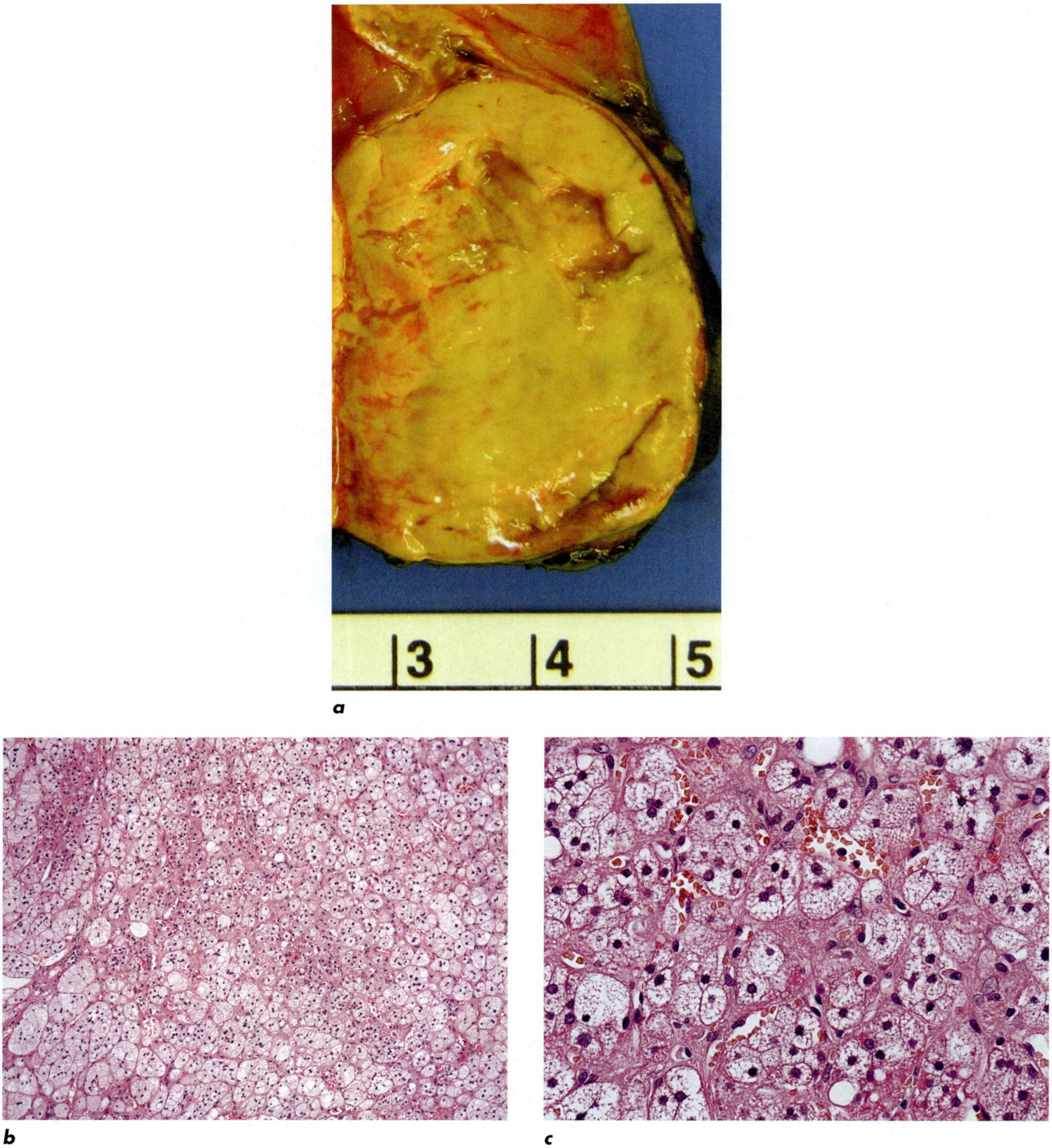

Figure 58-5.
Adrenal cortical adenoma exhibits a well-circumscribed nodule measuring 3.5 cm, with a solid homogenous bright yellow cut surface (*a*). Microscopically, the tumor is composed of sheets of cells with pale cytoplasm (*b*). High magnification shows that tumor cells contain fine lipid vacuoles in the cytoplasm and indented nuclei (*c*) similar to normal adrenal cortical cells.

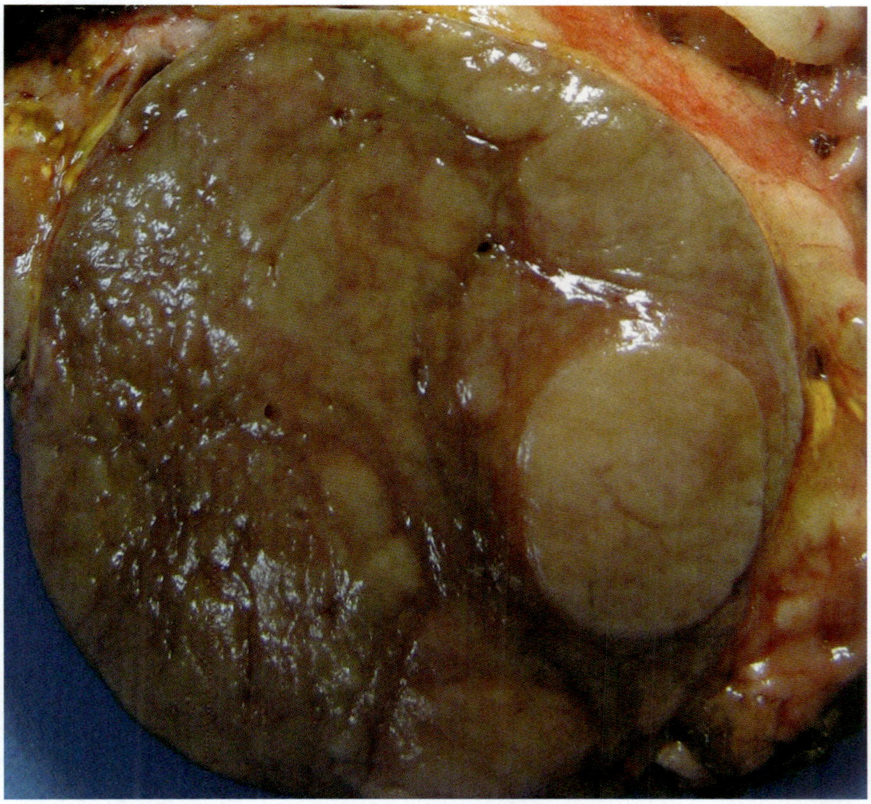

Figure 58-6.
A cortical adenoma, sc-called black adenoma, showing a gray tan cut surface.

Morphologic variants

- Black adenomas: have a distinctly dark brown or gray color grossly, due to the presence of either lipofuscin or neuromelanin (Fig. 58-6)
- Adrenocortical oncocytoma (Fig. 58-8): composed of cells with abundant, granular, pink cytoplasm due to the presence of abundant mitochondria
- Myxoid adenoma: myxoid changes are most often associated with malignant behavior, although rarely benign myxoid lesions have been described
- Not uncommonly, multiple neoplastic components can be present in one adrenal tumor such as corticomedullary mixed tumor (containing both cortical and medullary differentiation), adenoma with myelolipomatous component, adenoma with lipomatous component

Immunohistochemistry

Positive markers

- Inhibin, vimentin, melan A, synaptophysin
- Other makers such as BCL-2 and calretinin may be positive

Negative markers

- RCC markers such as AMACR, CA9
- Keratin markers such as AE1/AE3, Cam5.2, CK7, CK20
- Chromogranin

Differential diagnosis

Adrenocortical carcinoma

- Often larger (>100 g), prominent cytological atypia, atypical mitosis, necrosis, and invasive features

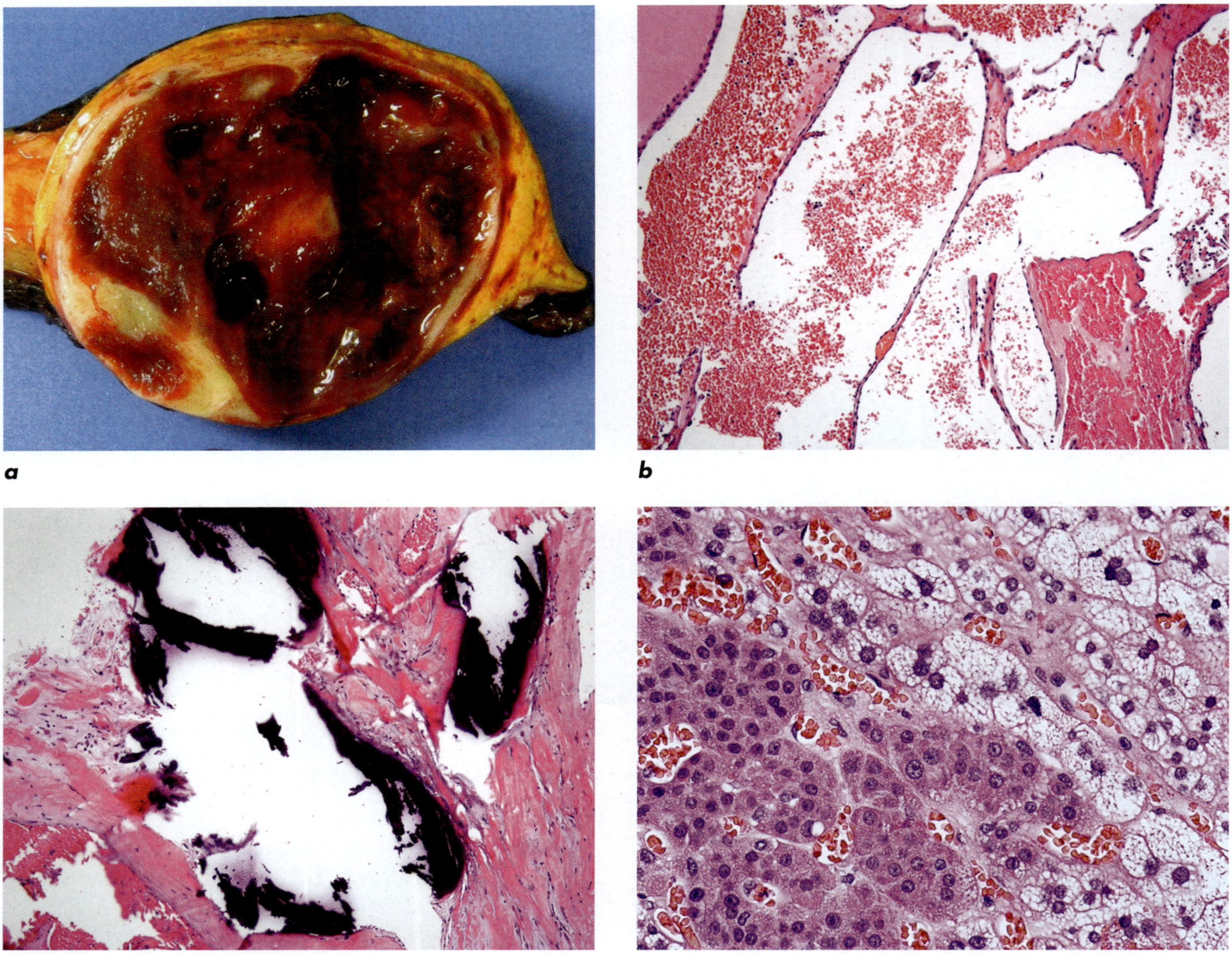

a b c d

Figure 58-7.
Hemorrhagic cortical adenoma displays a dark red cut surface (*a*). Microscopically, the tumor contains hemorrhage and blood-filled dilated channels (*b*) as well as fibrosis and calcification (*c*). Other areas show typical neoplastic cortical cells with eosinophilic or foamy cytoplasm (*d*).

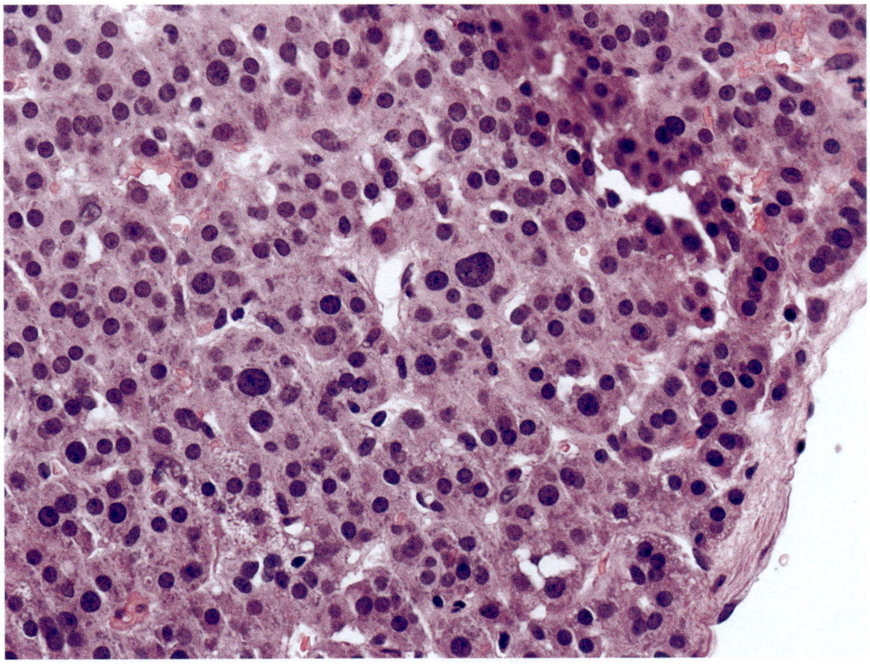

Figure 58-8.
Cortical adenoma consisting of tumor cells with abundant eosinophilic cytoplasm, occasional lipid vacuoles, and occasional enlarged nuclei.

Renal cell carcinoma, clear cell type

- Chicken-wire vascular pattern, more cytological atypia than a cortical adenoma. In difficult cases, IHC markers can be helpful. RCC positive for CA9, CD10, and epithelial markers, negative for inhibin and neuroendocrine markers

Pheochromocytoma

- Clear, eosinophilic, or amphophilic cytoplasm without lipid-rich foamy cytoplasm, Zellballen pattern. S100 demonstrates sustentacular cells

Molecular analysis

- Adenomas greater than 5 cm in size show activation of the Wnt/β-catenin pathway, with a proportion of cases containing a somatic mutation in the β-catenin gene (*CTNBB1*), resulting in aberrant immunohistochemical cytoplasmic or nuclear staining rather than the normal membranous staining

Clinical relevance (prognosis and treatment options)

- Indications for surgery include functional lesions and size greater than or equal to 6 cm (due to higher risk of tumor hemorrhage and potential for malignancy)
- Incidentalomas smaller or equal to 4 cm with benign imaging characteristics may be serially followed
- Management of lesions between 4 and 6 cm depends on radiographic appearance, growth, and patient concern

GANGLIONEUROMA

Definition

- Benign tumor of sympathetic nervous system composed of fully differentiated ganglion cells in a Schwannian stroma

Pathogenesis

- Arise from the primitive precursor cells of the sympathetic nervous system
- May represent a continuum of neuronal maturation: ganglioneuromas representing the most mature lesions, followed by ganglioneuroblastomas and neuroblastomas being the most immature
- May arise de novo or in neuroblastomas undergoing maturation

Clinical features

- Age at diagnosis usually between 5 and 10 years
- Most common sympathetic nervous system tumor in adults
- In addition to the adrenal gland, the other common sites include posterior mediastinum and retroperitoneum
- Elevated urine homovanillic acid (HVA) and vanilmandelic acid (VMA) levels
- Rarely cause symptoms (such as hypertension) related to catecholamine excess

Gross pathology

- Lobulated and well circumscribed
- Tan to white, fleshy cut surface with a golden yellow rim of normal cortical tissue can often be identified on the periphery of the tumor (Fig. 58-9)

Histology

- The tumor has a well-defined capsule without invasion (Fig. 58-10)
- Two components
  - Ganglion cells (Fig. 58-11). Mature-appearing ganglion cells in different sizes. Tumor cells may be binucleated
  - Schwannian-type stromal cells (Fig. 58-10). Spindle cells with wavy nuclei (Fig. 58-11)
- If neuroblasts are present in a ganglioneuroma, it is designated as ganglioneuroblastoma

Immunohistochemistry

- Ganglion cells positive for acetylcholinesterase, microtubule-associated protein, calretinin
- S100 stains Schwannian stroma and satellite cells surrounding ganglion cells

Differential diagnosis

Neurofibroma

- Lacking ganglion cell differentiation

Composite adrenal tumor

- Composite tumors may arise in the adrenal gland, which are composed of pheochromocytoma as the dominant component, intimately intermixed with a ganglioneuroma component. In 20% of cases, the patient has a history of neurofibromatosis

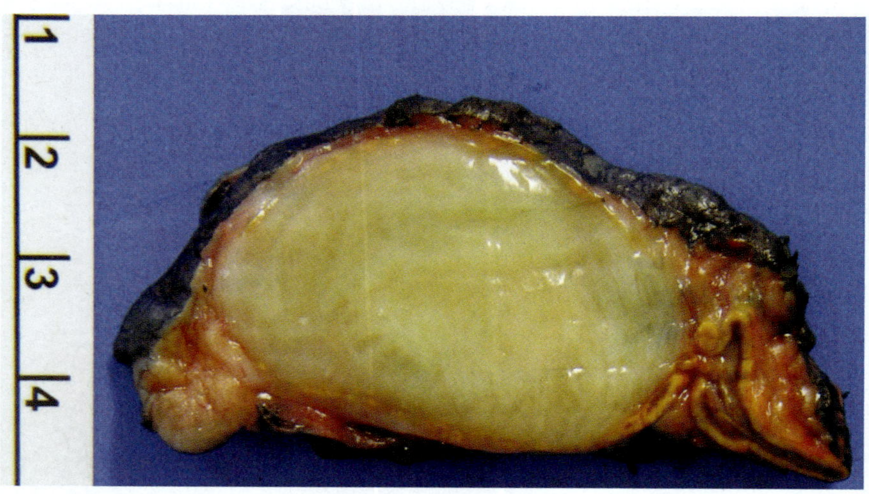

Figure 58-9.
Gross photo of adrenal ganglioneuroma demonstrated a well-circumscribed mass surrounded by the golden yellow cortical rim tissue. The tumor has a white-tan cut surface with somewhat fibrous appearance.

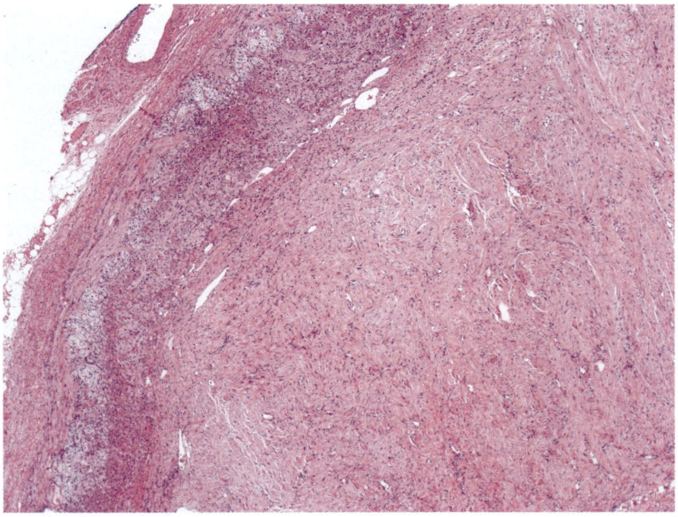

a

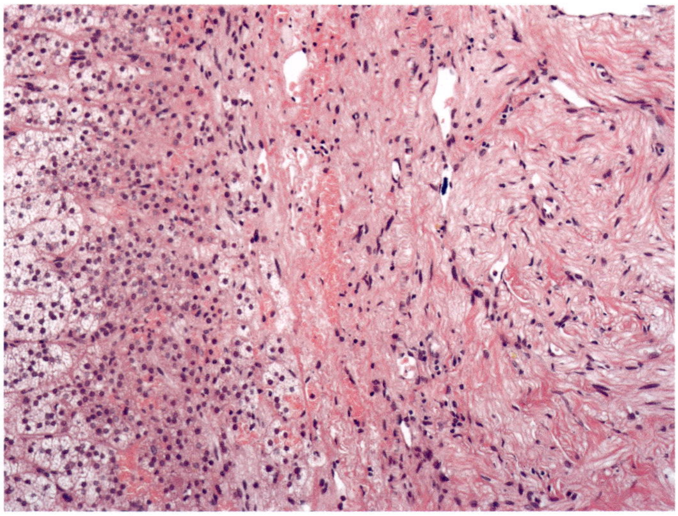

b

Figure 58-10.
Adrenal ganglioneuroma shows defined border between the tumor and adrenal cortical tissue (*a*). High magnification (*b*) demonstrates the interface between the adrenal cortical tissue (left) and the tumor (right) predominantly consisting of spindle cells with wavy nuclei.

Figure 58-11.
Adrenal ganglioneuroma is characterized by the presence of large ganglion cells in the background of spindle-shaped Schwannian-type neuronal cells (*a*). The neoplastic ganglion cells have abundant amphophilic cytoplasm and round or oval nuclei. Occasionally, binucleation can be seen, but no cytological atypia (*b*).

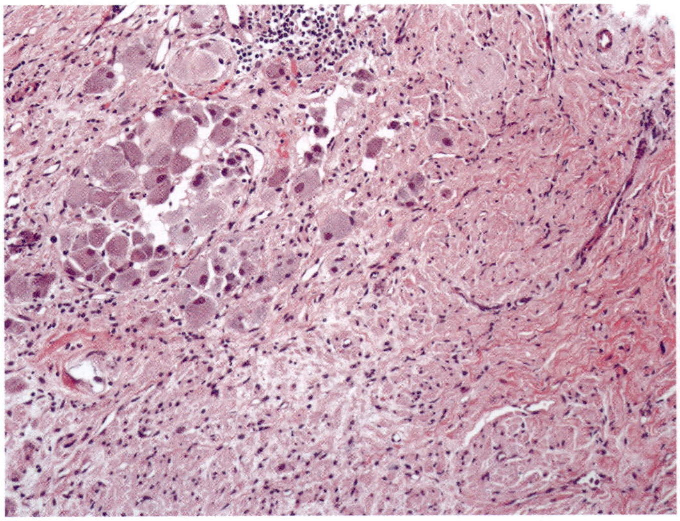

a

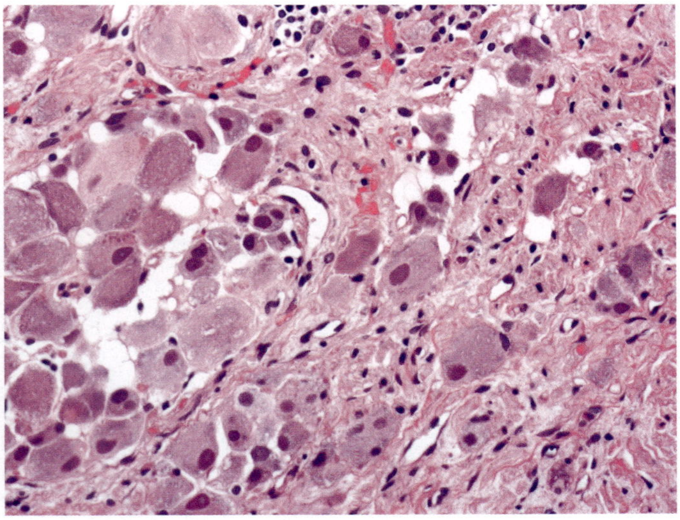

b

PHEOCHROMOCYTOMA

Definition

- Neoplasm derived from chromaffin cells of adrenal medulla
- The term pheochromocytoma (dusky colored tumor) is based on the color change when this tumor is immersed in chromate salts

Other terms

- Paraganglioma of the adrenal, chromaffinoma
- Strictly speaking, a paraganglioma is a pheochromocytoma in an extra-adrenal organ, although pheochromocytoma and paraganglioma have been used interchangeably

Pathogenesis

- Pheochromocytoma cells are morphologically very similar to the adrenal medullary cells
- Functionally, pheochromocytoma cells produce catecholamines. However, the production of catecholamines is unregulated, resulting in increased hormone production leading to clinical symptoms
- Malignant pheochromocytoma is defined by the presence of metastasis. Pathological diagnosis of a "benign" pheochromocytoma should be avoided in clinical practice because of its malignant potential

Clinical features

- The tumor occurs in wide age range, but most patients are in their forties or fifties
- Also known as a *10% tumor*: 10% are bilateral, 10% extra-adrenal, 10% occur in children, and 10% malignant
- Because of the excess of catecholamines, the classic triad of sweating attacks, headaches, and tachycardia are diagnostic
- Chest or abdominal pain may also develop
- Hypertension in the majority of cases, particularly in young patients. Hypertensive symptoms such as blurred vision and light-headedness may be associated with postural changes or exercises when the abdominal pressure is increased
- A small subset of patients may develop paraneoplastic syndromes such as diabetes mellitus due to peptide hormone production by the tumor
- May be a component of Multiple Endocrine Neoplasia type II in familial cases

Gross pathology

- Well-circumscribed mass, 3 to 5 cm in size (Fig. 58-12)
- Cut surface is white, gray, pink, fleshy, or tan (Fig. 58-13), the color of the tumor darkens when exposed to air
- Hemorrhage and necrosis may be present
- Normal adrenal cortex can be appreciated in most cases, as a bright yellow rim (Fig. 58-12) around the tumor

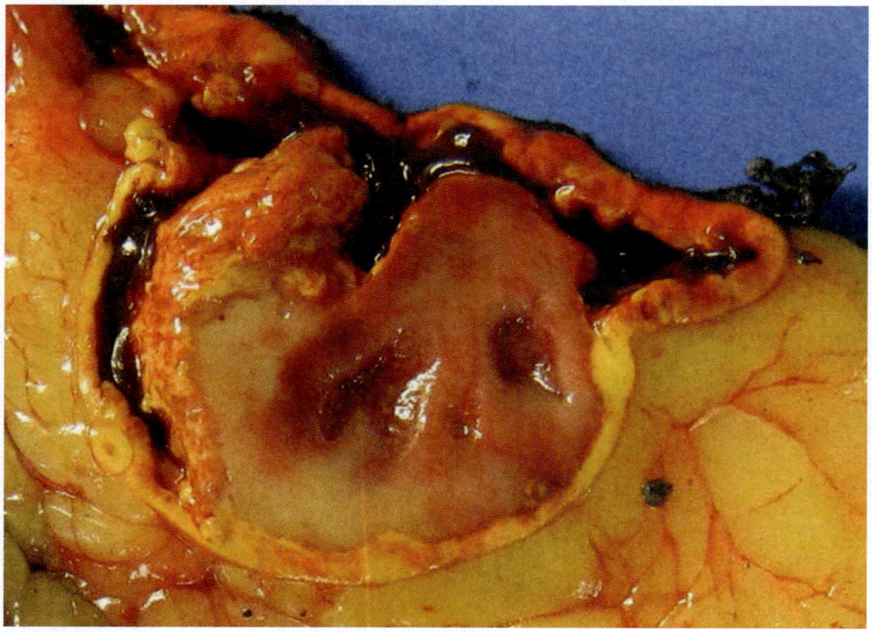

Figure 58-12.
A fleshy-colored pheochromocytoma located in the medulla and surrounded by bright yellow cortical tissue.

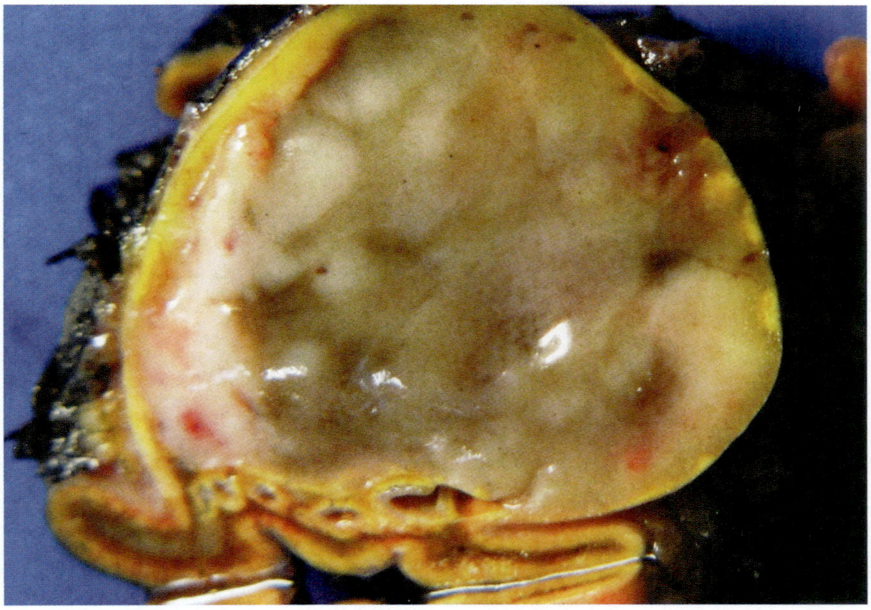

Figure 58-13.
Pheochromocytoma as a well-circumscribed mass with a white-tan cut surface, which is in sharp contrast to the bright yellow cortical tissue.

Histology

- Alveolar (Zellballen = cell ball) pattern or trabecular patterns are characteristic (Fig. 58-14)
- Tumor cells are large polygonal cells with abundant amphophilic cytoplasm (Figs. 58-15 to 58-17), similar to but larger than normal medullary cells
- Tumor nests are separated by thin-walled blood vessels (Fig. 58-16*b*)
- Isolated nuclear atypia, nuclear pleomorphism and nuclear pseudoinclusions are common (Fig. 58-16*b*), which is not an indication of malignancy
- Intracytoplasmic or extracellular hyaline globules (PAS positive) can be seen (Fig. 58-16*c*)
- Scattered ganglion cells are common. Uncommonly, small cells or spindle cells are seen
- The only true histological evidence of malignancy is the presence of metastasis, which should be carefully evaluated
- Weiss criteria such as cytological atypia, mitosis, or even invasion cannot be used reliably to predicate malignant behavior
- Pheochromocytoma is morphologically indistinguishable from a paraganglioma although it has a lower malignant potential (10%) than a paraganglioma of other GU organs (20% to 30%)

Immunohistochemistry

- Neuroendocrine markers such as chromogranin, synaptophysin, or NSE are positive (Fig. 58-16*d*)
- Patchy stellate-shaped sustentacular cells are positive for S100
- Epithelial markers such as AE1/ AE3, Cam5.2, CK20, HMWCK are negative

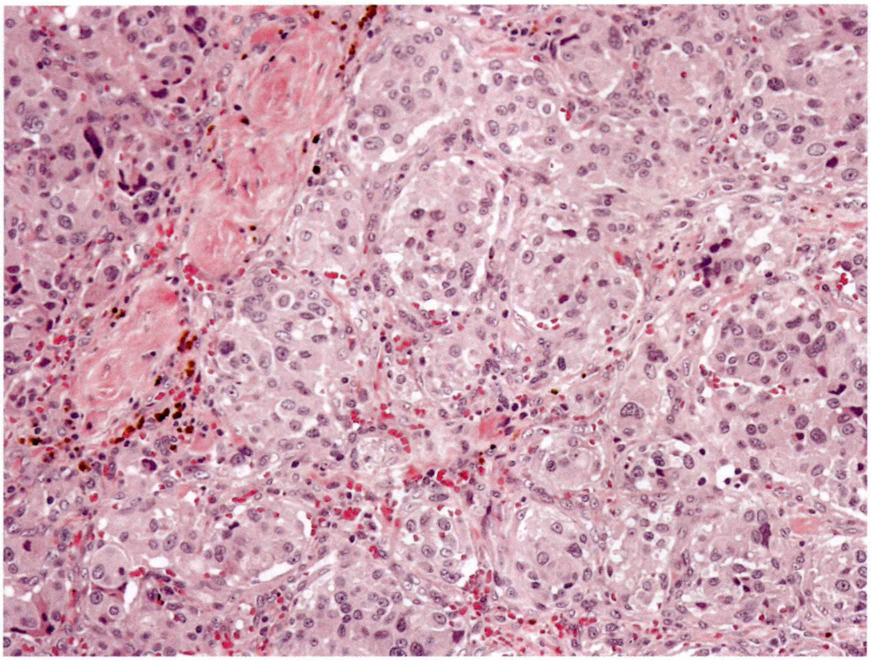

Figure 58-14.
Pheochromocytoma is composed of nests of tumor cells forming typical Zellballen patterns with thin fibrovascular septa between them.

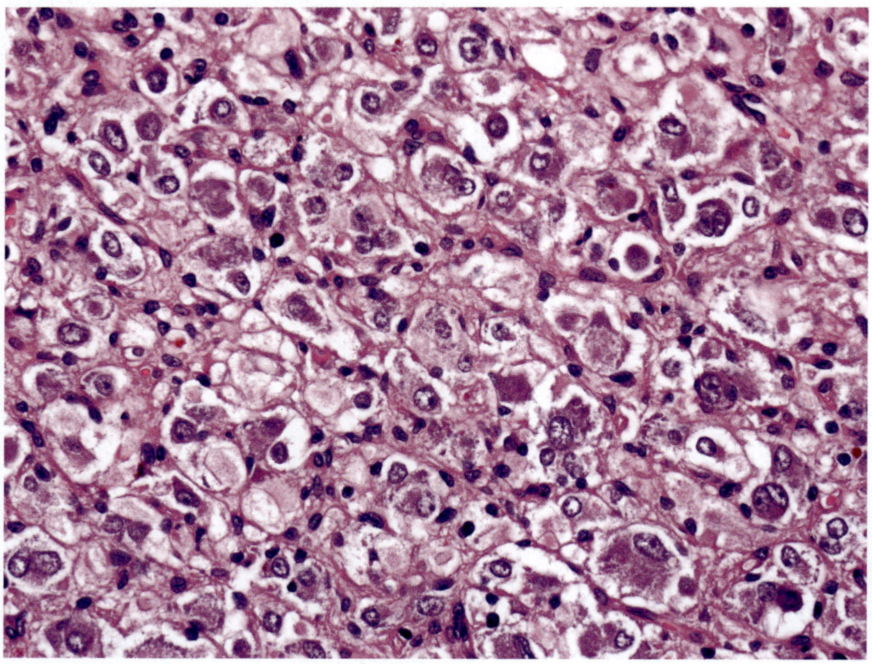

Figure 58-15.
Pheochromocytoma cells with abundant amphophilic granular cytoplasm and occasionally binucleation.

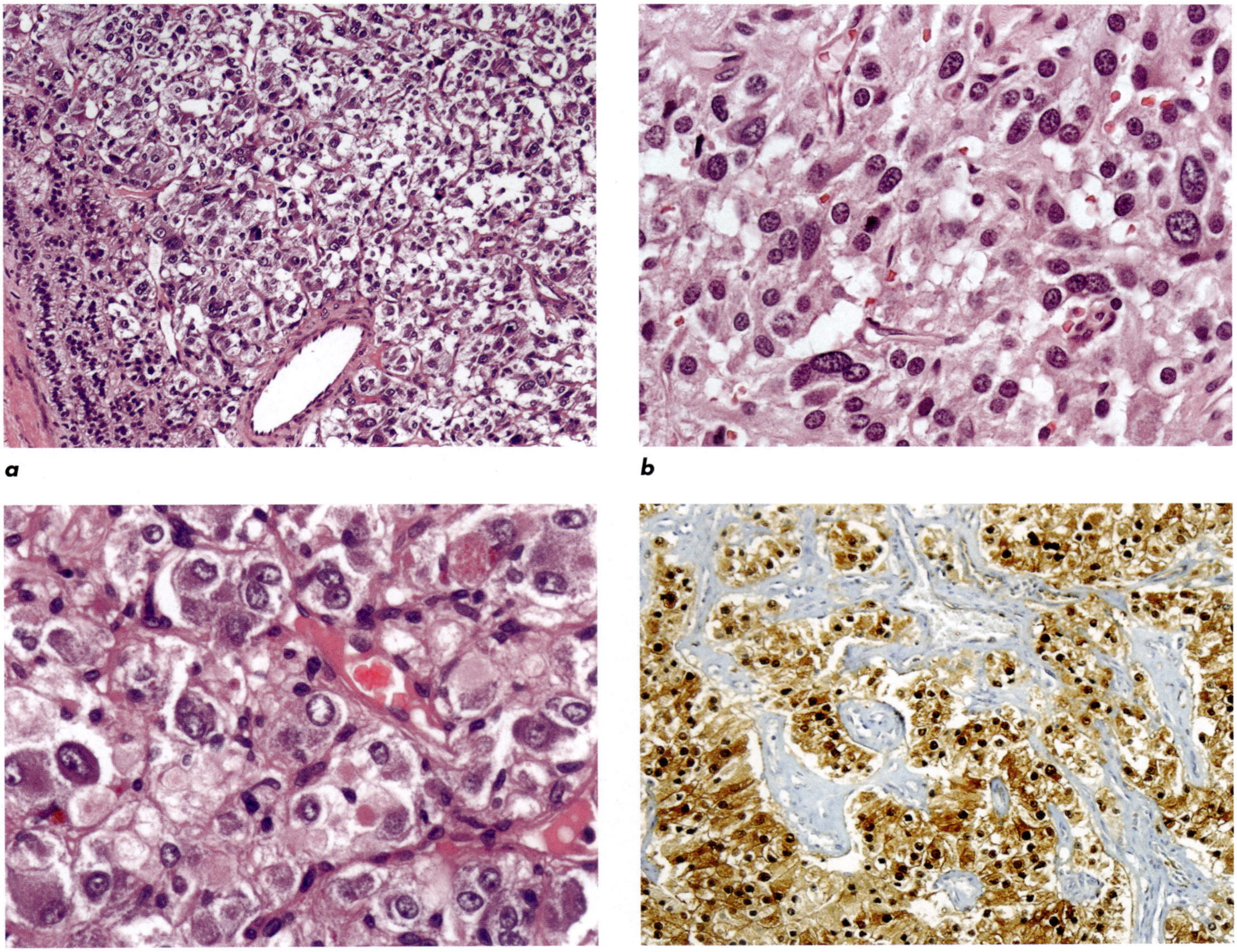

a b c d

Figure 58-16.

Pheochromocytoma cells show prominent granular cytoplasm (*a*) in contrast to the foamy cortical cells (left). Focal cytological atypia is present (*b*). An intracytoplasmic hyaline globule is seen in the lower middle portion of the photomicrograph (*c*). Tumor cells are positive for chromogranin (*d*).

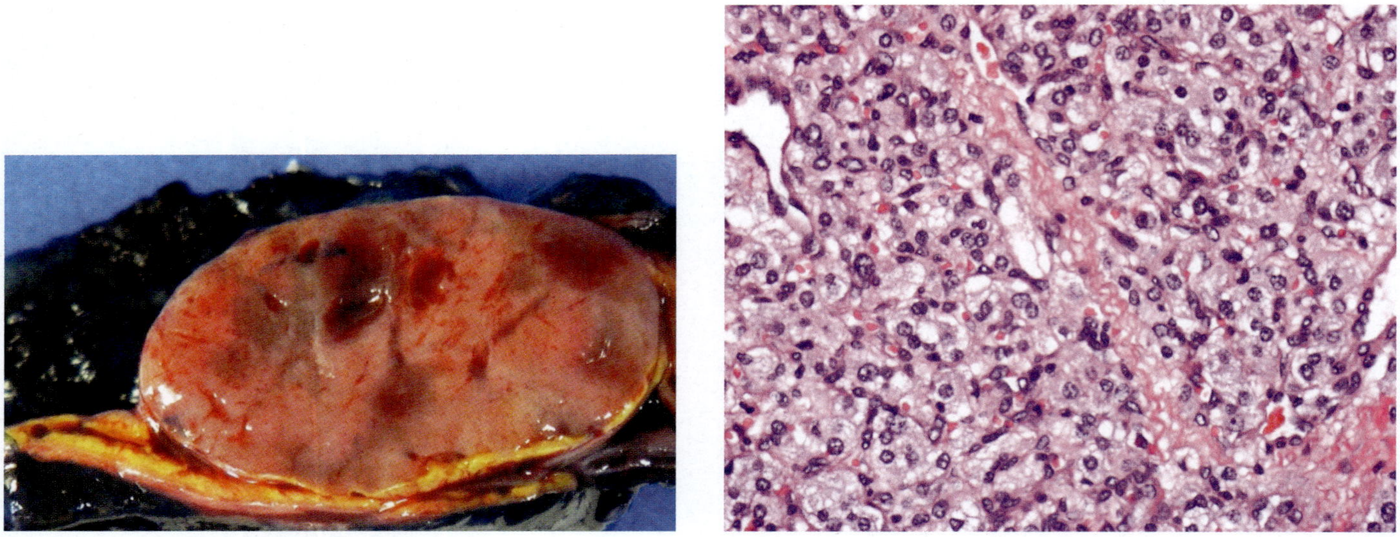

a b

Figure 58-17.
Pheochromocytoma in a patient with Von Hippel-Lindau syndrome displays a pink cut surface (*a*). Microscopically, the morphology of the tumor cells is identical to that of sporadic cases (*b*).

Differential diagnosis

Cortical adenoma

- Clinical symptoms reflect steroid hormone secretion; grossly bright yellow; tumor cells with foamy cytoplasm; S100 and neuroendocrine markers can be helpful

Metastatic carcinoma, particular metastatic RCC

- History of primary cancer; no typical symptoms such as hypertension; no Zellballen patterns; areas of clear cell may be seen in clear cell RCC; glandular formation is rare in pheochromocytoma

Molecular analysis

- Mutations of *SDHD* and *SDHB* genes have been demonstrated in the majority of familial cases; however, these mutations are rare in sporadic cases
- Not indicated for diagnosis

Clinical relevance (prognosis and treatment options)

- Morphological features cannot be reliably used to predict malignant or benign behavior
- Malignant pheochromocytoma can be diagnosed only if metastasis develops
- Surgical resection is the treatment of choice

COMPOSITE TUMOR OF THE ADRENAL

Definition

- Two or more tumor components coexisting in one adrenal mass

Other terms (typical combinations)

- Cortical adenoma with myelolipoma, cortical adenoma with pheochromocytoma, cortical carcinoma with myelolipoma, pheochromocytoma with ganglioneuroma, ganglioneuroma with myelolipoma
- A benign-benign composition is more common than benign-malignant or malignant-malignant composition

Pathogenesis

- Composite tumor is believed to be very rare with only case reports in the literature
- In reality, it is relatively more common in the adrenal than in other organs based on our experience

Clinical features

- Depend on the size of each component
- Hypertension in a patient with pheochromocytoma
- Cushing syndrome in a patient with cortical adenoma

Gross pathology

- Fleshy, yellow homogenous (Fig. 58-18) or heterogeneous appearance
- Hemorrhage and necrosis are rare

Figure 58-18.
Composite pheochromocytoma and ganglioneuroma. The cut surface of a well-circumscribed mass demonstrates homogeneous appearance (*a*). Microscopically, the tumor contains two components: pheochromocytoma (*b*) and ganglioneuroma (*c*).

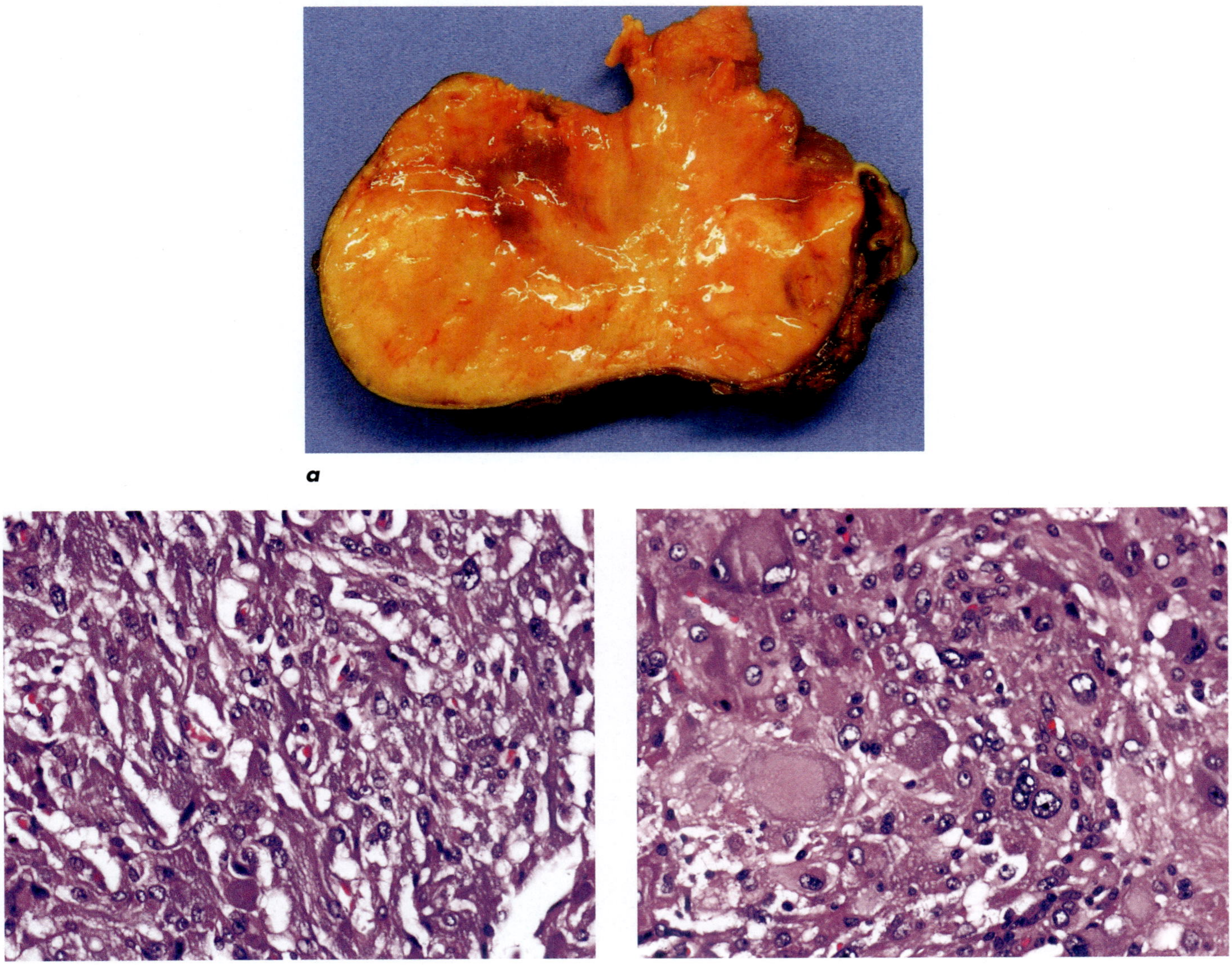

a

b

c

- Grossly, it is not possible to make a diagnosis of composite adrenal tumor
- Sufficient sampling is the key for diagnosis

Histology

- Adenoma with myelolipoma is the most common form, which is composed of adenomatous and myelolipomatous components (Fig. 58-19)
- A pheochromocytoma with ganglioneuroma (Fig. 58-18) is composed of both pheochromocytoma and ganglioneuroma features

Immunohistochemistry and molecular analysis

- Variable, dependent on tumor components

Clinical relevance (prognosis and treatment options)

- Different tumor components may have different biological behaviors, so that it is important to detect all different components by sufficient sampling
- If both components are benign such as adenoma and myelolipoma, it is treated as benign; surgical excision may be necessary if the tumor is large or symptomatic
- If one of the components is malignant or potentially malignant, follow-up or additional treatment may be necessary

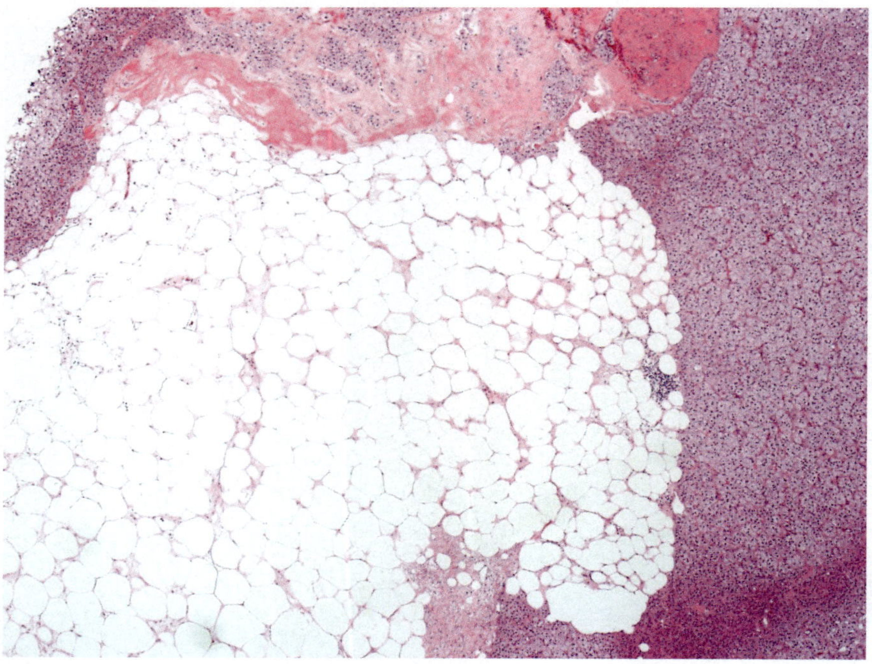

Figure 58-19.
Composite adenoma and myelolipoma. The tumor is composed of cortical adenoma (right) and myelolipomatous component (left).

CHAPTER 59

Malignant Neoplasms of the Adrenal

Celina Villa, Anjana Yeldandi, Ximing J. Yang

ADRENAL CORTICAL CARCINOMA

Definition

- Malignant epithelial neoplasm arising from the adrenal cortex

Pathogenesis

- Unclear if it derives de novo or it presents as a progression from an adrenocortical adenoma to malignancy

Clinical features

- It occurs most commonly in adults, very rarely in children
- May be functional, most are nonfunctional
- Patients usually present with symptoms related to mass effect or rarely due to hormone dysfunction
- If it is large and compressing or invading the kidney, it may be mistaken for a renal tumor by imaging studies
- Adrenocortical carcinoma in children and young adults should raise the suspicion of Li-Fraumeni syndrome, since an association has been found in more than half of cases regardless of family history. Molecular analysis reveals germ-line mutations in the *TP53* gene in this syndrome
- Increased frequencies are also seen in the Beckwith-Wiedemann syndrome and familial adenomatous polyposis

Gross findings

- May be encapsulated, although capsule frequently infiltrated by tumor (Fig. 59-1*a*)
- Usually solitary, but the tumor may have smaller satellite nodules (Fig. 59-1*b*)
- Cut surface shows variegated appearance, fleshy or white soft, friable, often with extensive hemorrhage and necrosis (Figs. 59-2 and 59-3)
- Invasion of the capsule, major veins, or adjacent organs may be seen grossly

Histology

- Microscopically, displays a wide range of differentiation, from well-differentiated lesions resembling adrenocortical adenoma to undifferentiated tumors
- Well-differentiated tumors may have resemblance to normal cortical cells
- Typically, cortical carcinoma is composed of sheets of tumor cells with a fine sinusoidal network, commonly with broad bands of fibrosis. Trabecular or nested patterns may be seen (Fig. 59-4*a*)
- Cortical carcinoma tends to have more diffuse pattern (Fig. 59-4*b*) than zonal patterns seen in adenoma

Figure 59-1.
Adrenal cortical carcinoma as a large tumor above the kidney with variegated cut surface and extensive hemorrhage and necrosis (*a*). Close-up photo demonstrates a tumor nodule with spotty yellow necrosis invading periadrenal fat (*b*, arrow).

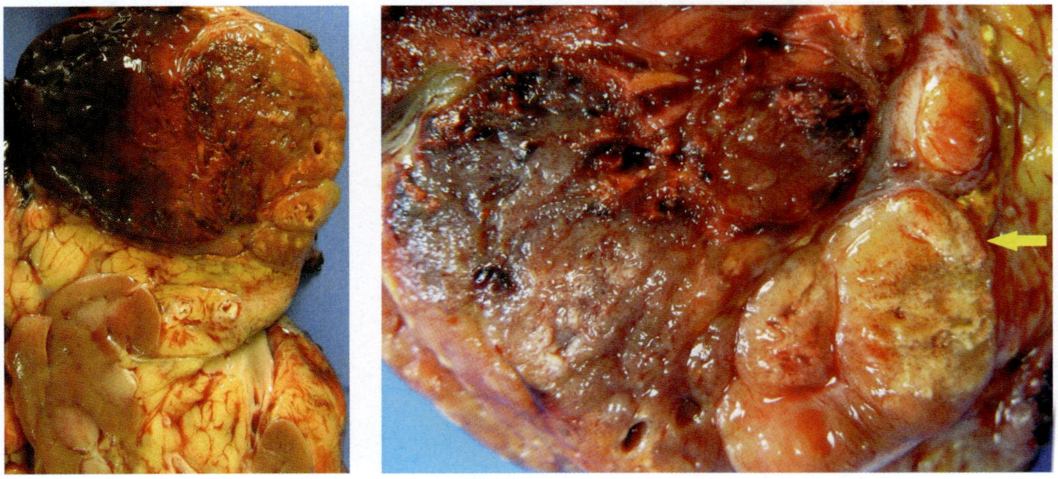

a b

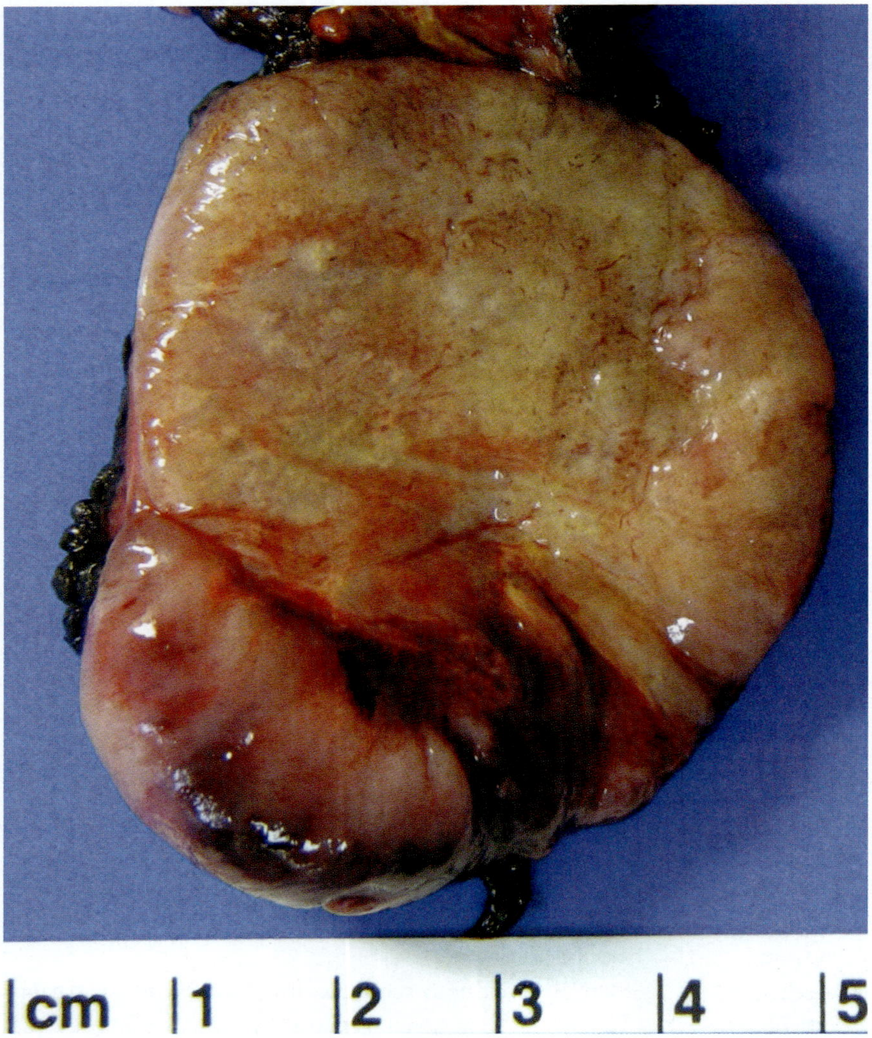

Figure 59-2.
Adrenal cortical carcinoma measuring 5 cm with spotty necrosis. Cortical rim is not seen, suggestive of tumor invasion.

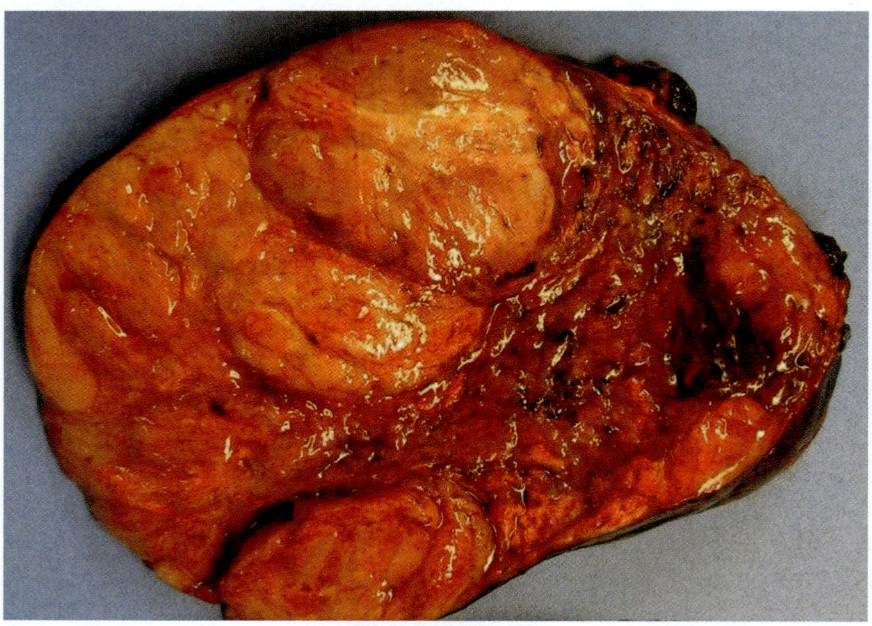

Figure 59-3.
Adrenal cortical carcinoma as a 10-cm mass replacing the entire adrenal displays a variegated cut surface with focal hemorrhage and necrosis

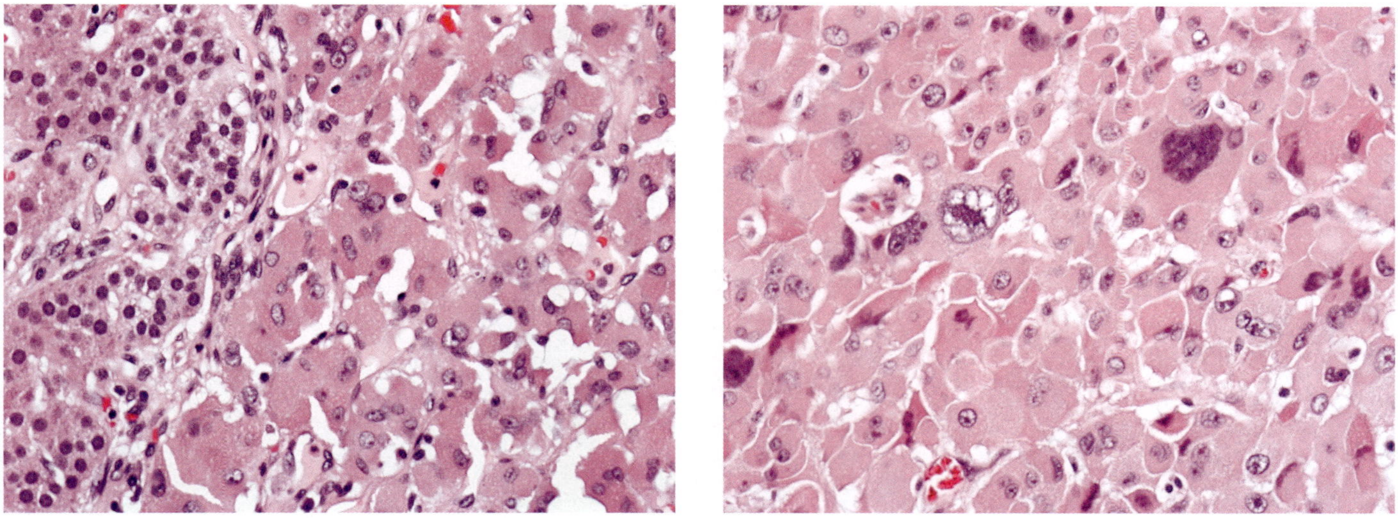

a b

Figure 59-4.
Comparison of benign cortical cells (*a*, left) with cortical carcinoma cells (*a*, right) that have nuclear enlargement and atypia with eosinophilic cytoplasm in a sinusoidal arrangement (*b*).

- Less differentiated tumor cells will have more eosinophilic cytoplasm (Fig. 59-4*b*) and less foamy (clear) cytoplasm
- Poorly differentiated tumor displays marked cytological atypia, resembles high-grade RCC (Fig. 59-5*a*)
- Mitotic figures are numerous and may include atypical ones
- Invasion to capsule, venous or sinusoidal, is often present (Figs. 59-5*b* and 59-6).
- Necrosis can be seen (Figs. 59-5*a* and 59-6*c*). Rarely may contain myxoid, oncocytic features or sarcomatous elements
- Tumor may be heavily infiltrated by neutrophils

The scoring criteria for adrenal cortical carcinoma

- This scoring system, also known as the Weiss criteria, is the most commonly used criteria to assess malignant potential of a cortical neoplasm
- The presence of three or more of the Weiss criteria features (Table 59-1) are highly correlated with malignant behavior of the cortical tumor
- For a cortical tumor greater than 10 cm and weighing more than 100 g, the likelihood of finding malignant features is very high

Caveats to Weiss diagnostic criteria

Pediatric adrenocortical tumors

- Commonly display high-grade nuclear atypia
- May contain atypical mitoses despite limited metastatic potential
- Reasonably good prognosis for children <5 years of age

Oncocytic adrenocortical neoplasms

- The majority of oncocytic adrenocortical neoplasms (Fig. 59-7) show benign behavior although these tumors can easily display three Weiss criteria: tumor contains cells with oncocytic cytoplasm (nonclear cells), diffuse architecture, and a subset of cells with high-grade nuclear atypia

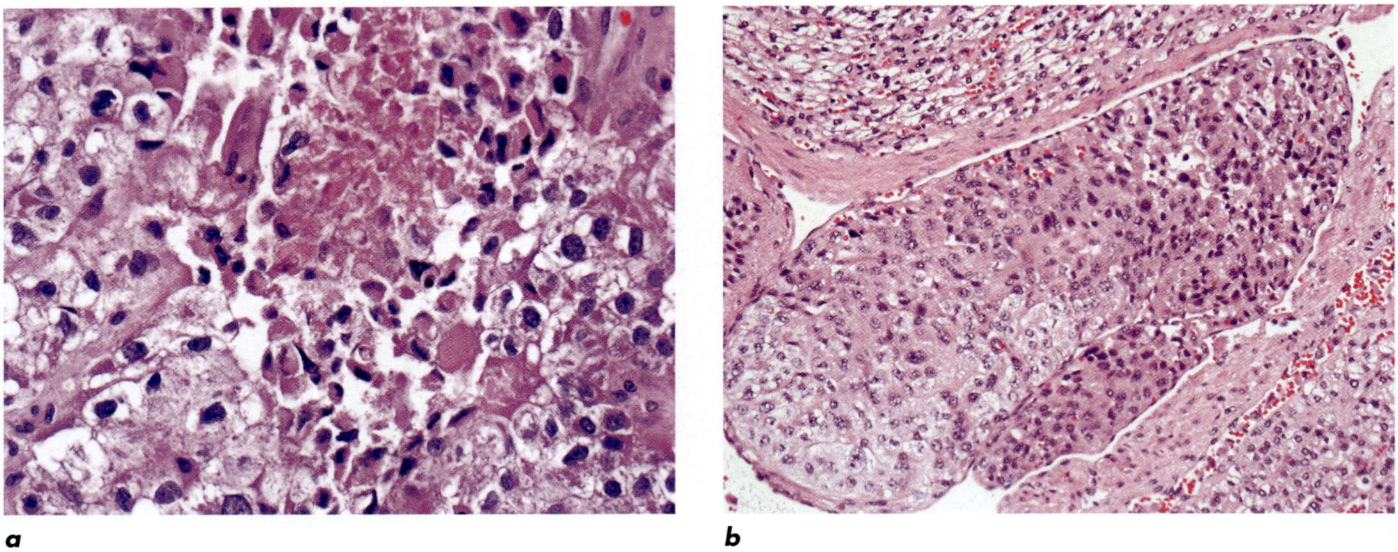

Figure 59-5.
Adrenal cortical carcinoma with focal necrosis (*a*) and vascular invasion (*b*).

Myxoid adrenocortical neoplasms

- Weiss criteria do not correlate well with biologic behavior, as lesions with a Weiss score less than three may display metastatic behavior

Sarcomatoid adrenal cortical carcinoma

- Adrenocortical carcinoma with a sarcomatoid component is associated with more aggressive behavior

Immunohistochemistry

- Markers positive in adrenal cortical carcinoma: vimentin, keratins, inhibin
- Other markers such as calretinin, melan A, synaptophysin (although not chromogranin)
- Insulin-like growth factor 2 (*IGF2*) and matrix metalloproteinase type 2 are expressed at higher rates in adrenocortical carcinomas compared with adrenocortical adenomas; however, the sensitivity and specificity of *IGF2* is not well known

Molecular analysis

- Most show loss of heterozygosity at 17p13 and 11q13
- Paternal disomy and loss of heterozygosity of the *IGF2* gene
- Activation of Wnt/β-catenin pathway

Clinical relevance

- Poor prognosis with overall 5-year survival rates between 10% and 40%
- Treatment is surgical excision, with possible chemotherapy
- A substantial number of patients with adrenocortical carcinomas present with advanced disease. Treatments for advanced disease are rarely curative (Table 59-2)

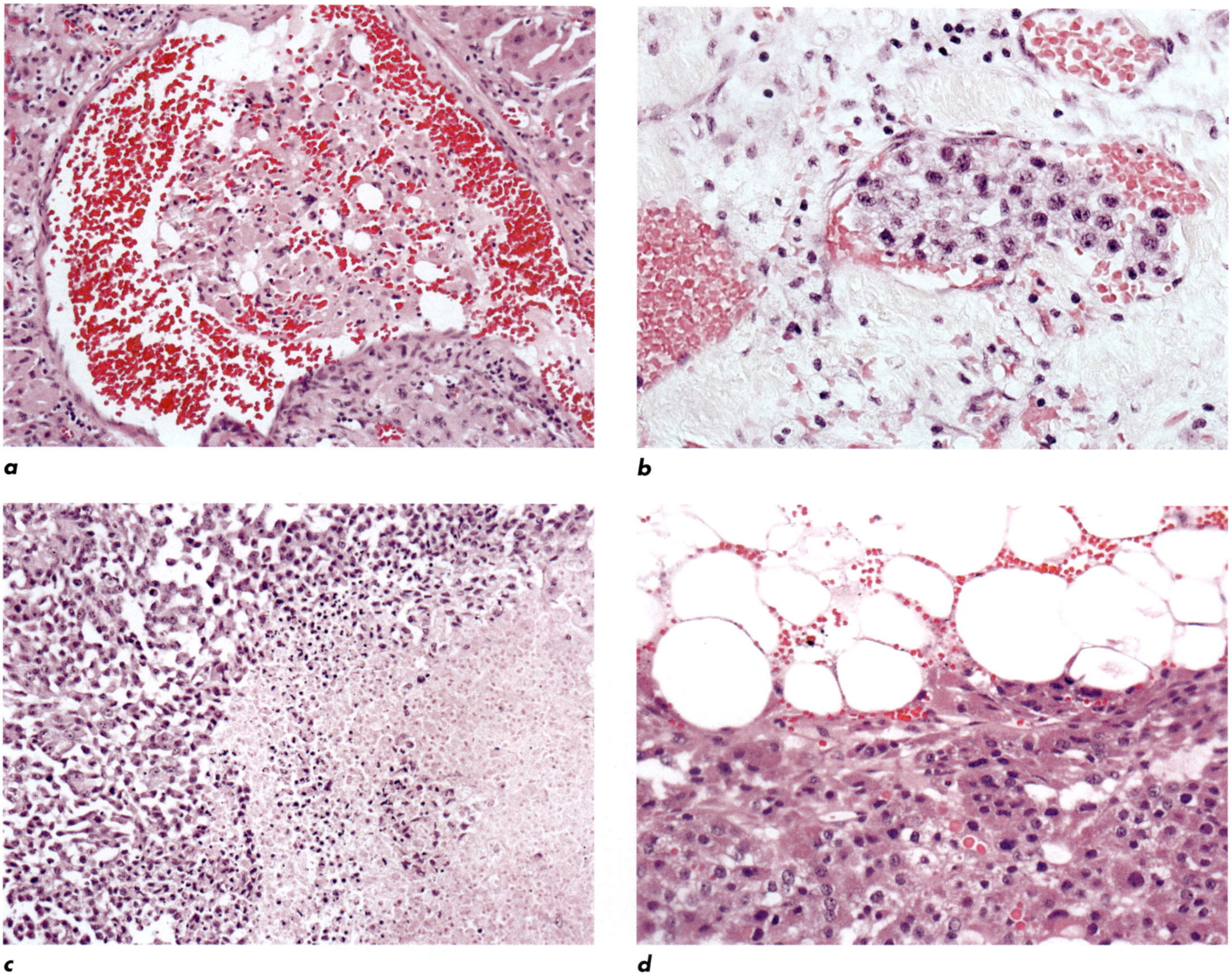

Figure 59-6.
Adrenal cortical carcinoma with multiple diagnostic features of carcinoma: a tumor thrombus in a larger vein (*a*), tumor cells with venous invasion (*b*), tumoral necrosis (*c*), and tumor cells invading periadrenal adipose tissue (*d*).

Table 59-1. Diagnostic Criteria of Adrenal Cortical Carcinoma

Category		*Features*
Cytological atypia	1	Mitotic rate ≥6/50 high power fields
	2	Atypical mitoses
	3	High nuclear grade (grade 3 or 4 based on Fuhrman criteria)
Invasive features	4	Capsular invasion
	5	Sinusoidal invasion
	6	Venous invasion
Growth pattern	7	Diffuse architecture (greater than one-third of tumor)
	8	Clear cells comprising 25% or less of tumor
	9	Necrosis

Figure 59-7.
Adrenal cortical oncocytic neoplasm, measuring 5 cm nodule with fleshy color (*a*). Low magnification shows tumor cells with oncocytic cytoplasm in a diffuse pattern (*b*). High magnification shows the high nuclear grade (*c*).

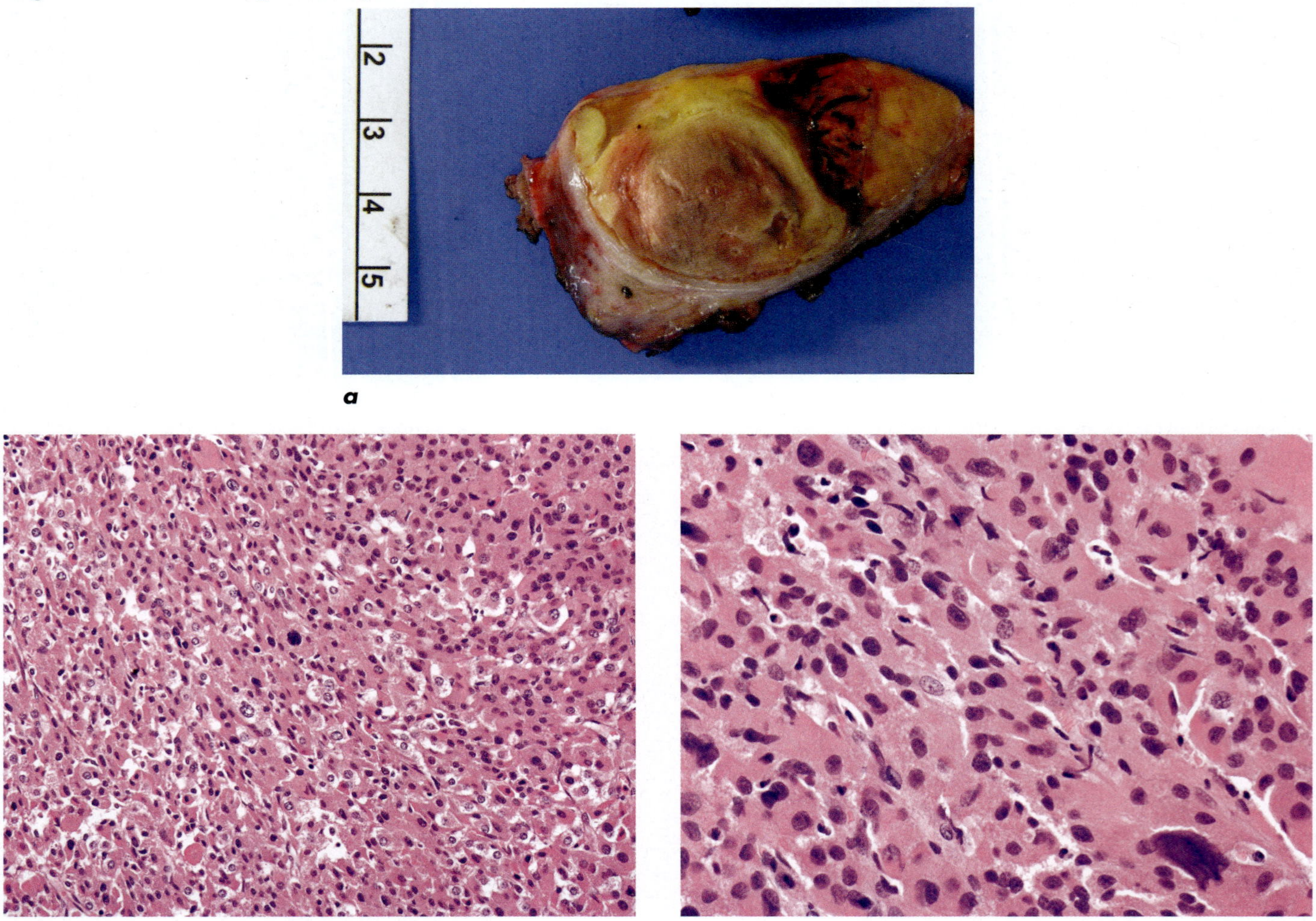

a **b** **c**

Table 59-2. Differential Diagnosis of Adrenal Tumors

	Step 1	*Step 2*	*Step 3*
Differential diagnosis of adrenal neoplasms	**Metastatic**	**Documented clinical history of neoplasm**	**Origin of the tumor**
	(history, histology)		RCC: CA9, PAX8; lung: TTF1
			Colon: CDX2; breast: ER/PR
			Liver: HepPar1
	Primary	**Cortical**	**Cortical adenoma**
		(foamy cytoplasm)	(small but >0.5 cm)
			Cortical carcinoma
			(Weiss criteria)
		Medullary	**Pheochromocytoma**
		(amphophilic cytoplasm)	(Zellballen pattern)
			Neuroblastoma neuroblasts
			Ganglioneuroma ganglion cells

NEUROBLASTOMA

Definition

- Malignant neoplasm of neural crest origin arising from the adrenal medulla and other sites

Clinical features

- Most common malignancy found in children, median age at presentation is 18 months, accounting for 10% of all childhood malignancies
- The adrenal medulla is the most common site. Other sites within the abdomen, along the sympathetic ganglia can also be involved
- Few cases arising in the posterior mediastinum or within the neck have been reported
- Laboratory studies reveal elevated urinary vanillylmandelic acid (VMA) and homovanillic acid (HVA)
- On imaging studies, a large suprarenal mass crossing the midline and showing heterogeneity and calcifications is characteristic
- MIBG scintigraphy is the imaging technique of choice to evaluate for tumor location, metastases, and staging

Gross pathology

- Fairly well circumscribed and encapsulated with a grayish, friable, and nodular cut surface. Areas of hemorrhage, necrosis, and calcifications are often seen.

Histology

- Neuroblastoma is composed of neoplastic neuroblasts with morphology of small round blue cells in sheets (Fig. 59-8*a*)
- Homer Wright rosettes in various stages of differentiation
- Tumor cells have "salt-and-pepper" chromatin (Fig. 59-8*b*)
- Sheets of tumor cells embedded in a fine neurofibrillary stroma (Fig. 59-9)
- Schwannian stroma comprises less than half of the tumor (Shimada classification)
- Extensive areas of necrosis may be seen

Histologic grading system based on Shimada classification

- Used to predict outcome, utilizing presence or absence of Schwannian stroma, degree of differentiation, and mitotic-karyorrhexis index

Neuroblastoma, undifferentiated

- Sheets of neuroblasts with no morphologic differentiation
- No ganglion cells or definite neurofibrillary stroma

Neuroblastoma, poorly differentiated

- Nests of neuroblasts with neurofibrillary stroma
- ganglion cells <5%

Neuroblastoma, differentiating

- Nests of neuroblasts with neurofibrillary stroma
- Ganglion cells >5%

Figure 59-8.
Adrenal neuroblastoma is composed of large nests of small round blue cells (*a*). Higher magnification shows the tumor cells with "salt-and-pepper" chromatin pattern in a pale neurofibrillary background (*b*).

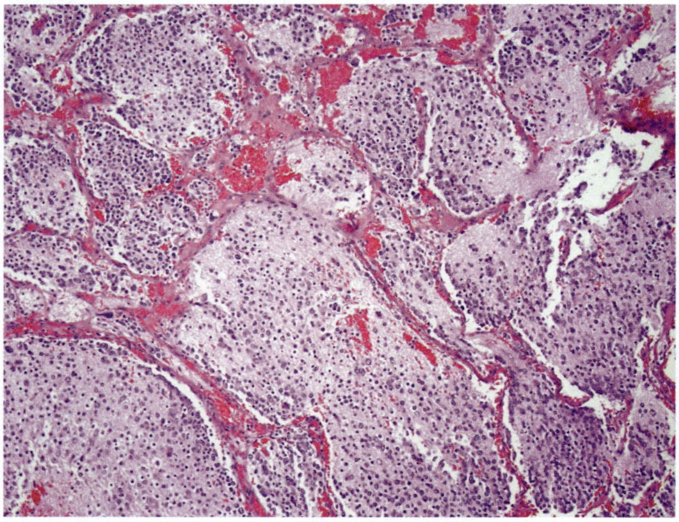

a

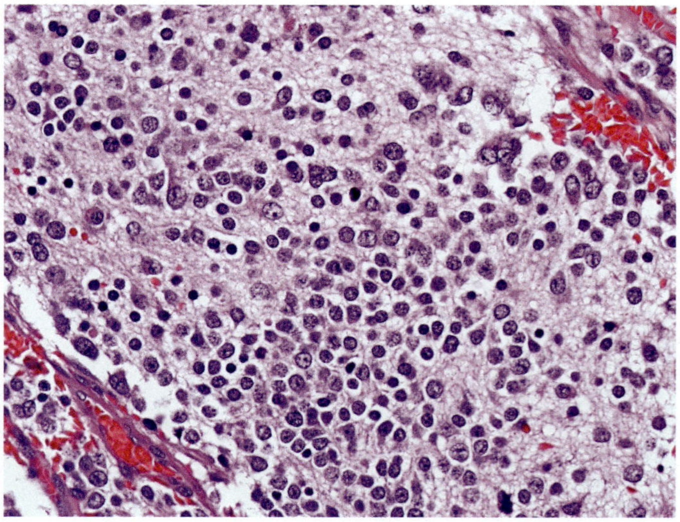

b

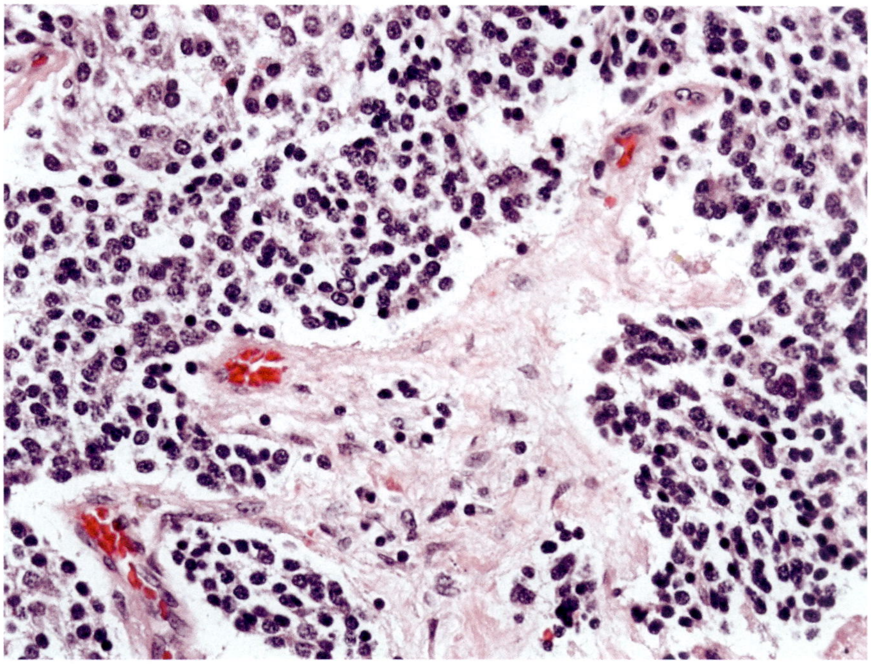

Figure 59-9.
Adrenal neuroblastoma with small primitive neuroblasts in fine neurofibrillary stroma.

Immunohistochemistry

- Small round blue cells show strong expression of neuron-specific enolase (NSE), CD56, chromogranin, and synaptophysin
- Schwannian stroma is S100 positive
- Negative for CD99

Differential diagnosis

Ewing sarcoma/PNET

- Small round blue cells may resemble neuroblasts; CD99 positive, chromogranin and synaptophysin negative. Characteristic t(11;22) by molecular studies or FISH analysis

Rhabdomyosarcoma

- Also, small round blue cells, rhabdomyocytes may be seen. MyoD-1 and myogenin positive, chromogranin and synaptophysin negative

Wilms tumor

- Blastema (small round blue cells) may resemble neuroblasts, also with stroma and epithelial components. Negative for synaptophysin, chromogranin, and NSE

Lymphoma

- Lymphoid cells may resemble neuroblasts, but no rosette formation or neurofibrillary background; CD45 positive, negative for neuroendocrine markers

Molecular analysis

- *N-MYC* amplification 11q, 1p aberrations, and 17q gain, which may be associated with unfavorable prognosis
- *TrK* gene expression is reportedly associated with favorable prognosis

Clinical relevance

- Over half of cases have metastatic disease at presentation, most commonly to bone and liver
- Age of <1 year associated with better prognosis, tumor may undergo spontaneous regression
- Although vast majority (>90%) have elevated catecholamines, only rarely are these symptomatic (ie, hypertensive encephalopathy or cardiac failure)
- May also present with paraneoplastic syndromes such as secretory diarrhea from vasoactive intestinal peptide secretion
- Increased serum levels of chromogranin A is associated with higher stage of disease
- Associations have been found with Hirschsprung disease, central hypoventilation syndrome, neurofibromatosis type I, Beckwith-Wiedemann syndrome, and DiGeorge syndrome

METASTATIC RENAL CELL CARCINOMA

Definition

- Renal cell carcinoma (RCC) metastatic to the adrenal

Pathogenesis

- Most textbooks state that lung cancer is the most common metastatic cancer in the adrenal
- However, metastatic RCC in the adrenal is by far the most common adrenal metastatic tumor in surgical specimens in our practice
- The adrenals harboring metastatic RCC are obtained from either radical nephrectomies or isolated adrenalectomy
- The incidence of adrenal metastasis in patients with RCC ranging from 2% to 10% in surgical specimens to 6% to 29% at autopsy

Clinical features

- Most commonly occurs in ipsilateral adrenal gland, although rarely can be contralateral or bilateral
- Mostly associated with higher RCC stage, often with RCC extending to perirenal tissues
- Imaging studies such as PET/CT can be helpful in identifying metastatic adrenal lesions, however, these modalities are not reliable in distinguishing benign adrenal lesions from metastasis
- Therefore, biopsy or resection of a large adrenal mass suspicious for metastatic carcinoma may be necessary to establish a definitive diagnosis

Gross pathology

- The metastatic RCC to the adrenal is usually solitary (Figs. 59-10 and 59-11), occasionally it can be multiple
- It is well circumscribed. Hemorrhage and necrosis (Fig. 59-10) are commonly present
- Invasion to the adrenal capsule or adjacent tissues may occur

Histology

- Morphologically, clear cell RCC (most common type) may resemble the adrenal cortex histologically
- The tumor cells are more pleomorphic than the normal adrenal cortical cells (Fig. 59-12)
- Other key distinguishing features include adrenal cortical cells with vacuolated cytoplasm that may indent the nucleus. Clear cell RCC has characteristic fine capillary vascular network (Fig. 59-13)

Immunohistochemistry

- RCC positive for PAX2/PAX8, vimentin, and CD10
- RCC, clear cell type stains for carbonic anhydrase IX (Fig. 59-11*d*); papillary RCC positive for AMACR
- Adrenal cortical cells are positive for inhibin, melan A, calretinin, and synaptophysin, while these markers are negative in RCC

Figure 59-10.
Metastatic renal cell carcinoma (RCC) of the adrenal is a large pink, fleshy mass with central necrosis. Residual cortical tissue is on the left (*a*). Microscopically, the tumor is a high-grade clear cell RCC (*b*).

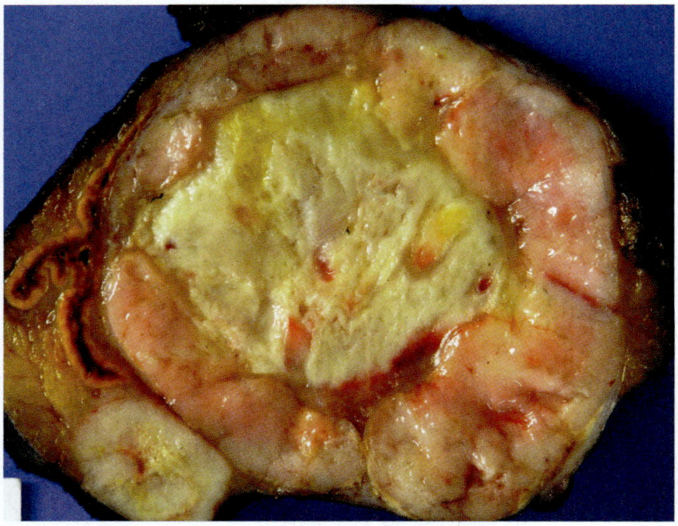

a

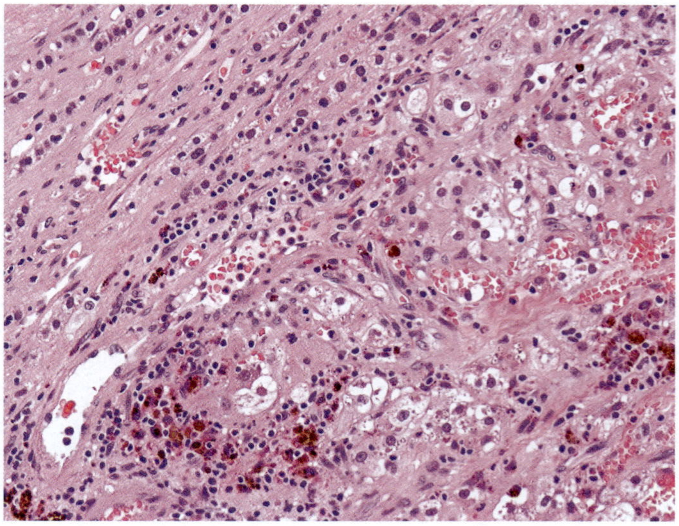

b

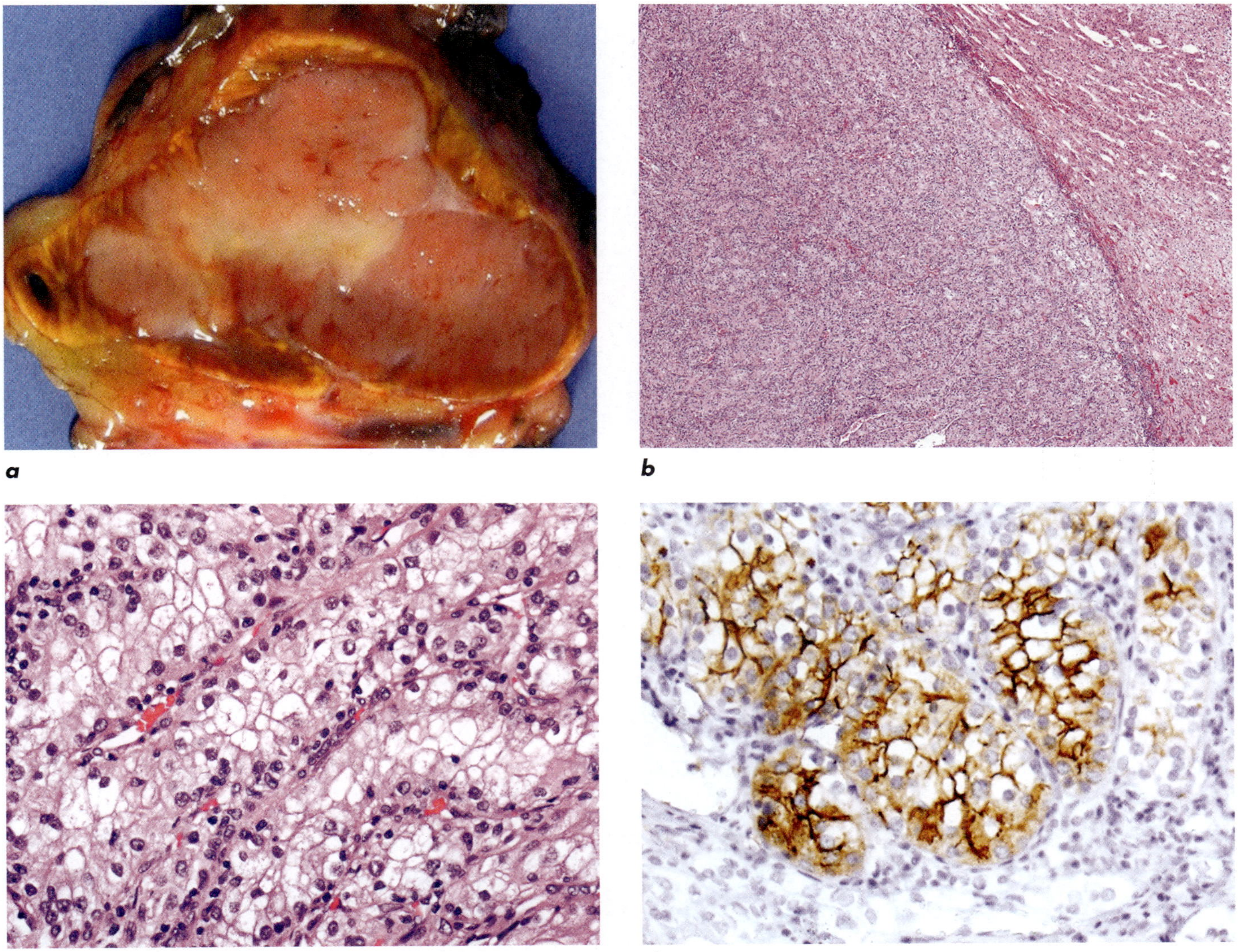

a b c d

Figure 59-11.
Metastatic RCC in the adrenal is a large mass replacing most of the adrenal with a rim of residual adrenal. The cut surface of the tumor is pink fleshy mimicking a pheochromocytoma (*a*). Microscopically, the tumor is sharply demarcated from adrenal tissue (*b*). High magnification shows the features of clear cells with Fuhrman grade 2 nuclei (*c*). The tumor cells are positive for CA9 (*d*).

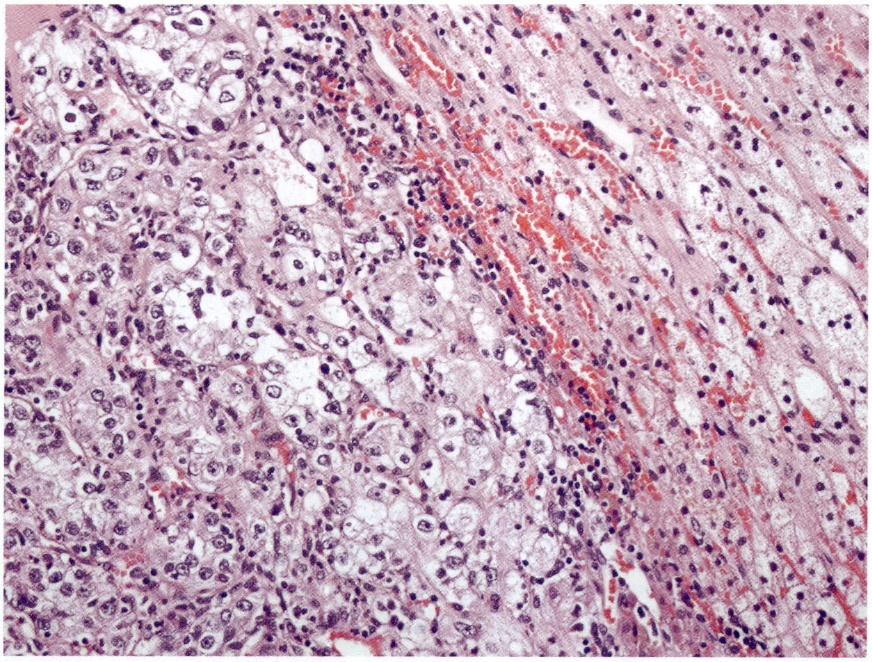

Figure 59-12.
Metastatic RCC in the adrenal. The tumor cells (left), distinct from adrenal cortical cells, display clear cytoplasm and atypical nuclei (Fuhrman grade 3).

Clinical relevance

- Metastatic RCC represents a high-stage disease
- Surgical resection of solitary adrenal metastasis of RCC, particularly a low-grade tumor, is effective to prolong survival, which is heavily dependent on the grade of RCC
- Therefore, we routinely report the histological type and Fuhrman grade of metastatic RCC because of their potential value in prognosis

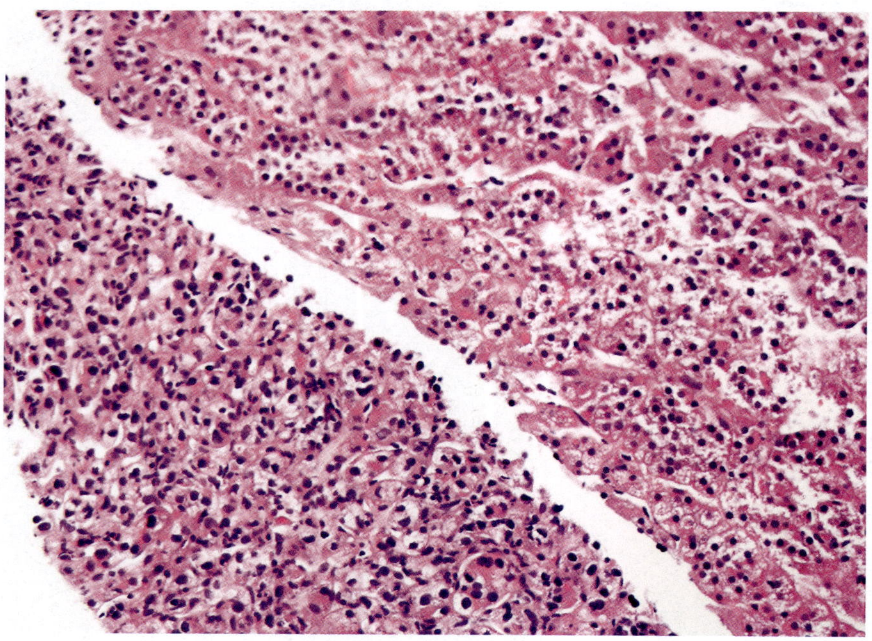

Figure 59-13.
Needle core biopsy of metastatic clear cell RCC. Carcinoma cells (lower left) are different from adrenal cortical cells (upper right) in their nuclear irregularity, higher N/C ratio, and "chicken-wire" vascular network.

OTHER METASTATIC NEOPLASMS IN ADRENAL

Definition

- Metastasis of malignant neoplasm in the adrenal

Pathogenesis

- Metastases are the most common malignant neoplasms found within the adrenal
- An adrenal mass in a cancer patient has a 50% to 75% probability of being a metastasis
- Although bilateral adrenal involvement may be more common in theory, unilateral adrenal metastasis is more common in surgical pathology specimens
- The adrenal gland represents the fourth most common site for metastases

Clinical features

- History of previous diagnosis of malignancy is important
- Again, kidney cancer is the most common metastatic carcinoma in the adrenal in surgical specimens
- Breast cancer and lung cancer have a 39% and 35% chance, respectively, of developing adrenal metastases
- Other common cancers from colon, liver, and melanoma can metastasize to the adrenals
- An ill-defined outline and heterogeneous density by imaging are suggestive of metastases, but never reliable
- Unlike adenomas, metastases show significant growth on interval imaging performed at 6 months, which is the most important feature if followed by imaging studies
- Adrenal metastases typically show high uptake on PET scan

Gross pathology

- Solitary or multiple, poorly defined nodule(s) in the adrenal, with invasion to the capsule or adjacent tissues (Figs. 59-14*a* and 59-15*a*)

Histology

- The histologic features of a metastatic tumor mostly resemble the primary tumor
- Because adrenal cortical carcinoma can also show significant variability in morphology, it is important to keep metastatic tumors in differential diagnosis particularly in a patient with a history of carcinoma
- Lung metastasis should be considered when an adrenal tumor with prominent glandular differentiation, but not clear cell type (Fig. 59-14*a* and *c*). TTF1 and other markers such as Napsin A can be used for confirmation
- Hepatocellular carcinoma cells may contain bile pigment (Fig. 59-15) and melanoma cells may contain melanin pigment (Fig. 59-16)

Immunohistochemistry

- TTF1 for lung adenocarcinoma (Fig. 59-14*d*) and small cell carcinoma
- GATA-3, mammaglobin, and ER/PR for breast adenocarcinoma
- HepPar1 for hepatocellular carcinoma
- CDX2 for colon adenocarcinoma
- ER/PR and PAX2/PAX8 for gynecological malignancies

Clinical relevance

- Clinical history of previously diagnosed cancer is very important for diagnosis, because adrenal carcinoma can mimic other carcinomas
- Generally, metastatic tumor in the adrenal is associated with very poor prognosis
- Low-grade tumors such as RCC can be treated by resection to improve survival

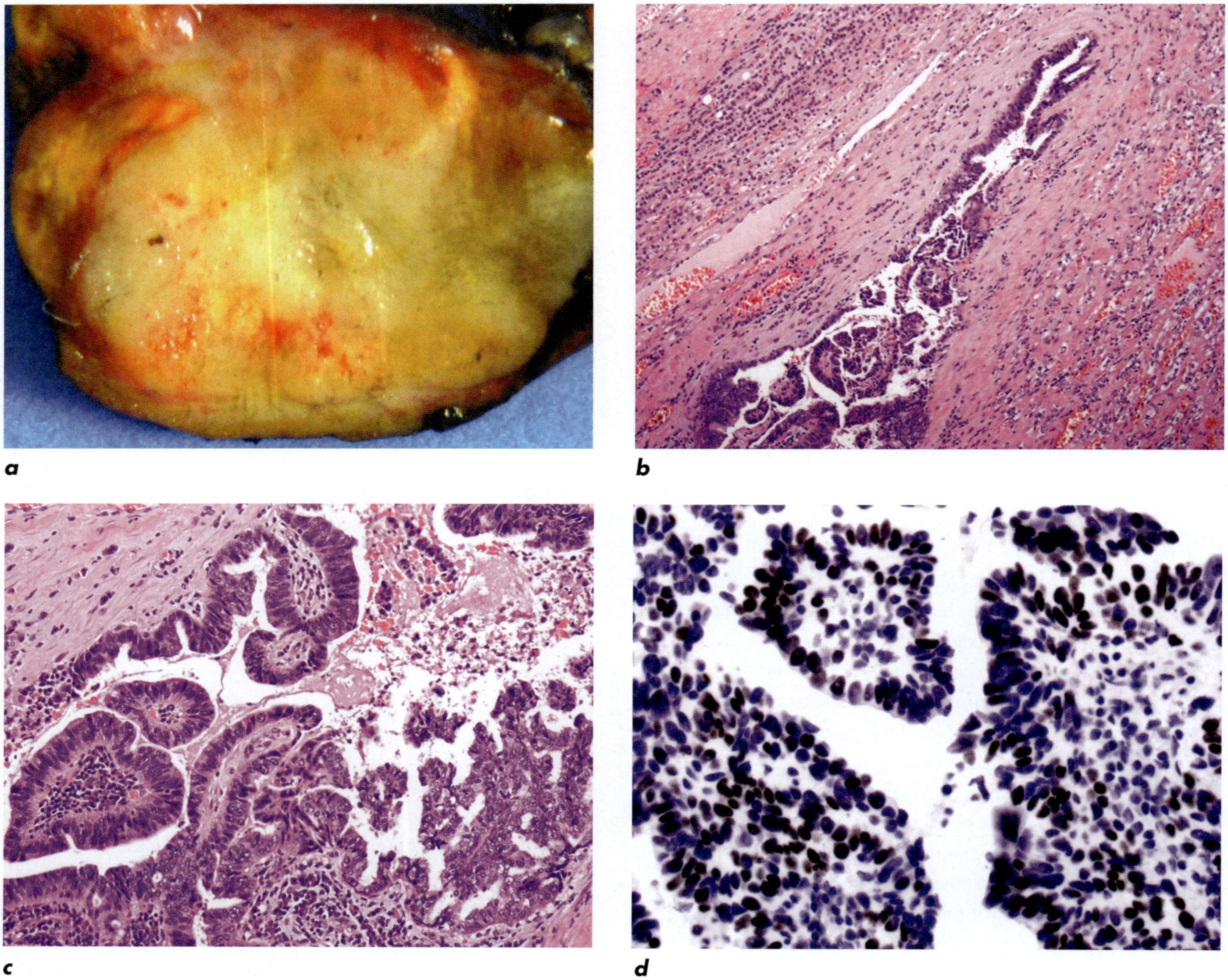

Figure 59-14.
Metastatic lung adenocarcinoma in the adrenal is a poorly defined mass (*a*). Microscopically, the tumor displays glandular (*b*) and papillary (*c*) configurations. Tumor cells are positive for TTF1 (*d*).

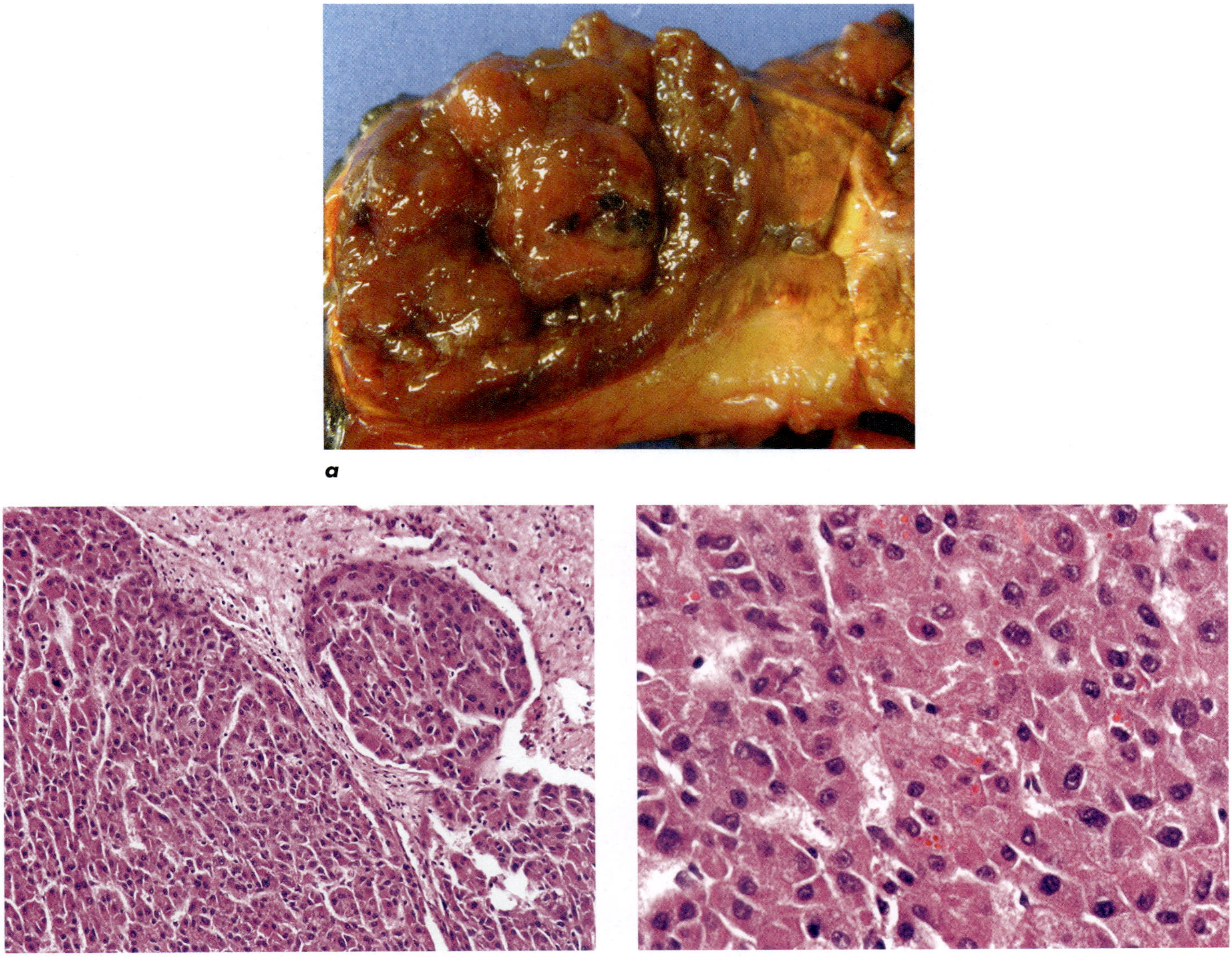

a **b** **c**

Figure 59-15.

Gross photo of metastatic hepatocellular carcinoma showing a large beefy-colored mass in the adrenal (*a*). Microscopically, the tumor is composed of large islands of cells with abundant eosinophilic cytoplasm (*b*). High magnification shows the granular cytoplasm and occasional bile particles in the tumor cells (*c*).

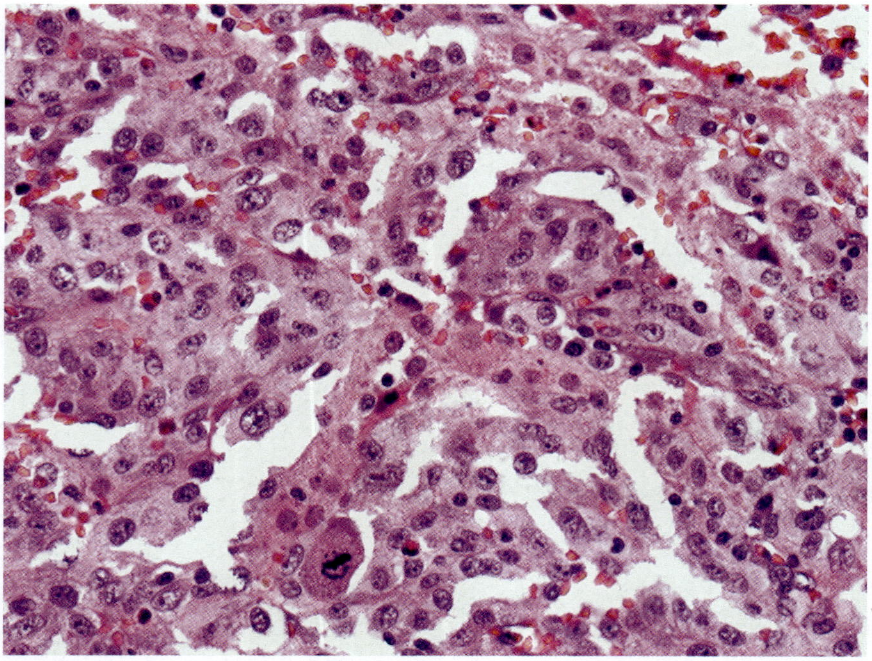

Figure 59-16.
Metastatic melanoma in the adrenal comprises of large cells with prominent nucleoli, dusty cytoplasm, and fine melanin.

SECTION 9
Special Structures

CHAPTER 60
Special Microscopic Structures in Genitourinary Pathology

Ximing J. Yang, Rajen Goyal

- These structures have specific morphological features
- They are generally associated with certain pathologic conditions
- Some of them are very specific or pathognomonic for defined pathologic conditions
- Recognition of these structures are important for diagnosis
- Most of these structures have been discussed in specific disease chapters
- However, they are discussed here for emphasis and easy reference since they are often being tested in different professional exams (see Table 60-1)

Table 60-1. Summary of Specific Microscopic Structures

Specific structure	*Specificity*	*Associated with condition*
Liesegang ring	Specific	Kidney tissue damage
Michaelis-Gutmann body	Pathognomonic	Malakoplakia
Schiller-Duval body	Pathognomonic	Yolk sac tumor
Crystal of Reinke	Specific for benign and neoplastic Leydig cells	Leydig cell tumor
Corpus amylacea	Relatively specific Also seen in lung or neuroglia	Prostate, benign
Dense corpus amylacea	Relative specific	Verumontanum
Crystalloid	Not specific, but more commonly seen in cancer than benign conditions	Prostatic adenocarcinoma
Glomeruloid body	Pathognomonic	Prostatic adenocarcinoma
Collagenous micronodule	Pathognomonic	Prostatic adenocarcinoma
Psammoma bodies	Relatively specific May be seen in benign conditions with papilla	Papillary carcinoma
Call-Exner body	Pathognomic	Granulosa cell tumor
Pustulo-ovoid bodies of Milian	Specific	Granular cell tumor
Keratin pearl	Pathognomic	Squamous cell carcinoma

LIESEGANG RING

Definition

- Round ring-like lamellated structures precipitated from a colloid solution
- Associated with tissue necrosis of the kidney

Pathogenesis

- Liesegang ring formation is a phenomenon by which ring-like structures are formed in colloids
- The term named after the German chemist Ralph Liesegang who first described this phenomenon
- The tissue necrosis in the kidney may lead to tissue liquidation and colloid formation, subsequently in certain pH conditions, the insoluble particles (Liesegang rings) will form

Histology

- Concentric lamellated structures (Fig. 60-1*a*)
- Most round or polygonal shaped
- Acellular
- Wide range in size from 20 to 50 μm (only microscopic findings) to 1 mm, which could be grossly seen (Fig. 60-1*b*)
- Most common in the kidney
- PSA and von Kossa and Masson stains are positive
- By electron microscopy, Liesegang rings are composed of fibrils with an adherent electron sense amorphous material
- Associated with necrotic tissue in inflammatory, benign, or neoplastic lesions

Differential diagnosis

Parasite eggs

- In the past, Liesegang rings were mistakenly identified as the ova of giant kidney worm (dioctophyma renale)
- Giant kidney worm is very rare, its eggs are cellular organisms
- While Liesegang rings are often associated with renal tissue necrosis without viable cellular structures
- Parasites are associated with marked inflammation, granuloma, and fibrosis

Clinical relevance (prognosis and treatment options)

- Found in necrotic tissue
- Can be seen in renal cell neoplasm or benign conditions
- Should not be considered organisms

Figure 60-1.
Liesegang ring in the background of macrophages (*a*). Another round Liesegang ring with a high refractile outrims (*b*).

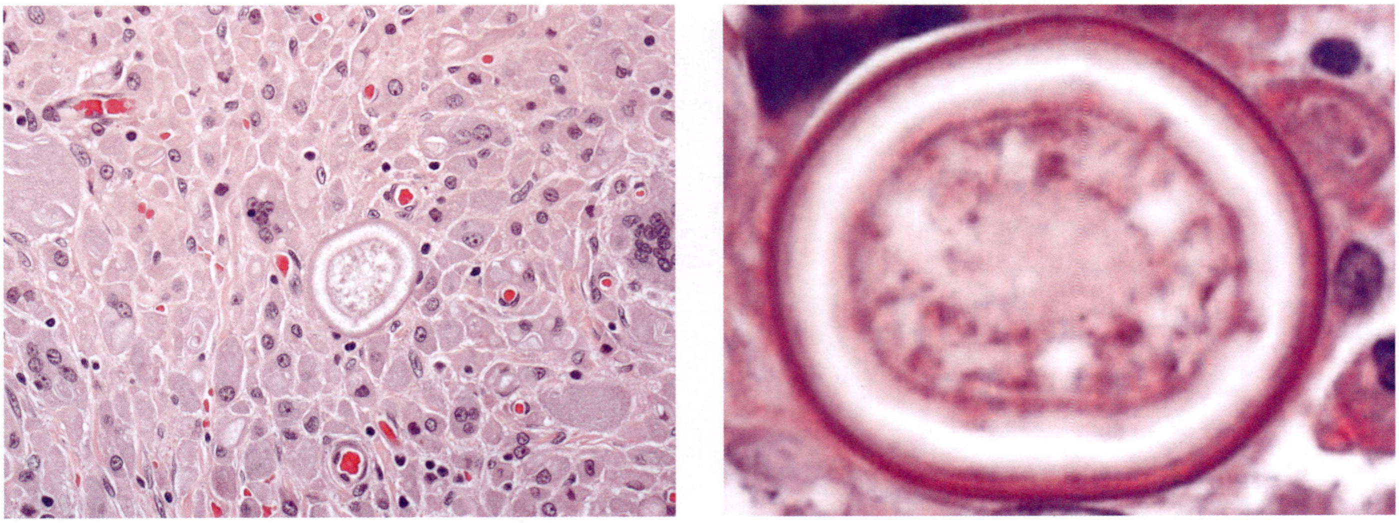

a **b**

MICHAELIS-GUTMANN BODY

Definition

- Special microscopic structures diagnostic for malakoplakia
- Presenting undigested bacteria in macrophages

Pathogenesis

Malakoplakia

- Malakoplakia is a reactive change associated with infection
- Accumulation of macrophages in the background of inflammation
- Because of insufficient killing, the gram-negative bacteria are ingested but not digested by macrophages. The partially digested or indigested bacterial material accumulated in the macrophages, leading to iron and calcium deposits
- Most commonly seen in the genitourinary tract, bladder, urethra, kidney, testis

Histology

- Michaelis-Gutmann body is characterized by the presence of basophilic inclusions as blue dots or targetoid structures inside foamy macrophages (Fig. 60-2)
- Background of inflammation and tissue destruction

Clinical relevance (prognosis and treatment options)

- Benign conditions
- Can be treated with antibiotics
- May be surgically removed if suspicious for neoplastic conditions

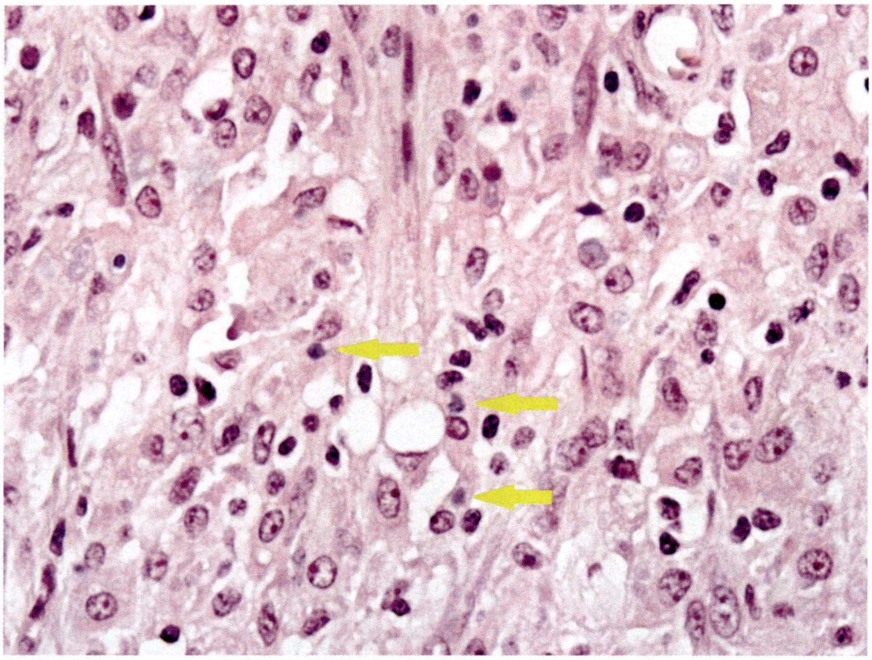

Figure 60-2.
Multiple Michaelis-Gutmann bodies are small blue dots indicated by arrows.

SCHILLER-DUVAL BODY

Definition

- A cellular structure specifically seen in yolk sac tumors (endodermal sinus tumor)

Pathogenesis

- Only present in less than 50% cases of yolk sac tumors

Histology

- Schiller-Duval body (Fig. 60-3), pathognomonic for yolk sac tumor is composed of
  - A vascular core
  - The core covered by one or multiple layers of tumor cells
  - Sitting in a sac surrounded by tumor cells

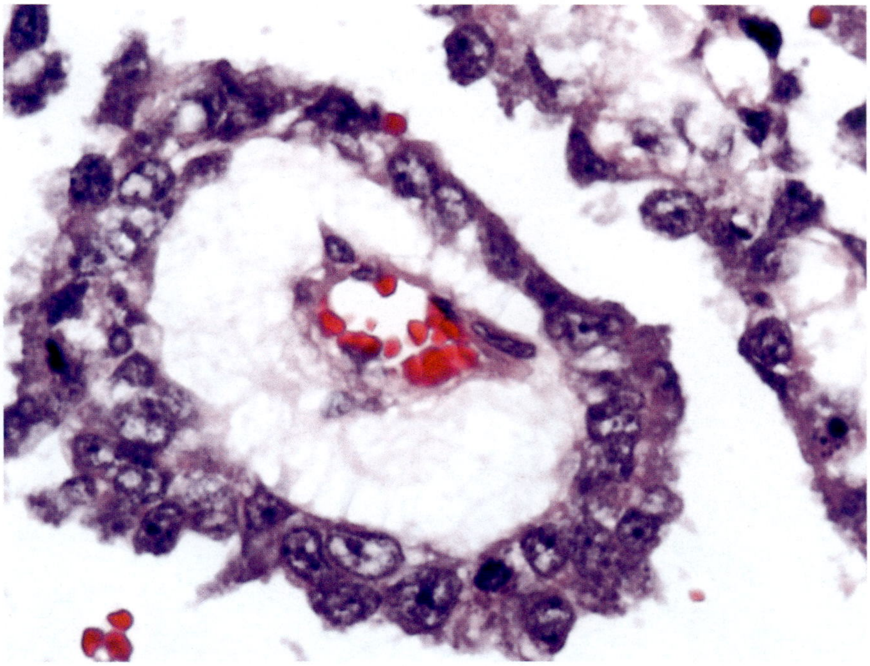

Figure 60-3.
Schiller-Duval body in yolk sac tumor of the testis is composed of fibrovascular core, covered by tumor cells and located in the sac formed by tumor cells.

CRYSTAL OF REINKE

Definition

- Specific crystal-like structures in Leydig cells

Pathogenesis

- Function unknown, not correlated with steroid hormonal production
- Possibly degenerative products

Histology

- Typically, crystal of Reinke is a rectangular or rod-shaped structure (Fig. 60-4)
- With refractile eosinophilc staining
- 3 to 20 μm in size, inside the cytoplasm of Leydig cells
- Can be seen in benign or neoplastic Leydig cells, more commonly seen in hyperplastic Leydig cells
- The number of crystals increases with ages
- By electron microscopy, crystal of Reinke appears to be regular grid spaces with a "parking lot" appearance

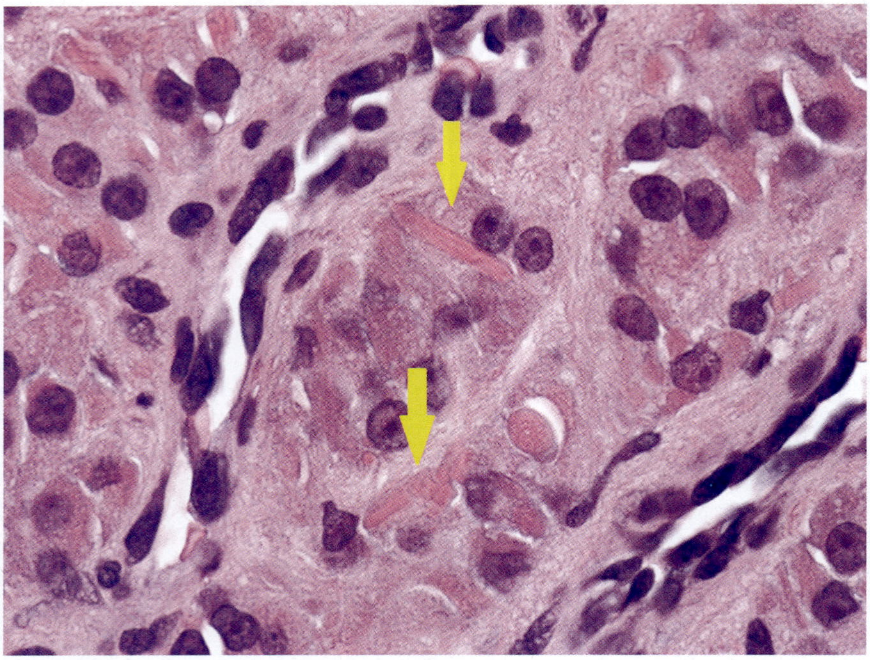

Figure 60-4.
Numerous crystals of Reinke indicated by arrows are seen in hyperplastic Leydig cells.

CORPUS AMYLACEA

Definition

- Small hyalinized concentric structures seen within the lumen of a benign prostatic gland
- May also be seen in the lung or neural glial tissue

Other term

- Prostatic concretions

Pathogenesis

- Function unknown, may be related to aging
- Possibly formed from condensed prostatic secretion
- Overtime, it may calcify and become a calculus

Clinical features

- No clinical significance
- Helpful in identifying prostatic identity in difficult situation such as necrotic tissue

Histology

- Round, oval, or polygonal-shaped structures (Fig. 60-5*a*)
- Eosinophilic with concentric ring appearance
- Located in the lumen of a prostatic gland
- More commonly seen in benign glands than in malignant glands
- May be seen in intraductal carcinoma
- In verumontanum, the corpus amylacea is condensed, brownish or yellowish in color (Fig. 60-5*b*)

Figure 60-5.
A corpus amylacea in the lumen of a benign prostatic gland (*a*). Multiple corpora amylacea in the lumens of verumontanum are dense and brownish in color (*b*).

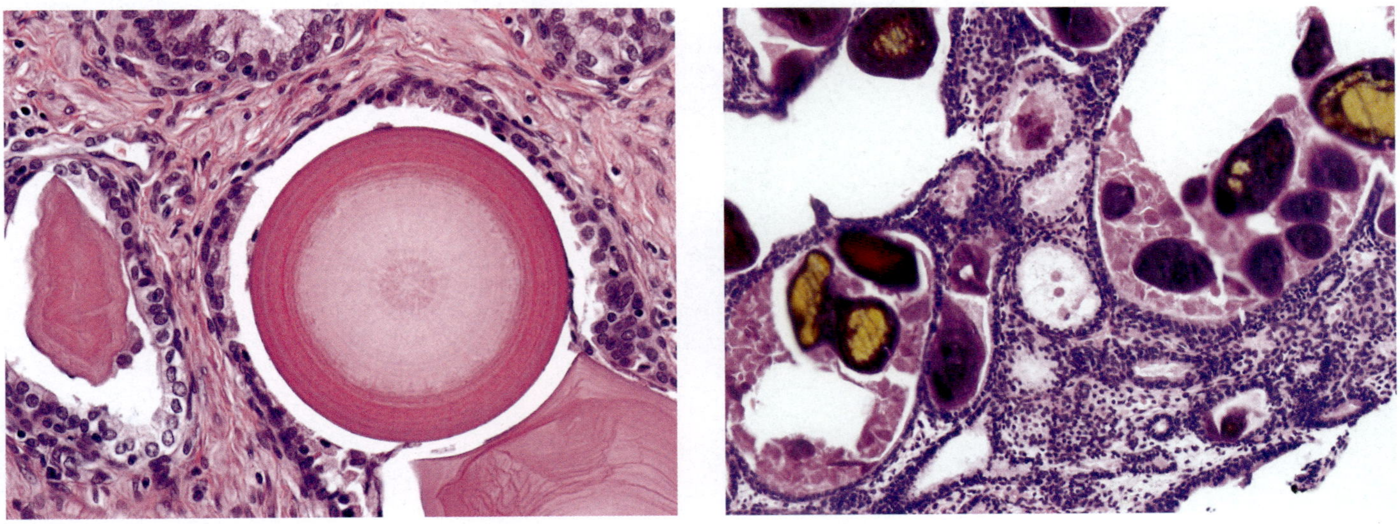

a **b**

CRYSTALLOIDS IN THE PROSTATE

Definition

- Crystalloids are intraluminal eosinophilic structures found in prostatic glands
- Although not highly specific, they are more commonly seen in adenocarcinoma than in benign glands

Histology

- Eosinophilic structures found with the lumen of malignant or benign prostatic glands (Fig. 60-6)
  - More commonly seen in malignant glands than in benign prostatic glands
  - More commonly seen in Gleason 2 or 3 patterns than in Gleason 4 or 5 patterns
- Crystalloids are not specific because they can be seen in adenosis, occasionally in high-grade PIN, atrophic glands, or benign glands adjacent to adenocarcinoma
- Rich in sulfur , function unknown
- Rarely seen in totally normal prostatic glands microscopically

Clinical relevance

- Helpful in identification of prostatic adenocarcinoma

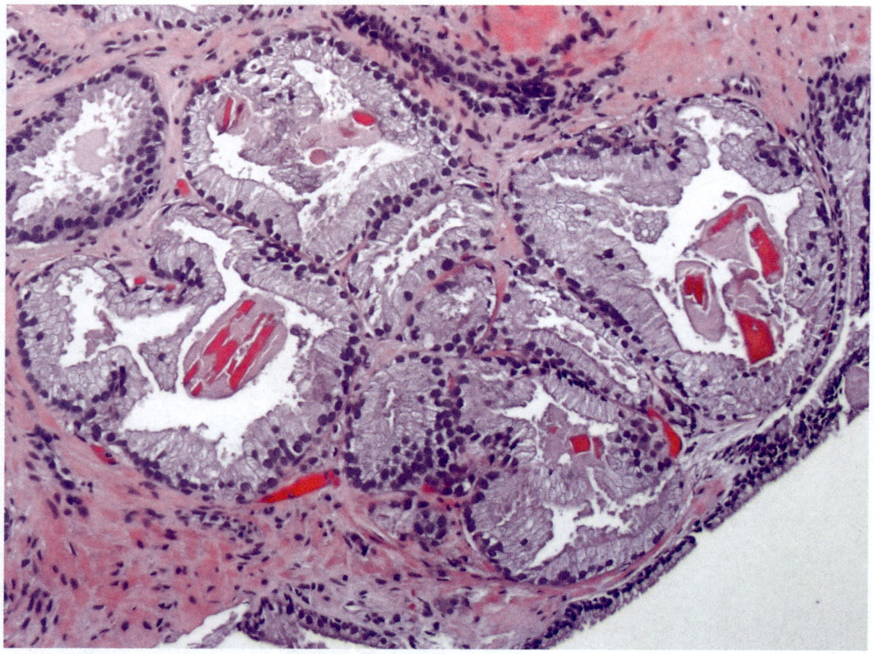

Figure 60-6.
Crystalloids are highly refractile eosinophilic material seen in the lumens of adenocarcinoma on needle core biopsy.

GLOMERULOID BODIES

Definition

- Specific structures resembling a glomerulus found in prostatic adenocarcinoma
- Pathognomonic for prostatic adenocarcinoma

Other terms

- Glomeruloid structures
- Glomerulation

Pathogenesis

- Possibly caused by proliferation of tumor cells within a glandular structure

Histology

- Resembles a glomerulus
- Characterized by the presence of a cluster of a typical epithelial cells within a glandular space (Fig. 60-7)
- The cytological atypia of carcinoma cells are evident

Differential diagnosis

Intraductal carcinoma of the prostate

- Similar to glomeruloid structure in prostatic adenocarcinoma
- The intraductal carcinoma displays a portion of benign prostatic epithelium in the gland involved

Figure 60-7.
Glomeruloid body can be seen in a malignant gland, surrounded by several malignant glandular structures (*a*). Intraductal carcinoma may have glomeruloid structures, but some of the cells within the gland are benign (*b*).

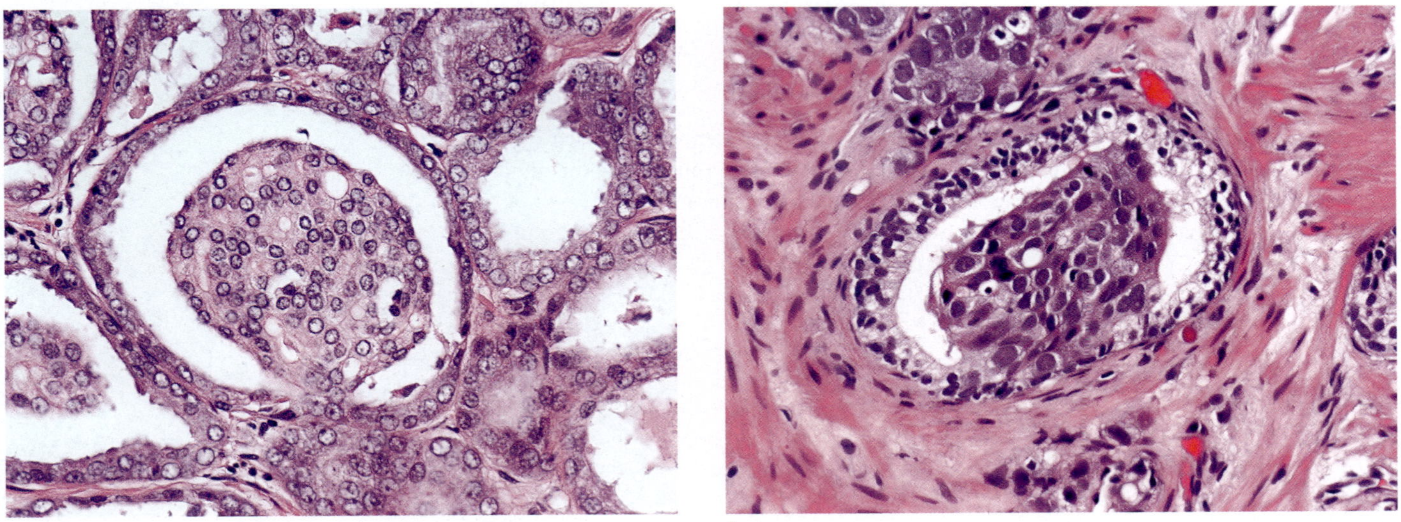

a b

COLLAGENOUS MICRONODULES

Definition

- Microscopic structures with fibrillar aggregate sounding prostatic adenocarcinoma
- It is pathognomonic and diagnostic of prostatic adenocarcinoma

Other term

- Mucinous fibroplasia

Pathogenesis

- Collagenous micronodules are composed of fragmented collagenous material
- Believed to be produced by the collagenase secreted by carcinoma cells
- Therefore, it is associated with the invasive nature of the prostatic adenocarcinoma
- Not always associated with mucinous production by the tumor cells as originally believed

Histology

- Extracellular material
- Eosinophilic and fibrillar material in nodular or dome-shaped structures (Fig. 60-8)
- Surrounded by the tumor cells with amphophilic cytoplasm (suggestive of active protein synthesis)
- Only seen in adenocarcinoma, not in any other benign conditions of the prostate
- Not associated with better or worse prognosis

Clinical relevance (prognosis and treatment options)

- One of the very few pathognomonic features of prostatic adenocarcinoma
- Highly specific, no other benign conditions in the prostate have exhibited this structure

Figure 60-8.
Two to three collagenous micronodules associated with prostatic adenocarcinoma are present in the middle of the field. They are nodular or dome-shaped structures surrounded by the tumor cells (*a*). Numerous collagenous micronodules are seen associated with adenocarcinoma (*b*).

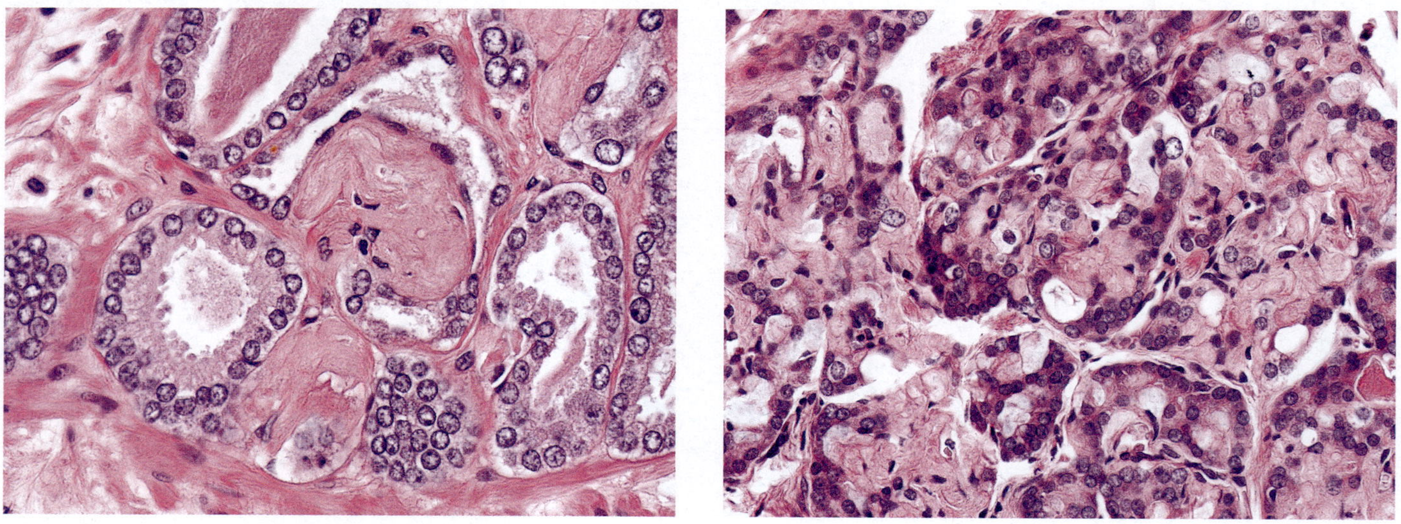

a *b*

PSAMMOMA BODY

Definition

- Psammoma (sand) bodies are round concentric layered calcified structures seen microscopically
- Often associated with papillary carcinoma

Pathogenesis

- Associated with papillary structures
- It arises from the calcification of the dead papillary tips

Histology

- Concentric layered structure (Fig. 60-9)
- Calcified, blue in color
- In the genitourinary system, it is most commonly seen in papillary renal cell carcinoma
- Can be seen in papillary urothelial carcinoma, prostatic ductal adenocarcinoma, or renal papillary adenoma

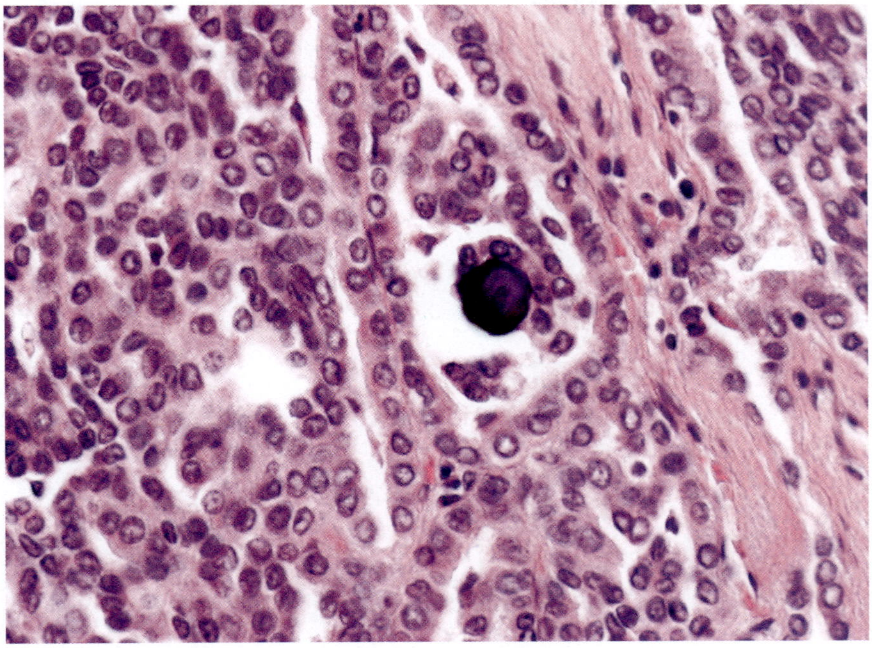

Figure 60-9.
Psammoma body in papillary renal cell carcinoma.

CALL-EXNER BODY

Definition

- Small spaces filled with eosinophilic fluid in granulosa cell tumor

Pathogenesis

- These structures represent the small incomplete primitive follicles formed by neoplastic granulosa cells

Histology

- Small spaces filled with eosinophilic fluid (Fig. 60-10)
- Surrounded by neoplastic sex cord stromal cells
- Indicative of granulosa cell tumor of the testis
- Granulosa cell tumors are more common in the ovary than testis

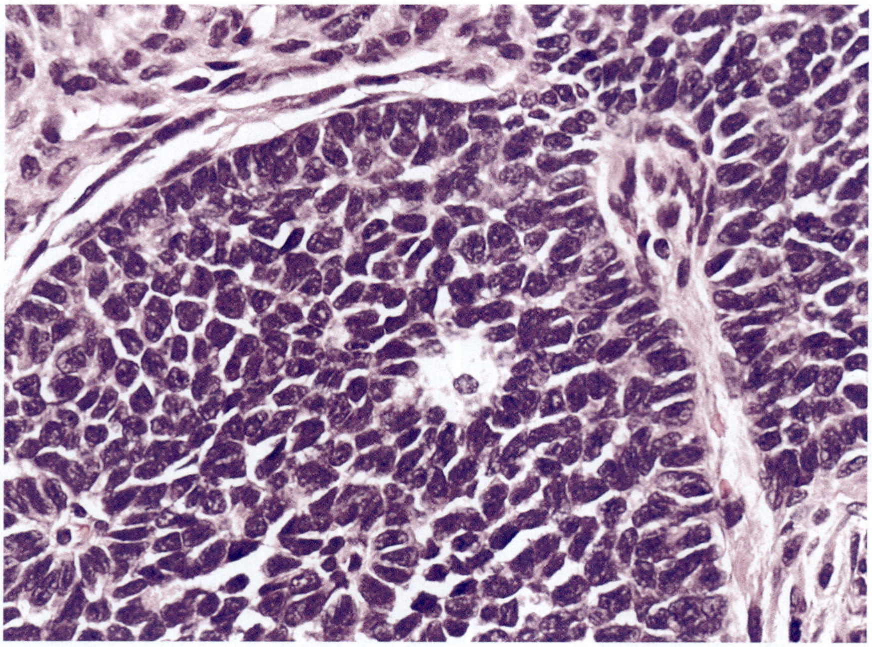

Figure 60-10.
Several Call-Exner bodies seen in a testicular granulosa cell tumor.

PUSTULO-OVOID BODIES OF MILIAN AND HYALINE GLOBULES

Definition

- Eosinophilic granules with a clear halo seen in granular cell tumor

Histology

- Small eosinophilic globules with a halo (Fig. 60-11)
- Typically seen in the cytoplasm of the tumor cells with many eosinophilic granules
- Size ranging 5 to 10 μm
- Seen in granular cell tumor, which is a benign neural tumor with prominent granular cytoplasm
- Similar eosinophilic (hyaline) globules can be seen in other GU neoplasms such as renal cell carcinoma, pheochromocytoma/paraganglioma, or basal cell hyperplasia of the prostate

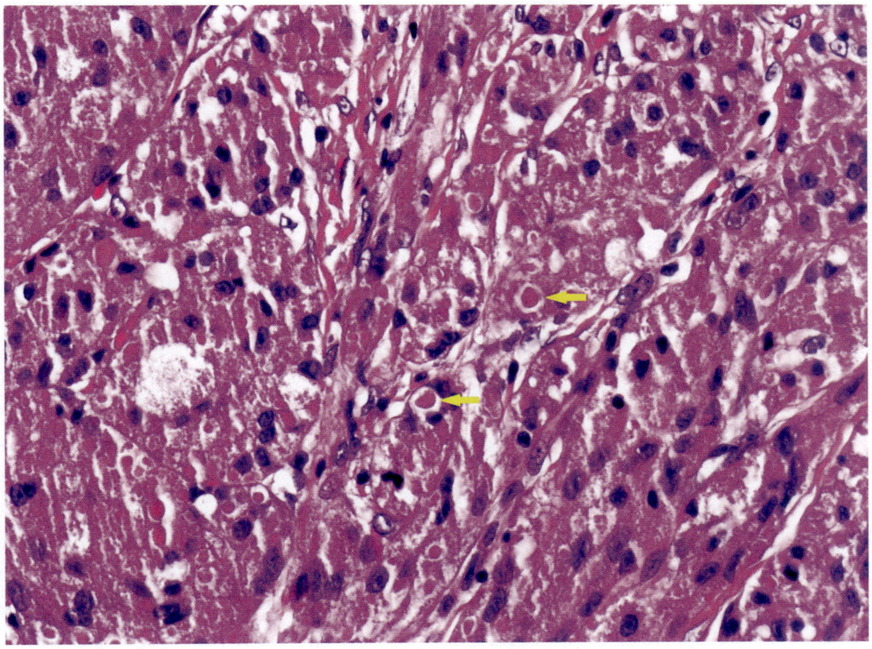

Figure 60-11. Hyaline globules with halo (Pustulo-ovoid bodies of Milian) indicated by arrows in a penile granular cell tumor.

KERATIN PEARL

Definition

- Special structures of keratin formation seen in squamous cell carcinoma

Histology

- Small focus of central keratinization with concentric layers of keratin surrounded by malignant squamous cells (Fig. 60-12)
- Seen in squamous cell carcinoma
- Also called epithelial pearl

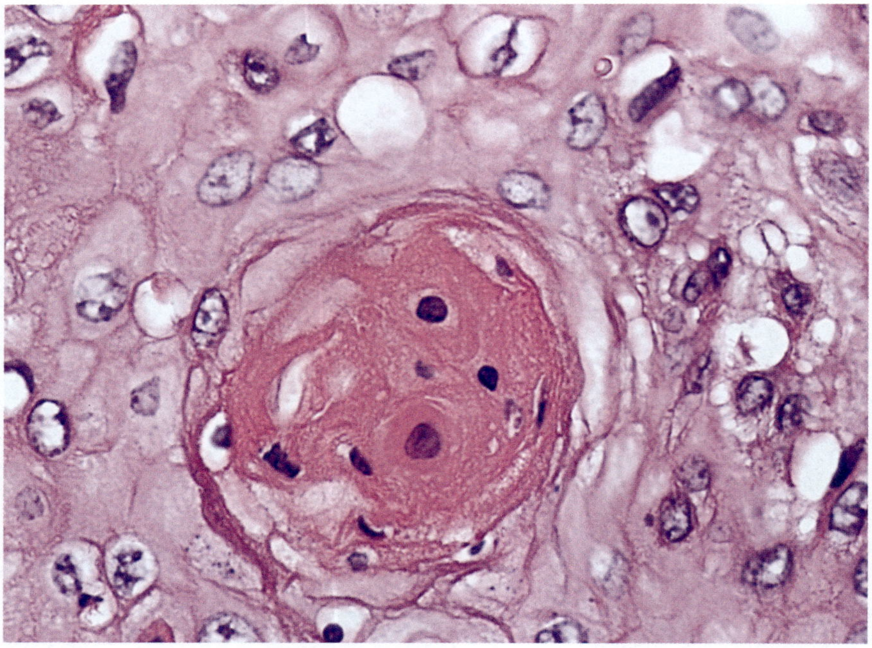

Figure 60-12.
Keratin pearl in an invasive squamous cell carcinoma.

Abbreviations

5αR	5-α-reductase
AAH	Atypical adenomatous hyperplasia
ACD-associated RCC	Acquired cystic (kidney) disease associated RCC
ACKD	Acquired cystic kidney disease
AFB	Acid fast bacilli (stain)
AFP	α-fetoprotein
AHRT	Adenomatous hyperplasia of the rete testis
AIS	Androgen insensitive syndrome
ALK/ALK-1	Anaplastic lymphoma kinase
AMACR	α-methylacyl-CoA racemase
AML	Angiomyolipoma
ANA	Antinuclear antibody
ANCA	Antineutrophilic cytoplasmic antibodies
ASAP	Atypical small acinar proliferation
ASO	Antistreptolysin O
BCG	Bacillus Calmette-Guérin
BCH	Basal cell hyperplasia
BHD	Birt-Hogg-Dube
BPH	Benign prostatic hyperplasia
CAH	Congenital adrenal hyperplasia
CAIX/CA9	Carbonic anhydrase 9
CC	Cystitis cystica
CCCH	Clear cell cribriform hyperplasia
CCSK	Clear cell sarcoma of the kidney
CDC	Collecting duct carcinoma
CEA	Carcinoembryonic antigen
CF	Cystic fibrosis
CFTR	Cystic fibrosis transmembrane conductance regulator
CG	Cystitis glandularis
ChRCC	Chromophobe renal cell carcinoma
CIS	Carcinoma in situ
CK20	Cytokeratin 20
CLL	Chronic lymphocytic leukemia
CMN	Collagenous micronodules
CMN	Congenital mesoblastic nephroma
CMV	Cytomegalovirus
CT	Computed tomography
DHT	Dihydrotestosterone
DN	Diabetic nephropathy
DPGN	Diffuse proliferative glomerulonephritis
EC	Eosinophilic cystitis
ED	Ejaculatory duct
EM	Electron microscope
EMA	Epithelial membrane antigen
EPE	Extraprostatic extension
ERG	ETS-related gene
ESRD	End-stage renal disease
FISH	Fluorescence in situ hybridization
FSGS	Focal segmental glomerulosclerosis
FSH	Follicle stimulating hormone
GBM	Glomerular basement membrane
GCT	Germ cell tumor
GI	Gastrointestinal
GIST	Gastrointestinal stromal tumor
GMS	Grocott methenamine silver (stain)
GPC3	Glypican 3
GTP	Guanosine-5′-triphosphate
GU	Genitourinary
H&E	Hematoxylin and eosin (stain)
HCG/β-HCG	Human chorionic gonadotropin (beta unit)
HHV8	Human herpesvirus 8
HIF	Hypoxia-inducible factor
HMWCK	High molecular cytokeratins
HPF	High power field
HPV	Human papilloma virus
HSV	Herpes simplex virus
HVA	Homovanillic acid
I(12p)	Isochromosome 12p
IC	Interstitial cystitis
IDC	Intraductal carcinoma (of the prostate)
IGF2	Insulin-like growth factor 2
IHC	Immunohistochemistry
ILNR	Intralobar nephrogenic rests
IMT	Inflammatory myofibroblastic tumor
ITGCNU	Intratubular germ cell neoplasias, unclassified
KIM-1	Kidney injury molecule
KS	Kaposi sarcoma

KW body	Kimmelstiel-Wilson body
LANA	Latency-associated nuclear antigen (of HHV8)
LCT	Leydig cell tumor
LDH	Lactate dehydrogenase
LN	Lupus nephritis
LOH	Loss of heterozygosity
LP	Lamina propria
LS	Lichen sclerosus
MCD	Minimal change disease
MEN	Multiple neuroendocrine neoplasia
MEST	Mixed epithelial and stromal tumor
MG body	Michaelis-Gutmann body
MGN	Membranous glomerulonephritis
MIA	Antimitochondrial antigen
MMP	Metalloproteinase
MP	Muscularis propria
MPGN	Membranoproliferative glomerulonephritis
MPO	Myeloperoxidase
MRI	Magnetic resonance imaging
mTOR	Mechanistic target of rapamycin
MTSCC	Mucinous tubular and spindle cell carcinoma
N/C ratio	Nuclear/cytoplasmic ratio
NE/NEC	Neuroendocrine cells
NGFR	Nerve growth factor receptor
NSE	Neuron-specific enolase
NSGO	Nonspecific granulomatous orchitis
NSGP	Nonspecific granulomatous prostatitis
OCT-4	Octamer-binding transcription factor 4
PAS	Periodic acid-Schiff
PAX2/PAX8	Paired box gene 2 or 8
PCR	Polymerase chain reaction
PDGFRA	Platelet-derived growth factor-α
PEC	Perivascular epithelioid cells
PECOMA	Perivascular epithelioid cell tumor
PET	Positron emission tomography
PIN	Prostatic intraepithelial neoplasia
PINATYP	High-grade PIN with atypia
PKD	Polycystic kidney disease
PKD1	Polycystic kidney disease gene 1
PKD2	Polycystic kidney disease gene 2
PLAP	Placental alkaline phosphatase
PLNR	Perilobar nephrogenic rests
PMN	Polymorphonuclear neutrophil
PNET	Primitive neuroectodermal tumor
PNI	Perineural invasion
PR3	Proteinase 3
PRCC	Papillary renal cell carcinoma
PSA	Prostate-specific antigen
PSAP	Prostate-specific alkaline phosphatase
PSGN	Poststreptococcal glomerulonephritis
PSMA	Prostate-specific membrane antigen
PTLD	Posttransplant lymphoproliferative disorders
PUNLMP	Papillary urothelial neoplasm of low malignant potential
RAT	Renal angiomyomatous tumor
RCC	Renal cell carcinoma
RMC	Renal medullary carcinoma
SCC	Small cell carcinoma
SLE	Systemic lupus nephritis
SLL	Small lymphocytic lymphoma
SMA	Smooth muscle actin
SqCC	Squamous cell carcinoma
SV	Seminal vesicle
TB	Tuberculosis
TBM	Tubular basement membrane
TML	Testicular microlithiasis
TS	Tuberous sclerosis
TTF1	Thyroid transcription factor
TUR	Transurethral resection
TURBT	Transurethral resection of bladder tumor
TURP	Transurethral resection of prostate
UC (UCa)	Urothelial carcinoma
UPJ	Ureteropelvic junction
VEGF	Vascular endothelial growth factor
VHL	Von Hippel-Lindau
VMA	Vanilmandelic acid
VMGH	Verumontanum mucosal gland hyperplasia
WT	Wilms tumor
WT1	Wilms tumor gene (protein) 1
XGPN	Xanthogranulomatous pyelonephritis
YST	Yolk sac tumor
ZF	Zona fasciculata
ZG	Zona glomerulosa
ZR	Zona reticularis

Index

B

C

D

E

F

I

J

K

N

Q

R

V

W

X

Y

Z